CANCER SYMPTOM MANAGEMENT

FOURTH EDITION

Edited by

Connie Henke Yarbro, RN, MS, FAAN
Adjunct Clinical Associate Professor
Sinclair School of Nursing
Editor, *Seminars in Oncology Nursing*
University of Missouri, Columbia
Columbia, Missouri

Debra Wujcik, PhD, RN, FAAN
Director, VICC Clinical Trials Shared Resource
Associate Professor, Vanderbilt School of Nursing
Vanderbilt Ingram Cancer Center
Nashville, Tennessee

Barbara Holmes Gobel, RN, MS, AOCN®
Operations Manager, Oncology Services
Northwestern Memorial Hospital
Adjuvant Faculty, Rush University College of Nursing
Chicago, Illinois

Past Editors
Margaret Hansen Frogge, RN, MS
Michelle Goodman, RN, MS

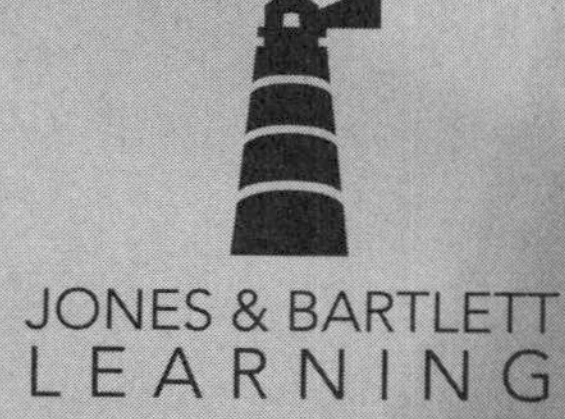

JONES & BARTLETT
LEARNING

World Headquarters
Jones & Bartlett Learning
5 Wall Street
Burlington, MA 01803
978-443-5000
info@jblearning.com
www.jblearning.com

Jones & Bartlett Learning books and products are available through most bookstores and online booksellers. To contact Jones & Bartlett Learning directly, call 800-832-0034, fax 978-443-8000, or visit our website, www.jblearning.com.

Substantial discounts on bulk quantities of Jones & Bartlett Learning publications are available to corporations, professional associations, and other qualified organizations. For details and specific discount information, contact the special sales department at Jones & Bartlett Learning via the above contact information or send an email to specialsales@jblearning.com.

Production Credits
Executive Publisher: William Brottmiller
Senior Acquisitions Editor: Nancy Anastasi Duffy
Editorial Assistant: Rebecca Myrick
Associate Production Editor: Sara Fowles
Marketing Communications Manager: Katie Hennessy
VP, Manufacturing and Inventory Control: Therese Connell
Composition: Lapiz, Inc.
Cover Design: Michael O'Donnell
Cover Image: © Ryan McVay/Photodisc/Getty Images
Printing and Binding: Courier Companies
Cover Printing: Courier Companies

To order this product, use ISBN: 978-1-284-02740-2

Library of Congress Cataloging-in-Publication Data
Cancer symptom management / [edited by] Connie Henke Yarbro, Debra Wujcik, Barbara Holmes Gobel. — 4th ed.
p. ; cm.
Includes bibliographical references and index.
ISBN 978-1-284-02553-8 (pbk.)
I. Yarbro, Connie Henke. II. Wujcik, Debra. III. Gobel, Barbara Holmes.
[DNLM: 1. Neoplasms—nursing. 2. Neoplasms—complications. 3. Oncologic Nursing—methods. 4. Patient Care Management—methods. WY 156]
616.99'40231—dc23

2013001117

6048

Printed in the United States of America
17 16 15 14 13 10 9 8 7 6 5 4 3 2 1

Contents

10 Diarrhea 185

Paula M. Muehlbauer, RN, MSN, AOCNS®; Rachael Christine Lopez, MPH, RD, CSO

11 Nausea and Vomiting 213

Janelle Tipton, MSN, RN, AOCN®

12 Malignant Ascites 241

Kim Slusser, RN, MSN, CHPN®

16 Effusions 331

Diane G. Cope, PhD, ARNP, BC, AOCNP®

Part VII Alterations in Nutrition 349

17 The Cancer Cachexia Syndrome 351

Regina S. Cunningham, PhD, RN, AOCN®

33 Spiritual Distress 683

Elizabeth Johnston Taylor, PhD, RN

34 Symptoms When Death Is Imminent 699

Marie Bakitas, DNSc, APRN, AOCN®, FAAN; Margaret Firer Bishop, MS, APRN; Margaret E. Hahn, MSN, FNP, APRN, ACHPN

Preface

When patients with cancer and their families are asked what bothers them most about their treatment or disease, they respond with examples of how the problems resulting from cancer or its treatment affect their daily activities. These problems often make life difficult and frustrating for the patient experiencing the problem.

The nurse assisting the patient and family needs up-to-date information about the problems that can occur, options for management of the problems, and information about how to teach the patient and family to provide care at home.

Cancer Symptom Management, Fourth Edition provides such information to the oncology nurse. The most common problems experienced by patients with cancer are addressed. Problems are identified as "symptoms" in this text. We recognize that some of the problems identified are not symptoms but signs or syndromes; however, rather than concern ourselves with the semantic distinctions among these terms we have focused on the important task of identifying the most common problems that individuals with cancer experience, describing how the problem affects the quality of the patient's life and identifying what the nurse can do to help relieve or diminish the patient's and family's suffering.

For the majority of individuals with cancer, their health care has shifted from the hospital to the ambulatory care setting and the home. The challenge to health professionals is to provide quality care and to meet the educational and care needs of patients within the dynamic environment of the ambulatory care setting and the home. Since family and caregivers now provide the majority of care in the home, nurses need a wide range of tools and ideas to offer the caregivers. *Cancer Symptom Management* is written by nurses and allied professionals who are recognized for their expertise as practitioners and who understand the challenges and the impact the symptoms have on the quality of life for a cancer patient and their family. The authors of the chapters provide creative approaches to evidence-based management of the most common problems experienced by cancer patients. These include symptoms of alterations in comfort, protective mechanisms, gastrointestinal function, genitourinary function, cardiopulmonary function, nutrition, neurological function, anatomical and surgical, and psychosocial function.

This fourth edition provides the reader with many new updates and revisions. We have 35 new authors that have completely rewritten the chapters or provided a comprehensive update. Four new chapters have been added to this fourth edition.

"Hypersensitivity Reactions to Antineoplastic Drugs" has been included to address problems related to allergic reactions, infusion reactions, and cytokine-release reactions, and provides the nurse with approaches to managing these reactions. The second new chapter is "Extravasation", which focuses on the prevention, early recognition, management, and patient education related to the extravasation of non-irritant, irritant, and vesicant agents.

The third new chapter is "Ocular and Otic Complications." Although these side effects are relatively uncommon, advances in treatment have resulted in longer survival for patients with cancer; thus we are seeing more adverse ocular and otic side effects secondary to treatment.

The fourth new chapter to this edition is entitled "Symptoms When Death Is Imminent." This chapter discusses the common cognitive, respiratory, and symptom management strategies (including palliative sedation) at the end-of-life stage. Family preparation for what to expect as death approaches and the postdeath period is a major part of the chapter.

Unique to this text are the patient self-care guides. For each problem discussed, at least one self-care tool is provided at the end of the chapter to assist in teaching the patient and family how to provide care at home. Feedback from our readers, patients, and family members have been incorporated in these updated self-care guides. They are written in a form that patients can understand and use. The reader is encouraged to adapt these self-care guidelines to their practice.

We acknowledge the challenges and opportunities faced by our readers and their patients who provide our purpose for this endeavor. We hope that this text will be helpful to both nurses and their patients and their families.

Connie Henke Yarbro
Debra Wujcik
Barbara Holmes Gobel

Acknowledgments

The editors would like to pay a special tribute to

Margaret Hansen Frogge, RN, MS
Michelle Goodman, RN, MS

Margaret and Michelle served diligently as editors since the inception of this text in 1996. Their leadership and dedication to the first three editions of *Cancer Symptom Management* have contributed to the continuing success of this text.

The Editors

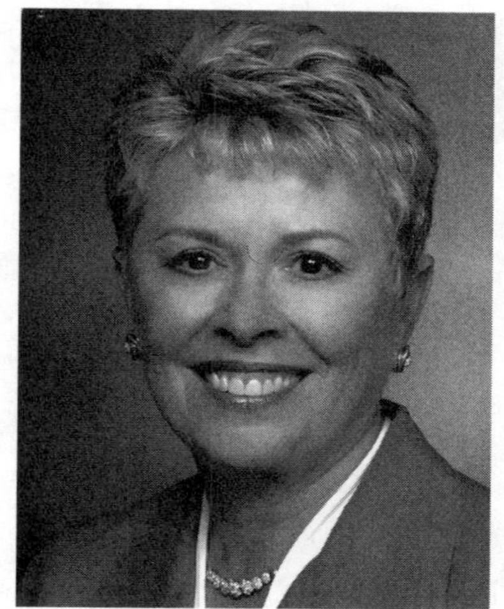
Connie Henke Yarbro

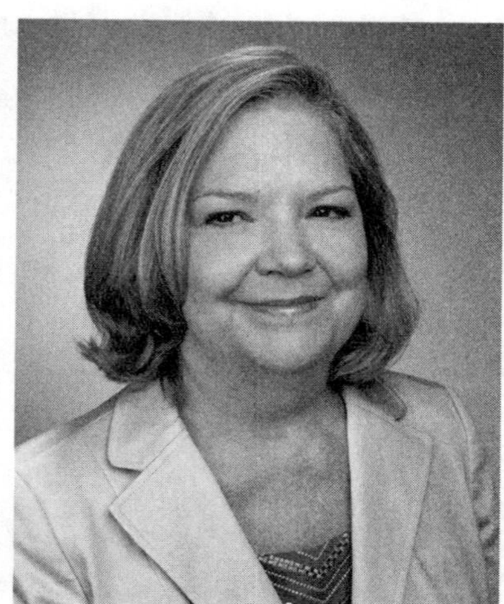
Debra Wujcik

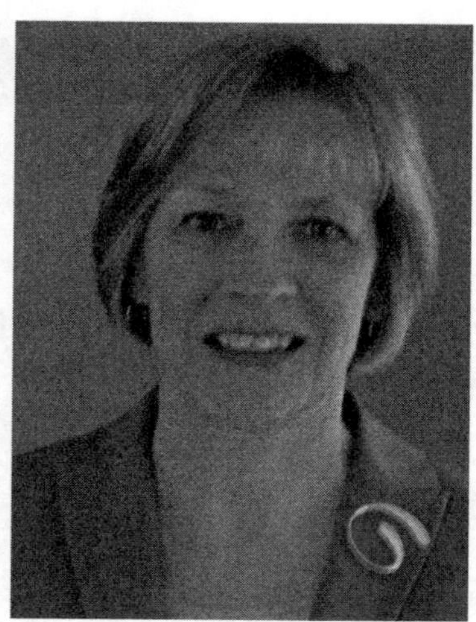
Barbara Holmes Gobel

Contributors

Terri S. Armstrong, PhD, ANP-BC, FAANP
Professor
John S. Dunn Distinguished Professorship in Oncology Nursing
Department of Family Health
University of Texas Health Science Center
Adjunct Professor, Department of Neuro-Oncology
MD Anderson Cancer Center
Houston, Texas

Marie Bakitas, DNSc, APRN, AOCN®, FAAN
Professor, Marie L. O'Koren Endowed Chair
University of Alabama School of Nursing
Birmingham, Alabama

Ann M. Berger, PhD, APRN, AOCNS®, FAAN
Professor and Dorothy Hodges Olson Endowed Chair in Nursing
Clinical Nurse Specialist, Oncology
Director, Doctoral Program
University of Nebraska Medical Center
Omaha, Nebraska

Donna L. Berry, PhD, RN, AOCN®, FAAN
Associate Professor, Department of Medicine
Harvard Medical School
Director, Phyllis F. Cantor Center for Research in Nursing and Patient Care Services
Dana-Farber Cancer Institute
Boston, Massachusetts

Margaret Firer Bishop, MS, APRN
Department of Anesthesiology, Section of Palliative Medicine
Dartmouth-Hitchcock Medical Center
Lebanon, New Hampshire

Jeannine M. Brant, PhD, APRN, AOCN®
Oncology Clinical Nurse Specialist/Research Scientist
Billings Clinic Inpatient Cancer Care
Montana State University College of Nursing
Bozeman, Montana

Cheryl Brohard, PhD, RN, AOCN®
Director of Education
Houston Hospice
Houston, Texas

Mary Callaghan, RN, MN, AOCNS®
Advanced Practice Nurse, Gynecological Oncology
Northwestern Memorial Hospital
Chicago, Illinois

Dawn Camp-Sorrell, MSN, FNP, AOCN®
Nurse Practitioner
Clinical Instructor
University of Alabama at Birmingham School of Nursing
Birmingham, Alabama

Kimberly Cantania, MSN, RN, CNS, AOCN®
Oncology Clinical Nurse Specialist
The Ohio State University Comprehensive Cancer Center
Arthur G. James Cancer Hospital
Richard J. Solove Research Institute
Columbus, Ohio

Marlene Z. Cohen, RN, PhD, FAAN
Professor and Kenneth E. Morehead Endowed Chair in Nursing
Associate Dean for Research
University of Nebraska Medical Center, College of Nursing
Omaha, Nebraska

Abby Cooper, RN, MSN, OCN®
Practice Manager, Oncology Services
Northwestern Memorial Hospital
Chicago, Illinois

Diane G. Cope, PhD, ARNP, BC, AOCNP®
Oncology Nurse Practitioner
Florida Cancer Specialists and Research Institute
Fort Myers, Florida

Regina S. Cunningham, PhD, RN, AOCN®
Associate Chief Nursing Officer for
Cancer Services
Abramson Cancer Center
University of Pennsylvania
Philadelphia, Pennsylvania

Carol Curtiss, MSN, RN-BC
Clinical Nurse Specialist Consultant
Curtiss Consulting
Adjunct Clinical Instructor
Tufts University School of Medicine
Boston, Massachusetts

Kerri A. Dalton, RN, MSN, OCN®
Clinical Nurse Specialist
Duke Cancer Institute
Durham, North Carolina

Mary Egger, RN, MSN, WHNP
Instructor, Breast Center Nurse Practitioner
The Vanderbilt Breast Center
Vanderbilt University Medical Center
Nashville, Tennessee

Margaret M. Fields, RN, MSN, ACNP-BC, AOCNP®
Nurse Practitioner
Neruo-Oncology
MD Anderson Cancer Center
Houston, Texas

Caryl D. Fulcher, MSN, RN, CNS-BC
Clinical Nurse Specialist and Team Leader
Department of Advanced Clinical Practice
Duke University Hospital
Durham, North Carolina

Barbara Holmes Gobel, RN, MS, AOCN®
Operations Manager, Oncology Services
Northwestern Memorial Hospital
Adjuvant Faculty, Rush University College of Nursing
Chicago, Illinois

Tracy Gosselin, RN, PhD, AOCN®
Associate Chief Nursing Officer
Duke Cancer Institute
Durham, North Carolina

Margaret E. Hahn, MSN, FNP, APRN, ACHPN
Instructor in Anesthesiology
Dartmouth-Hitchcock Medical Center
Lebanon, New Hampshire

Pamela J. Haylock, PhD, RN, FAAN
CEO, Association for Vascular Access
Medina, Texas

Margaret Joyce, PhD, ANP-BC, AOCN®
Assistant Professor
University of Medicine and Dentistry of New Jersey
Newark, New Jersey

Linda U. Krebs, PhD, RN, AOCN®, FAAN
Associate Professor
University of Colorado, College of Nursing
Aurora, Colorado

Rachael Christine Lopez, MPH, RD, CSO
Clinical Research Dietitian
National Institutes of Health
Bethesda, Maryland

Virginia R. Martin, MSN, RN, AOCN®
Clinical Director Ambulatory Care
Fox Chase Cancer Center
Philadelphia, Pennsylvania

Robert L. Massey, PhD, RN, CNNA
Assistant Professor, Department of Nursing,
Director, Clinical Nursing
The University of Texas
MD Anderson Cancer Center
Houston, Texas

Ellyn E. Matthews, PhD, RN, AOCN®, AOCNS®
Associate Professor
University of Colorado College of Nursing
Aurora, Colorado

Sandra A. Mitchell, PhD, CRNP, AOCN®
Research Scientist
National Cancer Institute, Outcomes Research Branch
Division of Cancer Control and Population
Sciences
Bethesda, Maryland

Linda Morse, RN, MSN
Clinical Research Nurse
The Lowe Center for Thoracic Oncology
Dana-Farber Cancer Institute
Boston, Massachusetts

Paula Muehlbauer, RN, MSN, AOCNS®
Clinical Nurse Specialist
San Diego Veterans Affairs Healthcare System
San Diego State University
San Diego, California

Colleen O'Leary, MSN, RN, AOCNS®
Clinical Nurse Specialist, Head and Neck Oncology
The Ohio State University Comprehensive Cancer Center
Arthur G. James Cancer Hospital
Richard J. Solove Research Institute
Columbus, Ohio

Sheryl Redlin Frazier, RN, MSN
Manager, Patient Care Services
The Vanderbilt Breast Center
Vanderbilt University Medical Center
Nashville, Tennessee

Sheila H. Ridner, PhD, RN, FAAN
Professor
Vanderbilt University School of Nursing
Nashville, Tennessee

Anna Liza Rodriguez, MHA, MSN, RN, OCN®
Director of Oncology Program
Presence Resurrection Medical Center
Chicago, Illinois

Yvonne A. Rucker, RN, MSN, OCN®
Performance Manager, Oncology Services
Northwestern Memorial Hospital
Chicago, Illinois

Nicole A. Shonka, MD
Oncologist
University of Nebraska Medical Center
Omaha, Nebraska

Kim Slusser, RN, MSN, CHPN®
Clinical Operations Director
Duke University Hospital
Durham, North Carolina

Susan S. Tavernier, PhD, RN, APRN-CNS, AOCN®
Post-Doctoral Fellow
University of Utah, College of Nursing
Salt Lake City, Utah

Elizabeth Johnston Taylor, PhD, RN
Associate Professor
Loma Linda University School of Nursing
Loma Linda, California

Janelle Tipton, MSN, RN, AOCN®
Oncology Clinical Nurse Specialist
University of Toledo Medical Center
Toledo, Ohio

Wendy H. Vogel, MSN, FNP, AOCNP®
Oncology Nurse Practitioner
Kingsport Hematology Oncology Associates
Kingsport, Tennessee

Jeffrey S. Wefel, PhD, ABPP
Chief *ad interim*, Section of Neuropsychology
Associate Professor, Department of Neuro-Oncology
MD Anderson Cancer Center
Houston, Texas

Gail M. Wilkes, MS, APRN-BC, AOCN®
Oncology Clinical Instructor
Kilauea, Hawaii

Debra Wujcik, PhD, RN, FAAN
Director, VICC Clinical Trials Shared Resource
Associate Professor, Vanderbilt School of Nursing
Vanderbilt Ingram Cancer Center
Nashville, Tennessee

Connie Henke Yarbro, RN, MS, FAAN
Adjunct Clinical Associate Professor
Sinclair School of Nursing
Editor, *Seminars in Oncology Nursing*
University of Missouri-Columbia
Columbia, Missouri

Laura J. Zitella, MS, RN, ACNP-BC, AOCN®
Lead Advanced Practice Provider, Inpatient Hematology/Oncology
Nurse Practitioner
Stanford University Medical Center
San Francisco, California

PART I

THE PROBLEM OF SYMPTOM DISTRESS

Chapter 1

Evidence-Based Symptom Management

Susan S. Tavernier, PhD, RN, APRN-CNS, AOCN®

The cancer experience, extending from screening and early detection to survivorship or death, involves a wide array of responses by the individual patient, his or her loved ones, and healthcare providers. The responses, most often referred to as symptoms, signs, or side effects, may have a positive, negative, or mixed impact on the person. When side effects of cancer or its treatment are negatively perceived, the person experiences distress. The experience of distress occurs in all patients with cancer,[1] making symptom management a clinical and ethical imperative.

Prolonged or ineffectual management of distress contributes to noncompliance with treatment, reduced quality of life, chronic psychosocial problems, and symptom worsening.[2] It is important to understand that distress is itself a symptom. Understanding distress and other symptoms and side effects of cancer and its treatment assists the oncology nurse caring for the patient to more accurately assess and diagnose the patient problem and intervene appropriately. To optimize patient outcomes, nursing assessments and interventions should be based on reliable and valid evidence. This chapter discusses evidence-based practice and theory and their application to nurse-sensitive outcomes using the symptom of distress as an exemplar.

EVIDENCE-BASED PRACTICE

Evidence-based practice (EBP) provides the rationale for nursing actions. The concept of providing nursing care based on the best available evidence stretches back to Florence Nightingale, who collected meticulous data about each patient and care setting.[3] Evidence-based practice comprises research findings, clinician expertise, patient preference, and practice setting culture and resources.[4] When each of these factors is maximally incorporated into nursing care, optimal patient outcomes are achieved.[5]

The task of analyzing the best available evidence can be overwhelming. Fortunately, there are many resources providing detailed outlines, helpful tools, and training in the EBP process. The reader is encouraged to use the list of sources in Table 1-1 for detailed information on the various models and steps, the commonly identified steps in the EBP process outlined in Table 1-2.

Evidence-based practice guidelines are developed when adequate, reliable, and valid evidence supports particular interventions or actions. Comprehensive and meticulous reviews of evidence are completed, which requires an excellent understanding of research methodology and statistics. However, the clinical utility, practicality, and cultural appropriateness must be evaluated by those healthcare providers in the setting where the research findings are to be implemented into practice. Implementation of evidence-based practice guidelines helps ensure high-quality and cost-effective oncology nursing care. Practice guidelines are available online from several organizations, including the Oncology Nursing Society,[6] National Comprehensive Cancer Network,[7] Agency for Research and Healthcare Quality,[8] and Joanna Briggs Institute.[9]

The implementation of an evidence-based guideline may be difficult due to the differences between the controlled environment in which research is conducted

TABLE 1-1

Sources of Information about EBP Models and Processes

- Larabee JH. *Nurse to Nurse: Evidence-Based Practice*. New York: McGraw-Hill; 2008.
- Barker J. *Evidence-Based Practice for Nurses*. Thousand Oaks, CA: SAGE Publications; 2009.
- Malloch K, Porter-O'Grady T. *Introduction to Evidence-Based Practice in Nursing and Health Care*. 2nd ed. Sudbury, MA: Jones & Bartlett Learning; 2009.
- Scott K, McSherry R. Evidence-based nursing: clarifying the concepts for nurses in practice. *Journal of Clinical Nursing*. 2009;18:1085–1095.
- Houser J, Oman KS. *Evidence-Based Practice: An Implementation Guide for Healthcare Organizations*. Sudbury, MA: Jones & Bartlett Learning; 2010.
- Newell R. *Research for Evidence-Based Practice in Healthcare*. 2nd ed. New York: John Wiley & Sons; 2010.
- Melnyk BM, Fineout-Overholt E. 2nd ed. Philadelphia: Wolters Kluwer Health/Lippincott Williams & Wilkins; 2011.
- Pearson A, Weeks S, Stern C. *Translation Science and the JBI Model of Evidence-Based Healthcare*. Philadelphia: Lippincott Williams & Wilkins/Joanna Briggs Institute; 2011.
- Schmidt NA, Brown JM. *Evidence-Based Practice for Nurses*. Sudbury, MA: Jones & Bartlett Learning; 2011.
- Dearhold S, Dang D. *Johns Hopkins Nursing Evidence-Based Practice Model and Guidelines*. 2nd ed. Indianapolis, IN: Sigma Theta Tau International; 2012.
- Rubin A. *Statistics for Evidence-Based Practice*., 3rd ed. Independence, KY: Cengage Learning; 2012.
- Iowa Model, http://www.nnpnetwork.org/ebp-resources/iowa-model
- Oncology Nursing Society, http://www.ons.org/Research/EBPRA/Process

Abbreviation: EBP: evidence-based practice.

TABLE 1-2

Process of Evidence-Based Practice

- Develop the clinical practice question
  - PICOT acronym often used to clarify the specific question/problem
    - **P**atient or population
    - **I**ntervention or issue of interest
    - **C**omparison intervention or group
    - **O**utcome desired
    - **T**ime frame
- Find relevant evidence
  - Research findings
    - Common system used for rating levels of evidence
      - Level I Systematic review or meta-analysis of randomized controlled studies
      - Level II Randomized, controlled clinical trials
      - Level III Controlled trials without randomization
      - Level IV Case control or cohort studies
      - Level V Systematic review of descriptive or qualitative studies
      - Level VI Single descriptive or qualitative study
      - Level VII Authoritative opinion or expert reports
  - Quality improvement data
  - Patient data
- Evaluate the evidence for quality, quantity, and consistency
- Develop a plan to incorporate the evidence into practice
  - Policy changes
  - Educational requirements
  - Procurement of supplies
  - Budgeting
- Evaluate the practice change on outcomes

TABLE 1-3

Phases in Translational Research

Phase	Description	Example
T_0	Identification of opportunities and approaches to health problems	Art therapy as an intervention to decrease distress.
T_1	Takes approaches identified in T_0 and applies them to a specific situation or population	Testing the use of art therapy in the oncology setting, exploring the optimal number and frequency of sessions to achieve a decrease in distress.
T_2	Evaluates the approach and results in an evidence-based guideline	Evaluate all evidence on decreasing distress in people being treated for cancer and develop a guideline for managing distress in patients being treated for cancer.
T_3	Moves evidence-based guidelines into practice	Tests the distress management guideline in the practice setting for feasibility and efficacy.
T_4	Evaluates the outcomes in the clinical setting	Measures the impact of using the distress management guideline on operational, provider and patient outcomes.

Source: Data from Khoury et al[11].

and the complex and real-life nature of clinical practice settings.[10] Organizations do not always implement evidence-based practices. If such practices or guidelines are implemented, they are often done so inconsistently or in a manner different than designed, leading to suboptimal benefits. Issues with adopting evidence-based practices into routine clinical care have recently brought about an emphasis on the translation and diffusion of evidence into practice. A growing body of literature addresses the clinical application of research, also known as translational research.

Translational research is defined as research that "transforms scientific discoveries arising from laboratory, clinical, or population studies into clinical applications to reduce cancer incidence, morbidity, and mortality."[11] There are five phases of translational health research (Table 1-3). When oncology nurses are implementing or changing practices due to evidence, they are most likely using level T_2 or T_3 study findings. If oncology nurses are involved in performance improvement activities related to the impact of using evidence in practice, level T_4 translational work is being conducted.

EVIDENCE-BASED PRACTICE AND DIFFUSION THEORY

Everett Rogers's Theory of the Diffusion of Innovation[12] has been applied to understanding the adoption of clinical practice guidelines by several authors.[13–15] Rogers's theory identifies five areas that determine the rate and success of adopting evidence-based practices: 1) perceived attributes of innovations; 2) type of innovation decision; 3) communication channels; 4) nature of the social system; and 5) extent of change agent's promotion efforts. In Rogers's theory, the speed at which evidence is incorporated into practice varies based on clinician and organizational perceptions of practice changes supported by the evidence. Adoption of evidence into practice is usually successful when positive perceptions of the change, involvement of stakeholders in key decisions, effective communication channels, and expectations are clear and a competent and respected person competently advocates for the changes.

NURSING IMPLICATIONS

Nursing is "the protection, promotion and optimization of health and abilities, prevention of illness and injury, alleviation of suffering through the diagnosis and treatment of human response, and advocacy in the care of individuals, families, communities, and populations."[16] The results of nursing care relative to the patient and his or her healthcare problems are called nursing sensitive outcomes. Requisites for determining whether an outcome is nurse sensitive include the intervention existing within the scope of nursing practice, evidence supporting the nursing intervention as contributing to the outcome, and the intervention being fundamental to the nursing process.[17] The Oncology Nursing Society identifies five categories of oncology nursing-sensitive outcomes: symptom experience, functional status, safety, psychological distress, and economic. The organization has used these categories as a framework for guiding the development of evidence-based practice guidelines and quality outcome initiatives.

Nursing care is based on the five steps of the nursing process: assessment, diagnosis, planning, implementation, and evaluation. Research has been conducted addressing each of the five steps within the nursing process. Within the realm of nursing assessment, tools for screening and assessment have been developed that reliably assess for many oncology nursing-sensitive outcomes, many of which are discussed in later chapters of this text. The diagnostic step of the nursing process is supported by research such as the work on symptom clusters.[18–23] Nursing interventions are critical to improving nursing-sensitive outcomes. A growing body of evidence has identified nursing interventions that can effectively improve symptom distress,[24–27] improve quality of life,[28–30] and improve cancer screening.[31,32]

Finally, the evaluation of nursing care is synonymous with outcomes and asks the question, "Were the goals of care achieved?" Evaluation occurs at the individual level, at which the patient perspective must be taken into account. Patient satisfaction surveys and focus groups are often used to collect such data. Evaluation may also occur at the aggregate level. Outcome measurements are often conducted using quality assurance, quality improvement, and research methods.

Nurses provide assessments of the cancer symptom experience throughout the cancer trajectory. Knowledge of the signs and symptoms of the tumor, treatments, and associated complications accounts for the vast majority of oncology nursing expertise. The diagnosis and treatment of cancer-related symptoms require the nurse to remain current with the variations among tumor and treatment types as well as the nuances that occur at the individual level. This responsibility can often seem overwhelming given the constantly changing clinical environment and the vast quantity of research that has been published. Fortunately, several organizations (identified earlier in this chapter) provide comprehensive reviews of the evidence and issue practice guidelines that can be used by the practicing nurse.

CASE EXAMPLE: DISTRESS MANAGEMENT

You work in a community outpatient cancer clinic that is a department within the hospital. The center is accredited through the American College of Surgeons. The center has three medical oncologists, one radiation oncologist, and one nurse practitioner. Your clinic provides radiation and chemotherapy treatments for adult patients only. Nursing staff provide patient care during physician visits and chemotherapy administration. The center also has a dedicated social worker and dietician. Other professional resources, such as counseling, chaplaincy, and physical therapy, are available by referral.

The Institute of Medicine identified distress management as a critical element of care in the report *Cancer Care for the Whole Patient*.[33] The American College of Surgeons recently made distress assessment and management a requirement for accreditation.[34] The hospital where you work has chosen to follow the National Comprehensive Cancer Network Distress Management Guideline.[35] This guideline uses the Distress Thermometer (DT), a vertically drawn depiction of a thermometer on which patients rate their distress level over the past week on a scale from 0 (bottom of thermometer, indicating no distress) to 10 (top of thermometer, extreme distress). They mark items on the problem list next to the Distress Thermometer that they feel contribute to their distress. The guideline has a decision tree for referrals and interventions, dependent upon the source(s) of distress.

Your clinic uses an electronic medical record (EMR), with computers located in each exam room, in the accelerator control room, and throughout the chemotherapy administration area. Current nursing assessment data required in the EMR focuses on physiologic symptoms, but not psychosocial needs. However, the hospital computer support department recently integrated the Distress Thermometer[35] into the nursing assessment page used by the nurses in the outpatient oncology areas.

You are a nurse working with one of the medical oncologists. Your manager has assigned you the task of developing the policy and procedure for distress management in the outpatient cancer center. He gave you level 3 accountability, which means you need only to keep him informed of your progress. Upon reviewing the guideline and decision diagrams, you realize implementation should involve several disciplines.[36] Using Rogers's Diffusion of Innovation Theory, you anticipate that adoption of the guideline into practice will be more successful if the staff most affected by the decisions are involved. Thus you decide to use a team approach for this project.

Your team members include the cancer center's social worker and dietician, a radiation therapist, a chemotherapy infusion nurse, the nurse educator responsible for patient and nurse cancer education for the hospital, a staff member of the quality improvement department, and a staff member from the computer support team. The medical oncologist you work with has agreed to champion the project among the physicians but will not attend the meetings. She has requested that you keep her informed of the project's progress and decisions. She has agreed to a team presentation of the completed project during the monthly physician meeting.

Your team meets to review the project. You review the guideline with the group.[35] Although the DT and problem list are already available on the EMR, the team has questions about who is responsible for the screening and referral process and the frequency of screening. Because the DT and problem list are to be completed by the patient, another question arises about how the patient is to complete the DT and problem list and how the responses should be entered into the EMR. After much discussion, the team identifies a need to review research related to the implementation of the guideline. You take the group through the PICOT process before requesting a literature search from the librarian at the hospital.

- **P**opulation: outpatient and/or office-based oncology clinic
- **I**ntervention/issue: implementation of a process for distress screening and management using EMRs
- **C**omparison intervention/group: none or pre/post implementation data
- **O**utcome desired: successful implementation of the guideline
- **T**ime frame: throughout the treatment phase of cancer

You take this information to the librarian at your hospital. She conducts a literature search and finds several articles.[37–44] She tells you there were very few research articles specific to your setting, so she broadened her search to include all clinical settings, reviews, and commentaries. The librarian notes that the entire April 2012 volume of the *Journal of Clinical Oncology* was dedicated to psychosocial care, with several articles covering distress management. You assign each team member to read and evaluate two articles each. You ask each team member to summarize each article using a table such as the one depicted in Table 1-4.

At the next team meeting, the summaries are reviewed and discussed for relevancy to your situation and setting. It is noted that the majority of articles found are anecdotal, case study, and quality improvement projects. The team summarizes the steps taken in each article that contributed to successful implementation as well as author recommendations. From this information you begin to develop a plan for implementing the National Comprehensive Cancer Network guideline. In your plan, you include education for all staff using several methods: self-study, online, and in-service programs. You work with the educator on the content and evaluation of learning. In addition, the educator helps draft the new policy using the required hospital format. This policy will be presented at the next Policy and Procedure Committee meeting for review and approval. The education effort requires a few resources such as paper, photocopying, and staff time. You work with your manager to develop the budget. You review the proposed policy and educational plan with the physician champion, and your team is scheduled to provide education and review of the project at the next physician meeting.

After the first week of implementing the policy for distress screening and management, your team meets again to celebrate the completion of this first phase of the project. The group also discusses how to monitor its ongoing use, resolve problems as they arise, and provide continual encouragement to the rest of the staff. At the meeting you suggest that the group publish their experiences of implementation to help others facing the same situation. Everyone enthusiastically agrees. You lead a discussion to outline which information each member should continue to collect during the initial implementation phase. The group agrees to meet each month to review problems, resolutions, staff comments and organizational issues affecting the implementation of the guideline. This information will be used in the article.

TABLE 1-4

Example of Literature Review Summary Table

Reference info (title, author, journal)	Study Design	Study Sample	Study Methods	Summary of Findings/ Key Factors to Implementation	Level of Evidence
• Educational intervention in cancer outpatient clinics on routine screening for emotional distress • Grassi, et al[39] • Psychooncology	Observational study	Newly diagnosed cancer patient	Compared the Distress Thermometer scores of patients referred to psychosocial services with those who were not	• Differences were identified between patients not referred and those who were • Routine screening of all new patients resulted in more accurate referrals • Routine screening resulted in more referrals • Acceptance by staff and patients was low	VI-single descriptive study

CONCLUSION

Evidence-based practice provides a rationale for nursing actions. Research findings are just one facet of such evidence. Empirical findings, clinician experience and expertise, cultural issues, available resources, and patient preferences must also be factored into making decisions about nursing care. The dissemination of evidence and its translation into practice are the responsibility of all oncology nurses. Oncology nurses are in an ideal position to assess and manage the effects of cancer and its treatment on individuals and caregivers, thereby reducing distress. The remainder of this text reviews and applies an evidence-based approach to the assessment and management of symptoms commonly experienced by people with cancer.

REFERENCES

1. Holland JC, Alici Y. Management of distress in cancer patients. *J Support Oncol.* 2010;8(1):4–12.
2. Jacobsen PB. Screening for psychological distress in cancer patients: challenges and opportunities. *J Clin Oncol.* 2007;25(29):4526–4527.
3. Aravind M, Chung KC. Evidence-based medicine and hospital reform: tracing origins back to Florence Nightingale. *Plast Reconstr Surg*; 2010;125(1):403–409.
4. Sackett DL, Straus SE, Richardson WS, Rosenbert W, Haynes RB. *Evidence-Based Medicine: How to Practice and Teach EBM.* London: Churchill Livingstone; 2000.
5. Melnyk B, Fineout-Overholt E. *Evidence-Based Practice in Nursing and Healthcare: A Guide to Best Practice.* 2nd ed. Philadelphia: Wolters Kluwer Health/Lippincott Williams & Wilkins; 2011.
6. Oncology Nursing Society. ONS PEP®: *Putting Evidence into Practice.* Oncology Nursing Society website. http://www.ons.org/Research/PEP. Accessed June 18, 2012.
7. *NCCN Evidence-Based Cancer Guidelines. Oncology Drug Compendium: Oncology Continuing Medical Education.* Fort Washington, PA: The Association, 2012.
8. Agency for Healthcare Research and Quality. National Guideline Clearinghouse. U.S. Department of Health and Human Services website. http://www.guideline.gov/. Accessed June 18, 2012.
9. Joanna Briggs Institute website. University of Adelaide, South Australia, Australia. The Association; 2011. http://www.joannabriggs.edu.au/. Accessed June 18, 2012.
10. Cochrane LJ, Olson CA, Murray, S, Dupuis M, Tooman T, Hayes S. Gaps between knowing and doing: understanding and assessing the barriers to optimal health care. *J Contin Educ Health Prof.* 2007;27(2):94–102.
11. National Cancer Institute. TRWG definition of translational research. National Institutes of Health website. http://www.cancer.gov/researchandfunding/trwg/TRWG-definition-and-TR-continuum/. Accessed June 18, 2012.
12. Rogers EM. *Diffusion of Innovations.* 4th ed. New York: Free Press; 1995.
13. Gale BV, Schaffer MA. Organizational readiness for evidence-based practice. *J Nurs Adm.* 2009;39(2):91–97.
14. Greenhalgh T, Robert G, MacFarlane F, Bate P, Kyriakidou O. Diffusion of innovations in service organizations: systematic review and recommendations. *Millbank Q.* 2004;83:581–629.
15. Leeman J, Jackson B, Sandelowski M. An evaluation of how well research reports facilitate the use of findings in practice. *J Nurs Scholarsh.* 2006;38(2):171–177.
16. American Nurses Association. http://www.nursingworld.org/EspeciallyForYou/What-is-Nursing. Accessed June 18, 2012
17. Given B, Beck S, Etland C, Gobel BH, Lamkin L, Marsee VD. Nursing-sensitive patient outcomes: description and framework. July 2004. http://www.ons.org/Research/NursingSensitive/Description. Accessed June 18, 2012.
18. Lopez V, Copp G, Brunton L, Molassiotis A. Symptom experience in patients with gynecological cancers: the development of symptom clusters through patient narratives. *J Support Oncol.* 2011;9(2):64–71.
19. Gilbertson-White S, Aouizerat BE, Jahan T, Miaskowski C. A review of the literature on multiple symptoms, their predictors, and associated outcomes in patients with advanced cancer. *Palliat Support Care.* 2011;9:81–102.
20. Esper P. Symptom clusters in individuals living with advanced cancer. *Semin Oncol Nurs.* 2010;26(3):168–174.
21. Karabulu N, Erci B, Ozer N, Ozdemir S. Symptom clusters and experiences of patients with cancer. *J Adv Nurs.* 2010;66(5):1011–1021.
22. Molassiotis A, Wengström Y, Kearney N. Symptom cluster patterns during the first year after diagnosis with cancer. *J Pain Symptom Manage.* 2010;39(5):847–858.
23. Kim E, Jahan T, Aouizerat BE, et al. Differences in symptom clusters identified using occurrence rates versus symptom severity ratings in patients at the end of radiation therapy. *Cancer Nurs.* 2009;32(6):429–436.
24. Payne C, Wiffen PJ, Martin S. Interventions for fatigue and weight loss in adults with advanced progressive illness. *Cochrane Database System Rev.* 2012;1:CD008427.
25. Rheingans JI. Pediatric oncology nurses' management of patients' symptoms. *J Pediatr Oncol Nurs.* 2008(6);25:303–311.
26. Wilkinson S, Barnes K, Storey L. Massage for symptom relief in patients with cancer: systematic review. *J Adv Nurs.* 2008;63(5):430–439.
27. Harris DJ, Eilers J, Harriman A, Cashavelly BJ, Maxwell C. Putting evidence into practice: evidence-based interventions for the management of oral mucositis. *Clin J Oncol Nurs.* 2008;12(1):141–152.
28. Rueda JR, Solà I, Pascual A, Subirana Casacuberta M. Non-invasive interventions for improving well-being and quality of life in patients with lung cancer. *Cochrane Database System Rev.* 2011;7:CD004282.
29. McCorkle R, Dowd M, Ercolano E, et al. Effects of a nursing intervention on quality of life outcomes in post-surgical women with gynecological cancers. *Psychooncology.* 2009;18(1):62–70.
30. Wanchai A, Armer JM, Stewart BR. Nonpharmacologic supportive strategies to promote quality of life in patients experiencing cancer-related fatigue: a systematic review. *Clin J Oncol Nurs.* 2011;15(2):203–214.
31. Menon U, Belue R, Wahab S, et al. A randomized trial comparing the effect of two phone-based interventions on colorectal cancer screening adherence. *Ann Behav Med.* 2011;42(3):294–303.
32. Kessler TA. Increasing mammography and cervical cancer knowledge and screening behaviors with an educational program. *Oncol Nurs Forum.* 2012;39(1):61–68.
33. Adler NE, Page EK, eds. *Cancer Care for the Whole Patient: Meeting Psychosocial Health Needs.* Washington, DC: National Academies Press; 2008. http://www.nap.edu/catalog.php?record_id=11993/. Accessed June 18, 2012.
34. Commission on Cancer. *Cancer Program Standards 2012: Ensuring Patient-Centered Care.* Chicago, IL: American College of Surgeons; 2011. http://www.facs.org/cancer/coc/cocprogramstandards2012.pdf. Accessed June 18, 2012.
35. National Comprehensive Cancer Network. *Distress Management Version 3.2012.* Fort Washington, PA: NCCN; 2012. http://www.nccn.org/professionals/physician_gls/pdf/distress.pdf. Accessed June 18, 2012.
36. Swihart D. *Shared Governance: A Practical Approach to Transform Professional Nursing Practice.* 2nd ed. Danvers, MA: HCPro, Inc.; 2011:9.
37. Loscalzo M, Clark KL, Holland J. Successful strategies for implementing biopsychosocial screening. *Psychooncology.* 2011;20(5):455–462.

38. Goncalves JJ, Rocha AM. A decision support system for quality of life in head and neck oncology patients. *Head Neck Oncol.* 2012;4;3. http://www.ncbi.nlm.nih.gov/pmc/articles/PMC3296664/?tool=pubmed. Accessed June 18, 2012.
39. Grassi L, Rossi E, Caruso R, et al. Educational intervention in cancer outpatient clinics on routine screening for emotional distress: an observational study. *Psychooncology.* 2011;20(6):669–674.
40. Bidstrup PE, Johansen C, Mitchell AJ. Screening for cancer-related distress: Summary of evidence from tools to programs. *Acta Oncol.* 2011;50(2):194–204.
41. Mitchell AJ, Vahabzadeh A, Magruder K. Screening for distress and depression in cancer settings: 10 lessons from 40 years of primary-care research. *Psychooncology.* 2011;20(6):572–584.
42. Fitch M. Screening for distress: a role for oncology nursing. *Curr Opin Oncol.* 2011;23(4):331–337.
43. Clark PG, Rochon E, Brethwaite D, Edmiston KK. Screening for psychological and physical distress in a cancer inpatient treatment setting: a pilot study. *Psychooncology.* 2011;20(6):664–668.
44. Jacobsen PB, Wagner LI. A new quality standard: the integration of psychosocial care into routine cancer care. *J Clin Oncol.* 2012; 30(11):1154–1159.

PART II

Alterations in Comfort

Chapter 2
Arthralgias and Myalgias

Chapter 3
Cancer-Related Fatigue

Chapter 4
Menopausal Symptoms

Chapter 5
Pain

Chapter 6
Sleep Disturbances

PART II

Chapter 2

Arthralgias and Myalgias

Virginia R. Martin, MSN, RN, AOCN®

THE PROBLEM

Newer chemotherapy drugs and biologic response modifiers and new combinations of these drugs have caused an increased incidence of side effects called arthralgias and myalgias in patients with cancer. *Arthralgia* is joint pain. *Myalgia* is diffuse muscle pain, usually accompanied by malaise. Both toxicities may be listed separately or alone or grouped with other neurotoxicities. Chemotherapy-induced peripheral neuropathy (CIPN) is very similar to arthralgia and myalgia in that it is pain caused by many of the same antineoplastic agents. However, CIPN has a sensory component, arising from nerve involvement that causes unusual or increased reaction to stimuli or loss of sensation.[1,2] The term *neuromuscular toxicity* is a more precise description of arthralgias and myalgias. Arthralgias and myalgias may also be grouped together with the side effect called flu-like symptoms or syndrome.

The impact of arthralgia and myalgia on the patient's quality of life can be significant. If the severity of the symptoms is great enough, patients' ability to perform their normal activities of daily living may be impaired. A review of several studies suggested anywhere from 23% to 40% of patients stop taking their aromatase inhibitor medication because of the side effects experienced including joint pain.[3] Most chemotherapy drugs have overlapping side effects. Fatigue, malaise, decreased appetite, and lack of energy are common complaints. CIPN also impacts quality of life and performance status. Nurses have an opportunity to educate patients about this potential problem and about strategies to manage the discomfort associated with it. Table 2-1 lists chemotherapy drugs and biologic response modifiers that may cause arthralgias and myalgias.

INCIDENCE

Arthralgias and myalgias have long been associated with chronic illnesses such as rheumatoid arthritis or fibromyalgia. *Fibromyalgia* is a term applied to persons who suffer from widespread musculoskeletal pain. Paclitaxel, a taxane, is one of the most useful active agents in antineoplastic therapy. Taxanes cause arthralgias and myalgias in as many as 58% of patients.[4] The intensity of these symptoms appears to be related to the dose of paclitaxel given; however, it is not a dose-limiting toxicity. Another frequently used taxane, docetaxel, also produces arthralgias and myalgias. The vinca alkaloid drugs are associated with arthralgias and myalgias as well, but the incidence is less frequent. Vinblastine, when used at high doses in the treatment of testicular cancer, causes severe myalgias—a clear dose-related phenomenon.[5] Colony-stimulating factors (CSFs) produce flu-like symptoms that include, but are not limited to, arthralgias and myalgias. The approach to mobilization of peripheral blood stem cells with granulocyte colony-stimulating factor (G-CSF) has produced as much as a 90% incidence of arthralgias and myalgias.[6] Although these effects appear to be dose related, they are usually mild and can be treated with analgesics.[6] Aromatase inhibitors (AIs), used in the treatment of breast cancer, are also responsible for arthralgia complaints in patients.[7] Other agents for which arthralgias or myalgias are listed as a side effect include interferon, topotecan, bryostatin,

TABLE 2-1

Chemotherapy/Biologic Response Modifiers that May Cause Arthralgias and Myalgias

Classification/Drugs	Comments
	Taxanes
Paclitaxel	Dose-related: mild discomfort at doses <170 mg/m²; more frequent and severe with doses >200 mg/m² Arthralgias and myalgias increase when colony stimulating factors added. Transient pain in muscles and joints, especially large axial, shoulder, and paraspinal muscles.
Docetaxel	Transient myalgias and arthralgias
	Vinca Alkaloids
Vincristine	Myalgias
Vinblastine	Myalgias; dose-related; severe muscle pain with high doses
Vinorelbine	Less severe than other vinca alkaloids
Vinflunine	Myalgias
	Biologic Response Modifiers
Denileukin diftitox	Flulike syndrome that includes myalgias and arthralgias
Bacillus Calmette-Guérin (BCG)	Same as above
Filgrastim	Flulike syndrome that includes arthralgias and myalgias; transient bone pain
Sargramostim	Skeletal pain
Interferon	Arthralgias and myalgias, involves proximal muscles of lower extremities
Interleukin-2	Arthralgias and myalgias; more significant at high doses
Rituximab	Myalgias
Tositumomab	Radioconjugate myalgias
	Miscellaneous Agents
Azacytidine	Muscle weakness and myalgia
Altremine	Flulike symptoms with fever, chills, malaise, myalgias, and arthraligas
Anastrozole	Myalgias and arthralgias
Bortezomib	Muscle cramps
Dacarbazine	Flulike symptoms with fever, chills, malaise, myalgias, and arthralgias
Exemestane	Arthralgias
Fludarabine	Causes fever that causes myalgias and arthralgias
Gemcitabine	Flulike symptoms with fever, chills, malaise, myalgias, and arthralgias
Isotretinoin (13 cis-retinoic acid)	Arthralgias and myalgias
Ixabepilone	Myalgias and arthralgias
Letrozole	Mild musculoskeletal pain and arthralgia is the most common adverse event.
Neulasta	Bone pain
Procarbazine	Flulike symptoms with fever, chills, malaise, myalgias and arthralgias
Topetecan	Same as above
Zoledronic acid	Myalgias

fludarabine, dacarbazine, altretamine, bacillus Calmette-Guérin, vinorelbine, gemcitabine, letrozole, procarbazine, isotretenoin (13-*cis*-retinoic acid), denileukin diftitox, vinflunine, exemestane, anastrozole, and ixabepilone.

ETIOLOGY

How chemotherapeutic agents cause joint and muscle pain is uncertain. It is interesting to note, however, that some agents associated with significant joint and muscle pains are agents that inhibit microtubular function (i.e., the vinca alkaloids, particularly vinblastine and vindesine, and the taxanes, paclitaxel and docetaxel). Microtubules play a critical role in cell division and mitosis. Although the vinca alkaloids and taxanes bind at different sites, they both disrupt the cell cycle and lead to cell death.[8] The antimicrotubule agents are among the most important anticancer drugs and have contributed significantly to the therapy of most curable neoplasms, such as Hodgkin's and non-Hodgkin's lymphomas, breast cancer, germ cell tumors, and childhood leukemias.[9,10] The aromatase inhibitors work differently. The AIs are used in hormone-responsive cancers that are altered by lower estrogen levels. As it has been suggested that estrogen helps to reduce pain and inflammation, AIs that work by lowering estrogen could contribute to the arthralgia symptoms.[11]

Vinca alkaloids

With the vinca alkaloids and taxanes, there is a clear dose-response relationship with arthralgias and myalgias. This association is most striking with vinblastine. The original Einhorn regimen employed vinblastine at a dose of 0.4 mg/kg administered in two equally divided doses (0.2 mg/kg) on the first and second days of therapy.[12] This high-dose program was associated with intense myelosuppression, as was to be expected, but two nonhematologic toxicities were also noted. The first was neurotoxicity, which was generally seen at lower doses; the second was severe muscle pain. The latter symptom developed a few days after drug administration and lasted for several days. It manifested as severe back and abdominal pain, and in its worse form, required opiate analgesics. Sometimes dose adjustments were required to convince patients to continue treatment.

Clinical trials investigating lower doses of vinblastine (0.1 to 0.2 mg/kg) revealed that the associated muscle pain was much milder with these doses, indicating that toxicity was dose related.[12,13] Now used at much lower doses, the vinca alkaloids are still associated with occasional muscle pain, but rarely, if ever, is the pain as severe as that which was seen with high-dose vinblastine.

A new vinca alkaloid in clinical trials is called vinflunine. Studies suggest that treatment-induced myalgia appears less severe with vinflunine than with other drugs in this class.[14]

Taxanes

Paclitaxel. As many as 58% of those patients treated with moderate to high doses of paclitaxel report transient arthralgias or myalgias.[4] Symptoms begin anywhere from 1 to 4 days after treatment and can last a week or longer.[15] As with vinblastine, this toxicity appears to be dose related, but rarely does it require dose adjustment. In contrast to the pain associated with high-dose vinblastine, less truncal pain and more pain in the distal muscles and joints are seen with paclitaxel. Large axial muscles—specifically, shoulder and paraspinal muscles—are involved, and patients report aching in the hips and thighs. Often the arthralgias and myalgias are referred to as flu-like symptoms without a fever, and occasionally patients may complain of abdominal pain as a component of the process.[16]

These side effects are diffuse and a self-limited process—characteristics that have led to a hypothesis that the symptoms may be a result of some inflammatory process. The development of the discomfort, usually more than 48 hours after the infusion, also supports the inflammation theory because all patients are premedicated with dexamethasone at the time of infusion to prevent the hypersensitivity reaction. Dexamethasone may simultaneously contain the inflammatory reaction until that premedication wears off. Elevations of muscle enzymes such as creatinine phosphokinase have not been observed in patients treated with paclitaxel.[9]

As no structural changes in muscles or joints have been shown, studies have begun to investigate the possibility that paclitaxel causes neuropathic injury. This pain syndrome is referred to as paclitaxel-associated acute pain syndrome (P-APS).[17] Laboratory research showed evidence of dorsal root ganglia and sciatic nerve damage after paclitaxel administration. Other studies support this idea by observing that patients with higher P-APS scores developed chemotherapy-induced peripheral neuropathy.[18] More research is needed to definitively determine the pathophysiology of paclitaxel. P-APS is characterized by severe arthralgias and mylagias, along with numbness and tingling.[17] Manifestation occurs 1 to 2 days after treatment and lasts a median of 4 to 5 days.

The dose-related nature of the toxicity suggests that the drug affects the muscle directly and—although it is speculation—influences the microtubular system, which is so critical to maintaining normal muscle function and physiology. Although these symptoms are usually mild at doses of paclitaxel less than 170 mg/m^2, they become more frequent and severe at doses greater than 200 mg/m^2.[19,20] Severe muscular complaints usually occur more often at paclitaxel doses greater than 250 mg/m^2.[19] Retrospective analysis of four phase II trials of paclitaxel at a dose of 210 mg/m^2 given as a 3-hour infusion concluded that the severity of the symptoms correlated with the total cumulative dose.[21] Thus the severity of this toxicity can be influenced by the treatment schedule, the single dose per course, and the cumulative dose. Age, sex, height, prior chemotherapy, renal or hepatic function, any pharmacokinetic parameters, and the metastatic sites did not show a significant correlation with neuromuscular toxicity.

Docetaxel. Docetaxel, a highly effective drug used in neoplastic therapy, causes myalgias and arthralgias, although the incidence of these effects appears to be lower than that associated with paclitaxel.[16,22] The side-effect incidence is proportional to the cumulative dose. After treatment with docetaxel revealed significant fluid retention toxicity and dermatologic toxicity, it was recommended that, to ameliorate toxicities, patients be given dexamethasone 8 mg PO bid starting 24 hours before treatment and continuing for as long as 5 days after administration. This prescribed premedication regimen may influence the incidence of myalgias. Two newer taxanes, nab-paclitaxel and cabazitaxel, have both been associated with neurotoxicity incidence.[23]

Miscellaneous agents

Azacytidine is an antimetabolite that is associated with muscle weakness and myalgia. Dacarbazine, topotecan, gemcitabine, and procarbazine are associated with flu-like symptoms that include myalgias and arthralgias. Fludarabine causes a fever that may cause myalgias and arthralgias. Letrozole lists mild musculoskeletal pain and arthralgia as a common adverse event. Bortezomib, a protease inhibitor, can cause myalgia, asthenia, and fever.[24,25] Vemurafenib, a multikinase inhibitor for patients with BRAF mutations, lists arthralgias as one of its more common side effects.[26] Ixabepilone, an epothilone, has a 2–10 times greater tubulin-polymerizing activity than paclitaxel.[27] Mylagias and arthralgias are observed as common side effects. Bisphosphonates are the mainstay of treatment for osteoporosis. There are four Food and Drug Administration (FDA)-approved agents: alendronate, risedronate, ibandronate, and zoledronic acid. Zoledronic acid is associated with myalgias.[28]

Aromatase inhibitors

Aromatase inhibitors have become an integral part of the treatment of postmenopausal women with breast cancer who have tumors that are estrogen receptor positive. The depletion of estrogen seen with AI therapy is clinically significant, as it has beneficial effects on the tumor, but it also exerts a negative effect on skeletal bone. Menopausal women have additional bone loss when using AIs. AIs have a profound estrogen-depletion effect, reducing the production of estrogen by more than 95%.[29] Thirty percent of patients receiving AIs report musculoskeletal problems, compared to approximately 24% of patients receiving tamoxifen.[29] Musculoskeletal pain associated with AI therapy presents a challenge for both the patient and the care team. There is little evidence to show how AIs cause muscle and joint pain. Endocrine therapy trials have identified the problem, but there is little guidance on how to predict which patients may experience these arthralgias and myalgias. A patient's history—such as preexisting musculoskeletal disorders, menopausal state, and cancer-related pain—may influence her ability to tolerate AIs.[30]

Biologic response modifiers

Toxicities associated with interferon include an acute syndrome characterized by arthralgias and myalgias.[31] This syndrome can occur in 80% to 90% of patients and may last as long as 8 to 9 hours. Most symptoms in the musculoskeletal system are related to the flu-like syndrome caused by interferon. The symptoms tend to be worse at the beginning of therapy, but usually improve over time. Symptoms consist of self-limited arthralgias and myalgias of transient duration. Severe myalgias were reported in 4 of 27 patients (15%) whose chronic myelogenous leukemia was treated with interferon.[31] The myalgias involved the proximal muscles of the lower extremities and were associated with limited movement. Treatment consisted of bed rest and therapy with steroids and opiate analgesics. Testing revealed a negative eletromyography (EMG) and no elevated muscle enzymes.

Colony-stimulating factors such as filgrastim, lenograstim, and pegfilgrastim provide protection for patients at risk for febrile neutropenia, a potentially fatal complication of cancer treatment. This group of drugs produce flu-like symptoms as side effects, and bone pain is a common reported side effect in 25% to 45% of patients.[32] Bone pain related to CSFs occurs secondary to the rapid growth of neutrophils in bone marrow before they are released to the periphery.[33] Mobilization of peripheral blood stem cells includes administration of G-CSF sequentially or simultaneously with interleukin-3 (IL-3) or as G-CSF alone; these methods have produced up to an 83% incidence of arthralgias and myalgias.[6] Pegfilgrastim is indicated for patients with nonmyeloid malignancies receiving myelosuppressive anticancer drugs associated with a clinically significant incidence of febrile neutropenia. In one study, bone pain and pain in extremities occurred at a higher incidence in pegfilgrastim-treated patients as compared with patients who received a placebo.[34]

Arthralgias and myalgias occur at high doses of interleukin-2 (IL-2) due to an accumulation of cytokine deposits in the joint spaces. Bacillus Calmette-Guérin (BCG) and denileukin diftitox cause a flu-like syndrome, with symptoms including arthralgias and myalgias being reported. Two monoclonal antibodies, rituximab and tositumomab radioimmunoconjugate, both list myalgias as a patient complaint.

A post-chemotherapy rheumatism syndrome was reported in eight patients treated with adjuvant therapy for breast cancer.[35] Symptoms appeared within a few months of completing combination chemotherapy and were collectively described as a musculoskeletal syndrome. Serologic tests for autoimmune markers and bone and joint scans were not remarkable, but there was noted mild periarticular swelling. Symptoms abated over several months for these patients. Nonsteroidal analgesics were ineffective in relieving pain, but one patient was treated effectively with low-dose steroids. Loprinzi et al.[35] concluded that the etiology was unclear for this syndrome.

Investigational agents

In a study of 33 patients receiving ABT-869, dose-limiting toxicities related to grade 3 fatigue were reported.[36] This group also reported significant treatment-related adverse events, including asthenia, hand and foot blisters, and myalgia. As the doses escalated, the symptoms of fatigue, myalgia, and skin toxicities increased.

A Japanese study linked the MAPK (MAP kinase) signal transduction pathway to myalgias.[37] This study addressed a link in which MAPK was activated and enhanced by the stimulation through induction of the mitochondrial reactive oxygen species production. Febrile attacks were reported and documented to last an average of 21 days. Patients experienced symptoms of myalgia, rash, abdominal pain, and arthralgia.

A phase I study of SU5416, a small-molecule inhibitor of the vascular endothelial growth factor receptor (VEGFR), reported the most serious drug-related toxicities were grade 3 liver enzyme abnormalities, arthralgia, and hallucinations.[38]

EMERGING ETIOLOGY

Cancer survivorship is an emerging area of new research. The number of cancer survivors now exceeds 10 million. One of the listed sequelae of cancer treatment is aprheumatologic condition. It is described as nonspecific, mild to moderate muscle and joint pain. Affected patients report a cluster of symptoms including mylagias and arthralgias. The syndrome is self-limited and responds to symptomatic treatment with nonsteroidal anti-inflammatory agents.[39]

PATHOPHYSIOLOGY

The pathophysiologic mechanisms of arthralgia and myalgia remain unclear, and a specific treatment is not available. *Microtubules* are polymers of tubulin believed to function as the major constituent of the mitotic spindle apparatus. The microtubules are also critical for maintenance of cell shape, motility, and anchorage; mediation of signals between cell surface receptors and the nucleus; and intracellular transport.[40] Microtubules are important in axonal transport and other vital neuron functions, and it is known that neurotoxicity is a major toxicity of antimicrotubule drugs.

Microtubule assembly and disassembly are in dynamic equilibrium. The vinca alkaloids induce microtubule disassembly, whereas the taxanes promote microtubule assembly and stabilization. The vinca alkaloids interact with the tubulin and disrupt the microtubules, inducing metaphase arrest in dividing cells.[41] The stabilization of the microtubules by paclitaxel inhibits mitosis in the G_2 and M phases of the cell cycle, inhibits fibroblast cell migration, and causes cell death.[10] The microtubules formed in the presence of paclitaxel are extraordinarily stable and dysfunctional, causing the death of the cell by disrupting the reorganization of the microtubule network.

Additionally, the diffuse and self-limited nature of the arthralgias and myalgias from chemotherapy and the lack of cumulative effects with multiple treatments lead to the hypothesis that the symptoms are possibly the result of some form of inflammatory reaction to paclitaxel.[42]

SYMPTOM ASSESSMENT

Arthralgia and myalgia following chemotherapy are not associated with physical findings. When these symptoms occur secondary to chemotherapy, they should be distinguished from fibromyalgia, viral infections, an overuse syndrome, neuropathies, and hypothyroidism. Joint symptoms may be due to trauma, infection, crystal-induced inflammation (gout), or primary inflammatory arthritis. Myalgia is sometimes associated with muscle tenderness and sometimes not. Myalgias may occur secondary to a localized problem (trauma or overuse) or a systemic disorder (acute or chronic infection, toxic or metabolic disorders), or, less commonly, may reflect a primary muscle disease. Differential diagnosis is based on the physical examination and history.

Muscle pain differs from cutaneous pain in several ways: (1) it is usually described as aching or cramping rather than stabbing or sharp; (2) it is poorly localized, whereas cutaneous pain is localized with great accuracy; and (3) it is generally referred to other deep somatic structures (muscles, fascia, tendons, ligaments, and joints), whereas cutaneous pain is not referred. Typical pain from arthralgias and myalgias develops in the large joints of the arms and legs 24 to 72 hours after treatment and disappears within 4 to 7 days. Patients report that the discomfort is constant; it does not wax and wane during those days but ends predictably within this time frame. Patients describe the pain as varying from a mild ache to a severe pain. It is similar to arthritic pain, as it is worse or more pronounced on movement and more relieved at rest. Many patients state that they do not feel the discomfort until they attempt to get out of bed in the morning. Others describe a feeling that comes over them, similar to a flu-like ache that begins the manifestation of the symptom. Myalgias generally involve shoulder muscles, the arms, and the leg joints. The weakness is greater in the lower extremities than in the upper extremities.

Arthralgias and myalgias are dose related and generally recur with repeated paclitaxel treatment, but they are not predictable. The discomfort also varies from cycle to cycle. The unpredictability and the fluctuation in severity of the symptoms contribute to anxiety in the patient. In addition, the joint and muscle aches can influence the patient's ability to function normally.

The muscle and bone pain experienced by patients receiving paclitaxel and aromatase inhibitors can be compared to that experienced with a bout of influenza or following administration of high doses of vinblastine or etoposide. Shoulder and paraspinal muscles are usually involved, and arthralgias in the large joints of the arms and legs are most frequently reported by patients.

Impaired physical mobility related to limitation of joint function and pain can have a deleterious effect on a patient's work, home, and leisure activities. Assessment of sociological and psychological factors is important in judging the strengths and resources the patient brings to coping with the condition. Functional changes can lead to depression, anxiety, and loss of confidence.

RISK FACTORS

The most important risk factor for developing arthralgias and myalgias is the dose of the chemotherapy. Risk factors for arthralgias and myalgias include the following[16]:

- Antecedent peripheral neuropathy
- History of diabetes
- Alcohol use
- High individual doses of paclitaxel (greater than 250 mg/m^2)
- High-dose vinblastine
- Concurrent administration of paclitaxel with cisplatin
- Administration of biologic response modifiers
- Age
- Full-time employment status[43]
- Prior neurotoxic chemotherapy
- History of arthritis
- History of neuromuscular disease
- For women receiving AIs, last menstrual period within 5 years of treatment[43]
- Sepsis[44]

Recognizing and treating any preexisting condition is an important first step in treatment, and the issue of toxic synergy should be addressed.[45] Once neuropathy occurs, continuing the same therapy may lead to progressive nerve damage and loss of function.

SELF-ASSESSMENT

Patients should be encouraged to report symptoms of arthralgias and myalgias at the onset of symptoms. Patient and caregiver education is the cornerstone of effective management of the patient's symptoms. Education on the use of analgesic medications and nonpharmacologic management of symptoms prior to onset is important in assisting the patient and caregivers to be able to manage these symptoms early. Patients should be encouraged to communicate and report symptoms to the nurse as well as relief measures that have proved effective in the past. Education on possible symptoms of myalgias or arthralgias related to the treatment should be undertaken during the initial discussion on potential side effects related to the chemotherapy plan. A diary can be used by the patient to self-report symptoms of arthralgia and myalgia as well as those interventions that proved to be most effective.

OBJECTIVE ASSESSMENT

Physical assessment

The first component of an assessment is a thorough history and physical examination with a focus on pain assessment. Details concerning the character of the pain, such as the location and quality of the discomfort or pain, its time of onset, and factors that make it worse or better, are important clues to the cause of pain. The patient may describe the severity of the pain using a numerical scale from 0 to 10 (0 = no pain, 10 = worst pain). Ask if the pain is present at rest or not, if it is present on movement or not, and the time of day when the pain occurs. The patient should be asked to localize the pain anatomically and to describe its character. Differentiation must be made from neurologic pain, which is described as numbness, "falling asleep," burning, shooting, or a pins-and-needles pain, which is often a neurologic rather than a neuromuscular toxicity. Important in the differentiation process is ascertaining whether the pain is described as an ache, which is often the case with arthralgias, versus a burning pain in an extremity, which may indicate neuropathy. Somatic pain is often described as aching, stabbing, throbbing, or pressure-like, whereas visceral pain is a gnawing or cramping pain and is poorly localizable. Forty percent of cancer pain syndromes are neuropathic, caused by the disease (cancer) or treatment.[44]

Many chemotherapy drugs also cause neurologic toxicity, including peripheral neuropathy affecting both sensory (pain and temperature) and motor pathways and/or autonomic pathways. Rowinsky et al.[19] suggest research aimed at identifying patients who are likely to develop complications, perhaps by using nerve conduction studies, quantitative sensory testing, or limited selective examinations. Patients should also be asked about accompanying stiffness or swelling in joints and any complaints of limited motion. Weakness and fatigue are common general complaints.

Careful listening during the assessment is essential. Encouraging the patient to call or come to the office when the symptom is present may be helpful. Trying to assess patients' limitations with the activities of daily living and trying to sort out the primary cause are important. Often neuromuscular pain is managed over the phone, so paying careful attention to what the patient is describing is most important. Confounding factors include patients receiving multiple drugs at one time with overlapping side effects and giving premedications to ameliorate the hypersensitivity reactions (i.e., decadron 20 mg IV). Corticosteroids can cause myopathy, for example, and their withdrawal may result in a rheumatologic syndrome that includes arthralgias and myalgias. Patients experience a "high" feeling from the steroid, which wears off in about 48 hours, precisely the time when the rheumatologic syndrome often may start. The authors who documented post-chemotherapy rheumatism in breast cancer patients concluded that the pulse administration of corticosteroids with chemotherapy did not seem to contribute to the post-chemotherapy rheumatism syndrome.[35]

Patients with cancer who have arthritis and a long history of aches and pains as well as a long history of medication use to manage their pain are a complicated group to assess. It is important to be aware of the signs and symptoms of arthritis. The symptoms include stiffness, pain, weakness, fatigue, and emotional depression or lability; the signs include tenderness localized over an afflicted joint, swelling, heat and erythema, crepitus, and bony spurs. Careful documentation of medication history and baseline data of functional status and pain are critical in the successful management of this group of patients. It is important to remember that the underlying cancer can cause additional symptoms or problems at any time, and those need to be ruled out as well. Usually the finite time that this symptom manifests itself makes it easy to rule out a new metastasis, because the pain associated with metastasis does not dissipate. Concomitant use of colony-stimulating factors may exacerbate the arthralgias and myalgias or may be the root cause of the symptoms, and differentiation of the cause is important.

Diagnostic evaluation

No specific diagnostic tests are recommended for making the diagnosis of cancer-related arthralgia or myalgia; it is made instead from a careful history and physical examination.

When evaluating a patient for arthralgias or myalgias, it is important to rule out contributing factors, such as medications, activity level, disease progression, or injury.[46] Evaluating the etiology of arthralgias and myalgias would include obtaining a temperature; if it is elevated, testing for bacterial, viral, or fungal infection as a possible cause should be undertaken. Erythrocyte sedimentation rate and C-reactive protein level are elevated with infection, inflammation, or malignancy. Negative antinuclear antibody eliminates systemic lupus erythematosus as a source of arthralgia. Rheumatoid factor and Lyme disease titer should be tested. A uric acid level is drawn to rule out gout. Coagulation studies would be appropriate to evaluate hemorrhagic synovial fluid; a synovial fluid exam may also be helpful. Further imaging could reveal multiple possibilities for causes of arthralgia.

DEGREES OF TOXICITY

Arthralgias and myalgias should be graded using the common terminology criteria for adverse events (CTCAE) published by the National Cancer Institute (Table 2-2).[47] This involves using a pain grading scale that ranges from no pain or normal to disabling.

SYMPTOM MANAGEMENT STRATEGIES

Patient education is an essential part of the nursing care plan for cancer-related arthralgias and myalgias. Patients must be prepared to recognize what is happening and have a plan to deal with the discomfort so that their quality of life is minimally affected.

TABLE 2-2

National Cancer Institute Common Terminology Criteria for Adverse Events (CTCAE): Arthralgia and Myalgia

	Grade 1	Grade 2	Grade 3	Grade 4	Grade 5
Arthralgia: A disorder characterized by a sensation of marked discomfort in a joint.	Mild pain	Moderate pain; limiting instrumental ADLs	Severe pain, limiting self-care ADLs		
Myalgia: A disorder characterized by marked discomfort sensation originating from a muscle or group of muscles	Mild pain	Moderate pain; limiting instrumental ADLs	Severe pain; limiting self-care ADLs		

Abbreviation: ADLs: activities of daily living.

Source: Data from National Cancer Institute Common Terminology Criteria for Adverse Events (CTCAE)[47].

Symptom management and reassessment are the most productive ways of treating this condition. Inform patients about what to expect, what can be prevented, and when and to whom to report the side effects. Nurses must educate patients regarding the potential for discomfort associated with arthralgias and myalgias. Patients may be reluctant to report adverse effects because of fear that their disease is progressing or that their treatment will be stopped. Reassurance can alleviate this concern. It is important to make patients understand that they may experience this side effect but that it is manageable and sometimes preventable with intervention. Providing concrete information about the finite period of time patients can expect to deal with this side effect can be reassuring.

A thorough nursing history and assessment must be done before the initiation of treatment as well as before each subsequent treatment, because a patient's history can have a great impact on the adverse effects experienced. For example, patients with a history of arthritis or rheumatoid arthritis will be more complicated to assess. As patients start therapy, provide them with a verbal and written explanation of this potential side effect, its delayed onset after the administration of the drug, the variation of discomfort (ranging from a mild ache to severe pain), and the duration of the side effect (i.e., it ends in 4 to 7 days), and inform them that the problem does not continue after therapy has been completed or discontinued. For most patients, it is not necessary to discontinue or modify the dose of drugs because of this side effect.

No evidence-based practices are available to treat musculoskeletal pain caused by AIs in patients with breast cancer. Clinically, the physician may choose to prescribe analgesics for the patient. The patient may also be given a treatment break, discontinue the drug, change to tamoxifen, or try another AI.[30]

THERAPEUTIC APPROACHES

Antihistamines, corticosteroids, nonsteroidal anti-inflammatory drugs (NSAIDs), and opiates have been helpful in managing arthralgias and myalgias. After 24% of patients experienced grade 3 arthralgias and myalgias, Schiller et al. started prednisone empirically in 10 patients at 40 mg/day for 2 to 5 days.[48] Patients reported a decrease in discomfort starting 2 to 4 hours after the first dose of the prednisone. In a phase I/II study to determine the maximum tolerated dose of paclitaxel, grade 1 and grade 2 arthralgias and myalgias were treated with nonsteroidal analgesics; grade 3 patients were given a 4-day course of dexamethasone at 4 to 8 mg bid.[49] In a study based on the hypothesis that the symptom is the result of some form of an inflammatory process, women were instructed to take ibuprofen 200–400 mg every 4 to 6 hours if needed for symptomatic relief. When these women presented for a subsequent cycle, they were queried about the arthralgia and myalgia symptoms. If their symptoms were inadequately controlled, they were offered treatment with oral prednisone 10 mg twice a day for 5 days starting 24 hours after the paclitaxel infusion. This study found that 80% of patients obtained substantial relief of symptoms with a low-dose oral prednisone regimen.[42]

Nonsteroidal analgesics are used because of their analgesic and anti-inflammatory effects; they work peripherally to decrease prostaglandin synthesis. The World Health Organization guideline suggests that a non-opioid—either an NSAID or paracetamol (acetaminophen)—be the first step in trying to relieve mild pain. Advantages of NSAID therapy include these agents' wide availability, familiarity to patients and families, and effectiveness for pain.[50] Corticosteroids are effective because of their ability to reduce the symptoms of inflammation reliably and rapidly. Corticosteroids inhibit a variety of pro-inflammatory genes and modify the leukocyte

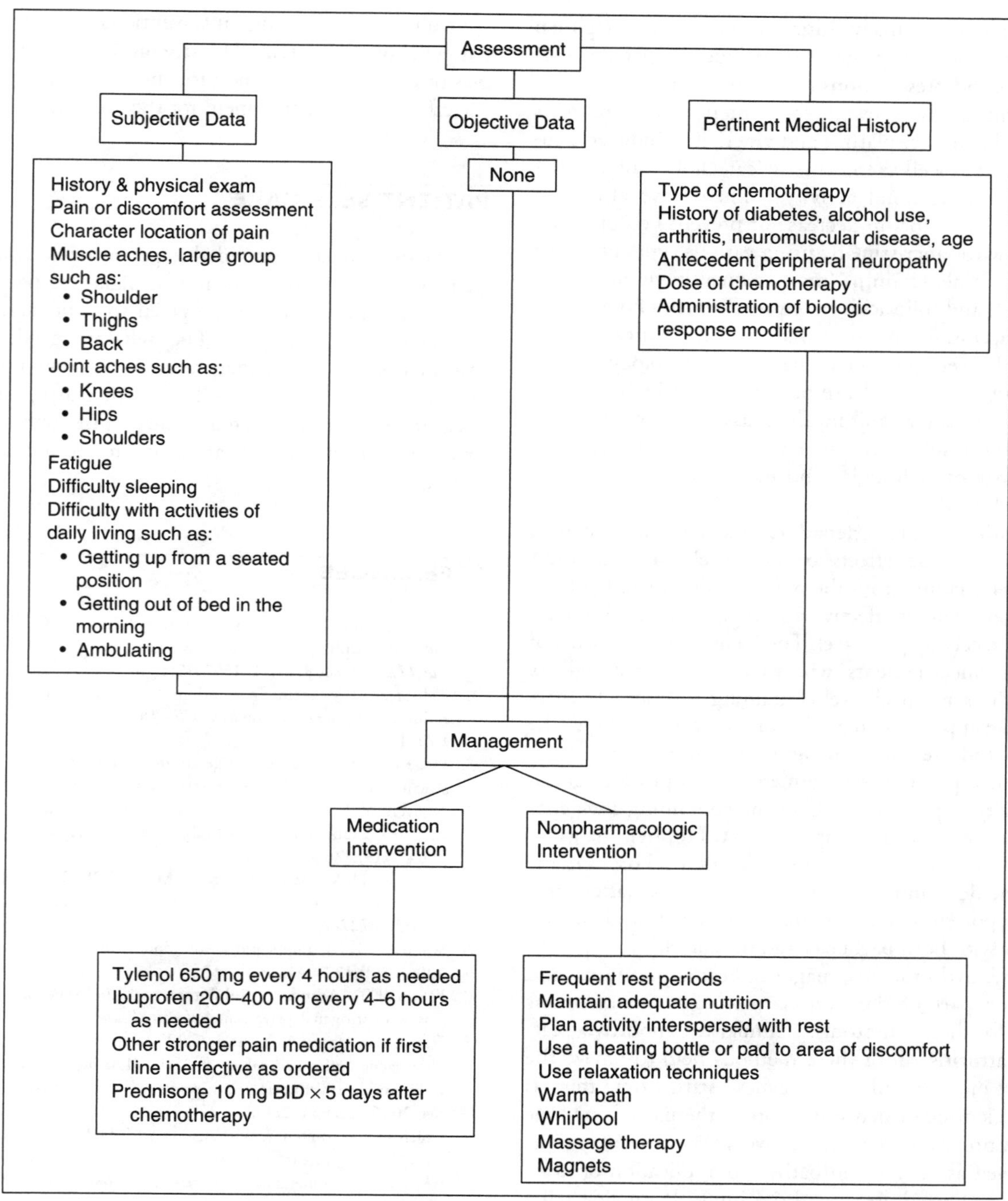

FIGURE 2-1

Treatment algorithm for arthralgias and myalgias.

Abbreviation: BID: twice daily.

number at the inflammation site. Although arthralgias and myalgias are not associated with muscle inflammation, corticosteroids are effective in relieving the aches and pains associated with these symptoms. With chronic high-dose use of corticosteroids, muscle weakness or steroid myopathy may occur.

Many institutions have found benefit in the prophylactic use of some nonsteroidal analgesics, with varying doses and schedules. Practitioners sometimes take a wait-and-see attitude, explaining to patients the possibility of the problem and providing instructions to call if this problem occurs. If the patient experiences arthralgias or myalgias, the practitioner will likely initiate a prophylactic regimen at the next cycle of treatment or provide the patient with instructions and prescriptions for intermittent use.

A recent study showed that interleukin-6 protects against paclitaxel-, cisplatin-, and vincristine-induced neuropathies just as well as four-methylcatechol without interfering with antitumoral activity.[51] There have also been unsuccessful attempts to decrease or prevent neurotoxicity associated with vincristine by using various types of agents such as thiamine, vitamins (most frequently vitamin B_6 or pyridoxine), and folic acid.[52] Despite the lack of documentation of success, when nurses were informally surveyed at a semiannual meeting of the Gynecologic Oncology Group, some reported anecdotal use of either vitamin B_6 or vitamin C for arthralgias and myalgias associated with taxane therapy. The results were mixed—some saw decreases in the incidence of arthralgias and myalgias, whereas others found no effect.

The antihistamine terfenadine was once used to help ameliorate the side effects of paclitaxel, but the FDA removed terfenadine from the market. Glutamate has been studied to evaluate its effectiveness in preventing side effects in patients receiving paclitaxel. The focus group consisted of 43 ovarian cancer patients, who were followed through six cycles of the same paclitaxel-containing regimen. Twenty-three were supplemented with glutamate throughout the trial. The study revealed no significant difference in signs or symptoms, proving the regimen fails to protect against neurotoxicity of paclitaxel.[53] Codeine-containing analgesics may lead to symptomatic improvement. Prophylactic gabapentin (300 to 400 mg three times daily for 24 or 48 hours prior to the dose and continued for 4 to 5 days afterward) has been reported to decrease the frequency of myalgias and arthralgias with both paclitaxel and docetaxel.[54]

Exercise, hydrotherapy, magnets, heat applications, and massage are part of the nonpharmacologic interventions suggested for these symptoms.[45] Similar to supportive treatment for arthritis, all of these methods help to relieve the discomfort of joint and muscle aches. At this time there is minimal scientific evidence to support the use of one type of intervention over another, but overall these interventions are perceived as safe. Warm baths and application of heating pads to affected areas for brief intervals provide relief to patients. Patients also report that remaining active and regular moderate walking are helpful to maintain normal activity function. Figure 2-1 provides a treatment algorithm for those patients with arthralgias and myalgias.

NURSING IMPLICATIONS

The nursing diagnosis associated with arthralgia or myalgia is discomfort or pain. The expected outcome is that the patient will be free from discomfort or have the pain controlled. The nursing interventions are to teach the patient about the potential for discomfort related to arthralgias or myalgias and to monitor the level of symptoms and the effectiveness of treatment for the problem.

PATIENT SELF-CARE

Information must be provided to patients receiving therapy that may cause arthralgias and myalgias. Appendix 2A is a self-care guide that can be given to patients at risk for arthralgias and myalgias. The self-care guide includes information on the management and follow-up care for arthralgias and myalgias. While an increasing number of chemotherapy and targeted agents cause arthralgias and myalgias, cancer patients can be assisted to minimize their negative impact.

REFERENCES

1. Wolf S, Barton D, Kottschade L, Grothey A, Loprinzi C. Chemotherapy-induced peripheral neuropathy: prevention and treatment strategies. *Eur J Cancer.* 2008;44(11):1507–1515.
2. Tofthagen C. Patient perceptions associated with chemotherapy-induced peripheral neuropathy. *Clin J Oncol Nurs.* 2010;14(3 suppl): E22–E28.
3. Hede K. Supportive care: large studies ease yoga, exercise into mainstream oncology. *J Natl Cancer Inst.* 2011;103(1):11–12.
4. Nguyen VH, Lawrence HJ. Use of gabapentin in the prevention of taxane-induced arthralgias and myalgias. *J Clin Oncol.* 2004;22(9):1767–1769.
5. Einhorn LH, Williams SD, Troner M, Birch R, Greco FA. The role of maintenance therapy in disseminated testicular cancer. *N Engl J Med.* 1981;305:727–731.
6. Winters JL. Complications of donor apheresis, *J Clin Apher.* 2006;21(2):132–141.
7. Felson DT. Aromatase inhibitors and the syndrome of arthralgias with estrogen deprivation. *Arthritis Rheum.* 2005;52(9):2594–2598.
8. Hande KR, Hagey A, Berlin J, Cai Y, Meek K, Kobayshi H, et al. The pharmacokinetics and safety of ABT-751, a novel, orally bioavailable sulfonamide antimitotic agent: results of a phase 1 study. *Clin Cancer Res.* 2006;12:2834–2840.
9. Coleman RE, Bolten WW, Lansdown M, Dale S, Jackisch C, Merkel D, et al. Aromatase inhibitor-induced arthralgia: clinical experience and treatment recommendations. *Cancer Treat Rev.* 2008;34(3):275–282.
10. Rowinsky EK, Cazenave LA, Donehower RC. Taxol: a novel investigational agent. *J Natl Cancer Inst.* 1990;82:1247–1259.
11. Rowinsky EK, Donehower RC. Paclitaxel (Taxol). *N Engl J Med.* 1995;332:1004–1014.
12. Einhorn LH, Donohue JP: Improved chemotherapy in disseminated testicular cancer. *J Urol.* 1977;117:65–69.
13. Vogelzang NJ, Fraley EE, Lange PH, et al. Stage II nonseminomatous testicular cancer: a 10-year experience. *J Clin Oncol.* 1983;1:171–178.
14. Ng J. Vinflunine: review of a new vinca alkaloid and its potential role in oncology. *J Oncol Pharm Pract.* 2010;17:209–224.
15. Bruera E, Portenoy RK. *Cancer Pain: Assessment and Management.* New York: Cambridge University Press; 2010.
16. Markman M. Managing taxane toxicities. *Support Cancer Care.* 2003;11:144–147.

17. Loprinzi C. The paclitaxel acute pain syndrome: sensitization of nociceptors as the putative mechanism. *Cancer J.* 2007;13(6) 399–403.
18. Pachman DR, Barton DL, Watson JC, Loprinzi CL. Chemotherapy-induced peripheral neuropathy: prevention and treatment. *Clin Pharmacol Ther.* 2011;90(3):377–387.
19. Rowinsky EK, Eisenhauer EA, Chaudhry V, Arbuck SG, Donehower RC. Clinical toxicities encountered with paclitaxel (Taxol). *Semin Oncol.* 1993;20(suppl 3):1–15.
20. Donehower RC, Rowinsky EK. An overview of experience with Taxol (paclitaxel) in the USA. *Cancer Treat Rev.* 1993;19(suppl C):63–78.
21. Kunitoh H, Saijo K, Furuse F, Noda K, Ogawa M. Neuromuscular toxicities of paclitaxel 210 mg/m^2 by 3-hour infusion. *Br J Cancer.* 1998;77:1686–1688.
22. Vasey PA. Survival and longer-term toxicity results of the SCOTROC study: docetaxel-carboplatin (DC) vs paclitaxel-carboplatin (PC) in epithelial ovarian cancer (EOC). *Proc Am Soc Clin Oncol.* 2002; 21:202a. (abstr)
23. Chu E, Obermiller A, Harrold LJ, Tiederman D, Sitki Copur M. Chemotherapeutic and biologic drugs, in Chu E, DeVita VT, eds. *Physicians Cancer Chemotherapy Drug Manual 2012.* Burlington, MA: Jones & Bartlett Learning; 2012:8–10 (albumin-bound paclitaxel), 59–62 (cabazitaxel).
24. Richardson PG, Briemberg H, Jagannath S, et al. Frequency, characteristics, and reversibility of peripheral neuropathy during treatment of advanced multiple myeloma with bortezomib. *J Clin Oncol.* 2006;24:3113–3120.
25. Badros A, Goloubeva O, Dalal JS, Can I, Thompson J, Rapoport AP, et al. Neurotoxicity of bortezomib therapy in multiple myeloma: a single center experience and review of the literature. *Cancer.* 2007;110:1042–1049.
26. Sosman JA, Kim KB, Schuchter L, Gonzalez R, Pavlick AC, Wber JS, et al. Survival in BRAF V600-mutant advanced melanoma treated with vemurafenib. *N Eng J Med.* 2012;366(8):707–714.
27. Ravnan M, Ravnan S, Wlaberg M. A review of current and novel pharmacotherapy. *Formulary 46.* 2011;4:130–144.
28. McBane S. Osteoporosis: a review of current recommendations and emerging treatment options. *Formulary 46.* 2011;10:432–438.
29. Viale PH. Aromatase inhibitor agenda in breast cancer: evolving practices in hormonal therapy treatment. *Oncol Nurs Forum.* 2005;32:343–353.
30. Winters L, Havin K, Gallagher J. Aromatase inhibitors and musculoskeletal pain in patients with breast cancer. *Clin J Oncol Nurs.* 2007;11:433–439.
31. Quesada JR, Talpaz M, Rois M. Clinical toxicity of interferons in cancer patients: a review. *J Clin Oncol.* 1986;4:234–243.
32. Kubista E, Glapy J, Holmes FA, et al. Bone pain associated with once-per-cycle pegfilgrastim is similar to daily filgrastim in patients with breast cancer. *Clin Breast Cancer.* 2003;3(6):391–398.
33. Polovich M, White J, Kelleher, eds. *Chemotherapy and Biotherapy Guidelines and Recommendations for Practice.* 2nd ed. Pittsburgh, PA: Oncology Nursing Society; 2005.
34. Green M, Koelbl H, Baselga J, et al. A randomized double-blind multicenter phase III study of fixed-dose single-administration pegfilgrastim versus daily filgrastim in patients receiving myelosuppressive chemotherapy. *Ann Oncol.* 2003;14:29–35.
35. Loprinzi CL, Duffy J, Ingle IN. Postchemotherapy rheumatism. *J Clin Oncol.* 1993;11:768–770.
36. Wong CI, Koh TS, Soo R, et al. Phase I and biomarker study of ABT-869, a multiple receptor tyrosine kinase inhibitor, in patients with refractory solid malignancies. *J Clin Oncol.* 2009;27:4718–4726.
37. Tsukamoto H, Ueda N, Horuchi T. Progress in classification and treatment for TNF receptor associated periodic syndrome. *Nihon Rinsho Meruki Gakkai Karshi.* 2011;34(5):361–368.
38. Kieran MW, Supko JG, Wallace D, Frusco R, Poussaint TY, Phillips P, et al. Phase I study of SU5416, a small molecule inhibitor of the vascular endothelial growth factor receptor (VEGFR) in refractory pediatric central nervous system tumors. *Pediatr Blood Cancer.* 2009;52(2):169–176.
39. Miller KD, Triano LR. Medical issues in cancer survivors: a review. *Cancer J.* 2008;14(6):375–387.
40. Rowinsky EK, Onetto N, Canetta RM, et al. Taxol: the first of the taxanes, an important new class of antitumor agents. *Semin Oncol.* 1992;19:646–662.
41. Rowinsky EK, Donehower RC. Antimicrotubule agents, in Chabner BA, Long DL, eds. *Cancer Chemotherapy and Biotherapy: Principles and Practice.* Philadelphia: Lippincott-Raven; 1996:263–296.
42. Markman M, Kennedy A, Webster K, et al. Use of low dose prednisone to prevent paclitaxel-induced arthralgias and myalgias. *Gynecol Oncol.* 1999;72:100–101.
43. Mao JJ, Stricker C, Bruner D, et al. Patterns and risk factors associated with aromatase inhibitor-related arthralgia among breast cancer survivors. *Cancer.* 2009;115(16):3631–3639.
44. Portenoy RK, Mathur G. Cancer pain, in Yeung S, Escalante CP, Gagel RF. *Medical Care of Cancer Patients.* Shelton, CT: People's Medical Publishing House USA; 2009:60–71.
45. Armstrong T, Almadrones L, Gilbert MR, et al. Chemotherapy-induced peripheral neuropathy. *Oncol Nurs Forum.* 2005;32(2):305–311.
46. Boyajian RN , Noonan KA. Arthralgia, in Sorrell DC, Hawkins RA. *Clinical Manual for the Oncology Advanced Practice.* 2nd ed. Pittsburgh, PA: Oncology Nursing Society; 2006:709–717.
47. National Cancer Institute. Common terminology criteria for adverse events (CTCAE), v 4.03. June 14, 2010. http://evs.nci.nih.gov/ftp1/CTCAE/CTCAE_4.03_2010-06-14_QuickReference_8.5x11.pdf. Accessed August 7, 2012.
48. Schiller JH, Storer B, Tutsch K, Arzoomanian R, Alberti D, Feierabend C, et al. Phase I trial of 3-hour infusion of paclitaxel with or without granulocyte colony stimulating factor in patients with advanced cancer. *J Clin Oncol.* 1994;12:241–248.
49. Natale RB. Preliminary results of Phase I/II clinical trial of paclitaxel and carboplatin in non-small cell lung cancer. *Semin Oncol.* 1996;23(suppl 16):51–54.
50. Impact of impaired access to controlled medications. World Health Organization website. 2012. http://www.who.int/medicines/areas/quality_safety/Impaired_Access/en/. Accessed June 18, 2012.
51. Callizot N, Anderiabeloson E, Glass J, Revel M, Ferro P, Cirillo R, et al. Interleukin-6 protects against paclitaxel, cisplatin and vincristine-induced neuropathies without impairing chemotherapeutic activity. *Cancer Chemother Pharmacol.* 2008;62(6):995–1007.
52. Jackson DV, Pope EK, McMahan RA, et al. Clinical trial of pyridoxine to reduce vincristine neurotoxicity. *J Neurooncol.* 1986;4:37–41.
53. Loven D, Levavi H, Sabach G, Zart R, Andras M, Fishman A, et al. Long-term glutamate supplementation failed to protect against peripheral neurotoxicity of paclitaxel. *Eur J Cancer Care.* 2009;18:78–83.
54. Nguyen VH, Lawrence HJ. Use of gabapentin in the prevention of taxane induced arthralgias and myalgias. *J Clin Oncol.* 2004;22:1767–1769.

Muscle Aches and Joint Pain

Patient Name: ______________________________

This guide will give you helpful hints to reduce muscle aches and pain in your joints.

Symptom and Description

Pain in your shoulders, hips, or knees can occur anytime from 24 to 72 hours after you receive chemotherapy. When it affects your joints, this pain is called arthralgia; when it is located in your muscles, it is called myalgia. The pain is a side effect of your treatment. It can range from a mild discomfort or ache to a severe pain. You may feel like you have the flu or you may have trouble moving around—for example, getting out of bed or a chair.

This muscle and joint pain may be more noticeable if colony-stimulating factors (such as the drug Neupogen or Neulasta) are part of your treatment.

This side effect may not occur with every treatment; you may experience the pain after one treatment and not feel any aches after the next treatment. You are at risk of having muscle aches and joint pain because of your cancer therapy. The drug(s) you are taking are called ______________________ is the cause. ______________________.

You may also be at risk for this side effect because

- You have a history of diabetes.
- You have a history of arthritis.
- You have a history of alcohol use.
- You have neuromuscular disease.

Prevention

The first thing to remember is that the symptoms may not appear for 24–72 hours after your treatment is given and that aches can last for as long as 4–7 days.

It is difficult to prevent muscle aches and joint pain because the drug you are getting for your cancer treatment causes it.

Medication may be prescribed by your clinician to reduce the discomfort from this side effect.

Management

These are some tips to manage the discomfort:

- Take the medication prescribed.
- Get plenty of rest and plan your activities to include rest periods.
- A heating pad or a hot water bottle may give comfort to an achy area.
- Keep the pad or bottle covered with a towel when putting it next to your skin.
- Use the heat for short periods of time 5–10 minutes several times a day.

- Elevate arms or legs when at rest. Relaxing in a recliner may give you comfort taking pressure off your muscles and joints.
- Position your legs with a pillow in between them or under them to give support or provide comfort.
- Massage may give comfort.
- A warm bath may provide comfort.
- Wear loose clothing.
- Exercise or walking around may relieve the restless feeling in the legs or muscles.
- Relaxation techniques such as guided imagery or biofeedback may help.
- Keep your nutrition up, eat a healthy diet, and eat regularly.

Follow-up

Keeping a record of your discomfort is helpful to take to your next appointment.

Write down the day the pain starts and the degree of pain you feel using a scale from 0 to 10.

Note also what you did to make yourself more comfortable and note whether it worked.

Bring all this information with you to your next appointment.

Phone Numbers

Nurse ______________________________

Physician ______________________________

Other ______________________________

Source: Martin VR. Arthralgias and Myalgias. In: Yarbro CH, Wujcik D, Gobel BH, eds. *Cancer Symptom Management*. 4th ed. Burlington, MA: Jones & Bartlett Learning; 2014.

Chapter 3

Cancer-Related Fatigue

Sandra A. Mitchell, PhD, CRNP, AOCN®

THE PROBLEM

Cancer-related fatigue (CRF) is a prevalent and disabling symptom experienced by both cancer patients and cancer survivors. It is a multifaceted condition characterized by diminished energy and an increased need to rest, disproportionate to any recent change in activity level, and accompanied by a range of other characteristics, including generalized weakness, diminished mental concentration, insomnia or hypersomnia, and emotional reactivity.[1] Decrements in physical, social, cognitive, and vocational functioning,[2,3] adverse mood changes,[4] sleep disturbances,[5] treatment noncompliance[6] and emotional and spiritual distress for both the patient and family members[7] are among the consequences of CRF.

Despite this degree of distress and functional loss associated with CRF, screening, evaluation, and treatment for CRF in clinical settings remain suboptimal. Reasons for this shortcoming may include clinicians' failure to offer interventions, patients' lack of awareness of effective treatments for fatigue, a desire on patients' part to treat fatigue without medications, and a tendency to be stoic about fatigue to avoid being labeled as a "complainer" or risk having the dose of anticancer treatment reduced.[8]

Although many different definitions of CRF have been proposed, the National Comprehensive Cancer Network (NCCN) defines CRF as a distressing, persistent, and subjective sense of tiredness or exhaustion related to cancer or cancer treatment that is not proportional to recent activity and interferes with usual functioning.[9] The clinical expression of CRF is multidimensional, making evaluation of a patient experiencing fatigue challenging.

An inherently subjective condition, fatigue may be experienced and reported differently by each individual. One qualitative study of fatigue underscored the fact that the cancer fatigue experience is unlike any other fatigue individuals have previously experienced, and suggested that its unpredictability and refractoriness to self-management strategies contribute to the distress associated with CRF.[10] Personality and coping style may also influence the experience of CRF.[11] Some patients identify the main features of their fatigue as a loss of efficiency, mental fogginess, inertia, and failure of sleep to be restorative, while others describe an excessive need to rest, the inability to recover promptly from exertion, and muscle heaviness and weakness. Further research is needed to determine whether these represent variable features of fatigue, suggest the presence of fatigue subtypes, or are the cause or sequelae of fatigue.[12] Efforts continue to be directed toward clarifying the defining features of fatigue, and determining how CRF may be distinguished from syndromes such as depression, cognitive dysfunction, or asthenia that have overlapping symptoms[13,14] or that may share neurophysiologic mechanisms.[15,16]

The varying estimates of the prevalence of CRF may be due in part to the fact that investigators use varying case definitions of cancer-related fatigue.[17] Progress in evaluating the effectiveness of new therapies for CRF is also hindered by the absence of a precise definition of the level of fatigue that must be present to define eligibility for trial participation. Establishing criteria for a diagnosis of cancer-related fatigue—that is, a case definition—will allow us to define clinically significant fatigue, will enable better classification of patients with CRF, and will facilitate comparisons across studies and populations.

Consensus criteria for a diagnosis of cancer-related fatigue syndrome were initially proposed in 1998[1] and are provided in Table 3-1. Based on these criteria, CRF is of a markedly different quality and severity from ordinary fatigue,

TABLE 3-1

International Classification of Diseases (10th Edition) ICD-10 Criteria for Cancer-Related Fatigue	
Six (or more) of the following symptoms have been present every day or nearly every day during the same two-week period in the past month, and at least one of the symptoms is (A1) significant fatigue.	
A1.	Significant fatigue, diminished energy, or increased need to rest, disproportionate to any recent change in activity level
A2.	Complaints of generalized weakness or limb heaviness
A3.	Diminished concentration or attention
A4.	Decreased motivation or interest to engage in usual activities
A5.	Insomnia or hypersomnia
A6.	Experience of sleep as unrefreshing or nonrestorative
A7.	Perceived need to struggle to overcome inactivity
A8.	Marked emotional reactivity (e.g., sadness, frustration, irritability) to feeling fatigued
A9.	Difficulty completing daily tasks attributed to feeling fatigued
A10.	Perceived problems with short-term memory
A11.	Post-exertional malaise lasting several hours
B.	The symptoms cause clinically significant distress or impairment in social, occupational, or other important areas of functioning.
C.	There is evidence from the history, physical examination, or laboratory findings that the symptoms are a consequence of cancer or cancer therapy.
D.	The symptoms are not primarily a consequence of comorbid psychiatric disorders such as major depression, somatization disorder, somatoform disorder, or delirium.

Source: Data from Cella D, Peterman A, Passik S, Jacobsen P, and Breitbart W. (1998). Progress toward guidelines for the management of fatigue. *Oncology (Williston Park), 12*(11A), 369–377[1]. Used with permission.

adversely impacts function, and is unrelieved by rest or sleep. It is also accompanied by symptoms such as an increasing need for rest, limb heaviness, diminished concentration, inertia, emotional lability, and post-exertional malaise. One must also be fairly certain that the underlying cause is cancer or its treatment. These criteria have been subjected to only limited empiric testing,[18] and more than one case definition may ultimately be needed to capture the features of clinically significant fatigue in varying populations.[12]

INCIDENCE

Fatigue is one of the most commonly reported symptoms experienced by patients receiving treatment for cancer, and it often persists beyond the conclusion of active treatment and at the end of life.[19,20] Depending on how CRF is defined and measured and the clinical characteristics of the population under study (e.g., tumor site, phase or stage on the cancer continuum, and type of anticancer therapy), prevalence estimates range from 25% to 99%.[20–24] Across all cancer types, fatigue was ranked as the most important symptom or concern in a survey of more than 500 patients and nearly 100 clinicians.[25] Longitudinal and comparative studies indicate that persistent fatigue may also be a significant problem for cancer survivors, even those free of disease.[26,27] In the setting of advanced cancer, almost 60% of patients experience fatigue, with one-fourth reporting severe fatigue.[28] Fatigue may occur as an isolated symptom, or as one component within a cluster of other symptoms, including depression, pain, sleep disturbance, and menopausal symptoms.[29–34]

ETIOLOGY

For a majority of patients, cancer and its treatment will be associated with the development of CRF, although patterns of fatigue onset, severity, daily fluctuations, and resolution vary widely depending on the type of treatment, and the site and stage of the underlying disease. Fatigue is reported in association with radiation, chemotherapy, hematopoietic stem cell transplantation, hormonal treatment, and biologic and molecularly targeted agents in patients receiving treatment in both outpatient and inpatient settings.[20,21,35–39] However, few direct relationships between treatment-related variables such as dose intensity, radiation fractionation schedule, and time since treatment completion have been seen.[19] Associations between the occurrence or severity of CRF and demographic variables such as gender, age, marital status, and employment status have also not been consistently identified.[40]

Direct and indirect biobehavioral mediators of CRF in patients on cancer treatment include pro-inflammatory cytokine release, anemia, mood disturbances, alterations in muscle metabolism, sarcopenia, hypothalamic-pituitary-adrenal

(HPA)-axis dysregulation, fluid and electrolyte disturbances, and deconditioning. Other potential etiologic factors for CRF include anxiety, depression, and psychological distress; concurrent symptoms such as pain and nausea/vomiting; sleep disturbances; cardiopulmonary, hepatic, or renal dysfunction; infection; malnutrition; and the side effects of drugs that act on the central nervous system, such as benzodiazepines and narcotics.[4,39–43] A number of metabolic and endocrine disorders can exacerbate CRF, including hypothyroidism, hypogonadism, adrenal insufficiency, hypercalcemia, hypomagnesemia, and dehydration[42] Cancer anorexia-cachexia and its resultant protein-calorie malnutrition lead to increased proteolysis in skeletal muscles, producing muscle wasting, weakness/asthenia, and reduced endurance.

PATHOPHYSIOLOGY

The pathophysiology of CRF likely involves the interaction of several biobehavioral mechanisms.[16,44] Accumulating evidence points to gene polymorphisms,[45] altered circadian rhythmicity,[46] and immune dysregulation and pro-inflammatory cytokine activity[47,48] as pathophysiologic mechanisms underlying CRF. Cancer and treatment-emergent side effects contribute to dysregulation of the HPA axis, adversely affecting the secretion of corticotrophin-releasing hormone.[48] Changes in this essential neuro-endocrine hormonal milieu can impair several aspects of sleep, including depth of sleep, slow-wave sleep, rapid-eye-movement sleep, and waking.[49] These adverse changes in sleep architecture act together with psychological stressors to produce significant sleep disturbances in patients with cancer[50] and may thereby contribute directly or indirectly to CRF.

Alterations in skeletal muscle energy metabolism have also been postulated to be a cause of CRF.[51] Accumulation of metabolites, nutrient deprivation, and the disruption of mitochondrial synthesis of adenosine-5'-triphosphate (ATP) or diminished oxygen delivery to muscle cells can all affect skeletal muscle energy metabolism, thereby influencing the ability of the muscle to perform mechanical work. It is through these and other mechanisms that cancer, cancer treatment, and treatment-emergent side effects such as anemia or cachexia alter skeletal muscle energy metabolism and reduce the capacity for muscle contraction.[39,52]

SYMPTOM ASSESSMENT

RISK FACTORS

Although CRF is experienced by patients almost universally across the continuum from diagnosis, through treatment, survivorship, and end of life, there is individual variability in its time course, severity, and extent to which it causes distress and interferes with daily activities. Risk factors for CRF[19,39,53–55] that may account for this variability are summarized in Table 3-2.

TABLE 3-2

Risk Factors for Cancer-Related Fatigue (CRF)

- Advanced/metastatic disease or cancer recurrence
- Cancer treatment (chemotherapy, radiation, surgery, biologic agents, hormonal agents, molecularly targeted agents)
- Anemia
- Neutropenia
- Hypothyroidism
- Adrenal Insufficiency
- Hypogonadism
- Infection
- Malnutrition
- Depletion of vitamins B_1, B_6, and B_{12}
- Electrolyte disturbances (calcium, magnesium, phosphorus)
- Cardiopulmonary, hepatic, or renal dysfunction
- Sarcopenia, asthenia, deconditioning
- Proinflammatory cytokine expression associated with generalized inflammation
- Medications with sedating side effects (e.g. narcotics, anxiolytics, antiemetics, antidepressants), or medications with a side effect profile that includes fatigue (e.g. beta-blockers)
- Concurrent symptoms (e.g. pain, dyspnea, nausea, diarrhea, urinary frequency)
- Impaired sleep quality
- Psychological distress (depression, anxiety)

SELF-ASSESSMENT

The etiology and clinical expression of CRF are multidimensional. An inherently subjective condition, fatigue may be experienced and reported differently by each individual. Qualitative studies of fatigue underscore the fact that the cancer fatigue experience is unlike the other fatigue individuals have previously experienced,[10] and patients emphasize that its unpredictability and refractoriness to self-management strategies make it a particularly distressing symptom. Personality and coping style may also influence the experience of CRF.[11] As noted earlier, some patients complain of a loss of efficiency, mental fogginess, inertia, and inability of sleep to have restorative effects, while others describe an excessive need to rest, the inability to recover promptly from exertion, and muscle heaviness and weakness. Efforts continue to be directed toward clarifying the defining features of fatigue,[56] and determining how CRF may be distinguished from syndromes such as depression, cognitive dysfunction, or asthenia that have overlapping symptoms[13,14,57–61] or may share neurophysiologic mechanisms.[15,62] Despite its complex etiology and often multifactorial presentation, fatigue may be defined quite simply as a persistent and subjective sense of tiredness that interferes with usual functioning.[9]

There are two aspects to symptom evaluation in the patient at risk for or experiencing CRF: (1) screening at regular intervals of all patients to identify the presence of CRF and gauge its severity, and (2) in patients with moderate or severe CRF, evaluating the characteristics, consequences, and potential contributing factors.

Brief screening measures for CRF are sensitive and can be applied efficiently in clinical settings to identify patients who could benefit from further evaluation.[63,64] The NCCN guidelines[9] recommend that every patient be screened for the presence of fatigue (yes/no). If present, CRF should be assessed quantitatively on a 0–10 scale (0 = no fatigue and 10 = worst fatigue imaginable). Those patients with a score of 4 or higher should be further evaluated by history and physical examination. Routine screening should occur at regular intervals during and following cancer treatment. Additional questions that may be useful in screening are provided in Figure 3-1.

Although a single-item measure may provide efficient screening for fatigue, evidence suggests that such measures do not fully capture all the dimensions of fatigue.[65] There is general consensus that the experience of fatigue can be separated into a sensory dimension (e.g., fatigue severity, persistence), a physiological dimension (e.g., leg weakness, diminished mental concentration), an affective dimension (e.g., sadness, loss of self-esteem), and a behavioral dimension (e.g., reduction in the performance of needed or valued activities). Multidimensional fatigue measures provide information about this full range of characteristics beyond fatigue presence and intensity. Measures available to evaluate CRF include (1) multi-item scales that assess fatigue as a unidimensional construct (e.g., presence, severity, interference, distress); (2) instruments designed specifically to evaluate CRF from a multidimensional perspective (e.g., physical, behavioral, and affective components of fatigue); and (3) single items or subscales measuring relevant aspects of the fatigue experience that have been drawn from existing measures of quality of life, psychosocial adjustment, mood or self-reported health status.[45] More than 20 self-report measures have been developed to measure fatigue in patients with cancer.[66–69] Examples of unidimensional measures of fatigue include the Functional Assessment of Cancer Therapy Fatigue (FACT-F),[70] Brief Fatigue Inventory,[71] Patient-Reported Outcomes Measurement Information System (PROMIS) Fatigue Scale,[14] and the fatigue subscale of the European Organization for Research and Treatment of Cancer Quality of Life Questionnaire (EORTC-QLQ-C-30).[72] Multidimensional measures of fatigue include the Multidimensional Fatigue Inventory,[73] Multidimensional Fatigue Symptom Inventory,[74] and Piper Fatigue Scale.[75] Measures of health, symptoms, emotional distress, or mood state such as the Medical Outcomes Study Short Form-36 (SF-36),[76] Profile of Mood States,[77] Rotterdam Symptom Checklist,[78] Brief Symptom Inventory,[79] and Symptom Distress Scale[80] also include single items that address fatigue or have subscales that reflect fatigue, vigor, or vitality.

To efficiently gather data to explore the factors that may contribute to CRF—specifically, sleep disturbance, distress, inactivity, and concurrent medications—the NCCN has recently proposed the Fatigue and Contributing Factors Inventory.[81] A new outcome measure to evaluate the construct of self-efficacy for fatigue management has also been recently developed and tested.[82] This measure may be useful in effectiveness studies of interventions that target self-efficacy, and in research to identify the mechanisms through which fatigue interventions exert their effects on intermediate and distal clinical outcomes.

When selecting a measure of fatigue, it is important to keep in mind that other descriptors of fatigue such as weakness, tiredness, or lack of vigor may not necessarily be equated with fatigue.[83] Considerations of reliability, validity, responsiveness to change, recall period, respondent burden, translation in multiple languages, and the availability of normative values to aid interpretation should guide decisions about the utility of a measure for specific clinical or research purposes.[84]

OBJECTIVE ASSESSMENT

History

As outlined in Table 3-3, a detailed history of the patient with CRF includes the presence, intensity, and pervasiveness of fatigue, its course over time, the factors that exacerbate or relieve fatigue, and the impact of fatigue on

1. In the past week, on a scale of 0 to 10, what is the 'worst' fatigue you have experienced?

None 0	1	2	3	4	5	6	7	8	9	Worst 10

2. On how many days in the past week have you felt somewhat to quite fatigued?

[ ] None [ ] 1–2 days [ ] 3–5 days [ ] More than 5 days

Within the past week, to what extent has fatigued interfered with:

	Not at all	A little bit	Somewhat	Quite a bit	Very much
3. Performing the activities you need or want to do..................................	0	1	2	3	4
4. Relationships with other people......	0	1	2	3	4
5. Mood.......................................	0	1	2	3	4

6. Have you been experiencing any of the following symptoms during the past 7 days? Select all that apply:

[ ] I have no symptoms

[ ] Pain [ ] Nausea [ ] Poor Appetite [ ] Difficulty Sleeping

[ ] Shortness of Breath [ ] Difficulty Moving Around

[ ] Problem with Bowels [ ] Other

7. Would you like to discuss your fatigue with a member of your healthcare team?

___No ___Yes

FIGURE 3-1

Screening questions for Cancer-Related Fatigue.

functioning and psychological distress. The consequences of CRF on mood, self-esteem, and the ability to perform activities of daily living; fulfill valued roles as a parent, spouse, and worker; and relate to family and friends are also evaluated. Inquiring about the self-management interventions the patient has tried for fatigue, including their effectiveness, can be helpful in tailoring recommendations for fatigue management.

A comprehensive history in a patient with CRF identifies etiologic or potentiating factors (as summarized in Table 3-3) that may contribute to CRF, including sleep disturbance, emotional distress, and uncontrolled symptoms. The medication profile should also be reviewed to identify specific classes of medications (including over-the-counter medications) with a sedative side-effect profile. Medications with sedating side-effects may include opioid analgesics, sedative-hypnotic agents such as secobarbital, benzodiazepines such as lorazepam, and anxiolytics such as buspirone. A number of antidepressant agents, antiemetics, antihistamines, and anticonvulsant agents (e.g., gabapentin, phenobarbital, tegretol) also have the potential to produce sedation, daytime sleepiness, and fatigue. Certain cardiac medications such as beta blockers may contribute to fatigue by causing bradycardia, while corticosteroids may

TABLE 3-3

Comprehensive Assessment of Cancer-Related Fatigue

Severity
- On a scale of 0–10 where zero is no fatigue and 10 is the worst fatigue imaginable, how severe has your fatigue been in the past 7 days?
- Would you say that your fatigue is mild, moderate, or severe?

Persistence/Frequency/Temporal Features
- When did the fatigue start?______________________________
- Frequency of fatigue: ____ days during past week or hours per day __________

Factors Associated with Fatigue
- What makes your fatigue better?
- What makes your fatigue worse?
- Does rest relieve your fatigue?
- Do you feel weak?
- Do you have any trouble sleeping?
- Do you have daytime sleepiness (likely to doze off during quiet activities such as reading, watching TV, sitting quietly after lunch)?
- Do you have other symptoms such as pain, difficulty breathing, nausea and vomiting?
- Do you experience anxiety? If yes, how often?
- Do you feel discouraged, blue or sad? If yes, how often?
- Do you feel bored? If yes, how often?

Interference/Distress
- As a result of fatigue, to what extent have you:
  - limited your social activity
  - had difficulty getting things done
  - felt like fatigue was making it difficult to maintain a positive outlook
- To what extent does fatigue interfere with relationships or fulfilling responsibilities at work or in the home?

Self-Management
- What do you do to help with fatigue or manage fatigue?
- Have you discussed your fatigue with anyone on your healthcare team?
- Have you ever been given any recommendations for managing your fatigue?

cause fatigue by disrupting sleep or by creating proximal muscle weakness. Coadministration of multiple agents with sedative, cardiac, or sleep-disrupting side effects may significantly compound fatigue symptoms.

Physical assessment and diagnostic evaluation

Physical examination of the patient with CRF may include clinical muscle strength testing; performance-based measures of physical function[2,85] such as the 6-minute walk, timed-up and go, and grip strength; and auscultation of heart and lungs for adventitious sounds.

Diagnostic evaluation in the patient with CRF is directed toward identifying the presence of hypothyroidism, hypogonadism, adrenal insufficiency, cardiomyopathy, pulmonary dysfunction, anemia, neutropenia, and electrolyte imbalance, as these conditions may cause or amplify CRF. Appropriate diagnostic tests will aid in determining whether disease progression or recurrence could be among the causes of fatigue.

DEGREES OF TOXICITY

The standard grading system for adverse events in cancer clinical trials is the National Cancer Institute's (NCI) Common Terminology Criteria for Adverse Events version 4.0 (CTCAE v.4.0).[86] Now in its fourth version, CTCAE toxicities are graded by healthcare providers, based on the clinician's review of systems, physical examination, and results review of laboratory and diagnostic studies. One of every eight adverse events included in the NCI CTCAE is a symptom or a side effect that could be validly and efficiently collected by direct patient report. Currently, research staff identify and grade toxicities that are reflected by the clinical staff in the health record, even though studies have demonstrated that health professionals tend to underestimate the onset, duration, and severity of symptoms such as fatigue and pain, compared to patients' own accounts.[87,88] Staff-based adverse event reporting also generally occurs at clinic visits, so adverse events that occur between visits may be missed. As a result of these gaps, we often lack a full understanding of the spectrum of toxicities associated with a new agent or a new regimen.[89] This incomplete picture of treatment-associated toxicities hinders the drug development process, and may restrict optimal treatment of toxicities for individual patients.

In response to these challenges, the NCI has recently developed the Patient Reported Outcomes—Common Terminology Criteria for Adverse Events (PRO-CTCAE). PRO-CTCAE comprises a psychometrically robust set of questionnaire items evaluating the presence, severity, and interference with usual activities of 81 symptoms drawn from the CTCAE.[90] The overall goal of PRO-CTCAE is to enhance the quality of adverse event data reporting in clinical trials, represent the patient perspective, and improve detection of potentially serious adverse events.[91] Incorporating the patient's self-report into the toxicity evaluation also has the potential to improve patients' satisfaction and communication with their clinicians and foster early detection of potentially serious adverse events.[92] PRO-CTCAE toxicity assessment and CTCAE grading for CRF are presented in Figure 3-2.

SYMPTOM MANAGEMENT STRATEGIES

THERAPEUTIC APPROACHES

Because fatigue typically has several different causes in any one patient, a multicomponent, individually tailored treatment plan is essential. Open communication between the patient, family, and caregiving team will facilitate discussion about the experience of fatigue and its effects on daily life, and promote collaborative goal setting. Deliberative selection of management strategies and tailoring of the program based on the patient's current level of energy, attention, motivation, and phases along the cancer continuum are important considerations, as at least one study suggests that too intensive or demanding intervention programs may actually worsen CRF.[93]

General supportive care recommendations for patients with fatigue include encouraging consumption of a balanced diet with adequate intake of fluid, calories, protein, carbohydrates, fat, vitamins, and minerals, and balancing rest with physical activity and attention-restoring activities such as exposure to natural environments and pleasant distractions such as music.[9]

There have been more than 190 empiric studies of pharmacologic and nonpharmacologic interventions to reduce or manage CRF, and several meta-analyses or systematic reviews are available.[94–104] For some interventions, there is strong and consistent evidence to support their effectiveness, while for other interventions only preliminary effectiveness data drawn from single-arm trials in small samples are available. Evidence-based interventions for CRF are summarized in Table 3-4.

Expert consensus indicates that patients with fatigue should be evaluated for potentially treatable etiologic factors contributing to fatigue, and managed as indicated.[9] Examples of such factors include endocrinopathies (e.g., hypothyroidism, hypogonadism, adrenal insufficiency), cardiopulmonary dysfunction, impaired sleep quality, medications with fatigue or sedation as side effects (e.g., opiates, antidepressants, antiemetics, antihistamines), deconditioning, asthenia, sarcopenia, and concurrent symptoms such as pain, nausea, or depression.

Deconditioning related to decreased activity is common among patients with cancer, and can cause or intensity fatigue from other causes. Meta-analyses of randomized trials support the benefits of exercise in the management of

As individuals go through treatment for their cancer they sometimes experience different symptoms and side effects. For each question, please check or mark an X in the one box O that best describes your experiences over the past 7 days...

1. FATIGUE, TIREDNESS OR LACK OF ENERGY				
What was the SEVERITY of your FATIGUE, TIREDNESS, OR LACK OF ENERGY at its WORST?				
O None	O Mild	O Moderate	O Severe	O Very severe
How much did FATIGUE, TIREDNESS, OR LACK OF ENERGY at its WORST INTERFERE with your usual or daily activities?				
O Not at all	O A little bit	O Somewhat	O Quite a bit	O Very much

FIGURE 3-2

Patient reported outcomes-common terminology criteria for adverse events (PRO-CTCAE) fatigue items[90].

TABLE 3-4

Evidence-Based Interventions to Manage Cancer-Related Fatigue

Evaluate All Patients For Fatigue

- Screen all patients for fatigue at regular intervals: On a scale of 0–10 where zero is no fatigue and 10 is the worst fatigue imaginable, how would you rate your fatigue over the past 7 days?
- If moderate (4–6) or severe (7–10), evaluate onset, pattern, duration, change over time, contributing factors, interference with function, and self-management strategies, and develop a tailored fatigue plan.

Exercise

- After appropriate medical clearances, recommend a program of physical activity such as walking, stretching, and cycling. Patient should begin with 5–10 minutes twice daily, and increase the time by 1 minute a day. They should avoid temptation to overdo in exercise, but rather strive for consistency.
- Consider referral to physical therapy, occupational therapy, exercise physiologist, or physiatrist to develop, tailor, and sustain an exercise program.

Improve Sleep Quality

- Provide behavioral interventions to improve sleep (e.g., go to bed only when sleepy and at approximately the same time each night; maintain a regular rising time each morning; avoid daytime napping, create a bedtime routine, avoid stimulants such as caffeine after noon, and eat dinner at least 3 hours before bedtime etc.).

Energy Conservation and Activity Management

- Instruct patient in energy conservation and activity management:
  - Set priorities to reduce or eliminate tasks that are less important
  - Schedule a daily routine to ensure pacing of activities and balance of rest and activity
  - Delegate or use labor-saving devices
  - Schedule activities for times of peak energy and mental concentration

Interventions to Manage Stress and Mood Disturbances

- Maintain open communication among patient, family, and healthcare professional about fatigue, its effects on daily life
- Offer information and referrals to counseling or support groups
- Consider treatment with an antidepressant for fatigue with depressive symptoms
- Teach diversional and relaxation techniques

Other Interventions

- Evaluate for treatable causes of fatigue (hypothyroidism, hypogonadism, adrenal insufficiency, cardiopulmonary dysfunction) and manage as indicated
- Optimize the management of concurrent symptoms (pain, depression, dyspnea)
- Consider referrals for structured rehabilitation, psychosocial and stress management interventions, or cognitive-behavioral therapy for sleep
- Consider massage, acupuncture, mindfulness-based stress reduction
- Consider levocarnitine supplementation or ginseng
- Consider treatment with a psychostimulant

Patient and Family Education about Fatigue

- Offer anticipatory guidance about possible patterns of fatigue onset occurrence (e.g., at nadir, with conclusion of radiotherapy, in association with muscle weakness/deconditioning, distress, excess activity, impaired sleep quality, sedating medications)
- Encourage patient to differentiate facets of the fatigue experience (fatigue, tiredness, weakness, cognitive slowing)
- Explain the multifactorial causes of fatigue including:
  - Side effects of treatment
  - Psychosocial stressors
  - Concurrent symptoms
  - Imbalance of rest and activity
  - Insufficient sleep
  - Inadequate nutrition
  - Muscle weakness/deconditioning
  - Sedating/fatiguing side effects of medications
  - Proinflammatory cytokine release
  - Anemia/neutropenia

TABLE 3-4

Evidence-Based Interventions to Manage Cancer-Related Fatigue (*Continued*)

- Explain that fatigue can develop or worsen as a direct result of treatment, and that this does not necessarily indicate that a treatment is ineffective or that the disease is progressing.
- Suggest a journal, log, or diary of activities, fatigue severity, associated feelings/symptoms, and an evaluation of self-care actions.
- Develop and tailor an individualized plan for fatigue management.
- Inform patient and family that interventions such as energy conservation, exercise, relaxation and stress management, psychosocial support, and measures to optimize sleep quality and reduce concurrent symptoms have been shown to be effective in limiting the severity of fatigue during treatment.
- Teach energy conservation strategies and principles of cognitive-behavioral self-management to improve sleep quality, and provide coaching to integrate these into daily patterns.
- Affirm the benefits of open communication between patient, family, and caregiving team to facilitate discussions about the experience of fatigue and its effects on daily life.
- Encourage attention restoring activities such as exposure to natural environments, and pleasant distractions such as music.
- Provide information concerning the importance of a balanced diet with adequate intake of fluid, calories, protein, carbohydrates, fat, vitamins, minerals.

fatigue during and following cancer treatment for patients with breast cancer, with solid tumors, or undergoing hematopoietic stem cell transplantation, although effect sizes are generally small and positive results for the outcome of fatigue have not been observed consistently across studies.[98,105–110] The exercise modalities that have been tested differ in content (walking, cycling, swimming, resistive exercise, or combined exercise), frequency (ranging from two times per week to two times daily), intensity (with most programs at 50% to 90% of the estimated VO_2 maximum heart rate), degree of supervision (fully supervised group versus self-directed exercise), and duration (from 2 weeks to 1 year). The type, intensity, and duration of physical exercise most beneficial in reducing fatigue at different stages of disease and treatment are not known,[107,108,111] and more research is needed to systematically assess the safety of exercise (both aerobic exercise and strength training) in cancer subpopulations. Patients require specific guidance about how to begin, maintain, and advance an exercise program. Referral to a rehabilitation professional such as physical therapist or an exercise trainer can be helpful in providing specific and detailed recommendations about the type, intensity, and frequency of exercise in which the patient should engage; in strengthening motivation and adherence; and in recommending advancements in the exercise program as functional capacity improves.

Several trials[112–115] and a systematic review[116] suggest that structured rehabilitation programs result in statistically significant and sustained improvements in fatigue, particularly in patients who have completed treatment and are in the survivorship phase. The rehabilitation interventions studied were multicomponent interventions consisting of a structured combination of intensive exercise, physical training, sports, psychoeducation, and physical modalities such as massage, mud packs, and manual lymph drainage. In some studies, these therapies were delivered over the course of a several-week inpatient rehabilitation hospital stay.

A growing body of evidence that includes several adequately powered randomized controlled trials suggests that educational interventions and psychological support play an important role in supporting positive coping in patients with fatigue.[117] Effective psychoeducational and self-management interventions include anticipatory guidance about patterns of fatigue, tailored recommendations for self-management of fatigue through activity/exercise and improved sleep hygiene, coaching to enhance motivation and empower self-care and active coping, and praise and encouragement to promote self-efficacy and augment feelings of control.

Energy conservation and activity management (ECAM) is a self-management intervention that teaches patients to apply the principles of energy conservation and activity management and provides coaching to integrate these activities into their daily lifestyle. ECAM has been found to have a modest but significant effect in a large, multisite randomized controlled trial (RCT) in patients (predominantly with breast cancer) initiating chemotherapy or radiation and in a small pilot study using historical controls[118,119]; however, a recent study did not find significant effects on fatigue outcomes when an energy and sleep self-management intervention was tested in patients receiving chemotherapy.[120]

Cognitive-behavioral interventions designed to improve sleep quality also have demonstrated a beneficial effect on fatigue.[121,122] These interventions to improve sleep quality can be delivered individually or in a group setting, and include relaxation training, sleep consolidation strategies (avoiding long or late-afternoon naps, limiting time in bed to actual sleep time), stimulus control therapy (going to bed only when sleepy, using the bed/bedroom for sleep and sexual activities only, lying down and getting up at a consistent time, avoiding caffeine and stimulating activity in the evening), and strategies to reduce cognitive-emotional arousal (keeping at least an hour to relax before going to bed, establishing a presleep routine to be used every night).

Cognitive-behavioral therapy (CBT) to treat fatigue and manage concurrent symptoms such as pain or depression has been shown to have beneficial effects on CRF.[99] Although outcomes of a randomized controlled trial of CBT for cancer pain in 131 patients demonstrated improvement in the outcomes of pain, the differences in fatigue were not statistically significant.[123] However, three RCTs (n = 200 cancer patients with major depressive disorder[124]; n = 83 cancer survivors with fatigue[125]; n = 45 women with metastatic breast cancer[126]) and a small case series (n = 6 women with metastatic breast cancer[127]) demonstrated that a CBT intervention targeted to fatigue and other symptoms resulted in statistically significant improvements in fatigue.

The use of erythropoiesis-stimulating agents (ESAs) to correct anemia characterized by a hemoglobin level less than 10 g/dL may result in increased vigor and diminished fatigue.[128–131] In contrast, only limited evidence supports the contention that erythropoietin improves fatigue outcomes when anemia is less severe. A target hemoglobin level of 11–12 g/dL is associated with the greatest gains in fatigue and other quality of life outcomes.[131] While both epoietin and darbepoietin are generally well tolerated, the use of these agents specifically for the management of fatigue must be considered in light of safety issues including a small increased risk of thrombotic events, hypertension, and pure red cell aplasia, and theoretical concerns that ESAs may support or extend tumor growth in certain disease tumor types.[132,133] Overall, better-quality evidence is needed to unequivocally support the use of ESAs solely to improve patient-reported outcomes such as fatigue. National clinical practice guidelines[134–136] and the recommendations of the Food and Drug Administration (FDA) should guide decisions about patient monitoring, treatment thresholds, dose reductions, treatment initiation and discontinuation, and the use of supplemental iron in patients receiving ESAs.

Paroxetine, donepezil, bupropion, methylphenidate, and modafinil have been evaluated for their effectiveness in reducing fatigue during and following cancer treatment. Several recent systematic reviews have concluded that only two pharmacologic treatments for CRF—treatment with psychostimulants (methylphenidate and dexmethylphenidate) and the wakefulness-promoting agent modafinil—are supported by evidence from adequately designed randomized trials.[97,101,102] Although additional evidence is needed, modafinil at a dose of 100 mg bid may be effective in treating fatigue and improving daytime wakefulness and cognitive function in patients during and following cancer treatment.[137–140] Randomized placebo-controlled trials of antidepressants do not appear to have a direct effect on fatigue outcomes, although improvement in mood has been observed.[97,141] In contrast, two small trials have demonstrated a trend toward a possible benefit for paroxetine in treating fatigue in two distinct subpopulations: women experiencing hot flashes and patients receiving interferon alpha.[141]

Several trials suggest that levocarnitine supplementation in patients who have low serum carnitine levels[142–145] and treatment with ginseng[146] are potentially efficacious in treating cancer-related fatigue. Levocarnitine is a naturally occurring amino acid that plays a vital role in the metabolism of fat by the mitochondria, and is thought to be essential for muscle contraction and endurance.[147] Systemic carnitine depletion is characterized by fatigue and muscle weakness, and has been described in association with cancer and its treatment.[148,149] Although interpretation of the results of the studies of levocarnitine or ginseng supplementation is complicated by small sample sizes, and in the case of levocarnitine by the absence of a double-blinded randomized controlled design, results are intriguing. The antioxidant effects of levocarnitine supplementation on treatment outcomes in patients receiving radiotherapy or chemotherapy also warrant further study.[150,151]

Complementary therapies such as yoga, relaxation, healing touch, massage, a mindfulness-based stress reduction intervention, acupuncture, acupressure and several combined modality interventions that include aromatherapy, lavender footsoak, and reflexology have demonstrated preliminary evidence of effectiveness in the management of CRF.[152] The design of these studies was open label and/or uncontrolled, with no random assignment, and with sample sizes that were extremely small, making it difficult to draw firm conclusions about efficacy. Of note, the studies evaluating acupuncture and the combined aromatherapy, footsoak, and reflexology intervention included patients with advanced cancer and at the end of life. If found to be effective in larger RCTs, these approaches may offer treatment options for patients with advanced cancer and those at the end of life for whom other fatigue interventions such as exercise may not be feasible.

In summary, although we have made gains in identifying interventions that are effective for this distressing symptom, the causative factors for CRF are distinct, and treatment approaches are evolving and largely empiric. The intervention approach for each patient is symptom oriented, and must be individualized and regularly revised. A multimodal approach that includes exercise, psychoeducational interventions, efforts to manage concurrent symptoms, and interventions to improve sleep quality, together with judicious use of medications such as modafinil, methylphenidate, and complementary therapies such as relaxation, massage, healing touch, or acupuncture, has the potential to improve clinical outcomes in CRF. An algorithm for fatigue screening, evaluation, and management is offered in Figure 3-3.

NURSING IMPLICATIONS

CRF outcomes sensitive to nursing intervention include a reduction in fatigue severity and improvements in the psychological distress and functional interference associated with fatigue. Other outcomes that reflect the effects of nursing

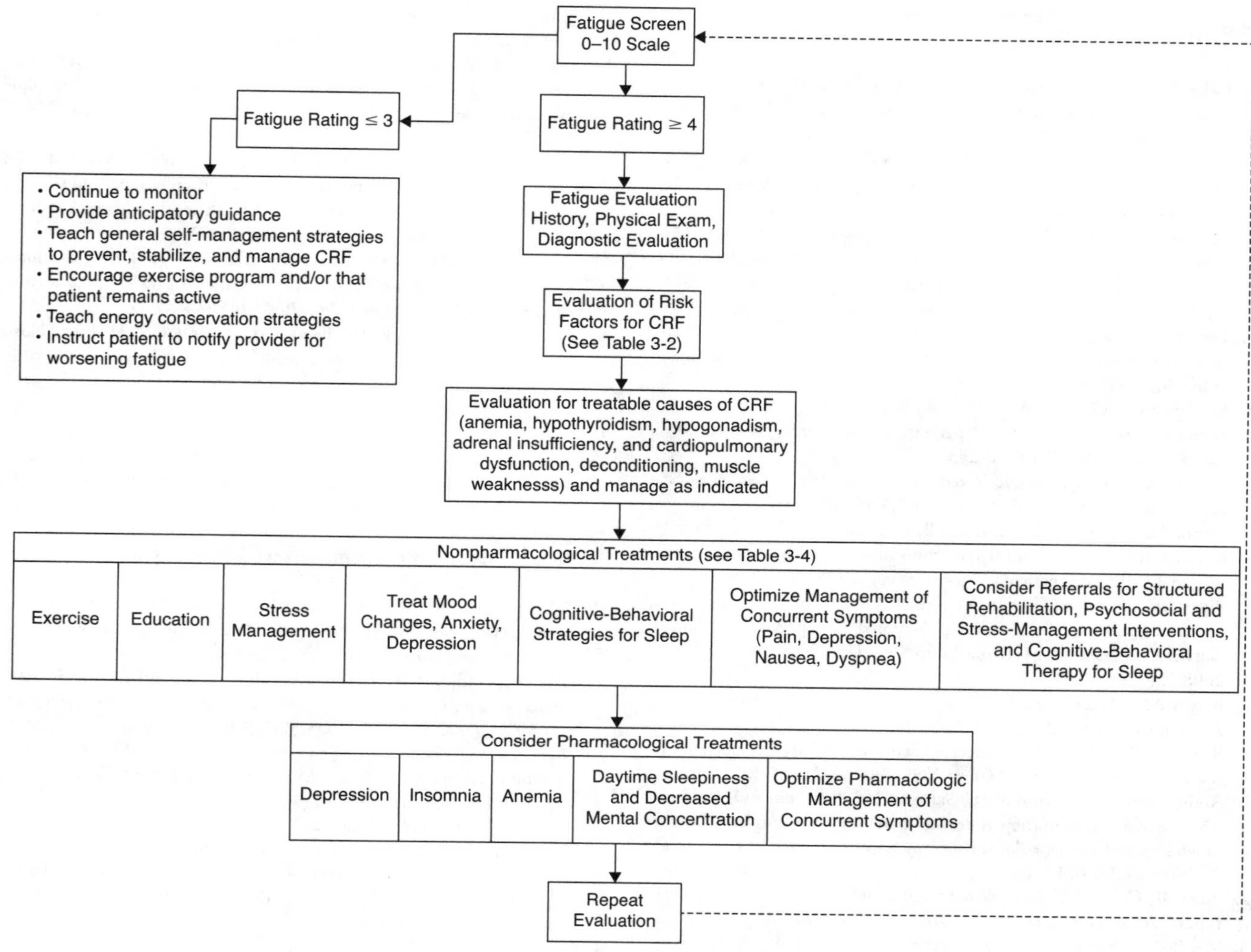

FIGURE 3-3

Algorithm for cancer-related fatigue (CRF) screening, evaluation, and management.

intervention include adequate knowledge of strategies for effective self-management, and self-efficacy for fatigue management. In some clinical situations (e.g., patients undergoing hematopoietic stem cell transplant or beginning a course of radiation therapy), reduction in fatigue severity, associated distress, and interference will not be achievable. In these circumstances, the clinical goal is to stabilize worsening of the fatigue severity, distress, and interference that would be expected across the course of treatment. Process outcomes that reflect implementation of an effective fatigue management program include that (1) all patients with cancer are screened for fatigue during each encounter with the health-care team while on active treatment and during long-term follow-up, and (2) in patients with moderate to severe fatigue, the health record documents the factors that contribute to cancer fatigue (concurrent symptoms, emotional distress, sleep disturbances, anemia, nutritional alterations, inactivity/deconditioning, and comorbidities such as hypothyroidism and cardiomyopathy) and the management plan to address these issues. Evidence-based guidelines to support the achievement of these outcomes have been published by the NCCN[9] and by the Oncology Nursing Society.[152]

PATIENT SELF-CARE

Evidence suggests that across the continuum from diagnosis, to treatment, survivorship, and the end of life, implementation of clinical guidelines and self-management interventions may reduce barriers to effective fatigue management,[153–155] contribute to reductions in fatigue severity, and improve the distress associated with CRF. A self-care guide that can be shared with patients to strengthen their knowledge of effective fatigue self-management is provided in Appendix 3A.

REFERENCES

1. Cella D, Peterman A, Passik S, Jacobsen P, Breitbart W. Progress toward guidelines for the management of fatigue. *Oncology (Williston Park).* 1998;12(11A):369–377.
2. Mallinson T, Cella D, Cashy J, Holzner B. Giving meaning to measure: linking self-reported fatigue and function to performance of everyday activities. *J Pain Symptom Manage.* 2006;31(3):229–241.
3. de Jong N, Candel MJ, Schouten HC, Abu-Saad HH, Courtens AM. Course of the fatigue dimension "activity level" and the interference of fatigue with daily living activities for patients with breast cancer receiving adjuvant chemotherapy. *Cancer Nurs.* 2006;29(5):E1–E13.
4. Brown LF, Kroenke K. Cancer-related fatigue and its associations with depression and anxiety: a systematic review. *Psychosomatics.* 2009;50(5):440–447.
5. Lindqvist O, Widmark A, Rasmussen BH. Meanings of the phenomenon of fatigue as narrated by 4 patients with cancer in palliative care. *Cancer Nurs.* 2004;27(3):237–243.
6. Rao AV, Cohen HJ. Fatigue in older cancer patients: etiology, assessment, and treatment. *Semin Oncol.* 2008;35(6):633–642.
7. Mystakidou K, Parpa E, Katsouda E, Galanos A, Vlahos L. The role of physical and psychological symptoms in desire for death: a study of terminally ill cancer patients. *Psychooncology.* 2006;15(4):355–360.
8. Piper BF, Borneman T, Sun VC, et al. Cancer-related fatigue: role of oncology nurses in translating National Comprehensive Cancer Network assessment guidelines into practice. *Clin J Oncol Nurs.* 2008;12(5 suppl):37–47.
9. Berger AM, Abernethy AP, Atkinson A, et al. Cancer-related fatigue. *J Compr Canc Netw.* 2010;8(8):904–931.
10. Wu HS, McSweeney M. Cancer-related fatigue: "It's so much more than just being tired." *Eur J Oncol Nurs.* 2007;11(2):117–125.
11. Andrykowski MA, Schmidt JE, Salsman JM, Beacham AO, Jacobsen PB. Use of a case definition approach to identify cancer-related fatigue in women undergoing adjuvant therapy for breast cancer. *J Clin Oncol.* 20 2005;23(27):6613–6622.
12. Piper BF, Cella D. Cancer-related fatigue: definitions and clinical subtypes. *J Natl Compr Canc Netw.* 2010;8(8):958–966.
13. Van Belle S, Paridaens R, Evers G, et al. Comparison of proposed diagnostic criteria with FACT-F and VAS for cancer-related fatigue: proposal for use as a screening tool. *Support Care Cancer.* 2005;13(4):246–254.
14. Lai JS, Cella D, Dineen K, et al. An item bank was created to improve the measurement of cancer-related fatigue. *J Clin Epidemiol.* 2005;58(2):190–197.
15. Bower JE, Ganz PA, Aziz N. Altered cortisol response to psychologic stress in breast cancer survivors with persistent fatigue. *Psychosom Med.* 2005;67(2):277–280.
16. Miller AH, Ancoli-Israel S, Bower JE, Capuron L, Irwin MR. Neuroendocrine-immune mechanisms of behavioral comorbidities in patients with cancer. *J Clin Oncol.* 2008;26(6):971–982.
17. Yeh ET, Lau SC, Su WJ, Tsai DJ, Tu YY, Lai YL. An examination of cancer-related fatigue through proposed diagnostic criteria in a sample of cancer patients in Taiwan. *BMC Cancer.* 2011;11:387.
18. Donovan KA, McGinty HL, Jacobsen PB. A systematic review of research using the diagnostic criteria for cancer-related fatigue. *Psychooncology.* 2012. (epub ahead of print)
19. Prue G, Rankin J, Allen J, Gracey J, Cramp F. Cancer-related fatigue: a critical appraisal. *Eur J Cancer.* 2006;42(7):846–863.
20. Weis J. Cancer-related fatigue: prevalence, assessment and treatment strategies. *Expert Rev Pharmacoecon Outcomes Res.* 2011;11(4):441–446.
21. Hofman M, Ryan JL, Figueroa-Moseley CD, Jean-Pierre P, Morrow GR. Cancer-related fatigue: the scale of the problem. *Oncologist.* 2007;12(suppl 1):4–10.
22. Spichiger E, Muller-Frohlich C, Denhaerynck K, Stoll H, Hantikainen V, Dodd M. Prevalence and contributors to fatigue in individuals hospitalized with advanced cancer: a prospective, observational study. *Int J Nurs Stud.* 2012; 49(9):1146–1154.
23. Skerman HM, Yates PM, Battistutta D. Cancer-related symptom clusters for symptom management in outpatients after commencing adjuvant chemotherapy, at 6 months, and 12 months. *Support Care Cancer.* 2012;20(1):95–105.
24. Spichiger E, Muller-Frohlich C, Denhaerynck K, Stoll H, Hantikainen V, Dodd M. Prevalence of symptoms, with a focus on fatigue, and changes of symptoms over three months in outpatients receiving cancer chemotherapy. *Swiss Medical Weekly.* 2011;141:w13303.
25. Butt Z, Rosenbloom SK, Abernethy AP, et al. Fatigue is the most important symptom for advanced cancer patients who have had chemotherapy. *J Natl Compr Canc Netw.* 2008;6(5):448–455.
26. Goldstein D, Bennett B, Friedlander M, Davenport T, Hickie I, Lloyd A. Fatigue states after cancer treatment occur both in association with, and independent of, mood disorder: a longitudinal study. *BMC Cancer.* 2006;6:240.
27. Shi Q, Smith TG, Michonski JD, Stein KD, Kaw C, Cleeland CS. Symptom burden in cancer survivors 1 year after diagnosis: a report from the American Cancer Society's Studies of Cancer Survivors. *Cancer.* 2011;117(12):2779–2790.
28. Johnsen A, Petersen M, Pedersen L, Groenvold M. Symptoms and problems in a nationally representative sample of advanced cancer patients. *Palliat Med.* 2009;23(6):491–501.
29. Glaus A, Boehme C, Thurlimann B, et al. Fatigue and menopausal symptoms in women with breast cancer undergoing hormonal cancer treatment. *Ann Oncol.* 2006;17(5):801–806.
30. Beck SL, Dudley WN, Barsevick A. Pain, sleep disturbance, and fatigue in patients with cancer: using a mediation model to test a symptom cluster. *Oncol Nurs Forum.* 2005;32(3):542.
31. Bender CM, Ergyn FS, Rosenzweig MQ, Cohen SM, Sereika SM. Symptom clusters in breast cancer across 3 phases of the disease. *Cancer Nurs.* 2005;28(3):219–225.
32. Chow E, Fan G, Hadi S, Filipczak L. Symptom clusters in cancer patients with bone metastases. *Support Care Cancer.* 2007; 11(4):591–600.
33. Francoeur RB. The relationship of cancer symptom clusters to depressive affect in the initial phase of palliative radiation. *J Pain Symptom Manage.* 2005;29(2):130–155.
34. Walsh D, Rybicki L. Symptom clustering in advanced cancer. *Support Care Cancer.* 2006; 20(11): 2837–2843.
35. Jereczek-Fossa BA, Marsiglia HR, Orecchia R. Radiotherapy-related fatigue. *Crit Rev Oncol Hematol.* 2002;41(3):317–325.
36. Storey DJ, McLaren DB, Atkinson MA, et al. Clinically relevant fatigue in men with hormone-sensitive prostate cancer on long-term androgen deprivation therapy. *Ann Oncol.* 2012;23(6):1542–1549.
37. Mosher CE, Redd WH, Rini CM, Burkhalter JE, DuHamel KN. Physical, psychological, and social sequelae following hematopoietic stem cell transplantation: a review of the literature. *Psychooncology.* 2009;18(2):113–127.
38. Cohen RB, Oudard S. Antiangiogenic therapy for advanced renal cell carcinoma: management of treatment-related toxicities. *Invest New Drugs.* 2012; 30(5):2066–2079.
39. Berger AM, Gerber LH, Mayer DK. Cancer-related fatigue: implications for breast cancer survivors. *Cancer.* 2012;118(8 suppl):2261–2269.
40. Oh HS, Seo WS. Systematic review and meta-analysis of the correlates of cancer-related fatigue. *Worldviews Evid Based Nurs.* 2011;8(4):191–201.
41. Morrow GR, Shelke AR, Roscoe JA, Hickok JT, Mustian K. Management of cancer-related fatigue. *Cancer Invest.* 2005;23(3):229–239.
42. Strasser F, Palmer JL, Schover LR, et al. The impact of hypogonadism and autonomic dysfunction on fatigue, emotional function, and sexual desire in male patients with advanced cancer: a pilot study. *Cancer.* 2006;107(12):2949–2957.
43. Kilgour RD, Vigano A, Trutschnigg B, et al. Cancer-related fatigue: the impact of skeletal muscle mass and strength in patients with advanced cancer. *J Cachexia Sarcopenia Muscle.* 2010;1(2):177–185.

44. Al-Majid S, Gray DP. A biobehavioral model for the study of exercise interventions in cancer-related fatigue. *Biol Res Nurs.* 2009;10(4):381–391.
45. Saligan LN, Kim HS. A systematic review of the association between immunogenomic markers and cancer-related fatigue. *Brain Behav Immun.* 2012:25(6):830–848.
46. Payne JK. Altered circadian rhythms and cancer-related fatigue outcomes. *Integ Cancer Ther.* 2011;10(3):221–233.
47. Barsevick A, Frost M, Zwinderman A, Hall P, Halyard M. I'm so tired: biological and genetic mechanisms of cancer-related fatigue. *Qual Life Res.* 2010;19(10):1419–1427.
48. Ryan JL, Carroll JK, Ryan EP, Mustian KM, Fiscella K, Morrow GR. Mechanisms of cancer-related fatigue. *Oncologist.* 2007;12 (suppl 1):22–34.
49. Parker KP, Bliwise DL, Ribeiro M, et al. Sleep/wake patterns of individuals with advanced cancer measured by ambulatory polysomnography. *J Clin Oncol.* 2008;26(15):2464–2472.
50. Akechi T, Okuyama T, Akizuki N, et al. Associated and predictive factors of sleep disturbance in advanced cancer patients. *Psychooncology.* 2007;16(10):888–894.
51. Yavuzsen T, Davis MP, Ranganathan VK, et al. Cancer-related fatigue: central or peripheral? *J Pain Symptom Manage.* 2009;38(4):587–596.
52. Jones LW, Eves ND, Haykowsky M, Freedland SJ, Mackey JR. Exercise intolerance in cancer and the role of exercise therapy to reverse dysfunction. *Lancet Oncol.* 2009;10(6):598–605.
53. Bower JE, Lamkin DM. Inflammation and cancer-related fatigue: mechanisms, contributing factors, and treatment implications. *Brain Behav Immun.* 2012.(epub ahead of print)
54. Mitchell SA. Cancer-related fatigue: state of the science. *Physical Med Rehab.* 2010;2(5):364–383.
55. Radbruch L, Strasser F, Elsner F, et al. Fatigue in palliative care patients: an EAPC approach. *Palliat Med.* 2008;22(1):13–32.
56. Jacobsen PB, Donovan KA, Weitzner MA. Distinguishing fatigue and depression in patients with cancer. *Semin Clin Neuropsychiatry.* 2003;8(4):229–240.
57. Capuron L, Gumnick JF, Musselman DL, et al. Neurobehavioral effects of interferon-alpha in cancer patients: phenomenology and paroxetine responsiveness of symptom dimensions. *Neuropsychopharmacology.* 2002;26(5):643–652.
58. Reuter K, Harter M. The concepts of fatigue and depression in cancer. *Eur J Cancer Care (Engl).* 2004;13(2):127–134.
59. Hinshaw DB, Carnahan JM, Johnson DL. Depression, anxiety, and asthenia in advanced illness.*J Am Coll Surg.* 2002;195(2):271.
60. Valentine AD, Meyers CA. Cognitive and mood disturbance as causes and symptoms of fatigue in cancer patients. *Cancer.* 2001;92 (6 suppl):1694–1698.
61. Traeger L, Braun IM, Greer JA, Temel JS, Cashavelly B, Pirl WF. Parsing depression from fatigue in patients with cancer using the fatigue symptom inventory. *J Pain Symptom Manage.* 2011;42(1):52–59.
62. Lee BN, Dantzer R, Langley KE, et al. A cytokine-based neuroimmunologic mechanism of cancer-related symptoms. *Neuroimmunomodulation.* 2004;11(5):279–292.
63. Butt Z, Wagner LI, Beaumont JL, et al. Use of a single-item screening tool to detect clinically significant fatigue, pain, distress, and anorexia in ambulatory cancer practice. *J Pain Symptom Manage.* 2008;35(1):20–30.
64. Alexander S, Minton O, Stone PC. Evaluation of screening instruments for cancer-related fatigue syndrome in breast cancer survivors. *J Clin Oncol.* 2009;27(8):1197–1201.
65. Banthia R, Malcarne VL, Roesch SC, et al. Correspondence between daily and weekly fatigue reports in breast cancer survivors. *J Behav Med.* 2006;29(3):269–279.
66. Mota DD, Pimenta CA. Self-report instruments for fatigue assessment: a systematic review. *Res Theory Nurs Pract.* 2006;20(1):49–78.
67. Minton O, Stone P. A systematic review of the scales used for the measurement of cancer-related fatigue (CRF). *Ann Oncol.* 2009;20(1):17–25.
68. Seyidova-Khoshknabi D, Davis MP, Walsh D. Review article: a systematic review of cancer-related fatigue measurement questionnaires. *Am J Hosp Palliat Care.* 2011;28(2):119–129.
69. Whitehead L. The measurement of fatigue in chronic illness: a systematic review of unidimensional and multidimensional fatigue measures. *J Pain Symptom Manage.* 2009;37(1):107–128.
70. Yellen SB, Cella DF, Webster K, Blendowski C, Kaplan E. Measuring fatigue and other anemia-related symptoms with the Functional Assessment of Cancer Therapy (FACT) measurement system. *J Pain Symptom Manage.* 1997;13(2):63–74.
71. Mendoza TR, Wang XS, Cleeland CS, et al. The rapid assessment of fatigue severity in cancer patients: use of the Brief Fatigue Inventory. *Cancer.* 1999;85(5):1186–1196.
72. Weis J, Arraras JI, Conroy T, et al. Development of an EORTC quality of life phase III module measuring cancer-related fatigue (EORTC QLQ-FA13). *Psychooncology.* 2012.(epub ahead of print)
73. Smets EM, Garssen B, Bonke B, De Haes JC. The Multidimensional Fatigue Inventory (MFI) psychometric qualities of an instrument to assess fatigue. *J Psychosom Res.* 1995;39(3):315–325.
74. Stein KD, Martin SC, Hann DM, Jacobsen PB. A multidimensional measure of fatigue for use with cancer patients. *Cancer Pract.* 1998;6(3):143–152.
75. Piper BF, Dibble SL, Dodd MJ, Weiss MC, Slaughter RE, Paul SM. The revised Piper Fatigue Scale: psychometric evaluation in women with breast cancer. *Oncol Nurs Forum.* 1998;25(4):677–684.
76. Ware JE Jr, Gandek B. Overview of the SF-36 health survey and the International Quality of Life Assessment (IQOLA) project. *J Clin Epidemiol.* 1998;51(11):903–912.
77. Baker F, Denniston M, Zabora J, Polland A, Dudley WN. A POMS short form for cancer patients: psychometric and structural evaluation. *Psychooncology.* 2002;11(4):273–281.
78. De Haes JC, Olschewski M, Fayers P, et al. *Measuring the Quality of Life of Cancer Patients with the Rotterdam Symptom Checklist: A Manual.* Groningen: Northern Center for Health Research; 1996.
79. Carlson LE, Angen M, Cullum J, et al. High levels of untreated distress and fatigue in cancer patients. *Br J Cancer.* 2004;90(12):2297–2304.
80. McCorkle R, Cooley ME, Shea JA. *A User's Manual for the Symptom Distress Scale.* Philadelphia: University of Pennsylvania School of Nursing; 1998.
81. Mortimer JE, Barsevick AM, Bennett CL, et al. Studying cancer-related fatigue: report of the NCCN scientific research committee. *J Natl Compr Canc Netw.* 2010;8(12):1331–1339.
82. Hoffman AJ, von Eye A, Gift AG, Given BA, Given CW, Rothert M. The development and testing of an instrument for perceived self-efficacy for fatigue self-management. *Cancer Nurs.* 2011;34(3):167–175.
83. Davis MP, Khoshknabi D, Yue GH. Management of fatigue in cancer patients. *Curr Pain Headache Rep.* 2006;10(4):260–269.
84. Agasi-Idenburg C, Velthuis M, Wittink H. Quality criteria and user-friendliness in self-reported questionnaires on cancer-related fatigue: a review. *J Clin Epidemiol.* 2010;63(7):705–711.
85. Kovalszki A, Schumaker GL, Klein A, Terrin N, White AC. Reduced respiratory and skeletal muscle strength in survivors of sibling or unrelated donor hematopoietic stem cell transplantation. *Bone Marrow Transplant.* 2008;41(11):965–969.
86. NCI. Common terminology criteria for adverse events (CTCAE) v.4.0. 2009. http://ctep.cancer.gov/protocolDevelopment/electronic_applications/ctc.htm#ctc_40. Accessed November 7, 2011.
87. Basch E, Iasonos A, McDonough T, et al. Patient versus clinician symptom reporting using the National Cancer Institute Common Terminology Criteria for Adverse Events: results of a questionnaire-based study. *Lancet Oncol.* 2006;7(11):903–909.
88. Bruner DW. Should patient-reported outcomes be mandatory for toxicity reporting in cancer clinical trials? *J Clin Oncol.* 2007;25(34):5345–5347.
89. Edgerly M, Fojo T. Is there room for improvement in adverse event reporting in the era of targeted therapies? *J Natl Cancer Inst.* 2008;100(4):240–242.

90. Patient-reported outcomes version of the Common Terminology Criteria for Adverse Events. 2012. http://outcomes.cancer.gov/tools/pro-ctcae.html. Accessed July 31, 2012.
91. Basch EM, Reeve BB, Mitchell SA, et al. Electronic toxicity monitoring and patient-reported outcomes. *Cancer J.* 2011;17(4):231–234.
92. Trotti A, Colevas AD, Setser A, Basch E. Patient-reported outcomes and the evolution of adverse event reporting in oncology. *J Clin Oncol.* 2007;25(32):5121–5127.
93. Brown P, Clark MM, Atherton P, et al. Will improvement in quality of life (QOL) impact fatigue in patients receiving radiation therapy for advanced cancer? *Am J Clin Oncol.* 2006;29(1):52–58.
94. Mitchell S, Beck S, Hood L, Moore K, Tanner E. Putting evidence into practice (PEP): evidence-based interventions for fatigue during and following cancer and its treatment. *Clin J Oncol Nurs.* 2007;11:99–113.
95. Kangas M, Bovbjerg DH, Montgomery GH. Cancer-related fatigue: a systematic and meta-analytic review of non-pharmacological therapies for cancer patients. *Psychol Bull.* 2008;134(5):700–741.
96. Jacobsen PB, Donovan KA, Vadaparampil ST, Small BJ. Systematic review and meta-analysis of psychological and activity-based interventions for cancer-related fatigue. *Health Psychol.* 2007;26(6):660–667.
97. Minton O, Richardson A, Sharpe M, Hotopf M, Stone P. Drug therapy for the management of cancer related fatigue. *Cochrane Database Syst Rev.* 2010;1:CD006704.
98. Cramp F, Daniel J. Exercise for the management of cancer-related fatigue in adults. *Cochrane Database Syst Rev.* 2008;2:CD006145.
99. Goedendorp MM, Gielissen MF, Verhagen CA, Bleijenberg G. Psychosocial interventions for reducing fatigue during cancer treatment in adults. *Cochrane Database Syst Rev.* 2009;1:CD006953.
100. Payne C, Wiffen PJ, Martin S. Interventions for fatigue and weight loss in adults with advanced progressive illness. *Cochrane Database Syst Rev.* 2012;1:CD008427.
101. Minton O, Richardson A, Sharpe M, Hotopf M, Stone PC. Psychostimulants for the management of cancer-related fatigue: a systematic review and meta-analysis. *J Pain Symptom Manage.* 2011;41(4):761–767.
102. Breitbart W, Alici Y. Psychostimulants for cancer-related fatigue. *J Natl Compr Canc Netw.* 2010;8(8):933–942.
103. Breitbart W, Alici-Evcimen Y. Update on psychotropic medications for cancer-related fatigue. *J Natl Compr Canc Netw.* 2007;5(10):1081–1091.
104. Portela MA, Rubiales AS, Centeno C. The use of psychostimulants in cancer patients. *Curr Opin Support Palliat Care.* 2011;5(2):164–168.
105. Kuchinski AM, Reading M, Lash AA. Treatment-related fatigue and exercise in patients with cancer: a systematic review. *Medsurg Nurs.* 2009;18(3):174–180.
106. Lowe SS, Watanabe SM, Courneya KS. Physical activity as a supportive care intervention in palliative cancer patients: a systematic review. *J Support Oncol.* 2009;7(1):27–34.
107. McMillan EM, Newhouse IJ. Exercise is an effective treatment modality for reducing cancer-related fatigue and improving physical capacity in cancer patients and survivors: a meta-analysis. *Appl Physiol Nutr Metab.* 2011;36(6):892–903.
108. Velthuis MJ, Agasi-Idenburg SC, Aufdemkampe G, Wittink HM. The effect of physical exercise on cancer-related fatigue during cancer treatment: a meta-analysis of randomised controlled trials. *Clin Oncol (R Coll Radiol).* 2010; 22(3):208–221.
109. Brown JC, Huedo-Medina TB, Pescatello LS, Pescatello SM, Ferrer RA, Johnson BT. Efficacy of exercise interventions in modulating cancer-related fatigue among adult cancer survivors: a meta-analysis. *Cancer Epidemiol Biomarkers Prev.* 2011;20(1):123–133.
110. Arnold M, Taylor NF. Does exercise reduce cancer-related fatigue in hospitalised oncology patients? A systematic review. *Onkologie.* 2010;33(11):625–630.
111. Humpel N, Iverson DC. Review and critique of the quality of exercise recommendations for cancer patients and survivors. *Support Care Cancer.* 2005;13(7):493–502.
112. van Weert E, Hoekstra-Weebers J, Otter R, Postema K, Sanderman R, van der Schans C. Cancer-related fatigue: predictors and effects of rehabilitation. *Oncologist.* 2006;11(2):184–196.
113. Strauss-Blasche G, Gnad E, Ekmekcioglu C, Hladschik B, Marktl W. Combined inpatient rehabilitation and spa therapy for breast cancer patients: effects on quality of life and CA 15-3. *Cancer Nurs.* 2005;28(5):390–398.
114. Korstjens I, Mesters I, van der Peet E, Gijsen B, van den Borne B. Quality of life of cancer survivors after physical and psychosocial rehabilitation. *Eur J Cancer Prev.* 2006;15(6):541–547.
115. Heim ME, v d Malsburg ML, Niklas A. Randomized controlled trial of a structured training program in breast cancer patients with tumor-related chronic fatigue. *Onkologie.* 2007;30(8–9):429–434.
116. van Weert E, Hoekstra-Weebers JE, May AM, Korstjens I, Ros WJ, van der Schans CP. The development of an evidence-based physical self-management rehabilitation programme for cancer survivors. *Patient Educ Couns.* 2008;4:4.
117. Jacobsen PB, Donovan KA, Vadaparampil ST, Small BJ. "Systematic review and meta-analysis of psychological and activity-based interventions for cancer-related fatigue": correction. *Health Psychol.* 2008;27(1):42.
118. Barsevick AM, Dudley W, Beck S, Sweeney C, Whitmer K, Nail L. A randomized clinical trial of energy conservation for patients with cancer-related fatigue. *Cancer.* 2004;100(6):1302–1310.
119. Barsevick AM, Whitmer K, Sweeney C, Nail LM. A pilot study examining energy conservation for cancer treatment-related fatigue. *Cancer Nurs.* 2002;25(5):333–341.
120. Barsevick A, Beck SL, Dudley WN, et al. Efficacy of an intervention for fatigue and sleep disturbance during cancer chemotherapy. *J Pain Symptom Manage.* 2010;40(2):200–216.
121. Zee PC, Ancoli-Israel S. Does effective management of sleep disorders reduce cancer-related fatigue? *Drugs.* 2009;69(suppl 2):29–41.
122. Ritterband LM, Bailey ET, Thorndike FP, Lord HR, Farrell-Carnahan L, Baum LD. Initial evaluation of an Internet intervention to improve the sleep of cancer survivors with insomnia. *Psychooncology.* 2012;21(7):695–705.
123. Dalton JA, Keefe FJ, Carlson J, Youngblood R. Tailoring cognitive-behavioral treatment for cancer pain. *Pain Manag Nurs.* 2004;5(1):3–18.
124. Strong V, Waters R, Hibberd C, et al. Management of depression for people with cancer (SMaRT oncology 1): a randomised trial. *Lancet.* 2008;372(9632):40–48.
125. Gielissen MF, Wiborg JF, Verhagen CA, Knoop H, Bleijenberg G. Examining the role of physical activity in reducing postcancer fatigue. *Support Care Cancer.* 2012;20(7):1441–1447.
126. Savard J, Simard S, Giguere I, et al. Randomized clinical trial on cognitive therapy for depression in women with metastatic breast cancer: psychological and immunological effects. *Palliat Support Care.* 2006;4(3):219–237.
127. Levesque M, Savard J, Simard S, Gauthier JG, Ivers H. Efficacy of cognitive therapy for depression among women with metastatic cancer: a single-case experimental study. *J Behav Ther Exp Psychiatry.* 2004;35(4):287–305.
128. Bohlius J, Schmidlin K, Brillant C, et al. Erythropoietin or darbepoetin for patients with cancer: meta-analysis based on individual patient data. *Cochrane Database Syst Rev.* 2009;3:CD007303.
129. Bohlius J, Tonia T, Schwarzer G. Twist and shout: one decade of meta-analyses of erythropoiesis-stimulating agents in cancer patients. *Acta Haematol.* 2011;125(1–2):55–67.
130. Tonia T, Bohlius J. Ten years of meta-analyses on erythropoiesis-stimulating agents in cancer patients. *Cancer Treat Res.* 2011;157:217–238.
131. Eton DT, Cella D. Do erythropoietic-stimulating agents relieve fatigue? A review of reviews. *Cancer Treat Res.* 2011;157:181–194.
132. Littlewood T, Collins G. Epoetin alfa: basic biology and clinical utility in cancer patients. *Expert Rev Anticancer Ther.* 2005;5(6):947–956.

133. Glaspy J, Crawford J, Vansteenkiste J, et al. Erythropoiesis-stimulating agents in oncology: a study-level meta-analysis of survival and other safety outcomes. *Br J Cancer.* 2010;102(2):301–315.
134. Cancer- and chemotherapy-induced anemia (version 1.2009). National Comprehensive Cancer Network; 2009. http://www.nccn.org/professionals/physician_gls/PDF/anemia.pdf. Accessed August 28, 2008.
135. Rizzo JD, Somerfield MR, Hagerty KL, et al. Use of epoetin and darbepoetin in patients with cancer: 2007 American Society of Hematology/American Society of Clinical Oncology clinical practice guideline update. *Blood.* 2008;111(1):25–41.
136. Lichtin AE. Clinical practice guidelines for the use of erythroid-stimulating agents: ASCO, EORTC, NCCN. *Cancer Treat Res.* 2011;157:239–248.
137. Blackhall L, Petroni G, Shu J, Baum L, Farace E. A pilot study evaluating the safety and efficacy of modafinal for cancer-related fatigue. *J Palliat Med.* 2009;12(5):433–439.
138. Cooper MR, Bird HM, Steinberg M. Efficacy and safety of modafinil in the treatment of cancer-related fatigue. *Ann Pharmacol.* 2009;43(4):721–725.
139. Kohli S, Fisher SG, Tra Y, et al. The effect of modafinil on cognitive function in breast cancer survivors. *Cancer.* 2009;115(12):2605–2616.
140. Spathis A, Dhillan R, Booden D, Forbes K, Vrotsou K, Fife K. Modafinil for the treatment of fatigue in lung cancer: a pilot study. *Palliat Med.* 2009;23(4):325–331.
141. Minton O, Richardson A, Sharpe M, Hotopf M, Stone P. A systematic review and meta-analysis of the pharmacological treatment of cancer-related fatigue. *J Natl Cancer Inst.* 2008;100(16):1155–1166.
142. Cruciani RA, Dvorkin E, Homel P, et al. L-carnitine supplementation for the treatment of fatigue and depressed mood in cancer patients with carnitine deficiency: a preliminary analysis. *Ann N Y Acad Sci.* 2004;1033:168–176.
143. Cruciani RA, Dvorkin E, Homel P, et al. Safety, tolerability and symptom outcomes associated with L-carnitine supplementation in patients with cancer, fatigue, and carnitine deficiency: a phase I/II study. *J Pain Symptom Manage.* 2006;32(6):551–559.
144. Gramignano G, Lusso MR, Madeddu C, et al. Efficacy of L-carnitine administration on fatigue, nutritional status, oxidative stress, and related quality of life in 12 advanced cancer patients undergoing anticancer therapy. *Nutrition.* 2006;22(2):136–145.
145. Graziano F, Bisonni R, Catalano V, et al. Potential role of levocarnitine supplementation for the treatment of chemotherapy-induced fatigue in non-anaemic cancer patients. *Br J Cancer.* 2002;86(12):1854–1857.
146. Barton DL, Soori GS, Bauer BA, et al. Pilot study of *Panax quinque folius* (American ginseng) to improve cancer-related fatigue: a randomized, double-blind, dose-finding evaluation: NCCTG trial N03CA. *Support Care Cancer.* 2009;18(2): 179–187.
147. Zammit VA, Ramsay RR, Bonomini M, Arduini A. Carnitine, mitochondrial function and therapy. *Adv Drug Delivery Rev.* 2009;61(14):1353–1362.
148. MacDonald N. Cancer cachexia and targeting chronic inflammation: a unified approach to cancer treatment and palliative/supportive care. *J Support Oncol.* 2007;5(4):157–162; discussion 164–156, 183.
149. Silverio R, Laviano A, Rossi Fanelli F, Seelaender M. L-carnitine and cancer cachexia: clinical and experimental aspects. *J Cachexia Sarcopenia Muscle.* 2011;2(1):37–44.
150. Block KI, Koch AC, Mead MN, Tothy PK, Newman RA, Gyllenhaal C. Impact of antioxidant supplementation on chemotherapeutic toxicity: a systematic review of the evidence from randomized controlled trials. *Int J Cancer.* 2008;123(6):1227–1239.
151. Khan HA, Alhomida AS. A review of the logistic role of L-carnitine in the management of radiation toxicity and radiotherapy side effects. *J Appl Toxicol.* 2011;31(8):707–713.
152. Mitchell SA, Beck SL, Eaton LH. ONS putting evidence into practice (PEP): fatigue. In: Eaton LH, Tipton JM, eds. *Putting Evidence into Practice.* Pittsburgh: Oncology Nursing Society; 2009; pp. 149–175.
153. American Cancer Society. Getting help for fatigue. 2012. http://www.cancer.org/acs/groups/content/@editorial/documents/document/acspc-031607.pdf. Accessed August 10, 2012.
154. Borneman T, Piper BF, Sun VC, Koczywas M, Uman G, Ferrell B. Implementing the fatigue guidelines at one NCCN member institution: process and outcomes. *J Natl Compr Canc Netw.* 2007;5(10):1092–1101.
155. Borneman T, Koczywas M, Sun V, Piper B, Smith-Idell C, Laroya B, Uman G, Ferell B. Effectiveness of a clinical intervention to eliminate barriers to pain and fatigue management in oncology. *Journal of Palliative Care.* 2011;14(2):197–205.

Fatigue

Patient Name: ______________________________

Symptom and Description

Fatigue is a common problem for patients during and often for many months following cancer treatment. It is one of the most difficult side effects of treatment and can be hard to describe to others. The symptoms of fatigue are different than "feeling tired." Fatigue can begin suddenly; it can affect all of your regular activities; naps may not help; and fatigue can be physically and emotionally draining on the patient as well as the family. General weakness may occur with a heavy feeling in your arms or legs, decreased ability to concentrate, trouble sleeping, and/or irritability. People sometimes think that patients with fatigue are just being lazy or depressed.

Many factors can contribute to the fatigue that a person with cancer experiences. Sudden changes in feelings of fatigue may mean that there is a serious problem. Slower, gradual development of fatigue can limit your ability to do everyday activities and enjoy life.

If you are experiencing this type of extreme tiredness, begin by speaking to your nurse or doctor about it. A few simple tests, including a blood count to check for anemia or infection, thyroid function tests, and a physical examination, will help your health provider find some causes that are treatable. Fatigue can be managed with a plan just for you and the factors that may be causing your fatigue.

Here are some ideas to think about:

Exercise

- With permission from your healthcare team, begin a program of physical activity such as walking, stretching, and cycling. Begin with 5–10 minutes twice daily, and increase the time by 1 minute per day. Do not be tempted to overdo the exercise, but be consistent.
- A moderate amount of exercise may help improve your energy level. Find a friend to walk with; he or she can encourage you to get out when you are tempted to stay in. An exercise trainer or physical therapist can also help with strengthening and building muscles and improving flexibility and balance.
- Think about asking your healthcare provider to refer you to physical therapy, occupational therapy, or an exercise specialist (such as a physiologist or physiatrist) to plan your own exercise program.

Gain Information about Fatigue

- Learn more about fatigue, and educate your family so they can be supportive.
- Consider the possible patterns of when fatigue occurs (e.g., related to muscle weakness/deconditioning, distress, excess activity, poor sleep quality, medications that make you sleepy) to see what makes fatigue better or worse.
- Learn the different aspects of the fatigue experience (fatigue, tiredness, weakness, cognitive slowing).
- Keep a journal or diary of activities, severity of fatigue, your feelings, symptoms, and the results of your self-care actions.

Improve Sleep Quality and Quantity

- Try to get undisturbed sleep. Go to bed at a regular time each day and follow a regular routine. The routine will begin to serve as a signal to your body that it is time for sleep.
- If you wake up at night because of pain or other symptoms, ask your doctor or nurse if your medication schedule can be changed to allow more hours of sleep at night.
- Try other activities rather than napping. Taking a daytime nap may cause you to have trouble sleeping at night. Try activities such as meditation, massage, or yoga instead. These activities can also help you avoid sleep troubles by reducing the anxiety and stress that play a part in sleep difficulties.

Energy Conservation and Activity Management

Energy conservation means looking at your daily routines to find ways to reduce the amount of effort needed to perform certain tasks and stopping other tasks. Sometimes switching rest periods with activities throughout the day can help. Although not every technique will work for you, these are suggestions that you can consider:

- Set priorities to reduce or stop tasks that are less important. Sort out the really important activities from those that can wait.
- Schedule a daily routine to help you balance rest and activity.
- Ask others to do some tasks such as laundry or meals or use labor-saving devices such as a robotic vacuum cleaner.
- Schedule activities for times of peak energy and mental concentration.
- Keep a journal to learn your energy patterns.
- Do not do jobs that do not need to be done every day, such as making beds.
- Ask your healthcare team about an occupational therapy evaluation to teach you energy-saving strategies.
- Keep a list of tasks that need to be done near your phone. When a neighbor, family member, or friend asks what they can do to help, tell them!

Seek Help in Managing Stress, Symptoms, and the Ups and Downs of the Cancer Experience

- Maintain open communication with family, friends, and healthcare professionals about fatigue and its effects on daily life.
- Ask your nurse or doctor if your fatigue or the other symptoms that are adding to your fatigue might be helped with medication.
- Make your team aware of the effects of your tiredness on your daily life.
- Consider joining a support group or talking with a counselor.

Phone Numbers

Nurse: ______________________________ Phone: ______________________

Physician: ___________________________ Phone: ______________________

Other: ______________________________ Phone: ______________________

Source: Mitchell SA. Cancer-Related Fatigue. In: Yarbro CH, Wujcik D, Gobel BH, eds. *Cancer Symptom Management.* 4th ed. Burlington, MA: Jones & Bartlett Learning; 2014.

Chapter 4

Menopausal Symptoms

Sheryl Redlin Frazier, RN, MSN
Mary Egger, RN, MSN, WHNP

THE PROBLEM

Menopause is the cessation of menses, a situation that may occur naturally as part of the female life cycle; as a result of surgery; or be induced by chemical treatment or radiation therapy. Natural menopause is a process that may take place over a period of time that is unique to each woman experiencing aging and the associated decline of the endogenous hormones that drive the menstrual cycle. Many physiologic symptoms are associated with this transition, such as vasomotor symptoms, predominately in the form of hot flashes (flushes) and night sweats; vulvovaginal atrophy; changes in the menstrual cycle; and other comorbid disease states. In healthy women, menopause can be troubling and disruptive to normal life, but for women who are cancer survivors, menopause can be especially difficult. Regardless of the origin of the onset of menopause, women with cancer may find the management of menopause and the management of their disease in direct conflict, causing increased physiologic and psychological distress. Nurses who care for women surviving cancer should familiarize themselves with the current state of knowledge regarding menopause and utilize the best evidence to partner with survivors in a collaborative effort to minimize the long-term effects of the menopausal state, improve quality of life, and encourage a life style that promotes long-term health.

INCIDENCE

According to the most recent U.S. Census, taken in 2010, nearly 53 million women in the United States are 50 years and older.[1] This number represents a continued increasing trend in the number of female healthcare consumers who are in or nearing menopause. In 2012, the American Cancer Society estimated that there were 226,870 new cases of breast cancer in women, and 88,750 new cases of gynecologic cancers: these disease sites account for the largest number of women who would likely be at risk for disease- or treatment-induced menopause.[2] The most recent Surveillance Epidemiology and End Results (SEER) data on incidence gathered between 2004 and 2008 reveal the median age at diagnosis for breast cancer to be 61 years of age; with the largest percentages, 22.6% and 24.4%, being between the ages of 45–54 and 55–64, respectively.[3] In gynecologic cancers, the median age at diagnosis ranges from 48 years of age in cervical cancer to 68 years of age in vulvar carcinoma.[4,5] It is important for nurses to remember that even though the median ages of diagnoses in these malignancies are near the age of menopause, treatments for breast, gynecologic, and other malignancies can induce menopause, either through surgery or via chemical and radiation therapies. Additionally, young women diagnosed with cancers may receive therapies that induce long-term amenorrhea or temporary ovarian suppression, and potentially induce a permanent state of menopause.

ETIOLOGY

Premenopause or the menopausal transition

As defined by the Stages of Reproductive Aging Workshop (STRAW) in 2001, and revised in 2011, there are 10 reproductive and menopausal stages in a woman's life[6,7]

Stage	Menarche −5	−4	−3b	−3a	−2	FMP (0) −1	+1a	+1b	+1c	+2
Terminology	REPRODUCTIVE				MENOPAUSAL TRANSITION		POSTMENOPAUSE			
	Early	Peak	Late		Early	Late	Early			Late
					Perimenopause					
Duration	*Variable*				*variable*	1–3 years	2 years (1+1)		3–6 years	*Remaining lifespan*
PRINCIPAL CRITERIA										
Menstrual Cycle	Variable to regular	Regular	Regular	Subtle changes in Flow Length	*Variable Length* Persistent ≥ 7-day difference in length of consecutive cycles	Interval of amenorrhea of ≥ 60 days				
SUPPORTIVE CRITERIA										
Endocrine FSH AMH Inhibin B			Low Low	Variable Low Low	↑ Variable Low Low	↑ >25IU/L* Low Low	↑ Variable Low Low		Stabilizes Very Low Very Low	
Antral Follicle Count			Low	Low	Low	Low	Very Low		Very Low	
DESCRIPTIVE CHARACTERISTICS										
Symptoms						Vasomotor symptoms *Likely*	Vasomotor symptoms *Most Likely*			*Increasing* symptoms of urogenital atrophy

*Blood draw on cycle days 2–5 ↑= elevated

FIGURE 4-1

The stages of reproductive aging.

Abbreviations: FMP: final menstrual period; FSH: follicle stimulating hormone; AMH: anti-Müllerian hormone.

Source: Reprinted from Harlow SD, Gass M, Hall JE et al., Executive summary of the Stages of Reproductive Aging Workshop + 10: Addressing the unfinished agenda of staging reproductive aging, Menopause 19(4): 387–395. 2012[7].

(Figure 4-1). Premenopause is defined as the time during which the menstrual cycle is variable and during which there are increases in the serum follicle-stimulating hormone (FSH), to 10 mIU/mL or greater (normal levels are 3–20 mIU/mL), and declining levels of estrogen (to less than 100 pg/mL), anti-Müllerian hormone (AMH), and inhibin,[6,7] The median age of premenopausal changes in menstruation is 47.5 years of age; however, the average range is from as early as 41 years to as late as 57 years.[6] Early menopause, before the age of 45, occurs in approximately 5% of women; premature menopause occurs in fewer than 1% of women younger than 40 years of age. In the United States, the average age of menopause is 51 years of age.[8] There are some ethnic differences in the onset of menopause: as compared to Caucasians, Chinese and Japanese American women experience a later onset and Hispanic and African American women have an earlier onset.[6] Other factors that are known to contribute to an earlier onset of menopause are cigarette smoking, a lower socioeconomic status, and hysterectomy without oopherectomy.[6]

Postmenopause

In postmenopause, the FSH level remains high (more than 25 mIU/mL) and there has not been a menstrual period for at least one year.[6,7] Estrogen levels may be in the range of 10–20 pg/mL, AMH may not be detected, and inhibin levels are less than 5 pg/mL, although the usefulness of inhibin in this setting is not fully appreciated at this time. The timeline of the transition from late reproduction to postmenopause can vary widely, from 5 to 8 years, and not all women follow this sequence of physiologic events.[7] There are relationships between fluctuations of estrogen, FSH, and inhibin and the increased incidence of somatic complaints of joint pain, stiffness, and aches.[9]

Male menopause

It is important to mention that while the natural state of hormonal decline in men is more gradual than the precipitous event observed in women, it is very similar in its physiologic effect. This state of decline is referred to as male menopause, andropause, or manopause. However, when there is an induction of male menopause due to oncologic therapies such as radiation, chemotherapy, or androgen deprivation therapy, the resulting loss of the bioavailability of testosterone, androgen deficiency, and hypogonadism is very distressing and results in an increase in comorbid conditions.[10] Both men and women respond to the diminishment of sex hormones in similar ways, evident by an increased risk of chronic disease.[10] It is important for nurses to know that men, as a result of this loss, will have changes in sexual function, sleep patterns, emotions, gynecomastia, osteoporosis, hot flashes, and other physical changes.[10]

PATHOPHYSIOLOGY

The reproductive tract of the woman is a complex integration of stimulation and suppression of substances involving mainly the hypothalamus, pituitary, and the ovary, known as the hypothalamic–pituitary–gonadal (HPG) axis.[11] The HPG axis is responsible for the regulation of the menstrual cycle. Other organs and glands, including the liver, thyroid, and adrenals, are peripherally involved. When considering the effects of menopause, it is important to remember the target tissues of the substances involved in the genesis of menstruation, which are subsequently—adversely—affected by their absence: the uterus, fallopian tubes, vagina, ovary, breast, and brain.

In the positive feedback loop, the ovary releases estrogen in response to the gonadotropins, luteinizing hormone (LH) and FSH, which stimulates the secretion of gonadotropin-releasing hormone (GnRH) from the hypothalamus and luteinizing hormone (LH) from the anterior pituitary.[6,11,12] There are three major estrogens in circulation: estrone (E1), estradiol (E2), and estriol (E3). Estradiol, which is primarily produced by the ovary, is the predominant estrogen in the premenopausal phase; estrone, a weaker form of estrogen, is the predominate estrogen produced during menopause by the aromatization of androstenedione. Progesterone is secreted from the ovary, initiating the negative feedback loop that suppresses further secretion of GnRH and LH.[6] It is the elevated estrogen and inhibin levels that provide the negative feedback to the pituitary to cease secretion of FSH.[6,11] As the ovaries begin to fail, there is a decline in circulating estrogen (normal levels are 50–400 pg/mL) and inhibin that results in rising levels of FSH.[6,11,12]

For the nurse to have some basic understanding of the role hormones play in the premenopausal, perimenopausal, and postmenopausal states can be helpful in providing education and support to women at risk for or diagnosed with cancers that may directly or indirectly induce menopause. For example, having some basic knowledge of the pathophysiology of estrogen conversion provides an understanding of the role of aromatase inhibition in breast cancer therapy. Because estrogen exerts effects on the central nervous system and neurotransmitters that result in impairment of thermoregulation, thereby causing hot flashes and other vasomotor symptoms, agents that block or mediate those effects are useful alternatives to hormone replacement therapy.[12,13] Similarly, it is important to understand that in menopause, even though estrogen levels are expected to decline, extraglandular production of estrogen occurs in fat cells, thereby creating a perpetuation of estrogen exposure in obese women long after the ovaries cease to function, leading to the risk of development of postmenopausal endometrial and breast cancers.[6,13] Nurses are ideally positioned to provide information and counseling on the benefits of a low-fat diet and maintenance of a healthy weight, combined with regular exercise to promote disease prevention, and to provide education on pharmacologic and nonpharmacologic interventions in the management of menopausal symptoms.

SYMPTOM ASSESSMENT

RISK FACTORS

Artificially induced menopause

Age is the most common cause or risk factor in developing menopause. However, there are a number of events or interventions that precipitate early menopause. Premature menopause is one of the most common complaints of cancer survivors.[14] The cause of the onset of menopause may be the result of surgery, chemotherapy, radiation treatment, or disease. The consequences of the inducement of early menopause are just beginning to be fully realized, and the evidence of its negative impact on long-term health is growing. Research is proving there is an increased risk of premature morbidity and mortality with the inducement of early menopause.[15,16] Some recent findings from this research have identified comorbid conditions such as cardiovascular and neurological disease, osteoporosis, symptoms related to menopause, impaired sexual function, psychological dysfunction, and even premature death as a consequence of early induced menopause.[15,16]

Hysterectomy

Nearly 600,000 women in the United States, undergo hysterectomy every year; in total, one-third of all U.S. women will have this surgery by the age of 60.[17] Nearly all gynecologic malignancies, including cervical, ovarian, and endometrial cancers, will result in hysterectomy, with or without salpingo-oophorectomy. Many women who are at risk for breast and ovarian cancer may also consider risk reduction surgeries that involve removal of the ovaries with or without hysterectomy. When possible, most providers will try to minimize the impact of treatment decision making on a woman's childbearing potential, but in these circumstances oophorectomy will often be done before the age of 40 and induce an early menopausal state.

Chemotherapy

The impact of single-agent chemotherapy on gonadal function is not fully understood, and the data on the more commonly used multiagent chemotherapy regimens are even less well understood. Chemical induction of menopause may occur following treatment with alkylating agents, procarbazine, and nitrosureas.[18] Other chemotherapeutic agents have been implicated in causing ovarian suppression that is temporary or otherwise results in chronic menstrual irregularities.[18,19]

Given that there is only a mediocre method of measuring ovarian reserve without conducting a primordial follicle count, age seems to be a predictive factor for ovarian failure when certain regimens are used.[18] When cyclophosphamide, methotrexate, and fluorouracil (CMF) are used, for example, 76% of women older than 40 years of age experience chemotherapy-induced ovarian failure (CIOF) compared to 40% of women younger than age 40.[18] Other evidence suggests that nearly 50% to 70% of premenopausal women with breast cancer will experience CIOF.[19] Chemotherapy treatments using nitrogen mustard, vincristine, procarbazine, and prednisone (MOPP) and bleomcyin, etoposide, doxorubicin, cyclophosphamide, vincristine, procarbazine, and prednisone (BEACOPP) regimens for Hodgkin's lymphoma have been implicated in damaging gonadal function. As many as 50% of women with Hodgkin's lymphoma have premature ovarian failure.[20]

Radiation therapy

Radiation of the pelvis, abdomen, brain, and spine, as well as total-body irradiation (TBI), all of which are used in a variety of therapeutic cancer modalities, will result in infertility, ovarian suppression, and premature menopause.[18] Typically, a dose of 24 Gy to the pelvis will result in ovarian failure, and most treatment planning will include higher doses.[21] While it might seem obvious that premature ovarian failure and menopause would occur in women receiving pelvic radiation therapy, it is important not to overlook the potential in those who receive radiation to the hypothalamic and pituitary regions or TBI. Doses from 20 to 30 Gy have contributed to ovarian failure.[18] When providing care to women undergoing chemotherapy and/or radiation therapies, it is important to have a complete understanding of the treatment plan to provide a comprehensive nursing plan of care.

Ovarian preservation

There are many options considered when young cancer patients are entering into treatment, and preservation of fertility is very important. However, just as fertility is considered, so should the prevention of premature ovarian failure be pondered, especially given the longevity of survivorship and the evidence of the morbidity and mortality associated with early menopause. Recognizing there is a limited tolerance of the ovary to the insults of chemotherapy and radiation therapies is just the first step and, in the rush to treatment, has great potential to be overlooked. Characteristics of the patient to be considered for ovarian preservation are age and type, dose, and intensity of chemotherapy and/or radiotherapy.[18,20] In as many as 56% of patients younger than age 40, there is greater likelihood of preserving ovarian function and regaining menstruation; by comparison, in the 40-and-older group there is a lower ovarian reservoir and, therefore, a higher rate of failure.[18,20]

Surgical transposition of the ovaries or oophoropexy is an option to be considered when pelvic or abdominal fields of radiation are necessary for treatment, as in Hodgkin's lymphoma, pelvic sarcomas, and gynecologic malignancies.[20,21] The goal of the surgery is preservation of ovarian function. After identifying the radiation field in conjunction with the radiation oncologist, the gynecologic surgeon will use a laparoscopic procedure to retrieve the ovaries from the pelvis and transpose them to a point at least 3 centimeters outside the radiation field, which may be in the paracolic gutters.[21] While this procedure seems to be fairly uncomplicated, it is important to verify adequate blood supply to the ovaries, and to secure them with non-absorbable suture. The surgeon places surgical clips at the site of the oophoropexy that enables the radiation oncologist to easily locate the ovaries during radiation simulation.[21]

The success rates of ovarian preservation have been reported to be as high as 90% in patients undergoing postoperative vaginal brachytherapy and 60% in patients treated with postoperative pelvic radiation, although the success rates vary widely.[21] Transpositions of the ovaries are not without complications, the least of which is ovarian failure. Such problems as chronic ovarian pain and reports of metastases to the transposed ovaries and to laparoscopic port sites (referred to as Sister Mary Joseph nodules) in cases of malignancies in the pelvis and lower abdomen have been reported.[21] There have been other successful attempts to relocate the ovaries outside of the pelvis such as to the upper extremity, axilla, and arm.[22] In these cases, oophoropexy was performed to preserve fertility, but the added benefit, if successful, would be to delay the onset of menopause, an equally valuable effort.

OBJECTIVE ASSESSMENT

Physical assessment and diagnostic evaluation

There is a collection of physiologic and psychological symptoms that characterize the transitional period of menopause. Some physiologic presentations include vasomotor symptoms (VMS), such as hot flashes and night sweats; irregular menses or amenorrhea; vaginal dryness; and diminished libido. Other symptoms are related to psychological function, such as changes in mood, insomnia, and cognitive function.[23] A thorough assessment will include a review of symptoms using the Menopause Rating Scale (MRS) or the Menopause-Specific Quality of Life Questionnaire (MENQOL). The MRS is an 11-question form with a 0–4 symptom rating (0 = none and 4 = severe symptoms).[24] The MENQOL contains 29 items in four domains: physical, psychosocial, vasomotor, and sexual.[25] The questions range from topics such as aches in muscles to difficulty sleeping in the physical domain to avoidance of intimacy in the sexual domain. The measurements are obtained through yes-and-no questions, with the yes answer expanding to include a Likert scale of 0 (not bothered at all) to 6 (extremely bothered). A recent factor analysis of the validity of the MENQOL resulted in the conclusion that the strength of the assessment continues to be relevant to today's women even though the tool was developed in 1996.[25]

The only way to diagnose menopause is to observe a lack of menstrual periods for 12 months. Other objective measurements of menopause include a history and physical examination with a focus on the medical and surgical history, and a specific focus on menstruation and gynecologic symptoms. Although there is no single blood test that reliably diagnoses menopause, the blood tests that are helpful are the FSH test, LH test, and estradiol levels. Low estradiol levels (<35 pg/mL) are found in postmenopausal women along with lower FSH and LH levels. During perimenopause, the levels of all of these biomarkers are quite variable.

Once this assessment is complete, interventions aimed toward mediating the symptoms of the menopausal state should be implemented and may include one or all of the following: medications, exercise, weight and diet management, and nonpharmacologic interventions.

SYMPTOM MANAGEMENT STRATEGIES

There are a number of symptoms associated with perimenopause and menopause, and each will be discussed separately here to distinguish the etiology and therapeutic interventions. Women with cancer and cancer-treatment-induced menopause may experience one or multiple symptoms.

VASOMOTOR SYMPTOMS

Incidence

Perhaps the most discussed phenomena of menopause, the hot flash (sometimes called a flush) and night sweats are undoubtedly the symptoms for which treatments and relief are most often sought.[9,23,26] These vasomotor symptoms (VMS) commonly present 5 to 10 years before the ending of the menstrual cycle or shortly after the removal of the ovaries or with the use of antiestrogenic compounds, all of which are related to the withdrawal of circulating estrogen and the role estrogen has in hypothalamic thermoregulatory homeostasis.[27] VMS occur in as many as 80% of menopausal women.[27] Although most women develop VMS during the perimenopausal and early postmenopausal periods, a minority of patients develop VMS while their menstrual cycles remain regular. A majority of women experience VMS, which may last for seconds to more than 1 hour; the duration of VMS may be for 1 to 2 years, but as many as 15% of women may have persistent hot flashes for as long as 30 years.[27,28] The scope of problem is staggering: nearly 27–37 million women in the United States may experience VMS over the next five decades.[28] As many as 7 million women will experience severe and intolerable symptoms.[27]

These common symptoms experienced by postmenopausal women, predominately in the late transition stage, affect women from most ethnic and racial groups.[27,29] African American women (46%) are more likely than other groups to express concerns about VMS symptoms, as compared with Hispanic (36%), Caucasian (31%),

Chinese (21%), and Japanese (18%) women.[27] These symptoms are associated with higher levels of distress, and the 15%–20% of women who report their hot flushes and night sweats as problematic also report higher levels of social impairment, work-related complications, and other difficulties such as anxiety, fatigue, and embarrassment.[30] Epidemiologic studies have found increased reports of sleep disturbance during the menopausal transition.[30,31] It has been assumed that this outcome reflects awakening effects of VMS.

Etiology

Physiologically, VMS are a result of peripheral vasodilation. As the temperature of the skin increases, blood flow and sweating increase within the first few seconds of the onset of the flash.[32] There are also increases in the metabolic and heart rates.[31]

Risk factors

Although the depletion of estrogen is a common factor for all women who experience VMS, other factors may place certain subsets of women at greater risk, such as certain ethnic differences identified in the Study of Women's Health Across the Nation (SWAN) trial.[33] SWAN, which began in 2001, was the first study to evaluate a sample of women from different racial and ethnic backgrounds and describe the multiple changes experienced by women during menopause.[33] The results of this study and others, in attempting to identify at-risk populations, have found some explanations for the variant nature of hot flashes.[27,33]

Obesity and body mass index. High body mass index (BMI) is directly related to hot flash frequency.[27] This may be due to the effect of increased insulation from body fat, resulting in elevated core body temperature and decreased dissipation of heat, which triggers hot flashes.[27,32] Increased incidence of VMS is also associated with the consumption of at least one high-fat meal per day when compared to diets that contain fewer meals high in fat content.[27]

Alcohol and cigarette smoking. Consumption of alcohol, in the form of one to five drinks per week, increases the incidence of VMS when compared to women who report consuming no alcohol.[27] Although the vasodilating effects of alcohol are understood and appreciated, the association of nicotine, a potent vasoconstrictor, with VMS effects are less understood. Cigarette smoking has also been found to increase the risk of VMS, possibly through the effect of estrogen metabolism or through the thermogenic effects of nicotine.[27,34] The odds of having VMS symptoms are 1.6 times higher among women who have ever smoked, and 4 times higher in heavy smokers, when compared with women who had never smoked cigarettes.[33] The effect of estrogen metabolism is hypothetical, but in addition to the evidence suggesting alterations in estrogen, progesterone, and androstenedione levels, it is theorized that nicotine accelerates ovarian aging.[27,32,34] Regardless of the mechanism, the association of cigarette smoking and the increased incidence of VMS is one of the most significant causes of VMS in menopausal women.[34]

Depression and alterations in mood. Although there is evidence that a history of depression places a woman at risk for perimenopausal depression, women who experience VMS clearly report a higher incidence of depression or depressed mood.[27] Less clear is the relationship between VMS and the incidence of other mood disorders, except for anxiety. Women with moderate to high anxiety levels are three to five times more likely to complain of VMS, respectively, even when adjusted for other risk factors such as high BMI, smoking, and race.[27] There is an association between the occurrence of abuse and neglect in childhood and VMS reporting.[27] This is an area where additional study needs to occur to help identify characteristics of risk for mental health issues and to implement early interventions such as hormone therapy (HT), other medications, or even exercise regimens to reduce VMS and to minimize the psychosocial effects.

Cancer-induced vasomotor symptoms. VMS are a distressing side effect of therapies for women treated for breast cancer and men treated for prostate cancer.[35] In women diagnosed with breast cancer, VMS are reported to be more frequent and severe. The rapid suppression of ovarian function that coincides with surgery and the use of drugs that target hormone receptor–positive breast cancers are directly associated with abrupt and severe hot flashes.[35]

Aromatase inhibitors and antiestrogenic agents have become widely used for the treatment of breast cancer in postmenopausal women. In the Breast International Group (BIG 1-98) clinical trial, hot flashes were more common among women who were randomized to a tamoxifen-containing regimen than among women who received letrozole alone (41.7%–44% versus 37.7%, p = .003).[36] Nurses caring for women who have a treatment-induced menopause should expect that their patients will experience more VMS than average women.

Men will experience VMS when treated with androgen-deprivation therapy (ADT) or after undergoing a surgical castration.[35] In a review of studies, VMS was found to be reported in 35%–80% of men treated for advanced prostate cancer with hormonally ablative therapies and surgical castration; VMS in these men have been reported to last as long as 8 years following treatment. The quality of life problems associated with VMS have been implicated as the cause of many men discontinuing hormonal therapies.[35]

Therapeutic approaches

Since the development of synthetic estrogen in the 1930s, the evolution of the replacement of hormones in menopausal women has traveled from an estrogen therapy (ET) alone model, to an estrogen plus progesterone therapy (EPT) model, to the current recommendations of an individualized care model.[35,37] Clinicians carefully address a benefit-to-risk ratio for each individual and, where appropriate, short-term use of hormone therapy (HT) in early menopause can be used to ameliorate the problems of severe menopausal symptoms and disease prevention. Hormonal therapies—estrogens and progesterones—are the most commonly utilized, well-known, and effective pharmacologic agents, with estrogen widely considered to be the most efficacious in alleviating hot flashes; nevertheless, the safety of these agents continues to be questioned and implicated in risky outcomes.[28,35,37]

Based on clinically relevant findings of the risks associated with HT, lifestyle modifications are proposed as the first step in the management of less severe hot flashes.[28,37] In addition, pharmacologic and nonpharmacologic agents have been studied and may show potential in treatment of VMS. Many complementary and alternative therapies, including herbal medications, exercise, acupuncture, and phytoestrogens, have been studied but none is clinically recommended at this time.[28] Consideration of alternatives to HT must be part of the management discussion between the clinician and the patient, particularly when HT is contraindicated.

Behavior modifications. Behavior modification is the safest, most reliably effective, and most broadly used management approach for VMS.[28] The North American Menopause Society (NAMS) recommends that women attempt to maintain a lower core body temperature by dressing in natural fibers such as cotton or linen, layering clothes to easily transition between periods of hot and cold, wearing open-neck shirts, consuming cool or cold food or drinks while avoiding spicy or hot foods, using a fan or air conditioning as needed, and avoiding smoking and alcohol.[38]

It is understood that hot flashes, which are activated by vasodilation and increased core temperature, occur more frequently in warm environments; therefore, interventions aimed at reducing core and ambient temperatures are recommended.[32,38] Many of the nonpharmacologic methods for reducing VMS are practical and reasonable lifestyle modifications. With as many as 40% of women reporting that they are negatively affected by the psychosocial and physiologic effects of VMS, many are motivated to reduce the impact on their quality of life.[39] Nurses understand that many patients want a quick fix for health problems, but altering health practices to reduce or minimize the negative effects of VMS, which may or may not include pharmacologics, can have overall health benefits such as maintenance of a healthy weight, consumption of low-fat diets, and stress reduction strategies.

Relaxation techniques. Stress, anxiety, and increased mental workload are all implicated as factors that increase VMS; efforts at reducing the effects of these factors may decrease the incidence and/or severity of VMS.[27] Slow-breathing techniques and meditation reduce the effects of the sympathetic nervous system, thereby reducing the frequency of VMS. Women should be taught to slowly inhale to a count of seven when the hot flash begins; the exhalation extends over a count of nine; then the cycle begins again. This concentrated effort at pacing respirations results in reducing stress and anxiety, which are both triggers and consequences of VMS. Relaxation may be combined with estradiol therapy to provide a more rapid reduction in VMS symptoms.[28] Mindfulness-based stress reduction (MBSR) is also to be considered in the management of VMS.[39]

Hypnosis. Hypnosis is another nonpharmacologic intervention that has some proven benefits. In a pilot study of 16 women, a scripted hypnosis intervention was used that focused on imagery of coolness and relaxation. The participants experienced a 69% reduction in VMS scores.[40] Based on these preliminary findings, the same authors are conducting a randomized clinical trial testing the hypnosis intervention in 180 postmenopausal women.[40]

Exercise. The therapeutic benefits of exercise are undeniable in postmenopausal women; however, there is some debate over whether exercise reduces the incidence of VMS. There is conflicting evidence that exercise increases the severity of VMS in overweight, postmenopausal women, an effect likely associated with increased core body temperature.[27,28]

Yoga has been suggested to be an effective exercise in the amelioration of VMS. The practice of yoga can range from a restorative, relaxation-based exercise to an aerobic, sweat-inducing dance-like Ashtanga-based Vinyasa flow or hot yoga practice. Again there is conflicting evidence and additional research is needed to further clarify the benefits.[28]

Peer counseling. Peer counseling has been demonstrated to have some beneficial effects in reducing VMS. In a small study, 60 African American women with breast cancer participated in a peer counseling group and experienced a reduction in symptoms.[34] Successful peer counseling can be achieved when peers are identified and trained in group facilitation methods.[41]

Acupuncture. Acupuncture—an ancient practice of using needles strategically placed in meridians to manipulate a variety of physiologic symptoms and diseases—has shown some beneficial effects on VMS in women and men.[28,35] Acupuncture is thought to stimulate beta-endorphin activity, may possibly exert an effect on serotonin and noradrenalin activity, and may influence the thermoregulatory center.[42] Kaplan et al. identified studies aimed at determining the effectiveness of using acupuncture alone or in combination with medications that have proved to be effective.[35] Studies continue to be developed in an effort to further clarify the benefits.

Pharmacologic agents

Hormone Therapy. The most effective treatment for alleviating VMS and other symptoms of menopause, including those related to quality of life, is hormone therapy, specifically estrogen. Numerous randomized trials have demonstrated that estrogen therapy (ET), even in very low doses, markedly reduces—by as much as 75% when compared to placebo—the frequency and intensity of hot flashes.[28,37] Progesterone therapy (PT), while not as effective as ET, has also been found to be effective in reducing VMS.[28,37] Megestrol acetate, medroxyprogesterone acetate, and transdermal progesterone cream are effective in the treatment of VMS and megestrol acetate is effective in both men and women.[28]

The results of one of the Women's Health Initiative (WHI) studies raised significant concerns about the long-term adverse effects associated with combined HT with medroxyprogesterone acetate and conjugated equine estrogens.[43] Suddenly, the risks of breast cancer, stroke, coronary heart disease (CHD), thromboembolism, and dementia outweighed other benefits, and there was a sharp decline in the use of HT.[44] Since 2004, there has been a gradual relaxing of opinion of ET based on additional findings that imply that short-term ET, tailored to the needs of the woman in early menopause, may be reasonable. Even more reassuring are the findings of a recent study in the same group of hysterectomized women who took the conjugated equine estrogens for a median length of time of 5.7 years.[45] After more than 10 years off of ET, these women have no more or less of the risks identified (CHD, stroke, thromboemboli, fracture, or other total mortality) in the early termination group, including what appears to be a decreased risk of breast cancer.[45] These results have helped to expand the level of comfort for women and their providers when considering the potential benefits of ET where there are no other contraindications.

In women who have their uterus, the choice of HT is a bit less clear. The risks linked to unopposed ET in women with uteri are endometrial hyperplasia and cancer; therefore ET must be balanced with progestin therapy in some form and sequence.[37,44] Results of a WHI trial identified that conjugated equine estrogen plus progestin (specifically medroxyprogesterone acetate) in a combined daily dose fashion (WHI E+P) was associated with a higher incidence of breast cancers that were of higher pathologic stage and that led to greater mortality.[43,45] Additionally, the WHI E+P trial and the Heart and Estrogen–Progestin Replacement Study (HERS) have provided clinicians with insight into the unreasonable risks associated with combination HT when used for menopausal symptom management.[43,45] Using the smallest doses of estrogen and progesterone therapies available in the shortest duration possible to achieve symptom relief is the current recommendation.[37,44] The progesterone choice, based on evidence suggesting that medroxyprogesterone acetate increases the risk for breast cancer, should be a micronized progestin or progestin-containing intrauterine device (IUD) with planned intervals of ultrasound surveillance of the uterine lining.[37,44,46]

It is worth mentioning that a retrospective review of the data gathered in the WHI E+P trial has uncovered an association between new-onset breast tenderness with an increase in breast cancer risk in women taking the WHI combination dose of conjugated equine estrogen and medroxyprogesterone.[47] This finding warrants a heightened awareness in clinicians who provide care for women on HT, as it describes a new onset of breast tenderness and the need for an expedited office visit for an assessment, clinical breast exam, and perhaps imaging to rule out any breast health problems.

Tibolone is a synthetic hormone widely used in other countries to manage menopausal symptoms and to prevent osteoporosis; however, it is not approved for use in the United States by the Food and Drug Administration (FDA).[48] In the LIFT (Long-Term Intervention on Fractures with Tibolone) trial, tibolone was found to reduce the risk of vertebral fracture in women with osteoporosis and to decrease the risk of breast cancer.[48] However, there was an increased risk of stroke in older women with osteoporosis.

Nonhormonal Prescription Alternatives. Clonidine is a central-acting alpha$_2$-adrenergic agonist used as an antihypertensive; it acts by relaxing blood vessels, improving blood flow, decreasing blood pressure, and lowering the heart rate.[49] The dosage is 0.1 mg/day, oral or transdermal.[50] The effect of clonidine on norepinephrine, which is thought to have a role in generating hot flashes, in the central nervous system may explain the drug's effect on reducing VMS. There may be a modest benefit in women with hot flashes, specifically women with breast cancer taking tamoxifen.[35,50] Clonidine has significant side effects such as dry mouth, dry eyes, constipation, and drowsiness.[49] It is common to encounter the use of clonidine for the treatment of VMS; however, its use is considered off-label and discontinuation of that use should be tapered over a few days.[50] In general, clonidine is not recommended for treating hot flashes.

Serotonin or 5-hydroxytryptamine (5-HT) is a monoamine neurotransmitter essential to many biological functions, however, circulating blood levels decrease by nearly 50% after menopause.[51] The role of serotonin in memory, anxiety, mood, sleep, eating, sexual behavior, and thermoregulation is undergoing vigorous exploration.[50–52] Because there is a direct association between serotonin levels and the severity of menopausal symptoms, the use of selective serotonin reuptake inhibitors (SSRIs) and serotonin–norepinephrine reuptake inhibitors (SNRIs) has been evaluated, mostly for their positive effect on mood disorders.[49,51] In an analysis of seven trials, Loprinzi et al. reported that venlafaxine and paroxetine were the most effective members of this class of drugs.[52] However, the use of SSRIs in patients on tamoxifen therapy must be evaluated with caution, due to the evidence that SSRI antidepressants, such as paroxetine, fluoxetine, and sertraline, inhibit the cytochrome P450 2D (CYP2D6) pathway and may be associated with a higher mortality rate from breast cancer in patients who are taking tamoxifen.[50,52] Other side effects of these agents that women may find unappealing are weight gain and sexual dysfunction.[50]

Gabapentin is an anticonvulsant that exerts an effect on the central nervous system.[53] The analysis by Loprinzi et al. noted that randomized controlled trials in women with breast cancer have demonstrated a decrease in the incidence of hot flashes, when compared with placebo and vitamin E. Other clinical trials have shown efficacy in the reduction of hot flashes at doses of 900 mg/day in women and in men with prostate cancer.[52]

Estrogen Agonists/Antagonists or Selective Estrogen Receptor Modulators. The selective estrogen receptor modulators (SERMs) are different from estrogens in their chemical structures, but act like estrogen by binding to the estrogen receptor sites in targets such as bone, breast, cardiovascular system (CVS), and uterine tissues.[54] SERMs act as estrogen receptor agonists or antagonists. Whereas estrogen is an agonist on receptor sites in the brain, breast, bone, CVS, uterus, and vagina, tamoxifen is an antagonist on receptor sites in the brain, breast, and vagina and an agonist in the uterus, bone, and CVS.[52] SERMs are not typically recommended for the management of VMS, but there are ongoing efforts to develop SERMs that will have beneficial effects on target tissue, reducing the comorbidities of the menopausal state while protecting other organs from disease development.

Nonpharmacologic agents

Diets rich in soy isoflavones have been hypothetically implicated in the reduced prevalence of breast cancers, osteoporosis, and fracture risks, and a lower incidence of cardiovascular disease (CVD) in Asian women—specifically, those who live in Asia.[55] Phytoestrogens are weakly estrogenic and exert antiestrogenic activity.[51] Clinical trials involving phytoestrogens such as black cohosh, soy supplements, and red clover have demonstrated mixed results, with most trials showing no improvement in hot flashes.[51,55]

Black cohosh is a perennial plant native to North America that has historical evidence of medicinal use by North American Indians for a wide variety of ailments.[56] It is available as a solution, tablet, or capsule. Its efficacy in reducing VMS is variable, although one trial in women taking tamoxifen showed a significant decrease in hot flashes.[57] Clinical trials evaluating black cohosh's efficacy continue, including one funded by the National Institutes of Health's (NIH) National Center for Complementary and Alternative Medicine (NCCAM).[56] According to the NIH's Office of Dietary Supplements, the American College of Obstetricians and Gynecologists (ACOG) states that short-term use of black cohosh may be helpful in reducing VMS.[56] Women with estrogen-sensitive cancers should not use black cohosh outside of a scientifically sound clinical trial.

Soy supplements have not been found to be of benefit in reducing the incidence of VMS.[55] In a randomized, double-blind, placebo-controlled trial of 248 women called the Soy Phytoestrogens as Replacement Estrogen (SPARE) trial, a daily dose of 200 mg of soy isoflavones for 2 years did not produce an improvement in menopausal symptoms.[55] In fact, the women who received soy supplementation reported more VMS than the placebo group.[58] This finding has been consistent in a trial of men with prostate cancer receiving androgen-deprivation therapy.[59]

Red clover, a phytoestrogen, has been used in the treatment of menopausal symptoms. A systematic review by Nelson et al. reported a modest improvement with few reported adverse events, with the exception of some gastrointestinal complaints.[58] The researchers noted that most clinical trials have used promensil, which contains biochanin and genistein in doses of 40 mg/day. Another red clover product, rimostil (57 mg/day), has been used in combination with promensil (82 mg/day) and results in decreased VMS symptoms.

Use of phytoestrogens must be weighed against the understanding that the estrogenic activity of these substances has the potential to cause an accumulation of endometrial tissue, leading to endometrial hyperplasia.[51,58] Nurses should be prepared to ask women who have menopausal complaints if they are supplementing their diets or taking herbal therapies, particularly if there is a recent onset of vaginal bleeding. Other areas of concern are the wide variation and lack of quality control measures among these products and the potential for serious adverse effects such as liver toxicity and failure.[51]

A variety of other agents are advertised as alternatives to traditional therapies for management of menopausal symptoms; some have undergone clinical investigation[60] (Table 4-1). Flaxseed may have some benefit in reducing VMS and may influence total and LDL cholesterol, but further trials are needed. Dong quai, used in traditional Chinese medicine (TCM) for the management of menstrual irregularities, has shown mixed results in clinical trials studying its usefulness in alleviating menopausal symptoms. Hops extract has been studied in the relief of menopausal symptoms with some evidence of benefit. Hops has been combined with other substances in a gel used to treat vaginal dryness with positive results. Wild yam, a rhizome native to North America, is widely available and advertised as a product effective in the relief of menopausal symptoms, but clinical trials have not been favorable. Wild yam is available in a cream that is applied to the skin. Likewise, ginseng, vitamin E, evening primrose oil, and ginkgo have all been studied and found to be ineffective in significantly reducing menopausal symptoms.[60]

Dehydroepiandrosterone (DHEA), a steroid hormone produced by the adrenal gland, which declines in women during aging, has been found to be effective when given as a supplement.[60] DHEA supplements have been shown to improve VMS, sexual functioning, bone density, and vaginal atrophy. There continues to be interest in further study of DHEA.

TABLE 4-1

Herbal Remedies Used in the Management of Menopause

Natural drug	Clinical evidence	Possible mechanism	Comments
Black cohosh	Six randomized, double blind controlled trials	Partial agonist at the 5HT1A and μ-opiate receptors	No clinical evidence of black cohosh efficacy in reducing climacteric symptoms although a beneficial effect in early climacteric women seems to occur
Dong quai	Randomized, double blind placebo-controlled trial	Enhanced endogenous estrogen production	No significant difference in KI, hot flash frequency, estrogen levels and vaginal cytology between active and placebo groups
Hops	Two randomized, double blind, placebo-controlled trials	Contains estrogen precursors	A significant difference in hot flushes, sweating, insomnia, heart palpitation, and irritability between active and placebo groups
Wild yam	Randomized, double blind placebo-controlled cross-over trial	Contains diosgenin, which is a precursor of progesterone	No significant difference in hot flash and night sweats between active and placebo groups
Ginseng	Randomized, double blind placebo-controlled multicenter trial	Estrogenic effects of triterpene saponin or a direct effect on the pituitary-hypothalamic axis	No significant difference in PGWB, WHQ, VAS, hot flash, and sweating episode frequency between active and placebo groups
Evening primrose	Randomized, double blind placebo-controlled trial	Mechanism unknown	No significant difference in KI, hot flash and sweating episode frequency between active and placebo groups
St John's wort	Randomized, double blind placebo-controlled trial	Mechanism unknown	No significant difference in hot flash frequency and intensity between active and placebo groups. Significant improvement in menopause-specific quality of life and sleep problems in St John's wort compared to placebo
Ginkgo	Two randomized, double blind placebo-controlled trials	Mechanism unknown	No significant effects of ginkgo on menopausal symptoms, mood, sleep disorders, memory, and sustained attention compared to placebo. Significant effect on the test of mental flexibility

Abbreviations: KI: Kupperman index; VAS: visual analogue scale; WHQ: women's health questionnaire; PGWB: psychological general well-being index.

Source: Reprinted from Borrelli F, Ernst E. Alternative and complementary therapies for the menopause, Maturitas, 66(4) 333–343, 2010[60].

Following the release of the WHI findings, there was a surge in efforts to develop "natural" alternatives to the pharmaceutical industry–produced conventional hormone replacement therapies. This drive led to compounding pharmacies' development of "bioidentical" hormone products, a term that is neither recognized by the FDA nor scientifically accepted.[61] In 2008, the FDA held a press conference regarding bioidentical products and launched enforcement action against several pharmacies that were providing bioidentical products and offering salivary testing of hormone levels.[61,62] Three authoritative organizations—ACOG, FDA, and NAMS—recommended against the use of hormone levels to measure response to therapy based on the lack of clinical or biologic meaning; response should be based on symptom management.[37,63] Compounded bioidentical products are promoted as "natural" alternatives but are not identical to human estrogens. Formulations of these hormones can be sold as creams, sprays (topical or nasal), suppositories, sublingual tablets, patches, and pellets.[61] It is important to convey to patients that these products are not FDA approved, typically do not undergo rigorous testing, do not have established indications, and are variable in efficacy.

UROGENITAL EFFECTS AND SEXUAL DYSFUNCTION

Incidence

Unlike hot flashes and VMS, which are well-known, annoying side effects of menopause, urogenital changes and sexual dysfunction are rarely discussed, even with providers. The urogenital effects of menopause are much more universal, reportedly occurring in 25% to 50% of women.[64] The effects of the loss of estrogen on the tissues of the urogenital tract may lead to atrophy, pain, dyspareunia, urinary tract infections, chronic irritation, and diminished quality of life. In women with cancer, the incidence is higher, reportedly as high as 75% among breast cancer survivors.[65] When menopause is combined with the effect of treatment with chemotherapy and an antiestrogen, the effect is more profound. It is essential that nurses understand the problem and its incidence, and assess their patients by asking questions that are directed at urogenital functionality.

Urogenital effects and sexual dysfunction are closely related. Sexuality is an important part of adult health, and the evidence suggests that maintaining an active sex life is important to both sexes, even as they age.[66–68] In spite of this, 43% of middle-aged women have low sexual desire and 39% have difficulty with lubrication.[66] Realistically, it is reasonable to assume that the prevalence of this problem is much greater due to lack of assessment by healthcare providers and low reporting by women. In a large cross-sectional study of 2207 women, higher rates of low sexual desire were found among women who became menopausal, either surgically or naturally, than among premenopausal women.[69] For women who undergo a surgically induced menopause, the level of distress about low sexual desire is nearly twice that of premenopausal women.[69]

Unfortunately, there is a paucity of science devoted to the assessment of menopause-induced urogenital problems other than in breast and gynecologic cancers, where the reported incidence of sexual dysfunction ranges from 30% to 100%.[64] In breast cancer survivors, 50% to 75% have one or more symptoms of urogenital dysfunction.[14,65] When chemotherapy and tamoxifen use are combined, the problems are more severe, and the use of aromatase inhibitors has further magnified symptoms.[65] In the Arimidex, Tamoxifen, Alone or in Combination (ATAC) trial, when arimidex was compared to tamoxifen, women experienced dyspareunia (17.3% versus 8.1%), decreased libido and loss of sexual satisfaction (34% versus 26.1%), and vaginal dryness (18.5% versus 9.1%) respectively after 5 years on therapy.[70] The incidence of urinary tract infections (UTIs) in women taking aromatase inhibitors and antiestrogens ranges from 3.5% to 10%, respectively.[64] Nurses know that cancer survivors who have received treatments that induce ovarian failure and loss of estrogen will be at risk for urogenital problems and, when indicated, should be counseled about symptom management and interventions.[65]

Pathophysiology

The loss of estrogen is the single greatest risk factor for urogenital symptoms in menopausal women. The bladder and urethra, pelvic floor musculature, vulva, vagina, and other organs of the pelvis are rich with estrogen receptors.[64,65] The decline of estrogen results in a cascade of changes in the epithelial cellular membranes of the urinary and vulvovaginal tissues that leads to diminishment of urethral resistance, bladder capacity, tissue elasticity, shortening of the urethra, and decreased bladder volumes. The other organs in the pelvis shrink in size, losing collagen, adipose tissue, and the ability to retain water as well as causing atrophic changes in the smooth muscles. The vagina gets shorter and narrower, tissues thin, and blood flow decreases. There is a decrease of vaginal secretions and a shift in the pH from acidic (3.8 to 4.5) to a more alkaline state, which in turn causes a loss of the protective lactobacilli, thereby creating an environment in which pathogens that increase the incidence of urinary tract infections and atrophic vaginitis will thrive. Vaginal atrophy is a syndrome where the vaginal walls dry, become inflamed, and appear pale and thin upon examination.[64,65] Cigarette smoking accelerates urogenital atrophy.[65]

Therapeutic approaches

Urogenital problems are reversible with treatment, and the goal is to alleviate symptoms and restore healthy tissues.[64] Although it might seem unlikely given the circumstances, regular sexual intercourse has been found to improve urogenital symptoms.[65,67] Avoiding scented soaps and lubricants, never using douches, and wearing loose, cotton underwear help manage tissue irritation.

Restoring estrogen levels is helpful, and 75% of women get relief from systemic ET, although it may not be the best option, and some women will need combined approaches.[64] In the face of concerns associated with ET, local treatment is an effective option. Systemic absorption is seen with the urogenital application of ET, although the degree of absorption varies, but the advantage is that lower doses of estrogen are effective.[65,67] This method of treatment in hormonally sensitive cancers should be reserved for clinical trials and administered under the close supervision of an oncologist.[64,65]

Estrogen therapy is available for urogenital application in suppositories, creams, vaginal rings, and pessaries.[64] The creams consist of estradiol or conjugated estrogens; vaginal tablets are estradiol hemihydrate; the rings are estradiol and estradiol acetate; and the pessaries contain estrogen preparations that are useful in women who have vaginal prolapse and vaginal atrophy.[71] There is some concern about the potential for inducement of endometrial hyperplasia or adenocarcinoma in women who use vaginal estrogen and who have an intact uterus.[64,71] The data regarding the risk are limited, but evidence suggests the occurrence is rare; however, treatment in this group should be closely monitored for vaginal bleeding. Surveillance should include a vaginal ultrasound to measure endometrial thickness and/or periodic progestin challenge to assess for endometrial hyperplasia.

There are drugs in development to treat these menopausal symptoms: two SERMs (ospemifene and lasofoxifene) that have shown benefits in urogenital health, and intravaginal application of a DHEA product.[54] DHEA has been shown to restore normal pH, reduce atrophy and dyspareunia, and improve sexual function and desire.[64]

There are a number of commercially available lubricants and vaginal moisturizers. It is important for women to avoid those products with an alcohol base, as further drying may occur as well as discomfort.[64] Nonhormonal products will not restore the tissues of the vulvovaginal areas. Oils such as olive, vegetable, coconut, and the oil squeezed from a vitamin E capsule are soothing alternatives to commercially prepared products. Women should be cautioned that these oils will stain sheets and clothing. In addition, oils will degrade latex condoms and should be used with caution or latex alternatives used. Hops extract in combination with hyaluronic acid, liposomes, and vitamin E in a gel has been shown to decrease vaginal dryness.[60]

It is important to initiate a conversation with all women with cancer who have the potential to be menopausal regarding urogenital health. Providing support and resources to assist women to live well by avoiding urogenital problems and sustain or improve sexual health is an important holistic effort.

OSTEOPOROSIS

Incidence

Bone health and osteoporosis represent a global problem, affecting an estimated 200 million women worldwide, and putting 40 million American men and women at risk.[72,73] After the age of 50, in developed countries, osteoporosis-related fractures will occur in approximately 33% of women and 20% of men.[72] When this incidence in the general population is combined with the increased fracture risk of cancer survivors, it becomes clear that nurses have a significant role in identifying, assessing, and providing education and intervention on behalf of their patients.[74]

Risk factors

Loss of bone mineral density (BMD) is part of the aging process and begins, typically, after age 35.[74,75] Primary osteoporosis is associated with aging and the shift in the dynamic process from a balanced bone lysis and resorption (bone remodeling) pattern to more resorption and less bone formation. Areas subject to the greatest change in BMD and, therefore, the greatest risk of fracture are the hip, long bones, femoral head, and vertebrae. In menopause, the rate of bone loss initially accelerates in the early years of estrogen depletion, particularly in an abrupt loss, and then slows after 5–10 years. Similarly, women who discontinue the use of ET or HT, after 3 years, will experience the same rate of fractures as women who have never been on HT.[37,75]

Other risk factors for women are being thin, inactive, low calcium intake, family history of osteopenia or osteoporosis, high caffeine consumption, alcohol abuse and cigarette smoking, and reduced exposure to sunlight.[6,74,75] Comorbid diseases such as rheumatoid arthritis, hyperthyroidism, and type 1 diabetes, as well as medications such as heparin, glucocorticoids, intramuscular medroxyprogesterone, proton pump inhibitors, and anticonvulsants, are other risk factors for osteoporosis.[74,75] Secondary osteoporosis results from causes other than aging, including cancer treatment–induced bone loss from chemotherapies, medications, radiation, and cancers such as leukemia, lymphomas, multiple myeloma, and bone cancer.[74]

An assessment of risk should be foremost in the minds of nurses caring for oncology patients who fit in any of these categories. The National Osteoporosis Foundation recommends screening for risk beginning at age 50, and where there are other high-risk comorbidities, clinical judgment on screening and intervention should be exercised.[74,76]

The World Health Organization (WHO) has a computer-based fracture assessment tool (FRAX) that calculates the probability of a fracture event and provides the clinician with decision-making procedures and interventions tailored to the individual[77] (Figure 4-2). Screening for BMD with dual-energy x-ray absorptiometry (DEXA) scan is considered the standard measurement tool, although there are many other tests available.[74,78] The recommendations are for routine screening in women 65 years and older and men 70 years and older who have only age as a risk factor; for those who are considered to be at high risk, such as cancer patients, screening is recommended based on the risk factor[76,78] (Figure 4-2). Men prescribed ADT and women on AIs should receive baseline screening before initiation of therapy and then periodically thereafter.[74,76,78] The results of the DEXA scan are interpreted based on a standard deviation (SD) from that of a young, normal adult and a T-score of −1.0 and greater. Osteopenia is defined as a BMD that is 1.0–2.5 SD below normal (T-score of −1.0 and −2.5); osteoporosis is defined as a BMD that is 2.5 SD or more below normal (T-score of −2.5 or greater).[72]

Therapeutic approaches

Regular exercise using weights and muscle strengthening at least twice per week is necessary for bone health and should be recommended.[74,76] Exercise must be sustained to achieve the benefits of improving BMD of the hip and spine.[60] Falls risk assessment and education on lifestyle modifications should be part of routine care for patients at risk.[74,76] Cancer survivors who have neuropathy, malnutrition, pain, polypharmacy, depression, weakness, and other risk factors should be considered at high risk for fractures, and efforts should be made to educate and raise awareness for patients and their caregivers.[76]

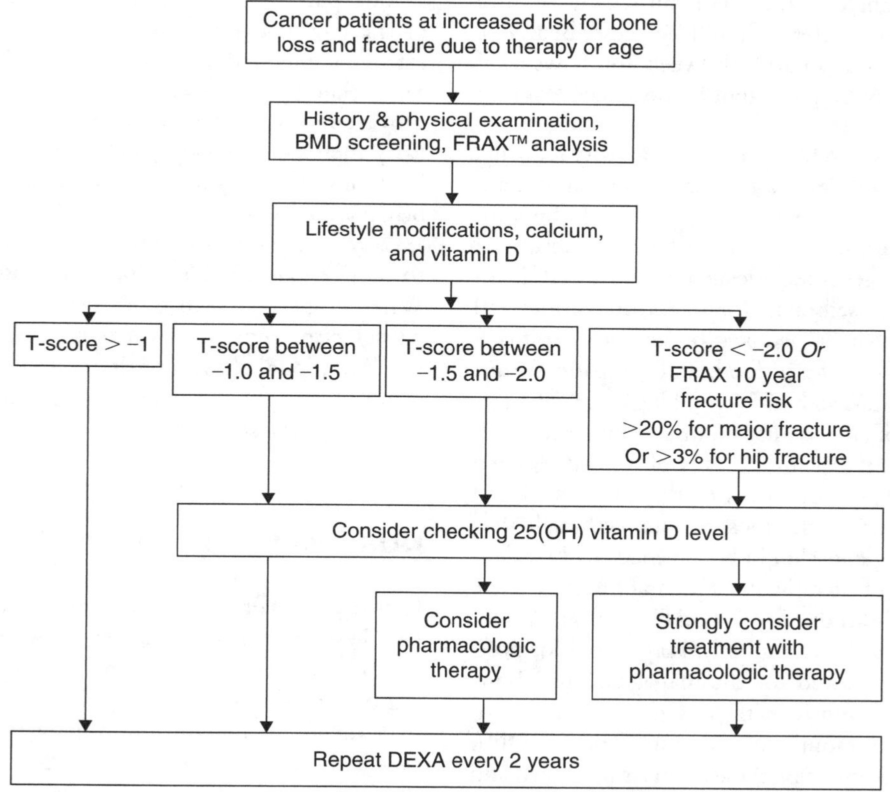

FIGURE 4-2

Algorithm for the management of bone health in cancer patients in the United States.

Abbreviations: 25(OH): serum hydroxyl; BMD: bone mineral density; DEXA: dual-energy x-ray absorptiometry; FRAX™: Fracture Risk Assessment Algorithm.

Source: Reprinted from Journal of the National Comprehensive Cancer Network. NCCN Task Force Report: Bone health in cancer care, 2009(7):S-1–S-32[78].

Calcium intake and supplementation with vitamin D is considered the safest, least expensive approach to maintaining bone health.[74,76] Nurses and nutritionists should assess their patients for adequate dietary calcium intake. Women older than age 50 should consume 1200 mg of calcium daily, and most women will need to supplement their diet with 600–900 mg/day of elemental calcium.[75,76] Consumption of more than the recommended amount may lead to the formation of renal calculi and cardiovascular disease. Additionally, vitamin D supplementation in the range of 800–1000 international units (IU) is recommended to facilitate the absorption of calcium. Measuring the serum 25(OH) vitamin D level is helpful in determining adequacy of the supplementation; this concentration should be 30 ng/mL or higher. Both calcium and vitamin D can be purchased as over-the-counter products.

There have been reports that soy isoflavones exert a protective effect on BMD loss.[60] The dose found to be most effective was 90 mg/day. DHEA has also shown some benefit in increasing BMD.

When the 25(OH) vitamin D level is less than normal, and the over-the-counter vitamin is insufficient, vitamin D in the form of ergocalciferol should be prescribed. The dose of ergocalciferol is 50,000 IU/week for 8 weeks.[76] The 25(OH) vitamin D level should be checked every 2–3 months for adequacy.

Bisphosphonates, which block osteoclast activity reducing bone resorption, are considered a first-line approach to management of bone loss and osteoporosis, and should be initiated with the incidence of a fracture or based on results of BMD loss.[74,76] These agents include alendronate (oral), ibandronate (oral and IV), risedronate (oral), and zoledronic acid (IV).[74] The oral agents must be taken on an empty stomach and require a delay in intake of food, and the patient must remain upright for at least an hour after taking them.[76] Unfortunately, nearly half of all patients will discontinue the use of these agents within one year for a variety of reasons. Among the many side effects, osteonecrosis of the jaw (ONJ) and atypical stress fractures are the most serious, although they occur only rarely.[74] Patients should be screened by their dentists before initiation of therapy; when dental procedures are necessary, a vacation from therapy should be initiated. Denosumab, a human monoclonal antibody, is approved for postmenopausal osteoporosis and for the management of bone metastasis in men and women with prostate and breast cancers.[74] It is given every 6 months and has a small risk for ONJ. The duration of treatment using these agents is unknown and the current recommendation in cancer is for indefinite use.[78]

CARDIOVASCULAR DISEASE

Cardiovascular disease is the leading cause of death in women, worldwide, according to the World Health Organization.[79] Generally, women develop CVD about 10 years later than men; however, after the age of 55, more women than men tend to have problems with CVD.[80,81] Surgically induced menopause increases the risk of vascular disease, stroke, and CVD.[82] The evidence suggests that there is an association, independent of the normal aging process, that may be related to the shift in the dominance of estrogen to the androgen hormone, between the menopausal state and the development of disease.[80,81] Postmenopausal women are more likely to have lower high-density lipoprotein cholesterol (HDL-C) levels, higher triglyceride levels, and central adiposity—all contributing to risks for CVD[81]—and early menopause is associated with a higher risk for stroke after the age of 50.[82,83] In addition, there is an increased risk for venous thromboembolic disease in women using estrogen.[37]

Therapeutic approaches

Contrary to the hypothesis advanced by the WHI, the combination of estrogen and progesterone used in the study showed an increase in the incidence of CVD among participants and resulted in an early termination of the trial.[81] Even though there are emerging data that estrogen may reduce CVD, currently estrogen replacement therapy, given alone, is not recommended for cardiovascular protection; however, in women who have early menopause or are younger than 59 years of age, the initiation of estrogen use should be considered based on other indications.[37]

Soy isoflavones and flavonoid extracts have been found to reduce diastolic blood pressure and LDL cholesterol.[60] When combined with other benefits in managing menopausal symptoms, isoflavones become even more intriguing. Additional clinical trials are needed in this population to be meaningful. Flaxseed has been found to reduce total and LDL cholesterol.[60]

NURSING IMPLICATIONS

Cancer survivorship is growing, and nearly 12 million people with a history of cancer are alive today in the United States, many of them women.[14] With more women surviving breast, gynecologic, and other cancers, many are living in a menopausal state induced by therapy, age, or both. Given the evidence of safety concerns regarding HT, and the small subset of women in whom therapy can be safely considered, many women with cancer will battle the challenges of menopause until research develops an ideal, safe substitute to manage each of the comorbid problems. It is possible that a SERM will be developed to protect the estrogen-sensitive tissues of the breast and gynecologic tract and exert positive benefits on the bone, heart, and brain, or some combination of these.

Consumers are plagued by claims of benefits of agents that are untried and unsafe, yet somehow appealing. Nurses must be sensitive to the inclination of patients to seek nonmedical interventions and be prepared to open dialogue in a safe, nurturing environment. By assisting in identifying menopausal symptoms such as those associated with VMS or the urogenital tract, nurses can reassure patients and help them make meaningful lifestyle adjustments using resources such as the Self-Care Guides included in this text. Discussing questions related to intimacy and sexual functions is essential to helping women understand and manage the effects of menopause. Educating patients who are at risk for osteopenia and osteoporosis is the first step in maintaining bone health. By accessing the resources identified in the "Osteoporosis: Maximizing the Health of Your Bones" Self-Care Guide and counseling, nurses can provide essential interventions that prevent loss of function and disability.

It is important for nurses to remember that there have been significant rates of physiologic decline associated with the postmenopausal state. This decline contributes adversely to physiologic and psychological functionality and significantly impacts aging comorbidities, hospitalization and institutionalization rates, and increased consumption of healthcare dollars.[15] Clearly, the implications for women who are at risk, particularly those who have cancer and early menopause, are concerning and must be addressed with certain interventions—namely, risk assessment, education, exercise, and surveillance. Armed with this knowledge, nurses must incorporate individualized clinical management and patient education focusing on optimizing functionality and overall well-being with pharmacologic, nonpharmacologic, and wellness planning.

PATIENT SELF-CARE

The Self-Care Guides that accompany this chapter can help patients manage the symptoms of menopause. These guides provide strategies to manage three important problems of menopause. "Hot Flashes and Night Sweats" (Appendix 4A) lists strategies to manage the vasomotor symptoms of menopause. Information related to intimacy and sexual function is essential to helping women understand and manage the effects of menopause and is found in Appendix 4B. The resources identified in "Osteoporosis: Maximizing the Health of Your Bones" (Appendix 4C) provide strategies that patients can use to prevent loss of function and disability. Women experiencing early-onset menopause due to their cancer treatment can be assisted in finding the evidence-based strategies they need to prevent, minimize, and manage unwanted symptoms.

REFERENCES

1. Department of Health and Human Services, Administration on Aging. U.S. population by age: July 1, 2010. National tables and trends. http://www.aoa.gov/aoaroot/aging_statistics/Census_Population/census2010. Accessed December 29, 2012.
2. American Cancer Society. Facts & figures 2012. http://www.cancer.org/acs/groups/content/@epidemiologysurveilance/documents/document/acspc-031941.pdf. Accessed December 29, 2012.
3. National Cancer Institute. Surveillance Epidemiology and End Results. SEER stat fact sheets: breast. http://seer.cancer.gov/statfacts/html/breast.html. Accessed December 29, 2012.
4. National Cancer Institute. Surveillance Epidemiology and End Results. SEER stat fact sheets: cervix uteri. http://seer.cancer.gov/statfacts/html/cervix.html. Accessed December 2012.
5. National Cancer Institute. Surveillance Epidemiology and End Results. SEER stat fact sheets: vulva. http://seer.cancer.gov/statfacts/html/vulva.html. Accessed December 2012.
6. Morelli S, Weiss G. Natural and surgical menopause. In: Santoro NF, Neal-Perry G, eds. *Amenorrhea: A Case-Based, Clinical Guide*. New York: Springer; 2010:141–170.
7. Harlow SD, Gass M, Hall JE, et al. Executive summary of the Stages of Reproductive Aging Workshop + 10: addressing the unfinished agenda of staging reproductive aging. *Menopause*. 2012;19(4):387–395.
8. National Institutes of Health. National Institute on Aging. Health and aging: menopause. 2011. http://www.nia.nih.gov/health/publication/menopause. Accessed December 29, 2012.
9. Freeman EW, Sammel MD, Lin H, et al. Symptoms associated with menopausal transition and reproductive hormones in midlife women. *Obstet Gynecol*. 2007;110(2, Part 1):230–240.
10. Horstman AM, Dillon EL, Urban RJ, Sheffield-Moore M. The role of androgens and estrogens on healthy aging and longevity. *J Gerontol A Biol Sci Med Sci*. 2012; 67(11):1140–1052.
11. Dicken C, Menke M, Neal-Perry G. The hypothalamic–pituitary–ovarian axis. In: Santoro NF, Neal-Perry G, eds. *Amenorrhea: A Case-Based, Clinical Guide*. New York: Springer; 2010:1–20.
12. Schorge JO, Schaffer JI, Pietz J, et al. Reproductive endocrinology. In: Schorge JO, Schaffer JI, Pietz J, Halvorson LM, Hoffman BL, Bradshaw KD, Cunningham FG, eds. *Williams Gynecology*. New York: McGraw-Hill; 2008:430–449.
13. Santoro N. Update in hyper- and hypogonadotropic amenorrhea. *J Clin Endocrinol Metab*. 2011;96(11):3281–3288.
14. Ganz PA. Survivorship: adult cancer survivors. *Prim Care Clin Office Pract*. 2009;36:721–741.
15. Hunter MS. Long-term impacts of early and surgical menopause. *Menopause*. 2012;19(3):253–254.
16. Tom SE, Cooper R, Patel KV, Guralnik JM. Menopausal characteristics and physical functioning in older adulthood in the National Health and Nutrition Examination Survey III. *Menopause*. 2012;19(3):283–289.
17. Department of Health and Human Services, Centers for Disease Control and Prevention. Women's reproductive health: hysterectomy. 2008. http://www.cdc.gov/reproductivehealth/WomensRH/Hysterectomy.htm. Accessed December 29, 2012.
18. Oktem O, Urman B. Options of fertility preservation in female cancer patients. *Obstet Gynecol Surv*. 2010;65(8):531–542.
19. Gordon AM, Hurwitz S, Shapiro CL, LeBoff MS. Premature ovarian failure and body composition changes with adjuvant chemotherapy for breast cancer. *Menopause*. 2011;18(11):1244–1248.
20. Thompson CA, Mauck K, Havyer R, Bhagra A, Kalsi, H, Hayes SN. Care of the adult Hodgkin lymphoma survivor. *Am J Med*. 2000;124(12):1106–1112.
21. Morris SN, Ryley D. Fertility preservation: nonsurgical and surgical options. *Semin Reprod Med*. 2011;29(2);147–154.
22. Laufer MR, Upton J, Schuster SR, Grier H, Emans SJ, Diller L. Ovarian tissue autologous transplantation to the upper extremity for

girls receiving abdominal/pelvic radiation: 20-year follow-up of reproductive endocrine function. *J Pediatr Adolesc Gynecol.* 2010;23(2):107–110.

23. Utian WH. Psychosocial and socioeconomic burden of vasomotor symptoms in menopause: a comprehensive review. *Health Qual Life Outcomes.* 2005;3:47.
24. Schneider HPG, Heinemann LAJ, Rosemeier HP, Potthoff P, Behre HM. The Menopause Rating Scale (MRS): reliability of scores of menopausal complaints. Climacteric. 2000;3:59–64
25. Van Dole KB, DeVellis RF, Brown RD, Jonsson ML, Gaynes, BN, Williams RE. Evaluation of the Menopause-Specific Quality of Life Questionnaire: a factor-analytic approach. *Menopause.* 2012;19(2);211–215.
26. Deecher DC, Dorris K. Understanding the pathophysiology of vasomotor symptoms (hot flushes and night sweats) that occur in perimenopause, menopause, and postmenopause life stages. *Arch Womens Ment Health.* 2007;10:247–257.
27. Ziv-Gal A, Flaws JA. Factors that may influence the experience of hot flushes by healthy middle-aged women. *J Women's Health.* 2010;19(10):1905–1914.
28. Morrow PKH, Mattair DN, Hortobagyi GN. Hot flashes: a review of pathology and treatment modalities. *Oncologist.* 2011;16(11):1658–1664.
29. Alexander IM. Harnessing the hot flash. *Adv Nurse Pract.* 2009;37(7):31–34.
30. Rendall MJ, Simonds LM, Hunter MS. The Hot Flush Beliefs Scale: a tool for assessing thoughts and beliefs associated with the experience of menopausal hot flushes and night sweats. *Maturitas.* 2008;60(2);158–169.
31. Ohayon MM. Severe hot flashes are associated with chronic insomnia. *Arch Intern Med.* 2006;166(12):1262–1268.
32. Freedman RR. Pathology and treatment of menopausal hot flashes. *Semin Reprod Med.* 2005;23(2):117–125.
33. Gold EB, Colvin A, Avis N, et al. Longitudinal analysis of the association between vasomotor symptoms and race/ethnicity across the menopausal transition: Study of Women's Health Across the Nation. *Am J Public Health.* 2006;96(7):1226–1235.
34. Cochran C, Gallicchio L, Miller S, Zacur H, Flaws J. Cigarette smoking, androgen levels, and hot flushes in midlife women. *Obstet Gynecol.* 2008;112(5):1037–1044.
35. Kaplan M, Mahon S, Cope D, Keating E, Hill S, Jacobson M. Putting evidence into practice: evidence-based interventions for hot flashes resulting from cancer therapies. *Clin J Oncol Nurs.* 2011;15(2):149–157.
36. Breast International Group (BIG) 1–98 Collaborative Group. A comparison of letrozole and tamoxifen in postmenopausal women with early breast cancer. *N Engl J Med.* 2005;353:2747–2757.
37. North American Menopause Society. The 2012 hormone therapy position statement of the North American Menopause Society. *Menopause.* 2012;19(3):257–271.
38. North American Menopause Society. Mayfield Heights: North American Menopause Society; 2012 http://www.menopause.org/for-women/menopauseflashes/breast-cancer-survivors-hot-flash-treatments. Accessed December 28, 2012.
39. Carmody JF, Crawford S, Salmoirago-Blotcher E, Leung K, Churchill L, Olendzki N. Mindfulness training for coping with hot flashes: results of a randomized trial. *Menopause.* 2011;18(6):611–620.
40. Elkins G, Fisher WI, Johnson AK. Hypnosis for hot flashes among postmenopausal women study: a study protocol of an ongoing randomized clinical trial. *BMC Complement Altern Med.* 2011;11:92–99.
41. Schover LR, Jenkins R, Sui D, Adams JH, Marion MS, Jackson KE. Randomized trial of peer counseling on reproductive health in African American breast cancer survivors. *J Clin Oncol.* 2006;24:1620–1626.
42. Spetz Holm AE, Frisk J, Hammar ML. Acupuncture as treatment of hot flashes and the possible role of calcitonin gene-related peptide. *Evid Based Complement Alternat Med.* 2012;1–9 [epub].
43. Hulley S, Grady D, Bush T, et al. Randomized trial of estrogen plus progestin for secondary prevention of coronary heart disease in postmenopausal women. *JAMA.* 1998;280(7):605–613.
44. Neal-Perry G. Hormone therapy in 2011: Rethinking the evidence. *Contemporary OB/GYN.* 2011;56(11):36–43.
45. LaCroix AZ, Chlebowski RT, Manson JE, Aragaki AK, Johnson KC, Martin L, et al. Health outcomes after stopping conjugated equine estrogens among postmenopausal women with prior hysterectomy: a randomized controlled trial. *JAMA.* 2011;305(13):1305–1314.
46. Simon JA. What's new in hormone replacement therapy: focus on transdermal estradiol and micronized progesterone. *Climacteric.* 2012;15(suppl 1):3–10.
47. Crandall CJ, Aragaki AK, Chlebowski RT, McTiernan A, Anderson G, Hendrix SL, et al. New-onset breast tenderness after initiation of estrogen plus progestin therapy and breast cancer risk. *Arch Intern Med.* 2009;169(18):1684–1691.
48. Cummings SR, Ettinger B, Delmas PD, et al. The effects of tibolone in older postmenopausal women. *New Engl J Med.* 2008;359:607–708.
49. Clonidine. Lexicomp. 2010. http://www.crlonline.com/lco/action/doc/retrieve/docid/250/413451#. Accessed December 29, 2012.
50. Rapkin, AJ. Vasomotor symptoms in menopause: physiologic condition and central nervous system approaches to treatment. *Am J Obstet Gynecol.* 207;92(2): 97–104.
51. Sturdee DW. The menopausal hot flush: anything new? *Maturitas.* 2008;60:42–49.
52. Loprinzi CL, Sloan J, Stearns V, Slack R, Iyengar M, Diekmann B, et al. New antidepressants and gabapentin for hot flashes: an individual patient pooled analysis. *J Clin Oncol.* 2009;27(17): 2831–2837.
53. Gabapentin. Lexicomp. 2012. http://www.crlonline.com/lco/action/doc/retrieve/docid/patch_f/6961?hl=GABA%20Analog#. Accessed December 29, 2012.
54. Komm BS, Chines AA. An update on selective estrogen receptor modulators for the prevention and treatment of osteoporosis. *Maturitas.* 2012;71:221–226.
55. Levis S, Strickman-Stein N, Ganjei-Azar P, Xu P, Doerge DR, Krischer J. Soy isoflavones in the prevention of menopausal bone loss and menopausal symptoms. *Arch Intern Med.* 2011;171(15):1363–1369.
56. Dietary supplement fact sheet: black cohosh. http://ods.od.nih.gov/factsheets/BlackCohosh-HealthProfessional/. Accessed July 21, 2012.
57. Hernández Muñoz G, Pluchino S. *Cimicifuga racemosa* for the treatment of hot flushes in women surviving breast cancer. *Maturitas.* 2003;44(suppl 1):S59–S65.
58. Nelson HD, Vesco KK, Haney E, et al. Nonhormonal therapies for menopausal hot flashes: systematic review and meta-analysis. *JAMA.* 2006;295(17):2057–2071.
59. Sharma P, Wisniewski A, Braga-Basaria M, et al. Lack of an effect of high dose isoflavones in men with prostate cancer undergoing androgen deprivation therapy. *J Urol.* 2009;182:265–2273.
60. Borrelli F, Ernst E. Alternative and complementary therapies for the menopause. Maturitas. 2010; 66:333–343.
61. Bhavnani BR, Stanczyk FZ. Misconception and concerns about bioidentical hormones used for custom-compounded hormone therapy. *J Clin Endocrinol Metab.* 2012;97(3):756–759.
62. U.S. Food and Drug Administration (FDA). Transcript of FDA press conference on FDA actions on bioidentical hormones. 2008. http://www.fda.gov/downloads/NewsEvents/Newsroom/MediaTranscripts/ucm122174.pdf. Accessed December 29, 2012.
63. U.S. Food and Drug Administration (FDA). Bio-identicals: sorting myths from facts. http://www.fda.gov/downloads/ForConsumers/ConsumerUpdates/ucm049312.pdf?utm_campaign=Google2&utm_source=fdaSearch&utm_medium=website&utm_term=bioidentical%20hormones&utm_content=9. Accessed December 29, 2012.
64. Sturdee DW, Panay N. Recommendations for the management of postmenopausal vaginal atrophy. *Climacteric.* 2010;13(6):509–522.

65. Trinkaus M, Chin S, Wolfman W, Simmons C, Clemons M. Should urogenital atrophy in breast cancer survivors be treated with topical estrogens? *Oncologist.* 2008;13:222–231.
66. Shifren JL. Increasing our understanding of women's sexuality at midlife and beyond. *Menopause.* 2011;18(11):1149–1151.
67. Avis NE, Zhao X, Johannes CB, Ory M, Brockwell S, Greendale GA. Correlates of sexual function among multi-ethnic middle-aged women: results from the Study of Women's Health Across the Nation (SWAN). *Menopause.* 2005;12(4):385–398.
68. Lindau ST, Schumm LP, Laumann EO, Levinson W, O'Muircheartaigh CA, Waite LJ. A study of sexuality and health among older adults in the United States. *N Engl J Med.* 2007;357:762–774.
69. West SL, D'Aloisio AA, Agans RP, Kalsbeek WD, Borisov NN, Thorp JM. Prevalence of low sexual desire and hypoactive sexual desire disorder in a nationally representative sample of US women. *Arch Intern Med.* 2008;168(13):1441–1449.
70. Cuzick J, Sestak I, Baum M, Buzdar A, Howell A, Dowsett M, et al. Effect of anastrozole and tamoxifen as adjuvant treatment for early-stage breast cancer: 10-year analysis of the ATAC trial. *Lancet Oncol.* 2010;11(12):1135–41.
71. North American Menopause Society. The role of local vaginal estrogen for treatment of vaginal atrophy in postmenopausal women: 2007 position statement of the North American Menopause Society. *Menopause.* 2007;14(3):359–369.
72. Baim S, Leslie WD. Assessment of fracture risk. *Curr Osteoporos Rep.* 2012;10:28–41.
73. National Institute of Health. National Institute of Arthritis and Musculoskeletal and Skin Diseases: osteoporosis. http://www.niams.nih.gov/Health_Info/Bone/Osteoporosis/default.asp. Accessed December 29, 2012.
74. Wickham R. Osteoporosis related to disease or therapy in patients with cancer: review and clinical implications. *Clin J Oncol Nurs.* 2011;15(6):E90–E104.
75. North American Menopause Society. Management of osteoporosis in postmenopausal women: 2010 position statement of the North American Menopause Society. *Menopause.* 2010;17(1):25–54.
76. National Osteoporosis Foundation (NOF). *Clinician's Guide to Prevention and Treatment of Osteoporosis.* Washington, DC: National Osteoporosis Foundation; 2010. http://nof.org/hcp/practice/practice-and-clinical-guidelines/clinicians-guide. Accessed December 29, 2012.
77. World Health Organization. Welcome to FRAX™. http://www.shef.ac.uk/FRAX/. Accessed December 29, 2012.
78. National Comprehensive Cancer Network (NCCN). NCCN Task Force Report: bone health and cancer care. *J Natl Compr Canc Netw.* 2009;7:S-1–S-32.
79. World Health Organization. Women's health 2009. http://www.who.int/mediacentre/factsheets/fs334/en/index.html. Accessed December 29, 2012.
80. Claassen M, Sybrandy KC, Appelman YE, Asselbergs FW. Gender gap in acute coronary heart disease: myth or reality? *World J Cardiol.* 2012;4(2):36–47.
81. Janssen I, Powell LH, Crawford S, Lasley B, Sutton-Tyrrell K. Menopause and the metabolic syndrome: the Study of Women's Health Across the Nation. *Arch Intern Med.* 2008;168(14):1568–1575.
82. Rexrode KM, Manson JE. Estrogens and stroke: disentangling a complex relationship. *Menopause.* 2012;19(3):247–249.
83. Rocca WA, Grossardt BR, Miller VM, Shuster LT, Brown RD. Premature menopause or early menopause and risk of ischemic stroke. *Menopause.* 2012;19(3):272–277.

Managing the Symptoms of Menopause: Hot Flashes and Night Sweats

Patient Name: ____

Symptom and Description

Many women recognize the symptoms of menopause by the onset of the hot flash. Decreasing levels or the total loss of estrogen is the primary reason for this problem. Menopause may happen gradually as a part of the aging process, or it may occur suddenly, immediately after the ovaries are removed during surgery or as a result of medication to treat breast cancer, or less quickly, during chemotherapy or radiation. Many women will have hot flashes and night sweats, whose frequency may range from rare occasions to several times a day. Hot flashes that occur at night disturb sleep, cause fatigue and changes in mood, and may affect thinking. It is not uncommon for women to feel anxious or depressed. These symptoms usually improve over time.

Management

The best way to manage these symptoms is to replace the estrogen through medication. Estrogen therapy is not recommended for all women; if it is recommended, it should continue only for the first few years of menopause. Estrogen is not used in women who have cancer that is sensitive to estrogen. In women who have a uterus, another hormone, progesterone, may be prescribed to reduce the chance of uterine bleeding. The doctor may want the patient to have ultrasounds of the uterus occasionally to monitor for uterine bleeding. Recommendations for medication used for the management of hot flashes are made with careful consideration and discussion between a woman and her healthcare provider. The following are suggestions that may help you manage the symptoms:

1. Wear clothes made of cotton, linen, or fabrics that can move sweat away from the skin. The fabric should be light and airy. Avoid materials such as nylon and polyester, as these may make you feel hotter and cause hot flashes.
2. Wear your clothes in layers that can be easily removed; neck scarves are good for cooler weather because they can be removed quickly in the event of a flash. Try to avoid turtlenecks or shirts with high necklines, tight clothing, and extra layers. Girdles, slips, and pantyhose may contribute to your hot flashes.
3. Use cotton sheets and sleepwear. Consider layering bed linen for comfort.
4. Keep your room temperature at a constant, moderately cool level and use fans to circulate air. You may find that small fans on your desk at work and your nightstand come in handy.
5. Avoid caffeine, alcohol, and smoking.
6. Drink water that is cold or with ice that can reduce your temperature when a hot flash occurs. Try to increase the amount of water you drink to hydrate and replace fluids lost during sweating.

7. Exercise even though it may raise your temperature and cause hot flashes. Exercise will make you feel better, reduce body fat, improve your mood, help you sleep better, and protect your heart and bones.
8. Women often benefit from counseling, consulting nutritionists, or seeking assistance from Integrative Health Centers in the management of hot flashes.

Follow-up

Consult your healthcare provider if you find these symptoms are intolerable or affecting your health. There are other medications and interventions that can be prescribed.

Phone Numbers

Nurse: ____________________ Phone: ____________

Provider: ____________________ Phone: ____________

Other: ____________________ Phone: ____________

Phone: ____________ Phone: ____________

Comments

Source: Frazier SR, Egger M. Menopausal Symptoms. In: Yarbro CH, Wujcik D, Gobel BH, eds. *Cancer Symptom Management.* 4th ed. Burlington, MA: Jones & Bartlett Learning; 2014.

Managing the Symptoms of Menopause: Changes in the Female Anatomy

Patient Name: ____

Symptom and Description

Menopause and the loss of estrogen cause changes in the bladder, vulva, and vagina. A woman's pelvic organs shrink, lose fat, and become less elastic. Many women experience problems with urination, bladder infections, or smaller bladder capacity. The vagina shortens and becomes dry. Changes in the vagina may make sexual intercourse difficult or painful, and some women lose sexual desire. The vulva may itch, burn, crack, and bleed.

Management

The best way to manage these symptoms is to replace estrogen through medication. Estrogen therapy is not recommended for all women. Estrogen is not used in women who have cancer that is sensitive to estrogen. In severe cases, providers may recommend estrogen be given by mouth or by a patch combined with estrogen applied directly to the vulva and the vagina with a cream, a vaginal insert, or a device placed in the vagina. The vaginal devices consist of a pliable ring or cube that contains estrogen. In women who have a uterus, another hormone, progesterone, may be prescribed to reduce the chance of uterine bleeding. Recommendations for management of these changes are made with careful consideration and discussion between a woman and her healthcare provider. The following are suggestions that may help you manage the symptoms:

1. Urinate frequently to avoid bladder infections. Urinate before and after intercourse.
2. Engage in sexual intercourse. Frequent intercourse keeps the tissues pliable and increases blood flow.
3. Use lubricants for sexual intercourse. Try water-based lubricants and avoid any that are scented, are flavored, or have an alcohol base.
4. Some oils, such as olive, vegetable, and coconut oils, are very pleasant lubricants. Oils will stain fabrics. Squeezing the oil from a vitamin E gel capsule and inserting it into the vagina is helpful.
5. Kegel exercises will strengthen the vaginal muscles, the bladder, and the muscles in the floor of the pelvis. This strengthening will improve blood flow, reduce incontinence, and may improve sexual pleasure. Ask your provider for Kegel exercise instructions.
6. There are a number of vaginal moisturizers available on the market. Consult your provider before choosing one.
7. If you are prescribed estrogen products that are applied directly to the skin of the vulva and vagina, follow the directions for usage. Avoid exposure to your male partner, as there is evidence that estrogen is absorbed through the skin.

Follow-up

Report any of the following symptoms to your provider:

1. Difficult or painful intercourse
2. Chronic vaginal discharge or bleeding
3. Problems with urinary frequency, burning, or difficulty voiding
4. Bleeding or ulcerations on the vulva

Phone Numbers

Nurse: ______________________________ Phone: ________________

Provider: ____________________________ Phone: ________________

Other: ______________________________ Phone: ________________

Phone: ________________ Phone: ________________

Comments

Source: Frazier SR, Egger M. Menopausal Symptoms. In: Yarbro CH, Wujcik D, Gobel BH, eds. *Cancer Symptom Management.* 4th ed. Burlington, MA: Jones & Bartlett Learning; 2014.

Osteoporosis: Maximizing the Health of Your Bones

Patient Name: ______________________________

This guide will help you maintain or restore bone strength.

Symptom and Description

Bone is a tissue that is constantly changing from birth to about 35 years. As we age, the body begins to lose the ability to rebuild bone. This change happens gradually for some individuals, but for people with certain illnesses, taking specific medications, and in menopause, it can occur rapidly. Bone changes are considered a "silent" disease because most people do not know they have a problem until they have a bone break or fracture. The most common areas for fracture are the wrist, hip, and spine.

When bones get thinner, it is called osteopenia. When holes develop in the bone, it is called osteoporosis. Low calcium and vitamin D intake, use of steroid medications, thyroid problems, and some cancer therapies will increase the risk for osteopenia and osteoporosis.

Some people are at higher risk for these problems than others. You should know your risk factors:

1. Women are at higher risk than men. White and Asian women who are thin and small are at higher risk than heavier women. African American women are at lower risk because their bones are denser.
2. Women who ate less than the recommended amounts of calcium-rich foods when they were growing, or who have had an eating disorder, or who have a family history of thinning bones, are at risk.
3. Men and women who consume large amounts of caffeine, smoke cigarettes, or drink three or more alcoholic drinks per day are at risk.
4. Poor exercise habits or sitting frequently will lead to poor bone health.

Management

1. If they do not have any risk factors, women 65 years or older and men 70 years or older should have bone mineral testing with a DEXA scan or other bone testing.
2. Anyone who has risk factors should see a healthcare provider and receive recommendations for their specific problem.
3. Calcium and vitamin D are good for bone building. Review your daily dietary intake of calcium and vitamin D. If you take in less than 1200 mg of calcium in your diet each day, you should supplement your diet to take in a total of 1200 mg of calcium each day. If you take in less than 600 IU of Vitamin D in your diet each day, you should supplement your diet to take in a total of 600 IU (for people over 70 years of age the amount increases to 800 IU) each day.
4. Good sources of calcium are green leafy vegetables such as spinach, collard greens, kale, and okra; dairy products such as milk, yogurt, and cheese; beans such as soy and white

beans; and some fish, including sardines, salmon, and trout. Some foods are fortified with calcium, such as orange juice, some breakfast cereals, and oatmeal.

5. It is harder to get enough vitamin D from foods, but good sources are from fish such as tuna and salmon; egg yolks; and foods that are fortified with vitamin D such as dairy products, cheese, orange juice, soy milk, and cereals. Vitamin D is produced in the skin by sunlight. Even though sun exposure is not recommended over time, it does help increase vitamin D.
6. If you have a history of kidney stones, do not take additional calcium without direction from your healthcare provider.
7. Regular exercise with muscle strengthening increases bone health. Consult your healthcare provider before beginning an exercise regimen, but once you do start a program, keep exercising.
8. Be especially wary of falling or hazards in your home or work that may cause you to fall. Exercise will help you maintain balance. Yoga and tai chi are good exercises for balance training.
9. If you smoke cigarettes or drink alcohol frequently, your healthcare team will help you learn ways to decrease the amount or quit.
10. A variety of medications can be prescribed if needed to help with your bone health. Your healthcare team will work with you to find the most effective treatment for you.

Follow-up

Consult your healthcare provider if you have any side effects from your medicines.

Phone Numbers

Nurse: ______________________________ Phone: ________________

Provider: ____________________________ Phone: ________________

Other: ______________________________ Phone: ________________

Phone: ________________ Phone: ________________

Comments

Source: Frazier SR, Egger M. Menopausal Symptoms. In: Yarbro CH, Wujcik D, Gobel BH, eds. *Cancer Symptom Management*. 4th ed. Burlington, MA: Jones & Bartlett Learning; 2014.

CHAPTER 5

Pain

Jeannine M. Brant, PhD, APRN, AOCN®

THE PROBLEM

Pain is a significant problem in patients with cancer and is often the most feared aspect of the disease. A multitude of pain guidelines exist to guide the management of cancer pain,[1–4] and the World Health Organization (WHO) estimates that its ladder for cancer pain can adequately manage pain in approximately 80%–90% of patients.[3] The healthcare team has a professional and ethical responsibility to assess and adequately manage pain in patients throughout the cancer trajectory. Being aware of the incidence and etiology of cancer pain is important to recognize how this problem impacts every aspect of the cancer illness. Appreciating the global aspects of pain enables clinicians to identify high-risk patients and obtain a comprehensive pain assessment. Recognizing that the assessment should focus on the patient's perspective of pain, however it is defined, is critical in pain assessment.[5] Finally, understanding the pathophysiology of pain enables healthcare professionals to use both pharmacologic and nonpharmacologic interventions that can interrupt pain signals along the pain pathway.

According to the International Association for the Study of Pain, pain is defined as "a sensory and emotional experience associated with actual or potential tissue damage or described in terms of such damage."[6] The definition reinforces the fact that pain is not just physical, but rather is a holistic experience. Total pain or global pain involves the interplay of physical, psychological, social, and spiritual factors that constructs each patient's unique pain experience. Total pain reinforces the inner-connectedness between the body, mind, and spirit.[7] Healthcare professionals commonly focus on the physical pain but should be reminded that pain is more than a physiologic process. Pain is psychological and can remind patients of their cancer and uncertainty of the future. Patients may even suppress pain in an effort to protect their family and deny pain due to fear of disease progression. Socially, patients may become isolated as pain keeps them from enjoying social activities and relationships. Spirituality can affect individual perception and intensity about pain, the significance of the meaning of pain, and the acceptance of the medical treatment plan. If total pain involves the physical, psychological, social, and spiritual domains, then the management of pain should likewise encompass all domains.[8–10]

Despite the full armamentarium of strategies available, cancer pain remains undertreated, and a multitude of barriers exist to its management. Data suggest that while a focus on cancer pain has existed for more than 20 years, pain is not adequately addressed, and misperceptions and limitations exist in pain-related knowledge and practice.[11] Barriers comprise healthcare professionals, healthcare systems, and patients and families.

First, healthcare professionals have inadequate knowledge about pain assessment and management. A recent study indicated that the most common physician-related barriers to adequate cancer pain management were insufficient knowledge and inadequate opioid prescribing.[12] A plethora of studies indicate that nurses' knowledge of pain assessment and management is also lacking, and only 49% of nurses in a recent study achieved a passing score of 80% or higher.[13] Lack of pain assessment is another major barrier, and has been considered the greatest barrier to adequate pain management.[4,11,12] For nurses, The Joint Commission frequently cites lack of pain assessment in the hospital setting as a problem. Pain cannot be managed if it is not assessed. Fears about addiction may lead to inadequate prescribing, and confusion still exists about the differences between addiction, tolerance, and physical dependence (Table 5-1).[14]

Second, healthcare and regulatory systems fuel the problem. Providers fear scrutiny from regulatory agencies and may be reluctant to prescribe opioid analgesics.[11] Most recently, risk evaluation and mitigation strategies (REMS) have added another layer to prescribing opioids for patients in need.[15]

Third, additional barriers have been noted throughout the last two to three decades for patients and families. Fears of addiction, failure to report pain, fear that pain is a sign of disease progression, perception that pain is an expected part of the disease, lack of knowledge about pain management options, lack of adherence due to side effects, and desire to be a "good" patient continue to prevail.[11,16–18] Barriers may be compounded in patients who are older,[19] female, of a minority race,[20] and have less education and lower socioeconomic status.[12,21]

TABLE 5-1

Glossary of Definitions

Term	Definition
Pain	• A sensory and emotional experience associated with actual or potential tissue damage or described in terms of such damage • Whatever the experiencing person says it is existing whenever he or she says it does
Somatic Pain	• Pain arising from skin, muscle, tendon, joints, fasciae, and bones
Visceral Pain	• Pain arising from visceral organs such as the lungs, GI tract, liver, gallbladder, kidneys, and bladder
Neuropathic Pain	• Pain arising from the peripheral or central nervous system
	Types of Pain
Acute Pain	• Pain that is self-limiting and resolves with healing of the underlying injury
Chronic Pain	• Persistent pain with pathology that is unable to explain the extension of pain beyond the expected period of healing
Persistent Pain	• Prolonged pain after a transient stimulus
Referred Pain	• Spread of pain to an uninjured tissue
Breakthrough Pain	• A transient exacerbation of pain that occurs either spontaneously, or in relation to a specific predictable or unpredictable trigger, despite relatively stable and adequately controlled background pain
End of Dose Pain	• Pain that occurs prior to the next dose of scheduled medication
	Characteristics Used to Describe Pain
Allodynia	• A painful response to a normally innocuous stimulus
Dysesthesia	• A spontaneous or evoked unpleasant and abnormal sensation
Hyperalgesia	• An increased response to a noxious stimulus
Hyperpathia	• Abnormal pain and exaggerated response, especially to a repetitive stimulus
	Opioid-Related Terms
Physical Dependence	• A state of adaptation that is manifested by a drug class specific withdrawal syndrome that can be produced by abrupt cessation, rapid dose reduction, decreasing blood level of drug and/or administration of an antagonist.
Tolerance	• A state of adaptation in which exposure to a drug induces changes that result in a diminution of one or more of the drug's effects over time.
Addiction	• Addiction is a primary, chronic, neurobiologic disease with genetic, psychosocial, and environmental factors influencing its development and manifestations. It is characterized by behaviors that include one or more of the following: impaired control over drug use, compulsive use, continued use despite harm, and craving.
Abstinence Syndrome	• Occurs with abrupt cessation or diminution of an opioid following chronic use

Abbreviation: GI: gastrointestinal tract.

INCIDENCE

A recent systematic review of more than 52 studies indicates that pain occurs in approximately 53% of patients with cancer, but the experience is highly variable and dependent on the stage of disease, goals of treatment, and type of cancer.[22] Pain is more common in the advanced stages of the disease, with 59% to 64% of patients with metastatic or terminal disease reporting pain. Higher rates, up to 70%, were reported in earlier studies where pain was rated by a family member and not by the patients themselves. Families have been recognized to overestimate the amount of pain the patient is experiencing. For patients undergoing cancer treatment, 59% experience pain, and pain is also found to occur in 33% of patients' post curative treatment, so that it is a growing concern for disease-free cancer survivors. In regard to type of cancer, 70% of patients with head and neck cancer experienced the most pain, followed by 60% of those with gynecologic malignancies, 59% with gastrointestinal cancer (colon, esophageal, pancreatic), 55% with lung cancer, 54% with breast cancer, and 52% with urogenital cancer (prostate, bladder). In those patients who had pain, more than one-third assessed the pain as moderate to severe; as many as 43% rated their pain as moderate, and 26% rated their pain as severe.[22]

A lack of consensus in the literature exists regarding which demographic characteristics predict the most pain. For example, the evidence on the prevalence of pain in older adults is conflicting. While some studies report an increased prevalence of pain in older adults,[21,23] others find no difference.[22] Research studies on gender differences in cancer-related pain have also yielded inconsistent results.[24]

ETIOLOGY

Cancer-related pain often results from three separate etiologies: from direct tumor involvement, diagnostic or therapeutic procedures, or cancer treatment. Cancer treatment-related pain can result from surgery, chemotherapy, biotherapy and targeted therapy, hormone therapy, and radiation therapy (Table 5-2). Patients may also experience pain that is unrelated to the cancer.[25] Examples include arthritic pain, fibromyalgia, and chronic low back pain.

Pain related to any of the causes can be somatic (e.g., bone pain), visceral (e.g., pancreas, liver), or neuropathic. Neuropathic pain can be peripheral or centrally mediated, and is usually caused by direct tumor invasion (approximately 64% of patients) or cancer treatment (approximately 20%).[26] Patients can also experience more than one type of pain. In a large international trial, 92.5% of the participating patients had one or more pains caused directly by the cancer and 20.8% of patients had one or more pains caused by cancer therapies.[27] A comprehensive assessment is critical to determine the etiology of the pain and to identify whether patients are experiencing more than one type of pain—information that can help guide treatment decisions.

Clinicians should recognize that pain can occur throughout the cancer trajectory. While pain is most prevalent during the advanced stages of the disease, as noted, it can occur at diagnosis and throughout treatment. Pain

TABLE 5-2

Cancer-Related Pain Syndromes

Etiology	Examples of Related Syndromes
Direct Tumor Involvement	Somatic pain • Bone pain – primary or metastases Visceral pain • Ascites • Lymphedema • Obstruction • Organ related pain – pancreas, liver, abdominal viscera Neuropathic • Brachial or lumbosacral plexopathies Headache
Therapeutic and Diagnostic Procedures	Therapeutic procedure-related • Pleurodesis • Post surgical pain Diagnostic procedure-related • Bone marrow aspirations • Lumbar puncture
Cancer Treatment	Surgical • Post surgical pain • Pain following access device placement Chemotherapy • Arthralgias from flare reactions • Avascular necrosis from corticosteroid administration • Hemorrhagic cystitis • Mucositis • Peripheral neuropathy Hormone therapy • Arthralgias • Gynecomastia Biotherapy/Targeted Therapy • Acneiform rash • Bone pain related to growth factor administration Radiation therapy • Dermatitis • Enteritis • Mucositis • Plexopathies

TABLE 5-3

Disease Specific Chronic Pain Syndromes in Cancer Survivors

Type of Cancer	Pain Syndromes	Characteristics
Anus	• Lumbosacral plexopathy	• Radiating pain from the pelvis down the associated lower extremity
Breast	• Phantom breast pain • Intercostobrachial neuralgia • Neuroma • Lymphedema • Post-radiotherapy-brachial plexopathy	• Location of pain can be arm, neck, shoulder, chest wall, or breast • Pain can be localized or can radiate down the affected arm • Sensations include paresthesias, dysesthesias, hyperalgesias, and allodynia
Head and Neck	• Neck and shoulder pain • Facial, mouth, dental, mandibular pain	• Can involve neck, shoulder, and myofascial pain • Pain includes loss of sensation and neuropathic pain syndromes
Lung	• Intercostal neuralgia	• Sensations include paresthesias • Decreases over the course of a year
Prostate	• Chronic pelvic pain	• Pain usually only present during urination or exacerbated during urination
Sarcoma	• Stump pain • Phantom limb pain (PLP)	• Stump pain can be related to a poorly fitting prosthesis • PLP decreases over the course of a year; pain present at 1 year is likely to persist chronically

Source: Data from Brant[25].

in cancer survivors is being increasingly recognized.[25] The most common cancer pain syndromes in cancer survivors are included in Table 5-3.

PATHOPHYSIOLOGY

The assessment and management of pain begins with an understanding of the pathophysiology of pain. While this process is more straightforward for acute pain, the mechanisms are less understood for chronic and cancer pain due to changes that occur within the nervous system over time, even without the pain stimuli.

Pain begins with transduction when a mechanical, thermal, or chemical stimulus triggers pain and initiates a cascade of events. At the time of injury, neuromediators such as prostaglandins, histamine, bradykinin, serotonin, and substance P flood the site of injury, initiating an inflammatory response.[28] Once the sensory nerve endings are stimulated, an action potential or depolarization occurs and transmits the painful message through primary afferent neurons in the peripheral nervous system and to the dorsal horn of the spinal cord. Within the spinal cord, neurotransmitters and other excitatory substances are released. Spinal neurons also release inhibitory amino acids such as gamma-aminobutyric acid (GABA) to inhibit presynaptic and postsynaptic nociceptive transmission, thereby modulating the pain sensation. Transmission continues to the brain stem and thalamus, eventually reaching higher centers in the brain. The painful message finally reaches the cortical level of the brain, where perception of pain occurs. The thalamus also relays information to the limbic system, where affective responses of pain are mediated.[28]

Past experience with pain, beliefs, and culture provide a contextual environment for interpretation of the pain. The brain, however, responds to the noxious stimuli to diminish perception through descending modulating mechanisms. Specifically, neurons within the pons and medulla descend to the dorsal horn and release serotonin, norepinephrine, and endogenous opioids at the dorsal horn of the spinal cord, which inhibit the transmission of pain impulses[29] (Figure 5-1).[30]

Both pharmacologic and nonpharmacologic modalities assist in managing pain during the transduction, transmission, perception, and modulation processes. For example, corticosteroids and nonsteroidal anti-inflammatory drugs (NSAIDs) inhibit prostaglandins in the periphery, disrupting transduction.[31] Topical capsaicin cream inhibits substance P.[32] Anticonvulsants such as gabapentin and pregabalin are nerve stabilizers and interrupt transmission of pain by preventing depolarization. Opioids work at the dorsal horn of the spinal cord by binding to receptors to prevent transmission to the higher brain centers. Psychosocial interventions and cognitive-behavioral therapy alter the amount of pain perceived by the brain.[33] Tricyclic antidepressants exert effects during modulation by blocking the reuptake of dopamine, serotonin, and norepinephrine within the synapse in the dorsal horn of the spinal cord.

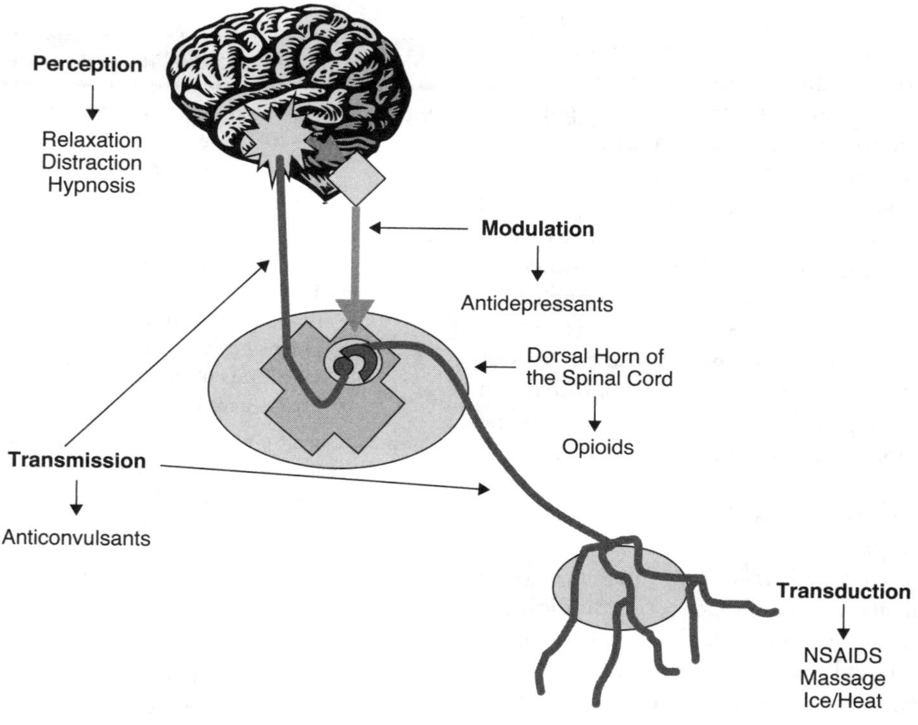

FIGURE 5-1

Pathophysiological mechanisms of pain and pharmacologic interventions.

Source: Data from Brant[30]. Used with permission.

CANCER PAIN PATHOPHYSIOLOGY

The pathophysiological mechanisms of cancer pain include both acute and chronic mechanisms. Acute pain can be described as pain that resolves with healing over time. Usually nociceptive, acute pain serves as a warning sign for impending injury. Psychological components are involved such as fear and depression, which can remodel the nervous system and provoke chronic pain.

Chronic pain, historically defined as pain that extends beyond 6 months of healing time, is now recognized as a complex phenomenon that no longer serves to protect function but rather disrupts sleep, activities of daily living, and quality of life. Chronic pain can be nociceptive, neuropathic, or both. In extreme situations, it can be accompanied by central sensitization, a state of spinal neuron excitability. "Wind-up" occurs as repeated stimulation of the nerve fibers causes an increase in dorsal horn neuron firing. When this occurs, pain progressively increases over time. Eventually, central inhibition is reduced in response to the pain, dorsal horn neuronal activity becomes spontaneous, and neurons that are usually mildly responsive are recruited to fire. This phenomenon can result in hyperalgesia, allodynia, persistent pain, and/or referred pain (Table 5-1). The potential for central sensitization calls for an aggressive plan to manage pain in its current state to prevent "wind-up" and further sequelae.[29]

SYMPTOM ASSESSMENT

Pain assessment begins with an understanding of patients who may be at risk for developing pain, an understanding of patients who may be at risk for the under-treatment of pain, and a comprehensive history and physical exam. While it may be helpful to diagnostically determine the etiology of the pain, it is never a requirement for the management of pain. Because the patient's report of pain is the most reliable indicator of its presence, it is the most significant assessment parameter.

RISK FACTORS

While pain is present in more than 50% of patients with cancer, some patients may be at greater risk.[22] As noted, a greater percentage of those patients with head and neck cancer have been found to have pain as well as those patients with gynecologic or gastrointestinal malignancies. Patients whose disease has metastasized are also at increased risk.[22] Recognition of the disease characteristics that are associated with greater risk allows clinicians to anticipate potential problems and include pain management education into the plan of care early, even prior to the onset of pain.

Some patient populations may also be at increased risk for under-treatment of pain, such as minority patients, older adults, and patients with a disease of addiction. Minority patients, especially those who speak English as a second language, may be at increased risk due to lack of communication and other biases. In one study, pain was underestimated in 64% of Hispanics and 74% of African Americans. Inadequate pain assessment was named as the primary gap for minority patients and linked to inadequate pain management.[20] Lay educators and others who speak the patient's language can assist with the overall assessment and education about pain.[21]

Older adults are another high-risk population. Loss of hearing and visual acuity may impede communication, as may dementia and memory loss. Despite these challenges, clinicians should recognize that self-assessment pain scales can often be used reliably in older patients with mild to moderate dementia, and even in some individuals with severe dementia. Behavioral scales should be used only in patients who cannot complete a self-assessment.[34] Behavioral scales can detect possible pain, but currently no standardized scale exists and existing tools are in early development.[35] Guidelines for assessing pain in older adults are included in Table 5-4.[1,35]

Patients with a disease of addiction are another high-risk population for under-treatment of pain and for misuse of opioid analgesics.[36] Lack of trust, provider lack of knowledge about addiction, and opiophobia may interfere with optimal management. Active substance abuse brings about additional challenges, as providers attempt to manage pain without contributing to the problem of addiction.[37] In addition to the pain assessment, clinicians will need to assess for risks of addiction. Behaviors that are less predictive of aberrancy include drug hoarding, aggressive demands for higher doses, occasional unsanctioned dose escalation, psychiatric side effects, and requests for specific drugs. Behaviors more predictive of aberrancy include selling and forging prescriptions, concurrent illicit drug use, multiple prescription losses, multiple dose escalations, stealing drugs, using a nonsanctioned route of administration, and repeated resistance to the recommended treatment plan.[38] Outcomes of opioid therapy in patients with a disease of addiction should include the four "A's": (1) **a**nalgesic response or pain relief, (2) **a**ctivities of daily living or physical, social, and emotional functioning, (3) **a**dverse effects of the prescribed analgesics, and (4) **a**berrant drug-seeking behaviors suggesting active addiction.[38] Ongoing communication and assessment are keys to maintaining comfort while preventing misuse, abuse, and diversion.

TABLE 5-4

Five Step Approach to Pain Assessment in Older Adults

Step 1	Attempt to obtain a self-report of pain. Options include: • "0–10" scale • Verbal descriptor scale • Vertical pain thermometer
Step 2	If unable to use a self-report, search for potential causes of the pain: • Trauma • Bladder distention • History of chronic pain • Decubitus ulcer • Progressive cancer
Step 3	Observe patient behaviors using a behavioral rating scale. Types of pain behaviors include: • Facial expressions • Verbal and vocal indicators • Body movements • Change in interpersonal interaction • Change in activity pattern or routine • Mental status change Nonverbal tool examples for use in older adults: • Assessment of Discomfort in Dementia Protocol (ADD) • Checklist of Nonverbal Pain Indicators (CNPI) • Doloplus 2 • Nursing Assistant-Administered Instrument to Assess Pain in Demented Individuals (NOPPAIN) • Pain Assessment Scale for Seniors with Severe Dementia (PACSLAC) • Pain Assessment in Advanced Dementia Scale (PAINAD)
Step 4	Ask family members to aid in the assessment. Ask about: • Typical behavior • Changes in behavior – families can detect subtle changes • Changes in cognition
Step 5	If Step 1 through Step 4 suggests the patient may be in pain: • ASSUME PAIN PRESENT • Use an analgesic trial and assess if there is a decrease in potential pain behaviors or improved cognition

Source: Data from American Geriatrics Society[1]; Herr et al[35].

SELF-ASSESSMENT AND PAIN HISTORY

The patient's report of pain is the most valuable component of a comprehensive pain assessment, and pain should be managed according to the patient's report of pain. Onset, location, duration, characteristics, aggravating factors, relieving factors, and treatment (OLDCART) can be used to systematically assess the physiological components of the pain (Table 5-5).[7] Information should be gathered for each

TABLE 5-5

Comprehensive Pain Assessment

Domain	Pain Assessment Components
Physical	• **O**nset – When did the pain start? • **L**ocation – Where is the pain located? Is there more than one location? • **D**uration – How often does the pain occur? Is it constant or intermittent? How long does the pain last? ○ Breakthrough pain (BTP) ■ Follow OLDCART assessment ■ Number of episodes per day ■ Incident versus idiopathic • Differentiate from end of dose pain ■ Onset and duration of BTP episodes ■ How the BTP responds to pharmacologic and nonpharmacologic interventions • **C**haracteristics – How does the pain feel? What words would you use to describe the pain? ○ Intensity ■ 0–10 scale preferred ■ Verbal descriptor scale (mild, moderate, severe) ■ Others: pain thermometer, visual analog scale, nonverbal scales as indicated ○ Patient descriptors can aid in diagnosing the pain syndrome. ■ Somatic pain (e.g. bone pain) – well localized, constant, dull, aching, gnawing ■ Visceral pain (e.g. abdominal pain) – poorly localized, can be referred, described as cramping, stretching, fullness ■ Neuropathic pain (e.g. peripheral neuropathy) – described as burning, numb, radiating, shock-like • **A**ggravating Factors – What makes your pain worse? ○ Movement – walking, other ○ Positional – sitting, standing, lying down ○ Miscellaneous activity – coughing, sneezing, urinating, moving bowels • **R**elieving Factors – What makes your pain better? ○ Analgesics ○ Positioning, splinting, modifying activity ○ Nonpharmacologic modalities – ice, heat, massage, TENS, cognitive behavioral strategies • **T**reatment – What treatments have you tried to control the pain? How are they working? How do the treatments affect the pain intensity? ○ Pharmacologic ○ Nonpharmacologic
Psychological	• The meaning of pain to the patient and family • History of anxiety, depression, or other psychological illness • Cognition, including confusion or delirium • Usual coping strategies in response to pain • Psychological responses to pain and illness such as depression, anxiety, and fear • Beliefs about opioids, addiction, and other concerns • Willingness to try complementary modalities such as cognitive behavioral therapy
Social	• Functional assessment: Interference of pain on daily living including physical or social withdrawal from activity • Family communication and response to illness • Support system • Economic impact of the pain and its treatment (e.g. ability to afford analgesics)
Spiritual/ Existential	• Spiritual beliefs related to pain and illness • Presence of a spiritual community and its role related to pain and illness • Influence of religion or spirituality on coping with pain • Use of traditional medicine in healing

Abbreviation: TENS: transcutaneous nerve stimulation.

Source: Data from Brant[7].

pain location. Aspects of the pain to be considered include both intensity and characteristics.

The pain intensity can be ascertained by asking the patient, "On a 0–10 scale, with 0 being no pain and 10 being the worst possible pain, what is your pain?" Quantifying the pain assists in communication between the patient, family, and healthcare team, and can measure the patient response to the interventions. The pain management plan of care can then be modified based on the patient's response. When patients are unable to provide a "0–10" response, alternative assessment tools are available, such as a verbal descriptor scale, pain thermometer, and pain faces scale. A nonverbal pain assessment scale should be used for patients who cannot provide a self-assessment of pain. Duration of the pain can determine whether controlled-release or immediate-release opioids should be employed.[4,39]

One type of intermittent pain—breakthrough pain (BTP)—requires individual assessment. Breakthrough pain is defined as "a transient exacerbation of pain that occurs either spontaneously, or in relation to a specific predictable or unpredictable trigger, despite relatively stable and adequately controlled background pain" (p. 332).[40] Onset, location, duration, characteristics, aggravating and relieving factors, and treatment response of the BTP episodes should be examined.[40]

Pain characteristics include the patient's description of the pain. Descriptors can help identify the etiology of the pain, which aids in the pharmacologic management. For example, if the patient complains of numbness and tingling of the feet following taxane therapy, the clinician assumes peripheral neuropathy and employs analgesics such as anticonvulsants. Aggravating and relieving factors as identified by the patient roll into the pain management plan of care. For example, if a patient complains of pain with movement and activity, analgesics should be given at the appropriate time prior to the activity so that comfort can be attained. Response to treatment should be evaluated on an ongoing basis as well so that therapy can be tailored accordingly. In addition to the physiological assessment, psychological, social, and spiritual influences on pain should be examined.[7,10]

A number of assessment tools are available to report the elements of the pain assessment. The Brief Pain Inventory (BPI) is a tool that can measure both pain intensity and interference of pain with daily functioning. The tool has established validity and reliability in measuring pain across cultures and has been translated in several different languages.[41] Additional scales such as the Edmonton Symptom Assessment Scale and the Rotterdam Symptom Checklist include the measurement of pain along with other global symptoms.[42]

Many healthcare settings are beginning to incorporate electronic pain assessment tools into practice. Electronic tools allow field prompts that guide the clinician through the assessment, ensuring consistency and comprehension. Electronic self-report tools are also available for patients to rate pain and other symptoms prior to clinic visits.[43]

OBJECTIVE ASSESSMENT

While self-assessment of pain is the most reliable indicator of its existence, objective assessment can further identify the etiology of the pain and guide treatment options. Both physical and diagnostic evaluations are critical in identifying and then treating the underlying causes of the pain.

Physical assessment

A physical assessment includes a head-to-toe examination with a focus on the neurological assessment. Initially, the clinician should observe the patient and identify overt signs of pain such as splinting or grimacing and more subtle signs of pain such as fatigue, exhaustion and sleep deprivation, and signs of depression that often cluster with pain.[44] The site of the pain should be assessed using observation, palpation, percussion, and, if indicated, auscultation. Color changes, edema, and tenderness with palpation and percussion assist in pinpointing the specific area.

Tests (brush, pinch, pin prick, and/or scratch) should be conducted to assess for allodynia, hyperalgesia, or hyperesthesia (see Table 5-1 for definitions). Sensory evaluation can detect different types of neuropathy. Reduced sensation to vibration as detected with a tuning fork or loss of proprioception can indicate large neuronal fiber damage. Small-diameter neuronal fiber damage is indicated by changes in temperature sensation and touch sensation using the pin-prick test.

Motor abnormalities or deficits and lack of coordination can also indicate neurologic problems. The musculoskeletal system should be observed, and causes of pain identified. Body posture, gait, and lack of symmetry can indicate compensation for pain and could lead to further sequelae. Patients may also limit range of motion when pain is severe. For example, women post-mastectomy can develop a painful frozen shoulder if range of motion is not maintained.[45]

Diagnostic evaluation

Radiographic exams can diagnose the underlying problem of the pain. Computed tomography (CT) scans can visualize tumor progression, magnetic resonance imaging (MRI) allows good visualization of nerve impingement and central nervous system involvement, and bone scans detect the extent of bony metastases. Laboratory analyses such as an increase in tumor marker levels and liver enzymes can also suggest pain related to progressive disease. The extent of the diagnostic work-up is related to the patient's goals of care. As goals move toward palliation, clinicians rely more on the patient's self-assessment and history. However, when pain can be ameliorated by radiation therapy or other cancer treatment modalities, the diagnostic evaluation is essential to obtain prior to the palliative treatment.[45]

DEGREES OF TOXICITY

The National Cancer Institute's Common Terminology Criteria for Adverse Events (CTCAE) includes comprehensive descriptive terminology to measure symptoms related to cancer and the manifestations of cancer treatment.[46] Within the CTCAE, which is often used to measure toxicity related to clinical trials, various types of pain are differentiated. While the overall CTCAE scale ranges from 0 to 5, pain is measured using a 0 to 3 scale where 0 is no pain, 1 is mild pain, 2 is moderate pain limiting instrumental activities of daily living (ADLs), and 3 is severe pain limiting self-care. One benefit of the criteria is the all-inclusive list of pain syndromes represented. The list reminds clinicians of the multitude of pain syndromes that can be experienced by patients with cancer. A limitation of the CTCAE is the lack of detail to each of the ratings, thereby limiting its usefulness. Clinicians should be reminded that these criteria are staging systems of pain but should not replace the pain assessment.

SYMPTOM MANAGEMENT STRATEGIES

PREVENTIVE STRATEGIES

A number of interventions can be employed to prevent pain in some patients. First, patients should be reminded to take analgesics as prescribed, often around the clock (ATC) to maintain a therapeutic blood level of the opioid and to prevent pain. Breakthrough pain medication should be taken, if possible, at the first indication of pain. For patients with predictable incident pain, the opioid analgesic should be employed at an appropriate interval according to the pharmacokinetics of the medication prior to the activity. This ensures that the opioid is peaking during the painful activity.

Novel strategies are also being investigated in the prevention of postoperative pain. For many patients with cancer, surgery is the initial painful experience. The use of preemptive analgesia is important to prevent peripheral and central sensitization, thereby preventing wind-up and postoperative injury. NSAIDs, gabapentin, and opioids are commonly used, but more research is needed to determine the optimal dose and schedule for these preemptive agents.[47,48]

Bone-modifying agents, which are now standard treatment in patients with lytic bone lesions, can prevent skeletal events such as fractures and subsequent bone pain related to bony metastases. Bisphosphonates such as pamidronate and zoledronic acid inhibit osteoclast-mediated bone resorption. Denosumab is a novel bone-modifying monoclonal antibody that binds to a protein called RANKL, which is responsible for the production, function, and survival of osteoclasts.[49]

THERAPEUTIC APPROACHES

Cancer treatment

Surgery, antineoplastic therapy, and radiation therapy can all be used to decrease tumor burden, thereby alleviating pain. While some cancer therapies can cause significant side effects and should be carefully weighed according to patient goals and disease status, other therapies are associated with few sequelae and may be considered even toward the end of life.

Surgery can be employed to resect tumor away from surrounding organs, bones, and nerves to prevent disease complications and alleviate pain. Specific surgical interventions for vertebral metastases include vertebroplasty and kyphoplasty. Both procedures can be performed with minimal invasion, are well tolerated, and can provide timely reduction in pain.[50,51] Bowel resection, decompression laminectomy, and renal stent placement are additional surgical procedures employed to manage pain caused by cancer.

Antineoplastic therapy such as chemotherapy, targeted therapy, biological therapy, and hormonal therapy may decrease tumor burden, thereby alleviating pain. However, the goal of antineoplastic therapy is rarely pain control, as the side effects of the treatment often outweigh benefits.

Radiation therapy is commonly employed to manage painful bone metastases. One study revealed that approximately 25% of patients achieved complete pain relief at 1 month and more than 50% at 4 weeks. The median duration of complete pain relief was 12 weeks.[52] Radioisotopes are another strategy for pain control in patients with disseminated bone metastases. Patients may experience a complete reduction in pain over 1 to 6 months. Pancytopenia is a common side effect and should be considered in terms of the risk–benefit ratio.[53]

Pharmacologic treatment

Pharmacologic therapy is the mainstay of cancer pain management. The approach is multimodal, using a variety of agents that interrupt the pain pathway and the transmission of pain to the brain. WHO has developed a three-step analgesic ladder that guides the pharmacologic management of pain (Figure 5-2).[3] The ladder suggests that when pain occurs, prompt administration of nonopioids should occur, followed by mild opioids (e.g., hydrocodone) as needed

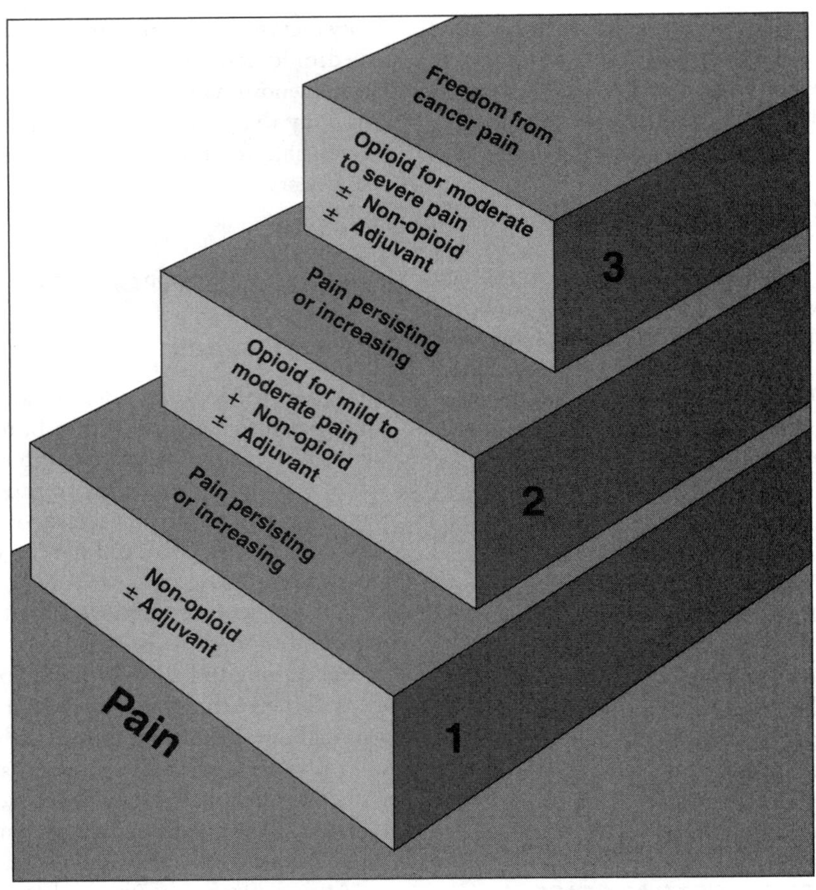

FIGURE 5-2

World health organization analgesic ladder.

Source: Data from World Health Organization, 1990[3]. Used with permission.

and then strong opioids (e.g., morphine) until the patient is comfortable. Adjuvants, also known as co-analgesics, should be used in all three steps to treat specific pain syndromes and the symptoms associated with pain such as anxiety and depression. To maintain freedom from pain, the WHO ladder recommends that analgesics be given ATC. Using the ladder with the right drugs and dosages is inexpensive and is 80%–90% effective.[3]

Nonopioids. Nonopioids, which include acetaminophen, aspirin, and NSAIDs, constitute Step 1 of the WHO ladder. Acetaminophen is often used in combination with opioids for cancer pain management. The mechanism of action for acetaminophen is poorly understood, but it appears to work primarily in the central nervous system. It has fewer adverse gastrointestinal (GI) effects compared to the NSAIDs and lacks antiplatelet effects. Studies suggest that acetaminophen may increase blood pressure[54] and may contribute to over anticoagulation[55,56] when administered with warfarin. Hepatotoxicity is a serious side effect of acetaminophen, and doses should not exceed 4000 mg per day.[2] Recent evidence suggests that even lower doses may be associated with an increased risk of hepatotoxicity.[57]

Aspirin, one of the oldest nonopioid analgesics, is rarely used in cancer pain management. It has been replaced with newer NSAIDs that have more favorable efficacy.

NSAIDs are widely used in cancer pain management and are especially indicated for inflammatory, bone, and joint-related pain.[31] Evidence suggests that using acetaminophen and NSAIDs together is superior compared to either drug alone.[58] They work by inhibiting cyclooxygenase (COX), a catalyst enzyme responsible for converting arachidonic acid (a cell-wall fatty acid) to prostaglandin (PGE_2), prostacyclin (PGI_2), and thromboxane A_2 (TXA_2). By blocking COX and subsequent prostaglandin production in the central and peripheral nervous systems, NSAIDs reduce inflammation. Two types of COX exist. Cyclooxygenase-1 is found in most human tissues, including the GI tract, platelets, and kidneys, whereas COX-2 is concentrated primarily in the kidneys, central nervous system, and peripheral tissues during painful and inflammatory states. Therefore, prostaglandins protect the gastrointestinal tract, allow for platelet aggregation, and provide vasodilation for adequate blood flow in the kidneys and other tissues. Inhibiting cyclooxygenase and subsequent prostaglandin production produces the significant side effects exhibited, including GI toxicity, bleeding, and renal compromise.[2]

NSAIDs are categorized according to their ability to inhibit both COX-1 and COX-2 (nonselective) or selectively COX-2. The majority of NSAIDs are nonselective, and celecoxib is the only selective COX-2 inhibitor currently approved by the Food and Drug Administration (FDA). While all NSAIDs can produce GI side effects including ulceration, bleeding, and perforation, evidence suggests that the COX-2 NSAIDs exhibit fewer GI effects compared to the nonselective NSAIDs. Patients should take NSAIDs with food to minimize these effects. In addition, COX-2 NSAIDs do not inhibit platelet function. One limitation is their increased risk of prothrombotic and related cardiovascular events. Central nervous system effects such as short-term memory loss, loss of concentration, decreased attention span, and confusion can also occur, likely due to prostaglandin inhibition in the central nervous system.[2,59]

Opioids. Opioids are the mainstay of cancer pain management and are included in both Step 2 and Step 3 of the WHO analgesic ladder. Opioids work by binding to mu (μ), kappa (κ), and delta (δ) receptors at the dorsal horn of the spinal cord and in the peripheral nervous system. While several opioids are available for use, agonist-antagonist opioids are not recommended for cancer pain control due to their psychomimetric effects and ceiling dose. These opioids that bind to κ and/or λ antagonize μ, which can precipitate withdrawal in patients taking pure μ agonists. Meperidine is one μ agonist that is not recommended in cancer pain management. Its toxic metabolite, normeperidine, can accumulate and cause central nervous system toxicity and seizures.[2]

Individual response to opioids occurs and can be explained by the polymorphic *OPRM1* gene that has multiple μ receptor subtypes. Approximately 20% to 30% of the population has heterozygous changes in alleles of the *OPRM1* gene, influencing pain sensitivity. Patients with the *OPRM1* GG genotype require higher doses of morphine compared to those patients with the *OPRM1* AA genotype.[60] Thus opioid therapy should be tailored per patient response. Patients also report better response from other opioids, but little is known about these individual variations. Following is a discussion of the opioids used to control cancer pain, and a summary of opioids is included in Table 5-6.

Morphine is the standard of comparison for all opioids and is efficacious in the management of cancer pain.[61] It is available via oral, suppository, and parenteral routes of administration, with the oral formulation being available in both controlled- and immediate-release preparations. Because of its poor oral bioavailability, the onset of effect for the immediate-release version is at least 30 minutes; it is 90 minutes for the controlled-release product.

Morphine is metabolized in the liver through glucoronidation to morphine-3-glucoronide (M3G) and morphine-6-gluconoride (M6G). M3G antagonizes morphine and is thought to be responsible for many of the adverse effects of the drug such as myoclonus, hallucinations, and hyperalgesia. M6G is more potent than the morphine itself and can add to the overall analgesic effect, which can increase over time with retention of the metabolites. Both metabolites can accumulate in patients with renal compromise, resulting in possible oversedation and an increase in other toxicities. The dose of morphine should be lowered in patients with renal insufficiency or an alternative opioid should be considered.[2]

Morphine is associated with additional side effects. It causes histamine release, which can lead to bronchospasm and hypotension. Anaphylaxis can also occur in patients with sulfa allergies when given morphine parenterally due to the presence of sulfites. Respiratory depression can occur and respiratory acidosis can result in increased morphine delivery to the brain and further respiratory compromise. Orthostatic hypotension, pruritus, and nausea and vomiting are additional side effects.

Oxycodone is 1.5 times stronger than morphine and is a useful oral opioid for the control of cancer pain. It is available in the pure form or combined with acetaminophen. Clinicians should use the pure form for BTP when the acetaminophen dose exceeds 4000 mg/day. Oxycodone is metabolized by CYP2D6 to oxymorphone, but the parent drug is responsible for the analgesic effect.[62]

Oxymorphone is a newer, synthetic and lipophilic opioid that is 10 times more potent than morphine. Drug–drug reactions with this agent are rare due to its lack of DYP2D6 or CYP3A4 metabolism. Its reduced histamine release can also be an advantage for patients who complain of histamine-related side effects such as pruritus and headache.[62]

Hydrocodone is a commonly used opioid but lacks usefulness in chronic cancer pain management due to its combination with acetaminophen. It is metabolized by CYP2D6 into hydromorphone. It is suggested in the literature that hydrocodone is a prodrug, so those patients who lack CYP2D6 may not achieve the full analgesic benefit; however, human studies of this effect are sparse.

Hydromorphone is a semi-synthetic opioid that is 7 to 10 times stronger than morphine. The recent approval of a sustained-release preparation has expanded the role of hydromorphone in managing cancer pain.

TABLE 5-6

Opioids Used to Manage Cancer Pain

Opioid	Preparations	Equianalgesic Ratios: Oral	Equianalgesic Ratios: IV	Common Side Effects	Comments
Morphine	• Oral: Controlled release (CR), Immediate release (IR), Oral solution • Rectal • Parenteral: Intravenous (IV) or subcutaneous (SC) • Intraspinal preservative free (PF)	30	10	• Respiratory depression • Nausea and vomiting • Pruritus • Orthostatic hypotension • Urinary retention • Constipation	• Standard for opioid comparison • Metabolites M3G and M6G can accumulate with renal compromise • Histamine release can cause bronchospasm and hypotension • Parenteral forms contain sulfites; patients with sulfa allergies may experience anaphylaxis
Fentanyl	• Transdermal (TD) • Transmucosal • Nasal • Parenteral: IV, SC • Intraspinal Preservative Free (PF)	–	0.1	• Similar to morphine	• Highly lipophilic • Onset and duration of action variable and dependent on route • TD onset 12 hours, peak 24–48 hours; potency of 25 ug TD fentanyl equal to approximately 30–75 mg morphine/day; remains in system approximately 24 hours after discontinuation • Transmucosal onset usually within 15 minutes • Nasal onset within 5 minutes • Parenteral onset within 5–10 minutes • Metabolized by CYP3A4 • Should not cut or tamper with the patch; heating the patch can cause overdose and death
Hydrocodone	• Oral: IR with acetaminophen or aspirin, oral solution	30	–	• Similar to morphine	• Proposed as a prodrug that must be metabolized by CYP2D6 enzyme prior to achieving an analgesic effect; patients who are CYP2D6 deficient may achieve less clinical benefit with hydrocodone, but studies are sparse
Hydromorphone	• Oral: CR, IR • Rectal • Parenteral: IV, SC • Intraspinal PF	7.5	1.5	• Similar to morphine • Not associated with histamine release	• May be preferred in patients with renal insufficiency • Extensive metabolism by the liver to primarily H3G and to some extent H6G; M3G accumulation can cause allodynia, myoclonus, and seizures in animal models
Oxycodone	• Oral: CR, IR with and without acetaminophen, oral solution	20	–	• Similar to morphine	• 1.5 times more potent than morphine • Parenteral preparation unavailable • Metabolized by CYP2D6; drug-drug interactions may occur with 2D6 inhibitors
Oxymorphone	• Oral: CR, IR • Parenteral: IV, SC • Rectal	10	1	• Similar to morphine • Reduced histamine effect	• To be administered on an empty stomach; food increases the maximum concentration • Do not administer with alcohol • No CYP450 drug-drug interactions

(continued)

TABLE 5-6

Opioids Used to Manage Cancer Pain (continued)

Opioid	Preparations	Equianalgesic Ratios: Oral	IV	Common Side Effects	Comments
					• Contraindicated in moderate and severe hepatic impairment • Dose reduce in patients with renal compromise and mild hepatic impairment • May be useful in patients with a morphine allergy or in those who experience itching or headache with other opioids
Methadone	• Oral: long acting • Rectal • Parenteral			• Similar to morphine • High risk of respiratory depression due to long half-life • QTc prolongation with doses > 100 mg/day	• Long half-life (up to 150 hours) allows for less frequent dosing but accumulation of drug • N-methyl-D-aspartate (NMDA) antagonism may be beneficial to prevent tolerance and manage neuropathic pain syndromes • Metabolized by P450 with potential for drug-drug interactions • Only experienced practitioners with substantial knowledge of methadone pharmacokinetics should prescribe methadone

While this agent has two metabolites (similar to morphine), hydromorphone-3-glucoronide (H3G) and hydromorphone-6-glucoronide (H6G), studies are sparse regarding the clinical effects of these metabolites. Hydromorphone lacks histamine release so is also helpful in patients who report histamine-related side effects.

Methadone is a synthetic, lipophilic, pure μ opioid agonist that has a long history in the management of cancer pain. It also has a role in addiction maintenance, which sometimes creates a stigma for this opioid. In addition to its pain-relieving properties, methadone demonstrates N-methyl-D-aspartate (NMDA) antagonism, which may confer benefits in the management of neuropathic pain syndromes[63]; however, a recent Cochrane review indicated that methadone was not superior to morphine.[64] Additional studies are needed in this area. Antagonizing the NMDA receptor has also been shown to prevent opioid tolerance, central nervous system desensitization, and hyperalgesia.

Although methadone has several advantages, its high affinity for protein and subsequently long half-life can lead to oversedation, respiratory depression, and fatal overdose when not accurately prescribed. The increased use of methadone over the last decade has resulted in a number of deaths that prompted the FDA to revise the package insert for methadone in 2006 to include clearer dosing guidelines.[65] Only clinicians with in-depth knowledge of methadone's pharmacokinetic profile should prescribe this opioid.

Fentanyl is a strong, lipophilic μ agonist commonly used for cancer pain management. Its pharmacokinetics varies significantly depending on the route of administration. When given transdermally (TD), fentanyl must first saturate the subcutaneous tissue prior to onset of pain relief, which usually occurs at approximately 12 hours. Short-acting analgesics should be used judiciously when initiating TD fentanyl because of this lag in onset. Titration should occur only at steady state, which is reached at 72 hours after administration. Some patients who experience end-of-dose failure prior to the three-day patch change may need to change the patch every two days. Transdermal fentanyl is contraindicated in opioid-naïve patients. Parenteral fentanyl, whose effect both peaks and dissipates rapidly, is used to manage acute and intractable cancer pain. Acute pain includes postoperative pain and mucositis-induced pain.[2]

Transmucosal fentanyl is an additional entry in the armamentarium for the management of breakthrough cancer pain. Its ease of use and rapid onset are especially beneficial for patients with idiopathic and sudden-onset BTP. Patients report a faster time to pain relief and greater reduction in pain compared to placebo and immediate-release opioids.[66,67] Several preparations exist, including a lollipop, buccal tablet, sublingual tablet, and buccal film. The products vary to some extent in their oral bioavailability, onset, and efficacy.[68]

Nasal fentanyl spray is the newest rapid-onset fentanyl product on the market. It demonstrates an even faster onset to pain relief (as early as 5 minutes) compared to the transmucosal fentanyl products. The product is designed using a pectin-based technology. When the drug comes into contact with mucosal surfaces (the nasal mucosa in this situation), it forms a gel that allows rapid absorption, yet prevents runoff.

Clinicians should keep in mind that dosing with these rapid-onset fentanyl products is unlike that other immediate-release opioids. Titration occurs by using the lowest dose available and titrating gradually upward to efficacy rather than basing the BTP dose on a percentage of the 24-hour opioid dose.[69,70]

Opioids can cause a variety of side effects. While tolerance occurs over time for some side effects such as respiratory depression, other effects, such as constipation, persist throughout treatment. Prevention of side effects is critical. Untoward side effects can affect patient adherence, pain control, and quality of life. The most common opioid-related side effects and strategies for management are included in Table 5-7.

TABLE 5-7

Opioid Side Effects: Pathophysiology and Management

Side Effect	Pathophysiology	Management Strategies
Constipation	• Decrease in normal bowel peristalsis, gastric and pancreatic secretions, increase in anal tone • Tolerance to constipation does not develop	• Prevention is the key • Bowel stimulant (e.g. senna) ± a stool softener for prophylaxis • Other options: polyethylene glycol, magnesium citrate, lactulose, dioctyl sodium sulfosuccinate • Methylnaltrexone – reverses opioid receptors in the gastrointestinal tract
Nausea and Vomiting	• Stimulation of the chemoreceptor trigger zone (CTZ) • Tolerance usually develops within one week.	• Antiemetics around the clock for up to one week if nausea/vomiting occurs with opioids • Rotate opioids if tolerance does not develop
Psychomimetric Effects: sedation, delirium, confusion, agitation, and restlessness	• Stimulation of the central nervous system. • May be related to co-analgesics and/or disease process; not always opioid-induced	• Attempt to identify the cause and modify pharmacologic agents as able • Psychostimulants to counteract sedation • Haloperidol or an antipsychotic for restlessness or agitation.
Pruritus	• Histamine release of some opioids, most commonly morphine	• Antihistamines to counteract pruritis • Nalbuphine may counteract pruritis if associated with intraspinal opioids • Rotate opioids if pruritis persists
Myoclonus	• Generalized or focal sudden, brief, involuntary movements caused by muscle contraction • Can result from the accumulation of the opioid metabolites such as the M_3G metabolite of morphine	• Opioid rotation may help • Administer agents to counteract myoclonus ○ Midazolam infusion starting at 1 mg/hour and titrate upward, shorter half-life than lorazepam and compatible with morphine ○ Lorazepam 1–4 mg q 4 hours as needed or via continuous infusion ○ Dantrolene 50–100 mg per day is an alternative to benzodiazepines that causes less sedation
Respiratory Depression	• Most common in opioid naïve patients and with opioid dose titration.	• Prevention is the key; individualize opioid therapy • Determine if respiratory depression is due to opioid, a co-analgesic, or the dying process. • For life-threatening respiratory depression related to the opioid: dilute 0.4 mg nalaxone in 10 cc normal saline and administer 1 cc every 2–5 minutes; do not administer naloxone too quickly as this can precipitate breakthrough pain and a pain crisis.

Co-analgesics. Co-analgesics are agents that have independent analgesic activity, enhance the efficacy of other pain-relieving agents, or counteract analgesic adverse events. These agents were initially approved for another indication but now have a role in the management of pain—often in the form of neuropathic pain, which can be difficult to control. Categories of some of the more common agents include alpha2-adrenergic agonists, antidepressants, anticonvulsants, benzodiazepines, corticosteroids, local anesthetics, muscle relaxants, NMDA antagonists, and stimulants.[2] A summary of co-analgesics is included in Table 5-8.

Alpha2-Adrenergic Agonists. Clonidine, an antihypertensive agent, can be used to alleviate neuropathic pain; however, limited data on this indication exist. Clonidine can be administered via the oral, transdermal, or intraspinal route but should be used only in refractory pain due to the limited evidence supporting its use as an analgesic.[2]

Antidepressants. Antidepressants are commonly used in the management of neuropathic pain syndromes such as chemotherapy-induced peripheral neuropathy, postherpetic neuralgia, and malignant nerve infiltration. They also are used as adjuvants in the management of depression and insomnia associated with pain. The agents are thought to work during pain modulation by blocking the reuptake of serotonin, norepinephrine, and/or dopamine at the dorsal horn of the spinal cord. Other theories suggest a role in nerve membrane stabilization and NMDA antagonism effects.[2] Studies suggest that one in three patients treated with a tricyclic antidepressant or venlafaxine will experience moderate relief. Limited evidence exists regarding the use of serotonin-specific antidepressants to manage pain.[71]

Anticonvulsants. Anticonvulsants have become first-line agents in the management of neuropathic pain, but are also helpful in a variety of other pain syndromes, including headaches. Gabapentin is used most commonly due to its cost, efficacy, and favorable toxicity profile. Adult dosing starts at 100 mg to 300 mg at bedtime and can be titrated every three days up to 3600 mg per day in three divided doses.[2] A novel once-daily long-acting gabapentin is now approved for postherpetic neuralgia. Carbemazepine is used less commonly, but some studies suggest it is as efficacious as gabapentin in the management of chronic neuropathic pain. Approximately two-thirds of patients report at least one adverse effect with this drug.[72] Pregabalin is the newest anticonvulsant used for neuropathic pain. Dosing is simpler than with gabapentin, and titration can occur more rapidly. As a result, the therapeutic effect may be reached earlier.[2]

Benzodiazepines. Benzodiazepines help relieve muscle spasm and anxiety associated with pain. They are commonly associated with oversedation and respiratory depression, especially when administered with opioids. While helpful in some patients, these agents should be used with caution due to their side-effect profile.

Corticosteroids. Corticosteroids work by inhibiting prostaglandins and decreasing inflammation caused by tumor or other causes. They are used in a variety of nociceptive and neuropathic pain syndromes, including pain caused by lymphedema, spinal cord compression, brain tumors, and bone metastases. Long-term side effects can be substantial and include hyperglycemia, fluid retention and weight gain, osteoporosis, Cushing syndrome, myopathy, and psychosis. Side effects should be carefully weighed against the benefits of treatment.[2,73]

Local Anesthetics. Local anesthetics are another useful type of co-analgesic for some pain syndromes. They are commonly employed in procedure-related pain such as bone marrow aspiration, pleurodesis, and lumbar puncture. Topical anesthetics such as EMLA are used to prevent pain associated with implantable port access and venipuncture procedures. The topical lidocaine 5% patch is approved for treating pain related to postherpetic neuralgia, but other uses exist, including management of postmastectomy pain and peripheral neuropathy. The patch should be worn for 12 hours and then removed for 12 hours. Several patches can be applied at once, and systemic effects are minimal.[74] Systemic administration of local anesthetics is also effective in relieving some neuropathic pain syndromes.[75]

Muscle Relaxants. Skeletal muscle relaxants are a helpful short-term strategy for pain related to musculoskeletal conditions. Treatment should not continue past a few weeks, as the efficacy of long-term treatment has not been established. Sedation is the most common side effect.[76]

NMDA Antagonists. Blocking the NMDA receptor suggests prevention of tolerance and hyperalgesia as well as efficacy in neuropathic pain management. Methadone has some NMDA antagonism. Other agents include dextromethorphan, which is combined with morphine in a novel agent. Ketamine, an anesthetic agent, is also an NMDA antagonist that can be given orally, intravenously, and intraspinally. Its therapeutic index is narrow, however, and side effects include sedation and hallucinations. NMDA antagonists are typically used for refractory neuropathic pain that is not responsive to opioids, antidepressants, and anticonvulsants.[77,78]

Stimulants. Stimulants are commonly used to counteract sedation caused by opioids and other pain-relieving agents. Methylphenidate is one option. Doses should be administered in the morning and before noon to prevent insomnia at night. Modafinil is a newer stimulant. Other options include caffeine, dextroamphetamine, and atomoxetine.[2] Other miscellaneous agents available as co-analgesics

TABLE 5-8

Co-Analgesics Used in Cancer Pain Management

Drug Class	Daily Adult Starting Dose (Range)	Routes of Administration	Adverse Effects	Indications
Alpha2-Adrenergic Agonists	Clonidine 0.1 mg qday	PO, TD, Intraspinal	Hypotension	Neuropathic pain
Tricyclic Antidepressants	Amitriptyline 10–25 mg hs Nortriptyline 10–25 mg hs Desipramine 10–25 mg hs	PO	Sedation, anticholinergic effects, cardiotoxicity, orthostatic hypotension, confusion, weight gain	Neuropathic pain, such as burning pain, poor sleep
Serotonin Norepinephrine Reuptake Inhibitor Antidepressants	Duloxetine 20 mg qday Venlafaxine 37.5 mg qday	PO	Duloxetine associated with nausea Venlafaxine associated with ECG changes	Neuropathic pain Treat depression and anxiety that exacerbate pain
Anticonvulsants	Gabapentin 100 mg qday or tid Gabapentin ER 300 mg qday Pregabalin 150 mg qday Carbamazapine 100–200 mg bid Clonazapam 0.5–1 mg hs, bid or tid	PO	Sedation, dizziness, ataxia, impaired concentration, peripheral edema Pregabalin associated with weight gain	Neuropathic pain, such as shooting pain Gabapentin for post-herpetic neuralgia
Benzodiazepines	Alprazolam 0.25 mg tid Clonazepam 0.5 mg tid Diazepam 1 mg bid Lorazepam 0.5 mg bid	PO, IV	Sedation, respiratory depression	Relieve anxiety and muscle spasm associated with pain
Corticosteroids	Dexamethasone: 2–4 mg tid, qid, or qday; may give up to 100 mg IV bolus for pain crises Methylprednisolone: 10 mg bid	PO/IV/SC	"Steroid psychosis," dyspepsia, hyperglycemia, Cushinoid syndrome long-term	Cerebral edema, spinal cord compression, bone pain, neuropathic pain, visceral pain
Local Anesthetics	Mexiletine 150 mg qday Lidocaine infusion: 2 mg/kg over 30 minutes Lidocaine 5% patch Capsaicin cream: 0.025% tid	PO IV TD Topical	Lightheadedness, arrhythmias	Neuropathic pain
Muscle Relaxants	Cyclobenzaprine 5 mg tid Carisoprodol 350 mg tid Tizanidine 2 mg hs Metaxalone 400 mg tid	PO	Sedation, dizziness,	Musculoskeletal pain, indicated short-term (2 weeks or less)
N-Methyl-D-asparate antagonists	Dextromethorphan: 15–20 mg tid Ketamine: 0.1 mg/kg	PO IV	Confusion, hallucinations, sedation	Neuropathic pain
Stimulants	Methylphenidate 2.5–5 mg qAM Dextroamphetamine 10 mg qday Modafinil 100 mg qAM	PO	Anxiety, agitation, insomnia	Counteract sedation caused by other analgesics
Antispasmodic	Baclofen 5 mg tid	PO	Muscle weakness, cognitive changes	Musculoskeletal pain and spasms
Bone Modifying Agents	Pamidronate 60–90 mg over 2 hours q 4 weeks Zoledronic acid 4 mg over 15 minutes q 3–4 weeks Denosumab 120 mg q 4 weeks	IV infusion SC	Pain flare, osteonecrosis of the jaw	Osteolytic bone pain, prevention of skeletal events

Abbreviations: PO: oral; TD: transdermal; IV: intravenous; SC: subcutaneous; BID: twice daily; TID: three times daily; HS: hour of sleep; q: every.

include antihistamines, antispasmodics, cannabinoids, and (as previously mentioned) bisphosphonate and radionucleotides. Treating the underlying cause of the pain and symptoms associated with the pain will increase success of the treatment plan.

Routes of administration. The simplest and most effective route of administration should be employed for each individual patient. The oral route is often the first choice for administration, but when it is not intact, other routes must be considered. Transdermal administration is another simple route and is especially helpful for patients who cannot take oral medications or cannot remember to take analgesics around the clock. Use of the transmucosal and nasal routes is becoming increasingly more common with greater use of the rapid-onset fentanyl products for breakthrough cancer pain. Their advantage is the fast onset that occurs following administration. Intravenous and subcutaneous routes can also be employed, especially for patients who have intractable pain uncontrolled with administration of pain relief via simpler routes.

Intraspinal routes of administration, including epidural and intrathecal routes, are additional options. Epidural administration can occur in the acute setting for postoperative pain or in patients with pain that is refractory to other routes. For refractory pain, the epidural catheter is usually tunneled at the waist line and attached to an infusion pump that delivers a continuous infusion of opioid and/or co-analgesic. An optional bolus dose can be programmed into the pump for patients who have BTP. The intrathecal route offers another option for refractory intractable pain. Due to the high risk of infection, this route often involves the placement of an intrathecal pump that delivers a continuous opioid dose to the patient. Because of the smaller doses required for intraspinal administration of opioids, side effects are minimal and patient satisfaction is high.[51,79] Intraspinal delivery poses some challenges, however. This route requires specialized care and resources that may not be available in all settings. The plan of care should be carefully weighed individually with the patient and family.

Analgesic prescribing principles. Analgesics should be administered starting at the lowest, most effective dose to treat the pain. Age, renal function, and other individual characteristics should be taken into consideration when choosing opioids and co-analgesics and when dosing and adjusting analgesics. Titration of opioids should be judicious according to patient response and side effects. Opioid dosing and titration guidelines are included in Table 5-9. For patients whose pain does not respond to escalating analgesic doses or when patients experience intolerable side effects, changing the route of administration or rotating opioids is recommended. Guidelines for opioid rotation are included in Table 5-10.

TABLE 5-9

Opioid Dosing and Titration Guidelines

- Individualize treatment based on personal characteristics and opioid tolerance.
- Initiate therapy at the lowest and most effective dose.
- Give each opioid a fair trial by titrating judiciously to therapeutic efficacy or until the patient experiences untoward side effects.
  - Titrate opioids by approximately 25%–33% for moderately controlled pain
  - Titrate opioids by up to 100% for intractable pain
- Administer analgesics around the clock if pain is constant.
- Administer shorter acting analgesics for breakthrough pain (BTP).
  - BTP dose should be 5%–15% of the 24 hour opioid dose (not applicable for rapid onset fentanyl products and methadone)
  - For patients established on methadone, 10% of the 24 hour methadone dose is recommended for BTP
- Use the simplest route of administration possible.
- Prevent and treat side effects.
- Consider opioid rotation with untoward side effects.
- Do not abruptly withdraw opioid as this will precipitate a withdrawal syndrome.
  - To discontinue opioids, decrease the dose by 10%–25% daily to prevent abstinence syndrome
- Consider an intraspinal route of administration with uncontrolled pain, especially pain that occurs at or below the waist.

Invasive therapeutic approaches

In addition to analgesics, nerve blocks, nerve stimulators, and other procedural interventions are options for the management of cancer-related pain. These interventions are often used as adjuncts to pharmacologic therapy.

A celiac plexus block is recommended as an option for patients with pain related to pancreatic cancer. The treatment involves neurolysis of the celiac plexus nerve, which innervates the pancreas. The procedure is most easily performed using an endoscopic ultrasound, which allows for better visualization of the celiac plexus. While results with this approach are mixed, many patients report better pain control and a reduction of opioid use.[80,81]

Transcutaneous nerve stimulation (TENS) is a noninvasive option but has produced mixed results. While some studies show little effect, others suggest a benefit with TENS.[82] The National Comprehensive Cancer Network (NCCN) guidelines recommend using TENS in addition to pharmacologic therapy.[4]

Sympathetic nervous system blockade and vertebroplasty are additional options for pain control.[51]

Nonpharmacologic management

A plethora of nonpharmacologic modalities exist to complement the pharmacologic management of pain. A growing body of evidence demonstrates the impact of

TABLE 5-10

Opioid Rotation

1. Calculate the current opioid dose:
   a. Add the amount of all opioids given over a 24 hour period for the past 2–3 days
      i. Morphine Day 1 total: 60 mg every 8 hours + MSIR 15 mg (6 doses) = 270 mg
      ii. Morphine Day 2 total: 60 mg every 8 hours + MSIR 15 mg (7 doses) = 285 mg
   b. Take the average from the past 2–3 days
      i. 270 mg + 285 mg = 555 mg ÷ 277.5 mg/day or approximately 280 mg
2. Calculate the equianalgesic dose of the new opioid based on the equianalgesic table.
   a. $\frac{30 \text{ mg morphine}}{20 \text{ mg oxycodone}} = \frac{280 \text{ mg morphine}}{x \text{ mg oxycodone}}$
   b. *Cross multiply: 30x = 5600, x = approximately 187 mg oxycodone per day*
3. Consider decreasing the dose of the new opioid by 25%–50% due to lack of cross tolerance
   a. Consider current degree of pain relief; may be unnecessary to reduce the dose if pain is intractable
   b. Consider 50% reduction with older age, minority race, comorbidities, and risk factors for oversedation; decrease dose if risk factors exist
   c. Consider 25% reduction if the patient does not have risk factors as stated above
      i. *Patient is opioid tolerant and 50 years old without comorbidities; pain control good but rotation performed due to confusion possibly related to morphine metabolites*
         - *187 mg × .75 (dose reduce by 25%) = 140 mg oxycodone/day*
4. Depending on the opioid, divide the 24 hour dose in every 12 hour or every 8 hour intervals; does not apply for transdermal fentanyl
   a. *140 mg ÷ 2 doses per day = 70 mg every 12 hours*
5. Increase breakthrough medication to equal 5%–15% of 24 hour dose
   a. *140 mg × .05 (5%) = 7 mg; oxycodone given in 5 mg increments so dose would equal 10–15 mg oxycodone immediate release every 3 hours as needed for breakthrough pain*
6. Methadone rotation:
   a. Calculate the 24 hour current opioid dose in morphine equivalents using an equianalgesic table (as above)
   b. Calculate the methadone dose based on the morphine equivalents:
      i. <90 mg morphine equivalents/day: 1:4 methadone to morphine
      ii. 90 mg to 300 mg morphine equivalents/day: 1:8 methadone to morphine
      iii. >300 mg morphine equivalents/day: 1:12 methadone to morphine
      iv. >800 mg morphine equivalents/day: 1:15–20 methadone to morphine
   c. Divide the methadone dose at 8 hour fixed intervals
   d. May use 10% the 24 hour methadone dose for breakthrough pain

Abbreviation: MSIR: morphine sulfate immediate release.

nonpharmacologic modalities such as institutional initiatives, educational interventions, cognitive-behavioral therapy, massage, and others. While the results of most of these studies are mixed, these modalities may provide some benefit and should be incorporated as able into practice.

Institutional quality initiatives have had mixed results in improving pain. Continued efforts are needed with studies that standardize the intervention and dose of various interventions so that improvement efforts can be replicated for improvement.[83] Patient education is a key component of nursing care. Evidence suggests that patient education has positive effects on pain intensity and patient knowledge about pain.[84] Cognitive-behavioral therapy such as that focusing on distraction, relaxation, and positive mood can decrease anxiety associated with pain and has been shown to improve pain intensity scores.[85] The NCCN guidelines recommend training in cognitive-behavioral therapy to improve pain and associated symptoms.[86] Music therapy in another complementary intervention that may improve pain intensity and decrease opioid requirements.[87] Therapeutic touch, massage, hypnosis, and exercise are additional measures that can be offered and employed based on patient preference.

NURSING IMPLICATIONS

Nurses play a direct role in the assessment and management of pain for patients across the cancer trajectory. Nursing interventions have a direct effect on pain care quality and pain outcomes, reinforcing pain as a nursing-sensitive patient outcome. These outcomes include changes in function, physical and psychosocial symptoms, safety, and costs. Pain is an important nursing-sensitive patient outcome in that nursing care can have a direct impact on the quality of pain assessment and management. The frequency of pain assessment, components of pain assessment, attitudes toward patients' pain, timeliness of analgesic administration, nonpharmacologic modalities, and patient education are all influenced by nursing care.[88] Quality measurement of pain care and nursing-sensitive patient outcomes related to pain management should occur on an ongoing basis. The Pain Care Quality Survey is one tool incorporating a subscale that measures the quality of nursing care.[89]

Overall, nurses have a primary responsibility to deliver quality pain care. Being armed with evidence-based information on the assessment and management of pain is the first step. However, knowledge alone does not ensure quality pain management. In addition, nurses have a responsibility to practice according to the best evidence available. Implementation of evidence-based strategies requires ongoing commitment and advocacy for patient comfort and well-being.

PATIENT SELF-CARE

Patient self-care is important in producing safe and efficacious pain management. Nurses have a primary responsibility in providing both written and verbal instructions to patients regarding when to report pain, what to report about their pain, and how the pain management plan of care works, including how to take medications safely. For example, differentiating between long-acting and short-acting opioids (which can be confusing for patients) and describing each analgesic's purpose is an important part of the pain management plan of care. The benefits of good pain management should be reinforced so that the patient and family are aware that comfort is an essential component of healing and quality of life. See Appendix 5A for a Self-Care Guide to assist patients in describing their pain to the healthcare provider and strategies for prevention and management of pain. Overall, the more that patients and families are informed about their care, the more likely they are to have positive pain outcomes.

REFERENCES

1. American Geriatrics Society. Pharmacological management of persistent pain in older persons. *Pain Med.* 2009;10(6):1062–1083.
2. American Pain Society. *Principles of Analgesic Use in the Treatment of Acute Pain and Cancer Pain* (6th ed.). Glenview, IL: APS Press; 2008.
3. World Health Organization. WHO's pain ladder. 2012. http://www.who.int/cancer/palliative/painladder/en/. Accessed July 28, 2012
4. Swarm R, Abernethy AP, Anghelescu DL, et al. Adult cancer pain. *J Natl Compr Canc Netw.* 2010;8(9):1046–1086.
5. Young JL, Davidhizar R. Attitude: impact on pain assessment. *J Pract Nurs.* 2008;58(2):6–10.
6. International Association for the Study of Pain. Pain Definitions. *IASP Taxonomy.* 2012. http://www.iasp-pain.org/Content/NavigationMenu/GeneralResourceLinks/PainDefinitions/default.htm#Pain. Accessed December 24, 2012.
7. Brant JM. The global experience of cancer pain. *Asian Pacific J Cancer Prev.* 2010;11(MECC supplement):7–12.
8. Ferrell B, Paice J, Koczywas M. New standards and implications for improving the quality of supportive oncology practice. *J Clin Oncol.* 2008;26(23):3824–3831.
9. Ferrell B, Virani R. National guidelines for palliative care: a roadmap for oncology nurses. *Oncology (Williston Park).* 2008;22(2 suppl nurse ed):28–34; discussion 34–25.
10. Ferrell B, Levy MH, Paice J. Managing pain from advanced cancer in the palliative care setting. *Clin J Oncol Nurs.* 2008;12(4):575–581.
11. Breuer B, Fleishman SB, Cruciani RA, Portenoy RK. Medical oncologists' attitudes and practice in cancer pain management: a national survey. *J Clin Oncol.* 2011;29(36):4769–4775.
12. Jacobsen R, Liubarskiene Z, Moldrup C, Christrup L, Sjogren P, Samsanaviciene J. Barriers to cancer pain management: a review of empirical research. *Medicina (Kaunas).* 2009;45(6):427–433.
13. Lewthwaite BJ, Jabusch KM, Wheeler BJ, et al. Nurses' knowledge and attitudes regarding pain management in hospitalized adults. *J Contin Educ Nurs.* 2011;42(6):251–257; quiz 258–259.
14. American Academy of Pain Medicine, American Pain Society, American Society of Addiction Medicine. *Definitions Related to the Use of Opioids for the Treatment of Pain.* Glenview, IL: American Pain Society; 2001.
15. Food and Drug Administration. Approved risk evaluation and mitigation strategies. 2012. http://www.fda.gov/Drugs/DrugSafety/PostmarketDrugSafetyInformationforPatientsandProviders/ucm111350.htm. Accessed March 30, 2012.
16. Cahana A, Arigoni F, Robert L. Attitudes and beliefs regarding the role of interventional pain management at the end-of-life among caregivers: a 4-year perspective. *Pain Pract.* 2007;7(2):103–109.
17. Cleeland CS. Barriers to the management of cancer pain. *Oncology (Williston Park).* 1987;1(2 suppl):19–26.
18. Glajchen M, Fitzmartin RD, Blum D, Swanton R. Psychosocial barriers to cancer pain relief. *Cancer Pract.* 1995;3(2):76–82.
19. Delgado-Guay MO, Bruera E. Management of pain in the older person with cancer. *Oncology (Williston Park).* 2008;22(1):56–61.
20. Anderson KO, Mendoza TR, Valero V, et al. Minority cancer patients and their providers: pain management attitudes and practice. *Cancer.* 2000;88(8):1929–1938.
21. Fairchild A. Under-treatment of cancer pain. *Curr Opin Support Palliat Care.* 2010;4(1):11–15.
22. van den Beuken-van Everdingen MH, de Rijke JM, Kessels AG, Schouten HC, van Kleef M, Patijn J. Prevalence of pain in patients with cancer: a systematic review of the past 40 years. *Ann Oncol.* 2007;18(9):1437–1449.
23. Desbiens NA, Wu AW, Broste SK, et al. Pain and satisfaction with pain control in seriously ill hospitalized adults: findings from the SUPPORT research investigations. For the SUPPORT investigators. Study to Understand Prognoses and Preferences for Outcomes and Risks of Treatmentm. *Crit Care Med.* 1996;24(12):1953–1961.
24. Miaskowski C. Gender differences in pain, fatigue, and depression in patients with cancer. *J Natl Cancer Inst Monogr.* 2004(32):139–143.
25. Brant JM. Pain and discomfort. In: Lester JL, Schmitt P, eds. *Cancer Rehabilitation and Survivorship.* Pittsburgh: Oncology Nursing Society; 2011:37–48.
26. Bennett MI, Rayment C, Hjermstad M, Aass N, Caraceni A, Kaasa S. Prevalence and aetiology of neuropathic pain in cancer patients: a systematic review. *Pain.* 2012;153(2):359–365.
27. Caraceni A, Portenoy RK. An international survey of cancer pain characteristics and syndromes. IASP Task Force on Cancer Pain. International Association for the Study of Pain. *Pain.* 1999;82(3):263–274.
28. Gold MS, Gebhart GF. Peripheral pain mechanisms and nociceptor sensitization. In: Fishman SM, Rathmell JP, eds. *Bonica's Management of Pain* (4th ed.). Hagerstown, MD: Lippincott & Williams; 2009:24–35.
29. Randich A, Ness T. Modulation of spinal nociceptive processing. In: Fishman SM, Rathmell JP, eds. *Bonica's Management of Pain* (4th ed.). Hagerstown, MD: Lippincott & Williams; 2009:48–60.

30. Brant JM. Strategies to manage pain in palliative care. In: O'Connor M, Lee S, Aranda S, eds. *Palliative Care Nursing: A Guide to Practice* (3rd ed.). Victoria, Australia: Ausmed; 2012:93–113.
31. McNicol ED. NSAIDs or paracetamol, alone or combined with opioids, for cancer pain. *Cochrane Database Syst Rev.* 2011;6:CD005180.
32. Head KA. Peripheral neuropathy: pathogenic mechanisms and alternative therapies. *Altern Med Rev.* 2006;11(4):294–329.
33. Osborn RL, Demoncada AC, Feuerstein M. Psychosocial interventions for depression, anxiety, and quality of life in cancer survivors: meta-analyses. *Int J Psychiatry Med.* 2006;36(1):13–34.
34. Pautex S, Herrmann F, Le Lous P, Fabjan M, Michel JP, Gold G. Feasibility and reliability of four pain self-assessment scales and correlation with an observational rating scale in hospitalized elderly demented patients. *J Gerontol A Biol Sci Med Sci.* 2005;60(4):524–529.
35. Herr K, Bjoro K, Decker S. Tools for assessment of pain in nonverbal older adults with dementia: a state-of-the-science review. *J Pain Symptom Manage.* 2006;31(2):170–192.
36. Hojsted J, Sjogren P. Addiction to opioids in chronic pain patients: a literature review. *Eur J Pain.* 2007;11(5):490–518.
37. Alford DP, Compton P, Samet JH. Acute pain management for patients receiving maintenance methadone or buprenorphine therapy. *Ann Intern Med.* 2006;144(2):127–134.
38. Passik SD. Issues in long-term opioid therapy: unmet needs, risks, and solutions. *Mayo Clin Proc.* 2009;84(7):593–601.
39. Brant JM. Thorough pain assessment: a nursing imperative. *Oncology (Williston Park).* 2010;24(10 suppl):18–20.
40. Davies AN, Dickman A, Reid C, Stevens AM, Zeppetella G. The management of cancer-related breakthrough pain: recommendations of a task group of the Science Committee of the Association for Palliative Medicine of Great Britain and Ireland. *Eur J Pain.* 2009;13(4):331–338.
41. Cleeland CS, Ryan KM. Pain assessment: global use of the Brief Pain Inventory. *Ann Acad Med Singapore.* 1994;23(2):129–138.
42. Khatcheressian J, Cassel JB, Lyckholm L, Coyne P, Hagenmueller A, Smith TJ. Improving palliative and supportive care in cancer patients. *Oncology (Williston Park).* 2005;19(10):1365–1376; discussion 1377–1368, 1381–1362, 1384 passim.
43. Brant JM, Beck SL, Dudley WN, Cobb P, Pepper G, Miaskowski C. Symptom trajectories during chemotherapy in outpatients with lung cancer colorectal cancer, or lymphoma. *Eur J Oncol Nurs.* 2011;15(5):470–477.
44. Barsevick AM, Whitmer K, Nail LM, Beck SL, Dudley WN. Symptom cluster research: conceptual, design, measurement, and analysis issues. *J Pain Symptom Manage.* 2006;31(1):85–95.
45. Berry PH, Covington EC, Dahl JL, Katz JA, Miaskowski C, eds. *Pain: Current Understanding of Assessment, Management, and Treatments.* Glenview, IL: American Pain Society; 2006.
46. U.S. Department of Health and Human Services. *Common Terminology Criteria for Adverse Events (CTCAE).* National Cancer Institute, Version 4.0. Bethesda, MD: U.S. Department of Health and Human Services; 2009.
47. Ip HY, Abrishami A, Peng PW, Wong J, Chung F. Predictors of postoperative pain and analgesic consumption: a qualitative systematic review. *Anesthesiology.* 2009;111(3):657–677.
48. Ho KY, Gan TJ, Habib AS. Gabapentin and postoperative pain: a systematic review of randomized controlled trials. *Pain.* 2006;126(1–3):91–101.
49. Van Poznak CH, Temin S, Yee GC, et al. American Society of Clinical Oncology executive summary of the clinical practice guideline update on the role of bone-modifying agents in metastatic breast cancer. *J Clin Oncol.* 2011;29(9):1221–1227.
50. Brogan S, Junkins S. Interventional therapies for the management of cancer pain. *J Support Oncol.* 2010;8(2):52–59.
51. Tay W, Ho KY. The role of interventional therapies in cancer pain management. *Ann Acad Med Singapore.* 2009;38(11):989–997.
52. McQuay HJ, Collins SL, Carroll D, Moore RA. Radiotherapy for the palliation of painful bone metastases. *Cochrane Database Syst Rev.* 2008;4:CD001793.
53. Roqué I, Figuls M, Martinez-Zapata MJ, Scott Brown M, Alonso-Coello P. Radioisotopes for metastatic bone pain. *Cochrane Database Syst Rev.* 2011;7:CD003347.
54. Forman JP, Rimm EB, Curhan GC. Frequency of analgesic use and risk of hypertension among men. *Arch Intern Med.* 2007;167(4):394–399.
55. Mahe I, Bertrand N, Drouet L, et al. Interaction between paracetamol and warfarin in patients: a double-blind, placebo-controlled, randomized study. *Haematologica.* 2006;91(12):1621–1627.
56. Parra D, Beckey NP, Stevens GR. The effect of acetaminophen on the international normalized ratio in patients stabilized on warfarin therapy. *Pharmacotherapy.* 2007;27(5):675–683.
57. Watkins PB, Kaplowitz N, Slattery JT, et al. Aminotransferase elevations in healthy adults receiving 4 grams of acetaminophen daily: a randomized controlled trial. *JAMA.* 2006;296(1):87–93.
58. Ong CK, Seymour RA, Lirk P, Merry AF. Combining paracetamol (acetaminophen) with nonsteroidal antiinflammatory drugs: a qualitative systematic review of analgesic efficacy for acute postoperative pain. *Anesth Analg.* 2010;110(4):1170–1179.
59. Agency for Health Research and Quality. *Comparative Effectiveness and Safety of Analgesics for Osteoarthritis.* Comparative Effectiveness Review No. 4. Rockville, MD: Author; 2006.
60. Reyes-Gibby CC, Shete S, Rakvag T, et al. Exploring joint effects of genes and the clinical efficacy of morphine for cancer pain: OPRM1 and COMT gene. *Pain.* 2007;130(1–2):25–30.
61. Wiffen PJ, McQuay HJ. Oral morphine for cancer pain. *Cochrane Database Syst Rev.* 2007;4:CD003868.
62. Trescot AM. Review of the role of opioids in cancer pain. *J Natl Compr Canc Netw.* 2010;8(9):1087–1094.
63. Mannino R, Coyne P, Swainey C, Hansen LA, Lyckholm L. Methadone for cancer-related neuropathic pain: a review of the literature. *J Opioid Manag.* 2006;2(5):269–276.
64. Nicholson AB. Methadone for cancer pain. *Cochrane Database Syst Rev.* 2008;4:CD003971.
65. Terpening CM, Johnson WM. Methadone as an analgesic: a review of the risks and benefits. *W V Med J.* 2007;103(1):14–18.
66. Zeppetella G, Ribeiro MDC. Opioids for the management of breakthrough (episodic) pain in cancer patients. *Cochrane Database Syst Rev.* 2008;1:CD004311.
67. Mercadante S. Managing breakthrough pain. *Curr Pain Headache Rep.* 2011;15(4):244–249.
68. Darwish M, Kirby M, Robertson P Jr, Tracewell W, Jiang JG. Absolute and relative bioavailability of fentanyl buccal tablet and oral transmucosal fentanyl citrate. *J Clin Pharmacol.* 2007;47(3):343–350.
69. Mystakidou K, Panagiotou I, Gouliamos A. Fentanyl nasal spray for the treatment of cancer pain. *Expert Opin Pharmacother.* 2011;12(10):1653–1659.
70. Fisher A, Watling M, Smith A, Knight A. Pharmacokinetics and relative bioavailability of fentanyl pectin nasal spray 100–800 microg in healthy volunteers. *Int J Clin Pharmacol Ther.* 2010;48(12):860–867.
71. Saarto T, Wiffen PJ. Antidepressants for neuropathic pain. *Cochrane Database Syst Rev.* 2010;11:CD005454.
72. Wiffen PJ, Derry S, Moore RA, McQuay HJ. Carbamazepine for acute and chronic pain in adults. *Cochrane Database Syst Rev.* 2011;1:CD005451.
73. Dy SM, Asch SM, Naeim A, Sanati H, Walling A, Lorenz KA. Evidence-based standards for cancer pain management. *J Clin Oncol.* 2008;26(23):3879–3885.
74. Moulin DE, Clark AJ, Gilron I, et al. Pharmacological management of chronic neuropathic pain: consensus statement and guidelines from the Canadian Pain Society. *Pain Res Manage.* 2007;12(1):13–21.

75. Challapalli V, Tremont-Lukats IW, McNicol ED, Lau J, Carr DB. Systemic administration of local anesthetic agents to relieve neuropathic pain. *Cochrane Database Syst Rev.* 2005;4:CD003345.
76. van Tulder MW, Touray T, Furlan AD, Solway S, Bouter LM. Muscle relaxants for non-specific low back pain. *Cochrane Database Syst Rev.* 2003;2:CD004252.
77. Okon T. Ketamine: an introduction for the pain and palliative medicine physician. *Pain Physician.* 2007;10(3):493–500.
78. Bell RF, Eccleston C, Kalso EA. Ketamine as an adjuvant to opioids for cancer pain. *Cochrane Database Syst Rev.* 2009;3:CD003351.
79. Ballantyne JC, Carwood C. Comparative efficacy of epidural, subarachnoid, and intracerebroventricular opioids in patients with pain due to cancer. *Cochrane Database Syst Rev.* 2008;1:CD005178.
80. Yan BM, Myers RP. Neurolytic celiac plexus block for pain control in unresectable pancreatic cancer. *Am J Gastroenterol.* 2007;102(2):430–438.
81. Arcidiacono PG, Calori G, Carrara S, McNicol ED, Testoni PA. Celiac plexus block for pancreatic cancer pain in adults. *Cochrane Database Syst Rev.* 2011;3:CD007519.
82. Robb K, Oxberry SG, Bennett MI, Johnson MI, Simpson KH, Searle RD. A Cochrane systematic review of transcutaneous electrical nerve stimulation for cancer pain. *J Pain Symptom Manage.* 2009;37(4):746–753.
83. Goldberg GR, Morrison RS. Pain management in hospitalized cancer patients: a systematic review. *J Clin Oncol.* 2007;25(13):1792–1801.
84. Bennett MI, Bagnall AM, Jose Closs S. How effective are patient-based educational interventions in the management of cancer pain? Systematic review and meta-analysis. *Pain.* 2009;143(3):192–199.
85. Kwekkeboom KL, Abbott-Anderson K, Wanta B. Feasibility of a patient-controlled cognitive-behavioral intervention for pain, fatigue, and sleep disturbance in cancer. *Oncol Nurs Forum.* 2010;37(3):E151–159.
86. National Comprehensive Cancer Network. NCCN clinical practice guidelines: adult cancer pain, version 1.2012. http://www.nccn.org/professionals/physician_gls/pdf/pain.pdfed 2012. Accessed August 9, 2012.
87. Cepeda MS, Carr DB, Lau J, Alvarez H. Music for pain relief. *Cochrane Database Syst Rev.* 2006;2:CD004843.
88. Green E, Zwaal C, Beals C, et al. Cancer-related pain management: a report of evidence-based recommendations to guide practice. *Clin J Pain.* 2010;26(6):449–462.
89. Beck SL, Towsley GL, Berry PH, Brant JM, Smith EM. Measuring the quality of care related to pain management: a multiple-method approach to instrument development. *Nurs Res.* 2010;59(2):85–92.

Pain

Patient Name: ______________________________

This guide provides suggestions on how to report, prevent, and treat your pain. It includes a log to record information about your pain. Keeping a pain diary will help your doctors and nurses better manage your pain.

Description

Pain is often feared by people with cancer, but good treatment is available to provide relief for most patients. Pain can contribute to many problems, such as sleep problems, depression, and a decrease in activity. Getting pain relief will allow you a better quality of life.

It is important to report your pain so that your doctor and nurse can treat it effectively. Here are the things you should report about your pain:

- Where the pain is located
- How much the pain hurts (try to rate your pain on a 0 to 10 scale with 0 being no pain and 10 being the worst possible pain)
- What kind of pain you have (e.g., aching, sharp, dull, numb)
- How your pain changes over time (e.g., constant, on and off)
- What makes the pain worse
- What makes the pain better
- What you have tried to manage the pain—both medicines and nonmedicines such as massage and ice

Sometimes patients and families do not report pain. Here are some reasons why:

- They may not want to bother the doctor.
- They may believe that pain is a part of having cancer.
- They may believe that pain is a sign that the cancer is getting worse and fear getting bad news.

Remember that your comfort is important to your doctor and nurse.

Prevention

The best way to treat pain is to prevent it from getting too bad. Here are some ways to prevent pain:

- Take your medicines as ordered.
  - Some pain medicines are scheduled. They work over a long period of time, and you should take them on time to keep the pain from coming back.
  - Some pain medicines can be taken as needed—for example, every 4 hours. Take the pain medicine before the pain gets too bad. Waiting too long will mean you will have to "catch up" on the pain medicine.

- Constipation is a side effect of opioid pain medicines. Take stool softeners and laxatives to prevent constipation. Constipation can make your pain worse. Report constipation to your doctor or nurse when it is not controlled.
- Report other side effects from the pain medicine. Most side effects can be treated.

Management

You are a partner in your pain management. Here are some tips for your comfort:

- Keep a pain diary. Include the items listed above in your diary.
- If you are having pain, be ready to discuss your pain at each office visit.
- Call the doctor or nurse if your pain is not controlled.
- Prevent constipation by taking stool softeners and laxatives.
- Try nondrug treatments for your pain. Relaxation, guided imagery, and distraction can help you to relax and take thoughts away from the pain. Massage may relieve muscle tension and stress that can increase pain. Warm rice bags or ice can help some patients.

Follow-up

Talk to your doctor and nurse when your pain is not controlled. Do not wait for your next office visit if your pain is not well controlled.

Phone Numbers

Nurse: ______________________________ Phone: ______________________________

Doctor: ______________________________ Phone: ______________________________

Source: Brant JM. Pain. In: Yarbro CH, Wujcik D, Gobel BH, eds. *Cancer Symptom Management*. 4th ed. Burlington, MA: Jones & Bartlett Learning; 2014.

Chapter 6

Sleep Disturbances

Ellyn E. Matthews, PhD, RN, AOCN®, AOCNS®
Ann M. Berger, PhD, APRN, AOCNS®, FAAN

THE PROBLEM

Sleep disturbances are a prevalent and distressing problem in patients with cancer. Difficulty falling asleep, maintaining sleep, and daytime sleepiness associated with cancer can become chronic in many patients, persisting for months or years after completion of cancer treatments. Both biological and behavioral factors influence the quality, quantity, and timing of sleep in patients with cancer. Factors include cancer pathophysiology, treatments, symptoms of pain, fatigue and depression, and sleep habits. Impaired sleep affects daytime activities, impacts quality of life (QOL), interferes with immune function, and may alter the response to treatment. Sleep disturbances are clearly detrimental to patients with cancer, yet evidence-based prevention and management strategies are underdeveloped and underused by oncology providers.[1]

Recognition of the nature and prevalence of cancer-related sleep disturbances can provide the basis of new approaches to supportive care, because many sleep problems can be treated effectively. Through better understanding of sleep problems and current therapies, oncology nurses are well positioned to improve sleep in patients with cancer. This chapter provides an overview of the biological and behavioral basis of sleep–wake disturbances that are most prevalent in people with cancer and discusses sleep evaluation and current treatment options.

Sleep disorders and sleep disturbances are prevalent in patients with cancer. These terms often are used interchangeably. Sleep disorders comprise the nearly 100 diagnostic entities identified by criteria in the International Classification of Sleep Disorders[2] and the *Diagnostic and Statistical Manual of Mental Disorders,* fourth edition (ICD-IV).[3] Common sleep disorders in general and in oncology populations include insomnia, sleep-disordered breathing (e.g., obstructive sleep apnea syndrome), movement disorders (e.g., restless legs syndrome), and circadian rhythm disorders. Sleep disturbances (also referred to as sleep–wake disturbances) are the perceived or actual alterations in nighttime sleep, both quantity and quality, with subsequent daytime impairment in the absence of a diagnostic label.[2,4] Oncology literature focuses primarily on sleep disturbance in terms of the symptoms of insomnia such as difficulty falling asleep (sleep latency), staying asleep (sleep maintenance), and nonrestorative sleep.

SLEEP DEFINITION, STATES, AND STAGES

Sleep is an active, biobehavioral process with essential health-promoting properties. Sleep experts define sleep as a behavioral state of temporary perceptual disengagement from and unresponsiveness to environmental surroundings.[5] Observable behaviors that indicate sleep are minimal movement, closed eyes, and reduced responsiveness to stimulation. Two basic states—non-rapid eye movement (non-REM) and REM—constitute sleep. The non-REM state contains lighter to deeper, more restorative sleep stages characterized by minimal brain activity and some body activity. Hallmarks of the REM state are muscle atonia and high levels of brain activity associated with dreaming. Typically sleep begins with light to deeper non-REM sleep stages, followed by alternating cycles of non-REM and REM sleep every 90–110 minutes.[5] Sleep and wakefulness alternate every 24 hours in a predictable circadian pattern.

Adequate sleep quantity, a regular sleep–wake schedule, and lifestyle behaviors in synchrony with the circadian pattern lead to healthy sleep and optimal daytime functioning.

Resting may resemble sleep, but patients with cancer may rest for long periods yet feel fatigued and function poorly due to lack of adequate sleep. Rest is characterized as a period of bodily inactivity without transitioning through the REM and non-REM stages that denote sleep.[5] Feeling refreshed upon awakening and the absence of sleepiness during wake periods are indications of restorative sleep.

Biological evidence suggests that sleep acts to conserve energy and metabolism, maintain homeostasis of physiological systems and immune functioning, and reverse or restore physiological processes that become degraded during wakefulness.[6] Polysomnography (PSG) quantifies the spectrum of wakefulness to deep sleep and includes the frequency and amplitude of electroencephalography (EEG) waves denoting sleep stages. PSG is routinely indicated for the diagnosis of sleep-related breathing disorders; for continuous positive airway pressure (CPAP) titration in sleep-related breathing disorders; with a multiple sleep latency test in the evaluation of suspected narcolepsy; and in certain atypical or unusual parasomnias.[7]

CHARACTERISTICS OF SLEEP DISTURBANCES

Sleep disturbances may occur at any time during the cancer trajectory and present with various features. Subjective reports of persons with cancer indicate common complaints that include difficulty in one or more of these areas: falling asleep, frequent awakenings with inability to resume sleep, nonrestorative sleep, and disruption of previous sleep patterns.[4,8] Excessive daytime sleepiness, which is experienced as a strong urge to sleep, is a different sensation than fatigue, but both are frequent consequences of disturbed sleep.[9] Even worry about a cancer diagnosis may contribute to sleep disturbances. In a cross-sectional study of American women (n = 1038; age range = 50–70 years) with no cancer history, more than half of the women with worries about breast cancer reported insomnia complaints that impaired daytime functioning.[10]

In the weeks immediately following a cancer diagnosis, sleep disturbance may be transient and remit spontaneously. Short-term sleep problems may be due to the anxiety and ruminative patterns that emerge in the wake of a cancer diagnosis or may reflect efforts to adjust to the disease. Persistent sleep problems may be due to the cancer itself, treatment, or other factors. For example, patients with newly diagnosed lung cancer reported marked sleep disturbances, excessive daytime sleepiness, and impaired quality of life when compared with a comparison group of noncancer patients with obstructive sleep apnea syndrome (OSAS).[11] The lung cancer patients were ambulatory and capable of all self-care activities, but were excluded from the study if they had any history of sleep disorders other than insomnia. Even before treatment, lung cancer patients' objective sleep data showed significantly lower sleep efficiency (defined as the percentage of time asleep/time in bed), greater number of awakenings during the night, and lower daytime activity compared with noncancer patients.[11]

Worsening sleep disturbances are associated with symptoms of tumor invasion such as pain, drainage, dyspnea, pruritus, fatigue, and gastrointestinal and genitourinary alterations.[12] Several studies describe sleep disturbances during chemotherapy treatments for breast cancer[13–15]; lung cancer, colorectal cancer, and lymphoma[16]; mixed-type cancer[17]; and gynecological cancers.[18] Complaints during treatment include waking up in the middle of the night, waking up earlier in the morning than intended, and being unable to fall asleep within 30 minutes. During radiotherapy, studies have revealed moderate to severe sleep problems in patients with breast and prostate cancer.[19–21] In 400 patients receiving palliative radiation for symptomatic bone metastases, 25% reported moderate sleep disturbance, while 36% patients reported severe sleep disturbance.[22]

Recent assessments of the duration of sleep disturbance demonstrate a trend toward persistent sleep problems. Sleep disturbances that begin or worsen during cancer treatment can become chronic in some patients. These disturbances often continue for many months or years after completing cancer therapy, indicating chronic sleep disturbance is a substantial problem in long-term cancer survivorship.[1] A qualitative analysis of cancer survivors with heterogeneous cancer types described disrupted sleep during and after cancer treatment.[23] The majority of a small sample of cancer survivors with chronic insomnia (n = 21) reported that active cancer treatment contributed to poor sleep quality via disruption of normal daily routines. Poor sleep patterns became persistent once active treatment ceased. Participants described becoming particularly concerned about their sleep during follow-up care. Insomnia affected mood, physical health, relationships, sleep quality, sleep-related behavior, and cognition.[23]

Although sleep disturbance and other common symptoms related to sleep may abate over time, breast cancer survivors continue to report moderate to severe sleep disturbances after cancer treatment has ended. In a recent cross-sectional study, women who completed primary breast cancer treatment (n = 182) reported symptom severity was highest for sleep disturbance in relation to four other common symptoms (i.e., fatigue, pain, distress, numbness/tingling).[24] The majority of participants were at least 5 years since diagnosis, and 20% were more than 10 years post diagnosis. In this study, disturbed sleep and distress interfered with general activity and enjoyment of life.[24] Thus sleep disturbance is a serious, ongoing concern for many cancer survivors.

Sleep disturbances are common in patients with advanced cancer. In one prospective study, more than one-fourth of terminally ill cancer patients presented with sleep disturbances at admission to a palliative care unit.[25]

In another study, patients with advanced lung cancer reported significantly worse sleep and more daytime sleepiness compared to healthy controls.[26] Those with advanced lung cancer described sleep impaired by breathing difficulty, cough, nocturia, and frequent awakenings. In a prospective chart audit, the prevalence and key causes of sleep disturbance were evaluated in a population of hospice patients (n = 74).[27] Fifty-two patients (70%) reported impaired sleep, deemed to be due to uncontrolled pain by most patients. Finally, a study of terminally ill patients (n = 102) suggested that poor sleep quality, hopelessness, and depression were among the strongest predictors of desire to hasten death.[28] Together, these studies highlight the burden of neglected sleep complaints throughout the cancer trajectory regardless of the cause or characteristics.

SLEEP DISTURBANCES AND SYMPTOM CLUSTERS

Cancer-related sleep disturbances often are part of a cluster of three or more interrelated symptoms, including pain, fatigue, mood disturbance, and loss of cognitive function.[20,21,29–32] Assessments of fatigue, pain, and sleep disturbance in 84 patients with mixed cancer diagnoses indicated that pain influences fatigue, both directly and indirectly, through its effect on sleep.[33] Another study of 93 women undergoing radiation therapy found that symptoms could be grouped into three distinct clusters: pain–insomnia–fatigue, cognitive disturbance–outlook, and gastrointestinal. The pain–insomnia–fatigue cluster was associated with reduced levels of optimism, self-transcendence, and positive mood.[21] Similarly, in breast cancer patients who were currently receiving chemotherapy or radiotherapy (n = 282), Kim and colleagues identified two symptom clusters—a psychoneurological symptom cluster (insomnia, depressed mood, cognitive dysfunction, fatigue, and pain) and a gastrointestinal cluster—that were stable across treatment.[34] Together, these studies suggest that sleep disturbance is an integral part of many symptom clusters. Their findings support the need to shift the clinical focus to the patient's symptom experience as a whole, and emphasize the importance of developing effective interventions for symptom clusters. Clinicians may need to consider all the symptoms in a cluster to provide the best management.

HYPERSOMNIA AND INSOMNIA

Most patients with cancer have sleep disturbances that take the form of either hypersomnia or insomnia. Hypersomnia is an abnormal increase in sleep duration (10 or more hours at a time) and difficulty staying awake during the day. Somnolence and excessive daytime sleepiness are other terms used to describe this troubling sleep disorder. Daytime napping typically does not relieve the excessive sleepiness. Hypersomnia is linked to specific cancers, treatment side effects, electrolyte imbalances, anemia, immune system functioning, and hormonal alterations.

In a study of 70 adults with brain tumors, sleepiness was assessed before, during, and after cranial radiotherapy.[35] Ninety percent of the patients initially experienced minimal somnolence accompanied by some tiredness that did not curtail activity. The score increased significantly from week 3 to week 12, with a peak occurring at the end of treatment. Somnolence scores decreased 6 weeks after treatment. Excessive sleepiness following cranial radiation (somnolence syndrome) coexists with distressing symptoms such as lethargy and slow mental processing.[35]

Evidence suggests that hypersomnia persists long after completion of cancer treatment. In a study of outpatients with mixed types of cancer (n = 219), fatigue and daytime sleepiness were the most prevalent and distressing symptoms reported at 1, 6, and 12 months after completion of adjuvant chemotherapy.[36] Nearly half of the outpatients reported daytime sleepiness up to a year post treatment, suggesting hypersomnia is a common and persistent problem that affects the quality of life long after completion of chemotherapy. Sleepiness can diminish or eliminate participation in daily activities such as work, school, and care of family members. Consequently, hypersomnia can isolate patients from social interactions and restrict the very activities that define their roles and identity.

Although hypersomnia and insomnia appear to be opposites, they share the negative consequence of significantly disrupting the pattern and quality of patients' lives. Sleep experts define insomnia as difficulty with sleep initiation or maintenance that occurs despite the opportunity for sleep, which causes clinically significant distress or impairment in social, occupational, or other relevant areas of functioning.[3] Insomnia may be a primary sleep disorder or it may be a co-occurring condition with a psychiatric, medical, or other sleep disorder. Insomnia can be situational, recurrent, or a persistent problem; thus it may be classified as acute or recurrent/chronic depending on its duration.[37] Acute insomnia symptoms can last days or weeks and often improve without an intervention. The criteria for the diagnosis of chronic insomnia disorder/syndrome is sleep disturbance that occurs at least three nights per week, lasts at least one month, and causes significant distress or impairment of daytime functioning.[2,3,37] Chronic insomnia disorder is often comorbid with medical conditions such as cancer and was previously referred to as "secondary" insomnia. Currently, sleep experts suggest that insomnia occurs on a spectrum (defined by duration and frequency) and is comorbid with—rather than secondary to—medical, surgical, or psychiatric conditions.[38]

In the past, healthcare professionals may have unwittingly contributed to the problem of cancer-related insomnia. Until recently, when patients complained of daytime fatigue, clinicians recommended rest and daytime naps.

This advice frequently increased sleep difficulties and fatigue by disrupting the normal 24-hour predictable sleep–wake circadian activity pattern.

CONSEQUENCES OF IMPAIRED SLEEP

Adequate sleep is essential for optimal human health and well-being. Sleep deprivation and disruption lead to a number of negative health, safety, cognitive, and psychosocial consequences in both healthy adults and persons with cancer.[4] Moreover, untreated sleep disturbance is associated with significant health costs across patient age groups.[39] Excessive daytime sleepiness is a serious public health problem leading to accidents, poor work performance, increased morbidity and mortality, and greater utilization of health resources.[40] Even without a diagnosis of cancer, evidence suggests that chronically inadequate sleep (less than 6–7 hours per night) is associated with increased blood pressure, reduced anabolic hormones needed for tissue repair, higher levels of inflammatory cytokines, and altered patterns of stress hormones.[41]

The physiological impact of poor sleep in patients with cancer may hinder recovery and contribute to fatigue.[24] Excessive daytime sleepiness and poor sleep can add to the distress caused by other cancer-related symptoms. For example, sleep disturbances may trigger or exacerbate other symptoms such as fatigue, pain, depression, anxiety, night sweats, and restless legs.[42,43] A growing body of evidence indicates sleep disturbance is positively correlated with cancer-related fatigue, and is more severe in fatigued patients than in nonfatigued patients, suggesting a common underlying etiology.[1] Moreover, impaired sleep in patients with cancer adversely affects daytime mood, daily functioning, and overall quality of life.[4,17,23] Sleep disturbances may even impact response to treatment. Recent research suggests that sleep disturbance has a consistent negative impact on immune functioning, and it may even have implications for tumor progression and survival.[44,45] There is an accumulating evidence base that sleep plays a supportive role in the functioning of the immune system, such that sleep loss is a risk factor for impaired immune function.[46,47] Diurnal rhythms of circulating immune blood cells have been identified under normal sleep–wake conditions, with lymphocyte levels peaking during the night.[46] In a recent study, Ackermann and colleagues reported that circulating granulocyte levels and diurnal rhythmicity are directly and negatively affected by the physical stress of acute sleep deprivation.[48] The health significance of these changes warrants further study to understand the role in development of long term-health conditions, such as cancer.

Family and friends who are involved in the care of patients with cancer also experience sleep disturbance. Between 36% and 95% of informal caregivers report disrupted sleep associated with poor sleep quality.[49] The sleep parameters most affected are short sleep duration, nocturnal awakenings, and daytime dysfunction. Caregivers describe "sleeping with one eye open" to indicate the vigilant nature of caregivers' sleep experience.[50] Alterations in usual sleep patterns pose a considerable threat to caregivers' quality of life.[49,50] Adequate, restorative sleep is vital for caregivers who attend to the needs of others.

INCIDENCE

Although the incidence of sleep disturbance reported in studies has varied because of differences in the populations studied, cancer stage, definition of sleep disturbance, and mode of assessment, it is estimated that one-third to one-half of cancer survivors experience sleep disturbance of some kind.[17,24,43,51,52] In contrast, sleep disturbances occur in 10% to 15% of the general population and are associated with today's 24/7 culture, situational stress, and aging.[4] In a landmark, large cross-sectional study of nearly 1000 adults with different types of cancer, fatigue (44%), leg restlessness (41%), insomnia symptoms (31%), and excessive sleepiness (28%) were the most common complaints related to sleep.[53]

A diagnosis of cancer with its associated psychological impact, time-consuming treatments, and distressing symptoms is known to disrupt sleeping patterns and quality, yet the true prevalence and incidence of sleep disturbances in the oncology population are not well established. Most studies of cancer-related sleep complaints employ a cross-sectional design using convenience samples with varied definitions and measures of sleep disturbance. In addition, cancer patients, family caregivers, and healthcare providers may believe that sleep problems are a normal and transient reaction to cancer and cancer treatment and, therefore, may underreport sleep disturbance. Other concerns, such as cancer-related morbidity and mortality, appear to take precedence over sleep assessment and management. Evidence suggests that the vast majority of patients with cancer do not report sleep problems to healthcare providers, even in palliative care settings where symptom management is a major focus.[27] In spite of inadequate communication of sleep symptoms, frequent use of hypnotics (22.6%) has been documented in large samples of patients with cancer, which provides evidence of the magnitude of the problem.[54]

Little is known about how sleep disturbances are affected by cancer site because much of sleep research in cancer has relied on small samples or combined cancer types. In some studies, the prevalence of sleep disturbances was greatest in breast cancer patients.[17,53] In a large-scale study of patients with cancer receiving chemotherapy ($n = 823$; mean age = 58 years; 72% female), breast cancer patients had the highest number of overall insomnia complaints, while lung cancer patients reported more severe insomnia.[17] The investigators speculated that differences in insomnia are affected by tumor biology, cancer treatments, and/or side effects.

Although older age is a significant risk for developing insomnia symptoms in the general population, younger patients with cancer may report greater insomnia than older patients.[17,51] Mao and colleagues analyzed data from the 2002 National Health Interview Survey, which included 1904 cancer survivors and a large sample of controls (n = 29,092)[51]. The 30% rate of insomnia among cancer survivors was significantly higher than the rate among controls without a history of cancer (17%). Compared with controls in the same age groups, younger survivors (age < 50 years) were more likely to report ongoing insomnia symptoms than older survivors (age > 64 years).[51] These results may be due to more aggressive tumors and treatments, as well as the expectations of better health among younger patients.[17,51] Studies have primarily been conducted months or years after completion of cancer treatment; therefore, it is difficult to determine the extent to which different cancers and specific treatments exacerbate sleep disturbances.

ETIOLOGY AND RISK FACTORS

Sleep disturbance in persons with cancer throughout the cancer trajectory is multidimensional in nature. A helpful framework to understand and categorize etiological factors is the "three P's" model of predisposing, precipitating, and perpetuating factors.[55] Table 6-1 presents a list of the factors that place patients at risk for developing insomnia.

Predisposing factors

Predisposing factors are enduring psychological or biological characteristics that make a patient predisposed and at risk to develop sleep problems during the course of the cancer experience (e.g., female gender, advanced age, anxiety-prone personality, family or personal history of insomnia, genetic factors).[37] Women and older adults in the general population are predisposed to more sleep disturbances. Persons with cancer may have underlying sleep disorders such as obstructive sleep apnea, restless leg syndrome, or circadian rhythm disorder. Poor sleep in patients with cancer may be

TABLE 6-1

Predisposing, Precipitating, and Perpetuating Factors (3 Ps) that Increase the Risk of Sleep Disturbance in People with Cancer

Factor	Examples
Predisposing: Enduring biological, psychological characteristics that increase the risk of developing sleep disturbances	• Female gender • Older age • Personal or family history of sleep difficulties • Personal or family history of mood or anxiety disorder • Current mood or anxiety disorder • Hyperarousal
Precipitating: Disease-related, psychological, and/or environmental factors and life events that trigger sleep disturbances	• Physiologic response to cancer or its treatments including chemotherapy, radiotherapy, hormone therapy, and supportive medications including: o Gastrointestinal symptoms (diarrhea, constipation, nausea) o Genitourinary symptoms (incontinence, retention) o Respiratory symptoms (dyspnea, orthopnea, coughing) o Menopausal symptoms (hot flashes, night sweats) o Pain, peripheral neuropathy o Immunologic changes o Thermoregulatory changes (fever) • Psychological distress in response to cancer diagnosis or treatment o Anxiety, depression, mood alterations • Change in environment o Disruptive noise/light, absence of usual light-dark cues, temperature
Perpetuating: Behaviors, beliefs, thoughts that maintain or exacerbate sleep difficulties	• Maladaptive behaviors o Excessive time in bed, daytime napping, reduced daily activity, irregular sleep-wake times, stimulant consumption, inappropriate use of sleep aids • Maladaptive beliefs o Unrealistic sleep expectations, false perception of sleep time and quality, fear of sleeplessness, difficulty discerning causes of daytime fatigue

Source: Data from Spielman et al[55].

related to the tendency to experience anxiety, depression, or other psychological symptoms.[56] Anxiety, characterized by heightened cortical and peripheral arousal, has been associated with complaints of disturbed sleep in a sample of women with ovarian cancer[57] and heterogeneous patients with cancer both at a preoperative visit and two months later.[52,57] In women with metastatic breast cancer, higher initial levels of depression were a risk factor for problems getting up in the morning, waking up during the night, and daytime sleepiness.[58] Increases in depression over 12 months were a risk factor for fewer hours of sleep, more problems with waking up during the night, and more daytime sleepiness.[58] It should be noted that some patients have insomnia independent of psychological distress.

Precipitating factors

Precipitating factors are the medical, environmental, and psychological factors and life events that trigger insomnia (e.g., cancer or other serious illness, medication, death of a significant other, familial or occupational stress). Risk factors that are likely to precipitate sleep disturbances in patients with cancer include the type of cancer, stage of cancer, and treatment side effects. Physical changes related to the type, location, and aggressiveness of cancer growth may increase pressure/pain in the tumor region, impair breathing, and obstruct major organs, leading to disrupted sleep. Chemotherapy, radiotherapy, and other therapies contribute to sleep disturbance, yet research examining the impact of different cancer treatments on sleep disturbances is needed.

Side effects of treatment that can affect the sleep–wake cycle include gastrointestinal disturbances (e.g., diarrhea, constipation, or nausea), genitourinary distress (e.g., incontinence, retention), and respiratory problems.[59] Unfortunately, the medications used for managing these side effects can put the patient at higher risk for disturbed sleep. Analgesics (e.g., opioids) and antiemetic medications (including corticosteroids) are known to disrupt sleep.[4,12]

Estrogen deficiency, whether induced by chemotherapy and hormone therapy, the abrupt cessation of hormone replacement therapy at cancer diagnosis, or ovary removal, may trigger or exacerbate preexisting menopausal vasomotor symptoms (hot flashes) that interfere with sleep. Nocturnal hot flashes occurring within the few months after adjuvant treatments for breast cancer have been associated with concurrent risk of increases in insomnia symptoms.[60] A limited body of evidence suggests that sleep problems due to nocturia and hot flashes are common in prostate cancer patients undergoing androgen deprivation therapy.[61,62]

Pain may cause sleep disruption in patients with cancer as well as patients with a multitude of medical conditions.[63] Sleep contributes to tissue recovery and repair, and may offer a temporary reprieve from the psychological awareness of pain. The relationship between pain and sleep is unclear; does pain contribute to poor sleep, do pain medications contribute to poor sleep, or are both effects seen? Several hypotheses have been proposed to explain this association. Pain causes the awakenings but then psychological distress prevents return to sleep, and poor sleep then leads to difficulty managing pain, thus creating a self-perpetuating cycle of pain and poor sleep.

Changes in cancer patients' usual sleeping environment can precipitate sleep disturbance. The sleep of hospitalized patients is frequently interrupted by treatment schedules and hospital routines, which alter the sleep–wake circadian cycle. Other factors that increase the risk of impaired sleep during hospitalization or treatment include pain, anxiety, medications, absence of daily light–dark cues, environmental noise, and temperature.[64,65]

Perpetuating factors

Perpetuating factors maintain or exacerbate sleep difficulties. They are typically behaviors (e.g., extending time spent in bed to try to sleep more, naps) and beliefs (e.g., fear of sleeplessness, excessive worries about daytime consequences) that people adopt as coping mechanisms. Other maladaptive behaviors that perpetuate sleep disturbances include poor sleep hygiene practices and lifestyle choices, such as irregular sleep schedule, poor nutrition, sedentary lifestyle, smoking, and lack of moderation in alcohol, caffeine, and other stimulant consumption.[59] Although some behaviors such as extensive napping can be useful in the short term, over time they tend to perpetuate insomnia. These factors may be difficult to alter during the stressful course of cancer treatment, and require education and counseling when patients are coping with many other lifestyle changes.

PATHOPHYSIOLOGY

Although the mechanisms by which chemotherapy and radiotherapy interfere with sleep are not fully understood, the co-occurrence of fatigue, depression, and sleep disturbance in cancer populations suggests that they may share common underlying physiological mechanisms.[66] There is growing interest in the possibility that these symptoms may be driven by activation of the pro-inflammatory cytokine network.[17,43] Administration of cytokines, particularly interferon, interleukin-2, and tumor necrosis factor, is associated with increases in depressed mood, fatigue, and sleep problems,[67] and inflammation is common among noncancer populations who have depression or sleep disorders.[68] Little is known about the role of cancer treatments as potential inducers of inflammation, yet chemotherapy has been associated with acute increases in inflammatory markers, which may persist long into survivorship.[69,70] Determining the mechanisms underlying these common and distressing symptoms of cancer treatment is critical for the development of effective interventions for prevention and treatment of sleep disturbances.

In addition to the physiological mechanisms, desynchrony of sleep–wake patterns may contribute to sleep disturbances in the context of cancer. Two main processes underlie the regulation of the sleep–wake cycle in humans: a homeostatic process determined by prior sleep and waking, and a clocklike circadian process that is largely independent of sleep and waking.[71] Circadian factors, both internal (e.g., immunologic, thermoregulatory) and external (e.g., light exposure), interact with homeostatic components to regulate the daily, 24-hour sleep–wake circadian rhythm.[5] Healthy sleep–wake rhythms occur when there is synchrony between homeostatic and circadian processes. Normal aging and lifestyle behaviors (e.g., shift work) can alter sleep–wake timing, circadian factors, and sleep architecture, leading to difficulty falling asleep, maintaining sleep, and excessive daytime sleepiness. Cancer and its treatment interfere with both processes by way of changes in patient behaviors, the environment (e.g., disrupted sleep patterns), and altered physiology (hypothalamic–pituitary–adrenal axis regulation).[4]

SYMPTOM ASSESSMENT

The high prevalence of disabling sleep disturbances in patients with cancer highlights the need for all healthcare providers to evaluate sleep during routine encounters. Healthcare providers, including nurses, often fail to ask patients about their sleep, which may lead to unnecessary morbidity. The scope of sleep assessments may vary according to the setting, health status, and developmental stage of the patients with cancer. Minimally, sleep-related questions could be included in a health history and medication review. Specialized sleep assessment methods for clinical practice include self-reported subjective measures (e.g., sleep diaries, questionnaires) and objective measures (e.g., polysomnography, actigraphy). The impact of sleep disturbances can be determined through clinical interview or questionnaire (e.g., sleepiness, functioning, mood).

SUBJECTIVE ASSESSMENT

Self-reports and clinician interviews offer a practical means of evaluating sleep quality and efficacy of sleep interventions. There are several self-report instruments that provide information about sleep disturbances from the patient's perspective. Using a patient's own appraisal of her or his sleep is desirable because the individual is able to compare usual sleep quality and quantity with sleep change during active treatment and beyond. Self-report daily sleep diaries, visual analog scales (VAS), questionnaires, and symptom or quality of life questionnaires with sleep items have been used in a variety of oncology settings. In addition, family members and friends may be an important source of information, as they can provide insight into etiological factors (e.g., fear over results of a diagnostic test) and possible relief measures to facilitate appropriate therapy. Patients may not be able to provide information about snoring or nocturnal limb movement. Therefore, clinicians need to obtain information from bed partners, although proxy reports may vary in reliability.[4]

Assessment is the first step in management of sleep disturbances (see Table 6-2 for examples of common subjective and objective measures). Minimally, assessment data should include predisposing factors, sleep patterns, symptoms, emotional status, activity levels, dietary stimulants, and medications. A good clinical interview guide for screening sleep disturbances is the Clinical Sleep Assessment for Adults.[72] On this instrument, seven questions assess employment status, examine sleep aid use, and screen for the following sleep parameters: sleep quality, total sleep time, sleep latency, awakenings, and daytime sleepiness. A shorter screening tool (four items) and a children's version are also available. This clinical sleep assessment alerts the clinician to the need to refer the patient to a sleep specialist, and may be used for research.[72] Another useful tool to organize sleep assessment in both children and adults is the mnemonic "BEARS,"[73] which covers the five domains of sleep: **B**edtime problems, **E**xcessive sleepiness, **A**wakenings, **R**egularity of sleep, and **S**leep-disordered breathing. This screening tool provides the basis for a more detailed sleep history and physical assessment if needed. The Pittsburgh Sleep Quality Index (PSQI) is a widely used research and screening tool that assesses general duration and quality of sleep, use of sleep medications, and other important sleep-related information in adults.[74]

Assessments that target specific sleep disturbances (e.g., insomnia, excessive daytime sleepiness, somnolence) may be indicated. The Insomnia Severity Index (ISI) is a seven-item evaluation and screening tool with established reliability and validity in the context of cancer.[74] The eight-item Epworth Sleepiness Scale is used to identify patients with excessive daytime sleepiness.[76] The Berlin Questionnaire is one of several widely used screening tools to evaluate risk for obstructive sleep apnea.[77] Sleep diaries are helpful in determining circadian rhythms and other sleep parameters.[78] The adoption of a standard sleep diary will facilitate comparisons across studies and is being tested, refined, and validated.[79]

Nurses must have a good understanding of developmental variations in sleep if they are to provide appropriate assessments, support, and education. The common misperception that poor sleep quality is a normal part of aging may prevent older adults from discussing sleep problems in general, but particularly in the context of cancer. It is critically important, therefore, to evaluate sleep and assist older adults to seek treatment for poor sleep. Age-adjusted assessment includes identifying any changes in circadian rhythms (e.g., phase advance) and increased daytime napping that interferes with ability to fall asleep.

TABLE 6-2

Assessments of Sleep Disturbance

Measure	Description
	Subjective - Clinical Interview
Basic questions	Basic clinical sleep evaluation (incorporated into a history/physical assessment) includes questions about predisposing factors, sleep patterns, symptoms, emotional status, sleep-related activity levels, diet, and medications.
Clinical Sleep Assessment for Adults[72]	The Clinical Sleep Assessment for Adults evaluates employment status, sleep aid use and screens for sleep quality, total sleep time, sleep latency, awakenings, and daytime sleepiness.
BEARS[73]	The mnemonic "BEARS" covers the five domains of sleep in children and adults: **B**edtime problems, **E**xcessive sleepiness, **A**wakenings, **R**egularity of sleep, and **S**leep-disordered breathing.
	Subjective - Patient Self-Report
The Pittsburgh Sleep Quality Index (PSQI)[74]	The PSQI is a 19-item, widely used research and screening tool that assesses general duration and quality of sleep, use of sleep medications, and other important sleep-related information in adults.
Insomnia Severity Index (ISI)[75]	The ISI is a 7-item evaluation and screening tool frequently used in the context of cancer. An ISI score of 8 or higher indicates insomnia symptoms (0–7 = no clinically significant insomnia, 8–14 = sub-threshold, 15–21 = moderate, 22–28 = severe insomnia).
Epworth Sleepiness Scale (ESS)[76]	ESS is comprised of 8-items that measure general propensity to fall asleep in various situations in recent times. Sleepiness scales provide information about circadian rhythms by tracking sleepiness and wakefulness throughout the day, allowing scheduling of patient activities during hours alert periods, and uninterrupted quiet time during periods of sleepiness. Sleepiness scales are brief and easy to use in the clinical setting, but patients must be able communicate of their sleepiness and fatigue.
Berlin Questionnaire[77]	Berlin Questionnaire is one of several widely used screening tools to evaluate risk for obstructive sleep apnea.
Daily sleep diaries, sleep log[78]	A self-report record of sleep and wake patterns with related information, usually over a period of several weeks. A sleep diary is useful in the diagnosis and treatment of insomnia, circadian rhythm sleep disorders, and in monitoring whether treatment is successful (e.g., CBTI). Sleep diaries may be used in conjunction with actigraphy.
	Objective
Polysomnography (PSG)	A diagnostic test typically conducted in a sleep lab involving simultaneous recording of multiple physiologic variables during sleep. Sensors measure brain activity, airflow, respiratory effort, oxygen saturation, EKG, eye, jaw, and leg muscle movement. Information is gathered, downloaded to computer, and outputted as waveform tracings which assist in the diagnosis of sleep disorders (e.g., sleep-related breathing disorders, movement disorders, parasomnias). The use of PSG in ICUs is possible but limited by access and cost.
Multiple Sleep Latency Test (MSLT)	An objective measure of the physiologic tendency to fall asleep in quiet situations to evaluate unexplained excessive daytime sleepiness or suspected narcolepsy. PSG is usually performed immediately before a MSLT.
	Objective-Behavioral
Wrist Actigraphy	A wristwatch-type device that records periods of activity and inactivity (rest or sleep) over days to weeks using sensors that detect movement. Actigraphs provide information about sleep latency, periods of nocturnal awakenings, total quantity of sleep and wake time. Limitations in ICU patients include decreased patient movement due to sedation, restraints, and weakness.

Abbreviations: CBTI: cognitive behavioral therapy for insomnia; EKG: electrocardiogram; ICU: intensive care unit.

Source: Data from Lee[72]; Owens[73]; Buysse[74]; Savard[75]; Johns[76]; Netzer[77]; Carney[78].

OBJECTIVE ASSESSMENT

A comprehensive health history and medication review provide key information about relevant medications and medical, surgical, and psychiatric conditions that may be associated with impaired sleep. A complete physical examination adds important supporting data about general health and physical signs of sleep disorders. For example, some anatomic abnormalities of the oropharynx are associated with increased likelihood of developing obstructive sleep apnea.[80]

Patients with suspected sleep disorders may be referred to a sleep disorders center or medical facility staffed by sleep specialists for an overnight diagnostic evaluation. The gold standard of objective sleep measurement is polysomonogram (PSG), which measures sleep parameters, stages, and architecture. The polysomnogram includes monitoring of brain waves, eye movement, breathing effort, air flow, oxygen saturation, electrocardiography, and body position. PSG is used to diagnose suspected sleep-related breathing disorders and movement disorders. Although it is not used to diagnose insomnia, PSG can rule out disorders that lead to insomnia symptoms.[80]

Actigraphy, in which a small wrist or leg accelerometer records gross motor activity and rest over long periods in home settings, can also be used to objectively evaluate activity–rest patterns. The activity and rest data are translated to quantitative values by a computer algorithm program. This device allows calculation of several important sleep parameters (e.g., total sleep time, number and length of awakenings). Actigraph monitoring has been used in the oncology setting to evaluate circadian rhythms[81–84] and response to sleep interventions in patients[13,85] and caregivers.[50]

DEGREES OF TOXICITY

Scoring systems for adverse events, toxicity, and performance status attempt to quantify the severity of symptoms such as insomnia or general health and/or ability to engage in daily activities. The Common Terminology Criteria for Adverse Events v 4.03 (CTCAE) is widely accepted as the standard classification and severity grading scale for adverse events in cancer therapy clinical trials and other oncology settings.[86] The CTCAE v 4.03 includes several sleep-related categories—insomnia, hypersomnia, somnolence, and sleep apnea—that are graded on a scale of 1–5, with 1 indicating a mild-grade event and 5 indicating death. CTCAE sleep-related categories are presented in Table 6-3.

TABLE 6-3

National Cancer Institute Common Terminology Criteria for Adverse Events (CTCAE): Sleep-related Assessment

Adverse Event	Grade				
	1	2	3	4	5
Insomnia	Mild difficulty falling asleep or waking up early	Moderate difficulty falling asleep or waking up early	Severe difficulty falling asleep or waking up early	-	-
A disorder characterized by difficulty falling asleep and/or remaining asleep.					
Hypersomnia	Mild increased need for sleep	Moderate increased need for sleep	Severe increased need for sleep	-	-
A disorder characterized by excessive sleepiness during the daytime.					
Somnolence	Mild but more than usual drowsiness or sleepiness	Moderate sedation; limiting instrumental activities of daily living (ADL)	Obtundation or stupor	Life-threatening consequences; urgent intervention indicated	Death
A disorder characterized by excessive sleepiness and drowsiness.					
Sleep apnea	Snoring and nocturnal sleep arousal without apnea periods	Moderate apnea and oxygen desaturation; excessive daytime sleepiness; medical evaluation indicated; limited instrumental ADL	Oxygen desaturation; associated with hypertension; medical intervention indicated; limited self-care ADL	Cardiovascular or neuro-psychiatric symptoms; urgent operative intervention indicated	Death
A disorder characterized by cessation of breathing for short periods during sleep.					

Source: Data from National Cancer Institute Common Terminology Criteria for Adverse Events (CTCAE)[86].

The impact of sleep on performance is important in both clinical settings and research studies. For example, the Karnofsky Performance Status (KPS) scale is designed to measure the level of patient activity and medical care requirements with scores ranging from 100 to 0.[87,88] A score of 100 indicates normal activity and no signs of disease; a score of 50 indicates daily help and frequent medical care are required; and a score of 0 is death. Sleep disturbance—one of the variables used to determine the initial validity of the scale—is moderately correlated with KPS, suggesting that sleep quality influences patient activity and medical needs.[89] The Eastern Cooperative Oncology Group (ECOG) score, also called the Zubrod, ranges from 0 to 5, with 0 denoting perfect health and 5 denoting death.[90] This scale is based on ability to ambulate and the percentage of time spent in bed during the day.

SYMPTOM MANAGEMENT STRATEGIES

THERAPEUTIC APPROACHES

Therapeutic approaches to prevent and manage the sleep disturbance of insomnia are the focus of this section. Figure 6-1 presents an insomnia management algorithm.

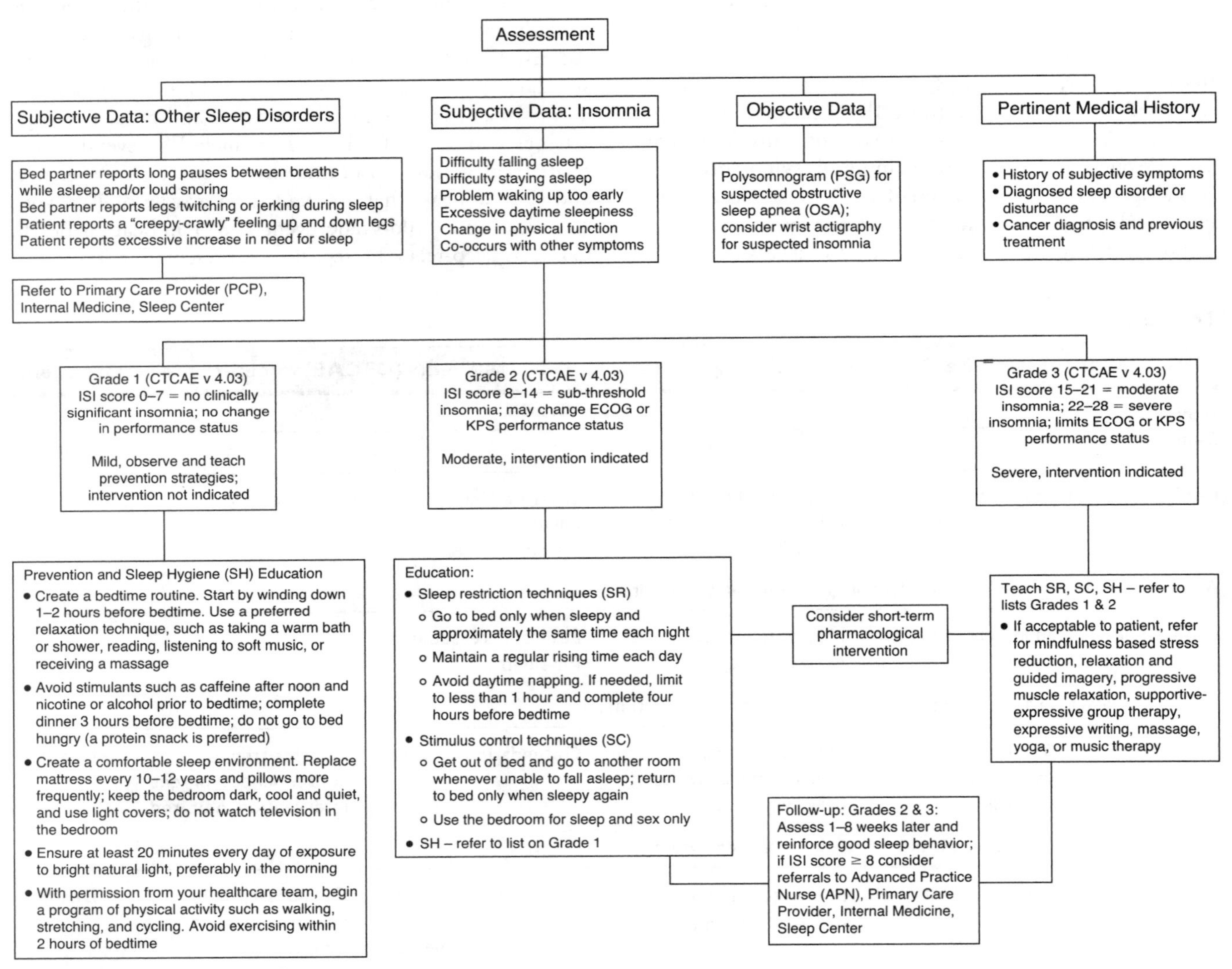

FIGURE 6-1

Insomnia management algorithm.

Abbreviations: CTCAE: common terminology criteria for adverse events; ECOG: eastern cooperative oncology group; ISI: insomnia severity index; KPS: karnofsky performance scale.

Source: Data from Morin[78]; Edinger and Carney[91]; Perlis, et al[92].

Management of other sleep disorders, such as obstructive sleep apnea, restless legs syndrome, and periodic limb movement disorder, occurs under the direction of a clinician who specializes in sleep medicine. Nurses need to screen for these prevalent sleep disorders and refer those patients who screen positive for further assessment.

When screening suggests the existence of insomnia, further assessment includes pertinent medical history and data related to insomnia and functioning. The Insomnia Severity Index (ISI) provides clinically useful ratings relative to the nature and severity of insomnia symptoms. Functional status may be evaluated using the ECOG or Karnofsky Performance Scale. Intervention strategies are individualized based on the ISI and function scores. Figure 6-1 includes strategies based on CTCAE Grades 1–3.

If the ISI score falls into the mild range (no clinical insomnia, Grade 1 CTCAE v 4.03), sleep hygiene (SH) education is recommended (Figure 6-1). Patients are educated about key sleep behaviors to prevent sleep disturbances, such as creating a bedtime routine and a comfortable sleep environment, maintaining a fixed sleep schedule, avoiding stimulants, and engaging in regular exercise. Follow-up includes routine clinical screening.

If the ISI score falls in the moderate range (subthreshold insomnia, Grade 2 CTCAE v4.03), additional education and behavior training pertaining to sleep restriction and stimulus control techniques may be indicated. Short-term (7–10 days) pharmacologic treatment can be considered, after weighing the risk–benefit ratio with the patient.

If the ISI score falls in the severe range and causes limitations in function (moderate to severe insomnia, Grade 3 CTCAE v4.03), insomnia management begins with the initial strategies for mild and moderate insomnia. If sleep problems are prolonged, patients may benefit from referral to clinicians with special training and experience in delivery of interventions that have shown positive benefits in patients with cancer. Follow-up assessments for moderate and severe insomnia are suggested 1–8 weeks later, depending on the circumstances and symptoms. If the patient's ISI score consistently remains 8 or greater, consider referral to an appropriate clinician for management of acute and chronic insomnia.

The next section summarizes current scientific knowledge about interventions found to improve sleep in patients with cancer.

Nonpharmacologic interventions

This summary synthesizes approximately 55 peer-reviewed, evidence-based studies that reported results of nonpharmacologic interventions to prevent or reduce sleep–wake disturbances in adults with cancer. The nonpharmacologic interventions are divided into four categories: cognitive-behavioral therapy for insomnia (CBTI), complementary therapies, education/information, and exercise. An Oncology Nursing Society (ONS) Putting Evidence into Practice (PEP) weight of evidence classification was assigned to each intervention category (e.g., "Recommended for Practice," "Likely to Be Effective," "Effectiveness Not Established").[93] This discussion updates the ONS-PEP Sleep–Wake Disturbances guidelines.[94]

Most of the recent studies supported prior findings and PEP classification for that category.[93] CBTI/behavioral therapy (BT) moved to the "Recommended for Practice" classification in patients receiving adjuvant treatment and in the off-treatment survivorship phase. Studies are needed to determine CBTI/BT's effects in patients with advanced disease and at the end of life. Complementary therapies, education/information, and exercise interventions remained in the "Effectiveness Not Established" classification, based on the evidence published to date. Additional large, randomized controlled trials (RCTs) are needed before concluding that these interventions can be "Recommended for Practice" to reduce sleep–wake disturbances in adults with cancer.

Cognitive-behavioral therapy for insomnia. CBTI is a multimodal approach aimed at eliminating perpetuating factors of insomnia by modifying sleep schedules, habits, and misconceptions about sleep that are responsible for chronic insomnia.[78,95,96] The most common components of CBTI (sleep restriction, stimulus control, sleep hygiene education, and cognitive therapy) are empirically supported treatments for insomnia in adults with persistent insomnia (Table 6-4).[78,91,92] Key educational and behavioral instructions for these components are presented in Figure 6-1 and Appendices 6A and 6B. Behavioral therapy interventions focus only on modifying the behavioral components that perpetuate insomnia. The goal of acute treatment is to reduce perpetuating factors below the insomnia threshold and to decondition the hyperarousal response. A positive response to treatment occurs when perpetuating factors are reduced below the threshold. CBTI therapies assist with sleep initiation and maintenance.

The 2006 American Academy of Sleep Medicine (AASM) practice parameters described psychological and behavioral interventions as effective, and recommended them as "standard" for treating chronic comorbid insomnia. AASM also recommended as "standard" three specific therapies for chronic insomnia: CBTI, stimulus control, and relaxation. Among the therapies rated by AASM as "guidelines" (indicating slightly lower strength of evidence than "standards" for treating chronic insomnia) were sleep restriction and multicomponent therapy.[97]

Examination of recent evidence reveals that five RCTs[13,98–102] and numerous quasi-experimental studies have reported positive results from CBTI or BT in patients with a variety of cancer diagnoses at various times along the continuum of care. Most studies reported improvement in several sleep outcomes using a variety of measures, most commonly perceived sleep quality using PSQI or the ISI. Two of the RCTs were conducted in the active phase of treatment; although the trials' inclusion criteria did not require current sleep disturbances, study participants reported improved sleep.[98,99]

TABLE 6-4

Cognitive Behavioral Therapy for Insomnia (CBTI) Components

Intervention	Description
Stimulus control (SC)	**SC** provides instructions that discourage sleep-incompatible behaviors, and reinforces a regular sleep-wake schedule, with the following instructions for patients: 1. Go to bed only when sleepy. 2. Do not use your bed for anything but sleep and sexual activity. 3. If you find yourself unable to fall asleep after 15–20 minutes, get up and go into another room, stay up until you feel sleepy and then return to the bedroom to sleep. 4. If you still cannot fall asleep within 15–20 minutes, repeat rule 3, do this as often as is necessary throughout the night. 5. Set your alarm and get up at the same time every morning regardless of how much sleep you got during the night. 6. Do not nap more than 45 minutes in the late afternoon.
Sleep restriction (SR)	**SR** curtails the amount of time spent in bed each night to the patient's estimated average total sleep time. This reduction in sleep time increases the homeostatic sleep drive through mild sleep deprivation, which results in improved quality of sleep and decreased time to fall asleep.
Cognitive therapy (CT)	**CT** modifies anxiety-producing and dysfunctional beliefs about sleep and sleep loss that perpetuate insomnia and helps patients develop realistic sleep expectations. Topics include realistic normative sleep requirements, the effects of mild sleep deprivation on sleep and daytime functioning, the influence of circadian rhythms, and the benefits of a regular sleep cycle. The CT process includes eliciting faulty cognitions, challenging their validity, and using restructuring strategies to replace them with more adaptive thoughts.
Sleep hygiene (SH) education	**SH** education promotes the following general practices: establish consistent bedtime and arise time, create a bedtime routine, avoid nicotine, foods, and beverages containing stimulants close to bedtime; light snack before bed; regular exercise; limited liquids in the evening; and initiate environmental modifications for a comfortable sleep environment including minimize noise, dim lights, maintain a cool bedroom temperature.

Source: Data from Morin[78]; Edinger and Carney[91]; Perlis et al[92].

Three RCTs were conducted with survivors who met study inclusion criteria for sleep disturbances, and all reported improved sleep.[100–102] The CBTI/BT interventions varied in content, length, frequency, and delivery, and measured sleep–wake outcomes in patients with varied diagnoses, though most participants had early-stage breast cancer. In a few recent studies, nurses with specialized sleep education and training delivered the CBTI/BT interventions.[13,100,101,103] Reports of CBTI/BT category studies were inconsistent regarding the impact of the intervention on functioning and other symptoms. Despite these limitations, effectiveness has been established: CBTI interventions improve sleep in cancer patients receiving adjuvant therapy and off-treatment survivors, and are ready for dissemination in clinical practice.

Complementary therapies. A variety of complementary therapies to relax the mind and body and improve sleep have been tested in adult patients with cancer. Types of complementary interventions delivered by specialized providers include Mindfulness-Based Stress Reduction (MBSR), autogenic training, supportive-expressive group therapy, expressive writing, progressive muscle relaxation (PMR), guided imagery, hypnosis, Healing Touch, and massage.

The results of only one large RCT have been reported. Breast cancer patients ($n = 170$) who were 2–12 months after surgery and adjuvant therapy were enrolled in this study; criteria for participation did not include the presence of insomnia. Cognitive therapy was compared to a combined relaxation and guided imagery (RGI) intervention; a control condition was included as a third group. Both interventions reduced psychological distress; but the RGI intervention was more effective in reducing levels of fatigue and sleep difficulties.[104]

In summary, investigations of complementary therapy interventions in cancer patients with mixed diagnoses have varied widely in terms of inclusion/exclusion criteria, content, frequency, and delivery as well as in the outcomes measured. The complementary therapy studies have rarely assessed the impact of the intervention on functioning, but have often reported on other symptoms. A growing body of evidence suggests that complementary therapies may improve sleep in cancer patients; however, results from several rigorous RCTs are needed before these interventions can be recommended for practice.

Education/Information. Favorable sleep outcomes resulting from an education/information intervention were found in only one RCT with a sample size greater than 100. An audiotaped educational intervention was effective in reducing problems with sleep in men receiving radiation for localized prostate cancer; however, criteria for participation did not include the presence of insomnia.[100] The education category studies rarely included the impact of the intervention on functioning, but often reported on other symptoms. More evidence is needed to evaluate the effects of education/information interventions in improving sleep in cancer patients before recommending such measures for oncology nursing practice.

Exercise. There are no published large RCTs that tested the benefits of exercise interventions on sleep–wake disturbances in patients with cancer. Evidence to date demonstrates a positive trend for exercise/activity interventions to improve sleep in patients with cancer, but the inclusion criteria for such studies have not required the presence of insomnia. The exercise category studies were inconsistent in including the impact of the intervention on functioning or other symptoms. More evidence from large RCTs is needed to evaluate the effects of exercise/activity interventions in improving sleep in cancer patients before exercise/activity can be recommended for practice.

Pharmacologic interventions

Despite a lack of evidence of effectiveness specific to cancer patients, there is widespread use of pharmacologic interventions to treat insomnia. Selection of medications to promote sleep is based on evidence from studies conducted in patients with primary insomnia. Current information about these medications are posted on the National Cancer Institute–PDQ website (www.cancer.gov/cancertopics/pdq/.../sleepdisorders/), and Table 6-5 outlines the various medication categories, names of medications within those categories, their doses, and comments about their use.

As can be seen in Table 6-5, several pharmacologic classes of medications are used to treat sleep disturbances: nonbenzodiazepine benzodiazepine receptor agonists, benzodiazepines, melatonin receptor agonists, antihistamines, antidepressants, and melatonin. Nurses need to become familiar with specific information about each class of medications.

Characteristics of these drugs that need to be taken into consideration by clinicians before selecting one to treat an individual patient include absorption, time to maximum concentration, elimination half-life, receptor activity, ability to cross the blood–brain barrier, dose and frequency, and short-acting versus long-acting formulation.

There are also safety issues to be considered by clinicians. In general, these include the potential for tolerance, abuse, dependence, and withdrawal (including risk of rebound insomnia), as well as medication interactions. Specific to cancer, concerns have been raised about potential interactions that may reduce the effectiveness of tamoxifen when it is taken with certain antidepressants.[107]

Despite their frequent use by the general public, over-the-counter (OTC) medications—most often antihistamines—have adverse effects on memory and performance and confer an increased risk of falls; thus they are not recommended.[108] Tolerance to the sedative effects of antihistamines can develop quickly. Medication interactions are possible and much remains unknown about the safety and effectiveness of OTC sleep aids.

Pharmacologic interventions had been rated using ONS-PEP as "Benefits Balanced with Harms"; current evidence does not support a change in this classification.[94] This category instructs clinicians to weigh the benefits versus the harmful effects of medications according to individual circumstances and priorities.

NURSING IMPLICATIONS

This chapter has presented information that confirms that sleep disturbances are common and distressing for people with various types of cancer and during several stages of disease. Sleep disturbances have been shown to result in a negative impact on physical, emotional, and social health and, therefore, on overall quality of life. With knowledge of sleep incidence, physiology, assessment, common disorders, and management strategies, oncology nurses are well positioned to intervene. Nurses play a key role in recognition of sleep disorders and general sleep disturbances at all phases of the continuum of care. Through routine sleep screening, nurses can identify patients with disrupted and insufficient sleep; referrals should be made for suspected primary sleep disorders (e.g., sleep apnea, restless legs syndrome). For general sleep disorders, nurses can provide and implement nonpharmacologic and pharmacologic interventions based on evidence-based recommendations for cancer patients. Nurses can make a difference in the quality of life of patients with cancer by recognizing the significant numbers of patients with sleep disturbances and by using available measures to accurately evaluate the severity and impact of sleep disturbance. In addition, nurses can become involved in research studies that build the science and lead to evidence-based recommendations and policies. Implementation and evaluation of these guidelines in community settings will assist nurses in adopting these interventions in specific practices.

PATIENT SELF-CARE

Appendices 6A and 6B outline self-care guidelines and monitoring strategies for patients. In addition to the information provided in the appendices, there are several patient-oriented

TABLE 6-5

Medications Commonly Used to Promote Sleep

Drug Category	Medication	Dose	Comments
Nonbenzodiazepine benzodiazepine receptor agonist	zaleplon (Sonata)	5–20 mg	Useful for problems falling asleep only.
	zolpidem tartrate (Ambien)	5–10 mg	Useful for problems falling asleep only.
	zolpidem tartrate extended-release (Ambien CR)	6.25–12.5 mg	Biphasic release; useful for problems both falling asleep and staying asleep; do not crush or split tablets.
	eszopiclone (Lunesta)	1–3 mg	Useful for problems both falling asleep and staying asleep; do not take with or right after meal.
Benzodiazepine	alprazolam (Xanax)	0.25–2 mg	Higher risk of withdrawal; side effects: lack of motor coordination, falls, and cognitive impairment.
	lorazepam (Ativan)	0.5–4 mg	Side effects: lack of motor coordination, falls, and cognitive impairment.
	clonazepam (Klonopin)	0.5–4 mg	Side effects: lack of motor coordination, falls, and cognitive impairment.
	temazepam (Restoril)	15–30 mg	Side effects: lack of motor coordination, falls, and cognitive impairment.
Melatonin receptor agonist	ramelteon (Rozerem)	8 mg	Little negative effect on cognition, somnolence, motor coordination, or nausea; useful for problems falling asleep only.
Antihistamine	diphenhydramine (Benadryl)	25–100 mg	Useful for problems falling asleep only; good side-effect profile.
	hydroxyzine (Vistaril, Atarax)	10–100 mg	Useful for problems falling asleep only; anticholinergic side effects.
Tricyclic antidepressant	doxepin (Sinequan)	10–25 mg	Lower doses used for treatment of primary insomnia when antidepressant effect not needed; risk of anticholinergic side effects and weight gain.
	amitriptyline (Elavil)	10–15 mg	Lower doses used for treatment of primary insomnia when antidepressant effect not needed; risk of anticholinergic side effects and weight gain.
	nortriptyline (Pamelor)	10–50 mg	Risk of anticholinergic side effects and weight gain.
Second-generation antidepressant	trazodone (Desyrel)	25–200 mg	Risk of orthostatic hypotension and falls.
	mirtazapine (Remeron)	7.5–45 mg	If depression not a concern, 7.5–15 mg best for sleep, hot flashes, increased appetite, and less morning sedation. Be aware of fall risk.
Antipsychotic	quetiapine (Seroquel)	25–100 mg	Risk of weight gain, metabolic syndrome, abnormal/involuntary movements; possible cardiovascular effects (e.g., prolonged QT interval).
	chlorpromazine (Thorazine)	10–50 mg	Risk of weight gain, metabolic syndrome, abnormal/involuntary movements; possible cardiovascular effects (e.g., hypotension).
Chloral derivative	chloral hydrate	0.5–1.0 g	Used mainly for sleep maintenance; risk of gastric irritation; risk of dependence and withdrawal; lethal in overdose.

Source: Data from National Cancer Institute. Sleep Disorders[106].

books specifically designed to provide general information about sleep that may aid in finding solutions to insomnia. A partial listing includes the following texts:

- *The Insomnia Workbook: A Comprehensive Guide to Getting the Sleep You Need* by Stephanie A. Silberman. Published by New Harbinger Publications, Inc., in 2008. ISBN13: 9781572246355.
- *Overcoming Insomnia: A Cognitive-Behavioral Therapy Approach Workbook (Treatments That Work)* by Colleen E. Carney. Published by Oxford University Press, Inc., in 2008. ISBN 978-0-19-536590-0.
- *Quiet Your Mind and Get to Sleep: Solutions to Insomnia for Those with Depression, Anxiety or Chronic Pain* by Colleen E. Carney and Rachel Manber. Published by New Harbinger Publications, Inc., in 2009. ISBN-10: 1572246278; ISBN-13: 978-1572246270.

Several websites provide helpful, current information about strategies to improve sleep for the general public and cancer patients:

- National Cancer Institute, Physician Data Query (PDQ): a comprehensive cancer database that contains summaries on a wide range of cancer topics, including information about sleep disorders for individuals with cancer. http://www.cancer.gov/cancertopics/pdq/supportivecare/sleepdisorders/Patient
- Cancer.net: oncologist-approved cancer information from the American Society of Clinical Oncology for managing sleep disturbances. http://www.cancer.net/all-about-cancer/treating-cancer/managing-side-effects/sleeping-problems-insomnia
- National Sleep Foundation: an educational, scientific not-for-profit organization dedicated to improving sleep health and safety through education, public awareness, and advocacy. http://www.sleepfoundation.org

REFERENCES

1. Roscoe JA, Kaufman ME, Matteson-Rusby SE, et al. Cancer-related fatigue and sleep disorders. *Oncologist.* 2007;12(suppl 1):35–42.
2. American Academy of Sleep Medicine. *The International Classification of Sleep Disorders: Diagnostic and Coding Manual.* 2nd ed. Westchester, IL: American Academy of Sleep Medicine; 2005.
3. American Psychiatric Association. *Diagnostic and Statistical Manual of Mental Disorders.* 4th ed. Washington, DC: American Psychiatric Association; 2000.
4. Berger AM. Update on the state of the science: sleep–wake disturbances in adult patients with cancer. *Oncol Nurs Forum.* 2009;36(4):E165–E177.
5. Carskadon MA, Dement WC. Normal human sleep: an overview. In: Kryger MH, Roth T, Dement WC, eds. *Principles and Practice of Sleep Medicine.* 5th ed. Philadelphia, PA: Elsevier Saunders; 2011:16–26.
6. Vassalli A, Dijk DJ. Sleep function: current questions and new approaches. *Eur J Neurosci.* 2009;29(9):1830–1841.
7. Kushida CA, Morgenthaler TI, Littner MR, et al. Practice parameters for the treatment of snoring and obstructive sleep apnea with oral appliances: an update for 2005. *Sleep.* 2006;29(2):240–243.
8. Parker KP, Bliwise DL, Ribeiro M, et al. Sleep/Wake patterns of individuals with advanced cancer measured by ambulatory polysomnography. *J Clin Oncol.* 2008;26(15):2464–72.
9. Neu D, Linkowski P, Le BO. Clinical complaints of daytime sleepiness and fatigue: how to distinguish and treat them, especially when they become 'excessive' or 'chronic'? *Acta Neurol Belg.* 2010;110(1):15–25.
10. Jean-Louis G, Magai C, Consedine N, et al. Cancer worry and insomnia complaints among American women. *Behav Sleep Med.* 2009;7(2):63–72.
11. Le Guen Y, Gagnadoux F, Hureaux J, et al. Sleep disturbances and impaired daytime functioning in outpatients with newly diagnosed lung cancer. *Lung Cancer.* 2007;58(1):139–143.
12. Ancoli-Israel S, Savard J. Sleep and fatigue in cancer patients. In: Kryger MH, Roth T, Dement WC, eds. *Principles and Practice of Sleep Medicine.* 5th ed. Philadelphia: Elsevier Saunders; 2011:1416–1421.
13. Berger AM, Kuhn BR, Farr LA, et al. Behavioral therapy intervention trial to improve sleep quality and cancer-related fatigue. *Psychooncology.* 2009;18(6):634–646.
14. Moore TA, Berger AM, Dizona P. Sleep aid use during and following breast cancer adjuvant chemotherapy. *Psychooncology.* 2011;20(3):321–325.
15. Savard J, Liu L, Natarajan L, et al. Breast cancer patients have progressively impaired sleep–wake activity rhythms during chemotherapy. *Sleep.* 2009;32(9):1155–1160.
16. Brant JM, Beck SL, Dudley WN, Cobb P, Pepper G, Miaskowski C. Symptom trajectories during chemotherapy in outpatients with lung cancer colorectal cancer, or lymphoma. *Eur J Oncol Nurs.* 2011;15(5):470–477.
17. Palesh OG, Roscoe JA, Mustian KM, et al. Prevalence, demographics, and psychological associations of sleep disruption in patients with cancer: University of Rochester Cancer Center–Community Clinical Oncology Program. *J Clin Oncol.* 2010;28(2):292–298.
18. Jim HS, Small B, Faul LA, Franzen J, Apte S, Jacobsen PB. Fatigue, depression, sleep, and activity during chemotherapy: daily and intraday variation and relationships among symptom changes. *Ann Behav Med.* 2011;42(3):321–333.
19. Garrett K, Dhruva A, Koetters T, et al. Differences in sleep disturbance and fatigue between patients with breast and prostate cancer at the initiation of radiation therapy. *J Pain Symptom Manage.* 2011;42(2):239–250.
20. Kim HJ, Barsevick AM, Beck SL, Dudley W. Clinical subgroups of a psychoneurologic symptom cluster in women receiving treatment for breast cancer: a secondary analysis. *Oncol Nurs Forum.* 2012;39(1):E20–E30.
21. Matthews EE, Schmiege SJ, Cook PF, Sousa KH. Breast cancer and symptom clusters during radiotherapy. *Cancer Nurs.* 2012;35(2):E1–E11.
22. Khan L, Uy C, Nguyen J, et al. Self-reported rates of sleep disturbance in patients with symptomatic bone metastases attending an outpatient radiotherapy clinic. *J Palliat Med.* 2011;14(6):708–714.
23. Fleming L, Gillespie S, Espie CA. The development and impact of insomnia on cancer survivors: a qualitative analysis. *Psychooncology.* 2010;19(9):991–996.
24. Berger AM, Visovsky C, Hertzog M, Holtz S, Loberiza FR Jr. Usual and worst symptom severity and interference with function in breast cancer survivors. *J Support Oncol.* 2012; 10(3):112–118.
25. Akechi T, Okuyama T, Akizuki N, et al. Associated and predictive factors of sleep disturbance in advanced cancer patients. *Psychooncology.* 2007;16(10):888–894.
26. Vena C, Parker K, Allen R, Bliwise D, Jain S, Kimble L. Sleep–wake disturbances and quality of life in patients with advanced lung cancer. *Oncol Nurs Forum.* 2006;33(4):761–769.

27. White C, McMullan D, Doyle J. "Now that you mention it, doctor . . .": symptom reporting and the need for systematic questioning in a specialist palliative care unit. *J Palliat Med.* 2009;12(5):447–450.
28. Mystakidou K, Parpa E, Tsilika E, Pathiaki M, Galanos A, Vlahos L. Depression, hopelessness, and sleep in cancer patients' desire for death. *Int J Psychiatry Med.* 2007;37(2):201–211.
29. Coleman EA, Goodwin JA, Coon SK, et al. Fatigue, sleep, pain, mood, and performance status in patients with multiple myeloma. *Cancer Nurs.* 2011;34(3):219–227.
30. Dirksen SR, Epstein DR, Hoyt MA. Insomnia, depression, and distress among outpatients with prostate cancer. *Appl Nurs Res.* 2009;22(3):154–158.
31. Donovan KA, Jacobsen PB. Fatigue, depression, and insomnia: evidence for a symptom cluster in cancer. *Semin Oncol Nurs.* 2007;23(2):127–135.
32. Liu L, Fiorentino L, Natarajan L, et al. Pre-treatment symptom cluster in breast cancer patients is associated with worse sleep, fatigue and depression during chemotherapy. *Psychooncology.* 2009;18(2):187–194.
33. Beck SL, Dudley WN, Barsevick A. Pain, sleep disturbance, and fatigue in patients with cancer: using a mediation model to test a symptom cluster. *Oncol Nurs Forum.* 2005;32(3):542.
34. Kim HJ, Barsevick AM, Tulman L, McDermott PA. Treatment-related symptom clusters in breast cancer: a secondary analysis. *J Pain Symptom Manage.* 2008;36(5):468–479.
35. Powell C, Guerrero D, Sardell S, et al. Somnolence syndrome in patients receiving radical radiotherapy for primary brain tumours: a prospective study. *Radiother Oncol.* 2011;100(1):131–136.
36. Skerman HM, Yates PM, Battistutta D. Cancer-related symptom clusters for symptom management in outpatients after commencing adjuvant chemotherapy, at 6 months, and 12 months. *Support Care Cancer.* 2012;20(1):95–105.
37. Morin CM, Benca R. Chronic insomnia. *Lancet.* 2012;379(9821): 1129–1141.
38. Roth T. Comorbid insomnia: current directions and future challenges. *Am J Manag Care.* 2009;15(suppl):S6–S13.
39. Ozminkowski RJ, Wang S, Walsh JK. The direct and indirect costs of untreated insomnia in adults in the United States. *Sleep.* 2007;30(3):263–273.
40. Ronksley PE, Hemmelgarn BR, Heitman SJ, et al. Excessive daytime sleepiness is associated with increased health care utilization among patients referred for assessment of OSA. *Sleep.* 2011;34(3):363–370.
41. Mullington JM, Haack M, Toth M, Serrador JM, Meier-Ewert HK. Cardiovascular, inflammatory, and metabolic consequences of sleep deprivation. *Prog Cardiovasc Dis.* 2009;51(4):294–302.
42. Flynn KE, Shelby RA, Mitchell SA, et al. Sleep-wake functioning along the cancer continuum: focus group results from the Patient-Reported Outcomes Measurement Information System (PROMIS). *Psychooncology.* 2010;19(10):1086–1093.
43. Miller AH, Ancoli-Israel S, Bower JE, Capuron L, Irwin MR. Neuroendocrine-immune mechanisms of behavioral comorbidities in patients with cancer. *J Clin Oncol.* 2008;26(6):971–982.
44. Blask DE, Hill SM, Dauchy R,T et al. Circadian regulation of molecular, dietary, and metabolic signaling mechanisms of human breast cancer growth by the nocturnal melatonin signal and the consequences of its disruption by light at night. *J Pineal Res.* 2011;51(3):259–269.
45. Innominato PF, Focan C, Gorlia T, et al. Circadian rhythm in rest and activity: a biological correlate of quality of life and a predictor of survival in patients with metastatic colorectal cancer. *Cancer Res.* 2009;69(11):4700–4707.
46. Lange T, Dimitrov S, Born J. Effects of sleep and circadian rhythm on the human immune system. *Ann N Y Acad Sci.* 2010;1193:48–59.
47. Mullington JM, Simpson NS, Meier-Ewert HK, Haack M. Sleep loss and inflammation. *Best Pract Res Clin Endocrinol Metab.* 2010;24(5):775–784.
48. Ackermann K, Revell VL, Lao O, Rombouts EJ, Skene DJ, Kayser M. Diurnal rhythms in blood cell populations and the effect of acute sleep deprivation in healthy young men. *Sleep.* 2012;35(7):933–940.
49. Kotronoulas G, WengstrÖm Y, Kearney N. Sleep patterns and sleep-impairing factors of persons providing informal care for people with cancer: a critical review of the literature. *Cancer Nurs.* 2012;36(1): E1–E15.
50. Hearson B, McClement S, McMillan DE, Harlos M. Sleeping with one eye open: the sleep experience of family members providing palliative care at home. *J Palliat Care.* 2011;27(2):69–78.
51. Mao JJ, Armstrong K, Bowman MA, Xie SX, Kadakia R, Farrar JT. Symptom burden among cancer survivors: impact of age and comorbidity. *J Am Board Fam Med.* 2007;20(5):434–443.
52. Savard J, Villa J, Ivers H, Simard S, Morin CM. Prevalence, natural course, and risk factors of insomnia comorbid with cancer over a 2-month period. *J Clin Oncol.* 2009;27(31):5233–5239.
53. Davidson JR, MacLean AW, Brundage MD, Schulze K. Sleep disturbance in cancer patients. *Soc Sci Med.* 2002;54(9):1309–1321.
54. Casault L, Savard J, Ivers H, Savard MH, Simard S. Utilization of hypnotic medication in the context of cancer: predictors and frequency of use. *Support Care Cancer.* 2011;20(6); 1203–1210.
55. Spielman AJ, Caruso LS, Glovinsky PB. A behavioral perspective on insomnia treatment. *Psychiatr Clin North Am* 1987 December;10(4): 541–53.
56. Bardwell WA, Profant J, Casden DR, et al. The relative importance of specific risk factors for insomnia in women treated for early-stage breast cancer. *Psychooncology.* 2008;17(1):9–18.
57. Price MA, Zachariae R, Butow PN, et al. Prevalence and predictors of insomnia in women with invasive ovarian cancer: anxiety a major factor. *Eur J Cancer.* 2009;45(18):3262–3270.
58. Palesh OG, Collie K, Batiuchok D, et al. A longitudinal study of depression, pain, and stress as predictors of sleep disturbance among women with metastatic breast cancer. *Biol Psychol.* 2007;75(1):37–44.
59. Ancoli-Israel S. Recognition and treatment of sleep disturbances in cancer. *J Clin Oncol.* 2009;27(35):5864–5866.
60. Savard MH, Savard J, Trudel-Fitzgerald C, Ivers H, Quesnel C. Changes in self-reported hot flashes and their association with concurrent changes in insomnia symptoms among women with breast cancer. *Menopause.* 2011;18(9):985–993.
61. Grunfeld EA, Halliday A, Martin P, Drudge-Coates L. Andropause syndrome in men treated for metastatic prostate cancer: a qualitative study of the impact of symptoms. *Cancer Nurs.* 2012;35(1):63–69.
62. Hanisch LJ, Gooneratne NS, Soin K, Gehrman PR, Vaughn DJ, Coyne JC. Sleep and daily functioning during androgen deprivation therapy for prostate cancer. *Eur J Cancer Care (Engl).* 2011;20(4):549–554.
63. Buffum D, Koetters T, Cho M, et al. The effects of pain, gender, and age on sleep/wake and circadian rhythm parameters in oncology patients at the initiation of radiation therapy. *J Pain.* 2011;12(3):390–400.
64. Boonstra L, Harden K, Jarvis S, et al. Sleep disturbance in hospitalized recipients of stem cell transplantation. *Clin J Oncol Nurs.* 2011;15(3):271–276.
65. Matthews EE. Sleep disturbances and fatigue in critically ill patients. *AACN Adv Crit Care* 2011;22(3):204–224.
66. Bower JE. Behavioral symptoms in patients with breast cancer and survivors. *J Clin Oncol.* 2008;26(5):768–777.
67. Eisenberger NI, Inagaki TK, Mashal NM, Irwin MR. Inflammation and social experience: an inflammatory challenge induces feelings of social disconnection in addition to depressed mood. *Brain Behav Immun.* 2010;24(4):558–563.
68. Howren MB, Lamkin DM, Suls J. Associations of depression with C-reactive protein, IL-1, and IL-6: a meta-analysis. *Psychosom Med.* 2009;71(2):171–186.
69. Liu L, Mills PJ, Rissling M, et al. Fatigue and sleep quality are associated with changes in inflammatory markers in breast cancer patients undergoing chemotherapy. *Brain Behav Immun.* 2012; 26(5): 706–713.
70. Mills PJ, Ancoli-Israel S, Parker B, et al. Predictors of inflammation in response to anthracycline-based chemotherapy for breast cancer. *Brain Behav Immun.* 2008;22(1):98–104.

71. Achermann P, Borbely AA. Sleep homeostasis and models of sleep regulation. In: Kryger MH, Roth T, Dement WC, eds. *Principles and Practice of Sleep Medicine*. 5th ed. Philadelphia: Elsevier Saunders; 2011:431–444.
72. Lee KA, Ward TM. Critical components of a sleep assessment for clinical practice settings. *Issues Ment Health Nurs.* 2005;26(7):739–750.
73. Owens JA, Dalzell V. Use of the "BEARS" sleep screening tool in a pediatric residents' continuity clinic: a pilot study. *Sleep Med.* 2005;6(1):63–69.
74. Buysse DJ, Reynolds CF III, Monk TH, Berman SR, Kupfer DJ. The Pittsburgh Sleep Quality Index: a new instrument for psychiatric practice and research. *Psychiatry Res.* 1989;28(2):193–213.
75. Savard MH, Savard J, Simard S, Ivers H. Empirical validation of the Insomnia Severity Index in cancer patients. *Psychooncology.* 2005;14(6):429–441.
76. Johns MW. A new method for measuring daytime sleepiness: the Epworth sleepiness scale. *Sleep.* 1991;14(6):540–545.
77. Netzer NC, Stoohs RA, Netzer CM, Clark K, Strohl KP. Using the Berlin Questionnaire to identify patients at risk for the sleep apnea syndrome. *Ann Intern Med.* 1999;131(7):485–491.
78. Morin CM. *Insomnia: Psychological Assessment and Management*. New York: Guilford Press; 1993.
79. Carney CE, Buysse DJ, Ancoli-Israel S, et al. The consensus sleep diary: standardizing prospective sleep self-monitoring. *Sleep.* 2012;35(2):287–302.
80. Ward TM. Conducting a sleep assessment. In: Redeker NS, McEnany GP, eds. *Sleep Disorders and Sleep Promotion in Nursing Practice*. New York: Springer; 2011:53–70.
81. Berger AM, Wielgus K, Hertzog M, Fischer P, Farr L. Patterns of circadian activity rhythms and their relationships with fatigue and anxiety/depression in women treated with breast cancer adjuvant chemotherapy. *Support Care Cancer.* 2009; 18(1): 105–114.
82. Grutsch JF, Ferrans C, Wood PA, et al. The association of quality of life with potentially remediable disruptions of circadian sleep/activity rhythms in patients with advanced lung cancer. *BMC Cancer.* 2011;11:193.
83. Hanisch LJ, Gehrman PR. Circadian rhythm of hot flashes and activity levels among prostate cancer patients on androgen deprivation therapy. *Aging Male.* 2011;14(4):243–248.
84. Miaskowski C, Lee K, Dunn L, et al. Sleep–wake circadian activity rhythm parameters and fatigue in oncology patients before the initiation of radiation therapy. *Cancer Nurs.* 2011;34(4):255–268.
85. Barsevick A, Beck SL, Dudley WN, et al. Efficacy of an intervention for fatigue and sleep disturbance during cancer chemotherapy. *J Pain Symptom Manage.* 2010;40(2):200–216.
86. National Cancer Institute. Common Terminology Criteria for Adverse Events (CTCAE), v 4.03. *National Cancer Institute* 2012 May 9; Available at: URL: http://evs.nci.nih.gov/ftp1/CTCAE/CTCAE_4.03_2010-06-14_QuickReference_8.5x11.pdf. AccessedMay 9, 2010.
87. Karnofsky DA, Burchenal JH. The clinical evaluation of chemotherapeutic agents in cancer. In: MacLeod CM, ed. *Evaluation of Chemotherapeutic Agents*. New York: Columbia University Press; 1949:196.
88. Mor V, Laliberte L, Morris JN, Wiemann M. The Karnofsky Performance Status Scale: an examination of its reliability and validity in a research setting. *Cancer.* 1984;53(9):2002–2007.
89. Yates JW, Chalmer B, McKegney FP. Evaluation of patients with advanced cancer using the Karnofsky Performance Status. *Cancer.* 1980;45(8):2220–2224.
90. Oken MM, Creech RH, Tormey DC, et al. Toxicity and response criteria of the Eastern Cooperative Oncology Group. *Am J Clin Oncol.* 1982;5(6):649–655.
91. Edinger JD, Carney CE. (2008). Overcoming Insomnia: A Cognitive-Behavioral Therapy Approach. New York: Oxford University Press.
92. Perlis M, Aloia M, Kuhn B. (2011). Behavioral Treatments for Sleep Disorders: A Comprehensive Primer of Behavioral Sleep Medicine Interventions. Burlington, MA: Academic Press.
93. Eaton LH, Tipton JM. *Putting Evidence into Practice: Improving Oncology Patient Outcomes*. Pittsburgh, PA: Oncology Nursing Society; 2009.
94. Page M, Berger A. Sleep–wake disturbances. In: Eaton L, Tipton J, eds. *Oncology Nursing Society Putting Evidence into Practice: Improving Oncology Patient Outcomes*. Pittsburgh, PA: Oncology Nursing Society; 2009:285–297.
95. Edinger JD, Carney CE. *Overcoming Insomnia: A Cognitive-Behavioral Therapy Approach*. New York: Oxford University Press; 2008.
96. Perlis M, Aloia M, Kuhn B. *Behavioral Treatments for Sleep Disorders: A Comprehensive Primer of Behavioral Sleep Medicine Interventions*. Burlington, MA: Academic Press; 2011.
97. Morgenthaler T, Kramer M, Alessi C, et al. Practice parameters for the psychological and behavioral treatment of insomnia: an update. An American Academy of Sleep Medicine report. *Sleep.* 2006;29(11):1415–1419.
98. Arving C, Sjoden PO, Bergh J, et al. Individual psychosocial support for breast cancer patients: a randomized study of nurse versus psychologist interventions and standard care. *Cancer Nurs.* 2007;30(3):E10–E19.
99. Berger AM, Kuhn BR, Farr LA, et al. One-year outcomes of a behavioral therapy intervention trial on sleep quality and cancer-related fatigue. *J Clin Oncol.* 2009;27(35):6033–6040.
100. Epstein DR, Dirksen SR. Randomized trial of a cognitive-behavioral intervention for insomnia in breast cancer survivors. *Oncol Nurs Forum.* 2007;34(5):E51–E59.
101. Espie CA, Fleming L, Cassidy J, et al. Randomized controlled clinical effectiveness trial of cognitive behavior therapy compared with treatment as usual for persistent insomnia in patients with cancer. *J Clin Oncol.* 2008;26(28):4651–4658.
102. Tremblay V, Savard J, Ivers H. Predictors of the effect of cognitive behavioral therapy for chronic insomnia comorbid with breast cancer. *J Consult Clin Psychol.* 2009;77(4):742–750.
103. Dirksen SR, Belyea MJ, Epstein DR. Fatigue-based subgroups of breast cancer survivors with insomnia. *Cancer Nurs.* 2009;32(5):404–411.
104. Cohen M, Fried G. Comparing relaxation training and cognitive-behavioral group therapy for women with breast cancer. *Res Soc Work Pract.* 2007;17(3):313–323.
105. Kim Y, Roscoe JA, Morrow GR. The effects of information and negative affect on severity of side effects from radiation therapy for prostate cancer. *Support Care Cancer.* 2002;10(5):416–421.
106. National Cancer Institute. Sleep Disorders. 2012. http://www.cancer.gov/cancertopics/pdq/supportivecare/sleepdisorders/HealthProfessional. Accessed July 13, 2012.
107. Sateia MJ, Lang BJ. Sleep and cancer: recent developments. *Curr Oncol Rep.* 2008;10(4):309–318.
108. Turner C, Handford AD, Nicholson AN. Sedation and memory: studies with a histamine H-1 receptor antagonist. *J Psychopharmacol.* 2006;20(4):506–517.

Managing Sleep Disturbances

Patient Name: ______________________________

This guide will help you learn how to get the sleep your body needs. It includes helpful hints about ways to help you to fall asleep and stay asleep through the night.

Symptom and Description

Insomnia is a sleep disturbance defined as difficulty falling asleep and/or staying asleep. Insomnia can occur at any time in your life. People often report that it occurs at times of higher than usual stress. Trouble falling asleep or staying asleep may improve when the stressful time passes, or it may become a chronic problem. Insomnia can range from mild to severe. When it is moderate to severe, it can limit your ability to function and make other symptoms worse. Improving your sleep restores function of your body and mind, reduces other symptoms, and allows you to function and to care for yourself and others.

Prevention

Insomnia can be prevented, or at least reduced, by learning how to manage stress in your busy life. Insomnia can also be prevented or reduced by trying methods to fall asleep and to stay asleep. Many adults are not setting aside the needed 7–9 hours for sleep every night. The following sleep tips will help you get the sleep your body needs:

- Keep the same bedtime and get-up time.
- Have a dark, cool, and quiet bedroom, and use light bed clothes and blankets.
- Deal with feelings of anxiety and depression when you are wake. Think of one thing you can do to help with the feelings the next day. Try not to take these feelings to bed with you.
- To help you fall asleep and stay asleep, relax your body and your mind. You may want to use a relaxing activity, such as a warm bath or reading a book, just before you turn out the light to fall asleep.
- Avoid stimulants, such as coffee and tea, after noon to prevent problems sleeping.
- If trips to the bathroom wake you up at night, stop drinking fluids 2 hours before bedtime and go to the toilet right before you go to bed.
- Alcohol can make you sleepy, but it may lead to a restless sleep. If you drink alcohol, it is best to stop drinking after your evening meal.
- After you check with your healthcare team, begin a workout program such as walking, biking, or lifting light weights.

Management

Keeping a record of your sleep (see Appendix 6B) for a week may help you find the root of your sleep problems. By finding the root of the problems, you may change behaviors that improve sleep. These ideas may help:

- Go to bed when sleepy and about the same time each night _______ (± 15 minutes) 7 nights a week.
- Get up at _______ (± 15 minutes) 7 days a week.
- If a nap is needed, limit each nap to less than 1 hour and complete naps at least 4 hours before bedtime.
- If you cannot fall asleep within 20–30 minutes when first trying to fall asleep, or after being awake 30 minutes during the night, get up and go to another room to sit, read, or listen to soft music and return to bed when sleepy (repeat as needed).
- Use your bed for sleep and sexual activity only.
- Treat your pain.
- Try to deal with your feelings of anxiety and or depression during the day, rather than during sleep times.
- Avoid eating a heavy meal or drinking alcohol within 3 hours of bedtime, and reduce or stop drinking fluids 2 hours before bedtime. Limit caffeine drinks during the day, and try not to drink them in the evening.
- Seek treatment for all health conditions that can get in the way of sleep. For example, treating fevers, pauses in breathing and loud snoring, many trips to the bathroom, and leg or arm movement can improve sleep. Also, treatment for heartburn, hot flashes, and high blood sugar can lead to better sleep. Ask your healthcare team about any of your medicines that get in the way of your job or chores and night sleep.

Follow-up

Let your healthcare team know if these ideas do not improve your ability to fall asleep and stay asleep. In addition, call them immediately if the following occurs:

- You experience any severe symptoms (pain, nausea, anxiety/depression, sleep disturbances).
- You have a sudden change in your ability to take care of yourself and others.

Phone Numbers

Physician: ______________________________ Phone: ______________________________

Nurse: ______________________________ Phone: ______________________________

Clinic number: ______________________________

Source: Matthews EE, Berger AM. Sleep Disturbances. In: Yarbro CH, Wujcik D, Gobel BH, eds. *Cancer Symptom Management*. 4th ed. Burlington, MA: Jones & Bartlett Learning; 2014.

Daily Sleep Diary

Sleep diaries are helpful to figure out sleep problems and keep your healthcare team informed.

Name: Date:	Example							
	5/21 Monday	Day 1	Day 2	Day 3	Day 4	Day 5	Day 6	Day 7
1. I napped from ____ to ____. (Note the times of all naps.)	2:00 to 2:45							
2. I took ____milligrams of medication and/or ____ounces ____ alcohol as a sleep aid.	Ambien 10 mg							
3. I went to bed at ____o'clock and turned the lights out at ____ o'clock.	10:30 11:15							
4. After turning the lights out, I fell asleep in ____ minutes.	10							
5. My sleep was interrupted ____ times. (List number of night awakenings.)	2							
6. My sleep was interrupted for ____ minutes. (List duration of each awakening.)	20; 30							
7. My sleep was interrupted by hot flashes. (0 = not at all, 1, 2, 3, 4 = a great deal.)	4							
8. I woke up at ____ o'clock. (Note time of last awakening.)	6:15							
9. I got out of bed at ____o'clock. (Specify the time.)	6:40							
10. When I got up this morning, I felt ____. (1 = exhausted, 2, 3, 4, 5 = refreshed.)	2							
11. Overall, my sleep last night was ____. (1 = very restless, 1, 2, 3, 4, 5 = very sound.)	1							

Instructions: Write on the diary each morning about the previous day and night. For example, on Monday, you will tell about Sunday's naps and sleep in the Sunday Column.

Adapted from: Morin CM. *Insomnia: Psychological Assessment and Management.* New York: Guilford Press; 1993.

Source: Matthews EE, Berger AM. Sleep Disturbances. In: Yarbro CH, Wujcik D, Gobel BH, eds. *Cancer Symptom Management.* 4th ed. Burlington, MA: Jones & Bartlett Learning; 2014.

PART III

Alterations in Protective Mechanisms

Chapter 7
Hypersensitivity Reactions to Antineoplastic Drugs

Chapter 8
Infection

Chapter 7

Hypersensitivity Reactions to Antineoplastic Drugs

Wendy H. Vogel, MSN, FNP, AOCNP®

THE PROBLEM

"Adverse drug reaction" is a broad term that covers any expected or unexpected negative response to a pharmacologic drug. A hypersensitivity reaction (as the term is used in this chapter) is a type of adverse drug reaction that could include allergic reactions, infusion reactions (both allergic and cytokine-release reactions), and pseudoallergic drug reactions. By definition, hypersensitivity is an exaggerated body response to a foreign substance (in this case, a drug) that may or may not be IgE mediated. Hypersensitivity reactions may affect any organ system and may have variable presentations.[1] Table 7-1 provides definitions of terms that will be utilized in this chapter and will further the understanding of the reader.[1–5]

INCIDENCE

The overall incidence of all hypersensitivity reactions, including anaphylaxis, allergic reactions, and infusion reactions, to antineoplastic drugs is difficult to determine. It is likely under-diagnosed and under-reported.[1] The greatest majority of hypersensitivity reactions are Type A reactions (85%–90%).[2] About 10%–15% of hypersensitivity reactions are Type B reactions.[2] It is estimated that the lifetime incidence of anaphylaxis in the general population is approximately 1%–2%.[6] There are certain oncologic drugs that are more commonly associated with hypersensitivity (allergic or cytokine) reactions (Table 7-2).[7]

ETIOLOGY

As noted previously, hypersensitivity reactions may be classified as Type A or Type B reactions (see Table 7-1). Type A reactions are predictable and related to drug pharmacology.[2,3] Type B reactions are unpredictable and occur only in susceptible patients.[2,3] Type B reactions may be classified as exaggerated responses, idiosyncratic reactions, or immunologic reactions. In an exaggerated response, the patient develops an exacerbated adverse reaction to a drug at low doses. An example of this type of hypersensitivity reaction is the patient with a dihydropyrimidine dehydrogenase (DPD) deficiency. A patient with this deficiency cannot adequately metabolize thymine or uracil. When given a drug such as fluorouracil (5FU) at usual doses, patients develop severe and even life-threatening toxicities such as neutropenia, diarrhea, and mucositis.[8]

Idiosyncratic reactions may include pseudoallergic reactions (see Table 7-1). The underlying pathology of these reactions is often unknown. These types of reactions may mimic true allergic reactions but do not worsen with repeated exposure and cannot be diagnosed with skin testing. Some idiosyncratic reactions may be caused by genetic aberrations that result in certain deficiencies such as the x-linked disorder of glucose-6-phosphate dehydrogenase (G6PD) deficiency. This deficiency causes severe hemolytic anemia when certain antimalarial drugs or other oxidizing chemicals are administered.[9] The previous example of a DPD deficiency could also be classified as an idiosyncratic reaction, as it is an autosomal recessive genetic disorder.[5]

TABLE 7-1

Hypersensitivity Reactions Definitions

Term	Definition
Adverse drug reaction	A broad term that refers to any expected or unexpected negative response to a pharmacologic agent.
Allergic reaction	A Type B (see below) adverse reaction that is due to an immunologic response (mediated by drug specific antibodies [such as IgE] or activated T lymphocytes) to a pharmacologic agent (may also be called an immune reaction).
Anaphylactic reaction	A severe, life-threatening, allergic, systemic reaction involving multiple organ systems with rapid onset and possibly fatal outcome. Does not usually occur with the first exposure to drug.
Anaphylactoid reaction	An adverse drug reaction resembling anaphylaxis but is not IgE-mediated, rather is mediated by a nonimmunologic mechanism. (This term is no longer recommended for use.)
Biphasic reaction	Resurgence of reaction symptoms after initial improvement, usually within 30 minutes up to 8 hours (but could recur within days).
Cytokine release reaction	An adverse drug reaction (often to a monoclonal antibody) that is mediated by a cellular immune response, which causes T lymphocytes to release cytokines thereby causing an inflammatory response. It may appear clinically similar to an allergic reaction usually with mild to moderate symptoms and is more likely with the first dose and risk decreases with subsequent doses.
Delayed reaction	An adverse drug reaction that occurs at least one hour after the last administered dose (typically 6 hours) up to days after treatment. Varied causes, but generally not IgE-mediated.
Hypersensitivity reaction	An exaggerated or overreaction of the body to a foreign substance; this reaction may or may not be IgE-mediated.
Immediate reaction	An adverse drug reaction that occurs within one hour of the last administered dose. Example: a Type I (See Table 7-3), IgE-mediated reaction with risk of anaphylaxis.
Infusion reaction	An adverse reaction to a drug administered intravenously, may be allergic (IgE-mediated) or anaphylactoid (not mediated by IgE).
Non-immune hypersensitivity reaction	A Type B adverse reaction that clinically resembles an allergic reaction but does not have a proven immunological basis (also called a non-allergic or pseudoallergic reaction). Example: reaction to NSAIDs.
Pseudoallergic reaction	A Type B adverse drug reaction that clinically resembles an allergic reaction but does not have a proven immunological basis (also called a non-immune hypersensitivity reaction or idiosyncratic reaction).
Type A reaction	Predictable adverse reaction based on the pharmacology of the drug that could occur in any patient, dependent upon dose and exposure; example: neutropenia or nausea occurring from a chemotherapeutic agent.
Type B reaction	An unpredictable hypersensitivity reaction unrelated to drug pharmacology that is not dose dependent and occurs in a small percentage of susceptible patients; example: anaphylaxis secondary to a pharmacologic agent or an exaggerated adverse reaction to fluorouracil due to DPD deficiency.

Abbreviations: NSAIDs: nonsteroidal anti-inflammatory drugs; DPD: dihydropyrimidine dehydrogenase.

Source: Data from Pillans[1]; Celik et al[2]; Gomes and Demoly[3]; Sampson et al[4]; Vogel[5].

TABLE 7-2

Antineoplastic Drugs Commonly Associated with Hypersensitivity Reactions
Alemtuzumab
Bleomycin
Carboplatin
Cetuximab
Cisplatin
Cytarabine
Docetaxel
Etoposide
Gemtuzumab
Ixabepilone
L-asparaginase
Oxaliplatin
Paclitaxel
Pegylated liposomal doxorubicin
Procarbazine
Rituximab
Trastuzumab

Source: Data from Lee et al[7].

Type B reactions also include allergic drug reactions (see Table 7-1). Allergic drug reactions are caused by an immunologic response mediated by IgE. Hypersensitivity reactions are immune-mediated responses but may or may not be mediated by immunoglobulin E (IgE). Allergic drug reactions may be distinguished by the rapidity of onset—that is, they may be classified as either immediate reactions or delayed reactions (see Table 7-1). There are different systems of classifying allergic drug reactions. One of the most common classification systems is the Gell and Coombs system,[10–20] which divides allergic reactions into four categories (I to IV). Table 7-3 gives a brief overview of this classification system and antineoplastic drugs that may produce these reactions. Some reactions may be difficult to classify due to inadequate knowledge about the predominant immunologic mechanism.[10] An example of a reaction that is difficult to classify is exfoliative dermatitis.[10]

PATHOPHYSIOLOGY

Type I reactions are always IgE mediated.[10] These reactions occur within minutes to hours after drug exposure. IgE-mediated reactions require previous exposure to the drug. Certain patients exposed to a drug will form drug-specific IgE complexes that bind to mast cells and basophils. Upon recognizing that drug again, the IgE complexes bind to the drug, activating the cell and thereby causing the release of histamine and inflammatory mediators. The onset of symptoms is rapid, usually within an hour after administration. The route of administration impacts the onset; intravenous administration may cause symptoms within seconds. Symptoms may include urticaria (wheal and flare), angioedema, flushing, bronchospasm, laryngeal spasms, wheezing, vomiting, diarrhea, hypotension, and, in severe cases, anaphylaxis. Fever is absent in Type I reactions.

Type II reactions are considered cytotoxic and are relatively rare. A drug binds to the surfaces of certain cells (called drug-hapten coated cells). Antibodies (usually IgG or rarely IgM) are produced in response to this antigen. These antibodies bind to the cell surface, which marks these cells for elimination by macrophages. Hematopoietic cells are the most commonly affected; thus Type II reactions may cause hemolytic anemia, neutropenia, and thrombocytopenia. Fludarabine and oxaliplatin are two chemotherapeutic drugs that can cause hemolytic anemia.[16] Heparin-induced thrombocytopenia (HIT) is a well-recognized syndrome that leads to the formation of antibodies against platelet factor IV.[21] Rituximab has been implicated in drug-induced neutropenia.[16] Some Type II reactions cause complement activation. During the immune response, antibodies (IgG and IgM) bind to the antigens that are part of the composition of the cell surfaces or other tissue. These antibody–antigen complexes activate the classical pathway of complement and cause inflammation. Opsonization of the cell surface or the resulting membrane defect causes cell lysis. Hemolytic anemia is an example of this complement activation reaction.[13] Type II reactions are more common in drugs given in higher doses, over a long period of time, or given in recurrent exposures.[10] Symptoms related to Type II reactions usually begin 5–8 days after exposure, but this can vary.

Type III reactions are rare, more often noted with higher doses and prolonged exposures. These reactions occur due to the formation of antigen–antibody complexes. The drug acts as the antigen and binds with drug-specific IgG. These complexes precipitate in tissues and activate inflammatory cells; they may also activate complement (as noted earlier) and may cause serum sickness, vasculitis, or fever. Type III reactions usually take more than a week to present. Numerous antigen–antibody complexes are required to initiate symptoms. Antithymocyte globulin and rituximab are two drugs used in oncology and hematologic diseases that are known to cause serum sickness.[13,22] Gemcitabine, infliximab, and levamisole have been implicated in vasculitis.[19,20] Case studies of persons receiving sirolimus and tacrolimus report drug-induced fevers.[11,15]

Type IV reactions are not antibody mediated, but rather cell mediated; specifically, they are mediated by T cells. Eosinophils, macrophages, and neutrophils may also be implicated in Type IV reactions. These reactions usually have a delayed onset and may occur as many as 2–7 days to weeks following drug exposure.[10] Reactions often involve the skin due to the large number of T cells located in the skin. T cells are memory-effect cells that respond rapidly to foreign agents and that penetrate the dermatologic layer either from the circulation or through the skin.[10] Drug-specific $CD4^+$ and $CD8^+$ T cells recognize drugs through

TABLE 7-3

Gell and Coombs Classification System of Allergic Responses

Type	Predominant Immune Mechanism	Onset	Example	Causative Neoplastic Drugs
I	IgE-mediated	Immediate	Anaphylaxis, angioedema, pruritus, urticaria	Carboplatin, cisplatin, L-asparaginase, oxaliplatin, procarbazine
II	Cytotoxic (IgG- or IgM-mediated)	Delayed, variable	Hemolytic anemia, neutropenia, thrombocytopenia	Fludarabine, heparin, oxaliplatin, rituximab
III	IgG, immune complex (antigen-antibody) deposition and complement activation	Delayed (1–3 weeks)	Arthralgias, fever, glomerulonephritis, lymphadenopathy, serum sickness, vasculitis	Antithymocyte globulin, cyclosporine, gemcitabine, infliximab, levamisole, procarbazine, rituximab, sirolimus, tacrolimus
IV	T cell-mediated	Delayed (2–7 days)	Allergic contact dermatitis, drug-induced hepatitis, interstitial nephritis, morbilliform eruptions, Stevens-Johnson syndrome, toxic epidermal necrolysis	Allopurinol, antiepileptics, anti-infection sulfonamides, bortezomib, carbamazepine, imatinib, lenalidamide, rituximab, phenytoin
IVa	Activation and recruitment of monocytes (macrophages)		Contact dermatitis, tuberculin reaction	
IVb	Activation and recruitment of eosinophils		Chronic asthma or allergic rhinitis, maculopapular exanthema	
IVc	Activation and recruitment of T cells		Contact dermatitis, bullous exanthema, maculopapular exanthema	
IVd	Activation and recruitment of neutrophils		Behcet's disease	

Source: Data from Riedle and Casillas[10]; Aires et al[11]; Allegra et al[12]; da Silva et al[13]; Hausmann et al[14]; Hochegger et al[15]; Mintzer et al[16]; Mockenhaupt[17]; Posadas and Pichler[18]; Radic et al[19]; Venat-Bouvet et al[20].

T-cell receptors relying on major histocompatibility complex presentation of drug molecules to the T cells. Drugs stimulate T-cell receptors by covalent binding to peptides or utilizing certain structural features to interact directly with T-cell receptors. The immune response is characterized by the release of cytokines and chemokines (such as interleukins) that serve to activate monocytes, eosinophils, or neutrophils.[14,18] Type IV reactions may be subclassified by the cytokine that is produced and the type of effector cells that are involved in the immune response.[18] The risk of a Type IV reaction may be higher during a viral infection, such as infection with the Epstein-Barr virus or human immunodeficiency virus (HIV).

Contact dermatitis, chronic rhinitis, and asthma are Type IV responses triggered by topical exposures. One of the most severe Type IV reactions is Stevens-Johnson syndrome, which can be life threatening.[17] Stevens-Johnson syndrome is characterized by cutaneous erythema—severe mucocutaneous, bullous lesions causing the skin to slough and necrose. Fever, severe conjunctivitis, and blepharitis may also occur.[17] This reaction may appear weeks after treatment with sudden development of immunologic symptoms. Several antineoplastic drugs have been linked to Stevens-Johnson syndrome, including allopurinol, bortezomib, imatinib, lenalidamide, and rituximab.[12] Another severe, potentially fatal Type IV reaction is drug rash with eosinophilia and system symptoms (DRESS), also called drug-induced hypersensitivity syndrome (DiHS). This syndrome consists of a rash, fever, hypereosinophilia, lymphadenopathy, and multiorgan failure.[23] Some of the most common drug culprits causing DRESS are allopurinol, antiretroviral agents, antiepileptic agents, NSAIDs, and antibiotics such as carbamazepine, vancomycin, and sulfusalazine.[23–25]

There is actually a fifth type of hypersensitivity reaction, which is often called a pseudoallergic or an idiosyncratic reaction. These reactions appear similar clinically to true allergic reactions. However, the complete pathophysiology of the reaction is unknown or difficult to classify by the Gell and Coombs classification system[26] (see Table 7-3). Cytokine-release syndrome is an example of a pseudoallergic reaction, generally classified as a Type B reaction (non-IgE mediated). Monoclonal antibodies (MOAs) are most often the drugs responsible for this type of adverse drug reaction. MOAs are utilized in the treatment of autoimmune disease, inflammatory disease, prevention of organ transplant rejection, and cancer.[27] It is believed that MOAs bind directly to T cells, B cells, natural killer cells (NK cells), granulocytes, antigen-presenting cells, or other immune cells and mediators such as cytokines, chemokines, growth factors, and complement components, acting to deplete or suppress their function or to induce immune activation.[27] The MOAs used in cancer management usually cause immune activation. The mechanism of action of MOAs is not completely understood but is believed to be related to complement-dependent cytoxicity (CDC), antibody-dependent cytoxicity, and/or anti-angiogenic effects.[27] The immunomodulatory effects of the MOA may have undesirable adverse effects because the molecules targeted by the MOA may also be expressed on normal cells and tissue types.[27] Adverse effects of MOAs could include reactions that mimic hypersensitivity reactions, such as cytokine-release reactions.[5,26]

Although rare, MOAs can cause true allergic (Type I) reactions including anaphylaxis.[4,27] As with any other IgE-mediated reaction, this kind of reaction requires prior exposure to the MOA and rarely occurs during the first infusion. An exception is when a patient has developed antibodies that cross-react with the MOA,[27] The incidence of MOA-induced allergic reactions has occurred with an abnormally high frequency related to cetuximab infusions in certain parts of Tennessee, North Carolina, and Arkansas.[28,29] This increased risk of reaction has been linked to the high incidence of tick bites in these geographic areas and to the development of IgE antibodies specific for galactose-α-1,3-galactose.[28,30]

Cytokine-release reactions are a result of immune stimulation and are considered an acute-phase response.[31,32] MOAs bind to target cells and other effector cells such as mast cells. This binding lyses the cell, resulting in the release of cytokines (such as interleukins, interferons, and tumor necrosis factor) from the tumor cell as well as the effector cell.[5,27,33,34] The severity of cytokine-release reactions appears to be related to tumor burden, and these reactions occur more often with the first infusion when tumor burden is the highest.[5] This effect can be predicted or anticipated based on the number of circulating lymphocytes or a baseline elevated lactic dehydrogenase (LDH).[35]

Cytokine-release syndrome leads to symptoms such as fever, flu-like symptoms, flushing, chills, fatigue, nausea, rash, myalgias, anorexia, vascular leak, shortness of breath, and hypotension[27] (Table 7-4). Most of these reactions are grade I–II (Table 7-5) and usually develop within 30–120 minutes after the infusion begins.[27,36] The incidence of infusion reactions varies for different MOAs (Table 7-6).[29,37–48] Most cytokine-release reactions occur with the first infusion, and the risk decreases with each subsequent infusion. For example, about 70% of patients receiving rituximab will experience an infusion reaction; however, this rate decreases to about 30% by the fourth infusion.[41] About 10% of patients receiving rituximab will experience a grade IV reaction.[41] About 44% of patients receiving their first infusion of ofatumumab will have an infusion reaction; 29% will have such a reaction with the second infusion.[43] Just like any other oncologic agent, any MOA confers a risk of infusion reaction. Even when administering radioimmunotherapy, it is important to know that infusion reactions may still occur.[47,48]

It may be difficult to clinically distinguish between a cytokine-release syndrome and a true allergic reaction. However, this is very important because retreatment is possible with cytokine-release reactions, but is contraindicated in anaphylactic reactions.[30] Table 7-7 examines the general differences between the two reactions. These reactions often have similar presentations, although signs of respiratory distress (especially bronchospasm and wheezing) and urticaria are more common with anaphylaxis, and fevers and myalgias are more common with cytokine-release reactions.[30] All of these symptoms can present in either an allergic (anaphylactic) or cytokine-release syndrome. For example, dermatologic symptoms may be absent in 10%–20% of anaphylactic cases.[49]

TABLE 7-4

Signs and Symptoms of Cytokine-Release Syndrome
Abdominal pain
Angioedema
Bronchospasm (rare)
Chills/rigors
Dizziness
Dyspnea
Fatigue
Fever
Headache
Hoarseness
Hypertension
Hypotension (usually mild)
Nausea
Pruritus
Rhinitis
Skin rash
Stridor
Sweating
Throat irritation
Tremor
Urticaria

TABLE 7-5

National Cancer Institute Common Terminology Criteria for Adverse Events (CTCAE): Allergic Reaction

Adverse Event	Grade I	Grade II	Grade III	Grade IV	Grade V
Allergic Reaction	Transient flushing or rash, drug fever <38 degrees C (<100.4 degrees F); intervention not indicated	Intervention or infusion interruption indicated; responds promptly to symptomatic treatment (e.g., antihistamines, NSAIDS, narcotics); prophylactic medications for clinical sequelae indicated for ≤24 hrs	Prolonged (e.g., not rapidly responsive to symptomatic medication and/or brief interruption of infusion); recurrence of symptoms following initial improvement; hospitalization indicated (e.g., renal impairment, pulmonary infiltrates)	Life-threatening consequences; urgent intervention indicated	Death

Definition: A disorder characterized by an adverse local or general response from exposure to an allergen.

Source: Data from National Cancer Institute Common Terminology Criteria for Adverse Events (CTCAE)[36].

TABLE 7-6

Monoclonal Antibodies and Incidence of Severe Infusion Reactions

Drug	Incidence of All Grades of Infusion Reactions	Incidence of Grade III–IV Infusion Reactions	Recommended Premedications
Alemtuzumab	90%	41%	Acetaminophen and diphenhydramine
Bevacizumab	<3%	<1%	None
Brentuximab	12%	<1%	None
Cetuximab	25%	2%–5%*	Diphenhydramine
Gemtuzumab	30%**	6%–8%	Acetaminophen and diphenhydramine
Ibritumomab	27%–50%	4%	Acetaminophen and diphenhydramine
Ofatumumab	44%	2%–5%	Acetaminophen, antihistamine, and corticosteroid
Panitumumab	4%	1%	None
Rituximab	77%	10%	Acetaminophen, antihistamine (usually diphenhydramine)
Tositumomab	29%	Less than 2%	Acetaminophen and diphenhydramine
Trastuzumab	40%	Less than 1%	None

*Varies according to geographical region (up to 20%)

**Gemtuzumab infusion reactions generally occurred at the end of the two hour infusion

Source: Data from O'Neil et al[29]; Amgen Inc.[37]; Bristol-Myers Squibb[38]; Genentech Inc.[39]; Genentech Inc.[40]; Genentech Inc.[41]; Genzyme Corporation[42]; GlaxoSmithKine[43]; GlaxoSmithKine[44]; Seattle Genetics Inc.[45]; Song et al[46]; Spectrum Pharmaceuticals Inc.[47]; Wiseman et al[48].

SYMPTOM ASSESSMENT

RISK FACTORS

Certain factors may increase the risk of hypersensitivity reactions (Table 7-8). Pharmaceutical factors that increase the risk of a reaction include the route of administration of the drug or higher doses of the drug.[7,50] Intravenous administration of an antineoplastic drug increases the risk of a hypersensitivity reaction. An increasing number of treatment cycles increases the risk for certain drugs such as carboplatin. In addition, patient factors may influence the risk for a hypersensitivity reaction, such as female sex and genetic polymorphisms in the human leukocyte antigen

TABLE 7-7

Difference between Anaphylaxis and Cytokine-Release Reaction

Sign/Symptom	Anaphylaxis	Cytokine-Release Reaction
Abdominal pain	Yes	Yes
Angioedema	Yes	No
Bronchospasm	Yes	No
Chills/Rigors	Yes	Yes
Fever	No	Yes
Flushing	Yes	Yes
Hypertension	No	Yes
Hypotension	Yes	Yes
Incidence with first infusion	No	Yes*
Myalgias	No	Yes
Nausea/Vomiting	Yes	Yes
Pruritus	Yes	No
Rash	Yes	Yes
Respiratory distress**	Yes	Yes (with severe reactions)
Severity dependent upon tumor bulk	No	Yes
Tachycardia	Yes	Yes
Timing of reaction	May occur within seconds	30–120 minutes into infusion
Urticaria	Yes	No

*May occur with subsequent infusions but less likely

**Respiratory symptoms such as cough, dyspnea, nasal congestion, chest tightness, wheezing, hoarseness, bronchospasm

(HLA).[7,50] There are also exogenous factors such as viral infections with HIV or Epstein-Barr virus (EBV).[50]

Some risk factors place the patient at risk for a negative outcome secondary to a hypersensitivity reaction. Any process or limitation that might impede the early recognition and reporting of symptoms of an adverse drug reaction or anaphylaxis would place that person at risk.[49] This could include very young age, ineffective communication, impaired vision or hearing, neurologic disorders, psychiatric disorders (including depression), use of sedating medications, substance abuse, impaired cognition, learning disability, or impaired mobility.[49]

SELF-ASSESSMENT

Hypersensitivity reactions—particularly those that occur during an infusion—may cause extreme stress and fear in persons experiencing these reactions. Physical symptoms may be described as a general sense of warmth coming from within, feeling flushed, or itching. Chest or throat tightness may occur. The nose or throat may feel "itchy." There are reports of urinary or bowel urgency, abdominal cramping, nausea, and vomiting. Some people may feel light-headed or faint. Patients may complain of headache or chest, neck, or back pain. The tongue may feel "thick" or swollen; there may be complaints of hoarseness and difficulty breathing or swallowing. The person having an infusion reaction may experience shaking chills or trembling. There may be an extreme feeling of fear, called a sense of "impending doom."

OBJECTIVE ASSESSMENT

History

During a hypersensitivity reaction, it may be difficult to obtain an accurate and thorough history. In an acute reaction, the healthcare provider may need to rely on the medical record for history; therefore it is imperative that the history is performed prior to drug administration. Patients must be screened for risk factors that could contribute to or exacerbate an infusion reaction (Table 7-8). Previous history of an allergy should be carefully characterized and documented. A current medication list should be maintained, including prescribed and over-the-counter medications, herbals, and supplements. Particular notation should be made of medications such as beta blockers and angiotensin-converting enzyme inhibitors, as these

TABLE 7-8

Factors Linked to Increased Risk of a Hypersensitivity Reaction

Pharmaceutical factors

- Certain concomitant medications such as β-adrenergic blockers, ACE inhibitors, NSAIDs, opioids
- Drug unique characteristics
- Frequent dosing
- Higher doses
- Intravenous route of administration
- Prolonged dosing
- Rapid speed of administration

Patient Factors

- Atopic dermatitis
- Comorbidities such as cardiac or pulmonary disease (e.g., asthma)
- Female gender
- Genetic polymorphisms in drug metabolism
- Hapten-forming drugs
- Hematologic malignancies
- Increased socioeconomic status
- Iodine or seafood allergies
- Macromolecular drugs
- Lowered levels of vitamin D
- Multiple allergies
- Older age
- Previous exposure to the agent
- Prior reaction to drug in same chemical class
- Treatment naïve patients

Exogenous Factors

- Epstein-Barr virus or HIV
- Geographic location

Abbreviations: ACE: angiotensin-converting enzyme inhibitors; HIV: human immunodeficiency virus; NSAIDs: nonsteroidal anti-inflammatory drugs.

Source: Data from Gomes and Demoly[3]; Lee and Vadas[7]; Breslin[32]; Chung and O'Neil[33]; Warrington and Silviu-Dan[50].

medications could increase the severity of an anaphylactic reaction.[49] Beta blockers may also inhibit the effectiveness of anaphylactic treatments.[49] Comorbidities such as cardiovascular or respiratory disorders might affect the ability to tolerate a hypersensitivity reaction, increasing the risk of death.

When taking a history of a previous adverse drug reaction, detailed information is useful.[50] The patient is queried about dose and route of the suspect drug, signs and symptoms, timing of a reaction in relation to suspect drug, medical treatment or hospitalization, response to treatment, concurrent medications around the time of the adverse reaction, and if the patient had taken the suspect medication at a time previous to the adverse event. In some instances, the use of premedications such as an antihistamine or corticosteroid might reduce the risk or severity of a hypersensitivity reaction. If this has been prescribed, documentation of patient adherence is required.

Physical assessment

A prompt, thorough physical examination during a hypersensitivity reaction will focus on (but is not limited to) the cardiovascular, dermatologic, and respiratory systems.[5] Any body system can be affected. Table 7-9 illustrates clinical signs per body system of a hypersensitivity reaction. The airway, breathing, and circulation are first assessed whenever there is a suspicion of an adverse drug reaction.[5,10] Ominous signs include urticaria, laryngeal or pharyngeal edema, wheezing, and hypotension.[10] The skin should be examined for any signs of rash, angioedema, or erythema, as this may help differentiate the type of reaction.[49] Characterization and documentation of any skin lesions are essential.[10] During an acute reaction, vital signs are assessed and compared to baseline (prior to drug administration). Vital signs are repeated every 2–5 minutes until the patient is stable.[5]

TABLE 7-9

Physical Exam Findings of a Hypersensitivity Reaction

Body System	Clinical Signs
Cardiovascular	Bradycardia, tachycardia, arrhythmia, non-pitting edema, hypotension, hypertension
Central nervous system	Confusion, change in level of consciousness, syncope
Dermatologic	Angioedema, conjunctival erythema, flushing, erythema, rash, tearing, urticaria
Endocrine	Diaphoresis, fever, warmth to skin touch, rigors
Gastrointestinal	Abdominal cramping and pain, bloating, diarrhea, dysphagia, vomiting
Genitourinary	Incontinence, pelvic discomfort, renal impairment
Musculoskeletal	Arthralgias, fatigue, generalized weakness, hypotonia, myalgias, piloerection
Psychiatric	Anxiety, fear, tearfulness, sense of impending doom
Respiratory	Acute respiratory distress, cough, cyanosis, hoarseness, hypoxemia, laryngeal or oropharyngeal edema, rhinitis, rhonchi, stridor, wheezing

Diagnostic evaluation

The diagnostic work-up is usually limited in an acute reaction and adds little to the management of the reaction.[49] However, pulse oximetry or cardiac enzymes may be among the diagnostic tests performed. An ECG for assessment of arrhythmias may be performed. Arterial blood gases and blood glucose may also be obtained. After the initial management of anaphylaxis and when the patient is stable, a plasma histamine level or serum total tryptase level may be ordered to confirm the diagnosis of anaphylaxis.[49] Histamine may be measured either in the blood or in the urine. The plasma histamine and serum total tryptase tests must be drawn within 15–60 minutes after onset of anaphylactic symptoms.[49] The plasma histamine test requires immediate special lab handling (wide-bore needle, sample placed on ice, prompt centrifuge, and then frozen).[49] The urine test for histamine and the histamine metabolite *N*-methylhistamine is collected over the next 24 hours following the possible anaphylactic episode. The diagnosis of anaphylaxis or cytokine-release syndrome is usually based on the history, physical examination findings, and clinical judgment.[10]

DEGREES OF TOXICITY

Assessment and documentation of the severity of the hypersensitivity reaction are imperative to future treatment decision making, including drug rechallenge. The National Cancer Institute (NCI) Common Terminology Criteria for Adverse Events (CTCAE) is the most commonly used and reliable way of accurately grading a hypersensitivity reaction.[51] Table 7-5 lists criteria for grading an allergic reaction; Table 7-10 demonstrates criteria for anaphylaxis grading, and Table 7-11, criteria for cytokine-release syndrome. Grade I reactions generally do not require any infusion interruptions

TABLE 7-10

National Cancer Institute Common Terminology Criteria for Adverse Events (CTCAE): Anaphylaxis

Adverse Event	Grade I	Grade II	Grade III	Grade IV	Grade V
Anaphylaxis	-	-	Symptomatic bronchospasm, with or without urticaria; parenteral intervention indicated; allergy-related edema/angioedema; hypotension	Life-threatening consequences; urgent intervention indicated	Death

Definition: A disorder characterized by an acute inflammatory reaction resulting from the release of histamine and histamine-like substances from mast cells, causing a hypersensitivity immune response. Clinically, it presents with breathing difficulty, dizziness, hypotension, cyanosis and loss of consciousness and may lead to death.

Source: Data from National Cancer Institute Common Terminology Criteria for Adverse Events (CTCAE)[36].

TABLE 7-11

National Cancer Institute Common Terminology Criteria for Adverse Events (CTCAE): Cytokine-Release Syndrome

Adverse Event	Grade I	Grade II	Grade III	Grade IV	Grade V
Cytokine release syndrome	Mild reaction; infusion interruption not indicated; intervention not indicated	Therapy or infusion interruption indicated but responds promptly to symptomatic treatment (e.g., antihistamines, NSAIDS, narcotics, IV fluids); prophylactic medications indicated for ≤24 hrs	Prolonged (e.g., not rapidly responsive to symptomatic medication and/or brief interruption of infusion); recurrence of symptoms following initial improvement; hospitalization indicated for clinical sequelae (e.g., renal impairment, pulmonary infiltrates)	Life-threatening consequences; pressor or ventilatory support indicated	Death

Definition: A disorder characterized by nausea, headache, tachycardia, hypotension, rash, and shortness of breath; it is caused by the release of cytokines from the cells.

Source: Data from National Cancer Institute Common Terminology Criteria for Adverse Events(CTCAE)[36].

or any intervention. Grade II reactions may often be managed by infusion interruption and/or infusion rate decrease, and/or supportive therapy. Grade III or IV reactions require infusion interruption and symptomatic, urgent management. Grade IV reactions require urgent intervention, possibly including vasopressor or ventilatory support.

SYMPTOM MANAGEMENT STRATEGIES

THERAPEUTIC APPROACHES

Prevention

Hypersensitivity reactions can occur with any treatment at any time in any individual. Reactions are difficult to predict and may occur despite prophylactic measures. Oncology healthcare professionals realize that being prepared is the basis for good outcomes when administering any treatment for cancer. Patient education is key for early recognition of signs of a hypersensitivity reaction.[5] Delayed reactions (see Table 7-1) may also occur, and patients and families must understand what symptoms to report promptly. Once an adverse drug reaction or drug allergy has been noted, patients must understand the level of risk for future anaphylaxis and avoidance measures. Instruction should be given regarding cross-reactivity between various pharmacologic agents. Cross-reactivity refers to the ability of an antibody to bind to an antigen that did not stimulate its production. This usually occurs among allergens (drugs) that are structurally similar. Persons who have a reaction to a drug in a certain class of drugs should avoid exposure to other drugs within that class. An example of cross-reactivity would be a hypersensitivity reaction to sulfamethoxazole. When the individual is first exposed to another agent within that class of drugs, such as sulfacetamide, a hypersensitivity reaction would then occur due to the antibodies previously developed against sulfamethoxazole. Some adverse drug reactions may require instruction on how to self-administer epinephrine. Table 7-12 lists key elements in patient education.

TABLE 7-12

Key Elements in Patient Education about Hypersensitivity Reactions
Need for prompt reporting
Emergent contact information
Self-administration of epinephrine (if indicated)
Early recognition of signs and symptoms of reaction
Include family/significant others in patient education
Treatment procedures for hypersensitivity reaction in clinic
Wearing of a MedicAlert bracelet or necklace (if indicated)

It is critical for oncology healthcare professionals to be aware of patient and pharmacologic risk factors for hypersensitivity reactions (Table 7-8). Identification of those patients at higher risk will allow closer assessment of these individuals. With certain medications, test doses may be given prior to the therapeutic dose to determine the individual's degree of hypersensitivity. Intradermal skin testing may also be utilized prior to the first dose. This is useful in patients receiving carboplatin after the sixth dose and prior to first dose of asparaginase.[51,52] When giving asparaginase, skin testing is recommended if doses are separated by more than a week.[52]

Premedications may decrease the risk of a hypersensitivity reaction and/or reduce the severity of a reaction. Anaphylaxis, however, is not usually prevented by premedications.[49] Premedications might include an antihistamine, corticosteroid, and acetaminophen. Table 7-6 lists recommended premedications for selected MOAs. It should be noted, however, that premedications do not take the place of vigilant nursing assessment.

Another method of preventing an infusion reaction is beginning the infusion rate slowly and titrating upward as tolerated. Subsequent infusions often may be given over shorter periods of time as the tumor bulk lessens and patient tolerance improves.[26]

Management

There are guidelines for the management of infusion reactions and anaphylaxis. The Oncology Nursing Society has recommendations for prevention, assessment, and nursing management of anaphylaxis and infusion reactions.[53] Other organizations such as the American Academy of Allergy, Asthma and Immunology; the American Heart Association; and the World Allergy Association also offer guidelines and recommendations.

It is vital that any facility that is administering drugs with the potential for infusion reactions or anaphylaxis have emergency medications and equipment as well as a thoroughly trained staff.[5] Written protocols or standing orders for emergent treatment should be in place. Staff who are trained in cardiopulmonary resuscitation are also vital.

Whenever an infusion reaction or anaphylaxis is suspected, the offending medication should be immediately discontinued but the intravenous line is maintained with normal saline.[10] Figure 7-1 is a suggested algorithm for the management of a suspected hypersensitivity reaction.[5] Airway patency is established if compromised. The patient is placed in a recumbent position with elevated lower extremities.[7] The first responder should request the help of a resuscitation team or emergency medical services (911 call). Supplemental oxygen may be given at a high rate (6–8 L/min).[49] Epinephrine is the drug of choice for a suspected anaphylatic reaction and should be administered

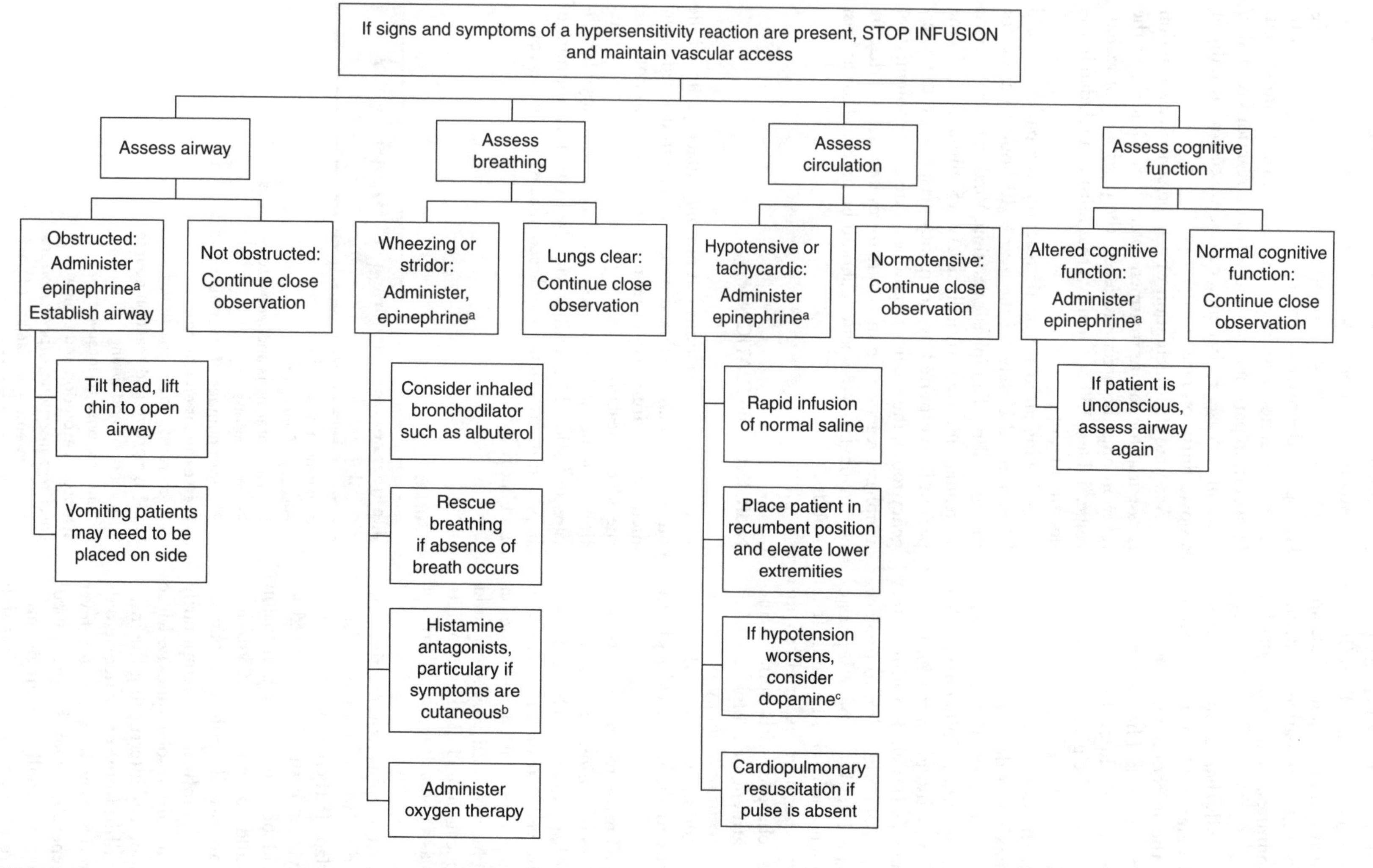

FIGURE 7-1

Suggested algorithm for the management of a hypersensitivity reaction.

Source: Adapted with permission from: Vogel WH. Infusion reactions: diagnosis, assessment, and management. *Clin J Oncol Nurs*. Apr 2010;14(2):E10–21.

[a]Epinephrine dosing is based on severity of the reaction. Epinephrine autoinjector intramuscularly (0.3 mg for adults) in lateral thigh may be given through clothing. Epinephrine 0.2–0.5 mg 1:1000 solution intramuscularly or subcutaneously may be repeated for five minutes as needed. Epinephrine also may be inhaled or given sublingually, via endotracheal tube, or via IV.

[b]Diphenhydramine is considered secondline to epinephrine and should never be administered alone in the treatment of anaphylaxis. Dosage is 25–50 mg IV. Combinations of H_1 and H_2 histamine antagonists are superior to single agent.

[c]Dopamine may be administered if hypotension is not controlled by epinephrine. Dosage is 400 mg in 500 mL of 5% dextrose at a rate of 2–20 mcg/kg per minute and titrated to patient's blood pressure.

promptly.[7,49,54] Other emergent medications may be indicated such as inhaled bronchodilators, H_1 or H_2 antihistamines, corticosteroids, and/or dopamine.[49] Vital signs are monitored every 2–5 minutes until the patient is stable, then every 5 minutes for 30 minutes, then 15 minutes for at least an hour.[55]

Epinephrine dosing is usually based on the severity of a reaction. Intramuscular (IM) administration is the preferred route, and the injection may be given through clothing in the lateral thigh.[7] The epinephrine auto-injector dose is 0.3 mg IM for adults. Epinephrine 0.2–0.5 mg of 1:1000 solution may be given IM or subcutaneously (SQ) and may be repeated every 15–20 minutes as needed. In children, the dose of epinephrine is given at 0.01 mg/kg to a maximum dose of 0.3 mg in a 30-kg child.[7] As many as one-third of patients will require a second dose of epinephrine.[7] Epinephrine also may be inhaled, given sublingually, given via endotracheal tube, or given intravenously. It is vital to administer epinephrine early in an anaphylactic reaction to prevent death.[7] This may reduce the likelihood of a biphasic reaction (see Table 7-1), which could also be fatal. It is recommended that patients who have experienced an anaphylactic reaction be discharged with epinephrine auto-injectors for prompt treatment of a biphasic reaction.[7] Biphasic reactions may occur in as many as 20% of anaphylactic reactions.[7] It should be noted that there are no absolute contraindications to the use of epinephrine in anaphylaxis.[54,56]

If the patient is not responsive to epinephrine and refractory bradycardia and hypotension are noted, the patient's current medication list should be checked for a beta blocker. It has been observed that beta blockers may decrease the efficacy of epinephrine.[7] Patients who are on beta blockers may require glucagon and aggressive fluid infusion.[7,49] The dose of glucagon is 1–2 mg in adults administered over 5 minutes as a bolus dose; this treatment may be repeated.[7]

Differentiating between an anaphylactic reaction and a cytokine-release reaction may not be possible, as signs of both reactions may overlap. If there is suspicion that the reaction may be anaphylaxis, it should be treated as such and epinephrine should be administered. Infusion reactions are most often mild to moderate. Cytokine-release syndrome reactions are usually mild to moderate and are managed by slowing the infusion or temporarily interrupting it.[28] Symptoms usually resolve quickly. More severe reactions require temporarily interrupting the infusion, and often additional antihistamine or corticosteroids may be indicated. Antipyretics may be given for fever and chills.[26] For rigors, meperidine may be prescribed. The infusion may be restarted (usually within 30 minutes) once symptoms have resolved, at a slower infusion rate. For severe reactions with life-threatening symptoms, epinephrine is recommended.[28] In cases of severe, life-threatening reactions, rechallenge is generally not recommended. With any decision to rechallenge, the underlying etiology of the reaction must be determined if possible. In an anaphylactic reaction, rechallenge is not recommended. However, in patients who had infusion reactions related to cytokine release, rechallenge can be successful, usually at a slower infusion rate.

Accurate documentation of a hypersensitivity reaction is essential for future treatment planning.[5] Grading of the reaction must be precise to assess the possibility of rechallenge. Table 7-13 lists elements that must be included in the documentation.

Following an anaphylactic reaction, the patient should be monitored closely for the next 8–12 hours to assess for the possibility of a biphasic reaction. Vital signs are assessed at regular intervals (usually every 15 minutes).[26] If the patient is transported by emergency personnel to the emergency room, the medics should be aware of the potential for a biphasic reaction. In moderate to severe reactions that are not anaphylaxis, the patient should be observed for at least 4 hours.[5]

NURSING IMPLICATIONS

Hypersensitivity reactions can not only affect quality of life but may also affect clinical outcomes due to delayed treatment or substitution of other medications that do not cause the adverse reaction. The most severe hypersensitivity reaction could be fatal. It is necessary that the oncology healthcare professional be familiar with the signs and symptoms of hypersensitivity reactions and recognize which agents confer a higher risk.

TABLE 7-13

Elements of Documentation of a Hypersensitivity Reaction
Pretreatment assessment
History of allergies
Baseline vital signs and laboratory values
Premedications
Previous number of treatment cycles
Pretreatment education
Infusion rates, doses, and timing
Initial symptoms and reaction course
Interventions and timing
Patient response to interventions
Symptom resolution and timing
Discharge instructions/prescriptions
Transfer to emergent facility (if performed)

Source: Data from Vogel[5].

The oncology nurse will ensure the safety of patients undergoing pharmacologic therapy for cancer in several ways. In the initial assessment, patients at risk for a hypersensitivity reaction are identified. These patients are monitored closely. A key to ensuring the safety of patients is the ongoing education of the patient and family about hypersensitivity reactions. The oncology nurse provides a setting in which patients feel encouraged and confident in reporting any early signs of a reaction.

The oncology nurse is skilled in safe administration of oncologic agents. The nurse is also adept in the early recognition and prompt management of a hypersensitivity reaction. Differentiating between Type I reactions and other reactions such as cytokine-release reactions is critical to decision making regarding possible retreatment. The grading of an adverse reaction is crucial to avoid undue subjectivity about the severity of the reaction. Prompt, skilled management of hypersensitivity reactions can avoid negative outcomes, including death. Follow-up and complete documentation allow future therapies to be completed safely. The assessment of psychological and coping mechanisms is another skill of oncology nurses intended to ensure ongoing safe therapy administration.

PATIENT SELF-CARE

Most oncologic treatments are given in an outpatient setting, so it is vital that patients and their support persons understand self-care strategies. It is vital that all of these parties be able to recognize early signs that indicate the need for urgent follow-up. Both verbal and written information must be provided to the patient and support persons. Appendix 7A provides a self-care guide for patients about hypersensitivity reactions to antineoplastic drugs. This guide may be copied and adapted for use in various facilities.

REFERENCES

1. Pillans PI. Clinical perspectives in drug safety and adverse drug reactions. *Expert Rev Clin Pharmacol.* 2008;1(5):695–705.
2. Celik G, Pichler WJ, Adkinson NF. Drug allergy. In: Adkinson NF, Bochner B, Busse W, Holgate S, Simons FE, Lemanske R, eds. *Middleton's Allergy Principles & Practice.* 7th ed. Philadelphia: Mosby Elsevier; 2009:1205–1226.
3. Gomes ER, Demoly P. Epidemiology of hypersensitivity drug reactions. *Curr Opin Allergy Clin Immunol.* 2005;5(4):309–316.
4. Sampson HA, Munoz-Furlong A, Campbell RL, et al. Second symposium on the definition and management of anaphylaxis: summary report—Second National Institute of Allergy and Infectious Disease/Food Allergy and Anaphylaxis Network Symposium. *J Allergy Clin Immunol.* 2006;117(2):391–397.
5. Vogel WH. Infusion reactions: diagnosis, assessment, and management. *Clin J Oncol Nurs.* 2010;14(2):E10–E21.
6. Lieberman P. Epidemiology of anaphylaxis. *Curr Opin Allergy Clin Immunol.* 2008;8(4):316–320.
7. Lee JK, Vadas P. Anaphylaxis: mechanisms and management. *Clin Exp Allergy.* 2011;41(7):923–938.
8. van Kuilenburg AB, Haasjes J, Richel DJ, et al. Clinical implications of dihydropyrimidine dehydrogenase (DPD) deficiency in patients with severe 5-fluorouracil–associated toxicity: identification of new mutations in the DPD gene. *Clin Cancer Res.* 2000;6(12):4705–4712.
9. Tripathy V, Reddy BM. Present status of understanding on the G6PD deficiency and natural selection. *J Postgrad Med.* 2007;53(3):193–202.
10. Riedl MA, Casillas AM. Adverse drug reactions: types and treatment options. *Am Fam Physician.* 2003;68(9):1781–1790.
11. Aires I, Carvalho D, Remedio F, et al. Sirolimus-induced drug fever in a renal transplant patient: a case report. *Transplant Proc.* 2009;41(3):957–958.
12. Allegra A, Alonci A, Penna G, et al. Stevens-Johnson syndrome after lenalidomide therapy for multiple myeloma: a case report and a review of treatment options. *Hematol Oncol.* 2012;30(1):41–45.
13. da Silva PS, Passos RM, Waisberg DR, et al. Serum sickness and severe acute renal failure after rabbit antithymocyte globulin treatment in aplastic anemia: a case report. *J Pediatr Hematol Oncol.* 2011;33(1):43–46.
14. Hausmann O, Schnyder B, Pichler WJ. Drug hypersensitivity reactions involving skin. *Handb Exp Pharmacol.* 2010;196:29–55.
15. Hochegger K, Rudnicki M, Auinger M, et al. Fever of unknown origin in renal transplant patients with tacrolimus. *Clin Transplant.* 2009;23(4):575–579.
16. Mintzer DM, Billet SN, Chmielewski L. Drug-induced hematologic syndromes. *Adv Hematol.* 2009;2009:495863.
17. Mockenhaupt M. The current understanding of Stevens-Johnson syndrome and toxic epidermal necrolysis. *Expert Rev Clin Immunol.* 2011;7(6):803–813; quiz 814–805.
18. Posadas SJ, Pichler WJ. Delayed drug hypersensitivity reactions: new concepts. *Clin Exp Allergy.* 2007;37(7):989–999.
19. Radic M, Martinovic Kaliterna D, et al. Drug-induced vasculitis: a clinical and pathological review. *Neth J Med.* 2012;70(1):12–17.
20. Venat-Bouvet L, Ly K, Szelag JC, et al. Thrombotic microangiopathy and digital necrosis: two unrecognized toxicities of gemcitabine. *Anticancer Drugs.* 2003;14(10):829–832.
21. Alberio L. Heparin-induced thrombocytopenia: some working hypotheses on pathogenesis, diagnostic strategies and treatment. *Curr Opin Hematol.* 2008;15(5):456–464.
22. Goto S, Goto H, Tanoshima R, et al. Serum sickness with an elevated level of human anti-chimeric antibody following treatment with rituximab in a child with chronic immune thrombocytopenic purpura. *Int J Hematol.* 2009;89(3):305–309.
23. Cacoub P, Musette P, Descamps V, et al. The DRESS syndrome: a literature review. *Am J Med.* 2011;124(7):588–597.
24. Hassan S, Wetz R, Zouein E. Allopurinol causing drug rash with eosinophilia and systemic symptoms syndrome: a challenging diagnosis. *Int J Gen Med.* 2011;4:789–792.
25. Jeung YJ, Lee JY, Oh MJ, et al. Comparison of the causes and clinical features of drug rash with eosinophilia and systemic symptoms and Stevens-Johnson syndrome. *Allergy Asthma Immunol Res.* 2010;2(2):123–126.
26. Gobel BH. Hypersensitivity reactions to biological drugs. *Semin Oncol Nurs.* 2007;23(3):191–200.
27. Brennan FR, Morton LD, Spindeldreher S, et al. Safety and immunotoxicity assessment of immunomodulatory monoclonal antibodies. *MAbs.* 2010;2(3):233–255.
28. Chung CH, Mirakhur B, Chan E, et al. Cetuximab-induced anaphylaxis and IgE specific for galactose-alpha-1,3-galactose. *N Engl J Med.* 2008;358(11):1109–1117.
29. O'Neil BH, Allen R, Spigel DR, et al. High incidence of cetuximab-related infusion reactions in Tennessee and North Carolina and the association with atopic history. *J Clin Oncol.* 2007;25(24):3644–3648.

30. Daguet A, Watier H. 2nd Charles Richet et Jules Hericourt workshop: therapeutic antibodies and anaphylaxis; May 31–June 1, 2011, Tours, France. *MAbs.* 2011;3(5):417–421.
31. Clarke JB. Mechanisms of adverse drug reactions to biologics. *Handb Exp Pharmacol.* 2010;196:453–474.
32. Breslin S. Cytokine-release syndrome: overview and nursing implications. *Clin J Oncol Nurs.* 2007;11(1 suppl): 37–42.
33. Chung CH, O'Neil BH. Infusion reactions to monoclonal antibodies for solid tumors: immunologic mechanisms and risk factors. *Oncology (Williston Park).* 2009;23(2 suppl 1):14–17.
34. Walker M, Makropoulos D, Achuthanandam R, et al. Recent advances in the understanding of drug-mediated infusion reactions and cytokine release syndrome. *Curr Opin Drug Discov Devel.* 2010;13(1):124–135.
35. Chung CH. Managing premedications and the risk for reactions to infusional monoclonal antibody therapy. *Oncologist.* 2008;13(6):725–732.
36. National Institutes of Health, National Cancer Institute. CTCAE: common terminology criteria for adverse events, version 4.03. http://evs.nci.nih.gov/ftp1/CTCAE/CTCAE_4.03_2010-06-14_QuickReference_8.5x11.pdf. Accessed August 12, 2012.
37. Amgen Inc. *Vectibix® (panitumumab) Prescribing Information.* Thousand Oaks, CA: Author; 2011.
38. Bristol-Myers Squibb. *ERBITUX® (cetuximab) Prescribing Information.* Indianapolis, IN: Author; 2012.
39. Genentech Inc. *AVASTIN (bevacizumab) Prescribing Information.* San Francisco, CA: Author; 2011.
40. Genentech Inc. *Herceptin (trastuzumab) Prescribing Information.* San Francisco, CA: Author; 2010.
41. Genentech Inc. *Rituxan (rituximab) Prescribing Information.* San Francisco, CA: Author; 2012.
42. Genzyme Corporation. *Campath® (alemtuzumab) Prescribing Information.* Cambridge, MA: Author; 2009.
43. GlaxoSmithKine. *ARZERRA (ofatumumab) Prescribing Information.* Research Triangle Park, NC: Author; 2011.
44. GlaxoSmithKline. *BEXXAR (tositumomab and Iodine I 131tositumomab) Prescribing Information.* Research Triangle Park, NC: Author; 2012.
45. Seattle Genetics Inc. *ADCETRISTM (brentuximab vedotin) Prescribing Information.* Bothell, WA: Author; 2012.
46. Song X, Long SR, Barber B, et al. Systematic review on infusion reactions associated with chemotherapies and monoclonal antibodies for metastatic colorectal cancer. *Curr Clin Pharmacol.* 2012;7(1):56–65.
47. Spectrum Pharmaceuticals Inc. *Zevalin (ibritumomab tiuxetan) Prescribing Information.* Irvine, CA: Author; 2011.
48. Wiseman GA, Gordon LI, Multani PS, et al. Ibritumomab tiuxetan radioimmunotherapy for patients with relapsed or refractory non-Hodgkin lymphoma and mild thrombocytopenia: a phase II multicenter trial. *Blood.* 2002;99(12):4336–4342.
49. Simons FE. Anaphylaxis. *J Allergy Clin Immunol.* 2010;125(2 suppl 2):S161–S181.
50. Warrington R, Silviu-Dan F. Drug allergy. *Allergy Asthma Clin Immunol.* 2011;7(suppl 1):S10.
51. Makrilia N, Syrigou E, Kaklamanos I, et al. Hypersensitivity reactions associated with platinum antineoplastic agents: a systematic review. *Met Based Drugs.* 2010: http://www.ncbi.nlm.nih.gov/pmc/articles/PMC2945654/.
52. Lee C, Gianos M, Klaustermeyer WB. Diagnosis and management of hypersensitivity reactions related to common cancer chemotherapy agents. *Ann Allergy Asthma Immunol.* 2009;102(3):179–187.
53. Polovich M, Whitford J, Olsen M, eds. *Chemotherapy and Biotherapy Guidelines and Recommendations for Practice.* 3rd ed. Pittsburgh, PA: Oncology Nursing Society; 2009.
54. Kemp SF, Lockey RF, Simons FE. Epinephrine: the drug of choice for anaphylaxis. A statement of the World Allergy Organization. *Allergy.* 2008;63(8):1061–1070.
55. Viale PH. Management of hypersensitivity reactions: a nursing perspective. *Oncology (Williston Park).* 2009;23(2 suppl 1):26–30.
56. Sheikh A, Shehata YA, Brown SG, Simons FE. Adrenaline for the treatment of anaphylaxis: Cochrane systematic review. *Allergy.* 2009;64(2):204–212.

Hypersensitivity Reaction to Antineoplastic Drugs

Definitions

A **hypersensitivity reaction** is an unwanted effect from a medication. It can occur during your treatment and may be mild or, in rare cases, life threatening.

An **anaphylactic reaction** is the most severe type of adverse drug reaction. It is a severe allergic reaction. This type of reaction can be caused by medicine, herbal products, supplements, and even foods. In some cases, anaphylaxis could be caused by an insect bite or sting or items such as latex gloves.

An **infusion reaction** is an unwanted effect from a medicine that is given through a vein (intravenously). An infusion reaction can vary from mild to severe. It may be an anaphylactic (or allergic) reaction or a cytokine-release reaction

A **cytokine-release reaction** is not an allergic reaction, but it may look and feel like one. This reaction may be stopped by slowing or stopping the infusion

Symptoms

If you experience any of the following reactions during your treatment, report right away to your oncology nurse:

- Fever
- Chills
- Itching
- Shaking
- Headache
- Rash, redness, hives
- Stomach pain, nausea, vomiting
- Feeling faint, dizzy, or light-headed
- Chest or throat tightness, hoarseness
- Trouble breathing, shortness of breath, wheezing
- Swelling of hands, feet, face, eyes, lips, or tongue

Prevention

Your Doctor or Nurse may give you medications to take before or after your treatment to help prevent a reaction. Not all reactions can be prevented.

Your medication to take to prevent a reaction: ______________________________

(continued)

Management

At times, a reaction can happen even if steps have been done to prevent it. If you have a reaction during treatment, your staff is trained to care for you during this time. It may seem scary, but remain calm. Some of the actions that your staff might take include these steps:

- Stop the treatment
- Oxygen therapy
- Run fluids in your IV line
- Take your blood pressure and pulse every few minutes
- Lie on your back in your chair or bed and raise your feet and legs up
- Medicine that may be given to treat your symptoms:
  - Epinephrine—for allergic reaction
  - Steroids—for allergic reaction
  - Antihistamines—for allergic reaction
  - Pain medicine—for any pain or hard, shaking chills
  - Antiemetics—for nausea or vomiting

If you are at home and feel any of the following symptoms, seek immediate medical care (call 911):

- Trouble breathing, wheezing, tightness in the chest or throat
- Trouble swallowing, swelling of the tongue or mouth
- Bad stomach pain, nausea and/or vomiting
- Feelings of dizziness, faintness or passing out
- Chest pain

After an Adverse Drug Reaction

Your Doctor or Nurse will help decide if this was an infusion reaction or an allergy. If this was an allergy, you may want to wear a MedicAlert bracelet or necklace. You will also want to inform all your other healthcare providers so that they could add this to your medical record.

If you have any questions, please do not hesitate to ask us!

Patient Name: ______________________________

Physician: ______________________________

Nurse: ______________________________

Contact Numbers: ______________________________ During office hours: ____________________

After office hours: ______________________________

Emergency: Call 911

Source: Vogel WH. Hypersensitivity Reactions to Antineoplastic Drugs. In: Yarbro CH, Wujcik D, Gobel BH, eds. *Cancer Symptom Management*. 4th ed. Burlington, MA: Jones & Bartlett Learning; 2014.

Chapter 8

Infection

Laura J. Zitella, MS, RN, ACNP-BC, AOCN®

THE PROBLEM

The patient with cancer is at increased risk of infection due to disease-related factors, treatment-related factors, and patient-related factors.[1] Cancer patients are a heterogeneous population, and the impact of infection varies based on the presence of these risk factors. Infectious complications affect the patient's quality of life, increase the risk of treatment-related morbidity and mortality, and contribute to dose reductions or dose delay, which may compromise the effectiveness of treatment.[2–6]

The type of cancer (solid tumor versus hematologic malignancy) increases the risk of neutropenia or other immune deficits such as those related to the number or function of lymphocytes. Treatment-related factors include the depth and duration of neutropenia or other immune deficits, disruption of the skin integrity due to surgery, the presence of indwelling catheters, and mucositis due to cytotoxic agents. Patient-related factors include age, nutritional deficiencies, and comorbidities such as chronic obstructive pulmonary disease (COPD) or diabetes. These factors should be considered when classifying patients into low risk, intermediate risk, and high risk categories. The prevention, diagnosis, and management of infectious complications are influenced by the overall risk of infection. Of these factors, neutropenia remains a significant risk factor; thus the prevention and management of neutropenia are critical in the care of patients with cancer. Patients who are hospitalized for febrile neutropenia have an estimated 6.8% to 20% mortality.[7]

This chapter reviews the current standards for the management of febrile neutropenia as well as the prevention and treatment of common infectious complications in patients with cancer. Strategies to prevent infection and effective management of infection can improve the delivery of optimal doses of cancer treatment, decrease disease burden and symptom distress, and enhance quality of life.

INCIDENCE

Febrile neutropenia (FN) occurs in 10% to 50% of patients after chemotherapy for solid tumors and in more than 80% of patients after chemotherapy for hematological malignancies.[8,9] Approximately 30% of patients on combination chemotherapy will experience either neutropenia, defined as an absolute neutrophil count (ANC) less than 500 cells/mm^3, or febrile neutropenia during their first cycle of chemotherapy.[10] Clinically documented infections occur in 20% to 30% of patients with FN; common sites of infection include bloodstream infections, gastrointestinal (GI) tract infections, pneumonia, and skin infections.[8] Bacteremia occurs in 10% to 25% of patients, generally in the setting of prolonged or profound neutropenia.[8] However, in the majority of cases of FN, no identifiable infection will be found, even though an estimated 50% of patients with febrile neutropenia have an infection.[11] In patients with solid tumors, the overall mortality associated with febrile neutropenia is 5%; this rate is approximately 1% in low-risk patients.[12] In contrast, overall mortality is as high as 11% in patients with hematologic malignancies, 18% in patients with microbiologically documented gram-negative infection, and 5% in patients with gram-positive bacteremia.[13]

ETIOLOGY

The etiology of infection in patients with cancer is multifactorial due to disease-related, treatment-related, and patient-related factors (Table 8-1).[1]

Disease-related factors

Hematologic malignancies, such as leukemia or lymphoma, inherently increase the risk of infection.[8] Infiltration of the bone marrow with tumor cells decreases normal white blood cell precursors or results in "functional neutropenia." Functional neutropenia is the term used to describe normal neutrophil counts accompanied by impaired neutrophil function, resulting in decreased microbicidal activity.[9] Involvement of the bone marrow was a significant risk factor for chemotherapy-induced febrile neutropenia in an analysis of patients with hematologic malignancies.[10]

Patients with leukemia experience prolonged periods of neutropenia, which correlates with the likelihood of sepsis or overwhelming infection.[11] Patients with chronic lymphocytic leukemia (CLL) or multiple myeloma are at increased risk of *Streptococcus pneumoniae, Haemophilus influenzae,* or *Neisseria meningitidis* infection due to

TABLE 8-1

Etiology of Infection in Patients with Cancer

Factor	Defect	Types of Infection
	Malignancy	
Acute leukemia	Neutropenia Qualitative defects	Bacterial, fungal, viral
Chronic lymphocytic leukemia, multiple myeloma	Humoral immunity	*Streptococcus pneumoniae* *Haemophilus influenzae* *Neisseria meningitidis*
Hodgkin's and non-Hodgkin's lymphoma	Cellular immunity	Viral, fungal
	Treatment	
Myelosuppressive chemotherapy	Neutropenia Altered mucosal barrier	Bacterial, fungal, viral Gram-negative colonization
Radiation	Neutropenia Altered skin integrity Altered mucosal barrier	Bacterial, fungal, viral Gram-negative colonization
Corticosteroids	Immunosuppression	Bacterial, fungal, viral *Pneumocystis jirovecii*
Bone marrow transplantation	Neutropenia Immunosuppression	Bacterial, fungal, viral Cytomegalovirus *Pneumocystis jirovecii*
Protein-calorie malnutrition	Immunosuppression	
Splenectomy	Humoral immunity	*Streptococcus pneumoniae* *Haemophilus influenzae* *Neisseria meningitidis*
	Nosocomial	
Tunneled central venous catheters, invasive procedures	Altered skin integrity	Coagulase-negative *Staphylococcus, Staphylococcus aureus*
Food	Colonization of exogenous organisms	*Escherichia coli, Salmonella, Listeria, Campylobacter jejuni*
Soil, decaying organic material, excavation or construction sites	Airborne fungal spores (can be inhaled)	*Aspergillus*

hypogammaglobinemia or functional hypogammaglobulinemia.[8,12,13] Patients with acute lymphocytic leukemia (ALL), CLL, Hodgkin's lymphoma, or non-Hodgkin's lymphoma typically have defects in cell-mediated immunity that predispose them to development of *Listeria, Salmonella,* mycobacterial, *Rhodococcus equi, Cryptococcus, Aspergillus,* and *Candida* infections; *Pneumocystis jiroveci* pneumonia; viral reactivation [herpes simplex virus (HSV), varicella zoster virus (VZV), cytomegalovirus (CMV), Epstein-Barr virus (EBV); adenovirus infections; and toxoplasmosis].[8,13,14]

Patients with advanced or refractory cancer are at higher risk of infection than patients who respond to therapy.[15] Tumor growth can alter normal anatomic structures and surgical procedures create wounds that are a site for potential infection.[16] Examples include head and neck cancers, which can erode through the neck or mouth; lung cancers, which predispose patients to post-obstructive pneumonia; tumors that obstruct the genitourinary tract and cause pyelonephritis; and tumors that obstruct the hepatobiliary tract and increase the risk of cholangitis.[16]

Treatment-related factors

Cancer treatments, such as chemotherapy, radiation, surgery, immunosuppressive therapy, or targeted agents, may influence the risk of infection through creation of immune dysfunction or disruption of the skin or mucosa. Disruption of the skin and mucosal barriers provides an opportunity for bacteria that colonize the skin, gastrointestinal tract, and mucosal membranes to invade the tissues and cause infection.[14] In particular, chemotherapy-induced mucositis and indwelling catheters create a significant breach in the skin and mucosal barriers, allowing direct access of pathogens to the bloodstream.[17–19] High-dose cytarabine is associated with severe mucositis that may predispose patients to life-threatening streptococcal infections, such as *Streptococcus viridans.*[20,21] Radiation therapy can also damage skin and mucosal integrity.

Chemotherapy regimens that result in severe myelosuppression are the main determinant of febrile neutropenia.[4,10] High dose chemotherapy, dose-dense chemotherapy regimens, and the use of chemotherapy agents such as anthracyclines, taxanes, or platinums are associated with an increased risk of neutropenia.[4,22,23]

Immunosuppressive agents, corticosteroids, and T-cell-depleting agents such as fludarabine and alemtuzumab impair T-cell function. Agents that impair T-cell function increase the risk for opportunistic infection such as invasive fungal infection, particularly *Aspergillus* and *Candida* spp., *Pneumocystis jiroveci, Listeria, Nocardia,* herpesviruses (cytomegalovirus, varicella zoster, and herpes simplex), and *Mycobacterium* spp. reactivation.[13] Temozolomide in combination with radiation is associated with increased susceptibility to *P. jiroveci,* as well as profound neutropenia.[24,25] Anti-CD20 monoclonal antibodies, such as rituximab, deplete B cells and increase the risk of hepatitis B reactivation.[26–28]

Splenectomy and functional asplenia increase the risk of sepsis from encapsulated bacteria such as *Streptococcus pneumoniae, Haemophilus influenzae,* and *Neisseria meningitidis.*[16] Functional asplenia refers to patients whose spleen is intact, but has reduced or absent function. Examples of conditions that result in functional asplenia include post-splenic irradiation, sickle cell anemia, or late complications of severe graft-versus-host disease (GVHD).[14,29,30] Anatomic asplenia occurs following splenectomy due to removal of the spleen or the congenital absence of a spleen from birth.

Patient-related factors

Patient-related factors that may influence infection include age, nutritional deficiencies, and comorbidities such as anemia, chronic obstructive pulmonary disease, and diabetes.[7,22] Patients with preexisting renal or hepatic dysfunction who are treated with chemotherapy have an increased risk of febrile neutropenia.[31] Malnourished patients are at increased risk of surgical site infections following tumor resection.[32,33] In patients with non-Hodgkin's lymphoma, an albumin level of 3.5 g/dL or less was associated with an increased risk of febrile neutropenia after the first cycle of cyclophosphamide, doxorubicin, vincristine, and prednisone (CHOP) chemotherapy.[34]

PATHOPHYSIOLOGY

The bone marrow, which is located in the medullary cavity of bone, is the site of effective hematopoiesis in adults. Hematopoietic stem cells in the bone marrow produce 6 billion cells per kilogram of body weight per day, including 1 billion neutrophils per kilogram of body weight per day. In adults, active sites of blood cell production include the bone marrow of the lower skull, sternum, ribs, vertebrae, pelvis, and proximal ends of the humerus and femur. Bone marrow dysfunction due to infiltration from hematologic malignancies or myelosuppressive effects of treatment can result in neutropenia. When bone marrow production of white blood cells is impaired by chemotherapy or radiation, there is a decrease in the number of circulating white blood cells, particularly neutrophils. Chemotherapy-induced neutropenia is relatively predictable, occurring 7 to 14 days after therapy and generally lasting for less than 7 days.[35,36] Patients undergoing hematopoietic cell transplantation (HCT) or induction therapy for acute leukemia have much longer periods of neutropenia and are at higher risk of infection.

SOURCES OF INFECTION

Infection occurs as a result of colonization by pathogenic bacteria, fungi, or viruses, particularly when host defenses are impaired. For this reason, the majority of initial infections in the neutropenic patient are due to endogenous bacterial and fungal flora and latent herpesvirus infections.[9,37] These pathogens include bacteria that routinely colonize the skin, such as *Staphylococcus aureus* and coagulase-negative staphylococci; oral microbes, such as *viridans* streptococci; and herpes simplex, as well as gram-positive bacteria and enteric gram-negative bacteria from the GI tract.[9] *Candida albicans* infections may be derived from the skin, the GI tract, or the female genital tract. Latent viral infections that may become reactivated during immunosuppression include those due to the herpes family of viruses, such as herpes simplex, varicella zoster virus, Epstein-Barr virus, and cytomegalovirus. Other pathogens that may become reactivated during periods of immunosuppression include hepatitis B and C viruses, *Mycobacterium* spp., and *Toxoplasma gondii*.[9]

Exogenous sources of infection from the home and hospital environment include contaminated water sources, contaminated blood products, contaminated hospital equipment, nosocomial infections due to spread of infection by healthcare workers, and spread of infection by family and friends. These types of infections may be due to pathogens including *Clostridium difficile,* respiratory viruses, vancomycin-resistant enterococci, multidrug-resistant bacteria, *Legionella*, *Klebsiella*, and *Enterobacter*. Foods can be a potential infection source; to counteract this risk, patients are advised to wash fresh fruits and vegetables thoroughly and to carefully cook meat, poultry, and eggs to the appropriate temperature. Potted plants, leaf blowers, and building or renovation sites should be avoided because aerosolization of *Aspergillus* and other molds found in organic decaying material and soil may cause disease.

SYMPTOM ASSESSMENT

RISK FACTORS

Major risk factors for the development of febrile neutropenia and its complications include age older than 65 years, the type and number of myelosuppressive chemotherapy agents used, planned dose intensity, comorbid conditions, previous chemotherapy, type of cancer, baseline leukopenia, liver function abnormalities, and renal dysfunction.[2,31,38] Although age is consistently identified as a significant risk factor, it is less important than the comorbidities that accompany increasing age. In fact, many studies have demonstrated that older patients are able to safely tolerate full doses of chemotherapy and that dose reductions compromise overall survival.[2,4,5,7] The risk of an initial episode of febrile neutropenia is greatest during the first cycle of treatment, presumably because growth factors or dose reductions are implemented with subsequent cycles after an episode of febrile neutropenia.[31,39]

The correlation between the depth and duration of neutropenia and the risk of infection has been recognized since 1966, when Bodey and colleagues published their sentinel data that demonstrated an increased risk of infection in patients with leukemia with an absolute neutrophil count (ANC) less than 1000 cells/mm^3 and a significantly increased risk of infection with an ANC less than 500 cells/mm^3.[11] The ANC is defined based on the number of segmented neutrophils and band neutrophils circulating in the bloodstream. It is calculated by multiplying the total white blood cell count by the percentage of neutrophils (Figure 8-1). The duration of neutropenia is also an important factor; the risk of infection increases when the ANC is less than 500 cells/mm^3 for more than 7 days, and it is in this setting that invasive fungal infections are likely to occur.

SELF-ASSESSMENT

Signs and symptoms of an infection may be muted or absent when neutropenia is present, but fever remains an early sign. Core body temperature is generally considered to be 37.0°C (98.6°F), yet it may vary in individuals by 0.5–1.0°C, according to circadian rhythm and menstrual cycle.[40] External variables also affect body temperature, such as heavy exercise, which can increase body temperature by 2–3°C.[40] The presence of mucositis can also artificially raise the oral temperature to 38°C.[41] Of the commonly available methods of measuring temperature, oral temperature measurements are recommended because they are safe, convenient, and accurate. Axillary measurements and chemical dot thermometers are not recommended because they are not as accurate; rectal temperature taking, which is the most accurate, should be avoided to decrease the risk of infection from enteric organisms.[40]

- Determine the white blood cell count (WBC) and percentage of neutrophils (segmented neutrophils and bands) from the complete blood cell count with differential.
- Use the following formula to determine the absolute neutrophil count (ANC).

$$\text{ANC} = \frac{(\%\ \text{segmented neutrophils} + \%\ \text{bands}) \times \text{WBC}}{100}$$

Example: $\text{ANC} = \frac{(24 + 1) \times 4000}{100} = 1000\ \text{cells/mm}^3$

FIGURE 8-1

Calculating the absolute neutrophil count (ANC).

OBJECTIVE ASSESSMENT

The Infectious Diseases Society of America (IDSA) and the National Comprehensive Cancer Network (NCCN) define febrile neutropenia as either (1) an ANC less than 500 cells/mm^3 or (2) an ANC less than 1000 cells/mm^3 predicted to decline to less than 500 cells/mm^3 over the next 48 hours.[1,9] Fever is defined as a core body temperature of 38.3°C (101°F) or for neutropenic patients, an oral temperature greater than 38°C (100.4°F) sustained for 1 hour or an isolated oral temperature greater than 38.3°C (101°F).[1,9,40,42] In some instances, a neutropenic patient may exhibit signs or symptoms of infection (e.g., abdominal pain, severe mucositis, perirectal pain) in the absence of a fever; he or she should be considered to have an active infection and started on empiric antibiotics. The concomitant administration of corticosteroids also may initially blunt the febrile response.

In contrast, noninfectious causes of fever in the setting of neutropenia are common and may include fever due to the underlying malignancy, administration of blood products, tumor lysis, hematomas, thrombosis, phlebitis, atelectasis, viscus obstruction, hematopoietic growth factors, or drug fevers.[43] It is not possible to distinguish between a noninfectious fever and an infectious fever, so all fevers must be treated as if there is an infection. Decades of research have demonstrated decreased infection-related mortality with the initiation of empiric antibiotics with the first observed fever.[43]

History

Febrile neutropenia requires prompt evaluation and intervention in the setting of neutropenia (Table 8-2).[1,9,44] The initial evaluation of a patient with fever should begin with a comprehensive history, physical examination, and assessment of the patient's level of risk for infection-related complications. The history includes a thorough site-specific review of systems as well as assessment of recent antibiotic therapy, recent surgery or other invasive procedures, chemotherapeutic agents given, concomitant steroid use, and possible exposure to infections from close contacts and household members, foods, animals, or travel. It is important to review previous positive microbiology—in particular, to identify prior infection with antibiotic-resistant organisms that might influence choice of therapy.

Physical examination

A complete physical examination is directed toward determining the possible sites of infection and causative organisms. However, typical clinical features of infection, such as induration, erythema, purulence, fluctuance, local pain, and tenderness, may be absent or muted in the absence of neutrophils and inflammation.[43] The absence of characteristic signs of infection contributes to the diagnostic challenge of documenting an infection, as it is not unusual for a patient to have pneumonia without a productive cough or evidence of pulmonary infiltrates on chest x-ray or to have an urinary tract infection without pyuria or dysuria.[43] The physical examination should include the oropharynx, which may reveal ulcers or white, plaque-like lesions due to herpes or thrush, respectively. Catheter sites should be assessed for erythema, tenderness, or discharge; of these, tenderness is the best predictor of infection because exudate may not be present in the absence of neutrophils. Gastrointestinal tract mucositis due to cytotoxic chemotherapy may cause a sore throat, oral ulcers, or diarrhea—conditions that are indistinguishable from the signs and symptoms of infection. Abdominal pain in neutropenic patients may be a sign of intestinal tumor necrosis or neutropenic enterocolitis. The perirectal area should not be overlooked because perirectal abscess, perirectal cellulitis, or anal fissures can occur in neutropenic patients.

Diagnostic evaluation

The initial laboratory evaluation should include a complete blood count with differential to determine the degree of neutropenia; complete metabolic panel with electrolytes, liver, and renal function tests; oxygen saturation; and urinalysis.[9] A chest x-ray should be performed when the patient presents with fever and neutropenia. Findings may not be conclusive in neutropenic patients with pneumonia, however, so a computerized tomography (CT) scan of the chest may be indicated to thoroughly assess for the source of infection.[1]

Culture specimens should be collected prior to the initiation of antibiotic therapy; there may be lower yields from cultures if antibiotics are administered prior to culture collection. Two sets of blood cultures should be obtained (one set of blood cultures generally consists of two blood culture bottles—one aerobic sample and one anaerobic sample), and each set of blood cultures should include at least 20 mL for a total of 40 mL of blood, given that an adequate volume of blood taken for culture enhances the likelihood of recovering a pathogen.[9,45] If a central venous catheter is present, one set of blood cultures should be obtained from the central venous catheter and one set from a peripheral vein for differential time to positivity testing. Differential time to positivity testing is a technique whereby cultures are drawn simultaneously from a central venous catheter and a peripheral vein. If the culture from the central venous catheter grows an organism 2 hours before the peripheral blood culture, it suggests that the infection is related to the central venous catheter. A meta-analysis of this technique showed an 81% to 85% sensitivity and specificity for identifying catheter-related bloodstream infections and more than a 99% negative predictive value.[46] In general, blood cultures from a peripheral vein are associated with a higher likelihood of identifying a causative organism.

TABLE 8-2

Nursing Assessment of Patients with Febrile Neutropenia

History
Previous cancer history, including dates of chemotherapy, biotherapy, and radiation
Review medications, including antimicrobial prophylaxis
Prior documented infections or pathogen colonization (e.g., MRSA, VRE)
Comorbidities
Recent surgical procedures
Infection exposures
Review of systems, including symptoms of infection
Physical Examination
Vital signs: Fever may be the only sign of infection, and hypotension or tachycardia suggests sepsis
Respiratory tract: Assess for abnormal breath sounds and cough
GI tract: Assess for abdominal tenderness, distention, firmness, or guarding
GU tract: Assess for lesions or breaks in the integrity of the perirectal area
Skin: Assess for lesions, breach of skin integrity, ulcers, erythema, or tenderness
Mucous membranes: Assess for redness, tenderness, ulceration, white patches, or plaques
Central nervous system: Assess for cranial nerve deficits or neurologic dysfunction
Catheter sites: Assess for erythema, exudate, inflammation, or tenderness
Laboratory Testing
CBC with differential
Comprehensive metabolic panel, including serum creatinine, blood urea nitrogen, electrolytes, hepatic transaminase enzymes, and total bilirubin
Blood cultures: obtained before administration of antibiotics from at least two separate sites, including one set from each lumen of a central venous catheter, if present, and from a peripheral vein. Differential time to positivity cultures can be helpful to determine if bacteremia is central line associated. A minimum of 40 mL of blood should be obtained to maximize diagnosis of bacteremia
Urinalysis
Chest radiograph
Site-Specific Testing
CSF: Lumbar puncture for culture of CSF if meningitis is suspected
Diarrhea: *Clostridium difficile* toxin assay
Dysuria: urine culture
Mucositis: HSV DFA
Rhinorrhea or nasal congestion: respiratory DFA for respiratory viruses
Productive cough: sputum culture
Skin or oral lesions: HSV/VZV DFA or biopsy of lesions

Abbreviations: CBC: complete blood count; CSF: cerebrospinal fluid; DFA: direct fluorescent antibody; GI: gastrointestinal; GU: genitourinary; HSV: herpes simplex virus; MRSA: methicillin-resistant Staphloccocus aureas; VRE: vacomycin-resistant enterococcus; VZV: varicella zoster virus.

Source: Data from National Comprehensive Cancer Network[1]; Freifeld et al[9]; Friese[44].

Routine cultures of the urine, stool, rectum, anterior nares, and oropharynx are rarely helpful in the absence of lesions or clinical signs and symptoms. However, cultures of suggestive sites of infection should be performed. For example, in the presence of diarrhea, stool cultures should be obtained for *C. difficile* toxin, and possibly rotavirus, norovirus, and adenovirus. Oral or perineal lesions should be tested for herpes simplex virus (HSV). Patients with symptoms of upper respiratory tract infections should be tested for respiratory viruses, such as influenza, respiratory syncytial virus, parainfluenza, adenovirus, and human metapneumovirus, using nasopharyngeal swab or nasal washing.[9] Urine culture should be performed in patients with dysuria or pyuria.

DEGREES OF TOXICITY

The Common Terminology Criteria for Adverse Events (CTCAE) [v.4.03], which is depicted in Table 8-3,[47] simply grades the depth of neutropenia after treatment. Clinically significant neutropenia, grade 4, is defined as

TABLE 8-3

National Cancer Institute Common Terminology Criteria for Adverse Events (CTCAE): Myelosuppression

Adverse event	Grade 0	Grade 1	Grade 2	Grade 3	Grade 4
Neutropenia (ANC, cells/mm³)	Normal ANC	< LLN–1500/mm³	<1500–1000/mm³	<1000–500/mm³	<500 mm³

Abbreviations: ANC: absolute neutrophil count; LLN: lower limit of normal.

Source: Data from National Cancer Institute Common Terminology Criteria for Adverse Events (CTCAE)[47].

a neutrophil count less than 500 cells/mm³. The CTCAE is used for grading response in cancer clinical trials, but is not useful for clinical management of febrile neutropenic patients.

Prediction of the risk for neutropenic complications guides the type of therapy (oral versus intravenous), the treatment setting (outpatient versus inpatient), and the duration of therapy. High-risk patients should be admitted to the hospital for intravenous antibiotics, whereas low-risk patients with no comorbidities may be considered for outpatient oral therapy.[9] Patients who are expected to have an ANC of less than 100 cells/mm³ for more than 7 days, including those undergoing allogeneic hematopoietic cell transplantation or induction therapy for acute leukemia, are considered to be at highest risk for infectious complications.[9] Febrile non-neutropenic patients with GVHD treated with corticosteroids also are considered to be at high risk for infections, particularly those due to encapsulated bacteria and invasive molds. The intermediate-risk group includes patients with solid tumors who have medical comorbidities, patients with lymphoma or CLL, and recipients of reduced-intensity conditioning allogeneic transplants, as they tend to have brief periods of neutropenia (less than 7 days). Although recipients of autologous hematopoietic cell transplants are generally neutropenic for 10 to 14 days, they are also considered to be at intermediate risk of infection. Any patient who presents with significant symptoms such as hypotension, abdominal pain, pneumonia, or neurological changes should be considered high risk and admitted to the hospital for evaluation and treatment.[9] Table 8-4 identifies high-risk and low-risk clinical features for neutropenic complications.[1,9,31]

The Multinational Association for Supportive Care in Cancer (MASCC) developed an index to predict the risk of serious neutropenic complications in febrile neutropenic cancer patients (Table 8-5).[15] Weighted numerical values are assigned to seven variables: (1) burden of illness (signs or symptoms at presentation); (2) hypotension; (3) COPD; (4) solid tumor or hematologic malignancy with no history of previous fungal infection; (5) dehydration; (6) outpatient status; and (7) age.

TABLE 8-4

Clinical Features of High Risk or Low Risk for Neutropenic Complications

High Risk
Neutropenia (ANC ≤100 cells/mm³) anticipated to extend more than 7 days Presence of any comorbid medical problems including, but not limited to: • Hemodynamic instability • Oral or gastrointestinal mucositis that interferes with swallowing or causes severe diarrhea • Abdominal pain or perirectal pain of new onset • Nausea and vomiting • Diarrhea (six or more loose stools daily) • Neurologic or mental status changes of new onset • Intravascular catheter infection, especially catheter tunnel infection • New pulmonary infiltrate or hypoxemia, or underlying chronic lung disease Evidence of hepatic insufficiency: • Aminotransferase values greater than 5 times normal values Evidence of renal insufficiency • Creatinine clearance less than 30 mL/min
Low Risk
• Neutropenia expected to resolve within 7 days • Absence of medical comorbidity • Adequate hepatic function and renal function

Source: Data from National Comprehensive Cancer Network[1]; Freifeld et al[9]; Lyman[31].

The maximal theoretical score is 26, and patients with a score of 21 or higher are considered low risk. Risk assessment should be performed as part of the initial evaluation of a patient with febrile neutropenia to determine whether the patient is high risk and requires admission to the hospital for intravenous antibiotics; low-risk patients may be candidates for outpatient management with oral antibiotics.[48] The MASCC risk index score has been validated in a

TABLE 8-5

Multinational Association of Supportive Care in Cancer (MASCC) Risk-Index Score

Characteristic	Weight
Burden of febrile neutropenia with no or mild symptoms	5
No hypotension (systolic BP > 90 mm Hg)	5
No chronic obstructive pulmonary disease	4
Solid tumor or hematological malignancy with no previous fungal infection	4
No dehydration requiring parenteral fluids	3
Burden of febrile neutropenia with moderate symptoms	3
Outpatient status	3
Age < 60 years	2

Note: Burden of febrile neutropenia refers to the general clinical status of the patient as influenced by the febrile neutropenic episode. It should be evaluated on the following scale:

1. No symptoms (score = 5 points)
2. Mild symptoms (score = 5 points)
3. Moderate symptoms (score = 3 points)
4. Severe symptoms (score = 0)
5. Moribund (score = 0)

Chronic obstructive pulmonary disease means active chronic bronchitis, emphysema, decrease in forced expiratory volume (FEV), and need for oxygen therapy and/or steroids and/or bronchodilators. Previous fungal infection means demonstrated fungal infection or empirically treated suspected fungal infection. The points attributed to the variable "burden of febrile neutropenia" are not cumulative.
The maximal theoretical score is therefore 26. The threshold for low risk is a score ≥ 21.
BP: blood pressure.

Source: Reprinted with permission from Klastersky J, Paesmans M, Rubenstein EB, et al. The Multinational Association for Supportive Care in Cancer Risk Index: a multinational scoring system for identifying low-risk febrile neutropenic cancer patients. *J Clin Oncol*. 2000;18:3038–3051[15].

number of trials; overall mortality is as low as 3% for low-risk patients with a MASCC score of 21 or higher, but as high as 36% if the MASCC score is less than 15.[48]

SYMPTOM MANAGEMENT STRATEGIES

THERAPEUTIC APPROACHES

Detection of a fever in a neutropenic patient is an oncologic emergency that requires an immediate evaluation and management (Figure 8-2).[1,9] There are no other specific clinical features, such as chills or hypotension, that can reliably distinguish between a fever due to infection and a fever due to a noninfectious cause. Therefore, all febrile neutropenic patients require empiric broad-spectrum antibiotics for initial therapy, ideally within 1 to 2 hours of the initial fever. The onset of the first neutropenic fever generally occurs 10 to 15 days following the start of chemotherapy, which coincides with the neutrophil nadir and the maximal cytotoxic effect on the intestinal mucosa.[43] Antimicrobials commonly used for the treatment of FN are listed in Table 8-6.

Initial empiric antibiotic therapy

The predominant cause of the initial neutropenic fever is bacteria.[43] In the past, gram-negative bacteria, including *Escherichia coli, Klebsiella* spp., and *Pseudomonas aeruginosa*, were the predominant causative organisms associated with febrile neutropenia. Currently, gram-positive pathogens, such as coagulase-negative *Staphylococcus, Staphylococcus aureus, Enterococcus* spp., and *viridians* group *Streptococcus*, are the most common source of neutropenic infections, presumably due to the increased use of central venous catheters and chemotherapeutic agents that cause mucositis.[49] Approximately 60% to 70% of positive blood cultures are reported to involve gram-positive pathogens.[9,43,50,51] However, antibiotic-resistant strains are emerging, such as extended-spectrum beta-lactamase (ESBL)–producing gram-negative bacteria, carbapenemase-producing organisms, vancomycin-resistant enterococcus (VRE), and methicillin-resistant *Staphylococcus aureus* (MRSA).[9,43] The initial empiric therapy for FN must include adequate gram-positive coverage as well as activity against gram-negative infections, particularly *Pseudomonas aeruginosa*, which are associated with a higher rate of mortality than gram-positive infections.[49] Despite numerous clinical trials to evaluate empiric antibiotic regimens, there is no empirical antibiotic therapy regimen that has demonstrated superiority over the others.[52,53] The choice of a specific regimen is based on the patient's risk factors for infection, the specific sites that may be sources of infection, and the prevailing institutional flora.

Monotherapy with a broad-spectrum antipseudomonal beta-lactam agent such as an extended-spectrum antipseudomonal cephalosporin (e.g., cefepime, ceftazidime), or piperacillin-tazobactam or a carbapenem (e.g., imipenem-cilastatin, meropenem), is recommended for the initial empiric therapy of febrile neutropenia.[1,9,50] Two meta-analyses reported an increased mortality with use of cefipime for the initial empiric treatment of febrile neutropenia,[52,53] but the Food and Drug Administration (FDA) performed an independent meta-analysis and determined that there was no increased risk of mortality associated with the use of cefipime.[54] An alternative initial approach is the use of combination therapy with an aminoglycoside plus either an extended-spectrum antipseudomonal cephalosporin or piperacillin-tazobactam or ciprofloxacin plus an

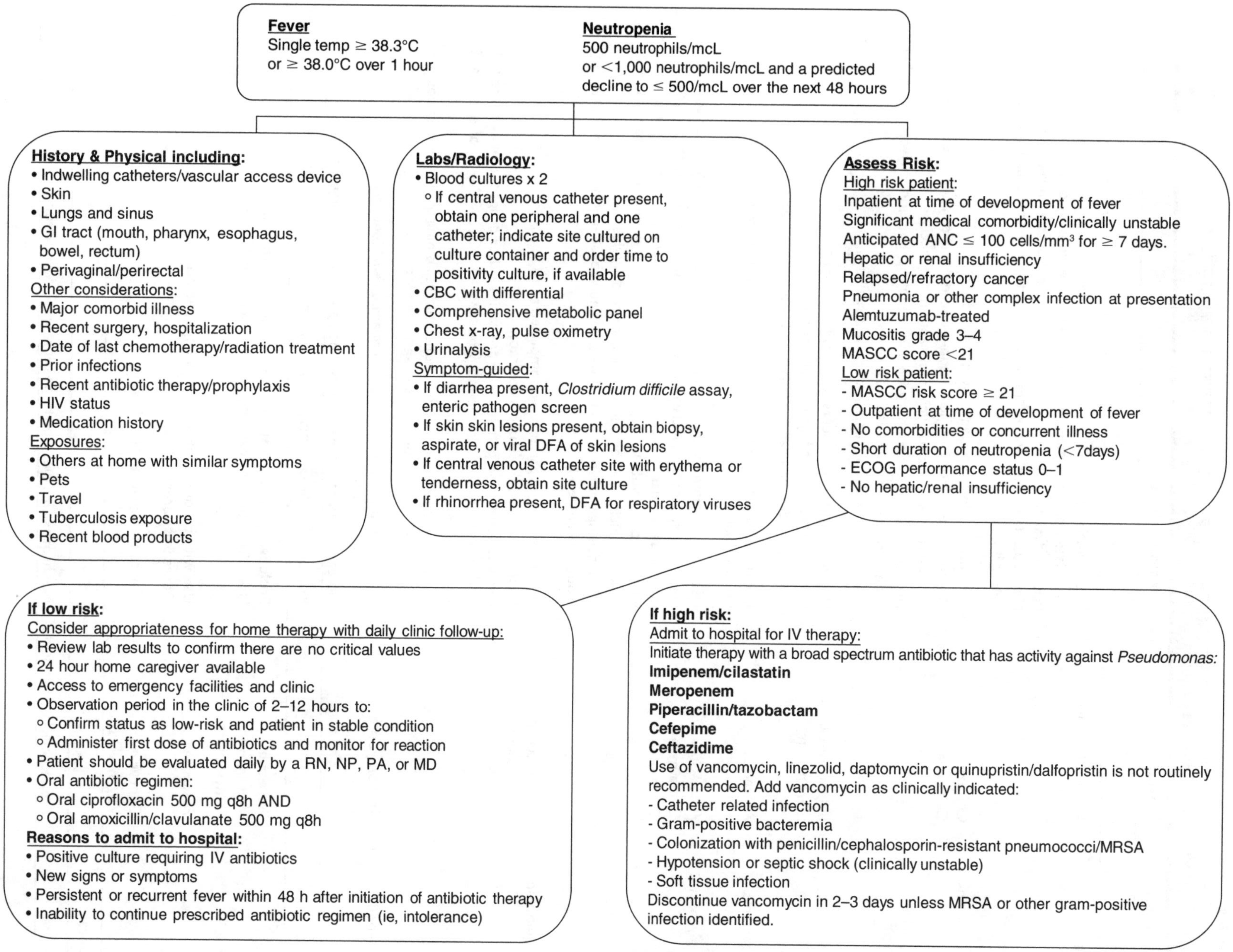

Fever
Single temp ≥ 38.3°C
or ≥ 38.0°C over 1 hour

Neutropenia
500 neutrophils/mcL
or <1,000 neutrophils/mcL and a predicted decline to ≤ 500/mcL over the next 48 hours

History & Physical including:
- Indwelling catheters/vascular access device
- Skin
- Lungs and sinus
- GI tract (mouth, pharynx, esophagus, bowel, rectum)
- Perivaginal/perirectal

Other considerations:
- Major comorbid illness
- Recent surgery, hospitalization
- Date of last chemotherapy/radiation treatment
- Prior infections
- Recent antibiotic therapy/prophylaxis
- HIV status
- Medication history

Exposures:
- Others at home with similar symptoms
- Pets
- Travel
- Tuberculosis exposure
- Recent blood products

Labs/Radiology:
- Blood cultures x 2
    - If central venous catheter present, obtain one peripheral and one catheter; indicate site cultured on culture container and order time to positivity culture, if available
- CBC with differential
- Comprehensive metabolic panel
- Chest x-ray, pulse oximetry
- Urinalysis

Symptom-guided:
- If diarrhea present, *Clostridium difficile* assay, enteric pathogen screen
- If skin skin lesions present, obtain biopsy, aspirate, or viral DFA of skin lesions
- If central venous catheter site with erythema or tenderness, obtain site culture
- If rhinorrhea present, DFA for respiratory viruses

Assess Risk:
High risk patient:
Inpatient at time of development of fever
Significant medical comorbidity/clinically unstable
Anticipated ANC ≤ 100 cells/mm^3 for ≥ 7 days.
Hepatic or renal insufficiency
Relapsed/refractory cancer
Pneumonia or other complex infection at presentation
Alemtuzumab-treated
Mucositis grade 3–4
MASCC score <21

Low risk patient:
- MASCC risk score ≥ 21
- Outpatient at time of development of fever
- No comorbidities or concurrent illness
- Short duration of neutropenia (<7days)
- ECOG performance status 0–1
- No hepatic/renal insufficiency

If low risk:
Consider appropriateness for home therapy with daily clinic follow-up:
- Review lab results to confirm there are no critical values
- 24 hour home caregiver available
- Access to emergency facilities and clinic
- Observation period in the clinic of 2–12 hours to:
    - Confirm status as low-risk and patient in stable condition
    - Administer first dose of antibiotics and monitor for reaction
- Patient should be evaluated daily by a RN, NP, PA, or MD
- Oral antibiotic regimen:
    - Oral ciprofloxacin 500 mg q8h AND
    - Oral amoxicillin/clavulanate 500 mg q8h

Reasons to admit to hospital:
- Positive culture requiring IV antibiotics
- New signs or symptoms
- Persistent or recurrent fever within 48 h after initiation of antibiotic therapy
- Inability to continue prescribed antibiotic regimen (ie, intolerance)

If high risk:
Admit to hospital for IV therapy:
Initiate therapy with a broad spectrum antibiotic that has activity against *Pseudomonas:*
Imipenem/cilastatin
Meropenem
Piperacillin/tazobactam
Cefepime
Ceftazidime
Use of vancomycin, linezolid, daptomycin or quinupristin/dalfopristin is not routinely recommended. Add vancomycin as clinically indicated:
- Catheter related infection
- Gram-positive bacteremia
- Colonization with penicillin/cephalosporin-resistant pneumococci/MRSA
- Hypotension or septic shock (clinically unstable)
- Soft tissue infection

Discontinue vancomycin in 2–3 days unless MRSA or other gram-positive infection identified.

FIGURE 8-2

Infection assessment and treatment.

Abbreviations: CBC: complete blood count; DFA: direct flourescent antibody; ECOG: Eastern Cooperative Oncology Group; GI: gastrointestinal; HIV: human immunodeficiency virus; MASCC: Multinational Association for Supportive Care in Cancer; MRSA: methicillin-resistant staphylococcus aureus

TABLE 8-6

Antibiotics Used to Treat Neutropenic Infection

Classification	Examples	Considerations
Beta-lactams		
Penicillins	Amoxicillin-clavulanate Piperacillin-tazobactam	Hypersensitivity. Associated diarrhea may be decreased with twice-daily dosing. Platelet dysfunction may occur, especially in patients with renal failure. May cause false-positive serum antigen test for galactomannan, a test for aspergillosis.
Cephalosporins	Ceftazidime Cefepime	Use with caution in patients on low-salt diets. May increase risk of *C. difficile* toxin-induced diarrhea and increase risk of colonization with vancomycin-resistant enterococci. Use with caution in patients with impaired renal function, if given with other nephrotoxic drugs, or if age >50 years. Contraindicated in patients with penicillin allergy.
Carbapenems	Imipenem-cilastatin Meropenem	Use with caution in patients with penicillin allergy. Can cause seizures at high concentrations. Risk of pseudomembranous colitis and hemorrhagic colitis.
Monobactams	Aztreonam	Contraindicated in patients with cephalosporin or penicillin allergy. Risk of toxic epidermal necrolysis.
Aminoglycosides	Amikacin Gentamycin Tobramycin	Use with extreme caution in patients with impaired renal function or hearing impairment; ototoxic; increased renal impairment if given with cisplatin. May cause tubular necrosis and renal failure; deafness due to cochlear toxicity; vertigo from vestibular organ damage; and (rarely) neuromuscular blockade. Risk of toxicity may be decreased by once-daily dosing. Initial dosing is based on actual weight, and subsequent doses are based on trough serum levels.
Fluoroquinolones	Ciprofloxacin Levofloxacin	Decrease dose in patients with impaired renal function. Gastrointestinal side effects common. Use with caution in patients who are taking other drugs that may cause QT interval prolongation; in patients who have low K^+, low Mg^{++}, or bradycardia; and in women. Tendon rupture can occur with concomitant administration of corticosteroids. Can cause false-positive urine drug screen for opiates.
Glycopeptides	Vancomycin	Use with caution in patients with impaired renal function. Risk of ototoxicity. Increased risk of nephrotoxicity when given with aminoglycosides.
Antivirals		Risk of kidney/liver damage and deafness.
	Acyclovir Valacyclovir Famciclovir	Prolonged use may result in emergence of resistant organisms. Use with caution in patients with impaired renal function.
	Foscarnet	Use with caution in patients with impaired renal function. Decreases serum calcium.
	Gancyclovir Valgancyclovir	May cause myelosuppression.
Antifungals		
	Amphotericin B products	Nephrotoxicity, electrolyte wasting, fever, chills, rigors.

TABLE 8-6

Antibiotics Used to Treat Neutropenic Infection (*continued*)

Classification	Examples	Considerations
Azoles	Fluconazole Itraconazole Posaconazole Voriconazole	Nausea and vomiting Hepatotoxicity Drug interactions Ocular toxicity (changes in color perception, blurred vision) with voriconazole Posaconazole should be administered with food to ensure adequate absorption
Echinocandins	Anidulafungin Caspofungin Micafungin	Excellent safety profile Rare hepatotoxicity

antipseudomonal penicillin, but there is no clear benefit to combination therapy and there is less toxicity associated with monotherapy.[1,9] If the patient is at risk for specific infections, such as MRSA infection, the addition of vancomycin is prudent. If the patient has pneumonia, the addition of an antipseudomonal fluoroquinolone (i.e., ciprofloxacin or levofloxacin) ensures a broadened spectrum against potentially resistant gram-negative or atypical pathogens, such as *Legionella*.[55] If an ESBL infection is identified, a carbapenem provides more effective coverage than a beta-lactam antibiotic.[9] When a culture demonstrates a causative organism, sensitivities should be performed to identify appropriate antibiotic therapy for the infection.[9]

Patients with FN who are clinically unstable, such as those with hypotension, or those who have a history of *P. aeruginosa* colonization or invasive disease, should receive multidrug therapy with an antipseudomonal beta-lactam (cephalosporin, carbapenem, or penicillin, depending on local susceptibilities) plus an aminoglycoside or ciprofloxacin, and vancomycin or another gram-positive active agent. Broad coverage is warranted in view of the high mortality rate in neutropenic patients with systemic inflammatory response syndrome.[56] Table 8-7 lists signs and symptoms seen with sepsis and septic shock. The standard management with sepsis or septic shock includes fluid resuscitation, oxygen, invasive hemodynamic monitoring, vasopressor support and stress-dose steroids.[56]

Despite the predominance of gram-positive pathogens in patients with febrile neutropenia, vancomycin is not routinely recommended for the initial treatment of febrile neutropenia.[9,57] The common antibiotics used for the initial treatment of FN provide adequate gram-positive coverage in most circumstances, and concern has arisen that the widespread routine empirical use of vancomycin will potentiate the prevalence of vancomycin-resistant organisms, especially enterococci. However, vancomycin should be considered for specific clinical situations such as suspected catheter-related infection in institutions with a high prevalence of MRSA infections.[58] Other indications for vancomycin include hemodynamic instability, skin or soft-tissue infection, pneumonia, or prophylaxis with fluroquinolones.[9] If the patient is known to be colonized with MRSA, vancomycin may be included in the initial regimen until blood and

TABLE 8-7

Progressive Organ Dysfunction in Septic Shock

Organ System	Severe Sepsis	Septic Shock
Central nervous system	Disorientation, agitation	Obtundation, coma
Cardiovascular	Sinus tachycardia	Dysrhythmias
	Decreased systemic vascular resistance	Systemic vascular resistance increases or decreases Acrocyanosis
Pulmonary	Tachypnea, hypoxia on room air	Refractory hypoxemia Pulmonary edema Acute respiratory distress syndrome
Renal	Decreased urine output	Oliguria
	Increased osmolality	Increased blood urea nitrogen, increased creatinine Acute renal failure
Metabolic and electrolyte	Lactic acidosis	Decreased albumin, potassium, sodium, calcium, magnesium, and phosphate
Integument	Dry, warm, and flushed skin	Cold, pale, and clammy skin
Gastrointestinal	Decreased motility	Increased liver function tests, jaundice

other cultures are proved negative.[9] Likewise, if a patient is known to be colonized with VRE, linezolid or daptomycin may be added to the initial regimen until cultures are proven negative.[9] Vancomycin may also be considered in patients who are at high risk of *viridans* streptococci infections given that approximately 10% to 25% are beta-lactam resistant.[9] If vancomycin was added initially for empirical coverage, it should be discontinued after 2 to 3 days if no evidence of a gram-positive pathogen is found.[9]

Outpatient management with oral antibiotics is a safe alternative for low-risk patients based on a meta-analysis of randomized controlled trials in adults and children with febrile neutropenia.[59] Oral ciprofloxacin plus amoxicillin-clavulanate (or clindamycin for patients who are allergic to penicillin) is a common outpatient regimen that is recommended by the NCCN and the IDSA based on several randomized controlled trials that demonstrated it is as effective as intravenous monotherapy.[1,9] Ciprofloxacin as a single agent does not provide adequate coverage for certain gram-positive organisms and, therefore, should not be used without an additional antibiotic directed toward those pathogens. Levofloxacin oral monotherapy has not been adequately studied.

Persistent neutropenic fever. The response to treatment is defined by resolution of fever or defervescence, and the median time-to-defervescence for high-risk patients treated with appropriate empirical antibacterial regimens is 5 to 7 days.[60] Therefore, at least 3 to 4 days of the initial antibiotic regimen should be continued in stable patients, regardless of persistent fever.[9] If there is a documented infection, it may take longer for the patient to respond to antimicrobial therapy, particularly if the infection is tissue based, such as pneumonia. Frequent and arbitrary antibiotic changes for persistent fever, in an otherwise stable patient, are not recommended.

Although fever resolution may be slow, persistent fever may suggest the emergence of an invasive fungal infection, a resistant bacterial infection, the emergence of a secondary infection, a closed-space infection, inadequate antimicrobial serum levels, or drug fever. Additional diagnostic testing, such as CT chest scan, may be considered to evaluate for the source of infection. Modification of the antibacterial antibiotics may be warranted to include increased gram-negative coverage. However, the addition of vancomycin, without specific indications, has not been shown to be effective.[9]

Patients with persistent fever after 4 to 7 days of initial broad-spectrum antimicrobial therapy without an identifiable site or source of infection should be treated with empiric antifungal coverage, as the risk of fungal infection increases with prolonged neutropenia.[9] Fungi are rarely the cause of the initial neutropenic fever; instead, they are associated with prolonged neutropenia. The most common fungal pathogens are *Candida* spp., which tend to colonize the mucosal tissue, and *Aspergillus*, which is inhaled through the respiratory tract and tends to cause sinus or pulmonary infection.[9] Liposomal amphotericin B preparation, caspofungin, itraconazole, voriconazole, and fluconazole are considered acceptable choices for empiric antifungal therapy.[1,9]

Duration of antibiotic therapy. It generally is recommended that empirical antibiotic therapy be continued for a clinically stable, afebrile patient until recovery of the ANC to more than 500 cells/mm^3 on one occasion.[1,9] In a stable patient who remains febrile despite resolution of neutropenia, it usually is safe to discontinue antimicrobials and look for a source of the fever. In patients who are afebrile and clinically stable but have continued neutropenia, some clinicians recommend completion of a 2-week course of antibiotics, followed by either close observation or fluoroquinolone prophylaxis.[9] Documented infections should be treated for a minimum duration of 7 to 14 days with an antibiotic regimen based on the particular organism.[1,9]

Central line–associated bloodstream infections. Central line–associated bloodstream infections (CLABSI) are common in cancer patients who have long-term central venous catheters. Differential time to positivity blood cultures that demonstrate growth from the culture drawn from the central line more than 120 minutes sooner than growth from a culture drawn from a peripheral vein suggests a CLABSI. If the CLABSI is caused by *S. aureus*, *P. aeruginosa*, fungi, or mycobacteria, the central line should be removed and antimicrobial therapy should be administered for at least 14 days.[9]

For clinically apparent catheter-related tunnel or pocket infection or septic phlebitis, vancomycin should be added to the initial empiric therapy. If there is no response to antibiotic therapy within 72 hours and/or there is hemodynamic instability or sepsis, the catheter should be removed.[1]

Prevention of infection

Colony-stimulating factors. Colony-stimulating factors (CSFs) such as granulocyte colony-stimulating factor (G-CSF) regulate the production, maturation, and function of neutrophil cells and result in an increase in circulating neutrophils.[61] Research has consistently shown that CSFs reduce the severity and duration of neutropenia, febrile neutropenia, and infection in adults and children who receive chemotherapy for cancer; however, there is no infection-related mortality or overall survival advantage.[62–66] Three consensus groups—the National Comprehensive Cancer Network (NCCN), the American Society of Oncology (ASCO), and the European Organisation of Research and Treatment of Cancer (EORTC)—recommend the primary use of CSFs in patients who are treated in the curative or adjuvant setting with regimens that carry a 20% or greater risk of febrile neutropenia.[22,23,42] CSFs may be considered as primary prophylaxis with regimens that have a 10% to 20% risk of febrile neutropenia if there are patient-specific risk factors, such as age, prior extensive chemotherapy, comorbid conditions, performance status, bone marrow involvement, and pretreatment blood counts.[22,23,42] Table 8-8[42] lists recommended doses and adverse events for CSFs. Figure 8-3 provides an algorithm for the use of CSFs.

TABLE 8-8

Colony-Stimulating Factors

Drug	Adverse Reactions
Filgrastim 5 mcg/kg (rounded to 300 mcg or 480 mcg) SC daily starting 24–72 hours after chemotherapy until ANC recovery	Allergic reactions: rash, pruritus, hypotension, tachycardia Splenic rupture ARDS Sickle cell disease crisis Bone pain Vasculitis Reversible increases in uric acid, lactate dehydrogenase and alkaline phosphatase; spontaneously reversible
Pegfilgrastim 6 mg SC once given 24–72 hours after the completion of chemotherapy and at least 14 days prior to the next cycle of chemotherapy	Splenic rupture ARDS Allergic reaction including anaphylaxis Bone pain
Sargramostim 250 mcg/m^2/day IV over 4 hours starting on day 11 or 4 days after completion of induction therapy in acute leukemia, if the bone marrow biopsy contains $<$ 5% blasts; continue until ANC $>$ 1500 cells/mm^3 for 3 consecutive days	Fluid retention Pleural or pericardial effusion Dyspnea Transient supraventricular arrhythmias (use with caution in patients with cardiac comorbidities) Diarrhea Rash Abdominal pain, chest pain, diarrhea, nausea, vomiting, hemorrhage, bone pain, high BUN, high cholesterol, insomnia (particularly after allogeneic HCT)

Abbreviations: ANC: absolute neutrophil count; ARDS: acute respiratory distress syndrome; BUN: blood urea nitrogen; HCT: hematopoietic cell transplantation; IV: intravenous; SC: subcutaneous.

Source: Data from National Comprehensive Cancer Network. *NCCN Clinical Practice Guidelines in Oncology: Myeloid Growth Factors* [v.1.2012][42].

Antibiotic prophylaxis. Antibiotic prophylaxis is defined as the administration of antibiotics to patients undergoing chemotherapy so as to decrease the risk of infection during chemotherapy-induced neutropenia. Antibiotic prophylaxis with fluoroquinolones significantly decreases the risk of infection, fever, and overall mortality in high-risk patients.[67–69] The majority of patients in clinical trials that evaluated the use of antibiotic prophylaxis have been high-risk patients with acute leukemia or undergoing HCT.[67,69] Patients who are at lower risk of infection do not derive as much benefit from the use of prophylactic antibiotics, and concern has arisen that the widespread use of broad spectrum antibiotics may promote antibiotic resistance.[1,70] Therefore, the use of antibiotic prophylaxis is recommended only for high-risk patients who are expected to have an ANC of 100 cells/mm^3 or less for more than 7 days.[1,9] Fluoroquinolones (e.g., ciprofloxacin 500–750 mg orally twice daily for 7 days or levofloxacin 500 mg orally daily for 7 days) are the recommended agents for antibacterial prophylaxis.[1,9] Levofloxacin is preferred for patients who are at risk of mucositis because it provides better coverage of mucositis-related *Streptococcus viridans* infections.[9] Table 8-9 lists the recommended antimicrobial prophylaxis based on the level of risk.[1,9]

Antiviral prophylaxis. Reactivation of latent human herpes viruses, such as HSV, VZV, and CMV, is common in patients with hematologic malignancies, particularly when such patients are treated with T-cell–depleting agents or HCT.[71] HCT recipients are at highest risk for viral infection, and seropositive patients who are not treated with prophylactic antiviral agents have an 80% risk of HSV infection, 20% to 30% risk of CMV infection, and 20% to 50% risk of VZV infection.[71]

Most HSV infections result from reactivation of latent virus. The patient populations at highest risk for HSV reactivation are patients with hematologic malignancies, patients undergoing HCT, patients with prolonged neutropenia, and patients treated with high-dose corticosteroids, T-cell–depleting agents, alemtuzumab, or bortezomib.[1] Patients in these high-risk groups who are HSV seropositive should receive prophylaxis against HSV infection with acyclovir, valacyclovir, and famciclovir.[1,8,48,49] In addition, if a patient has a HSV reactivation requiring treatment, HSV prophylaxis should be considered during all future episodes of neutropenia.

The principal risk factor for VZV infection is impaired cellular immunity, often associated with allogeneic HCT or therapy with a T-cell–depleting agent, such as fludarabine, alemtuzumab, or bortezomib. VZV prophylaxis is recommended in these patients using oral acyclovir 800 mg twice daily, oral valacyclovir 500 mg twice daily, or oral famciclovir 250 mg twice daily.

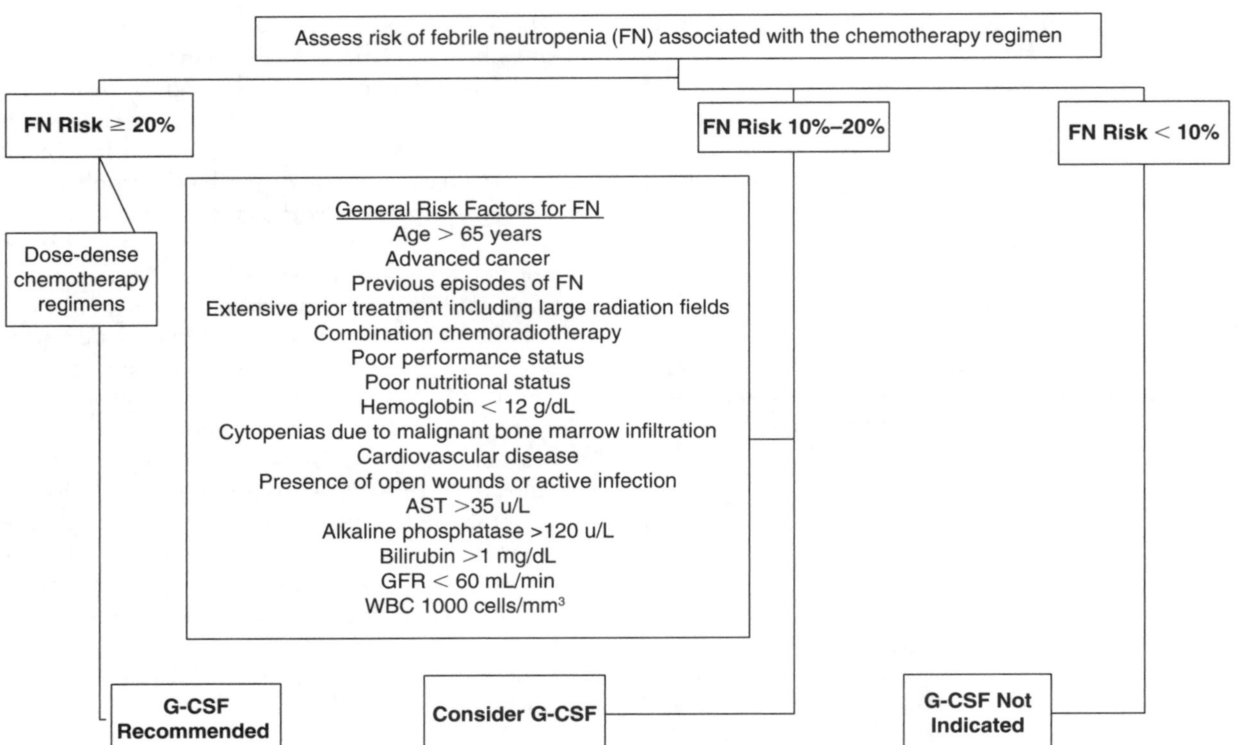

AST: aspartate aminotransferase; FN: febrile neutropenia; G-CSF: granulocyte-colony-stimulating factor; GFR: glomerular filtration rate; WBC: white blood count.

FIGURE 8-3

Prophylactic use of G-CSF to prevent febrile neutropenia (FN).

The individuals at highest risk for CMV reactivation are patients undergoing allogeneic HCT and patients with CLL treated with alemtuzumab.[1] CMV infection generally results from reactivation of the latent virus, yet there is a low risk of CMV transmission through blood products. The risk of CMV transmission can be prevented by the use of blood products from CMV-seronegative donors or the use of leukocyte-reduced, filtered blood products.[72] There is no recommended prophylaxis for CMV. Instead, a preemptive antiviral strategy is used for patients at high risk of CMV infection.[1,29,72] CMV viremia is monitored by CMV DNA polymerase chain reaction (PCR) technology; when CMV is detected, antiviral treatment with foscarnet, ganciclovir, or valganciclovir is initiated.[1,72]

Hepatitis B virus reactivation may occur with immunosuppression or B-cell depletion, so the patients at greatest risk of HBV reactivation are HCT recipients and patients with B-cell lymphoid malignancies treated with anti-CD20 monoclonal antibodies (rituximab or ofatumumab).[1] Fulminant hepatitis due to hepatitis B reactivation has been documented in patients treated with rituximab, and the product label carries a black box warning. The presence of the hepatitis B surface antigen (HBsAg) suggests active HBV infection or recent infection prior to the development of immunity. Hepatitis B surface antibody (HBsAb) is associated with protective immunity, such as with vaccination, and hepatitis B core antibody (HBcAb) is associated with immunity after previous hepatitis B infection.[1] Patients with a positive HBsAg serology are at highest risk of HBV infection, but patients who have protective immunity, as suggested by the presence of HBcAb, may lose their immunity when the lymphocytes that produce hepatitis B antibody are eliminated by lymphocytotoxic therapy.[28,73–75]

HBV serology tests should be performed prior to starting therapy with rituximab, or other anti-CD20 antibodies. HBV testing is also recommended for patients undergoing HCT and patients who are at high risk of HBV disease, such as intravenous drug users, patients with HIV, and patients from areas where HBV is endemic.[1,29] If the HBsAg test is positive, a baseline quantitative PCR for HBV DNA should

TABLE 8-9

Recommended Antimicrobial Prophylaxis

Type of Prophylaxis	Indications	Examples of Medications
Antibacterial	Patients at high risk of infection: • Anticipated prolonged neutropenia with ANC < 100 cells/mm^3 for more than 7 days • Autologous and allogeneic HCT • Acute leukemia induction/consolidation • GVHD treatment with high-dose steroids • Therapy with alemtuzumab or purine analogs (fludarabine, clofarabine, nelarabine)	Levofloxacin 500 mg PO daily × 7–10 days Ciprofloxacin 500–750 mg PO twice daily × 7–10 days
Antifungal	• Autologous and allogeneic HCT • Therapy for acute leukemia • Previous fungal infection • Significant GVHD treated with steroids	Fluconazole 400 mg PO daily Itraconazole suspension 400 mg PO daily Voriconazole 200 mg PO twice daily Posaconazole 200 mg PO three times daily with food Micafungin 50 mg IV daily
Antiviral (HSV)	HSV-seropositive patients: • Autologous or allogeneic HCT • Acute leukemia • Treatment with bortezomib, alemtuzumab, or purine analogs • Significant GVHD treated with steroids • Prior HSV reactivation during treatment	Valacyclovir 500 mg PO daily Acyclovir 400 mg PO twice daily
Antiviral (CMV)	• Allogeneic HCT • Treatment with alemtuzumab	Surveillance with CMV PCR testing for 1–6 months after HCT or 2 months after alemtuzumab
Antiviral (HBV)	• Hepatitis B surface Ag–positive patients	Entecavir 0.5 mg PO daily Lamivudine 100 mg PO daily Tenofovir 300 mg PO daily
Pneumocystis jirovecii pneumonia (PCP)	• Autologous and allogeneic HCT • ALL receiving induction therapy • Treatment with alemtuzumab • Prolonged corticosteroid use • Treatment with purine analogs	Trimethoprim/sulfamethoxazole double-strength tablet (160/800 mg) one tablet Monday, Wednesday, Friday Alternative therapy could include: • Dapsone 100 mg PO daily • Inhaled (aerosolized) pentamadine 300 mg/month • Atovaquone 1500 mg PO daily (suspension) taken with food

Abbreviations: ALL: acute lymphoblastic leukemia; ANC: absolute neutrophil count; CMV: cytomegalovirus; GVHD: graft-versus-host disease; HBV: hepatitis B virus; HCT: hematopoietic cell transplantation; HSV: herpes simplex virus; IV: intravenous; MDS: myelodysplastic syndrome; PCP: *Pneumocystis jirovecii* pneumonia; PCR: polymerase chain reaction; PO: oral.

Source: Data from National Comprehensive Cancer Network[1]; Freifeld et al[9].

be performed and antiviral prophylactic therapy is advised during cancer chemotherapy or immunosuppressive therapy, and for 6 months afterwards.[1,9,75]

Antifungal prophylaxis. Antifungal prophylaxis should not be routinely prescribed for all cancer patients, although it is recommended for selected high-risk patients. Invasive fungal infections may occur in high-risk neutropenic patients; they are associated with high rates of mortality and are often difficult to diagnose. Patients with acute leukemia, patients undergoing hematopoietic cell transplantation, and patients with GVHD treated with immunosuppressive therapy are at highest risk due to prolonged neutropenia and immunosuppression. Azoles (e.g., fluconazole, itraconazole, voriconazole, posaconazole) and echinocandins (e.g., caspofungin and micafungin) are acceptable options for antifungal prophylaxis.[9] Patients who are receiving therapy for acute leukemia or myelodysplastic syndrome (MDS) and those undergoing autologous HCT should receive antifungal prophylaxis until neutrophil recovery. In patients receiving an allogeneic HCT, antifungal prophylaxis should be continued until 75 days post transplant.[1]

The most common fungal pathogens are *Candida albicans* and *Aspergillus fumigatus*. Fluconazole, the most commonly used agent for antifungal prophylaxis, is well tolerated and effective against *Candida* infection, but does not have activity against *Aspergillus*. Patients who are at high risk of *Aspergillus* infection, such as those with acute leukemia, MDS, or GVHD, should be treated with posaconazole, which is effective against both *Candida* and *Aspergillus*.[76] Posaconazole is dosed at 200 mg orally three times daily and must be taken with food to achieve adequate serum levels, as it is best absorbed with a high-fat meal.[76]

***Pneumocystis jiroveci* pneumonia.** *Pneumocystis jiroveci* pneumonia, formerly known as *pneumocystis carinii* pneumonia (PCP), occurs nearly exclusively in immunocompromised hosts as a result of cellular immune dysfunction.[77] Patients with T-cell dysfunction should be treated with trimethoprim/sulfamethoxazole, or an alternative, as prophylaxis for PCP. Patients with T-cell dysfunction include those with a CD4 count less than 200 cells/mm^3, patients treated with T-cell–depleting agents or prolonged corticosteroid therapy, patients with ALL, and patients undergoing HCT.[1]

Oral candidiasis. Antifungal drugs that are absorbed from the gastrointestinal (GI) tract (e.g., fluconazole, ketoconazole, and itraconazole) and antifungal drugs that are partially absorbed from the GI tract (e.g., miconazole and clotrimazole) are effective to prevent oral candidiasis.[80] In contrast, the antifungal drugs that are not absorbed from the GI tract (amphotericin B, nystatin, chlorhexidine, nystatin plus chlorhexidine, thymostimulin, amphotericin B plus nystatin, polyenes, natamycin, and norfloxacin plus amphotericin B) have not shown any significant benefit in preventing oral candidiasis.[78] Most patients with cancer can be advised to perform oral care,[79,80] and clotrimazole troches may be added if candidiasis is observed. High-risk patients, such as those on T-cell–depleting chemotherapeutic agents or corticosteroids or those undergoing HCT, may be benefit from prophylactic oral fluconazole.[1]

Vaccinations. Patients with cancer are at risk for vaccine-preventable disease, such as influenza or pneumococcal disease. Vaccines in immunocompromised patients may be less effective; moreover, live vaccines, which have the potential to cause disease, should be avoided until immune function has recovered.[1,81] Despite the muted response to vaccines, 30% to 60% of patients with cancer have been shown to mount a protective response to the influenza vaccine.[82] The optimal timing of vaccination for patients receiving chemotherapy is more than 2 weeks prior to the start of chemotherapy, or at least 7 days after their last treatment.[9,81] Administration of vaccines on the same day as cytotoxic chemotherapy may decrease the efficacy of vaccination.[1] Household contacts of patients who are immunocompromised may receive all age-appropriate vaccines, with the exception of smallpox; measles, mumps, and rubella (MMR); varicella; and rotavirus—the latter are considered live viruses and should be administered only if clinically indicated.[1] All household contacts should receive influenza vaccines, but the intranasal preparation should be avoided.[1]

Patients with functional or anatomic asplenia require additional vaccination because they are at increased risk for infection from encapsulated bacteria, especially *Streptococcus pneumoniae* (pneumococcus), *Neisseria meningitidis* (meningococcus), and *Haemophilus influenzae* type b (Hib). Patients undergoing splenectomy should receive triple vaccination (pneumococcal, meningococcal, and Hib vaccination) at least 2 weeks prior to splenectomy.[1,81] Table 8-10 lists vaccination recommendations for patients with cancer.[81]

Nonpharmacologic measures

Hand hygiene is the most effective tool to prevent infection. The body's first line of defense against infection is the skin and mucous membranes, which provide a physical barrier against microorganisms. Colonization of the hands with microorganisms is associated with increased transmission of infection; likewise, effective hand hygiene significantly decreases the risk of infection.[83–85] Despite the strong evidence that hand hygiene prevents infection, clinicians and patients are not universally compliant, so patient and staff education should emphasize the importance of effective hand hygiene. Either warm soap and water or an alcohol-based hand rub may be used for hand hygiene; with either method, the key to effective removal of microbes is friction during hand hygiene and thorough drying of the hands. Wet hands remain colonized with microorganisms and significantly increase the risk of transmission of microorganisms.[83,85] Alcohol-based hand rubs have been implemented in many healthcare settings because they reduce microbe counts more effectively than soap and water, cause less dermatitis than soap and water, and require less time to complete.[83,85] The two circumstances in which soap and water are preferred are when the hands are visibly soiled or contaminated with proteinaceous material, or when caring for patients with *C. difficile* infection. Alcohol-based hand rubs are not sporicidal against *C. difficile*.[83,85]

Protective isolation has not been shown to decrease the risk of infection in neutropenic patients.[86] Thus the Centers for Disease Control and Prevention (CDC) does not recommend protective isolation.[84] Nevertheless, it is prudent to continue to recommend that neutropenic patients avoid or minimize exposure to potentially infectious people. Visitors should be screened for symptoms indicating potential respiratory infection and instructed not to visit the patient.

In the 1970s, research established that foods, particularly fresh fruits and vegetables, may contain *Escherichia coli, Pseudomonas aeruginosa,* and other gram-negative

TABLE 8-10

Vaccination Recommendations for Cancer Patients

Recommended Vaccines	Vaccines Used for Specific Circumstances	Vaccines to Avoid
Influenza annually (inactivated vaccine). Pneumococcal vaccine (repeat once 5 years after initial vaccination if initial vaccination was administered at age < 65 years). Tetanus, diphtheria, and acellular pertussis (Td/Tdap): Administer a one-time dose of Tdap to adults < 65 years of age who have not received Tdap previously or for whom vaccine status is unknown to replace one of the 10-year Td boosters. Subsequently, administer Td every 10 years.	Splenectomy, splenic irradiation or functional asplenia: Vaccination against encapsulated bacteria including pneumococcal polysaccharide vaccine (PPSV), meningococcal conjugate vaccine quadrivalent (MCV4), and *Haemophilus influenzae* type b (Hib) vaccine, administered at least 2 weeks prior to splenectomy or splenic irradiation. Revaccinate with PPSV 5 years after first dose and revaccinate with MCV4 2 months after first dose and every 5 years thereafter. Hepatitis B vaccine.	Live, attenuated virus vaccines. Influenza live vaccine (FluMist). Smallpox. Measles, mumps, rubella vaccine (MMR). Varicella zoster. Rotavirus. Yellow fever. Oral typhoid vaccine (TY21a). BCG. Oral poliovirus vaccine.

Note: Except for inactivated influenza vaccine, vaccination during chemotherapy or radiation therapy should be avoided if possible because the antibody response might be suboptimal. Patients vaccinated within 14 days before starting immunosuppressive therapy or while receiving immunosuppressive therapy should be considered unimmunized and should be revaccinated at least 3 months after therapy is discontinued if immune competence has been restored.
BCG: bacille Calmette-Guérin.

Source: Data from Centers for Disease Control and Prevention[81].

bacilli.[87] Based on these observations, it became common practice to recommend specific dietary restrictions for neutropenic cancer patients, commonly referred to as a low-microbial or "neutropenic" diet. Nearly all healthcare institutions surveyed in the 2000s recommended a neutropenic diet to their patients with cancer, and the most common recommendation was to avoid uncooked fruits and vegetables.[88,89] Current research, however, suggests that dietary restrictions beyond customary food safety practices are unlikely to decrease the risk of infection. Several small trials demonstrated that there was no difference in infection rates between patients on a neutropenic diet and patients on a general diet.[90,91] The largest trial to date evaluated 153 patients who underwent induction chemotherapy for either acute myelogenous leukemia (AML) or myelodysplastic syndrome (MDS); no significant difference was found in the rates of infection for those patients who were randomized to a diet with fresh fruits and vegetables compared to those who consumed a diet that restricted raw fruits and vegetables.[87] Therefore, "neutropenic" or low-microbial diets that restrict uncooked fruits and vegetables are not recommended to prevent infection in neutropenic cancer patients.

Basic food safety principles are recommended, however—for example, avoiding uncooked meats, seafood, eggs, and unwashed fruits and vegetables. The U.S. Department of Agriculture offers an informative, easy-to-read guide, "Food Safety for People with Cancer," that provides practical food safety advice to help patients reduce their risk of food-borne illness.[92] The four basic steps to ensure food safety are as follows:

1. *Clean.* Thoroughly clean hands, surfaces, and raw fresh fruits and vegetables.
2. *Separate.* Separate raw meat, poultry, seafood, and eggs from other foods.
3. *Cook.* Cook food to the proper temperature.
4. *Chill.* Refrigerate foods promptly at the appropriate temperature.[92]

To date, no research studies have evaluated the potential for infection from exposure to flowers and plants. However, the CDC recommends that no flowers and plants be allowed in the rooms of neutropenic patients. Its guidelines permit flowers and plants in the rooms of immunocompetent patients, but recommend that the water in the vase be changed every two days and discarded outside the patient's room.[84] Outpatients do not need to remove plants or flowers from their home, but it is recommended that family members care for them and that patients avoid gardening, leaf blowing, raking, or other outdoor activities that involve contact with vegetation.

NURSING IMPLICATIONS

The Oncology Nursing Society (ONS) developed evidence-based recommendations for the prevention of infection as part of its initiative called Putting Evidence into Practice, or ONS-PEP. Interventions are classified as recommended for practice, likely to be effective, benefits balanced with harms, effectiveness not established, effectiveness unlikely, and not recommended for practice. Strategies related to the prevention of infection, classified into these categories, can be found in Table 8-11[1,17,42,81,83,89], and neutropenic precautions can be found in Table 8-12.

TABLE 8-11

Summary of Interventions to Prevent Infection

Recommended for Practice

- Hand hygiene—the single most important nursing intervention to prevent infection.
- Oral care, including frequent oral care with gentle tooth brushing, flossing (if tolerated), and oral rinse with a bland solution such as saline or baking soda mouth rinses.
- Food safety advice to prevent food-borne infection.
- Colony-stimulating factors for patients with 20% or greater risk of febrile neutropenia.
- Avoid placement of catheters when the patient is functionally or quantitatively neutropenic; may not always be possible based on clinical circumstances.
- Aseptic practice and full barrier precautions during placement of central venous catheters.
- Injection ports on intravenous tubing or vascular catheters should be scrubbed (like "juicing an orange") with an appropriate antiseptic (e.g., 70% alcohol) before access.
- Sterile dressings should be applied to vascular access devices.
- Catheter sites should be inspected and palpated for tenderness at every visit.
- Implantable port needles (noncoring) should be changed every 7 days. Needle and dressing changes should be timed to be simultaneous.
- IV administration sets should be changed every 96 hours or when compromised or soiled. IV administration sets for blood products and lipids should be changed every 24 hours.
- Yearly influenza vaccine.
- Administer 23-valent pneumococcal polysaccharide vaccine for patients older than the age of 5 years (revaccination is needed 5 years after the initial vaccination; if possible, provide vaccination at least 2 weeks before cytotoxic or immunosuppressive therapy; otherwise, provide vaccination during treatment and revaccination 3 months after therapy is discontinued).
- Limit visitors with symptoms of respiratory infection.
- Oxygen humidifiers (prevents drying of mucous membranes).
- Prophylaxis with fluoroquinolones for high-risk patients.
- Penicillin prophylaxis to prevent pneumococcal infection for functionally asplenic or otherwise high-risk patients.
- Contact precautions when caring for patients with multidrug-resistant organisms.
- Negative-pressure rooms for patients with documented or suspected airborne infections.
- High-efficiency particulate air (HEPA) filters for immunocompromised patients.

Likely to Be Effective

- Private rooms to decrease transmission of infection.
- Neutropenic patients should avoid close contact with plants and flowers.
- Avoid ice bins if an automated ice dispenser is available, check for cleanliness; avoid handling ice by hand.

Unlikely to Be Effective

Low-microbial diet ("neutropenic diet").

Routine use of gowns upon entering a high-risk unit (e.g., HCT unit).

Abbreviations: CSF: colony-stimulating factor; HCT: hematopoietic cell transplantation; IV: intravenous.

Source: Data from O'Grady et al[17]; National Comprehensive Cancer Network[42]; Centers for Disease Control and Prevention[81]; Boyce and Pittet[83]; Zitella et al[89].

TABLE 8-12

Neutropenic Precautions

Precaution	Principle
Strict hand washing by all persons before and after contact with patients.	Decreases the amount of bacteria transported to patients.
Provide additional instruction regarding personal hygiene.	Aids in preventing self-infection. Increases the patient's participation in care.
Instruct patients in preventive oral care.	Decreases oral colonization.
Thoroughly wash uncooked fruits and vegetables, and cook meat, poultry, and eggs to the appropriate temperature.	Minimizes bacterial colonization.
Avoid contact with fresh flowers, live plants, and sources of stagnant water.	Minimizes bacterial colonization.
Instruct patients in preventive pulmonary hygiene.	Promotes ventilation and decreases respiratory colonization.
Avoid contact with anyone who has symptoms of infection.	Protect patients from potentially life-threatening infections.
Nothing per rectum (including suppositories, thermometers, enemas). Initiate bowel regimen with daily stool softeners to avoid constipation.	Prevents fissure and infection.
Vital signs every 4 hours and complete assessment every 12 hours for hospitalized patients.	Detects fever and early signs of pending septic shock.

PATIENT SELF-CARE

Patient education should focus on providing the patient and family with the knowledge needed to prevent infection and recognize signs of infection. The National Cancer Institute publishes a free booklet for patients, *Chemotherapy and You: Support for People with Cancer*, which provides useful advice for patients about chemotherapy and the management of side effects. This booklet can be downloaded from http://www.cancer.gov/cancertopics/coping/chemotherapy-and-you.

In addition, many healthcare providers develop their own patient education materials. Comprehensive patient education should include the following elements: (1) measures to prevent infection; (2) signs and symptoms of infection; (3) when and how to call the healthcare team; and (4) measures to manage infection. The self-care guides included in the appendix to this chapter can be used for patient education; they cover prevention of infection (Appendix 8A), food safety (Appendix 8B), and hand washing (Appendix 8C).

REFERENCES

1. National Comprehensive Cancer Network. *NCCN Clinical Practice Guidelines in Oncology: Prevention and Treatment of Cancer-Related Infections* [v.1.2012]. 2012. http://www.nccn.org/professionals/physician_gls/pdf/infections.pdf. Accessed February 5, 2013.
2. Lyman GH. Impact of chemotherapy dose intensity on cancer patient outcomes. *J Natl Compr Canc Netw.* 2009;7(1):99–108.
3. Khan S, Dhadda A, Fyfe D, Sundar S. Impact of neutropenia on delivering planned chemotherapy for solid tumours. *Eur J Cancer.* 2008;17(1):19–25.
4. Shayne M, Culakova E, Poniewierski MS, et al. Dose intensity and hematologic toxicity in older cancer patients receiving systemic chemotherapy. *Cancer.* 2007;110(7):1611–1620.
5. Shayne M, Culakova E, Wolff D, et al. Dose intensity and hematologic toxicity in older breast cancer patients receiving systemic chemotherapy. *Cancer.* 2009;115(22):5319–5328.
6. Pettengell R, Schwenkglenks M, Leonard R, et al. Neutropenia occurrence and predictors of reduced chemotherapy delivery: results from the INC-EU prospective observational European neutropenia study. *Support Care Cancer.* 2008;16(11):1299–1309.
7. Kuderer NM, Dale DC, Crawford J, Cosler LE, Lyman GH. Mortality, morbidity, and cost associated with febrile neutropenia in adult cancer patients. *Cancer.* 2006;106(10):2258–2266.
8. Almyroudis NG, Battiwalla M, Segal BH. Modulation of immune function. In: Kleinberg M, ed. *Managing Infections in Patients with Hematological Malignancies: Contemporary Hematology.* New York City: Springer; 2009:235–258.
9. Freifeld AG, Bow EJ, Sepkowitz KA, et al. Clinical practice guideline for the use of antimicrobial agents in neutropenic patients with cancer: 2010 update by the Infectious Diseases Society of America. *Clin Infect Dis.* 2011;52(4):427–431.
10. Moreau M, Klastersky J, Schwarzbold A, et al. A general chemotherapy myelotoxicity score to predict febrile neutropenia in hematological malignancies. *Ann Oncol.* 2009;20(3):513–519.
11. Bodey GP, Buckley M, Sathe YS, Freireich EJ. Quantitative relationships between circulating leukocytes and infection in patients with acute leukemia. *Ann Intern Med.* 1966;64(2):328.
12. Dearden C. Disease-specific complications of chronic lymphocytic leukemia. 2008;2008:450–456.
13. Morrison VA. Infectious complications of chronic lymphocytic leukaemia: pathogenesis, spectrum of infection, preventive approaches. *Best Pract Res Clin Haematol.* 2010;23(1):145–153.
14. Rolston KVI. Lymphomas and chronic lymphocytic leukemia. In: Kleinberg M, ed. *Managing Infections in Patients with Hematological Malignancies: Contemporary Hematology.* New York City: Springer; 2009:173–187.
15. Klastersky J, Paesmans M, Rubenstein EB, et al. The Multinational Association for Supportive Care in Cancer Risk Index: a multinational scoring system for identifying low-risk febrile neutropenic cancer patients. *J Clin Oncol.* 2000;18(16):3038–3051.
16. Rapoport BL. Management of the cancer patient with infection and neutropenia. *Semin Oncol* 2011;38(3):424–430.

17. O'Grady NP, Alexander M, Burns LA, et al. Guidelines for the prevention of intravascular catheter-related infections. *Clin Infect Dis.* 2011;52(9):e162–e193.
18. Vescia S, Baumgärtner AK, Jacobs VR, et al. Management of venous port systems in oncology: a review of current evidence. *Ann Oncol.* 2008;19(1):9–15.
19. Kosmidis CI, Chandrasekar PH. Management of gram-positive bacterial infections in patients with cancer. *Leuk Lymphoma.* 2012;53(1):8–18.
20. Kern W, Kurrle E, Schmeiser T. Streptococcal bacteremia in adult patients with leukemia undergoing aggressive chemotherapy: A review of 55 cases. *Infection* 1990;18(3):138–145.
21. Engelhard D, Elishoov H, Or R, et al. Cytosine arabinoside as a major risk factor for *Streptococcus viridans* septicemia following bone marrow transplantation: a 5-year prospective study. *Bone Marrow Transplant.* 1995;16(4):565–570.
22. Aapro MS, Bohlius J, Cameron DA, et al. 2010 update of EORTC guidelines for the use of granulocyte-colony stimulating factor to reduce the incidence of chemotherapy-induced febrile neutropenia in adult patients with lymphoproliferative disorders and solid tumours. *Eur J Cancer.* 2011;47(1):8–32.
23. Smith TJ, Khatcheressian J, Lyman GH, et al. 2006 update of recommendations for the use of white blood cell growth factors: an evidence-based clinical practice guideline. *J Clin Oncol.* 2006;24(19):3187–3205.
24. De Vos FY, Gijtenbeek JM, Bleeker-Rovers CP, van Herpen CM. *Pneumocystis jirovecii* pneumonia prophylaxis during temozolomide treatment for high-grade gliomas. *Crit Rev Oncol Hematol.* 2013:85(13):373–382.
25. Stupp R, Dietrich P-Y, Kraljevic SO, et al. Promising survival for patients with newly diagnosed glioblastoma multiforme treated with concomitant radiation plus temozolomide followed by adjuvant temozolomide. *J Clin Oncol.* 2002;20(5):1375–1382.
26. Evens AM, Jovanovic BD, Su Y-C, et al. Rituximab-associated hepatitis B virus (HBV) reactivation in lymphoproliferative diseases: meta-analysis and examination of FDA safety reports. *Ann Oncol.* 2011;22(5):1170–1180.
27. Kusumoto S, Tanaka Y, Ueda R, Mizokami M. Reactivation of hepatitis B virus following rituximab-plus-steroid combination chemotherapy. *J Gastroenterol.* 2011;46(1):9–16.
28. Koo Y, Tay M, Teh Y, et al. Risk of hepatitis B virus (HBV) reactivation in hepatitis B surface antigen negative/hepatitis B core antibody positive patients receiving rituximab-containing combination chemotherapy without routine antiviral prophylaxis. *Ann Hematol.* 2011;90(10):1219–1223.
29. Tomblyn M, Chiller T, Einsele H, et al. Guidelines for preventing infectious complications among hematopoietic cell transplantation recipients: a global perspective. Recommendations of the Center for International Blood and Marrow Transplant Research (CIBMTR®), the National Marrow Donor Program (NMDP), the European Blood and Marrow Transplant Group (EBMT), the American Society of Blood and Marrow Transplantation (ASBMT), the Canadian Blood and Marrow Transplant Group (CBMTG), the Infectious Disease Society of America (IDSA), the Society for Healthcare Epidemiology of America (SHEA), the Association of Medical Microbiology and Infectious Diseases Canada (AMMI), and the Centers for Disease Control and Prevention (CDC). *Biol Blood Marrow Transplant.* 2009;15(10):1143–1238.
30. Spelman D, Buttery J, Daley A, et al. Guidelines for the prevention of sepsis in asplenic and hyposplenic patients. *Intern Med J.* 2008;38(5):349–356.
31. Lyman GH, Kuderer NM, Crawford J, et al. Predicting individual risk of neutropenic complications in patients receiving cancer chemotherapy. *Cancer.* 2011;117(9):1917–1927.
32. Ma CY, Ji T, Ow A, et al. Surgical site infection in elderly oral cancer patients: is the evaluation of comorbid conditions helpful in the identification of high-risk ones? *J Oral Maxillofac Surg.* 2012;70(10): 2445–2452.
33. Antoun S, Rey A, Béal J, et al. Nutritional risk factors in planned oncologic surgery: what clinical and biological parameters should be routinely used? *World J Surg.* 2009;33(8):1633–1640.
34. Intragumtornchai T, Sutheesophon J, Sutcharitchan P, Swasdikul D. A predictive model for life-threatening neutropenia and febrile neutropenia after the first course of CHOP chemotherapy in patients with aggressive non-Hodgkin's lymphoma. *Leuk Lymphoma.* 2000;37(3–4):351–360.
35. Kloft C, Wallin J, Henningsson A, Chatelut E, Karlsson MO. Population pharmacokinetic-pharmacodynamic model for neutropenia with patient subgroup identification: comparison across anticancer drugs. *Clin Cancer Res.* 2006;12(18):5481–5490.
36. Friberg LE, Henningsson A, Maas H, Nguyen L, Karlsson MO. Model of chemotherapy-induced myelosuppression with parameter consistency across drugs. *J Clin Oncol.* 2002;20(24):4713–4721.
37. Wisplinghoff H, Seifert H, Wenzel RP, Edmond MB. Current trends in the epidemiology of nosocomial bloodstream infections in patients with hematological malignancies and solid neoplasms in hospitals in the United States. *Clin Infect Dis.* 2003;36(9):1103–1110.
38. Lyman GH, Lyman CH, Agboola O. Risk models for predicting chemotherapy-induced neutropenia. *Oncologist.* 2005;10(6):427–437.
39. Crawford J, Dale DC, Kuderer NM, et al. Risk and timing of neutropenic events in adult cancer patients receiving chemotherapy: the results of a prospective nationwide study of oncology practice. *J Natl Compr Canc Netw.* 2008;6:109–118.
40. O'Grady NP, Barie PS, Bartlett JG, et al. Guidelines for evaluation of new fever in critically ill adult patients: 2008 update from the American College of Critical Care Medicine and the Infectious Diseases Society of America. *Crit Care Med.* 2008;36(4):1330.
41. Ciuraru NB, Braunstein R, Sulkes A, Stemmer SM. The influence of mucositis on oral thermometry: when fever may not reflect infection. *Clin Infect Dis.* 2008;46(12):1859–1863.
42. National Comprehensive Cancer Network. *NCCN Clinical Practice Guidelines in Oncology: Myeloid Growth Factors* [v.1.2012]. 2012. http://www.nccn.org/professionals/physician_gls/pdf/myeloid_growth.pdf. Accessed February 5, 2013.
43. Bow EJ. Neutropenic fever syndromes in patients undergoing cytotoxic therapy for acute leukemia and myelodysplastic syndromes. *Semin Hematol.* 2009;46(3):259–268.
44. Friese CR. Prevention of infection in patients with cancer. *Semin Oncol Nurs.* 2007;23(3):174–183.
45. Cockerill FR, Wilson JW, Vetter EA, et al. Optimal testing parameters for blood cultures. *Clin Infect Dis.* 2004;38(12):1724–1730.
46. Safdar N, Fine JP, Maki DG. Meta-analysis: methods for diagnosing intravascular device-related bloodstream infection. *Ann Intern Med.* 2005;142(6):451–474.
47. Department of Health and Human Services, National Cancer Institute. *Common Terminology Criteria for Adverse Events* [v.4.03]. Bethesda, MD: National Cancer Institute Cancer Therapy Evaluation Program; 2010. http://ctep.cancer.gov/protocolDevelopment/electronic_applications/ctc.htm#ctc_40. Accessed February 5, 2013.
48. Innes H, Lim S, Hall A, Chan S, Bhalla N, Marshall E. Management of febrile neutropenia in solid tumours and lymphomas using the Multinational Association for Supportive Care in Cancer (MASCC) risk index: feasibility and safety in routine clinical practice. *Support Care Cancer.* 2008;16(5):485–491.
49. Feld R. Bloodstream infections in cancer patients with febrile neutropenia. *Int J Antimicrob Agents.* 2008;32(suppl 1):S30–S33.
50. de Naurois J, Novitzky-Basso I, Gill MJ, et al. Management of febrile neutropenia: ESMO clinical practice guidelines. *Ann Oncol.* 2010;21 (suppl 5):v252–v256.
51. Klastersky J, Ameye L, Maertens J, et al. Bacteraemia in febrile neutropenic cancer patients. *Int J Antimicrob Agents.* 2007;30(suppl 1):51–59.
52. Paul M, Yahav D, Bivas A, Fraser A, Leibovici L. Anti-pseudomonal beta-lactams for the initial, empirical, treatment of febrile neutropenia: comparison of beta-lactams. *Cochrane Database Syst Rev.* 2010;11:CD005197.

53. Yahav D, Paul M, Fraser A, Sarid N, Leibovici L. Efficacy and safety of cefepime: a systematic review and meta-analysis. *Lancet Infect Dis.* 2007;7(5):338–348.
54. Food and Drug Administration. Information for healthcare professionals: cefepime (marketed as Maxipime). June 17, 2009. http://www.fda.gov/Drugs/DrugSafety/PostmarketDrugSafetyInformationforPatientsandProviders/DrugSafetyInformationforHeathcareProfessionals/ucm167254.htm. Accessed February 5, 2013.
55. Mandell LA, Wunderink RG, Anzueto A, et al. Infectious Diseases Society of America/American Thoracic Society consensus guidelines on the management of community-acquired pneumonia in adults. *Clin Infect Dis.* 2007;44(suppl 2):S27–S72.
56. Dellinger RP, Levy M, Carlet J, et al. Surviving Sepsis Campaign: international guidelines for management of severe sepsis and septic shock: 2008. *Crit Care Med.* 2008;36(1):296–327.
57. Paul M, Borok S, Fraser A, Vidal L, Cohen M, Leibovici L. Additional anti-gram-positive antibiotic treatment for febrile neutropenic cancer patients. *Cochrane Database Syst Rev.* 2005;3:CD003914.
58. Mermel LA, Allon M, Bouza E, et al. Clinical practice guidelines for the diagnosis and management of intravascular catheter-related infection: 2009 update by the Infectious Diseases Society of America. *Clin Infect Dis.* 2009;49(1):1–45.
59. Teuffel O, Ethier MC, Alibhai SM, Beyene J, Sung L. Outpatient management of cancer patients with febrile neutropenia: a systematic review and meta-analysis. *Ann Oncol.* 2011;22(11):2358–2365.
60. Bow EJ, Rotstein C, Noskin GA, et al. A randomized, open-label, multicenter comparative study of the efficacy and safety of piperacillin-tazobactam and cefepime for the empirical treatment of febrile neutropenic episodes in patients with hematologic malignancies. *Clin Infect Dis.* 2006;43(4):447–459.
61. Page AV, Liles WC. Colony-stimulating factors in the prevention and management of infectious diseases. *Infect Dis Clin North Am.* 2011;25(4):803–817.
62. Bohlius J, Herbst C, Reiser M, Schwarzer G, Engert A. Granulopoiesis-stimulating factors to prevent adverse effects in the treatment of malignant lymphoma. *Cochrane Database Syst Rev.* 2008;4:CD003189.
63. Kuderer NM. Meta-analysis of randomized controlled trials of granulocyte colony-stimulating factor prophylaxis in adult cancer patients receiving chemotherapy hematopoietic growth factors in oncology. In: Lyman GH, Dale DC, eds. Hematopoietic Growth Factors in Oncology Vol. 157. New York, Springer; 2011:127–143.
64. Kuderer NM, Dale DC, Crawford J, Lyman GH. Impact of primary prophylaxis with granulocyte colony-stimulating factor on febrile neutropenia and mortality in adult cancer patients receiving chemotherapy: a systematic review. *J Clin Oncol.* 2007;25(21):3158–3167.
65. Lyman GH, Kuderer NM, Djulbegovic B. Prophylactic granulocyte colony-stimulating factor in patients receiving dose-intensive cancer chemotherapy: a meta-analysis. *Am J Med.* 2002;112(5):406–411.
66. Sung L, Nathan PC, Alibhai SM, Tomlinson GA, Beyene J. Meta-analysis: effect of prophylactic hematopoietic colony-stimulating factors on mortality and outcomes of infection. *Ann Intern Med.* 2007;147(6):400–411.
67. Bucaneve G, Micozzi A, Menichetti F, et al. Levofloxacin to prevent bacterial infection in patients with cancer and neutropenia. *N Engl J Med.* 2005;353(10):977–987.
68. Cullen M, Steven N, Billingham L, et al. Antibacterial prophylaxis after chemotherapy for solid tumors and lymphomas. *N Engl J Med.* 2005;353(10):988–998.
69. Gafter-Gvili A, Fraser A, Paul M, et al. Antibiotic prophylaxis for bacterial infections in afebrile neutropenic patients following chemotherapy. *Cochrane Database Syst Rev.* 2012;1:CD004386.
70. Wingard JR, Eldjerou L, Leather H. Use of antibacterial prophylaxis in patients with chemotherapy-induced neutropenia. *Curr Opin Hematol.* 2012;19(1):21–26.
71. Yahav D, Gafter-Gvili A, Muchtar E, et al. Antiviral prophylaxis in haematological patients: systematic review and meta-analysis. *Eur J Cancer.* 2009;45(18):3131–3148.
72. Boeckh M, Ljungman P. How we treat cytomegalovirus in hematopoietic cell transplant recipients. *Blood.* 2009;113(23):5711–5719.
73. Niitsu N, Hagiwara Y, Tanae K, Kohri M, Takahashi N. Prospective analysis of hepatitis B virus reactivation in patients with diffuse large B-cell lymphoma after rituximab combination chemotherapy. *J Clin Oncol.* 2010;28(34):5097–5100.
74. Yeo W, Chan TC, Leung NW, et al. Hepatitis B virus reactivation in lymphoma patients with prior resolved hepatitis B undergoing anticancer therapy with or without rituximab. *J Clin Oncol.* 2009;27(4):605–611.
75. Hwang J, Vierling J, Zelenetz A, Lackey S, Loomba R. Hepatitis B virus management to prevent reactivation after chemotherapy: a review. *Support Care Cancer.* 2012;20(11):2999–3008.
76. Cornely OA, Maertens J, Winston DJ, et al. Posaconazole vs. fluconazole or itraconazole prophylaxis in patients with neutropenia. *N Engl J Med.* 2007;356(4):348–359.
77. Carmona EM, Limper AH. Update on the diagnosis and treatment of *Pneumocystis* pneumonia. *Ther Adv Respir Dis.* 2011;5(1):41–59.
78. Clarkson JE, Worthington HV, Eden OB. Interventions for preventing oral candidiasis for patients with cancer receiving treatment. *Cochrane Database Syst Rev.* 2007;1:CD003807.
79. Rubenstein EB, Peterson DE, Schubert M, et al. Clinical practice guidelines for the prevention and treatment of cancer therapy–induced oral and gastrointestinal mucositis. *Cancer.* 2004;100(S9):2026–2046.
80. Worthington HV, Clarkson JE, Bryan G, et al. Interventions for preventing oral mucositis for patients with cancer receiving treatment. *Cochrane Database Syst Rev.* 2011;4:CD000978.
81. Centers for Disease Control and Prevention. General recommendations on immunization: Recommendations of the Advisory Committee on Immunization Practices (ACIP). *MMWR Recomm Rep.* 2011; 60(RR02):1–60.
82. Pollyea DA, Brown JM, Horning SJ. Utility of influenza vaccination for oncology patients. *J Clin Oncol.* 2010;28(14):2481–2490.
83. Boyce JM, Pittet D. Guideline for hand hygiene in health-care settings: recommendations of the Healthcare Infection Control Practices Advisory Committee and the HICPAC/SHEA/APIC/IDSA Hand Hygiene Task Force. *Infec Control Hosp Epidemiol.* 2002;23(12suppl):S3–40.
84. Sehulster L, Chinn RY, CDC, HICPAC. Guidelines for environmental infection control in health-care facilities: rRecommendations of CDC and the Healthcare Infection Control Practices Advisory Committee (HICPAC). *MMWR Recomm Rep.* 2003;52(RR-10):1–42.
85. Kampf G, Kramer A. Epidemiologic background of hand hygiene and evaluation of the most important agents for scrubs and rubs. *Clin Microbiol Rev.* 2004;17(4):863–893.
86. Mank A, van der Lelie H. Is there still an indication for nursing patients with prolonged neutropenia in protective isolation? An evidence-based nursing and medical study of 4 years experience for nursing patients with neutropenia without isolation. *Eur J Oncol Nurs.* 2003;7(1):17–23.
87. Gardner A, Mattiuzzi G, Faderl S, et al. Randomized comparison of cooked and noncooked diets in patients undergoing remission induction therapy for acute myeloid leukemia. *J Clin Oncol.* 2008;26(35):5684–5688.
88. Zitella LJ, Friese CR, Hauser J, et al. Putting evidence into practice: prevention of infection. *Clin J Oncol Nurs.* 2006;10(6):739–750.
89. Zitella L, Gobel BH, O'Leary C. Prevention of Infection. In: Eaton LH, Tipton JM, eds. *Putting Evidence into Practice: Improving Oncology Patient Outcomes.* Pittsburgh: Oncology Nursing Society; 2009:267–283.
90. DeMille D, Deming P, Lupinacci P, Jacobs LA. The effect of the neutropenic diet in the outpatient setting: a pilot study. *Oncol Nurs Forum.* 2006;33(2):337–343.
91. van Tiel F, Harbers MM, Terporten PH, et al. Normal hospital and low-bacterial diet in patients with cytopenia after intensive chemotherapy for hematological malignancy: a study of safety. *Ann Oncol.* 2007;18(6):1080–1084.
92. U.S. Department of Agriculture. Food safety for people with cancer. 2006. http://www.fda.gov/downloads/Food/ResourcesForYou/Consumers/SelectedHealthTopics/UCM312761.pdf. Accessed February 5, 2013.

Prevention of Infection

Patient Name: ____

Symptom and Description

Cancer and certain types of cancer treatment can increase the risk of infection. Infections are caused by germs, such as bacteria, viruses, and fungi. The body's defense against these germs is the skin and mucous membranes (the moist pink tissue that lines the inside of your mouth, nose, digestive system, urethra, and vagina). They provide a physical barrier to prevent organisms from entering the body. If there is an opening in the skin or mucous membranes, such as a cut or a mouth sore, germs can enter your body and cause infection.

If germs enter your body, it is the function of the white blood cells of the immune system to destroy them. Chemotherapy and other cancer treatments can destroy the white blood cells, causing low numbers of white blood cells in the blood around one week later. When the number of white blood cells is low, it is harder for you to fight infections. It is important to know the signs of infection and to call your healthcare team immediately if you have any signs of infection. You may need to be admitted to the hospital for antibiotics to prevent a serious infection.

Prevention

- Hand washing with soap and water or alcohol-based gel is effective unless the hands are very soiled. If hands are very soiled, use soap and water.
- Wash your hands frequently, but especially before eating, after using the bathroom, after contact with animals, after going outside, and before preparing food.
- Perform frequent oral care, including gentle tooth brushing and flossing (as tolerated).
- Keep your body clean by bathing every day.
- Avoid people who are sick.
- Food safety advice:
  - Clean hands and food preparation surfaces well.
  - Wash fresh fruits and vegetables carefully and avoid raw meat, poultry, fish, and eggs.
  - Separate raw meat, poultry, seafood, and eggs from other foods.
  - Cook food to the proper temperature.
  - Refrigerate foods promptly at the appropriate temperature.
- Avoid constipation and straining to have a bowel movement by eating a diet high in fiber and drinking at least 8 to 10 glasses of fluids daily. You may also need to use medications such as stool softeners or laxatives. Do not use enemas or suppositories, as they can increase your risk of infection.
- Do not change cat litter or clean up excreta from animals.
- Obtain the influenza vaccine every year.

- Signs and symptoms of infection—when to call your healthcare provider:
  - Body temperature >100.4°F
  - Chills
  - Sore throat, shortness of breath, cough, or sinus tenderness
  - Pain or burning with urination
  - Diarrhea
  - Mouth sores
  - Rectal discomfort
  - Abdominal pain
  - Pain, redness or swelling at any catheter site

Management

Take your temperature anytime you feel sick. If your temperature is more than 100.4°F or you have any signs of infection, call your healthcare provider immediately. You may need to go to the hospital or the clinic for blood counts and examination. If your white blood cell count is low and you have a fever, you may be admitted to the hospital for treatment.

Follow-Up

If you have a fever or any signs of infection, call your healthcare provider immediately. Be prepared to tell them:

- Date and type of last treatment
- Highest temperature in 24 hours
- Signs of infection

Phone Numbers

Listed below are the people to contact if you develop a fever of signs of infection.

Doctor: ______________________________

Nurse Practitioner: ______________________________

Nurse: ______________________________

Other: ______________________________

Source: Zitella L. Infection. In: Yarbro CH, Wujcik D, Gobel BH, eds. *Cancer Symptom Management*. 4th ed. Burlington, MA: Jones & Bartlett Learning; 2014.

Food Safety

Patient Name: ______________________________

Symptom and Description

Bacteria and other germs can contaminate food and increase the risk of infection. You can decrease the chance of getting a food-borne illness by carefully handling and preparing your food using the four basic steps for food safety. These four steps are clean, separate, cook, and chill.

Prevention/Management

When using the four basic steps to food safety, keep in mind the most common routes of food contamination, which include uncooked food, unpasteurized milk and juices, hot dogs, lunch meats, ground meats, undercooked eggs, contaminated fruits and vegetables, and other animal products.

The Four Basic Steps to Ensure Food Safety

1. **Clean.** Wash your hands and surface areas frequently and thoroughly. Wash your hands in warm soapy water for 20 seconds before and after handling foods. Wash surfaces such as cutting boards, dishes, and countertops with hot soapy water. Rinse fruits and vegetables under running tap water, and clean the lids of canned foods before opening the cans.
2. **Separate.** Keeping foods separate is important to the safe handling of food. Keep raw meat, poultry, seafood, eggs, and their juices away from ready-to-eat food. It is also important to keep these items separate in your shopping carts, bag, and refrigerator. Another way to help keep foods separate is to use two cutting boards: one for meat, and another for fresh produce.
3. **Cook.** Cook your foods to the proper temperatures, and use a food thermometer to measure the internal temperature of your food. Refer to the chart below for proper cooking temperatures. Also, cook eggs and yolks until whites are firm, and reheat luncheon meats, bologna, and other deli meats until steaming hot.
4. **Chill.** Cold temperatures slow the growth of harmful bacteria. Keep your refrigerator at a temperature of 40°F or below; keep your freezer at a temperature of 0°F or below. After shopping, refrigerate or freeze meats, poultry, seafood, eggs, and other perishables within 2 hours of cooking or purchasing. If the temperature outside is above 90°F, freeze or refrigerate these foods within 1 hour. Frozen foods should be thawed in the refrigerator, in cold water, or in the microwave. Refer to the chart below for proper food storage temperatures.

Product	Refrigerator (40°F)	Freezer (0°F)
Eggs	3–5 weeks	Do not freeze
Deli and vacuum-packed products	3–5 days	Do not freeze
Hot dogs (opened)	1 week	1–2 months
Luncheon meats (opened)	3–5 days	1–2 months
Hamburger or other ground meats	1–2 days	3–4 months
Fresh poultry	1–2 days	9 months–1 year
Seafood (fatty fish—tuna or salmon)	1–2 days	2–3 months
Cooked meats	3–4 days	2–6 months

Follow-Up

Despite your best efforts, it is still possible to get a food-borne illness. Food-borne illnesses often present with flu-like symptoms such as nausea, vomiting, diarrhea, and fever. If you suspect you have a food-borne illness, follow these four simple steps:

1. Contact your healthcare provider and seek medical advice or treatment immediately.
2. Preserve the food if a portion of the suspect food is available. Wrap the food securely, label it as dangerous, and place it in the freezer. The remaining food might help your healthcare provider provide treatment.
3. Save all the packaging materials, cans, or cartons. Don't forget to write down the food type, date, time consumed, and time of the onset of symptoms. If possible, save identical unopened products. Report contaminated food to the USDA meat and poultry hotline (1-888-674-6854).
4. Call your local health department if you believe that you became ill after eating at a restaurant. Visit http://healthguideusa.org/local_health_departments.htm.

The complete food safety guide can be found at http://www.fda.gov/downloads/Food/ResourcesForYou/Consumers/SelectedHealthTopics/UCM312761.pdf

Source: Zitella L. Infection. In: Yarbro CH, Wujcik D, Gobel BH, eds. *Cancer Symptom Management.* 4th ed. Burlington, MA: Jones & Bartlett Learning; 2014.

Hand Washing

Patient Name: ______________________________

Symptom and Description

Hand washing is the most important way to prevent an infection. The body's first line of defense against foreign invaders is the skin; the skin provides a physical barrier to prevent germs from entering the body. Your hands come into contact with many types of germs, so washing your hands helps prevent the spread of infection. In general, either soap and water or an alcohol-based rub can be used for hand hygiene. it is more important that hands are rubbed vigorously during hand washing and that they are dried carefully after hand washing.

Management

If hands are *not* visibly dirty:

- Use regular soap and water, antimicrobial soap and water, or an alcohol-based hand rub.

If hands are visibly dirty:

- Wash hands with a non-antimicrobial soap or antimicrobial soap and water.

When washing hands with soap and water:

- Wet hands with water.
- Apply soap to hands and rub hands together vigorously for at least 15 seconds, covering all surfaces of the hands and fingers.
- Rinse hands with water and dry thoroughly.
- Use a towel to turn the faucet off.

When washing hands with an alcohol-based hand rub:

- Apply the product to the palm of one hand and rub hands together, covering all surfaces of hands and fingers, until hands are dry.
- Antimicrobial wipes (i.e., towelettes) may be considered as an alternative to washing hands when you are away from home.

When to wash your hands:

- Before eating or preparing food
- After using the bathroom
- After going outdoors or to a public place
- After touching plants or dirt
- After touching animals
- After collecting or depositing garbage
- Before touching a wound
- Before giving yourself an injection

You may find it helpful to carry an alcohol-based hand rub with you so you can periodically disinfect your hands when you are out in public places.

Source: Zitella L. Infection. In: Yarbro CH, Wujcik D, Gobel BH, eds. *Cancer Symptom Management*. 4th ed. Burlington, MA: Jones & Bartlett Learning; 2014.

PART IV

Alterations in Gastrointestinal Function

CHAPTER 9

Constipation

Pamela J. Haylock, PhD, RN, FAAN
Carol Curtiss, MSN, RN-BC
Robert L. Massey, PhD, RN, CNAA

THE PROBLEM

Constipation, which is simply defined as "having a bowel movement fewer than three times per week,"[1] is an exceedingly common problem among otherwise healthy people. It is a more frequent and compelling problem for people with cancer, causing distress rivaling that related to pain.[2]

Constipation is not a new concern: I. Phillips Frohman, vice-chairman of the American Medical Association in 1955, noted that constipation as a disorder of humans is at least as old as recorded history.[3] The Ebers Papyrus—dating to 3000 BC—references consumption of dates and olive oil to promote bowel elimination.[3,4] Early Chinese medical records described preparation of an animal horn to be "inserted and used as a funnel to instill water into the rectum"—the invention of the enema.[3]

Constipation has also been noted as a long-standing vexation for nurses and patients in their care. Kate Williams, writing in a 1901 issue of *The American Journal of Nursing*, noted: "Constipation is one of the ills from which no small proportion of mankind suffers, and any therapeutic measure which will mitigate or cure it is not to be lightly considered."[5(p718)] In the classic 1967 *American Journal of Nursing* series, "Hazards of Immobility," constipation is noted as a consequence of immobility-induced interference with skeletal and smooth muscle activity, visceral reflex patterns, reduced expulsive power, and loss of the defecation reflex.[6]

In the mid-1950s, the American public spent $85 million for over-the-counter laxatives and another $20 million for prescribed laxatives.[1] Today, an estimated $725 million is spent annually for over-the-counter and prescribed laxative products in America.[1]

For patients at the end of life, constipation is one of the most common problems, causing much needless pain and suffering. The prevalence of constipation throughout the cancer trajectory leads to the undeniable conclusion that evidence for practice is generally poor and further research on all aspects of constipation in cancer care is imperative. Constipation may cause physical and emotional distress, alter social interactions, and thereby influence a person's overall sense of well-being.[7] The effect of constipation on individual suffering is an important reason for nurses to aggressively research and develop nursing interventions for its management. The European Consensus Group on Constipation in Palliative Care concluded, "The current evidence base is poor and further research is required on many aspects of the assessment, diagnosis and management of constipation in palliative care."[8]

Anecdotally, nurses' efforts to bring attention to the multitude of issues relating to constipation are often met with snickers and indifference among colleagues. Constipation is not a glamorous or exciting aspect of nursing care: it does not involve new, high-technology, complicated, and expensive devices, nor, for the most part, do assessment and management involve new breakthrough medications and other interventions. Bowel elimination is a basic and normal physiologic function. Assessment, diagnosis, identification of outcomes, planning, implementation, and evaluation of interventions are essential elements of nurses' scope of practice.[9] Despite the fundamental premise that potential and actual compromise of bowel elimination is a concern for nurses, the prevalence of constipation in various populations remains alarming and is suggestive of misplaced priorities and focus in nursing education and practice.

PREVALENCE

Frequent constipation affects more than 4 million Americans—between 2% and 28% of the general North America population—and accounts for 2.5 million physician visits each year.[1] A 1955 review of constipation indicated that men suffered more from constipation than women, with the etiology being linked to "psychic tension"[3]—the occupational hazards of strain and worry that were assumed to confront more men than women. Current data reveal that constipation is actually more common among women.[1,10] In 2009, the worldwide prevalence of functional constipation among children was estimated at 7% to 30%.[11,12] Constipation accounts for nearly 5% of all pediatric outpatient visits and more than 25% of referrals to gastroenterology specialists.[12,13] An estimated 30% to 75% of children with long-standing functional constipation experience fecal impaction, with this condition becoming severe in 90% of affected children.[14,15]

Constipation among people with cancer, particularly among specific subgroups—notably, patients receiving certain classes of cytotoxic agents and opioid analgesics—is documented in the medical and nursing literature as a common adverse effect of cancer and cancer treatment. Nevertheless, Cimprich noted in 1985 that "the true extent of this symptom in patients with various types of cancer and in varying stages of illness has not been fully explored. . . ."[16(p39)] She went on to assert, "In practice, constipation may be one of the least anticipated and most overlooked symptoms experienced by the patient with cancer."[16(p39)] Wright and Thomas labeled constipation and diarrhea as neglected symptoms,[17] noting that "pain, nausea, vomiting, and lethargy resulting from constipation and diarrhea are distressing to the patient with cancer."[17] Accurate present-day estimates of prevalence remain elusive, but the rate is variously reported to range from 40% to 100%,[2,8] affecting patients at different points throughout the disease continuum, relating to treatment modalities, management of comorbidities, cancer and treatment-related symptoms, diet, and mobility.[17,18]

ETIOLOGY AND PATHOPHYSIOLOGY

The etiology and mechanisms of constipation among persons with cancer are most often multifactorial, complex, and only partially understood.[19] Constipation rarely stands alone as an isolated symptom, but is instead most often a component of a cluster of symptoms.[19–24] Among children, the pathogenesis of constipation can be linked to dietary changes, recent infection, stressful events, and purposeful avoidance. Pain, poor appetite, and encoporesis often lead to emergency care.[25,26]

Two forms of constipation are distinguished. With *idiopathic constipation*, the etiology is unknown and the problem does not respond to standard treatment.[1] *Functional constipation* occurs in bowel that is healthy but not working properly, often as the result of poor dietary habits and lifestyle.[1] This type of constipation occurs in both children and adults.

Colonic inertia, delayed transit, and pelvic floor dysfunction are three types of functional constipation. Colonic inertia and delayed transit are caused by decreased colonic muscle activity affecting the entire colon; alternatively, they may be confined to the sigmoid colon.[1] Pelvic floor dysfunction is caused by weakness of muscles surrounding the anus and rectum. Anal and rectal structural problems cause anorectal dysfunction or anismus, resulting in inability of rectal and anal muscles to relax, thereby preventing expulsion of stool, and development of functional constipation.[1]

NORMAL INTESTINAL PHYSIOLOGY

Thorough understanding of normal digestive and elimination physiology are essential for identification and planning around potential and actual deviations from normal and, in turn, the pathophysiology that contributes to development of constipation. Gastrointestinal function and dysfunction occur as a result of neural, endocrine, and luminal forms of cellular communication that collectively form the enteric nervous system (ENS).[27,28] The small bowel and colon are responsible for digestion and assimilation of nutrients from food, regulation of secretion and absorption of water and electrolytes, and storage and subsequent forward transport of intraluminal intestinal contents.[28,29] The gastrointestinal (GI) tract has its own intrinsic nervous system—the myenteric and submucosal plexi—as well as innervation by the autonomic nervous system.[28,30] Interstitial cells of Cajal provide pacemaker activity to generate rhythmic electrical activity.[30] The GI tract is richly innervated with mu and kappa opioid receptors and serotonin receptor subtypes.[28,30] More than 80% of the body's serotonin resides in the GI tract, where it affects GI motility.[29] The bowel produces segmental contractions to mix luminal contents in place. Propulsive peristaltic contractions move stool forward through the GI tract.[27–29]

MECHANISMS OF CONSTIPATION

Alterations in peristalsis

Peristalsis is stimulated when fecal mass stretches the bowel wall. When peristalsis is sluggish, stool moves through the colon more slowly. This diminished transit time allows more fluid to be absorbed from stool, resulting in hard, dry stool that is confined in the sluggish colon. At the same time, segmental contractions continue to churn, breaking stool into small, hard pieces.[31] Bowel sounds may still appear normal.[29] Immobility, decreased dietary intake of fluids and fiber, stress, depression, and many medications may all contribute to slowing of the gut.[31–33]

Changes in motor control of the anal sphincter and rectal capacity

Sphincter control maintains fecal continence and regular defecation. Normally, the internal sphincter is contracted and controlled by the autonomic nervous system.[10,15] When the rectal wall is distended by stool mass, the internal sphincter relaxes to allow rectal contents to move farther toward the anus. The external sphincter is a voluntary muscle that contracts to retain feces and relaxes to expel feces. The rectum must be able to retain and store stool to function properly. The normal rectum accommodates approximately 300 cc of stool and gas.[1,10]

Under normal circumstances, gut contents remain in the small bowel for 2 to 4 hours; normal transit time through the colon ranges from 24 to 48 hours, but can be much longer:[19] nearly 50% of a hospice population had transit times between 4 and 12 days.[29] Normal defecation requires a series of orchestrated actions, starting with relaxation of the puborectalis muscles, descent of the pelvis floor with straightening of the anorectal angle by as much as 15 degrees, inhibition of segmental peristalsis, contraction of the abdominal wall muscles, and relaxation of the external anal sphincter with expulsion of feces.[27]

Bowel function depends on normal peristalsis, sensory awareness of rectal filling, motor control of the anal sphincter, adequate rectal capacity, recognition of and compliance with the urge to defecate, and physical and emotional environments conducive to defecation.[19,27] Disruptions in these complex processes can lead to diarrhea or constipation. Notably, the presence of tumor in or around the rectum, hemorrhoids, anal fissures causing pain, surgical reduction of rectal capacity, radiation-induced fibrosis of the anorectum, and changes in innervation to the sphincters or rectum may result in constipation.

CONSTIPATION IN THE PERSON WITH CANCER

Sykes groups potential changes in bowel function among people with cancer into four general categories:[19] (1) interrelationships of cancer, cancer therapy, and comorbidities and their management; (2) factors arising directly from the cancer; (3) factors arising from cancer treatment; and (4) factors associated with cancer.

The effects of advanced age and the side effects of many medications increase the risk of constipation for people with cancer. Any decrease in dietary intake of fluids and fiber increases the risk of constipation.[12,19] These factors include anorexia, dysphagia, stomatitis, mucositis, changes in taste, early satiety, fatigue, depression, poorly controlled nausea and vomiting, tumor affecting intake and digestion, and a general decline in overall health status.[22–24] Decreases in mobility, ambulation, and exercise caused by fatigue and physical limitations that occur as effects of illness and therapy can also alter normal bowel function.[6,21] Alterations in patterns of elimination may occur because of changes imposed by a hospital or other institutional or unfamiliar environments. Lack of privacy and comfort during defecation may contribute to constipation by encouraging the person to ignore the urge to defecate, thus altering normal bowel routines.[31,33] The use of bedpans rather than commodes or toilets and the restrictions imposed by diagnostic tests or treatments can affect patients' ability to eliminate when convenient or when the urge is present.[33] Stress, mental confusion, depression, sedation, loss of consciousness, and confusion can also affect sensory awareness of the need to defecate.[34] The psychological effects of constipation often result in diminished activity levels and social isolation.[33]

Comorbidities

People with cancer often have other acute and chronic deviations from health—that is, comorbidities—that increase their risk of developing constipation. A partial list of these diseases or conditions is provided in Table 9-1. Persistent stretching of the pudendal nerves from chronic constipation may result in complications such as hemorrhoids, rectal prolapse, rectal fissures, and incontinence. Constipation is common among people who resist the urge to defecate. Pain caused by hemorrhoids and rectal fissures contributes to delayed defecation and, therefore, increases the risk for constipation. Use of laxatives to prevent hemorrhoids increases the likelihood of constipation secondary to laxative overuse. The medical management of comorbid conditions could contribute to the development of constipation. Agents known to cause constipation in the general population are listed in Table 9-2.[31]

Cancer-related factors

Age. The major risk factor for development of cancer is increasing age.[33] In fact, the older population throughout the world accounts for the majority of people treated for cancer.[34] Reports have identified associations between advancing age, constipation, and increased use of laxatives, but the link between age and constipation remains controversial.[19] A number of structural bowel changes occurring

TABLE 9-1

Partial List of Diseases or Conditions that Cause Constipation

Diet and Nutrition
- Lack of fiber
- Milk
- Dehydration

Changes in Life or Routine
- Pregnancy
- Aging
- Travel
- Lack of physical activity

Pelvic Causes
- Pregnancy & puerperium
- Endometriosis

Neuromuscular Disorders
- Multiple sclerosis
- Parkinson's disease
- Pseudo-obstruction
- Stroke
- Spinal cord injuries
- Hirschsprung's disease
- Chagas' disease

Metabolic and Endocrine Conditions
- Diabetes mellitus
- Uremia
- Hypercalcemia
- Hypokalemia
- Poor glycemic control
- Hypothyroidism

Systemic Disorders
- Amyloidosis
- Lupus
- Scleroderma

Colon, Rectal & Anal Problems
- Intestinal obstruction
- Scar tissue (adhesions)
- Perianal abscess
- Rectocele
- Anal fissure
- Anal stenosis
- Hemorrhoids
- Diverticulosis
- Colorectal stricture
- Anorectal dysfunction (anismus)

Intestinal Dysfunction
- Irritable bowel syndrome (IBS)
- Chron's Disease
- Ulcerative colitis
- Diverticulitis
- Amoebiasis
- Hernia
- Pelvic floor dysfunction

Medications (see Table 9.2)

Source: Data from National Digestive Diseases Information Clearinghouse[1].

TABLE 9-2

Agents Causing Constipation and Percent Distribution as a Causative Factor for Constipation

Analgesics
- Opioids (2.6%)
- NSAIDs

Anticholinergics
- Tricyclic antidepressants (8.2%)
- MAO inhibitors
- Antipsychotics (phenothiazines, clozapine, risperidone, haloperidol) (1.9%)
- Antiparkinsonian medications
- H1 antihistamines (9.2%)
- Antispasmodics (dicyclomine) (11.6%)

Anticonvulsants (2.5%)

Antihypertensives
- Calcium channel blockers
- Diuretics (5.6%)
- Clonidine

Cytotoxic Chemotherapeutic Agents (vinca alkaloids)

Cation Containing Agents
- Aluminum-based antacids (3%)
- Calcium-based antacids
- Bismuth subsalicylate
- Iron salts (2.8%)
- Lithium

Miscellaneous
- Amidarone
- Bile acid sequestrants
- 5-HT3 antagonists
- Adrenergics

Source: Data from Deepak and Ehrenpreis[31].

in older people have been noted, including the loss of enteric neurons, changes in calcium handling in colonic muscle, and changes in rectal sensitivity.[35,36]

Exercise. The links between bed rest, immobility, and constipation have been recognized for more than 60 years.[6,37] Colonic mass movements are associated with physical activity, such that reduced mobility is likely to impair propulsive contractility in the large bowel.[37,38] There is evidence of faster bowel transit time and more colonic propulsive activity after aerobic exercise.[39] Exercise, or lack of it, among people with cancer is an important assessment factor for risk of or actual constipation, depending on the degree of disability and immobility imposed by cancer and its treatment.[38,40]

Diet. It is readily accepted that adequate bowel function depends on sufficient intake of dietary fiber and fluids. The question then becomes, what amount is "sufficient"? People with cancer, and particularly those undergoing many forms of treatment or using various symptom control measures, experience changes in GI function, including postoperative ileus, anorexia, nausea, and vomiting, any of which can interfere with adequate dietary intake.[19,40] Reduced food consumption contributes to diminished gastric distention, decreased colonic activity and reflex, and subsequent constipation.[19] Disease progression is often accompanied by decreased consumption of fluids. In this case, fiber is less effective as a colonic stimulant. Without adequate fluid, fiber supplements may produce a gelatinous mass in the GI tract, resulting in intestinal obstruction.[41]

Alterations in anatomy and physiology. Sensory awareness depends on intact neural pathways between the anorectum and the brain, and is affected by the individual's level of consciousness. External intestinal compression or internal obstructions by tumor are the most common factors contributing to development of constipation among people with cancer.[19] Pressure from ascites is often associated with constipation. Constipation occurs as a result of narrowing of the intestinal lumen or functional obstruction caused by damage to enteric nerves and muscles.[19]

Spinal cord injury disrupts sympathetic and parasympathetic control of intestinal function.[19,42] The precise clinical effects experienced depend on the level of the lesion. Compression of the spinal cord between the T8–L5 levels and subsequent interrupted neural transmission are often responsible for constipation.[42,43] Although occurring less often among people with cancer, high cord compression (C4–C7), which is often associated with quadriplegia, causes reduced colonic activity and constipation.[19] Cauda equina, caused by sacral lesions at any level, produces lower bowel atonicity, severe constipation, and overflow incontinence.[19,42]

Paraneoplastic syndromes. Paraneoplastic constipation is generally accompanied by other neurologic symptoms—gut-related symptoms such as dysphagia and gastroparesis—and sensory neuropathies indicative of damage to the nervous system.[19] Sykes asserts that "autonomic dysfunction is an under-recognized, nonmetastatic manifestation of cancer that may exacerbate constipation," a point verified by studies finding impaired autonomic function in 50% to 63% of people with advanced cancer.[19 (p215)]

Intestinal nerve damage can occur as a result of paraneoplastic syndromes, especially those associated with small-cell lung cancer (SCLC) and carcinoid tumors.[45,46] Research findings suggest an autoimmune mechanism and link between polyclonal immunoglobulin G (IgG) antibodies (anti-Hu) that react with neuronal nuclear proteins in the central nervous system and GI paraneoplastic syndromes.[43,44] Damage occurs as a result of the immune response to tumor antigens present in neural cells. Antigens exposed by tumor apoptosis stimulate antibody formation and activation of cytotoxic T cells, reflected in damage to normal neural tissue.[19,45]

Biochemical and neuroendocrine disturbance. Case studies suggest that cancer-related constipation could result from secretion of chemical mediators that inhibit peristalsis as well as the pathologic effects of cytokines produced by intestinal endothelium.[19] Constipation associated with SCLC has been corrected by a somatostatin analogue, octreotide, contributing support for a theory of oversecretion of an intrinsic mediator of intestinal motility.[46]

Constipation is associated with hyperkalemia and hypokalemia in malignant disease. Calcium is known to play a role in the excitation and contraction of muscle and stimulus of exocrine and endocrine glands in the gut. The mechanism of action is not fully known, but it is clear that changes in extracellular calcium levels affect tissue excitability, intestinal contractility, and management of fluid levels.[19] Likewise, hypokalemia alters nerve and muscle activity in the gut, leading to constipation.

Cancer treatment-related factors

Surgical alteration of the gastrointestinal tract, disruption of nerve pathways in the gut, irradiation involving pelvic fields, medications (including cytotoxic agents, antiemetics, and anticholinergics), and immobility and debility of disease contribute to the high frequency of constipation in this population.

Chemotherapy agents. Neurotoxicity from medications such as vincristine, vinblastine, oxaliplatin, and thalidomide inhibits transmission of impulses controlling bowel function and contributes to constipation. Neurotoxicity triggered by vinca alkaloid cytotoxic agents occurs as a result of direct damage to the myenteric plexus and subsequent paralysis of the gut.[47–50] Faller and Pandit[51] note that vinorelbine induces cytotoxicity by inhibiting the transition of tubulin dimers into microtubules, thereby disrupting mitotic spindle formation. Vinorelbine is selective for mitotic microtubules, demonstrating only minimal activity in atonal or other microtubule classes; thus it is less likely to cause neurotoxicity (and constipation) than the nonselective microtubule inhibitors, vincristine and vinblastine.[51]

Radiation therapy. Constipation is sometimes induced intentionally among patients undergoing brachytherapy for gynecologic and prostate cancers. In these situations, a low-residue diet and antidiarrheal agents are prescribed to prevent bowel movements while implants are in place. Normal bowel activity may not return for several days after completion of therapy. Increased dietary fiber and hydration are usually sufficient to reverse this side effect of therapy, allowing patients to return to normal bowel patterns. However, these patients often receive opioid analgesics and, therefore, are prone to the constipating effects of opioids. Additional complicating factors of radiation therapy that contribute to constipation when the pelvis lies within the radiated field include fatigue, proctitis, erythema, rectal irritation, and bowel damage.[23,24,52,53]

Patients receiving brachytherapy of the head and neck often experience stomatitis and mucositis, requiring use of alternative methods of feeding such as gastric tubes. These dietary changes can contribute to constipation through diminished dietary fiber and fluid intake in any patient population, but may be particularly problematic among patients undergoing head and neck brachytherapy. Brachytherapy is an increasingly common treatment option for patients with gynecological, prostate, and head and neck cancers, so oncology nurses often face the dilemma of constipation and diarrhea that accompanies this treatment modality.[54]

Opioid-induced constipation. The most common cause of constipation among people with cancer is the use of opiates (compounds that contain the morphine or thebaine structure, and have affinity for any or all opioid receptors) and opioids (compounds that do not contain the basic morphine or thebaine structure, but still possess some affinity for opioid receptors) in the management of pain.[55–57] Indeed, most contemporary literature citations for cancer-related constipation relate to that induced by opioids. An accurate estimate of the prevalence of opioid-induced constipation among people with cancer is difficult to obtain because of other disease-related factors that also induce this condition. People with cancer often experience constipation relating to opioid use, and existing disease-related constipation can worsen with opioid therapy. Constipation occurs in more than 85% of people with cancer being treated with opioids.[58,59]

Opioid analgesics act primarily on mu, kappa, and delta opioid CNS receptors, although mu receptors are responsible for decreased gastrointestinal motility, sedation, and analgesia.[55,58] Opioids slow the transit of stool through the colon by decreasing peristalsis, stimulating segmental non-propulsive motility, and increasing the tone of the ileocecal and anal sphincters via effects on enteric neurons.[19,55,58] In addition to increased transit time in the gut, increased fluid absorption due to opioids stimulates mucosal sensory receptors to activate a reflex arc that promotes additional fluid absorption.[19,55,58]

SYMPTOM ASSESSMENT

As is generally the case, prevention, early diagnosis, and intervention for constipation necessitate use of a consistent terminology for this condition. Despite centuries-old awareness of constipation as a distressing and common condition, a consensus-derived and universally accepted definition has yet to be devised. The *Rome Criteria* constitute "a system developed to classify the functional gastrointestinal disorders (FGIDs), disorders of the digestive system in which symptoms cannot be explained by the presence of structural or tissue abnormality, based on clinical symptoms."[60] Table 9-3 outlines the Rome III Diagnostic Criteria for Functional Constipation. The validity of the Rome criteria has been questioned due to a recognized disparity between self-reported and criteria-based definitions.[61] It is also noteworthy that for the Rome criteria to apply, constipation symptoms must be present for 3 months,[60] rendering these criteria largely unsuitable for the cancer patient population.

Timing of bowel habits, given that defecation can vary from one or more times per day to more than once weekly or even less often, is commonly used to define constipation.[62] The sensation of incomplete evacuation of stool after defecation is used as both a symptom and a definition of constipation.[18,58] Attempts to qualify and quantify constipation have met with reliability and validity issues.[63,64]

TABLE 9-3

Rome III Diagnostic Criteria* for Functional Constipation

1 Must include 2 *or more* of the following:
   a. Straining during at least 25% of defecations
   b. Lumpy or hard stools (scybala) in at least 25% of defecations
   c. Sensation of incomplete evacuation for at least 25% of defecations
   d. Sensation of anorectal obstruction or blockage for at least 25% of defecations
   e. Manual maneuvers needed to facilitate at least 25% of defecations
   f. Fewer than 3 defecations per week (daily stool weight less than 35 g/day)

2 Loose stools rarely present without use of laxative

3 Prolonged whole gut or colonic transit

**Criteria fulfilled for the last 3 months with symptom onset at least 6 months prior to diagnosis.*

Source: Data from Drossman[60].

As a result, confusion continues to exist, there is no definitive definition or operationalized measure of constipation, and implementation of assessment tools and prevention and management strategies remains inconsistent at best.[17,54,61–63]

SELF-ASSESSMENT

Failure to anticipate and adequately manage constipation is an unnecessary cause of discomfort and pain that affects quality of life for individuals with cancer and their caregivers.[65–67] Fortunately, even in the face of cancer and cancer treatment, constipation is a preventable problem for most people. Prevention of constipation does require paying close attention to one's body functions, exercise, routine efforts to use complementary modalities, diet and fluid intake to maintain and/or improve bowel function, and at times, use of medications to soften stool and promote regular bowel movements.

Any person with cancer needs to be made aware of his or her risks for developing constipation. Completion of a constipation risk assessment scale, such as that devised by Richmond and Wright[64] (Figure 9-1) can sensitize both patient and caregiver to risk factors, and can initiate all-important communication relevant to constipation risks, prevention, and self-management and other changes in bodily functions. Individuals at risk will benefit from starting a constipation prevention plan—sometimes called a "bowel protocol"—at diagnosis but especially

Circle risk factors in table and total

GENDER:

Male	1
Female	2

MOBILITY:

Independently mobile	0
Dependent on walking aids/assistance from others	1
Restricted to bed/chair	2
Spinal cord injury/spinal cord compression	3

FIBER INTAKE:

5 pieces fruit/veg or more consumed daily	0
3 or 4 pieces fruit/veg consumed daily	1
2 pieces fruit/veg or less consumed daily	2
Bran products consumed daily Yes	0
No	2

FLUID INTAKE:

10 cups/glasses or more consumed daily	0
6 to 9 cups/glasses consumed daily	1
5 cups/glasses or less consumed daily	2

PERSONAL BELIEFS:

Does patient believe they are prone to constipation? **Yes/No**

Have laxatives ever been used for constipation? **Yes/**

Current bowel habit:__________

SECTION SUB TOTAL [ ]

WARD PATIENTS ONLY:

Does patient have difficulty evacuating bowels in hospital toilets?

No	0
Yes	2

PATIENTS REQUIRING COMMODE/BEDPAN:

Does patient anticipate problems using a commode or bedpan?

No	0
Yes	2

SECTION SUB TOTAL [ ]

Conditions which increase risk of constipation.

From medical notes, patient history and blood results, assess presence of the following:

PHYSIOLOGICAL CONDITIONS

Metabolic disorders: Hypokalemia/uremia/lead poisoning	2
Pelvic conditions: Hysterectomy/ovarian tumor/uterine prolapse/pregnancy	3
Neuromuscular disorders: Parkinson's Disease/Multiple Sclerosis/Systemic Sclerois/Hirsprungs's Disease Cerebrovascular Accident/Spina Bifida/Rheumatoid Arthritis/cerebral tumor	3
Endocrine disorders: Diabetes Mellitus/hypothyroidism/hypopituitarism/hypercalcaemia	3
Colorectal/abdominal disorders: Irritable Bowel Syndrome/Crohn's disease/Diverticulitis/Ulcerative Colitis/ Colorectal tumor/anorectal stricture/anorectal fissure/anorectal prolapse/ hemorrhoids/hernias	3

PSYCHOLOGICAL CONDITIONS

Psychiatric illness: Depression/Anorexia Nervosa/Bulimia Nervosa	2
Learning disabilities or dementia (as evidenced by lack of understanding of speech or situations)	2

SECTION SUB TOTAL [ ]

Medications which increase risk of constipation

Is patient presently taking any of the following medication on a regular basis?

Antiemetics	2
Calcium channel blockers	2
Iron supplements	2

Analgesics:

Non-opioid analgesia	3
OR continuous opioid therapy	3

Anticholinergic containing medication:

Anticonvulsants	2
Antidepressants	2
Antiparkinson drugs	2
Antispasmodics	2

Cytotoxic chemotherapy

Cytotoxic chemotherapy	3
OR Vinca alkaloid agents	5

SECTION SUB TOTAL [ ]

Low risk for constipation <10
Medium risk for constipation 11–15
High risk for constipation >16

TOTAL SCORE [ ]

FIGURE 9-1

Constipation risk assessment.

Source: Reprinted from Journal of Orthopaedic Nursing, Richmond JP, Wright ME, Establishing reliability and validity of a constipation risk assessment scale. 2008;12:139–150, with permission from Elsevier[64].

at the initiation of treatment. An important piece of the self-managed bowel protocol is use of a patient diary, similar to the one depicted in Figure 9-2. If and when constipation is suspected, use of McMillan's Constipation Assessment Scale (CAS), Figure 9-3, helps to determine the severity of the problem and the need for additional diagnostic testing.[63]

OBJECTIVE ASSESSMENT

The incidence of under-diagnosis of constipation is indicative of inconsistencies in definition, lack of knowledge of underlying conditions and failure to initiate preventive interventions, lack of appropriate assessment, and underuse of diagnostic tests. Many patients do not volunteer information about bowel symptoms to their physicians and nurses.[69–71] Vigilant assessment and regular and consistent reassessment are essential to identification of risks for constipation among persons with cancer.[72]

Studies demonstrate lack of congruence between patients and caregivers in recognizing and reporting cancer-related symptoms and symptom intensity.[73] Agreement between patients and nurses is reported to be stronger than agreement between patients and physicians.[73] Disagreements between the Rome criteria and patient self-report and between the Rome criteria and physician assessment have been reported.[71] A qualitative study by Jacobsson et al.[74] describes how cancer-related symptoms are assessed and managed in a cancer care setting. This study generated four themes relating to the symptom management process:

- Creating a relationship with each patient
- Understanding the ways in which patients are affected by the symptom management process, while integrating clinicians' competence and values

- Assessing the symptom: assessment methods, identifying symptoms using signs, and symptom clusters
- The importance of care by an interdisciplinary team, emphasizing availability and knowledge about each team member, communication, and role assignments within the team

The Constipation Risk Assessment Scale developed by Richmond and Wright[64] (Figure 9-1) is useful for conducting baseline assessment at diagnosis, initiation of therapy, and introduction of new medication and other treatment modalities. McMillan's Constipation Assessment Scale (Figure 9-3) has demonstrated validity and reliability, and

Date & Time	B.M.	Consistency	Color	Strain	Pain or Discomfort	Medication
July 22	None	–	–	–	Some abdominal fullness	1 colace
July 23 9:30 AM	Small	Hard	Dk brown	Yes	Rectal pain	2 dulcolax
2:45 PM	Medium	Hard	Dk brown	Yes, but less than earlier	Rectal pain	None
9 PM	None				Abdominal cramps	Senekot
July 24 8 AM	Medium	Normal	Dk brown	No	No	Senekot & Metamucil

FIGURE 9-2

Sample bowel activity diary.

Directions: Circle the number that indicates whether, during the past three days, you have had "no problem", "some problem", or a "severe problem" with each item on this list.			
Item	**No Problem**	**Some Problem**	**Severe Problem**
Abdominal distention or bloating	0	1	2
Change in amount of gas passed rectally	0	1	2
Less frequent bowel movements	0	1	2
Oozing liquid stool	0	1	2
Rectal fullness or pressure	0	1	2
Rectal pain with bowel movement	0	1	2
Small stool size	0	1	2
Urge but inability to pass stool	0	1	2
Total scores can range between 0 (no constipation) to 16 (the most severe constipation). If the patient indicates a problem with item 4 (oozing, liquid stool), consider possibility of impaction.			

FIGURE 9-3

Constipation assessment scale.

Source: Courtesy of Susan C. McMillan, PhD, ARNP, FAAN.

is useful in evaluating constipation status.[63] Asking the patient to define constipation, describe symptoms, and explain the symptoms' effect on quality of life and activities of daily living allows the nurse to understand constipation from the patient's perspective: Inquiring about onset, severity, and duration of symptoms is essential. A patient diary, such as that depicted in Figure 9-2, is helpful in understanding patients' perspectives about bowel habits before and after initiation of medications, including analgesics, and other medical and surgical interventions.

History

An objective assessment of suspected or actual constipation begins with a detailed patient history that includes the assessment factors outlined in Table 9-4.

Physical assessment

The complete physical examination, including a detailed neurological examination, may help identify systemic diseases that can cause constipation. The abdomen is carefully examined for the presence of stool, especially in the left quadrant. It is important to rule out an intestinal mass.[75]

1. Assess for nutritional and hydration status. Measures of hydration include thirst level, vein filling and emptying times, skin turgor and resiliency, mucosal moisture, vital signs, fluid intake and output, osmolality and specific gravity of urine.
2. Assess the abdomen for tenderness and auscultate for bowel sounds.
3. Evaluate the perianal region and perform a rectal or stoma exam to rule out hemorrhoids, impaction, or rectal tumor.

Diagnostic evaluation

After physical examination, additional diagnostic evaluation for constipation is a stepwise process, initiated with a digital rectal exam (DRE) followed by plain abdominal radiography.[75,76] In a prospective cross-sectional study of 50 patients with advanced cancer admitted to a palliative care unit, Nagaviroj and colleagues[76] found no strong correlation between scores of the CAS and plain abdominal radiographs. Based on these findings, the authors recommend that constipation in patients with advanced-stage cancer be assessed both clinically and radiographically.[76]

Clinicians' ability to perform DRE is an underappreciated skill. In surveys of final-year medical students, only 40% felt confident in basing an opinion on their own DRE findings.[77] In another survey of senior medical students and house officers, fewer than 20% had performed more than 10 procedures.[78] A multicenter study involving medical students, primary care and internal medicine physicians, and gastroenterologists showed that gastroenterologists performed the most DREs annually, followed by primary care physicians and internal medicine subspecialities.[79] There is no similar study in the available literature assessing nurse-performed DRE. Nevertheless, thorough perianal and digital rectal examination is often the most telling piece of the clinical evaluation for constipation.[75]

The DRE begins as the clinician assesses for external hemorrhoids, skin tags, rectal prolapse, warts, anal fissure and evidence of pruritus. A patient's experience of excruciating pain as the DRE begins is indicative of anal fissure.[75] High resting sphincter tone may result in difficult evacuation.[75] Palpation of the rectal walls can identify polyps, masses, rectocele, and intussusception.[75] A finding of stool in the rectal vault, its consistency, and a patient's lack of awareness of it is suggestive of rectal hyposensitivity.[75]

Pelvic floor function is assessed during the DRE by asking the patient to push and bear down as if to defecate.[75] The examiner places a hand over the abdomen to assess the push effort. The normal response occurs when the anal sphincter and puborectalis relax and the perineum descends. If, instead, the muscles contract or there is no perineal descent, pelvic floor dyssynergia is suggested and indicates the need for additional diagnostic evaluation.[75]

The complete diagnostic evaluation progresses from DRE through more complex, precise, and costly procedures, as outlined here:[75,76]

1. Digital rectal exam.
2. Fecal occult blood test.
3. Radiographs in supine and upright positions (differentiate mechanical obstruction from decreased motility associated with ileus); abdominal and pelvic ultrasound and/or computed tomography (CT) scan if extraluminal obstruction is suspected.
4. Laboratory tests to assess metabolic status (electrolytes, complete blood count, renal and liver tests, thyroid-stimulating hormone).
5. Electronic measuring (manometric) techniques are useful examinations in situations in which neurophysiologic mechanisms are potential causes of constipation.
6. Endoscopic exam if intraluminal obstruction is suspected.

The more complex manometric diagnostics best practice recommendations offered by Rao and Meduri[75] provide guidance for accurate determination of underlying physiologic mechanisms of constipation, and are useful when patients do not respond to simple dietary (fiber and fluid) interventions, increased physical activity, and use of stool softener and laxatives.

TABLE 9-4

Evaluation of Constipation—History and Physical Assessment

Assessment	Individual Characteristics
	History
Usual pattern of elimination	• Frequency, consistency, amount • Usual routine, including time for elimination and rituals followed • Last bowel movement • Elimination aids (raised toilet seat, laxative use, etc.) • Individual's definitions of regularity and constipation • Changes since diagnosis or treatment
Previous experience with constipation and responses	• Interventions that have worked in the past • Current or past laxative use and response to laxative therapy • Underlying conditions that increase constipation
Usual and current dietary patterns	• Amounts and types of fluid daily—identify recent changes • Intake of bulk and fiber—identify recent changes • 3-day recall of dietary intake • Changes in appetite, taste, dentition, energy
Recent changes in lifestyle	• Changes in activity, mood, increased stress, changes in mobility • Physical changes affecting defecation
Symptoms of constipation/obstipation	• Flatus, bloating, cramping • Oozing stool in the presence of symptoms of constipation/obstipation • Straining of defecation, difficult passage of stool; hard, dry stool • Abdominal pain, fullness, anorexia, other symptoms
Current medications	• Identify medications that increase risk of constipation • Identify laxative use
Other risk factors for constipation	• Recent and past cancer and cancer therapy • Other underlying health problems
Knowledge of individual	• Subjective understanding of constipation and therapy for constipation
Evaluate laboratory findings	• Identify presence of thrombocytopenia or leukopenia, or metabolic conditions that cause constipation (hypercalcemia, hypokalemia)
	Physical Assessment
Examine	• Visualize abdomen for visible peristalsis, masses, distention, bulges
Palpate	• For tenderness, decreased muscle tone, presence of palpable tumor, nodes, or stool
Percuss	• For dullness in an otherwise tympanic area of the abdomen
Auscultate	• For presence and character of bowel sounds
Examine	• Rectal area (or stoma) for irritation, hemorrhoids, fissures, lesions, or rashes
Perform rectal exam	• Evaluate external sphincter tone, rule out obstipation, and evaluate for internal hemorrhoids or tumor • *Rectal exam is contraindicated in presence of leukopenia or thrombocytopenia* • Signs of systemic conditions related to hydration, overall performance status, and underlying conditions related to constipation (e.g., skin tugor)
Evaluate	• Assess lower-extremity strength, sensation, and reflexes for possible spinal cord compression

DEGREES OF TOXICITY

The National Cancer Institute (NCI) Common Terminology Criteria for Adverse Events are useful in determining and communicating necessary levels of intervention based on adverse event criteria.[80] Toxicity grades (Table 9-5) range from 1 to 5 on a scale that rank-orders the level of adversity and constipation.

SYMPTOM MANAGEMENT STRATEGIES

THERAPEUTIC APPROACHES

The basic goal in therapeutic approaches to constipation is to maintain or reestablish the patient's normal bowel pattern and habits (time of day for normal bowel movement, consistency, color and amount).[8,33,81,82] Figure 9-4 provides a bowel management protocol.

Prevention

Evidence-based prevention of constipation and management of existing constipation employ a combination of nonpharmacologic and pharmacologic interventions. Identification of the cause and its relationship to the individual's cancer diagnosis are essential to matching etiology to intervention. Unlike many distressing symptoms that occur among people with cancer, constipation is a pervasive symptom that is largely preventable. Anticipation and aggressive assessment of constipation among people with cancer and prophylactic implementation of bowel management protocols to prevent constipation are critical to quality nursing care for this high-risk population. Constipation is also a problem that can be prevented or relieved by relatively simple and autonomous nursing interventions, or through nurses' participation in interdisciplinary planning and intervention.[74]

Identifying persons at risk is essential to prevention. Monitoring bowel function and preventing constipation are much easier than treating constipation, obstipation, or obstruction that has already developed.[18] A prevention program for individuals at risk for constipation consists of use of prophylactic medications, increasing dietary fiber and fluid intake, and promoting exercise. Almost every person using opioids without preventive measures will develop constipation.[19,24] Given this fact, prevention strategies, including diet, fluid, activity considerations and prophylactic medications, must accompany introduction and use of opioid analgesics.[2,19,33] The National Comprehensive Cancer Network (NCCN) guideline for management of adult cancer pain[83] includes principles of management of opioid adverse effects; similarly, the palliative care guideline[84] identifies prevention and management of constipation as priority concerns. In addressing constipation in the palliative setting, NCCN recommends that opioid-induced constipation "be anticipated and treated prophylactically with a stimulating laxative to increase bowel motility with or without stool softeners."[84(MS-10)]

Nonpharmacologic interventions

Hospitalized patients, people living in unfamiliar and/or subacute care settings other than home, people forced to use bedpans, and those who lack privacy are at risk for constipation.[32,33] Prevention and management of this symptom includes implementation of programs that provide a regular schedule for toileting, privacy, exercises to strengthen and tone abdominal muscles, and routine reminders to respond to the urge to defecate.

Nutrition. People with cancer often experience anorexia, fatigue, and other symptoms, and have difficulty increasing fluids and tolerating dietary bulk and fiber. After assessing a patient's current dietary status, including fiber and fluid intake, the nurse, patient, and caregiver, perhaps

TABLE 9-5

National Cancer Institute Common Terminology Criteria for Adverse Events (CTCAE): Constipation

Adverse Event	Grade 1	Grade 2	Grade 3	Grade 4	Grade 5
Constipation	Occasional or intermittent symptoms; occasional use of stool softeners, laxatives, dietary modification or enema	Persistent symptoms with regular use of laxatives or enemas; limiting instrumental activities daily living (ADL)	Obstipation with manual evacuation indicated; limiting self-care ADL	Life-threatening consequences; urgent intervention indicated	Death

Definition: A disorder characterized by irregular and infrequent or difficult evacuation of the bowels

Source: Data from National Cancer Institute Common Terminology Criteria for Adverse Events (CTCAE)[77].

Prevention

- Perform Constipation Risk Assessment
- Initiate prevention process consistent with identified risks
  - Increase fluid intake if no fluid restrictions
  - Increase fiber if patient has adequate fluid intake and physical activity level
  - Active or passive exercise: 30 minutes 3/week
- Identify available expert resources: nutritionist, physical therapist
- Instruct patient and caregiver in prevention and early identification measures
- Prophylactic medications: stimulant laxative ± stool softener; polyethylene glycol
- Increase laxative dose with increased dose of opioids

↓

Adverse Event = 1
(Occasional/Intermittent Symptoms)

- Administer Constipation Assessment Scale (determine severity)
- Assess for cause and treat as indicated
- Rule out obstruction
- Diet modifications: increase fluid and fiber intake
- Initiate stool softener, laxative, enema
- Titrate stool softener/laxative as needed: goal of one non-forced bowel movement every 1–2 days
- Consider altered opioid dose or protocol to allow reduced opioid dose

↓

Adverse Event = 2
(Persistent symptoms with regular use of laxatives or enemas; limits instrumental ADL)

- Administer Constipation Assessment Scale (Reassess for cause and severity)
- Rule out obstruction
- Check for impaction/obstipation
- Add additional agents – magnesium hydroxide (30–60 mL/day); biscacodyl (2–3 tablets PO/day; 1 rectal suppository daily; lactulose (30–60 (30mL/day); sorbitol (30mL every 2h x 3) then as needed; magnesium citrate (8 oz PO daily); PEG (1 cap/8 oz water PO 2/day)
- Fleet, saline or tap water enema
- Consider prokinetic agent (i.e., metoclopramide 10–20 mg PO qid – long-term use limited by potential for neurologic side effects)
- With unsatisfactory response to laxative therapy for opioid-induced constipation in patients with advanced disease, consider methylnaltrexone (0.15 mg/kg SQ – qod: maximum 1 dose/day)

↓

Adverse Event = 3 & 4
(Obstipation with manual evacuation indicated; limiting self-care ADL)

- DRE
- Rule out obstruction
- Additional diagnostic evaluation
- Administer glycerin rectal: one PRN

  OR
- Bisacodyl 5–10 mg rectal suppository: one PRN
- Sodium/Potassium enema: 133 mL (21.3 gm)
- Apply topical anesthetic to decrease pain
- Lubricate rectal area with water-soluble lubricant
- Insert glycerin suppository or mineral or olive oil retention enema
- Perform manual evacuation
- Soap suds or tap water enema until clear
- Initiate Senna protocol and determine response

  OR
- Initiate aggressive constipation management plan
- With unsatisfactory response to laxative therapy for opioid-induced constipation in patients with advanced disease, consider methylnaltrexone (0.15 mg/kg SQ – qod: maximum 1 dose/day)
- Consider opioid rotation to fentanyl or methadone
- Consider neuraxial analgesics, neuroablative techniques – interventions to decrease pain, relieve constipation, reduce opioid dose

FIGURE 9-4

Management of constipation: A step-wise approach.

Abbreviations: ADL: activities daily living; DRE: digital rectal exam; PEG: poly ethylene glycol.

in collaboration with a dietician, can develop nutritional interventions aimed at increasing fiber and fluid to optimal dietary levels. Increasing dietary fiber is contraindicated for patients with inadequate fluid intake due to the risk of obstruction. For patients who are able to maintain proper fluid intake, dietary fiber can be slowly titrated upward, initially adding 3–4 g of fiber per day, increasing to 6–10 g daily.[33] As fiber intake increases, patients may initially experience abdominal discomfort, flatulence, and erratic bowel habits. Foods rich in dietary fiber include whole-grain cereals (3 tablespoons of wheat bran provides 10 g of dietary fiber), breads, legumes, root vegetables, fruits with seeds and skins (prunes, figs, applesauce), nuts, peanut butter, and popcorn.[33,82]

Maintaining optimal fluid intake can be challenging for people experiencing nausea, vomiting, anorexia, or fatigue. Although efficacy data are lacking,[20] expert opinion supports intake of 6–8 glasses (1–2 liters) of water daily as a measure to promote soft stool.[20,33] This amount may seem overwhelming to people struggling with fluid intake—particularly when confronting a full liter container. Having a water bottle close-by at all times, however, can encourage routine and frequent sipping. Coffee, tea, and grapefruit juice act as diuretics and should be discouraged when hydration is a concern.[82]

Activity and exercise. Mobility and regular exercise within the limits of individual tolerance, including passive range-of-motion and abdominal isometric exercises, help maintain bowel function.[33] Brisk walking for at least 30 minutes three times per week is conducive to a more normal bowel routine.[33] However, fatigue, advanced disease, poor pain control, fractures due to bone metastasis, or decreased endurance may impair mobility.

Massage. Writing from the Illinois Training School for Nurses in 1901, Kate Williams offered guidance for using massage for constipation.[5] She noted that not all cases of constipation are amenable to massage, and that in some cases it is contraindicated. Williams described a variety of massage techniques—vibration, kneading, friction, hacking, and clapping—to be adapted to the treatment to each individual patient.[5] In 1915, Chapman provided a detailed review of the physiological effects of massage, defined as "any specific manipulation executed on the human body with a curative, palliative or hygienic object in view." [85(p635)] She noted the effect of abdominal massage on voluntary muscles of the walls of the colon, the influence on smooth muscle fibers of the alimentary canal, and stimulation of glands connected to the digestive tract. From these effects, colon function is improved and constipation is relieved.[85] More recently, Billhult and Dahlberg showed physical and emotional benefits of massage for cancer patients.[86] Other studies suggest the combination of aromatherapy (the therapeutic use of specially prepared essential or aromatic oils[87]) and massage can help relieve constipation.[87,88] Although not specific to the cancer patient population, growing evidence indicates that abdominal massage can stimulate peristalsis, decrease colonic transit time, increase frequency of bowel movements, and decrease discomfort and pain.[89]

Pharmacologic interventions

The NCCN Guidelines for Management of Opioid Adverse Effects[83] and Palliative Care[84] include preventive and management measures that employ medications. Suggested prophylactic medications include stimulant laxatives with or without stool softener (e.g., senna with or without docusate) and polyethylene glycol (PEG), with the laxative dose being increased as the opioid dose increases.[83,84,90]

The Oncology Nursing Society's *Putting Evidence into Practice* (PEP) resource identifies interventions for preventing and treating constipation in people with cancer that are deemed "likely to be effective."[33] Among the pharmacologic interventions for adults, the efficacy and safety of PEG, with or without electrolytes, is supported by a high level of incidence in non-oncology populations.[90] Expert opinion offered in PEP for prophylaxis of opioid-induced constipation is that "not enough evidence exists to identify the most effective regimen."[33(p93)]

The use of daily stool softeners and peristaltic stimulators to soften and propel feces through the colon facilitates evacuation of feces. Concurrent administration of senna (Senokot) with opioid doses decreases the constipating effects of opioid analgesics. Use of lactulose and sorbitol shows promise in hospice programs and in older people with chronic laxative abuse.[19,69,81] Use of low-dose naloxone (2 mg or 4 mg orally three times per day) as treatment for opioid-induced constipation has been suggested, a strategy that has the potential to disrupt the overall analgesia plan of care.[91–93] An alternating schedule of prolonged-release naloxone and prolonged-release oxycodone has been used with mixed outcomes.[91,92] Offering choices for specific products and regimens for maintaining bowel function will help ensure acceptable options.

Fecal obstipation (impaction). Failure to manage bowel function adequately can result in fecal impaction, now often referred to as obstipation.[7,8,80] In this condition, large amounts of hard, dry feces accumulate in the rectum and cannot be eliminated normally. As stool collects, seepage of liquid stool around the impacted stool may present as diarrhea. Other symptoms of obstipation include rectal discomfort, lower abdominal pain, tenesmus, lower back pain, and urinary incontinence and retention. If unrelieved, nausea, vomiting, hypotension, confusion, respiratory and circulatory compromise, or death may occur. Assessment and physical examination are similar to that for constipation, with the possible addition of a flat or upright abdominal x-ray to rule out impaction.[75] Rectal examination reveals large amounts of hard stool in the rectum, unless obstipation is higher, in the sigmoid colon.

Once obstipation is recognized, the therapeutic goal is to soften the stool and lubricate the bowel so that the fecal mass can be removed with minimal injury to surrounding rectal mucosa. A glycerin suppository (placed between the rectal mucosa and stool), oil retention or hypertonic phosphate enemas, or nonstimulating laxatives may be helpful, allowing stool to pass without causing fissures or increasing the chance of hemorrhoid development.[94] Laxatives that increase peristalsis or cause cramping are contraindicated until the impaction is removed and stool is able to pass through the bowel.[12,26]

After assessing the patient for thrombocytopenia, neutropenia, rectal fissure, the possibility of latex sensitivity, and the need for premedication with opioids and/or an anxiolytic to reduce physical and psychological discomfort, manual removal of obstipation is performed after applying a topical anesthetic (2% lidocaine ointment) and a water-soluble lubricant to the rectal area below the stool mass.[94,95] Care providers with long or sharp fingernails should not perform rectal examination or manual removal of impaction because of the risk of trauma and tears to the anal and rectal mucosa. Removal of obstipation requires caution to prevent mucosa or rectal tearing. After the mass of stool is lubricated and softened, perform a rectal exam using a single finger lubricated with 2% lidocaine ointment. After several minutes, the sphincter should relax, and a second finger can be inserted. The two fingers are then gently and slowly moved apart to dilate the anal sphincter. The two fingers gently "slice apart" the impacted mass of stool. After most of the fecal material is removed, follow with a cleansing enema. An aggressive, well-monitored bowel management program is then instituted to prevent recurrence of impaction.[94,95]

Laxative therapy. The goal of laxative therapy is to promote normal elimination patterns and prevent constipation and obstipation. Restoration of water in feces is the desired physiologic outcome. Fecal water content is increased with osmotic and stimulant laxatives, reducing bowel transit time (with exercise, stimulants, or osmotic laxatives) and increasing the ability of feces to retain water with fiber, docusate, and osmotic laxatives.[96] Effects of laxatives are dose related, with the softener effect followed by a laxative effect: high doses act as cathartics. A laxative regimen titrated to an individual's need promotes regular bowel function without swings from constipation to diarrhea.

Laxatives are divided into seven classes: (1) bulk-producing agents, (2) lubricants, (3) saline laxatives, (4) osmotic laxatives, (5) detergent laxatives, (6) stimulants, and (7) suppositories and enemas. Table 9-6 lists common laxatives. Oral laxatives are contraindicated with suspected or actual intestinal obstruction or obstipation, due to the risk of bowel perforation by increasing peristalsis in the presence of obstruction.

Bulk laxatives are natural or synthetic polysaccharides or cellulose that increase peristalsis by causing water retention in the stool, thereby increasing stool size and weight.[7,8,18] They are not recommended to counteract opioid-induced constipation or in the setting of palliative care.[8,41,84] Bulk laxatives are of limited use for severe constipation and in individuals who are unable to tolerate at least 3000 cc (3 liters) of fluid per day.[8,41,53] Individuals with anorexia, early satiety, fluid restrictions, food aversions, and other alterations in nutrition that compromise appetite require a focus on adequate nutritional intake as opposed to simply increasing fluids.[53]

Lubricants coat and soften stool, decreasing friction as stool moves through the colon. Excess doses can lead to rectal seepage and perianal irritation. Long-term use can cause malabsorption of fat-soluble vitamins, making lubricants of limited use in a prophylactic bowel management program.

Saline and osmotic laxatives are high-osmolarity compounds that combine with saline to attract water into the intestines, soften stool consistency and distend the bowel to stimulate peristalsis.[46] Frequent use of these compounds can lead to fluid and electrolyte imbalance, and these medications are contraindicated in patients with impaired renal function, megacolon, congestive heart failure, hypertension, and edema.

Osmotic laxatives include magnesium salts, saccharine, alcohols, and macrogols. Lactulose, a synthetic disaccharide, passes through the colon undigested. As it is broken down in the colon, lactic acid, formic acid, acetic acid, and carbon dioxide are formed, increasing osmotic pressure and water retention in the stool.[81] Bacteria in the colon metabolize lactulose; osmotic pressure in the colon increases, as does the amount of water in the colon; and subsequent softening of stool improves the frequency of defecation. Lactulose binds with ammonia, lowering ammonia levels and reducing colon pH. The side effects most often associated with lactulose use include flatulence, bloating, and abdominal cramping. Sorbitol, another osmotic laxative, increases water absorption in the colon. Macrogols, such as oral PEG, do not alter pH or bowel flora.[81,90] Instead, PEG softens stool and increases stool volume, decreases bowel transit time, and dilates the bowel wall to trigger the defecation reflex. PEG has been studied extensively, including meta-analyses to determine its efficacy compared to placebo and lactulose: PEG was found to be more effective than either placebo or lactulose, with fewer side effects.[81,90]

Detergent laxatives act directly on the intestines by reducing surface tension, allowing water and fats to penetrate dry stool and thereby causing the stool to soften and

TABLE 9-6

Common Laxatives Used to Prevent and Manage Constipation

Preparation	Action/Onset	Special Considerations	Contraindications
		Bulk-Forming Laxatives	
Methylcellulose Psyllium Mucilloids Malt soup extracts Carboxymethyl cellulose	Increase peristalsis by causing water retention in the stool. Increase size and weight of stool. Onset is from 12h to several days.	Must be accompanied by a full (8 oz) glass of water. Daily fluid intake must be increased to at least 3 liters. Failure to increase fluids decreases efficacy and may cause intestinal or esophageal obstruction.	Not appropriate for person with fluid restrictions, or for those unable to drink increased volume of fluid. Should not be used with suspected or actual bowel obstruction. Psyllium is not recommended for individuals taking salicylates, nitrofurantoin, or digoxin. Psyllium decreases the action of these medications.
		Lubricants	
Mineral oil Liquid petrolatum	Coat and soften stool and decrease friction as stool moves through the colon. Onset is between 24 and 48h.	Chronic use can result in rectal seepage and malabsorption of oil-soluble vitamins and medications. Systemic absorption of mineral oil is increased when taken with docusate.	May cause aspiration pneumonia in persons with reflux, dysphagia, or confusion. Do not administer at bedtime or to debilitated patients. Also contraindicated in pregnant women and persons on anticoagulant therapy. Mineral oil decreases the availability of vitamin K and thus alters coagulation.
		Saline laxatives	
Magnesium citrate Sodium biphosphate Magnesium hydroxide	Draws water into the gut and increases water absorption into the stool. Alters stool consistency, increasing weight of stool, distending the bowel, and increasing peristalsis. Onset is dose dependent. High doses produce watery stool within 1–2h. Lower doses produce semifluid stool in 6–12h.	Of little to no use in prevention of constipation. Primary use is in the acute evacuation of the bowel.	Magnesium-containing laxatives should not be used with aluminum-containing antacids. Sodium salts should not be used in individuals with cardiac or renal disease, hypertension, or edema.
		Osmotic laxatives	
Lactulose Sorbitol	Bacteria in the colon metabolize osmotic laxatives. increasing osmotic pressure and water retention in the stool. Lactulose also lowers serum ammonia levels and decreases colon pH.	Sweet taste of products may be unpalatable to persons with anorexia, taste changes, or nausea. Excessive amounts will result in watery diarrhea. Lactulose is more expensive than most laxatives.	Not appropriate for individuals with acute abdomen, fecal impaction, or obstruction.

(continued)

TABLE 9-6

Common Laxatives Used to Prevent and Manage Constipation (*continued*)

Preparation	Action/Onset	Special Considerations	Contraindications
		Detergent laxatives	
Docusate Docusate sodium Docusate potassium	Act directly on the colon to reduce surface tension and allow water and fats to penetrate the stool. Decrease electrolyte and water absorption from the colon. Onset is 12–24h with oral preparations, 2–15 min with rectal preparations.	Docusate increases systemic absorption of mineral oil and danthron. Enteric coated medications such as docusate must be taken whole for correct absorption. Do not split, crush. chew, or alter. Of little value in a prophylactic bowel management program for long-term constipation. Appropriate for short-term use when straining is to be avoided.	Daily use of docusate sodium and oxyphenisatin acetate for more than 8 months may produce chronic active liver disease, including jaundice.
		Stimulant laxatives	
Diphenylmethanes Phenothalein Bisacodyl	Act directly on the colon to stimulate motility via local irritation and stimulation of intramural nerve plexus. Onset Diphenylmethanes 6–10h PO 15–60 min rectally	Often the mainstay of a prophylactic bowel management program for opioid-induced constipation. May cause cramping.	Avoid bisacodyl within 1h of using antacids, milk, or cimetidine (tablet dissolves prematurely). Phenothalein and bisacodyl are not effective in the presence of biliary obstruction (must be excreted in the bile to be effective). Avoid bisacodyl with actual or suspected ulcerative lesions of the colon.
		Anthraquinones	
Senna products Casanthrol Cascara Danthron	Activated by bacterial degradation in the intestines. Onset Anthraquinones 6–12h PO May require up to 24h 15–60 min rectally	Prolonged use results in loss of normal bowel function and dependence. Some products may tint urine pink or red.	Avoid use in intestinal obstruction, Chrohn's disease, colitis, and abdominal pain of unknown origin, and children under 12 years old.
		Suppositories	
Glycerin Bisacodyl Senna Phenothalein	Stimulate intestinal plexus and cause rectal emptying due to local irritation. Glycerin exerts an osmotic effect. Onset is within 15 min to 1 h.	Suppositories must be placed between the rectal mucosa and the stool to be effective. If placed in stool, suppository will not dissolve properly. Rectal irritation may occur with repeated use.	Rectal manipulation, including the use of suppositories and enemas, is contraindicated in individuals with neutropenia, thrombocytopenia, or rectal fissures.

increase in bulk. The colon stretches to initiate receptors that increase peristalsis.

Stimulant laxatives act directly on the colon to degrade bacteria that stimulate intestinal motility. A common stimulant laxative recommended for use in people receiving opioids is senna. Senna, in combination with a stool-softening agent given at the same time the patient receives an opioid, is effective in reducing opioid-induced constipation.[96]

Suppositories stimulate the intestinal nerve plexus to induce evacuation of stool from the rectal vault. These agents are potentially useful as a second step when oral laxatives are ineffective, but are not useful in long-term bowel management due to their induction of tolerance, or when the patient is constipated or experiencing obstipation.

Enemas are useful to cleanse the bowel after removal of impaction but are not useful for long-term bowel management. The composition of the enema fluid determines the mechanism of action. Tap water and normal saline increase fluid volume and bulk in the colon. Vegetable oils and lubricants lubricate and soften stool. Soap is an irritant that stimulates peristalsis. The disadvantage of enemas is that they cleanse only the distal colon and do not prevent recurrent constipation. Enemas and suppositories in individuals with neutropenia or thrombocytopenia are generally contraindicated, due to increased risk of injury, bleeding, and perirectal abscesses secondary to rectal manipulation.

When constipation is apparent, and after appropriate assessments, stool softener and laxative doses are titrated with the goal of one nonforced bowel movement at a minimum of every two days.[83,84] Recommendations to treat persistent constipation include adding another agent—magnesium hydroxide (30–60 mL daily), bisacodyl (2–3 oral tablets or 1 rectal suppository daily), lactulose (30–60 mL daily), sorbitol (30 mL every 2–3 hours and then as needed), magnesium citrate (8 oz orally daily), or PEG (1 capful in 8 oz water orally two times daily).[83,84] Fleet, saline, or tap water enemas are included among the interventions for persistent constipation.[83,84] A prokinetic agent (metoclopramide 10–20 mg orally four times daily) can be considered, but long-term use of such products is limited by the potential for neurologic complications.[84]

Oral naloxone can reverse opioid-induced constipation, but in doing so, is likely to reverse the analgesic effect of the opioid. A naloxone protocol typically begins with 4 mg oral naloxone daily, with titration to a maximum dose of 12 mg.[57,81] Dosing intervals of 6 hours or longer are suggested if multiple daily doses are required. For patients taking morphine, the dose of naloxone may also be calculated as 20% of the 24-hour morphine dose.[55] Close monitoring of patients on a naloxone protocol is essential to avoid opioid withdrawal.[56] Dose reduction or an increased interval of naloxone dosing seems to prevent this complication.[56] Oral naloxone is an expensive alternative to other medications used to manage constipation.

Most recently, methylnaltrexone (0.15 mg/kg subcutaneously, maximum one dose per day) has been suggested to relieve opioid-induced constipation that is resistant to laxative therapy.[97] Use of methylnaltrexone (MNTX) represents an important milestone in the management of constipation; it is an evidence-based, effective, and mechanism-based therapy.[97–99] MNTX reduces side effects in an agonist–antagonist combination.[98,99] Because of its inability to cross the blood–brain barrier, MNTX exerts peripheral inhibition of opioid-related effects but does not influence opioid-induced central effects; thus the analgesic effect of opioids is not affected.[98,99] Preliminary data from clinical trials suggest that MNTX could have pharmacoeconomic advantages, and could offer additional clinical benefits including improved gastric emptying, relief of nausea and vomiting, and reduced risks of regurgitation and pulmonary aspiration.[97]

NURSING IMPLICATIONS

Nursing care of the person at risk for or with actual changes in bowel elimination—that is, constipation—should be guided by empirical evidence. While a growing body of evidence is available to guide many aspects of clinical practice and patient care, there is a paucity of such guidance relating to constipation. Yet, quality of life among both patients and caregivers[17,66] continues to be affected by this distressing, painful, sometimes life-threatening, though mostly preventable symptom of cancer and adverse effect of cancer treatment, supportive care, and palliative care.[17,61,62,65] Data are beginning to demonstrate financial costs, above and beyond the costs of pain and suffering, linked to unplanned emergency department visits[100,101] and treatment and management of constipation.[102,103] A retrospective analysis of costs of managing constipation among 58 patients receiving palliative care in England found the mean cost of such care to be slightly more than $48 (£29.81) per admission and staff time accounted for 85% of the costs. Staff discussion about bowel management occurred once or twice daily and involved as many as eight staff members at a time.[102] These authors concluded that earlier and more effective intervention could have both clinical and economic benefits.[102]

Another retrospective study analyzed insurance claims of more than 1 million individuals throughout Brazil—3% of Brazil's insured population—who received opioid therapy over a 35-month period in 2007.[103] The analysis compared the costs associated with opioid-treated patients with and without constipation, including both patients with cancer pain and those with noncancer-related chronic pain conditions. The average monthly cost for opioid-induced constipation was 787.84 BRL (approximately $388). Twenty-seven percent of cancer patients receiving opioids had constipation-related claims and higher average costs than noncancer patients. The findings from this study suggest that patients with opioid-induced constipation, but particularly those with cancer, produce a higher economic burden compared to patients who do not have constipation, indicating that reducing opioid-induced constipation could lead to cost savings at the healthcare system level.[103]

Multidisciplinary documentation must reflect elimination patterns, effects of therapy on elimination, and progress toward the desired outcome of maintaining or reestablishing the patient's normal bowl pattern and habits.

Documentation will include assessment of patients' abilities to comply with recommended interventions. A tool such as the Bowel Activity Diary (Figure 9-2) provides a record of bowel function and can be reviewed by the nurse and patient, and shared with other healthcare providers, so that preventive and management interventions can be planned, initiated, and evaluated.

Effective prevention, correction, and management of constipation affecting people with cancer must move to the imperative level in cancer nursing considerations. There is no viable excuse for this largely preventable symptom—a symptom management concern that that falls squarely within the autonomous domain of nursing—to continue taking its enormous emotional and psychosocial toll on patients, family caregivers, and healthcare professionals, while simultaneously placing an unnecessary but significant economic burden on the healthcare delivery system.

PATIENT SELF-CARE

Appendix 9A provides a self-care guide to help people with cancer prevent and manage constipation. Any person at risk for constipation—or that individual's family and friends enlisted to help in caregiving—can benefit from learning about ways to prevent or manage this very common problem. Learning is most helpful when information begins as the need is first apparent—when the person is identified as being at risk for constipation—and continues throughout treatment and the remainder of that person's life. This guidance is most useful when it is tailored to each patient's needs and changed as the risk of constipation changes. With the nurse's wise guidance, the person with cancer (and his or her caregiver) can take a proactive stance: at the start of any course of treatment and when starting any new medicine, ask the doctor or nurse if a proposed plan for cancer treatment or symptom control can cause constipation. Certain chemotherapy medicines and pain medicines increase the risk of developing constipation. If cancer treatment and the prescribed pain control medicines are known to increase the risk of developing constipation, follow-up questions can cover simple measures to prevent this problem.

A good bowel management program will include active and passive exercise, plenty of fluids, foods that are high in fiber content, a comfortable and private toileting routine, complementary modalities such as massage to stimulate peristalsis, and use of stool softeners and laxatives to ease movement of stool through the bowel. The record provided by use of the bowel activity diary offers a way for individuals at risk for constipation, and their caregivers, to become aware of subtle changes in bowel function before serious constipation occurs. Any bowel care program will work best when the doctor, nurse, and nutritionist or dietician work with the patient and caregiver to create a plan that is unique to the needs and lifestyle of each individual patient.

REFERENCES

1. National Digestive Diseases Information Clearinghouse (NDDIC). Constipation. http://digestive.niddk.nih.gov/ddiseases/pubs/constipation. Accessed May 25, 2012.
2. Dunlop GM. A study of the relative frequency and importance of gastrointestinal symptoms and weakness in patients with far advanced cancer: student paper. *Palliat Med.* 1990;4(1):37–43.
3. Frohman IP. Constipation. *Am J Nurs.* 1955;55(1):65–67.
4. University of Indiana. Egyptia: Ebers Papyrus. www.indiana.edu/~ancmed/egypt.htm. Accessed May 28, 2012.
5. Williams KW. Massage for constipation. *Am J Nurs.* 1901;1(10):708–714.
6. Olsen EV, Thompson LF, McCarthy J, et al. Immobility: effects on gastrointestinal function. *Am J Nurs.* 1967;67(4):785–787.
7. Economou DC. Bowel management: constipation, diarrhea, obstruction, and ascites. In: Ferrell BR, Coyle N, eds. *Oxford Textbook of Palliative Nursing.* 3rd ed. New York: Oxford University Press; 2010:269–290.
8. Larkin PJ, Sykes NP, Centeno C, et al. The European Consensus Group on Constipation in Palliative Care. The management of constipation in palliative care: clinical practice recommendations. *Palliat Med.* 2012;22(7);796–807.
9. White KM, O'Sullivan A, eds. *The Essential Guide to Nursing Practice: Applying ANA's Scope and Standards in Practice and Education.* Silver Spring, MD: American Nurses Association; 2012.
10. Higgins PD, Johanson JF. Epidemiology of constipation in North America: a systematic review. *Am J Gastroenterol.* 2004;99:750–759.
11. McCrea GL, Miaskowski C, Stotts NA, Macera L, Varma MG. A review of the literature on gender and age differences in the prevalence and characteristics of constipation in North America. *J Pain Symptom Manage.* 2009;37(4);737–745.
12. Blackmer AB, Farrington EA. Constipation in the pediatric patient: an overview and pharmacologic considerations. *J Pediatr Health Care.* 2010;24(6):385–399.
13. van den Berg MM, Benninga MA, Di Lorenzo C. Epidemiology of childhood constipation: a systematic review. *Am J Gastroenterol.* 2006;101(10):2401–2409.
14. Bekkali, N, van den Berg M, Dijkgraaf M, et al. Rectal fecal impaction treatment in childhood constipation: enemas versus high doses of oral PEG. *Pediatrics.* 2009;124(6):e1108–e1114.
15. Abi-Hanna A, Lake A. Constipation and encopresis in childhood. *Pediatr Rev.* 1998;19(3):23–31.
16. Cimprich B. Symptom management: constipation. *Cancer Nurs.* 1985;8(suppl 1):39–42.
17. Wright PS, Thomas SL. Constipation and diarrhea: the neglected symptoms. *Semin Oncol Nurs.* 1995;11(4):289–297.
18. Plaisance L, Ellis JA. Opioid-induced constipation: management is necessary but prevention is better. *Am J Nurs.* 2002;102:72–73.
19. Sykes NP. The pathogenesis of constipation. *J Support Oncol.* 2006;4:213–218.
20. Eaton LH, Tipton JM, eds. *Putting Evidence into Practice: Improving Oncology Patient Outcomes.* Pittsburgh, PA: Oncology Nursing Society; 2009:85–92.
21. Walsh D, Rybicki L. Symptom clustering in advanced cancer. *Support Care Cancer.* 2006;14:831–836.
22. Esper P. Symptom clusters in individuals living with advanced cancer. *Semin Oncol Nurs.* 2010;26(3):168–174.
23. Zucca AC, Boyes AW, Linden W, Girgis A. All's well that ends well? Quality of life and physical symptom clusters in long-term cancer survivors across cancer types. *J Pain Symptom Manage.* 2012;43(4):720–731.

24. Kumar NB. Dysfunction of the bowel/constipation. In: Kumar NB. *Nutritional Management of Cancer Treatment Effects.* Berlin/Heidelberg: Springer-Verlag; 2012:221–244.
25. Loening-Baucke V. Constipation as a cause of acute abdominal pain in children. *J Pediatr.* 2007;151:666–669.
26. Reynolds SL, Jaffe DM. Diagnosing abdominal pain in a pediatric emergency department. *Pediatr Emerg Care.* 1992;8:126–128.
27. Camilleri M, Murray JA. Diarrhea and constipation. In: Longo DL, Fauci AS, Kasper DL, Hauser SL, Jameson JL, Loscalzo J, eds. *Harrison's Principles of Internal Medicine.* 18th ed. New York: McGraw-Hill; 2012, 308–319.
28. Grundy D, Al-Chaer ED, Aziz Q, et al. Fundamentals of neurogastroenterology: basic science. *Gastroenterology.* 2006;130:1391–1411.
29. Sykes NP. Methods of assessment of bowel function in patients with advanced cancer. *Palliat Med.* 1990;4:287–292.
30. Sanders KM. A case for interstitial cells of Cajal as pacemakers and mediators of neurotransmission in the gastrointestinal tract. *Gastroenterology.* 1996;111:492–515.
31. Deepak P, Ehrenpreis ED. Constipation. *Dis Mon.* 2011;57:511–517.
32. Tally NJ, Jones M, Nuyts G, et al. Risk factors for chronic constipation based on a general practice sample. *Am J Gastroenterol.* 2003;98:1107–1111.
33. Bisanz AK, Woolery MJ, Eaton LH. Constipation. In: Eaton LH, Tipton JM, eds. *Putting Evidence into Practice.* Pittsburgh, PA: Oncology Nursing Society; 2009:93–104.
34. Lichtman SM, Balducci L, Aapro M. Geriatric oncology: a field coming of age. *J Clin Oncol.* 2007; 25(14):1821–1823.
35. Lichtman SM, Brain E. The International Society of Geriatric Oncology Conference: Paris 2011. *Aging Health.* 2012;8(2):123–126.
36. Gomes OA, deSouza RR, Liberti EA. A preliminary investigation of the effects of aging on the nerve cell number in the myenteric ganglia of the human colon. *Gerontology.* 1997;43:210–217.
37. Asher R. The dangers of going to bed. *Br Med J.* 1947;2:967–968.
38. Holdstock DJ, Misiewicz JJ, Smith T, Rowlands EN. Propulsion (mass movements) in the human colon and its relationship to meals and somatic activity. *Gut.* 1970;11:91–99.
39. Cordain L, Latin RW, Behnke JJ. The effects of an aerobic running program on bowel transit time. *J Sports Med Phys Fitness.* 1986;26:101–104.
40. Massey RL. A randomized trial of rocking-chair motion on the effect of postoperative ileus duration in patients with cancer recovering from abdominal surgery. *Appl Nurs Res.* 2010;23:59–64.
41. Waud SP. Fecal impaction due to a hygroscopic gum laxative. *Am J Dig Dis.* 1940;7(7):297–298.
42. Schiff D. Spinal cord compression. *Neuro Clin North Am.* 2003;21:67–86.
43. Winge K, Rasmussen D, Werdelin LM. Constipation in neurological diseases. *J Neurol Neurosurg Psychiatry.* 2003;74:13–19.
44. Walsh D, Nelson KA. Autonomic nervous system dysfunction in advanced cancer. *Support Care Cancer.* 2002;10:523–528.
45. Ahmed MN, Carpenter S. Autonomic neuropathy and carcinoma of the lung. *Can Med Assoc J.* 1975;113:410–412.
46. Sorhaug S, Steinshamn SL, Waldum HL. Octreotide treatment for paraneoplastic intestinal pseudo-obstruction complicating SCLC. *Lung Cancer.* 2005;48:137–140.
47. Hertz R, Lippett MB, Moy RH. Effect of vincaleukoblastine on metastatic choriocarcinoma and reticular trophoblastic tumors in women. *Cancer Res.* 1960;20:1050–1053.
48. Bleehen NM, Jelliffe AM. Vinblastine sulphate in the treatment of malignant disease. *Br J Cancer.* 1965;19:268–273.
49. Bradley WG. Side effects of vinca alkaloids. (letter). *BMJ.* 1968;3(5609):58.
50. Smith B. The myenteric plexus in drug-induced neuropathy. *J Neurol Neurosurg Psychiatry.* 1967;30(6):506–510.
51. Faller BA, Pandit TN. Safety and efficacy of vinorelbine in the treatment of non small cell lung cancer. *Clin Med Insights: Oncol.* 2011;5:131–144.
52. Knapp K, Cooper B, Koetters T, et al. Trajectories and predictors of symptom occurrence, severity, and distress in prostate cancer patients undergoing radiation therapy. *J Pain Symptom Manage.* 2012;44(4):486–507.
53. Roszak A, Wareńczak-Flforczak Z, Bratos K, Milecki P. Incidence of radiation toxicity in cervical cancer and endometrial cancer patients treated with radiotherapy alone versus adjuvant radiotherapy. *Rep Prac Oncol Radiother.* 2012; 17(6):332–338..
54. Robbins MA, Gosselin TK. Symptom management in radiation oncology: acute and long-term side effects. *Am J Nurs.* 2002;102(suppl 4):32–36.
55. Trescot AM, Datta S, Lee M, Hanson H. Opioid pharmacology. *Pain Physician.* 2008:11(2 suppl):133–153.
56. Camilleri M. Opioid-induced constipation: challenges and therapeutic opportunities. *Am J Gastroenterol.* 2011;106:835–842.
57. Strassels SA, Maxwell TL, Iyer S. Constipation in persons receiving hospice care. *J Pain Symptom Manage.* 2010;40(6):810–820.
58. Panchal SJ, Müller-Schwefe P, Wurzelmann JI. Opioid-induced bowel dysfunction: prevalence, pathophysiology and burden. *Int J Clin Pract.* 2007;61(7):1181–1187.
59. Twycross RG, Lack SA. *Symptom Control in Far Advanced Cancer: Pain Relief.* London: Pittman; 1983.
60. Drossman DA. Rome III: the new criteria. *Chin J Dig Dis.* 2006;7:181–185.
61. Ferreira KASL, Kimura M, Teixeira MJ, et al. Impact of cancer-related symptom synergisms on health-related quality of life and performance status. *J Pain Symptom Manage.* 2008;35(6):604–616.
62. Stark LL, Tofthagen C, Visovsky C, McMillan SC. The symptom experience of patients with cancer. *J Hosp Palliat Nurs.* 2012;14(1):61–70.
63. McMillan SC, Williams FA. Validity and reliability of the Constipation Assessment Scale. *Cancer Nurs.* 1989;12(3):183–188.
64. Richmond JP, Wright ME. Establishing reliability and validity of a constipation risk assessment scale. *J Ortho Nurs.* 2008;12:139–150.
65. McMillan SC, Small BJ, Weitzner M, et al. Impact of coping skills intervention with family caregivers of hospice patients with cancer: a randomized clinical trial. *Cancer.* 2006;106(1):214–222.
66. Valeberg BT, Grov EK. Symptoms in the cancer patient: of importance for their caregivers' quality of life and mental health? *Eur J Oncol Nurs.* 2013;17(1):46–51.
67. Nourissat A, Vasson MP, Merrouche Y, et al. Relationship between nutritional status and quality of life in patients with cancer. *Eur J Cancer.* 2008;44:1238–1242.
68. Kwon G, Ryu E, Noh GO, Sung YH. Health-related quality of life in cancer patients between baseline and a three-year follow-up. *Eur J Oncol Nurs.* 2012;16:131–136.
69. Strassels SA, Maxwell TL, Iyer S. Constipation in persons receiving hospice care. *J Pain Symptom Manage.* 2010;40(6):810–820.
70. McMillan SC, Small BJ, Haley, WE. Improving hospice outcomes through systematic assessment. *Cancer Nurs.* 2011;34(2):89–97.
71. McMillan SC, Moody LE. Hospice patient and caregiver congruence in reporting patients' symptom intensity. *Cancer Nurs.* 2003;26(2):113–118.
72. Rhondali W, Nguyen L, Palmer L, Kang D-H, Hui D, Bruera E. Self-reported constipation in patients with advanced cancer: a preliminary report. *J Pain Symptom Manage.* 2012 epub ahead of print.
73. Cirillo M, Venturini M, Ciccarelli L, Coati F, Bortolami O, Verlato G. Clinician versus nurse symptom reporting using the National Cancer Institute—Common Terminology Criteria for Adverse Events during chemotherapy: results of a comparison based on patient's self-reported questionnaire. *Ann Oncol.* 2009;20:1929–1935.
74. Jakobsson S, Ekman T, Ahlberg K. Components that influence assessment and management of cancer-related symptoms: an interdisciplinary perspective. *Oncol Nurs Forum.* 2008;35(4):691–698.
75. Rao SSC, Meduri K. What is necessary to diagnose constipation? *Best Pract Res Clin Gastroenterol.* 2011;25:127–140.

76. Nagaviroj K, Yong WC, Fassbender K, Zhu G, Oneschuk D. Comparison of the Constipation Assessment Scale and plain abdominal radiography in the assessment of constipation in advanced cancer patients. *J Pain Symptom Manage.* 2011;42(2):222–228.
77. Lawrentschuk N, Bolton DM. Experience and attitudes of final-year medical students to digital rectal examination. *Med J Aust.* 2004;181: 323–325.
78. Turner KJ, Brewster SF. Rectal examination and urethral catheterization by medical students and house officers: taught but not used. *Am J Gastroenterol.* 2000;86:422–426.
79. Wong RK, Drossman DA, Bharucha AE, et al. T1029 the utility of the Digital Rectal Exam (DRE) amongst physicians and students: a multicenter study. *Am J Gastroenterol.* 2010;138:S472.
80. U.S. Department of Health and Human Services. Common terminology criteria for adverse events (CTCAE) version 4.0. May 28, 2009. (v. 4.02: September 15, 2009). http://www.acrin.org/Portals/0/Administration/Regulatory/CTCAE_4.02_2009-09-15_QuickReference_5x7.pdf. Accessed August 5, 2012.
81. Librach SL, Bouvette M, De Angelis C, et al. Consensus recommendations for the management of constipation in patients with advanced progressive illness. *J Pain Symptom Manage.* 2010;40(5): 761–773.
82. Engelking C. Diarrhea and constipation. In: Gates RA, Fink RM, eds. *Oncology Nursing Secrets.* 3rd ed. Philadelphia, PA: Mosby; 2008: 372–397.
83. National Comprehensive Cancer Network. NCCN guidelines version 1.2012. Adult cancer pain. 2012. www.nccn.org/professionals/physician_gls/pdf/pain.pdf. Accessed August 7, 2012.
84. National Comprehensive Cancer Network. NCCN guidelines version 1.2012. Palliative care. 2012. www.nccn.org/professionals/physician_gls/pdf/palliative.pdf. Accessed September 23, 2012.
85. Chapman AQ. Massage: its physiological effects. *Am J Nurs.* 1915;15(8):635–639.
86. Billhult A, Dahlberg K. A meaningful relief from suffering: experiences of massage in cancer care. *Cancer Nurs.* 2001;24(3):180–184.
87. Fellowes D, Barnes K, Wilkinson S. Aromatherapy and massage for symptom relief in patients with cancer. *Cochrane Database Syst Rev.* 2004;3:CD002287.
88. Lai TKT, Cheung MC, Lo CK, et al. Effectiveness of aroma massage on advanced cancer patients with constipation: a pilot study. *Comp Ther Clin Pract.* 2011;17:37–43.
89. Sinclair M. The use of abdominal massage to treat chronic constipation. *J Bodywork Movement Therapies.* 2011;15:436–445.
90. Belsey JD, Geraint M, Dixon TA. Systematic review and meta analysis: polyethylene glycol in adults with non-organic constipation. *Int J Clin Pract.* 2010;64(7):944–955.
91. Bennett M, Cresswell H. Factors influencing constipation in advanced cancer patients: a prospective study of opioid dose, dantron dose and physical functioning. *Palliat Med.* 2003;17(5):418–422.
92. Becker G, Galandi D, Blum HE. Peripherally acting opioid antagonists in the treatment of opiate-related constipation: a systematic review. *J Pain Symptom Manage.* 2007;34(5):547–565.
93. Leppert W. The role of opioid receptor antagonists in the treatment of opioid-induced constipation: a review. *Adv Ther.* 2010;27(10): 714–730.
94. Powell M, Rigby D. Management of bowel dysfunction: evacuation difficulties. *Nurs Stand.* 2000;14(47):47–54.
95. Winney J. Constipation. *Nurs Stand.* 1998;13(11):49–53, 55–56.
96. Twycross R, Sykes N, Mihalyo M, Wilcock DM. Stimulant laxatives and opioid-induced constipation. *J Pain Symptom Manage.* 2012;43(2);306–313.
97. Thomas J, Karver S, Cooney GA, et al. Methylnaltrexone for opioid-induced constipation in advanced illness. *N Engl J Med.* 2008;358:2332–2343.
98. Gatti A, Sabato AF. Management of opioid-induced constipation in cancer patients: focus on methylnaltrexone. *Clin Drug Invest.* 2012;32(5):293–301.
99. Berde C, Nurko S. Opioid side effects: mechanism-based therapy. *N Engl J Med.* 2008;358(22):2400–2402.
100. Livingston PM, Craike M, Considine J. Unplanned presentations to emergency departments due to chemotherapy induced complications: opportunities for improving service delivery. *Australasian Emerg Nurs J.* 2011;14:62–68.
101. Pirie J. Management of constipation in the emergency department. *Clin Pediatr Emerg Med.* 2010;11(3):182–188.
102. Wee B, Adams A, Thompson K, Percival F, Burslem K, Jobanputra M. How much does it cost a specialist palliative care unit to manage constipation in patients receiving opioid therapy? *J Pain Symptom Manage.* 2010;39(4):644–654.
103. Takemoto MLS, Fernandes RA, Almeida GR, Monteiro RDC, Colombini-Neto M, Bertola-Neto A. Health care resource use and costs in opioid-treated patients with and without constipation in Brazil. *Value in Health.* 2011;14:S78–S81.

Prevention of Constipation

Patient Name: ______________________________

Symptom and Description

Constipation are stools that are too hard, too small, too difficult to expel, and not regular. This means being unable to move your bowels as you normally would. If you are passing dry or hard stool, passing small amounts of stool, having to push harder to move your bowels, or moving them less often than usual, you may be suffering from constipation.

You are at risk for constipation if you:

- Have a decrease in the amount you eat and drink each day
- Have a decrease in your activity or exercise
- Take medicines that cause constipation
- Resist the urge to pass stool
- Try to pass stool on a bedpan rather than get up to the toilet
- Are taking pain medications
- Are receiving chemotherapy

Keeping your bowel routine regular and your bowel movements easy to pass is important. Your bowels should move as they normally did before you got sick with little or no strain. Your physician or nurse may ask you to keep a diary of your bowel activity. This diary will ask you to describe the frequency, amount, and type of stool you pass or when the last time it was that you were able to pass a stool.

What can you do to prevent constipation?

Prevention

You can help prevent constipation if you:

- Do not resist the urge to pass stool
- Sit in an upright position when passing stool
- If possible, sit on the toilet or bedside toilet
- Drink at least 8–10 glasses of fluid each day
- Have a warm or hot drink (senna tea) 30 minutes before usual bedtime
- Eat foods that are high in dietary fiber, at least 20–35 grams per day, especially whole grains, fruits, vegetables, legumes, seeds, and nuts
- Exercise daily (if you are unable to increase your exercise, tighten and relax the muscles in your abdomen and move your legs often while sitting or in bed)
- Take medications as instructed to prevent constipation

(continued)

- Try to move your bowels at your usual times (many people find that after breakfast is a good time to try to have a bowel movement)
- Tell your doctor or nurse about things that have worked for you in the past to prevent constipation

Tips on increasing fiber in your diet:

- Eat fiber rich beans as the primary source of protein in a meal once or twice a week
- Eat five fruits or vegetables each day
- Eat 2–3 servings of whole grains
- Choose high fiber cereals and snacks that identify whole grains as one of the first ingredients
- Read food labels to determine fiber content
- Select whole fresh and dried fruits rather than juices

Examples of types of fiber:

- Grains: brown rice, corn bread, whole wheat grains, wheat bran cereals, barley, oat bran, oatmeal, soybean fibers
- Nuts/seeds: almonds, sesame seeds, sunflower seeds, peanuts, pecans, walnuts
- Fruits/vegetables: apples, bananas, berries, broccoli, cherries, green peppers, pears, red cabbage, spinach, sprouts

Examples of natural or home preparations to promote regular bowel function include:

- Option #1 Fiber Pudding

  1 part bran
  2 parts prune juice
  3 parts applesauce

Mix all ingredients together, bran with 1⁄8 to 1⁄4 cup (30 to 60 ml), one to two times daily. Increase or decrease as needed to regulate bowel function.

- Option #2 Senna Tea

  1 ounce (28 g) of senna leaves
  1 quart (approximately 1 liter) water

Boil senna leaves gently in water. Strain off leaves and drink as tea as needed to regulate bowel function.

Management

You can treat mild constipation by following the steps just listed in prevention. When your bowels have not moved or if you are at risk for severe constipation, you will need to use medications to help your bowels move regularly.

1. *Using medications to prevent constipation.* Preventing and managing constipation are easy when you work together with your healthcare provider. You may need to increase or decrease doses of medicine to achieve easy and regular bowel movements. Please follow these directions carefully, and feel free to call to ask questions or to let us know if your bowels are not regular.
2. *Goal.* To have a bowel movement as you did prior to your being sick. You should:
   - Increase level of exercise as tolerated
   - Drink at least 8–10 glasses of fluids per day (preferably water)
   - Eat as much fiber in your diet as you can tolerate but attempt to eat at least 20–35 grams per day

- Never resist the urge to pass stool and do so on the toilet
- Take medications as ordered by your doctor
- Take laxative at bedtime.
- If you do not have a bowel movement in the morning, take another laxative dose after breakfast.
- If you do not have a bowel movement by evening, take another laxative dose at bedtime.
- If you do not have a bowel movement by the following morning, take a laxative dose after breakfast.

3. If your bowels have not moved in 48 hours, call your doctor or nurse.
4. Once you begin to have regular bowel movements, use the morning and evening doses of medicines you were taking when you had a bowel movement as your regular dose.
5. If you are unsure of what to do, please call your doctor or nurse.

Follow-Up

If you are having trouble with your bowel movements, call your doctor or nurse. Be ready to tell them the following:

1. When you last had a bowel movement (Bowel Activity Diary can help you recall)
   - Was it normal in size, color, and firmness?
   - Was it difficult to pass?
   - Have you had diarrhea?
2. The amount and kinds of fluid and food you are eating and drinking
3. The names and amounts of medicine you are taking for your bowels
4. Any changes in your health
5. Any new medications or treatments since your last visit
6. What you are doing to manage your bowels on your own

It is important to call your doctor or nurse if your pain medications are increased, so your bowel management plan can be checked.

If you need help in learning about foods that help prevent constipation, call the nutritionist.

Phone Numbers

Doctor: ______________________________

Nurse: ______________________________

Physician: ______________________________

Nutritionist: ______________________________

Comments

Source: Haylock PJ, Curtiss C, Massey RL. Constipation. In: Yarbro CH, Wujcik D, Gobel BH, eds. *Cancer Symptom Management*. 4th ed. Burlington, MA: Jones & Bartlett Learning; 2014.

Chapter 10

Diarrhea

Paula M. Muehlbauer, RN, MSN, AOCNS®
Rachael Christine Lopez, MPH, RD, CSO

THE PROBLEM

Diarrhea is not only highly prevalent among patients undergoing cancer treatment but is also debilitating and can be life threatening if left untreated.[1] Though it is not a disease itself, diarrhea is both a sign, or objective measure that can be identified during medical professionals' assessments, and a symptom, or subjective measure identified by the patient, indicative of a change in the patient's clinical status. Because of the prevalence of diarrhea in the oncology population, as well as the potential negative impact on treatment course and/or patients' clinical status, oncology nurses must be familiar with and attentive to the identification, assessment, and management of diarrhea.

Though a universal definition of diarrhea does not exist, many sources define diarrhea using the National Cancer Institute's Common Terminology Criteria for Adverse Events (CTCAE v 4.03), which classifies diarrhea by the increase in number of stools per day over baseline. For the purpose of this review, diarrhea is defined as an abnormal increase in both the liquidity and the frequency of stools. This definition is used to capture a broader array of the signs and symptoms of diarrhea, beyond those captured in the CTCAE criteria. However, the CTCAE criteria will be referenced throughout this review when referring to the grade of diarrhea. See Table 10-1 for a description of the CTCAE criteria.[2]

In addition to the increase in number of stools per day, diarrhea is further classified by the length of time it persists (i.e., acute or chronic) as well as by its severity. Acute diarrhea resolves within 14 days. Diarrhea persisting longer than 14 days is classified as chronic diarrhea. The severity of diarrhea is most commonly assessed using the CTCAE criteria in addition to accompanying signs and symptoms. The signs and symptoms indicating severe or complicated diarrhea, as described by an expert multidisciplinary panel of oncology and gastrointestinal (GI) specialists, are listed in Table 10-2.[3]

TABLE 10-1

National Cancer Institute Common Terminology Criteria for Adverse Events (CTCAE): Diarrhea[a,b]

Grade	Description
1	Increase of <4 stools/day over baseline; mild increase in ostomy output compared to baseline
2	Increase of 4–6 stools/day over baseline; moderate increase in ostomy output compared to baseline
3	Increase of ≥7 stools/day over baseline; incontinence; hospitalization indicated; severe increase in ostomy output compared to baseline; limiting self-care ADL
4	Life-threatening consequences; urgent intervention indicated
5	Death

Source: Data from National Cancer Institute Common Terminology Criteria for Adverse Events (CTCAE)[2].

Abbreviation: ADL: activities of daily living.

[a]*Definition: A disorder characterized by frequent and watery bowel movements.*

[b]*Self-care ADL refers to bathing, dressing and undressing, feeding self, using the toilet, taking medications, and not bedridden.*

TABLE 10-2

Assessing the Severity of Diarrhea

Severity of Diarrhea*	
Classification	**Criteria**
Uncomplicated diarrhea	Common Toxicity Criteria grades 1–2 with no complicating signs or symptoms
Complicated diarrhea	Common Toxicity Criteria grades 3–4 OR grades 1–2 with one or more of the following signs or symptoms: 1. Abdominal cramping 2. Nausea/vomiting (CTCAE grade 2–5) 3. Decreased performance status 4. Fever 5. Sepsis 6. Neutropenia 7. Frank bleeding 8. Dehydration

Source: Data from Benson et al[3].

*(Note: the grades refer to the National Cancer Institute's Common Terminology Criteria for Adverse Events (CTCAE) as outlined in Table 1.)

As indicated in Tables 10-1 and 10-2, the magnitude of diarrhea can vary significantly, ranging from very mild to severe, debilitating, and even life threatening. Complicated diarrhea can be life threatening due to the loss of fluids and electrolytes, resulting in dehydration, renal insufficiency, electrolyte imbalances and subsequent cardiovascular morbidities, and/or infectious complications leading to sepsis in immunocompromised patients.[3] Patients incontinent of stool are also at risk of impaired skin integrity and pressure ulcer formation.[4,5]

Because of the myriad of complications, diarrhea can also cause delays or cessation in cancer treatment, which ultimately impacts the disease course.[6,7] For example, in a retrospective study of 100 patients with colorectal cancer, 22% of patients required a dose reduction, 8% of patients required a dose delay, 15% of patients had to discontinue treatment, and 11% of patients had to change treatment regimens due to chemotherapy-induced diarrhea.[7,8] Patients may receive suboptimal treatment when dose reductions are necessary.[6]

Not surprisingly, diarrhea can also have a profound impact on patients' quality of life.[3,7] Acute diarrhea can lead to electrolyte and fluid losses, causing fatigue, weakness, and lethargy; chronic diarrhea can cause significant fatigue, malnutrition, changes in skin integrity, sleep disturbances, discomfort, and anxiety leading to social isolation.[9] Furthermore, persistent diarrhea affects activities of daily living, limits patients' ability to travel outside the home or clinical setting, decreases sexual activity, decreases work attendance, alters self-image, and increases caregiver burden.[7]

INCIDENCE AND ETIOLOGY

The etiology and incidence of diarrhea vary according to location of disease, treatment modality, treatment course, and use of medications. Though a full discussion of the incidence of diarrhea by each possible cause is beyond the scope of this chapter, the following text provides a summary discussion of the myriad of factors that can cause diarrhea in the oncology population. Table 10-3 provides a summary of the factors that may result in diarrhea in the oncology population.[10–12]

Incidence of diarrhea by diagnosis

Diagnoses with a higher incidence of diarrhea include pancreatic adenocarcinomas,[7] carcinoid tumors,[10] vasoactive intestinal protein-secreting tumors (VIPomas),[5] small intestinal lymphomas,[13] medullary carcinoma of the thyroid,[10] pheochromocytoma,[10] colon cancer,[10] and other gastrointestinal cancers. See Tables 10-3 and 10-4[14] for information on the cancer diagnoses most likely to cause diarrhea, as well as the characteristics and underlying physiological mechanisms causing diarrhea.

Incidence of diarrhea by treatment modality

Diarrhea has long been recognized as a side effect of many cancer treatments. Treatment modalities that are most likely to cause diarrhea are discussed next.

Chemotherapy. Chemotherapy causes damage to both cancer cells and to normal, rapidly dividing intestinal crypt cells. As a result, the epithelial lining of the GI tract is susceptible to damage from chemotherapy, thus disrupting the normal fluid balance. Fluid reabsorption into the body from the GI tract decreases, and fluid and electrolyte secretion into stool increases, resulting in watery bowel movements that can lead to life-threatening conditions.[6,15]

Chemotherapy-induced diarrhea is reported in 50%–80% of patients, with more than 30% experiencing grade 3 to grade 5 diarrhea per the CTCAE criteria.[3] A grade 5 classification is given if death is the result from diarrhea complications. The incidence of diarrhea increases with the use of specific chemotherapy regimens, including fluorouracil (5-FU) and irinotecan.[3] Table 10-3 lists specific chemotherapy agents most likely to cause diarrhea.

Radiation therapy. Radiation-induced diarrhea results when radiotherapy to the abdomen or pelvis damages intestinal mucosa. When the intestinal mucosa is damaged, the intestinal villi are denuded, which decreases the absorptive surface area. Mucosal ulcerations may also be present and can inhibit digestion by decreasing absorptive surfaces, causing intestinal perforation, fistulae, or abscesses, and/or causing the intestinal wall to narrow or obstruct as

TABLE 10-3

Summary of Possible Factors Contributing to Diarrhea in the Oncology Population

Cancer-related	Carcinoid syndrome
	Colon cancer
	Lymphoma
	Medullary carcinoma of the thyroid
	Pancreatic cancer, particularly islet cell tumors (Zollinger-Ellison syndrome)
	Pheochromocytoma
Surgery- or procedure-related	Celiac plexus block
	Cholecystectomy, esophagogastrectomy
	Gastrectomy, pancreaticoduodenectomy (Whipple procedure)
	Intestinal resection (malabsorption due to short bowel syndrome)
	Vagotomy
Chemotherapy-related	Capecitabine, cisplatin, cytosine arabinoside, cyclophosphamide, daunorubicin, docetaxel, doxorubicin, 5-fluorouracil, irinotecan, leucovorin, methotrexate, oxaliplatin, paclitaxel, topotecan
Biological and Targeted Related Therapy	Interleukin-2, interferon alpha, ipilumumab, lapatinib, erlotinib, gefitinib, sorafenib, sunitinib, imatinib, bortezomib, everolimus, sirolimus, pertuzumab.
	Note: This list provides an example of agents and is not comprehensive. It is recommended that the reader check for diarrhea as a side effect as new agents become Food and Drug Administration (FDA) approved.
Radiation therapy–related	Irradiation to the abdomen, para-aortics, lumbar, and pelvis
Bone marrow transplantation–related	Conditioning chemotherapy, total-body irradiation, graft-versus-host disease after allogeneic bone marrow or peripheral blood stem cell transplants
Drug adverse effects	Antibiotics, magnesium-containing antacids, antihypertensives, colchicine, digoxin, iron, lactulose, laxatives, methyldopa, metoclopramide, misoprostol, potassium supplements, propranolol, theophylline
Concurrent disease	Diabetes, hyperthyroidism, inflammatory bowel disease (Crohn's disease, diverticulitis, gastroenteritis, HIV/AIDS, ulcerative colitis), obstruction (tumor-related)
Infection	Clostridium difficile, Clostridium perfringens, Bacillus cereus, Giardia lamblia, Cryptosporidium, Salmonella, Shigella, Campylobacter, Rotavirus
Fecal impaction	Constipation leading to obstruction
Diet-related	Alcohol, milk, and dairy products (particularly in patients with lactose intolerance)
	Caffeine-containing products (coffee, tea, chocolate); specific fruit juices (prune juice, unfiltered apple juice, sauerkraut juice)
	High-fiber foods (raw fruits and vegetables, nuts, seeds, whole-grain products, dried legumes); high-fat foods (deep-fried foods, high fat–containing foods)
	Lactose intolerance or food allergies
	Sorbitol-containing foods (candy and chewing gum); hot and spicy foods; gas-forming foods and beverages (cruciferous vegetables, dried legumes, melons, carbonated beverages)
Psychological factors	Stress

Source: Data from National Cancer Institute[10]; Stein et al[11]; Cherny[12].

ulcers harden. This damage induces prostaglandin release and bile salt malabsorption, leading to increased intestinal peristalsis and, therefore, diarrhea.[12,15] The decrease in the reabsorptive surface can also impair absorption of fat, carbohydrate, protein, bile salt, and vitamin B_{12}, leading to loss of water, electrolytes, and protein in the small intestine, resulting in malabsorptive diarrhea.[16]

Radiation to the abdominal or pelvic region causes diarrhea in approximately 50% of patients, with increased incidence noted among patients receiving concurrent chemotherapy.[3] Diarrhea usually peaks 1–2 weeks after initiation of radiation.[1] Radiation-induced diarrhea is classified as acute radiation enteritis if it occurs within 6 weeks of therapy; acute radiation enteritis usually resolves without

TABLE 10-4

Types of Diarrhea and Causative Factors that Occur in the Oncology Population

Type of Diarrhea	Characteristics	Underlying Mechanism	Common Causes
Secretory	Large volume of watery stools; output not alleviated by fasting; stools may appear greenish	Overstimulation of intestines, leading to increased secretion of fluids and electrolytes. Secretion of water into the intestinal lumen exceeds absorptive capacity and results in diarrhea.	• Endocrine tumors • Bacterial infections (e.g., cholera) • Graft-versus-host disease • Short gut syndrome has a secretory component • Unabsorbed bile acids in the colon
Exudative	Increase in the frequency of stools; variable volume	Disturbed intestinal epithelium, allowing excess mucus, serum, protein, or blood into the GI tract, causing inflammation	• Pelvic irradiation • Inflammatory bowel disease • Gastrointestinal (GI) tumors • Compromised gut integrity
Osmotic	Large volume of watery stools; symptoms alleviated when individual fasts or stops consuming the poorly absorbed solute	Excessive solute load in intestinal lumen draws fluid into the lumen. High flux of fluid and electrolytes entering intestinal lumen results in impaired absorption of fluids and watery diarrhea.	• Intake of poorly absorbed solutes such as carbohydrate (e.g., lactose-when there is a deficiency of lactase in the brush border) • Sorbitol containing products (e.g., candies, gum, mints) • Hyperosmolar enteral formula • Use of magnesium containing laxative products
Dysmotility	Increase in frequency and volume of stools	Hyper-peristaltic activity causing substances and fluids to move rapidly through the gut	• Fecal impaction • Peristaltic stimulants • Irritable Bowel Syndrome • Damaged vagus nerve • Bowel resection
Chemotherapy or biological therapy or targeted therapy induced	Frequent watery and semisolid stools occurring 24–96 hours after treatment	Sloughing of epithelial mucosa causing superficial ulceration and inflammation to the bowel	Most common include: capecitabine, cisplatin, cytosine arabinoside, cyclophosphamide, daunorubicin, docetaxel, doxorubicin, 5-fluorouracil, interferon, irinotecan, leucovorin, methotrexate, oxaliplatin, paclitaxel, topotecan, lapatinib, interleukin-2, erlotinib, sorafenib, sunitinib, imatinib, bortezomib, ipilumumab ***Note:*** This list is not comprehensive.
Malabsorptive	Large volume of foul-smelling stool that may be accompanied by cramping, bloating, gas, and weight loss; stool may appear yellowish, oily, and float in the toilet; if bile is not entering the small bowel, movements may be gray or white	Incomplete digestion and/or absorption of macronutrients results in a high flux of hyperosmolar substances entering the colon	• Gastroinestinal resection (e.g. resection resulting in short gut syndrome, or Whipple surgery resulting in exocrine pancreatic insufficiency) • Exocrine pancreatic insufficiency • Intake of high fat diet when lipolysis is defective or a biliary obstruction prevents bile from reaching gut • Certain medications • Radiation enteritis

Source: Reprinted with permission from: 2010 Oncology Nutrition Connection, Oncology Nutrition, a dietetic practice group of the Academy of Nutrition and Dietetics[14].

specific therapy within 2–6 months. Chronic radiation enteritis, though less common, appears and persists months to years after the initial exposure.[12] Fecal incontinence (FI) has been reported to occur in as many as 53% of cancer survivors treated with pelvic radiation therapy.[17]

Hematopoietic stem cell transplantation. Diarrhea is a common side effect following hematopoietic stem cell transplantation (HSCT), primarily due to acute graft-versus-host-disease (GVHD). The exact mechanism remains uncertain, but the following three conditions must be present to generate GVHD: (1) the introduction of immunologically competent T cells with the graft; (2) a host that has antigenic differences to the graft, which therefore stimulates donor T cells; and (3) a host immune system response that is insufficient to completely reject the graft.[18] The development of GVHD is known to correlate with the severity of diarrhea during the conditioning regimen as well as with the serum levels of many inflammatory cytokines released during the conditioning regimen and early-phase post-transplantation.[18,19] Of note, the conditioning regimen prior to the HSCT involves chemotherapy and/or radiation therapy, so it causes diarrhea via the mechanisms mentioned in the preceding discussion.

Acute GVHD occurs in approximately 20%–50% of HLA-matched sibling transplants, and in as many as 60%–80% of HLA-mismatched sibling transplants or transplants from unrelated donors; 50% of cases of acute GVHD will have GI involvement, manifested as diarrhea.[18] Based on the number of transplants and the ratio of related to unrelated donor transplants, these percentages translate to a predicted 5500 cases of grade II–IV acute GVHD per year.[20]

Targeted therapy and biotherapy. Diarrhea is a frequent side effect among patients treated with some tyrosine kinase inhibitor (TKI) drugs, specifically those directed against the epidermal growth factor receptor (EGFR), such as erlotinib and gefitinib. Onset is about 3 weeks after the start of treatment. Diarrhea occurs less frequently with monoclonal antibodies directed against EGFR, such as cetuximab and panitumumab. The cause of diarrhea with use of these agents is not completely understood. EGFR signaling pathways are tightly controlled in normal cells, including intestinal mucosa. In contrast, these pathways are unregulated in some cancers such as colorectal cancer, causing a proliferation of tumor cells, tumor metastasis, and increased angiogenesis. Inflamed mucosa has increased levels of EGFR, especially in goblet cells, which appear to factor into the initiation of chemotherapy-induced diarrhea.[21,22]

Tyrosine kinase inhibitors that target multiple signaling pathways including EGFR, tyrosine kinase signaling pathways, apoptosis, and angiogenesis cause diarrhea in 30%–50% of patients, with severe diarrhea occurring less than 10% of the time.[11] Examples of multikinase targeted therapies include sorafenib and sunitinib. An additional potential reason for diarrhea caused by these agents is the high expression of the protein tyrosine kinase Kit in the interstitial cells of Cajal. The Cajal cells function as electrical pacemakers in the intestine, affecting intestinal motility or peristalsis. Another targeted therapy, imatinib, which inhibits the Bcr-Abl protein tyrosine kinase, is associated with a 30% occurrence rate of diarrhea, although severe diarrhea is uncommon.[11]

Inhibitors of the mammalian target of rapamycin (m-TOR) include everolimis and temsirolimus, which are used to treat renal cell carcinoma. Diarrhea occurs in as many as 40% of patients receiving everolimis, but the rate of severe diarrhea is less than 5%.[11]

The incidence of diarrhea during treatment with anti-EGFR agents ranges from 21% to 72% depending on the treatment agent and whether it is combined with other treatment modalities.[21] Further research is needed to fully understand diarrhea using targeted therapies and appropriate treatment strategies.[11]

Diarrhea also occurs with some biologic agents such as aldesleukin, more commonly referred to as interleukin-2 (IL-2). Diarrhea incidence related to IL-2 is 67% for all grades, but less than 2% for grade 4.[23,24] Incidence of grade 3 and 4 diarrhea has declined as clinical management has improved. The etiology of IL-2–induced diarrhea is not clearly understood and the onset varies, but it is recognized that diarrhea can occur either within 24 hours after the start of therapy or later in the treatment cycle.[23–25]

The biologic agent ipilumumab is a monoclonal antibody that interferes with anti-cytotoxic T-lymphocyte–associated antigen 4. Diarrhea due to ipilumumab can be significant and could lead to immune-related colitis. Beck et al.[26] identified three separate mechanisms with histopathologic evidence of enterocolitis: neutrophilic alone (46%), lymphocytic inflammation (38%), and combined neutrophilic and lymphocytic inflammation (38%). Pathology showed that neutrophilic inflammation was distinguished by cryptitis and crypt cell abscesses in 33% of cases. Eosinophils were prominent in crypts, especially when lymphocytic inflammation was present.

The prescribing information for ipilumumab states that diarrhea of all grades occurs in as many as 37% of people receiving this drug. Colitis is reported among 8% of all patients receiving this drug. Median time to the development of moderate or severe enterocolitis is reported to be 6–7 weeks.[27]

Surgical resection. Gastrointestinal surgery can also cause diarrhea, but the incidence of diarrhea following gastrointestinal surgery varies significantly, depending on the amount and location of intestinal resection. Resection of more than 100 centimeters of ileum is likely to cause diarrhea due to impaired reabsorption of bile acids and/or a resultant disaccharidase deficiency, causing carbohydrate malabsorption and osmotic diarrhea.[5] Extensive resection of the small intestine leads to inadequate functional bowel to support nutrient and fluid absorption, which is termed short bowel syndrome (SBS) or short gut syndrome; it also results in diarrhea. Of note, any resection leading to inadequate functional bowel can be referred to as SBS, but SBS is also more specifically defined as a small intestinal length of 100–120 centimeters without a colon, or 50 centimeters of small intestine with a colon.[13] The mechanisms causing SBS-associated diarrhea include the following: changes in GI motility, increased gastric secretions, hyperosmotic content within the intestinal lumen from fatty acids, deconjugated bile salts and carbohydrates, bacterial overgrowth, lactose intolerance, and fatty acid irritation of the colon.[28] Resection of the colon is also likely to result in diarrhea due to the reduction in the water absorption capacity of the colon, which is not fully compensated for by the small intestine.[5]

Patients who have undergone a Whipple procedure (pancreaticoduodenectomy) or a partial or total gastrectomy with Roux-en-Y reconstruction may develop bacterial overgrowth in the efferent loop, leading to diarrhea secondary to malabsorption.[5] Patients who have undergone a Whipple procedure or a partial or total gastrectomy are also at risk of diarrhea due to dumping syndrome, with an estimated 25%–50% of gastric surgery patients experiencing symptoms of this syndrome. Dumping syndrome is attributed to (1) the alteration of gastrointestinal anatomy, resulting in a reduced gastric reservoir; (2) the removal or bypass of the pylorus; and (3) the interference with gastric innervations and gastrointestinal hormone secretion. Due to the reduced reservoir and faster pyloric emptying, osmotically active solids and liquids are rapidly delivered to the small intestine, provoking fluid shifts into the intestinal lumen, which stimulates bowel contractility and distention, resulting in urgent, liquid stools.[29]

Surgical alteration of the GI tract can also cause diarrhea due to dysfunctional intestinal motility. This is often categorized as dysmotility-associated diarrhea. Dysmotility-associated diarrhea may either slow GI transit time, which allows for small bowel bacterial overgrowth and subsequent diarrhea, or accelerate GI transit time, which reduces enteral absorption and subsequently leads to diarrhea.[7]

Additional causes of diarrhea following surgical resection of the intestine include disruption of the mucosal membrane and changes in digestive enzyme production. The latter leads to malabsorption and the release of osmotically active substances into the bowel lumen, which then draws fluid into the lumen, resulting in large volume, liquid stools.[7]

Additional causes of diarrhea

An additional cause of diarrhea in the oncology population is colonization with infectious agents. *Clostridium difficile* is the most common cause of infectious diarrhea in hospitalized patients.[1,30] The incidence of *C. difficile*–associated diarrhea (CDAD) among oncology patients is partly attributable to their frequency of hospitalization, as *C. difficile* is one of the most common nosocomial pathogens.[30,31] In addition, oncology patients receiving chemotherapy have an increased risk of contracting CDAD.[32]

In addition to hospitalization and immunosuppression, risk factors for CDAD include use of antibiotics, repeated enemas, prolonged nasogastric tube insertion, bowel surgery, and any form of suppression of the normal GI flora, including the use of chemotherapy.[1,12] Patients receiving chemotherapy are at a higher risk of CDAD even without antibiotic therapy.[33] Once a patient is infected with *C. difficile*, the risk of relapse is 10%–25% for all patients; relapses are usually attributable to the failure to eradicate the organism during the initial treatment regimen.[1]

Diarrhea can also occur as a side effect of many medications that are required during cancer treatment. Categories of medications known to induce diarrhea include, but are not limited to, the following: magnesium-containing medications, phosphate-containing medications, antihypertensives, nonsteroidal anti-inflammatory agents, antibiotics, theophyllines, antiarrhythmics, liquid medications containing sorbitol, lactulose, and prokinetic agents.[34] As noted earlier, the use of antibiotics also increases the risk of CDAD. A summary of medications that increase the risk of diarrhea can be found in Table 10-3.

PATHOPHYSIOLOGY

Diarrhea is identified by its underlying cause; many times, there is more than one contributing mechanism. In normal digestion, the small intestine and colon absorb 99% of fluid from oral secretions and intake daily, which is roughly equal to 9–10 liters. A small reduction (1%) of intestinal absorption or an increase in gastrointestinal secretions may be enough to cause diarrhea.[35] The discussion in this section reviews how aberrations in normal digestion can cause diarrhea. Mechanisms include osmotic, secretory, exudative, and motility disorders. Table 10-4 provides a summary of these mechanisms along with underlying causes common in the oncology population.[14]

Osmotic diarrhea is the result of increased intake or decreased absorption of water-soluble solutes that remain in the bowel and retain water. Substances such as mannitol, sorbitol, lactulose, and magnesium salts found in antacids and laxatives pull water across the mucosa, resulting in diarrhea. Osmotic diarrhea resolves during periods of fasting, or when the aggravating agent is discontinued.[6,15,35]

Secretory diarrhea occurs when secretions of fluid and electrolytes into the intestinal lumen exceed what can be absorbed. Causes include infections, malabsorption syndromes, surgery such as ileal resection, and drugs.

Endocrine tumors—including vasoactive intestinal peptide tumors (VIPomas), medullary carcinoma of the thyroid, and carcinoid tumors—secrete hormones, which also cause secretory diarrhea. Characteristics of secretory diarrhea include large stool volumes, lack of red or white blood cells in the stool, and fever or systemic symptoms. Secretory diarrhea persists despite lack of food or fluid intake.[6,15,35]

Exudative diarrhea is a consequence of direct damage to the small or large intestinal mucosa. Epithelial damage leads to leakage of excessive mucus, serum protein, blood, and fluids into the bowel. Once the intestinal barrier of the epithelium is damaged, hydrostatic pressure in the blood and lymphatic system causes water, electrolytes, mucus, and protein to amass in the intestinal lumen. This type of diarrhea is seen with some bacterial infections, such as *Salmonella*, and with inflammatory disorders of the gut such as Crohn's disease and ulcerative colitis. Other causes include chemotherapy-induced and radiation-induced enteritis.[6,15] Motility disorders may reduce intestinal transit time, thereby reducing absorption and increasing stool volume. As previously mentioned, conditions related to increased transit time include small and large bowel resection or bypass, gastric resection, and inflammatory bowel disease. Other causative factors include medications that may stimulate intestinal smooth muscle, magnesium-containing antacids, laxatives, and selective serotonin reuptake inhibitors. Decreased motility disorders stimulate bacterial overgrowth and induce bile acid deconjugation, resulting in diarrhea. Mucosal damage and fat malabsorption may also cause diarrhea.[6,35]

SYMPTOM ASSESSMENT

RISK FACTORS

Patients with any of the risk factors discussed in the preceding sections should be monitored for the onset of diarrhea. Geriatric patients must be educated about and assessed for additional risk factors. These patients may be taking noncancer drugs that can cause diarrhea, such as digitalis, beta blockers such as propranolol, angiotensin-converting enzyme inhibitors, and oral hypoglycemic agents. Elderly patients are more susceptible to fecal impaction, which can cause diarrhea. The older adult patient may also present with leakage of mucus or fecal matter due to rectal irritation or impaired anal sensation.[36,37]

Fecal incontinence has been reported in specific populations, including long-term gynecological cancer survivors who underwent pelvic radiation therapy and patients with diarrhea from GVHD.[17,38] Other risk factors for FI include increasing age, obesity, neurologic conditions, and injuries to the perineal area. FI causes stress and embarrassment in those persons experiencing it and, therefore, is an underreported symptom.[17,38–40]

The following section discusses self-assessment tools for patients to utilize as well as the healthcare professional's assessment of diarrhea.

SELF-ASSESSMENT

Patients must be educated on the signs and symptoms of diarrhea, the signs and symptoms of dehydration, and the consequences of untreated diarrhea, because vigilant and timely management of diarrhea can significantly improve treatment course and outcome, as well as decrease the negative impact on patients' quality of life. Patients at risk of or already experiencing diarrhea should be encouraged to keep a log or diary indicating the number of daily stools, the volume of liquid stools, the time of day of defecation, the presence of fecal incontinence, sensations or alterations in the perianal area, intake of known diarrhea stimulants, dietary intake, fluid intake, herbal or supplement practices, and medication use, with specific attention to laxative or bowel regimen use. Patients with ongoing diarrhea should weigh themselves daily, as daily weight fluctuations are an indicator of fluid imbalance. Any febrile episodes, orthostatic changes in heart rate, dizziness, abdominal cramps, presence of bloody stool, or excessive thirst should also be reported.[36] Appendix 10A provides a sample diary for the patient.

Older adults become dehydrated quickly and may present with lethargy, delirium, or weakness. Dehydration can quickly lead to electrolyte imbalances, especially hypokalemia with dysrhythmias, which need to be assessed in the context of both hydration status and medication use, particularly in cases where patients are also taking cardiac medications. The elderly adult patient needs to be treated promptly when severe diarrhea persists for 24 hours or more or if the patient has a history of dehydration and electrolyte imbalance.[36]

OBJECTIVE ASSESSMENT

The history and physical assessment includes both subjective and objective data. It consists of a detailed medical history, history of recent travel, diet history, medication review (including antibiotic use within 3 months), normal bowel habits, current stool description (color, consistency, smell, and frequency), duration and severity of diarrhea, and presence of additional GI symptoms such as cramping or pain. Fecal incontinence can occur with diarrhea, and patients should be asked about its presence—especially patients at high risk of diarrhea, as fecal incontinence can lead to incontinence-associated dermatitis causing perineal skin breakdown.[17,38–40]

The directed questions found in Table 10-5 may be helpful to the clinician when obtaining a history for the person presenting with diarrhea. To assist patients in identifying characteristics of their stools or changes in stool consistency, the Bristol Stool Chart (Figure 10-1) provides a visual reference that helps to more accurately describe stool quality and consistency.[3,12,14,35] Liquid stool should be measured by volume if possible, and the frequency of bowel movements must be noted. As discussed previously, the most common tool used to assess diarrhea is the National Cancer Institute's Common Terminology Criteria for Adverse Events (CTCAE), Version 4.03, found in Table 10-1.[2]

The physical assessment must include an evaluation for the signs and symptoms of dehydration, which are outlined in Table 10-6, as well as abdominal and rectal abnormalities. Findings that indicate a serious etiology of diarrhea include blood or pus, fever, signs of dehydration, chronic diarrhea, and unintentional weight loss. Patients with diarrhea that requires repetitive cleaning should be examined for perineal breakdown or peristomal breakdown. Assessment includes risk factors for perineal breakdown—the form of diarrhea (i.e., increased risk with liquid versus soft but formed stool), the duration of time skin is exposed to diarrhea, the appearance of skin (i.e., increased risk for denuded or eroded skin, with dermatitis, or erythema), and the presence of other contributing factors such as low albumin, *C. difficile* infection, and antibiotic use.[4,36] Abdominal assessment must include evaluation for distention, auscultation of bowel sounds, and palpation for tenderness.[41,42]

TABLE 10-5

Medical History: Diarrhea Assessment Questions

Category	Questions
Previous Health History	• History of sensitive gastrointestinal (GI) tract or irritable/inflammatory bowel syndrome? • Previous bowel resection? Segment of bowel? Length or extent? With or without diversion? Reason for surgery? • Current medications including over-the-counter and herbal supplements? Recent changes to medications? • Recent history of antibiotic use? • Are family members or housemates currently experiencing diarrhea? • Recent travel outside the United States?
Bowel Pattern (usual and current)	• What is your usual bowel pattern (number of stools per day or week)? • What is your current bowel pattern? • Describe the stools (Formed? Semisolid? Soft? Liquid?) • Do any symptoms accompany the diarrhea (e.g., bloating, cramps, fever, flatus, nocturnal stooling, etc)? • Are you experiencing any fecal incontinence? • What aggravates and alleviates your diarrhea? • What do you use at home to manage your diarrhea? Do you take special home remedies? Are you using any of these now? If so, how often?
History of Cancer	• Diagnosis? This includes specific type of tumor, duration, and association of malignancy with hormonal hypersecretion. Does this type of cancer interfere with bowel function or enzyme production? • What is your extent of disease?
Prescribed Antineoplastic Regimen	• Receiving chemotherapy, biologic or targeted therapies? If so, what agents, the dose and regimen? • What is your previous experience with chemotherapy? • Receiving radiation therapy now or in the past? Was it abdominal or pelvic? • Is therapy multimodal? • Have you had a stem cell transplant or total body irradiation?
Planned Supportive Care Interventions	• Is anticipated neutropenia significant enough to put patient at risk for opportunistic infection, *Clostridium difficile* or other? • Is antibiotic therapy anticipated? • Will any diarrhea-producing supportive medications be ordered (e.g. Mesna, metoclopramide?) • Are enteral supplements or parenteral nutrition anticipated?

Source: Data from Engelking[41].

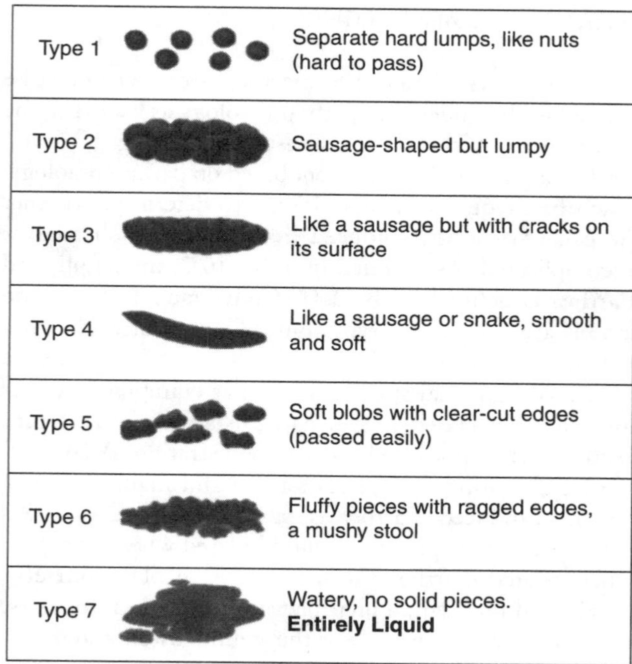

FIGURE 10-1

Bristol stool chart.

Source: Data from Conlon[14]. Reprinted with permission.

When evaluating cancer treatment–induced diarrhea of uncertain etiology, clinicians should also include an evaluation of dietary intake to identify foods or fluids that may be contributing to or exacerbating diarrhea.[3,7,45] A registered dietitian (RD) should be consulted to assist with the evaluation and to provide counseling for the management of symptoms.

In addition to the history and physical assessment and diet evaluation, further clinical work-up may be required, depending on the clinical course of the patient. Supplementary evaluation tools may include, but are not limited to, the following: (1) stool analysis to evaluate for fecal leukocytes or infectious causes such as *C. difficile, Salmonella*, and *E. coli*; (2) blood analysis for complete blood count and electrolyte abnormalities suggestive of dehydration or renal impairment; (3) abdominal radiographic imaging studies to evaluate for gastrointestinal obstruction or fecal impaction[5]; (4) endoscopy and/or colonoscopy with biopsy to evaluate for gastrointestinal abnormalities, inflammation, GVHD, or other etiology[46]; (5) endocrine evaluation for abnormal hormone secretion if there is suspicion of a vasoactive intestinal protein-secreting tumor or other neuroendocrine tumor; and (6) absorption studies to evaluate for pancreatic exocrine insufficiency, intestinal villous atrophy, or other malabsorptive etiology.[47]

TABLE 10-6

Signs and Symptoms of Dehydration

System	Symptom
General	• Sunken eyeballs • Unintentional weight loss • Fever • Malnutrition • Increased thirst (may not always be present in older people)
Integumentary	• Poor skin turgor • Skin may be cool and clammy • Pallor • Dry mucous membranes • Cracked lips and/or tongue, licking of lips • Saliva may be thick, and viscous • Perianal irritation
Neurologic	• Lethargy • Headache • Confusion • Change in mentation • Dizziness • Lightheadedness
Respiratory	• Rapid, shallow breathing
Circulation	• Rapid, weak and thread pulse • Delayed capillary refill (>3 seconds) • Decreased blood pressure or orthostatic blood pressure changes • Elevated blood urea
Elimination	• Decreased urine output • Dark, concentrated and/or foul smelling urine • Imbalanced intake and output

Source: Data from Richardson and Dobish[6]; Schmelzer[42]; Kornblau et al[43]; Welch[44].

SYMPTOM MANAGEMENT STRATEGIES

Strict monitoring of diarrhea toxicity should be applied to all cancer treatment regimens but particularly to those treatments known to have a high incidence of diarrhea. Strict monitoring is also indicated for any patient receiving cancer therapy who has a history of developing diarrhea with prior treatments. The healthcare provider needs to be aware of any bowel surgery and subsequent sequelae as outlined in the previous section. Patients should be closely observed during the first cycle of chemotherapy as well as in the 48–72 hours before the next cycle of chemotherapy.[41] Lab work, including an electrolyte panel and complete blood cell count with differential, should be obtained to watch for electrolyte imbalances and/or neutropenia.[3]

All patients and caregivers need to understand when diarrhea is most likely to occur, which will vary according to the treatment agent. The oncology nurse should provide information specific to each patient's treatment plan. For example, patients receiving irinotecan-based chemotherapy experience early-onset diarrhea that can occur during administration and late-onset diarrhea that may occur 5–11 days after dosing. It is imperative that these patients and their families are able to identify and report diarrhea, and that the diarrhea is managed aggressively.[3,6] Therefore, patients and caregivers must be educated on the appropriate medication regimen for the treatment of diarrhea. Patients should be instructed not to mix over-the-counter antidiarrheal agents, as this can further aggravate the gastrointestinal system, thereby exacerbating concomitant nausea and vomiting.[3,6,36] Additional strategies to manage chemotherapy-based diarrhea are discussed in the symptom management and therapeutic approaches sections of this chapter.

Among patients undergoing colorectal surgery, diarrhea is common in the first 3 weeks postoperatively. Strategies to manage diarrhea during the initial postoperative period include changes in diet and use of antidiarrheal agents. Over time, patients tend to incorporate their own practices, which may include further diet modification, exercise, and alternative therapies. Distress due to diarrhea is greater in patients with more than six stools daily in the initial week after surgery but gradually decreases over time.[48]

People who have undergone sphincter-sparing bowel surgery for colorectal cancer generally report a change in bowel habits 6–24 months postoperatively, and this may continue for years. Nikoletti et al.[49] conducted a study (n = 101) to describe bowel problems, self-care practices, and information needs of patients 6–24 months after recovering from sphincter-sparing bowel surgery. More than 70% of participants reported a change in bowel habits, including incomplete evacuation, excessive flatus, urgency, straining, perianal itchiness or soreness, and bloating. The most common change was increase in frequency of bowel movements, and more than two-thirds stated their stool was soft or liquid. Nearly 40% of patients reported fecal incontinence. Primary self-care practices included a change in diet and taking antidiarrheal medications to manage diarrhea. Other self-care practices included protective pads for fecal leaking, seeking advice from the physician, and, to a lesser degree, the use of complementary and alternative therapies.

Regardless of the cause or risk of diarrhea, the oncology nurse should be knowledgeable about the time frame for expected onset of diarrhea and about the tools and strategies patients can employ to manage the diarrhea. Patients should be reassessed on an ongoing basis for presence, type, and duration of diarrhea as well as for additional risk factors such as dietary intake.

THERAPEUTIC APPROACHES

Due to the myriad causes of diarrhea, treatment must be tailored to the underlying pathophysiology as well as to the specific needs of the patient. Benson and colleagues[3] developed an algorithm for treatment based on pathophysiology, which first requires the practitioner to determine whether the cancer-treatment–induced diarrhea is complicated or uncomplicated. As outlined in Table 10-2, uncomplicated diarrhea is defined by NCI CTCAE grade 1–2 with no complicating signs or symptoms. Complicated diarrhea is defined by NCI CTCAE grade 3–4 or grade 1–2 with additional signs and symptoms such as cramping, nausea/vomiting, decreased performance status, fever, sepsis, neutropenia, frank bleeding, and dehydration. A comprehensive algorithm for the assessment and management of treatment-induced diarrhea is shown in Figure 10-2. An interprofessional approach should be used when managing cancer-related diarrhea, to include the oncology nurse(s), a registered dietitian, a pharmacist, the physician or nurse practitioner, and, if necessary, the wound, ostomy, and continence nurse (WOCN).

Dietary management of diarrhea

Although dietary factors are not usually the primary cause of diarrhea in the oncology population, diet modification can often alleviate or help manage diarrhea symptoms. Per a review of the expert clinical guidelines, and as indicated in the treatment algorithm shown in Figure 10-2, evaluation of dietary intake to identify foods or fluids that may exacerbate diarrhea is one of the first steps in assessing and managing treatment-induced diarrhea. General diet guidelines to promote resolution of diarrhea are also listed in Table 10-7.[3,45,50–52] Specific guidelines for foods to choose and foods to avoid are provided in Appendix 10C. When diet modification is necessary, a registered dietitian (RD) should be consulted to assist the patient in achieving both diet tolerance and nutritional adequacy while remaining sensitive to patients' individual and cultural food preferences. This consideration is especially important in cases of persistent diarrhea, which increase the risk of nutritional deficiencies due to decreased oral intake during treatment and/or illness and due to impaired nutrient absorption with diarrhea, leading to chronic nutrient losses in the stool.

In cases of gastrointestinal GVHD, patients must begin with a period of bowel rest and then transition to oral feedings with diet modification as the GI symptoms resolve. Table 10-8 outlines the diet transition for patients with gastrointestinal GVHD. Due to damage to the GI tract, patients with gastrointestinal GVHD require a period of bowel rest. During bowel rest, nutrition support in the form of parenteral nutrition is recommended to prevent compromised nutrition status. As symptoms begin to resolve, oral

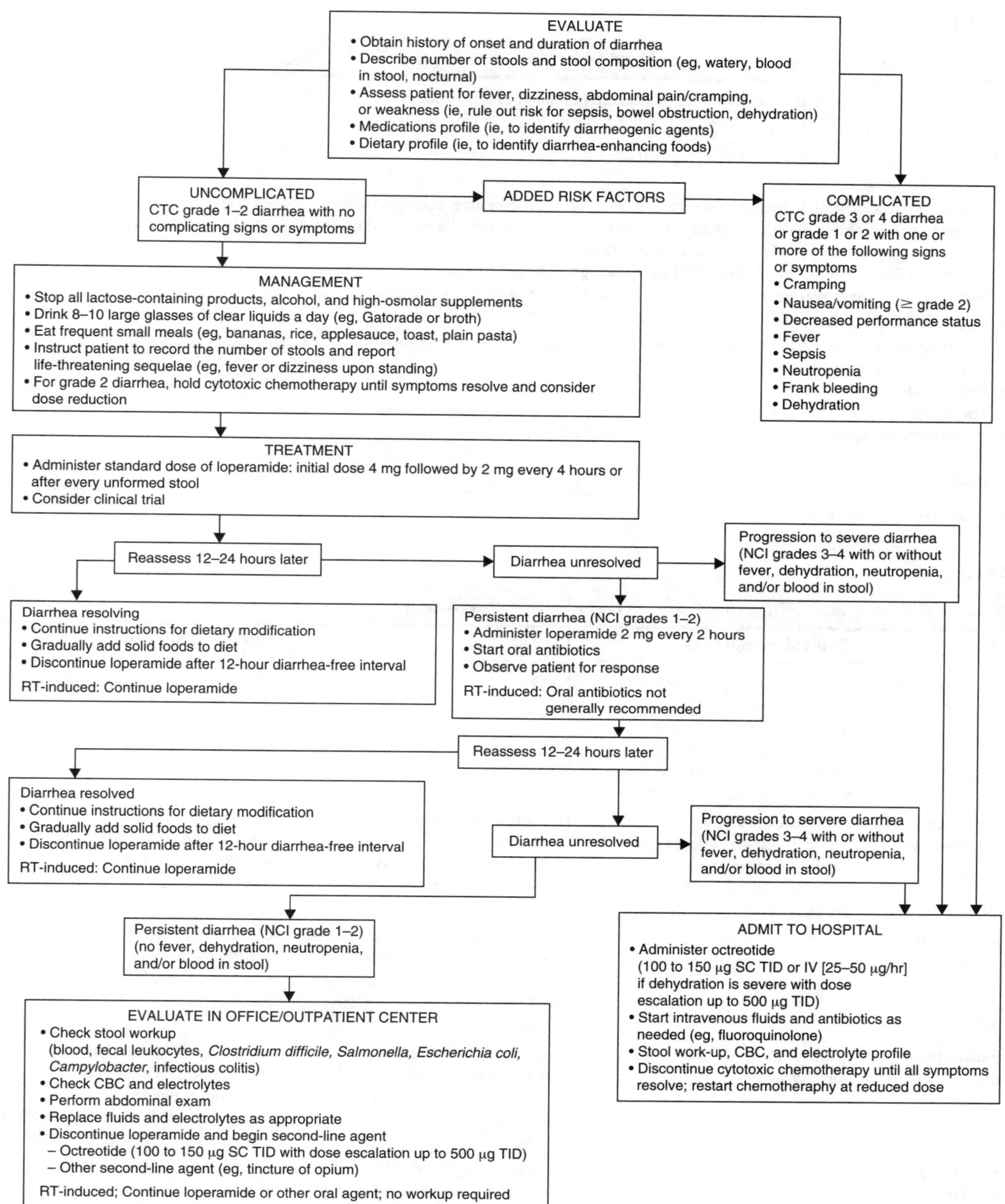

FIGURE 10-2

Proposed algorithm for the assessment and management of treatment-induced diarrhea.

Abbreviations: CTC: Common Toxicity Criteria; NCI: National Cancer Institute; RT: radiotherapy; SC: subcutaneous; tid: three times per day; IV: intravenous; CBC: complete blood count; CID: chemotherapy-induced diarrhea.

Source: Used with permission from Benson et al[3]; Kornblau et al[43].

TABLE 10-7

General Diet Strategies for Treatment-Induced Diarrhea

Increase fluid intake to a minimum of 8 ounces per episode of diarrhea stool; consume at least 8–10 eight-ounce servings of fluid per day

Drink liquids at room temperature

Eat 5–6 small, frequent meals instead of 3 large meals

Choose the following:

- Foods high in soluble fiber (pectin-containing) foods, such as applesauce, oatmeal, bananas, cooked carrots, peeled potatoes, and rice
- Foods low in insoluble fiber, such as rice, noodles, well-cooked eggs, bananas, white toast, canned or cooked fruit without skin, skinned turkey or chicken, fish, and mashed potatoes
- Foods and fluids that replenish electrolytes, including foods high in sodium and potassium, such as commercially prepared broths and soups, bananas, peach nectar, apricot nectar, oranges, and peeled potatoes.

Avoid the following:

- Foods high in insoluble fiber (examples: raw fruit and vegetables, whole grain bread, nuts, popcorn, skins, seeds, legumes)
- Greasy, fried and/or high-fat foods
- Spicy foods
- Foods and beverages that contain lactose (or supplement with lactase enzyme)
- Hyperosmotic liquids (examples: fruit juice, sweetened fruit drinks)
- Caffeinated beverages
- Alcohol

Source: Data from Muehlbauer et al[55].

TABLE 10-8

Gastrointestinal Graft-Versus-Host-Disease (GVHD) Diet Progression

Phase	Clinical Symptoms	Diet	Nutrition Support
1. Bowel rest	GI cramping, large volume of watery diarrhea or active GI bleeding, severely reduced transit time, small-bowel obstruction or diminished bowel sounds, nausea and vomiting	NPO	TPN with multivitamins and minerals, trace elements, supplemental zinc, consideration of copper
2. Introduction of oral feeding	Minimal GI cramping, diarrhea <500 mL/day, guaiac-negative stools, improved transit time (minimum of 1.5 hours), infrequent nausea and vomiting	Isotonic, low residue, low-lactose fluids; initially 60 mL every 2–3 hours for several days with monitoring of tolerance	TPN; Introduction of trophic enteral feeds of semi-elemental formula if patient unable to take fluids by mouth.
3. Introduction of solids	Minimal or no GI cramping; formed stools	Introduction of solid foods every 3–4 hours; minimal lactose, low-fiber, low-fat (20–40 grams/day); avoid high-acid foods, no gastric irritants	Cycle and/or wean TPN; advance enteral feeds if patient unable to take food/fluids by mouth.
4. Expansion of diet	Minimal or no GI cramping; formed stool	Low-lactose, low-fiber, no gastric irritants, avoid high-acid foods. If stool studies indicate fat malabsorption, continue low-fat diet.	Nocturnal TPN if oral intake inadequate or if patient is unable to maintain weight due to malabsorption. Enteral feeding PRN, depending on oral diet tolerance.
5. Resumption of regular diet	No GI cramping, normal stool, normal transit time	Progress to regular diet by introducing one restricted food per day. If no evidence of steatorrhea, fat restriction liberalized slowly.	Discontinue TPN and/or supplemental enteral feeds if patient able to meet nutrient needs via PO intake alone.

Abbreviations: GI: gastrointestinal; NPO: nothing by mouth; PO: orally; PRN: as necessary; TPN: total parenteral nutrition.

Source: © Academy of Nutrition and Dietetics (formerly the American Dietetic Association). Adapted with permission[51].

intake begins with small volumes (60 mL every 2–3 hours) of isotonic, low-lactose, nonfat, clear liquids to minimize osmotic diarrhea. Once the patient tolerates isotonic clear liquids, the diet can be advanced to include easily digested foods. More specifically, the diet should include only low-lactose, low-fiber, low-fat, low-acidity foods and fluids without gastric irritants, before advancing to a regular diet.[51] Nutrition support should be weaned as oral intake increases. Table 10-8 provides specific recommendations based on the trajectory of patients' GI symptoms.

When diarrhea results from surgical resection of the intestine, additional or alternative diet strategies may be required based on the location of the resection, any resulting dysmotility, and complications such as ileus or small bowel obstruction. In the case of short bowel syndrome, the primary goal is to maximize absorption within the remaining gut while providing adequate nutrition, fluid, and electrolytes to maintain lean body mass, support recovery, and promote optimal health status.[28,52] Patients with SBS often require supplementation with intravenous fluids, electrolytes, or total parenteral nutrition (TPN), but the goal is to transition to a full oral diet. The diet considerations for patients with SBS are outlined in Table 10-9. These guidelines aim to increase transit time so as to facilitate maximal absorption within the remaining small bowel. The diet also emphasizes the need for adequate fluids due to the risk of dehydration. It is important to note the specific site and extent of intestinal resection and to identify whether

TABLE 10-9

Diet Considerations for Patients with Short Bowel Syndrome

Management of rapid transit time	Consume at least 6 small meals per day (versus 3 large meals)
	Eat slowly and relax while eating
	Chew foods completely before swallowing
	Avoid fiber supplementation unless stool volume exceeds 3 liters per day; then add 5–10 grams soluble fiber
	Limit fluids with meals; instead, consume fluids between meals to maintain adequate hydration
Management of carbohydrate malabsorption	Avoid concentrated/simple carbohydrates
	Choose complex carbohydrates
	Eat protein at each meal to balance carbohydrate intake
	For patients with a colon: increase complex carbohydrate intake to 50%–60% of total calories
	For patients without a colon: complex carbohydrate intake should be 20%–50% of total calories
	For patients with a colon: may require low lactose fluids if signs of lactose intolerance
Management of fat malabsorption	For patients with a colon: limit fat to 20%–30% of total calories, primarily as essential fats
	For patients without a colon: limit fat to ≤60% of total calories
	If steatorrhea occurs, consider pancreatic enzyme replacement with each meal
	If steatorrhea persists despite pancreatic enzymes, consider very low fat diet and supplementation with medium-chain triglyceride (MCT) oil or MCT-containing supplements
	Monitor and replace fat-soluble vitamins (vitamins A, D, E and K) as needed
	Monitor need for calcium supplementation
Management of protein malabsorption	Consume 20%–30% of calories from protein
Management of dehydration	Consume oral rehydration solutions as needed
	Choose isotonic or hypo-osmolar fluids (instead of hyperosmolar fluids)
	For patients without a colon: may require high-sodium, isotonic, carbohydrate-containing rehydration solutions
Additional considerations	For patients with a colon: limit foods/fluids that contain oxalate to prevent calcium oxalate kidney stones (no oxalate restriction required for patients without a colon)
	Choose foods/fluids that contain sodium and/or add salt at meals
	Limit enteral stimulants such as alcohol and caffeine
	Choose a liquid or chewable multivitamin supplement if necessary

Source: Data from Gottschlich et al[13]; Parrish[28].

the colon remains intact, and then to individualize the diet recommendations accordingly.[52] For example, patients with a colon intact should consume a higher percentage of calories in the form of carbohydrates than patients without a colon, because the colon can ferment a percentage of carbohydrates for energy. An RD should be consulted to assist with patient education and menu planning and to determine whether additional nutrition supplements are needed.

In cases of partial or total gastrectomy, Whipple procedure (pancreatoduodenectomy), or other resection involving manipulation of the stomach or pyloric valve, an anti-dumping syndrome diet may be required. Guidelines to prevent diarrhea due to dumping syndrome are outlined in Table 10-10. This diet also aims to slow transit time to maximize enteral absorption of nutrients. Therefore, patients must avoid simple carbohydrates to prevent osmotic diarrhea, eat small but frequent meals, and separate fluid consumption from consumption of solids. In some cases of gastrectomies, and in the case of a small bowel resection, particularly resection of the jejunum where the lactase enzyme is produced, temporary lactose intolerance may occur and patients may require a low-lactose diet.[13,51] See Table 10-11 for guidelines on a low-lactose diet.

When diarrhea results from *C. difficile* infection, the primary treatment is to discontinue the inciting antibiotic as soon as possible and to begin medical and symptom management of the infection.[53] The patient should continue a regular diet as tolerated, with monitoring of hydration status.

Hydration

Fluid needs are based on the age and activity level of the patient, and must be modified to account for additional variables such as fever, infection, volume of diarrhea, or

TABLE 10-10

Guidelines for Management and Prevention of Diarrhea Secondary to Dumping Syndrome

Management of rapid transit time	Consume at least 6 small meals per day (versus 3 large meals)
	Eat slowly and relax while eating
	Chew foods completely before swallowing
	Limit fluids to ½ cup at meals
	Drink additional fluids at least 30–45 minutes before or after meals
	Remain supine for 30 minutes after meals
	Choose foods high in soluble fiber such as peeled apples, bananas, oatmeal, rice, peeled potatoes
	Consider supplementation with soluble fiber (pectin, gaur gum, etc) to slow GI transit time
Management of carbohydrate malabsorption	Avoid concentrated/simple carbohydrates
	Choose complex carbohydrates
	Eat protein at each meal to balance carbohydrate intake
	For at least two weeks after surgery, dilute juice 1:1 with water
Management of fat malabsorption	Avoid large amounts of dietary fat per meal
	If steatorrhea occurs, limit fat intake to 40–60 grams of fat per day
	If steatorrhea persists, consider pancreatic enzyme replacement with each meal
	If steatorrheal persists despite pancreatic enzymes, consider very low fat diet and supplementation with medium-chain triglyceride (MCT) oil
	Monitor and replace fat-soluble vitamins (vitamins A, D, E and K) as needed
	Monitor need for calcium supplementation
Management of dehydration	For at least two weeks after surgery, choose low-lactose, low osmolality fluids such as juice diluted 1:1 with water and sports drinks
	Limit fluids to ½ cup at meals
	Drink additional fluids at least 30–45 minutes before or after meals.
	Total daily fluid intake should be at least 8 eight-ounce glasses per day; adjust goal as needed per the individual's fluid needs

Source: Data from Conlon[14]; Ukleja[29]; Elliot et al[51].

TABLE 10-11

Diet Guidelines for a Low-Lactose Diet
Limit or avoid non-fermented dairy products such as milk and foods/fluids containing dairy milk
Choose fermented dairy products such as yogurt or buttermilk
Read food labels closely for ingredients containing lactose
Try supplemental lactase enzymes to aid in digestion of lactose
Consider calcium and/or Vitamin D supplementation if unable to tolerate other dietary sources of calcium and Vitamin D

Source: Data from Gottschlich et al[13]; Elliot et al [51].

other causes of increased insensible fluid losses. Maintenance fluid needs per day for adults are as follows:[51]

- Age 16–30 years, active: 40 mL/kg
- Age 31–55 years: 35 mL/kg
- Age 56–75 years: 30 mL/kg
- Age 76+ years: 25 mL/kg

Fluid goals need to be adjusted upward to account for fluid losses—specifically, losses via diarrhea. For most adult patients, minimum fluid needs are approximately 2–3 liters per day. Patients should be instructed on their specific fluid goals. They should also be instructed on the appropriate electrolyte-repleting fluids to choose, such as sports drinks, broths, gelatin, diluted fruit juice (50:50 juice and water), broth, and noncaffeinated drinks. See Table 10-7 and Appendix 10C for additional recommendations regarding appropriate fluids for diarrhea management.

It is essential to educate patients and families on the signs and symptoms of dehydration as listed in Table 10-6. Patients with severe, complicated diarrhea need to receive intravenous hydration to prevent cardiovascular collapse.[3,6,48,54]

Skin care

Detailed skin care is described in the patient self-care guide in Appendix 10D. Meticulous skin care is indicated for people experiencing diarrhea with or without the presence of fecal incontinence. Instruct patients to thoroughly cleanse their perineal area daily and as needed. Mild, nondrying soap and water can be used; in addition, over-the-counter products are available that are designed to maintain the skin's pH balance and not over-dry the skin. Cleansing should be followed with application of a protective barrier cream, ointment, or paste, all of which shield the skin from exposure to irritants and moisture. The active ingredients in skin barriers generally include petrolatum, dimethicone, lanolin, or zinc oxide.[4] Instruct patients to avoid vigorous scrubbing with soap, water, and a washcloth, as this practice may exacerbate skin breakdown and increase the risk of irritation and infection. Some patients find sitting in a warm bath or sitz bath alleviates discomfort. The perianal area should be inspected by the healthcare provider for skin breakdown or signs of infection.[4,6,36] Incontinence increases the risk of pressure ulcer formation; thus skin barriers need to be used to prevent skin irritation from fecal matter. For patients with full-thickness skin breakdown, a prescriptive ointment containing balsam of Peru, castor oil, and trypsin is available.[4,5]

Fecal incontinence

Uncontrolled diarrheal episodes or FI is embarrassing, which can lead to social isolation; thus emotional support for patients with these conditions is indicated. Patient and family education are instrumental in identifying and treating FI. Patients, especially women, experiencing FI tend to restrict what they eat and may skip meals before going out to avoid embarrassment, which can lead to malnutrition, dehydration, or other adverse consequences.[17] Treatment of FI includes diet modifications, antidiarrheal medications, determining warning signals of FI, pelvic floor muscle training, and use of containment products such as pads.

Fecal incontinence is medically managed with the antidiarrheal loperamide, which increases sphincter tone, thereby diminishing FI. Patients may find that using loperamide prophylactically before social occasions decreases the risk of FI in public. Loperamide needs to be taken in sufficient dosages (2–4 mg doses, with a total of 16 mg daily) at least 30 minutes before meals. Other antidiarrheal agents suggested for FI include amitriptyline, which reduces rectal urgency, and diphenoxylate, which prolongs gastrointestinal transit time.[40]

Nurses can help patients determine the warning signals of FI by discussing symptom patterns, which will vary from patient to patient. Urgency along with FI indicates a loose stool or weakness of the external anal sphincter. Patients will state they have a strong urge to defecate and cannot delay more than a couple of minutes. Some patients have no warning signals and may have passive soiling.[39]

Pelvic floor exercises are done by squeezing the muscles adjacent to the anal canal without contracting the abdominal wall and holding for 10 seconds. These exercises are performed alternately in sitting and standing positions multiple times daily. Biofeedback has shown some effectiveness in treating FI once medical management fails, but this technique is used in patients with weak sphincters or impaired rectal sensation.[17,37,39,40]

Providing practical tips, such as the use of incontinence pads in undergarments, gives the patient some control and may reduce embarrassment. Containment pads have a permeable upper layer allowing watery stool to flow through to the absorbent layer underneath without coming into skin contact. For larger volumes of FI, containment underpants may be necessary to avoid pad leakage and contact of fecal matter with the skin.[38] In the geriatric population, assessment for and removal of fecal impaction needs to be performed.[37]

Medications

Many pharmacologic strategies exist for the treatment of diarrhea. This section primarily covers the most common strategies that have the best evidence to support their use according to the Oncology Nursing Society's *Putting Evidence into Practice* guidelines. However, some medications used based primarily on expert opinion are included here as well.[50,55] Benson et al.[3] include medication recommendations in their algorithm for evaluating and managing cancer treatment induced diarrhea, which is shown in Figure 10-2. This algorithm is cited frequently for the management of all cancer treatment related diarrhea.

Chemotherapy-induced diarrhea. A loading dose of 4 mg of loperamide, an oral opiate agonist, followed by 2 mg orally every 4 hours is the standard first-line therapy for chemotherapy-induced diarrhea (CID) in grades 1 and 2 diarrhea.[3,6] High-dose loperamide has shown moderate effectiveness in controlling CID associated with irinotecan. High-dose loperamide consists of 2 mg orally every 2 hours (4 mg every 4 hours at night) or after every unformed stool or until the patient is diarrhea free for 12 hours. Loperamide should not be taken for longer than 48 hours, and the maximum recommended dose of loperamide is 16 mg daily.[3,6,56]

Another agent that has shown good efficacy is octreotide acetate, a somatostatin analog, which is administered subcutaneously at a standard dose of 100–150 micrograms three times daily.[3,57] Octreotide reduces the secretion of some pancreatic and intestinal hormones, thereby increasing the transit time and promoting intestinal reabsorption of fluids and electrolytes. It is recommended for use in complicated diarrhea or diarrhea that is unresolved after using loperamide.[6]

Atropine at a dose of 0.25–1 mg administered IV or subcutaneously has been used as prophylaxis or for treatment of early-onset diarrhea in patients receiving irinotecan. Atropine suppresses the cholinergic effects associated with irinotecan. Its total dose should not exceed 1.2 mg per day, and it is recommended to monitor heart rate and blood pressure during atropine treatment.[6]

Tincture of opium is a widely used antidiarrheal agent and may be a reasonable alternative as second-line therapy for CID. Two preparations are available; because of the difference in their morphine content, care must be taken not to confuse them.[3,6,50] Deodorized tincture of opium, the preferred preparation, contains the equivalent of 10 mg/mL morphine; its recommended dose is 10–15 drops in water every 3–4 hours. Camphorated tincture of opium (paregoric), a less concentrated preparation, contains the equivalent of 0.4 mg/mL morphine; its recommended dose is 1 teaspoon (5 mL) in water every 3–4 hours.[3] These agents should be used with caution, as they can slow GI function to the point where an ileus may form. Tincture of opium should be discontinued if a patient complains of abdominal pain and a work-up should ensue.

Targeted therapy-induced diarrhea. Similar loperamide dosing guidelines for chemotherapy have been used in clinical practice for patients receiving anti-EGFR therapies who experience mild to moderate diarrhea. Patients experiencing more severe diarrhea may need to be hospitalized for fluid and electrolyte replacement. More research is needed to determine the best antidiarrheal medications and optimal dosing to treat diarrhea caused by these newer chemotherapeutic agents.[11,21]

Biotherapy-induced diarrhea. Interleukin-2 is known to trigger significant diarrhea in many patients. Although the etiology is unknown, clinical practice has been to try several different antidiarrheal agents until the desired results are achieved. Loperamide dosing, as described previously for chemotherapy-induced diarrhea, is the first line of treatment for diarrhea.[23] Other agents that have been used include lomotil, codeine, and deodorized tincture of opium. Interleukin-2 is associated with a low incidence of ileus and bowel perforation; however, caution must be exercised when using codeine and deodorized tincture of opium during interleukin-2 treatment.[23,25]

Another immunotherapy agent that causes diarrhea is ipilumumab, an immune-modulating monoclonal antibody that is FDA approved for advanced melanoma. Treatment for mild diarrhea (grade 1–2) includes stopping ipilumumab and initiating loperamide and electrolyte replacement. If grade 2 diarrhea persists for 5–7 days, corticosteroid therapy (e.g., prednisone 0.5 mg/kg daily or equivalent) should be administered.[58,59] Budesonide (9 mg oral daily), which targets the colon, has been used by some practitioners in clinical trials.[58] More severe and prolonged diarrhea requires a work-up using a stool sample to rule out other possible causes including GI infection or inflammatory bowel disease. Colitis should be confirmed or excluded by endoscopy. Bowel perforation or peritonitis needs to be ruled out when patients present with abdominal pain and diarrhea. Opioids may mask symptoms of perforation, so these agents should be used with caution. Ipilumumab is permanently discontinued in patients with grade 3 or 4 diarrhea and high-dose steroids are administered (e.g., methylprednisone 1–2 mg/kg IV daily). Steroids can be tapered over 4 weeks if symptoms improve. Unresolved symptoms after 5–7 days, or a relapse in symptoms after steroid taper, indicate the need for further immunosuppressants. A single dose of infliximab at 5 mg/kg as second-line therapy has been shown to provide resolution of symptoms. Infliximab is contraindicated in the presence of bowel perforation or sepsis. No decrease in ipilumumab effectiveness occurred with the administration of corticosteroids.[26,58,59]

Radiation therapy-induced diarrhea. Current clinical practice guidelines recommend the use of loperamide and diphenoxylate as the standard of practice for patients with mild diarrhea symptoms related to radiation therapy. Mild symptoms are generally classified as grade 1 or 2 with no added risk factors such as cramping, nausea/vomiting, impaired performance status, fever, sepsis, neutropenia, dehydration, or frank bleeding.[3]

Octreotide has also been studied as an intervention for radiation-induced diarrhea. In a study of patients receiving concomitant 5-FU with pelvic radiation therapy for rectal carcinoma, patients with grade 2 or 3 diarrhea who were refractory to loperamide were given 150 mcg of octreotide subcutaneously 3 times per day with nearly complete resolution of their symptoms.[60] In a similar study of patients who were receiving radiation therapy only, the researchers found that subcutaneous administration of 100 mcg 3 times per day produced better results than diphenoxylate 10 mg per day in patients with grade 2 or 3 diarrhea. Issues raised for discussion during the literature review for octreotide and the treatment of radiation-induced diarrhea include significant concerns about the cost of the drug and difficulties in obtaining insurance authorization for treatment of diarrhea because the research is still in the early stages.[50,61]

Diarrhea due to short bowel syndrome. Medications are used in conjunction with dietary modifications to treat diarrhea associated with SBS; see Table 10-9 for these dietary modifications. Antidiarrheal agents increase intestinal transit time, thus increasing absorption of nutrients.[52] Different agents used include loperamide, codeine, tincture of opium, and diphenoxylate; doses of these medications should be maximized. The greatest effect is achieved when antidiarrheal agents are administered 30–60 minutes before meals. Patients may benefit from taking antimotility agents every 6 hours if they are willing to do so. Oral elixirs containing sorbitol further aggravate diarrhea and should be avoided.[52,62]

Patients with a proximal jejunostomy may benefit from clonidine, an alpha$_2$-adrenergic receptor agonist. Clonidine works by inhibiting GI motility, increasing sodium and water absorption, and decreasing bicarbonate secretion. Hence, diarrhea and sodium loss are reduced.[62]

Because significant resection of the small bowel results in increased gastric secretions, the increased acid load is corrosive to the proximal small bowel and the increased secretion volume contributes to total stool output. Treatment comprises both histamine-2-receptor antagonists and proton pump inhibitors (PPIs). Histamine-2-receptor antagonists include cimetidine (40 mg twice daily); famotidine (40 mg twice daily), and ranitidine (300 mg twice daily.)[28] These medications should be taken on an empty stomach 1 hour before consuming food. PPIs are effective only if greater than 50 cm of jejunum is present for absorption; the liquid form of PPIs may be better absorbed. PPIs include esomeprazole (40 mg twice daily), omeprazole (40 mg twice daily), lansoprazole (30 mg twice daily), and pantoprazole (40 mg twice daily).[28]

Octreotide is another agent that has shown efficacy in treating secretory diarrhea by increasing absorption of water and sodium, and decreasing the need for electrolyte and fluid replacement. Octreotide can be given to those patients requiring greater than 3 liters daily of fluid replacement. However, this treatment should be undertaken only with careful consideration, as octreotide increases the risk of cholelithiasis, compromises intestinal adaptation, and reduces luminal transport activity.[52,62]

Pancreatic enzyme supplementation can improve digestion in patients who have a history of pancreatic insufficiency and in patients experiencing malabsorption due to rapid transit time. Patients with SBS—specifically with less than 100 cm of remaining ileum—have diminished ability to complete bile salt absorption, resulting in watery diarrhea and impaired fat absorption. Administration of synthetic bile salts is then indicated to facilitate fat and fat-soluble vitamin absorption.[28,50]

GVHD-induced diarrhea. Management of GVHD diarrhea is focused on the underlying cause. Electrolyte replacement, hydration, and skin care are paramount. If appropriate, antidiarrheal agents may be administered.[63] Treatment includes systemic corticosteroids, and patients with acute GVHD may benefit from the addition of oral budesonide. For patients with steroid-refractory GVHD, infliximab has been shown to be effective. The practitioner must be aware of the potential for an increased rate of infections when infliximab is used. Octreotide has reported to be effective in symptom relief of diarrhea related to GVHD.[18,20]

Probiotics

Probiotics are defined as live microorganisms that, when administered in adequate amounts, confer a health benefit on the host; one potential benefit to the host is management or prevention of diarrhea. Probiotics produce antimicrobial substances including hydrogen peroxide, organic acids, and bacteriocins. Probiotic bacteria also lower the intestinal intraluminal pH by secreting acetic and lactic acids, which create an antagonistic environment to aggressive bacteria in the intestinal luminal and produce cytoprotective qualities. Probiotics replace pathogenic organisms by coating the mucosal layer of the gut, so there is no room for other organisms. Subsequently, the intestine secretes anti-inflammatory cytokines and reduces pro-inflammatory cytokine production. Probiotics modulate immune activity and epithelial function in the large and small intestines. They induce the heat-shock protein expression in intestinal epithelial cells, and prevent cytokine-induced epithelial damage.[64] The gut is then able to distinguish different types of microbials, which has led to the increased reliability of probiotics as clinical therapies.[65,66]

Interest in the use of probiotics to alleviate antibiotic-associated diarrhea (AAD) and other gastrointestinal diseases is increasing. A meta-analysis of 25 randomized controlled trials showed that probiotics significantly decreased the risk of AAD and may have efficacy in *C. difficile*–associated diarrhea.[67] A variety of probiotics were included, but the ones that showed the most promise for AAD were *Saccharomyces boulardii*, *Lactobacillus rhamnosus* GG, and probiotic mixtures. The only organism showing effectiveness for CDAD is *S. boulardii*.

At the time of this book's publication, the Cochrane Library was conducting a review of the efficacy of probiotics for diarrhea prevention and management in people receiving chemotherapy or radiation therapy.[68] The use of probiotics for chemotherapy-induced diarrhea is now being studied actively as well. Österlund et al.[64] randomized 97 patients receiving 5-FU chemotherapy (bolus or continuous infusion) to receive the probiotic *Lactobacillus rhamnosus* GG; another 51 patients received no probiotics. The incidence of grade 3 or 4 diarrhea was lower in the *Lactobacillus rhamnosus* GG group versus the non-probiotic group, and the decrease in diarrhea was statistically significant ($p = 0.027$). The group who received *L. rhamnosus* GG also reported less abdominal discomfort and had fewer chemotherapy dose reductions. Although no reports of *L. rhamnosus* being identified in blood cultures occurred during the study, it is important to note that lactobacilli may infrequently cause septicemia in severely immunocompromised patients.

The probiotics VSL #3 and *Lactobacillus acidophilus* have demonstrated some effect on radiation-induced diarrhea. There are some positive studies on these agents indicating their administration may result in a decrease in diarrheal episodes or a decreased incidence in watery diarrhea.[66] The Yale Workshop on Probiotics[69] is a group of leaders in gastroenterology who updated their recommendations on probiotics in radiation-induced diarrhea based on available literature. This group rates the efficacy of interventions using a scale of A, B, and C, where "A" equals strong, positive studies found in the literature. The group give probiotics—specifically, VSL #3 and *Lactobacillus acidophilus*—a "C" grade, meaning there are some positive studies, but more work needs to be done to establish confidence in their effectiveness.

Ohigashi and colleagues[70] reviewed the effects of probiotics on patients and their quality of life (QOL) status post surgery for colorectal cancer. These researchers stratified patients according to the location of resection: rectal or colon, right or left. Seventy-seven patients who consented to answer QOL questionnaires agreed to take a probiotic product called "The Guard" that contains *Bacillus natto* and *Lactobacillus acidophilus* for 3 months. At the 3-month mark, the QOL questionnaires were administered again. The outcomes examined were (1) functional outcomes and QOL after surgery for rectal versus colon cancer and right colon versus left colon and (2) the effects of administration of probiotics on changes in functional outcome and QOL. The researchers defined "functional outcome" as defecation frequency, anal pain, daytime versus nighttime defecation, urgency, use of a pad, and incontinence.

Forty of the 60 patients taking probiotics (63.5%) described improvements in bowel habits. Patients in the rectal and right colon resection groups experienced greater improvements. Those in the right colon resection group chose to continue taking probiotics after the study was completed. Ohigashi et al.[70] reported improvements in functional QOL in all groups taking probiotics. Frequency of defecation decreased with improvements in soft stool in the patients who underwent right-sided colon resection. Constipation decreased in the group with left colon resection, and both constipation and diarrhea episodes decreased in the rectal group. The authors postulate that these results may reflect changes in intestinal flora with the use of probiotics. More specifically, intestinal flora change after resection of the ileolcecal valve, leading to a loss of regulation of intestinal contents and irregular influx of hyperosmotic small intestinal fluid into the large intestine. As a result, aerobes in the large intestine increase and the distribution of anaerobes found in a significant portion of bacteria in the large intestine changes to a noticeable extent. Subsequently, the changes in intestinal flora are improved with administration of probiotics and affect postoperative intestinal motility disorder.

Probiotics are live bacterial organisms; therefore precautions need to be taken when administering probiotics to immunocompromised patients. There have been case reports of infections with some probiotic strains such as *L. rhamnosus* GG and *S. boulardii*, but the risk is difficult to assess. Type, dosing, frequency, and duration of probiotic therapy depend on the probiotic being used. *Lactobacillus casei* DN-114-001 is recommended for prophylaxis of radiation-induced diarrhea at a dose of 96 mL of 10^8 CFU/g three times daily. The probiotic mixture VSL #3 is also proposed for prophylaxis at a dose of one capsule three times per day. Strict hand hygiene is required when handling probiotics.[65,66]

NURSING IMPLICATIONS

Nursing interventions are paramount in the management and treatment of diarrhea, and can significantly improve patients' physical symptoms, minimize the psychological and psychosocial distress related to diarrhea, prevent exacerbation of symptoms, and ultimately decrease healthcare costs. Nurses play a key role in the assessment and education of patients and families to help maintain adequate hydration and electrolyte balance, to help prevent unnecessary hospitalizations for severe dehydration, and to avoid cardiovascular collapse. Tools that assist the provider in evaluating fluid status include the patient's self-maintained diary (Appendix 10A), weight, and directed questions designed to elicit adequate information to treat the patient (Table 10-5).

Early identification of and intervention to prevent complicated diarrhea may reduce healthcare costs.[71] Grades 3 and 4 chemotherapy-induced diarrhea are reported at a rate as high as 58%, and current guidelines recommend hospital admission for grades 3 and 4 diarrhea or other factors contributing to complicated diarrhea as described in Figure 10-2. A Canadian study ($n = 63$) examining the cost of severe diarrhea in patients with colorectal cancer found that the mean increase in cost was approximately U.S.$8377 (C$8230) per patient, and the median hospital stay was 8 days.[71]

Nursing interventions are also paramount in improving patients' QOL and minimizing their psychological and psychosocial distress by addressing personal and private issues such as bowel habits and fecal incontinence. Patients may be uncomfortable talking about their bowel habits, especially FI. FI is not commonly reported by patients, as it is perceived to be an off-limits subject. Most patients rely on trial and error to treat FI because of the limited research conducted in this area. Stool leakage may be loose or liquid with varying frequency and amounts ranging from small amounts, which can be contained in an absorbent pad or underwear, to larger amounts, which may soil outer garments. No matter the amount, embarrassment and a negative impact on quality of life cause anxiety about future episodes. Actively screening patients for presence of FI allows the nurse to address reversible or treatable causes of FI, provide symptom management, and reduce psychological distress.[39,40]

Additional physical symptoms requiring nursing intervention include skin care. Excellent perineal skin care is essential to minimize risk of skin breakdown and infection. Nurses are experts at providing good skin hygiene and teaching the important aspects of skin hygiene, as outlined previously in this chapter. Skin breakdown can arise when perineal cleansing is inadequate. This issue is of particular concern when FI occurs with diarrhea. Incontinence-associated dermatitis may progress to ulceration and secondary infections involving bacteria (*Staphylococcus*) and/or yeast (*Candida albicans*), thereby impacting the patient's comfort, quality of life, and treatment costs.[4]

Molassiotis and colleagues[72] conducted a randomized, controlled trial to assess the effectiveness of a symptom-focused home care program for patients diagnosed with breast cancer ($n = 110$) or colorectal carcinoma ($n = 54$) receiving oral capecitabine. Patients were randomized to either a standard care arm for six cycles of chemotherapy (18 weeks) or to receive home care visits by a nurse (experimental arm). Overall, the researchers found significantly less toxicity in the experimental arm in relation to the symptoms of diarrhea, pain, oral mucositis, constipation, fatigue, and insomnia. These improvements were more pronounced in the first 6 weeks (2 cycles) of therapy and were maintained after that period. Effectiveness decreased with some symptoms (i.e., vomiting) as the symptom plateaued. The authors of this study suggest that the home care nursing intervention may be best utilized early on in treatment. This finding is due in part to the fact that patients are overwhelmed with the amount of education they receive and, therefore, are unable to synthesize and absorb all of the information during admission or prior to starting chemotherapy. The home care visit arm addressed this information on a more routine basis.

Molassiotis et al.[20] also looked at service utilization in both groups, including number of visits to physicians, calls to the hospital emergency hotline, additional visits to the hospital, and inpatient days. Physician visits were similar in both arms, but other service utilization decreased; for example, patients receiving the intervention had a lower number of inpatient days and lower usage of other healthcare services. The authors suggest that home care nursing visits may be beneficial to certain groups such as the elderly and frail individuals as the use of oral chemotherapeutics increases.

Cancer-related diarrhea remains a complex side effect to manage. As discussed previously, there are many interventions available to facilitate the best care and education for the patient and families. However, the optimal approach is one that is interprofessional in nature, including not only the oncology nurse but also the physician or nurse practitioner, registered dietitian, pharmacist, and specialty nurses such as radiation oncology and possibly the wound, ostomy, and continence nurses.

PATIENT SELF-CARE

Patient education is essential in managing and treating cancer-related diarrhea. Appendices 10A, 10B, and 10C provide information for patients to help with self-care. Appendix 10A is a self-reported diary to help the patient identify factors that may be aggravating diarrhea, such as food or beverage consumption, as well as identify symptoms associated with diarrhea, such as fever, fecal incontinence, and abdominal pain. The healthcare team, including the physician, oncology nurse, and dietitian, should review these diaries with patients when discussing symptom management. Appendix 10B provides a summary of self-care guidelines, including signs and symptoms alerting the patient to notify the healthcare team, and general information on diarrhea. Appendix 10C provides dietary guidelines to prevent exacerbation of treatment-induced diarrhea. Appendix 10D details essential skin care guidelines to prevent skin breakdown and to minimize the risk of infection.[73] These self-care guides are intended to provide cancer patients with information that allows them to manage their diarrhea proactively and help them to identify potential complications and subsequent treatment.

REFERENCES

1. Davila M, Bresalier RS. Gastrointestinal complications of oncologic therapy. *Nature Clin Pract Gastroenterol Hepatol.* 2008;5(12):682–696.
2. U.S. Department of Health and Human Services. Common terminology criteria for adverse events, version 4. June 14, 2010. http://evs.nci.nih.gov/ftp1/CTCAE/CTCAE_4.03_2010-06-14_QuickReference_8.5x11.pdf Accessed January 3, 2012.
3. Benson A, Ajani J, Catalano R, et al. Recommended guidelines for the treatment of cancer treatment-induced diarrhea. *J Clin Oncol.* 2004;22(14):2918–2926.
4. Nix D, Haugen V. Prevention and management of incontinence-associated diarrhea. *Drugs Aging.* 2010;27(6):491–496.
5. Soloman R, Cherny NI. Constipation and diarrhea in patients with cancer. *Cancer J.* 2006;12(5):355–364.
6. Richardson G, Dobish R. Chemotherapy induced diarrhea. *J Oncol Pharmacy Pract.* 2007;13:181–198.
7. O'Brien BE, Kaklamani VG, Benson AB. The assessment and management of cancer treatment-related diarrhea. *Clin Colorect Cancer.* 2005;4(6):375–381.
8. Arbuckle RB, Huber SL, Zacker C. The consequences of diarrhea occurring during chemotherapy for colorectal cancer: a retrospective study. *Oncologist.* 2000;5:250–259.
9. Esper P, Kuebler K, eds. *Palliative Practices from A–Z for the Bedside Clinician.* 2nd ed. Pittsburgh, PA: Oncology Nursing Society; 2008.
10. National Cancer Institute. *Gastrointestinal Complications (PDQ®).* Bethesda, MD: National Cancer Institute; June 30, 2011. http://www.cancer.gov/cancertopics/pdq/supportivecare/gastrointestinalcomplications/HealthProfessional/page5. Accessed January 31, 2012.
11. Stein A, Boigt W, Jordan K. Chemotherapy-induced diarrhea: pathophysiology, frequency and guideline-based management. *Ther Adv Med Oncol.* 2010;2(1):51–63.
12. Cherny, NI. Evaluation and management of treatment-related diarrhea in patients with advanced cancer: a review. *J Pain Symptom Manage.* 2008;35(4):413–423.
13. Gottschlich MM, DeLegge MH, Mattox T, Mueller C, Worthington, P, eds. *The A.S.P.E.N. Nutrition Support Core Curriculum: A Case-Based Approach—The Adult Patient.* Silver Spring, MD: American Society for Parenteral and Enteral Nutrition; 2007.
14. Conlon, B. Malnutrition and malabsorptive diarrhea in pancreatic cancer. *Oncol Nutr Connect.* 2010;19(4):10–21.
15. Bisanz A, Tucker AM, Amin DM, et al. Summary of the causative and treatment factors of diarrhea and the use of a diarrhea assessment and treatment tool to improve patient outcomes. *Gastroenterol Nurs.* 2010;33:268–281.
16. Yeoh E, Horowitz M, Russo A, et al. Effect of pelvic irradiation on gastrointestinal function: a prospective longitudinal study. *Am J Med.* 1993;95:397–406.
17. Dunberger G, Lind H, Steineck G, Waldenström A-C, Onelöv E, Ävall-Lundqvist E. Loose stools lead to fecal incontinence among gynecological cancer survivors. *Acta Oncologica.* 2011;50:233–242.
18. Ross WA, Couriel D. Colonic graft-versus-host disease. *Curr Opin Gastroenterol.* 2005;21:64–69.
19. Liu D, Yan C, Xu L, et al. Diarrhea during the conditioning regimen is correlated with the occurrence of severe acute graft-versus-host disease through systemic release of inflammatory cytokines. *Am Soc Blood Marrow Transplant.* 2010;16:1567–1575.
20. Jacobsohn DA, Vogelsang GB. Acute graft versus host disease. *Orphanet J Rare Dis.* 2007;2:35. http://www.OJRD.com/content/2/1/35. Accessed January 31, 2012.
21. Ouwerkerk J, Boers-Doets C. Best practices in the management of toxicities related to anti-EGFR agents for metastatic colorectal cancer. *Eur J Oncol Nurs.* 2010;14:337–349.
22. Wujcik D. Targeted therapies. In: Yarbro CH, Wujcik D, Gobel BH, eds. *Cancer Nursing Principles and Practice.* 7th ed. Burlington, MA: Jones & Bartlett Learning; 2011:561–583.
23. Schwartzentruber DJ. Guidelines for the safe administration of high-dose interleukin-2. *J Immunotherapy.* 2001;24(4):287–293.
24. *Proleukin (Aldesleukin) for Injection, for Intravenous Infusion* [package insert]. San Diego, CA: Prometheus Laboratories; 2011.
25. Muehlbauer PM. Biotherapy. In: Yarbro CH, Wucjik D, Gobel Holmes B, eds. *Cancer Nursing Principles and Practice.* 7th ed. Burlington, MA: Jones & Bartlett Learning; 2011:530–560.
26. Beck KE, Blansfield JA, Tran KQ, et al. Enterocolitis in patients with cancer after antibody blockade of cytotoxic T-lymphocyte–associated antigen 4. *J Clin Oncol.* 2006;24:2283–2289.
27. *Yervoy (Ipilumumab) Injection for Intravenous Infusion* [package insert]. Princeton, NJ: Bristol-Myers Squibb; 2011.
28. Parrish CR. The clinician's guide to short bowel syndrome. *Practical Gastroenterol.* 2005;29:67–106.
29. Ukleja A. Dumping syndrome: pathophysiology and treatment. *Nutr Clin Pract.* 2005;20:517–525.
30. McDonald LC, Owings M, Jernigan DB. *Clostridium difficile* infection in patients discharged from short-stay US hospitals, 1996–2003. *Emerg Infect Dis.* 2006;12(3):409–415.
31. Bartlett, JG. Narrative review: the new epidemic of *Clostridium difficile*–associated enteric disease. *Ann Intern Med.* 2006;145(10):758–764.
32. Loo VG, Bourgault AM, Poirier L, et al. Host and pathogen factors for *Clostridium difficile* infection and colonization. *N Engl J Med.* 2011;365:1693–1703.
33. Shafi MS, Bresalier RA. The gastrointestinal complications of oncologic therapy. Gastroenterol Clin North Am. 2010;39(3):629–647.
34. Makic MB. Management of nausea, vomiting and diarrhea during critical illness. *AACN Adv Crit Care.* 2011;22(3):265–274.
35. Bharucha A. Diarrhea. In: Porter RS, Kaplan JL, eds. *The Merck Manual for Healthcare Professionals,* 19th ed. 2007. http://merckmanuals.com/professional.print/gastrointestinal_disorders/approach_to_the_patient_with_lower_gi_complaints/diarrhea.html. Accessed March 7, 2012.
36. Ackley BJ. Diarrhea. In: Ackley BJ, Ladwig GB, eds. *Nursing Diagnosis Handbook An Evidence-Based Guide to Planning Care.* 8th ed. St. Louis, MO: Mosby Elsevier; 2008:311–315.
37. Roach M, Christie JA. Fecal incontinence in the elderly. *Geriatrics.* 2008;63(2):13–22.
38. Woodward S. Management of faecal incontinence in graft-versus-host disease. *Brit J Nurs.* 2012;21(2):84–88.
39. Bliss DZ, Norton C. Conservative management of fecal incontinence. *Am J Nurs.* 2010;110(9):30–38.
40. Bharucha AE. Management of fecal incontinence. *Gastroenterol Hepatol.* 2008;4(11):807–817.
41. Engelking C. Diarrhea. In: Yarbro CH, Frogge MH, Goodman M, eds. *Cancer Symptom Management.* 3rd ed. Sudbury, MA: Jones and Bartlett; 2004:528–557.

42. Schmelzer M. Nursing management: lower gastrointestinal problems. In Lewis SL, Hietkemper MM, Dirksen SR, et al, eds. *Medical–Surgical Nursing Assessment and Management of Clinical Problems.* 7th ed. St. Louis, MO: Mosby Elsevier; 2007:1036–1040.
43. Kornblau S, Benson AB, Catalano R, et al. Management of cancer treatment-related diarrhea: issues and therapeutic strategies. *J Pain Symptom Manage.* 2000;19:118–129.
44. Welch K. Fluid balance. *Learning Disabil Pract.* 2010;13:33–38.
45. Maroun JA, Anthony LB, Blais N, et al. Prevention and management of chemotherapy-induced diarrhea in patients with colorectal cancer: a consensus statement by the Canadian Working Group on chemotherapy-induced diarrhea. *Curr Oncol.* 2007;14(1):13–20.
46. Shen B, Khan K, Ikenberry O, et al. The role of endoscopy in the management of patients with diarrhea. *J Gastrointest Endosc.* 2010;71(6):887–892.
47. Fine KD, Schiller LR. AGA technical review on the evaluation and management of chronic diarrhea. *Gastroenterology.* 1999;116:1464–1486.
48. Pan LH, Tsai YF, Chen ML, Tang R, Chang CJ. Symptom distress and self-care strategies of colorectal cancer patients with diarrhea up to 3 months after surgery. *Cancer Nurs.* 2011;34(1):E1–E9.
49. Nikoletti S, Young J, Levitt M, King M, Chidlow C, Hollingsworth S. Bowel problems, self-care practices, and information needs of colorectal cancer survivors at 6 to 24 months after sphincter-saving surgery. *Cancer Nurs.* 2008;31(5):389–398.
50. Muehlbauer PM, Thorpe D, Davis AB, Drabot, RC, Kiker, ES, & Rawlings, BL. Oncology Nursing Society PEP resource: Diarrhea. In: Eaton LH, Tipton JM, eds. *Putting Evidence into Practice: Improving Oncology Patient Outcomes.* Pittsburgh, PA: Oncology Nursing Society; 2009:125–134.
51. Elliot L, Molseed L, McCallum P, Grant B, eds. *The Clinical Guide to Oncology Nutrition.* 2nd ed. USA: Oncology Nutrition Dietetic Practice Group; 2006.
52. Matarese LE, Steiger E. Dietary and medical management of short bowel syndrome in adult patients. *J Clin Gastroenterol.* 2006;40:S85–S93.
53. Kachrimanidou M, Malisiovas, N. *Clostridium difficile* infection: a comprehensive review. *Crit Rev Microbiol.* 2011;37(3):178–187.
54. Pellat G. Clinical skills: bowel elimination and management of complications. *Brit J Nurs.* 2007;16(6):351–355.
55. Muehlbauer PM, Thorpe D, Davis AB, et al. Putting evidence into practice: evidence-based interventions to prevent, manage and treat chemotherapy- or radiation therapy-induced diarrhea. *Clin J Oncol Nurs.* 2009;13(3):1–6.
56. *Imodium (Loperamide Hydrochloride) Capsule* [package insert]. Ft. Washington, PA: McNeil Consumer Healthcare; 2008.
57. Zidan J, Haim N, Beny A, Stein M, Gez E, Kuten A. Octreotide in the treatment of severe chemotherapy-induced diarrhea. *Ann Oncol.* 2001;12(2):227–229.
58. Kähler KC, Hauschild A. Treatment and side effect management of CTLA-4 antibody therapy in metastatic melanoma. *J Dtsch Dermatol Ges.* 2011(4):277–285.
59. Rubin K. Managing immune-related adverse events to ipilumumab: a nurse's guide. *Clin J Oncol Nurs.* 2012;16:E69–E75.
60. Topkan E, Karaoglu A. Octreotide in the management of chemoradiotherapy-induced diarrhea refractory to loperamide in patients with rectal carcinoma. *Oncology.* 2006;71:354–360.
61. Yavuz AA, Aydin F, Can G, Kavgaci H. The efficacy of octreotide in the therapy of acute radiation-induced diarrhea: a randomized controlled study. *Int J Radiat Oncol Biol Physics.* 2002;54(1):195–202.
62. Efsen E, Jeppesen PB. Modern treatment of adult short bowel syndrome patients. *Minerva Gastroenterol Dietol.* 2011;57:405–17.
63. Anderson-Reitz L. Complications of hematopoietic cell transplantation. In: Yarbro CH, Wujcik D, Gobel, BH. eds. *Cancer Nursing Principles and Practice.* 7th ed. Burlington, MA: Jones & Bartlett Learning; 2011:514–529.
64. Österlund P, Routsalainen T, Korpela R, et al. *Lactobacillus* supplementation for diarrhoea related to chemotherapy of colorectal cancer: a randomised study. *Brit J Cancer.* 2007;97:1028–1034.
65. Morrow LE, Gogineni V, Malesker M. Probiotics in the intensive care unit. *Nutr Clin Pract.* 2012;27:235–241.
66. Visich KL, Yeo TP. The prophylactic use of probiotics in the prevention of radiation therapy-induced diarrhea. *Clin J Oncol Nurs.* 2010;14(4):467–473.
67. McFarland LV. Meta-analysis of probiotics for the prevention of antibiotic associated diarrhea and the treatment of *Clostridium difficile* disease. *Am J Gastroenterol.* 2006;101:812–822.
68. Wang T, Ma L, Luo L, Wu T, Zhou Q. Probiotics for the prevention or treatment of chemotherapy or radiotherapy related diarrhoea in cancer patients (protocol). *Cochrane Database Syst Rev.* 2010;11:CD008831.
69. Floch MH, Walker A, Madsen K, et al. Recommendations for probiotic use—2011 update. *J Clin Gastroenterol.* 2011;45:S168–S171.
70. Ohigashi S, Hoshino Y, Ohde S, Onodera H. Functional outcome, quality of life, and efficacy of probiotics in postoperative patients with colorectal cancer. *Surg Today.* 2011;41:1200–1206.
71. Dranitsaris G, Maroun J, Shah A. Estimating the cost of illness in colorectal cancer patients who were hospitalized for severe chemotherapy-induced diarrhea. *Can J Gastroenterol.* 2005;19(2):83–87.
72. Molassiotis A, Brearley S, Saunders M, et al. Effectiveness of a home care nursing program in the symptom management of patients with colorectal and breast cancer receiving oral chemotherapy: a randomized controlled trial. *J Clin Oncol.* 2009; 27(36):6191–6198.
73. MedlinePlus. Skin care and incontinence [Web page]. U.S. National Library of Medicine, National Institutes of Health website. http://www.nlm.nih.gov/medlineplus/ency/article/003976.htm. Accessed April 10, 2012.

Weekly Bowel Pattern Diary

Please keep track of your bowel movements (BM) using this diary. Bring this diary with you to your next appointment. Do not hesitate to call with any concerns before your appointment.

Patient Name: ______________________________

What to Record	**Day**	**Day**	**Day**	**Day**	**Day**	**Day**	**Day**
Time(s) of day for BM							
How many stools did you have per day?							
What did your stools look like? (Please use Bristol Stool Chart)							
Was there any blood in your stool?							
Did you have any abdominal cramps?							
Did you have a fever? Is yes, what was your temperature?							
Did you have any incontinence?							
Did you have any change in your diet or consume any foods that may contribute to diarrhea? (Refer to diet sheet)							
Which medications did you take to control diarrhea?							
Do you have any pain, itching, or tenderness around your rectal area?							
Did you have any dizziness?							
Did you notice any changes in thirst?							
What was the total volume of liquid you drank per day? (see diet list for suggestions)							
Daily weight							

Please share with us any additional comments or concerns:

Source: Muehlbauer PM, Lopez RC. Diarrhea. In: Yarbro CH, Wujcik D, Gobel BH, eds. *Cancer Symptom Management.* 4th ed. Burlington, MA: Jones & Bartlett Learning; 2014.

Diarrhea from Cancer Treatment

☐ Radiation Therapy

☐ Chemotherapy

☐ Targeted or Biological Therapy

☐ Bowel Surgery

Regimen: ______________________________

Patient Name: ______________________________

Symptom and Description

Diarrhea is defined as an abnormal increase in both the liquidity and the frequency of stools over what is normal for you. It can be caused when radiation is directed to your abdomen or lower back. Diarrhea may be worse if you are also receiving chemotherapy or certain targeted or biological therapies. These loose or watery stools may start 1–2 weeks after your treatments begin or during the treatment. Left untreated, diarrhea can result in dehydration, weakness, weight loss, electrolyte imbalance, skin soreness, and poor nutrition.

You can act to control your diarrhea, but need to know what you can handle on your own and when you need to call your doctor or nurse.

Prevention

Choosing certain foods before and during treatment may help to reduce the number of loose stools per day. Please refer to the dietary suggestions provided.

Management

- Choose foods from the recommended food list supplied with this self-care guide.
- Use an over-the-counter anti-diarrheal medicine for loose stools, as directed by your physician or healthcare provider.
- Drink at least eight to ten 8-ounce glasses of fluid per day (unless told not to do so by your doctor).

Skin Care

If you are having several stools daily or have some incontinence, you will need to take care of the skin around your rectum. See the Skin Care and Incontinence Guidelines.

(continued)

Follow-up

Let your doctor or nurse know if these measures do not control your diarrhea. In addition, you should call them immediately in the following situations:

- You have a temperature of 100.5°F (38°C) or greater.
- You have bloody stools or severe abdominal pain.
- You are unable to keep down liquids for more than 12 hours.
- You become suddenly dizzy, weak, and dry, or feel disoriented.
- Your urine becomes dark yellow in color, indicating that it is more concentrated.
- You have diarrhea that does not stop after 24 hours of treatment with loperamide.

Phone Numbers

Physician: ______________________________

Registered Dietitian: ______________________________

Oncology Nurse: ______________________________

After Hours: ______________________________

Source: Muehlbauer PM, Lopez RC. Diarrhea. In: Yarbro CH, Wujcik D, Gobel BH, eds. *Cancer Symptom Management.* 4th ed. Burlington, MA: Jones & Bartlett Learning; 2014.

Dietary Guidelines to Prevent Exacerbation of Treatment-Induced Diarrhea by Food Group

Food Group	Foods to Choose	Foods to Avoid
Grains and starches	**Breads:** enriched white, French, rye without seeds, corn, potato, any other bread made from white or refined flour	**Breads:** whole-wheat or whole-grain bread, bran, breads with seeds or nuts such as poppy, sesame, rye, or nut breads
	Baked goods: plain muffins, corn muffins, plain pancakes, plain waffles, plain rolls without seeds	**Baked goods:** products made with nuts, seeds, fruit skins, or whole grains such as whole wheat or brain
	Cereals: hot or cold cereals made from white or refined flour such as oatmeal, buckwheat, cream of wheat, cream of rice, corn flakes, Rice Krispies®, Rice Chex®, and Cheerios®	**Cereals:** hot or cold cereals made from whole grain or bran; high-fiber cereals; cereals with nuts, seeds or dried fruit
	Other starches: white rice, brown rice, plain pasta, potatoes without the skin, sweet potatoes without the skin	**Other starches:** wild rice, whole-wheat pasta, potato skins, corn, popcorn, fried starches such as french fries
Dairy and dairy substitutes	**Milk**[1]: • Evaporated, skim, and low-fat milk • Buttermilk • Powdered milk • Low-fat soy milk, almond milk, rice milk or other nondairy alternative	**Milk:** high-fat milk products such as whole milk, half-and-half, cream
	Yogurt and ice cream: • Plain or blended yogurt with live active cultures[2] • Low-fat frozen yogurt, low-fat ice cream	**Yogurt and ice cream:** • Yogurt with berries, dried fruit, or nuts • Regular (whole-milk) ice cream
	Cheese: low-fat cheeses such as low-fat cottage cheese, low-fat cream cheese, skim-milk cheese, part-skim mozzarella, part-skim ricotta, string cheese, parmesan and any other cheese with less than 5 grams of fat per serving	**Cheese:** high-fat cheeses (more than 5 grams of fat per serving)
Protein	**Meat/poultry/fish:** stewed, boiled, baked, lean meat (remove visible fat), poultry without the skin, or fish	**Meat/poultry/fish:** fried meat, poultry or fish, luncheon meats (cold cuts), sausage, bacon, hot dogs, fatty meats, cured meats, poultry skin
	Eggs: nonfried eggs such as omelets, scrambled eggs, hard-boiled eggs	**Eggs:** fried eggs
	Plant proteins: soy foods made without added fat, smooth nut butters	**Plant proteins:** nuts, chunky nut butters, beans, legumes, lentils, seeds

(continued)

Fruit	**Fresh or frozen fruit:** • Ripe bananas • Melon without seeds **Canned fruit:** applesauce, all canned fruit (packed in natural juice) without seeds **Fruit juice:** fruit juice without pulp, except prune juice **Dried fruit:** none	**Fresh or frozen fruit:** all raw or frozen fruit except bananas and melon without seeds **Canned fruit:** canned fruit in heavy syrup or sweetened with sorbitol, fruit preserves (with seeds) **Fruit juice:** all fruit juice with pulp, fruit juice sweetened with sorbitol, prune juice **Dried fruit:** all, including prunes and raisins
Vegetables	**Fresh vegetables:** no raw vegetables **Cooked vegetables:** well-cooked vegetables without seeds or skins such as well-cooked green beans, beets, squash, pumpkin, potatoes without the skin, carrots, spinach, asparagus, strained tomatoes, mushrooms **Vegetable juice:** strained vegetable juice	**Fresh vegetables:** all raw vegetables **Cooked vegetables:** • Broccoli, Brussels sprouts, cabbage, cauliflower, onions, corn, olives, pickles, potato skins • Vegetables cooked in added fat such as creamed vegetables or fried vegetables such as french fries **Vegetable juice:** all vegetable juice with pulp
Added fats	• Total of 8 or fewer teaspoons per day • Fats include oil, butter, cream, cream cheese, margarine, gravy, mayonnaise	Limit fats to less than 8 teaspoons per day
Other beverages	• Decaffeinated tea or coffee • Soft drinks without caffeine such as ginger ale • Sports drinks or rehydration beverages such as Gatorade®	• Caffeinated beverages (regular coffee or tea, colas, energy drinks) Limit beverages containing high-fructose corn syrup to 12 ounces per day • Beverages sweetened with sorbitol • Alcoholic beverages
Mixed dishes	Dishes made with allowed ingredients, such as broth-based soups with allowed foods, casseroles made with refined starch and allowed protein and vegetables	Dishes made with foods to avoid such as cream-based soups made with whole milk and casseroles made with high-fiber grains
Desserts	Popsicles, sherbet, water ice, Jell-O, angel food cake, vanilla wafers, ginger snaps, plain cake (without nuts or fruit seeds), hard candy, jelly beans, low-fat pudding, frozen yogurt, low-fat frozen desserts	High-fat desserts, desserts with seeds such as fruit pies, frosting made with added fat or whole milk, desserts with coconut, nuts, or fruit seeds
Other		• Hot pepper, white or black pepper • Spicy foods • Sugar alcohols such as xylitol and sorbitol • Sugar-free gum and candy made with sorbitol

[1]People with lactose intolerance should avoid dairy milk products, which may exacerbate diarrhea. Nondairy alternatives and/or supplementation with lactase enzymes may be needed. Fermented products such as cheese and yogurt are likely to be well tolerated, even for individuals with lactose intolerance.
[2]Unless contraindicated due to neutropenia or other precautions.

Source: Muehlbauer PM, Lopez RC. Diarrhea. In: Yarbro CH, Wujcik D, Gobel BH, eds. *Cancer Symptom Management*. 4th ed. Burlington, MA: Jones & Bartlett Learning; 2014.

Taking Care of Your Skin

Skin Care and Incontinence

People who have problems controlling their urine or bowels (a condition called incontinence) are at greater risk for skin problems around the buttocks, hips, genitals, and the area between the pelvis and rectum (perineum). Excess moisture in these areas makes skin problems such as redness, peeling, irritation, and yeast infections more likely. Bedsores (pressure sores) may also develop if you:

- Have not been eating well (are malnourished)
- Have received radiation therapy to the area
- Spend most or all of the day in a wheelchair, regular chair, or bed

Using diapers and other products may actually make skin problems worse. Although they may keep bedding and clothing cleaner, these products tend to keep the urine or stool in constant contact with the skin. Over time, the skin can break down. Special care must be taken to keep the skin clean and dry.

- After urinating or having a bowel movement, clean and dry the area right away.
- Clean the skin with mild, dilute soap and water. Rinse well, and gently pat dry.
- Look for skin cleansers that do not cause dryness or irritation. These products include foams, nonaerosol sprays, and wet wipes (individual disposable towelettes). Be sure to follow the product's instructions. Some of the products do not require rinsing. Be aware that some people may have allergies to the fragrances used in these cleansers.
- You may use moisturizing creams to keep the skin moist. Avoid products that have alcohol in them, because thealcohol may irritate the skin. If you are receiving radiation therapy, ask your healthcare provider if it is okay to use any creams or lotions.
- Consider using a skin sealant or moisture barrier. Creams or ointments that contain zinc oxide, lanolin, or petrolatum form a protective barrier on the skin. Some skin care products (often in the form of a spray or a towelette) can create a clear, protective film over the skin. A doctor or nurse can recommend barrier creams to help protect the skin.
- Even if you use these products, you must still clean the skin after each episode of incontinence. Reapply the cream or ointment after cleaning and drying the skin.

People who often have incontinence problems may develop a yeast infection on the skin. An itchy, red, pimple-like rash appears, and the skin may feel raw. There are several products (both over-the-counter and prescription) that can be used to treat such yeast infections. If the skin is moist most of the time, you may use a powder with antifungal medication (such as nystatin powder). A moisture barrier or skin sealant may be applied over the powder. If severe skin irritation develops, see your healthcare provider.

(continued)

The National Association for Continence (NAFC) publishes a resource guide of continence products and services, which includes a listing of the manufacturers and distributors of specific products. To get a copy of this resource guide, call 1-800-BLADDER or go to the website www.nafc.org.

Source: MedlinePlus. Skin care and incontinence [Web page]. U.S. National Library of Medicine, National Institutes of Health website. http://www.nlm.nih.gov/medlineplus/ency/article/003976.htm

Source: Muehlbauer PM, Lopez RC. Diarrhea. In: Yarbro CH, Wujcik D, Gobel BH, eds. *Cancer Symptom Management*. 4th ed. Burlington, MA: Jones & Bartlett Learning; 2014.

Chapter 11

Nausea and Vomiting

Janelle Tipton, MSN, RN, AOCN®

THE PROBLEM

Despite the advances in the management of nausea and vomiting (N&V) in the past two decades, patients and healthcare providers continue to be challenged with this problem. The issues related to nausea and vomiting are often complex and multifaceted. During the cancer journey, many patients with cancer experience nausea and/or vomiting during curative therapy or palliative cancer care. Nausea is often more frequent, and may be the more significant problem because it is under-assessed and is more poorly controlled than vomiting. Unfortunately, healthcare providers may underestimate the incidence of delayed nausea and vomiting in patients receiving chemotherapy and radiation therapy.[1–3]

Several reasons have been suggested for the failure to adequately control chemotherapy-induced nausea and vomiting (CINV), as shown in Table 11-1.[4–7] Duration of N&V, relative to severity, has been shown to have the greatest impact on quality of life (QOL), despite the many effective antiemetic agents.[8] Assessment of risk and individualized treatment planning may help to improve nausea and vomiting prophylaxis and management. Nausea and vomiting can have a significant impact on QOL in a growing population of patients who are surviving a considerable length of time. When the N&V is severe or long-lasting, interferes with activities of daily living (ADLs), or impacts other toxicities of treatment, there are consequences that can lead to poor QOL, including effects on nutritional status, physical functioning, and increased anxiety.[9] Physiologic complications and the stated effects on QOL can lead to interruption or delay in therapy, or refusal of treatment.

There are also considerable costs to uncontrolled CINV. Table 11-2 lists potential consequences and costs of uncontrolled CINV.[10–13] While the physiological consequences of N&V are of utmost concern for patient safety and tolerance, these consequences can affect the overall treatment-related consequences such as dose delay, dose reduction, and response. Other consequences that have been reported that are more immediate to the patient include unplanned office visits, emergency room visits, and hospitalizations. Patients may also experience significant costs due to uncontrolled N&V such as missed work, financial burdens due to prescriptions, and transportation. Additionally, the costs of inadequate control of N&V to the healthcare system may affect efficiency and financial outcomes.

TABLE 11-1

Potential Reasons for Failure to Control Chemotherapy Induced Nausea and Vomiting (CINV)
Lack of knowledge of physiology of CINV
Lack of knowledge of mechanism of action of antiemetic agents
Reimbursement and expense of newer agents
Availability of agents on formularies
Underestimation of the magnitude of CINV
Lack of knowledge and adherence to national antiemetic guidelines
Poor communication of symptoms between patients and providers

Source: Data from Kurtin[4]; Viale et al[5]; Hesketh[6]; Herrstedt[7].

TABLE 11-2

Potential Consequences and Costs of Uncontrolled Chemotherapy Induced Nausea and Vomiting (CINV)

Physiological Consequences

- Dehydration
- Electrolyte imbalance
- Poor oral intake: anorexia, mouth sores, malnutrition
- Fatigue
- Depression
- Aspiration pneumonia
- Esophageal irritation

Treatment-Related Consequences

- Delay/interruption in chemotherapy schedule
- Dose reductions
- Response to therapy and survival
- Refusal to continue treatment

Patient Social/Financial Consequences

- Office and Infusion Center visits, ER visits, and hospitalizations
- Missed work and lost productivity
- Costs for antiemetic medications
- Diminished quality of life: effect on everyday activities, eating, socializing
- Strain on family/caregiver resources: home life, transportation, social activities

Healthcare System Costs/Consequences

- Infusion chair and nursing time
- Lack of reimbursement if diagnosis/documentation not adequate
- Pharmacy costs: fluids and antiemetics
- Outpatient, ER, hospitalization costs

Source: Data from Tina Shih et al[10]; Burke et al[11]; Craver et al[12]; Haiderali et al[13].

Because symptoms do not typically appear in isolation, nausea and vomiting often occur with each other, and within other symptom clusters. Symptom clusters are defined as three or more simultaneous symptoms that are related to each other, but do not necessarily have the same cause.[14] Symptom clusters including nausea or vomiting vary and depend on disease and treatment, or both. Some symptom clusters have a common cause, while others may influence one another.[15] For example, patients who have lung cancer may concurrently have nausea, appetite loss, fatigue, weight loss, taste changes, and vomiting. Assessment of the dimensions of symptom clusters is relevant, as severity and distress may impact QOL and patient outcomes. Symptom clusters are relevant because they may predict changes in patient function, treatment failures, and post-therapy outcomes. There may be greater therapeutic benefit to treat the symptom cluster rather than individual symptoms.[14]

Additionally, guidelines are readily available for assessment, prophylaxis, and management of nausea and vomiting. Nevertheless, many patients continue to receive suboptimal prophylaxis and coverage of this side effect. Due to this inconsistency and lack of adherence to national guidelines, many patients receive less than adequate care.[16]

INCIDENCE

Approximately 70%–80% of patients receiving chemotherapy experience nausea and/or vomiting, despite receiving the best available antiemetics.[4] Patients with cancer may also experience N&V after radiation therapy, with rates of 50%–80% reported in the literature.[2,3] More than 30% of patients with advanced cancer may experience nausea, and approximately 60% have both N&V, often causing distress to patients and their families.[14] Anticipatory nausea and vomiting (ANV) occurs in approximately 10%–44% of patients.[4] Anticipatory nausea is more common than anticipatory vomiting, and develops within three or four cycles of chemotherapy when CINV has been inadequately controlled—regardless of the degree of emetogenicity.

The incidence and severity of radiation-induced nausea and vomiting (RINV) is dependent on the irradiated site, single and total dose, fractionation, irradiated volume, and radiotherapy techniques. RINV is most likely to occur if the treatment field includes the abdomen. Total-body irradiation (TBI) and hemibody RT to the upper body most predictably cause N&V. Other patient-related factors that may impact RINV are gender, general health, age, concurrent or recent chemotherapy, psychological state, and tumor stage.[17]

ETIOLOGY

Chemotherapy, radiation therapy, other emetogenic drugs and therapies, another cancer-related condition or problem, or the disease itself may cause N&V. Chemotherapy can cause acute, delayed, and anticipatory CINV. Moderately to highly emetogenic agents are most likely to induce acute CINV as well as delayed and persistent CINV.[16] Anticipatory nausea and vomiting occur by classical conditioning, as the events and cues surrounding chemotherapy (e.g., odors, tastes of drugs, visual cues such as the chemotherapy nurse) become linked with subsequent acute and delayed CINV.[18,19] Nausea and vomiting of progressive cancer are often multicausal, therefore, are mediated via more than one pathway.

Nausea and vomiting (intermittent or constant) are common in terminally ill cancer patients (pain and dyspnea are more frequent).[20] Nausea and vomiting are most likely with advanced cancers of any type, and may result from intestinal obstruction, impaired liver or kidney function, hypercalcemia, dehydration, or brain metastases.[20]

PATHOPHYSIOLOGY

The pathogenesis of N&V is not fully understood, but emesis occurs by one or more of several different mechanisms. Most research has focused on acute vomiting from chemotherapy; less is known about the pathogenesis of nausea, as well as about N&V from other causes. Nausea and vomiting are different entities and may exist along a continuum or may be mediated by different mechanisms. Vomiting is a highly conserved normal physiological reflex that is a protective mechanism to rid a human being or animal of accidental poisons or toxic substances, whether orally ingested or intravenously administered.

The two phases of N&V are pre-ejection and ejection. Nausea—an unpleasant feeling of the need to vomit (feeling sick to one's stomach)—occurs in the pre-ejection phase. Nausea involves a gut–brain connection, including the cerebral cortex and autonomic nervous system, and may be accompanied by salivation, tachypnea, tachycardia, and cold sweat and pallor. With the onset of nausea, the stomach relaxes, and gastric acid secretion is inhibited.[21] A single retrograde giant contraction (RGC) of the small intestine propels alkaline small bowel contents back into the stomach, which further decreases the acidity of stomach contents and confines ingested material to the stomach. Retching (dry heaves), the first ejection phase event, occurs when the RGC reaches the stomach. While retching is a related symptom where there is no expulsion of stomach contents, it still entails abdominal and respiratory muscle contractions. Ultimately, vomiting ensues when coordinated contractions of the abdomen and diaphragm compress stomach contents and force them up through the mouth and nose (throwing up).[22] Figure 11-1 depicts the proposed chemotherapy-induced nausea and vomiting pathways.[23]

NEURAL STRUCTURES, TRANSMITTERS, AND RECEPTORS INVOLVED IN EMESIS

Understanding of the physiology, structures, and neurotransmitters and receptors involved in emesis has evolved and is relevant in understanding the actions of newer antiemetic agents. The vomiting center (VC) is located in the medulla and is a cluster of neurons with a loose network of neural connections among several brain stem and somatic nuclei. It is the final common pathway for emesis; that is, vomiting does not occur unless the VC is stimulated by afferent input from the periphery (e.g., vagus or other

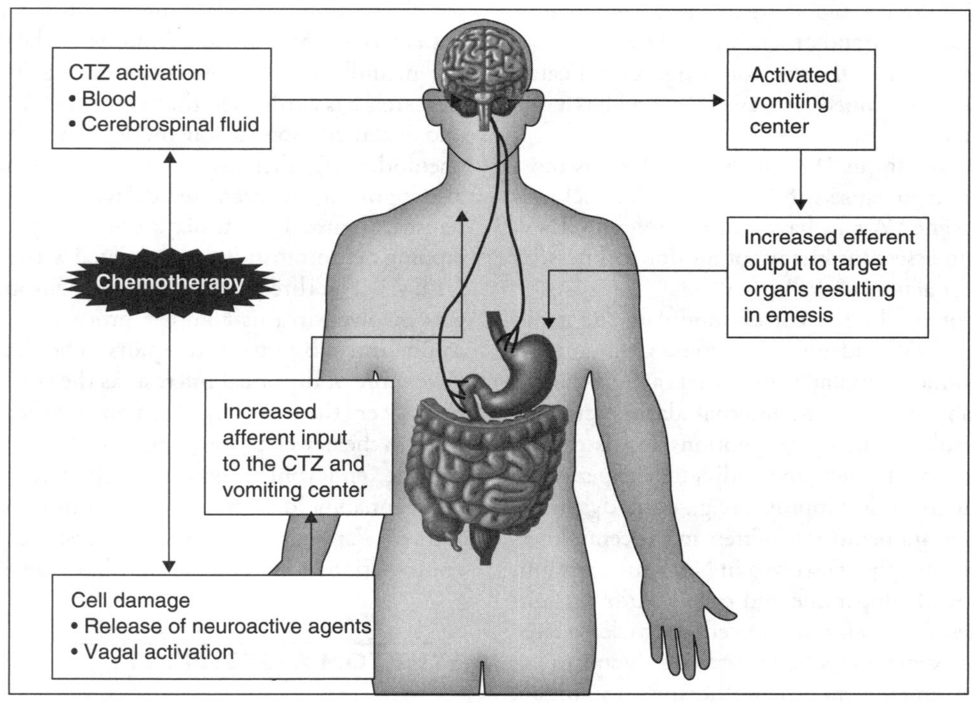

FIGURE 11-1

Proposed chemotherapy-induced nausea and vomiting (CINV) pathways.

Abbreviation: CTZ: chemotherapy trigger zone.

Source: Data from slide presentation for CINV Regional Oncology Nursing Society (ONS) program "Advocating for Optimal Management of CINV" Copyright 2006 ONS. Reprinted with Permission[23].

visceral nerves) or central nervous system (CNS) structures (e.g., chemoreceptor trigger zone (CTZ), higher cortical centers, vestibular apparatus). Therefore, the VC remains the control and integration center of the action of vomiting. The nervous system is characterized by plasticity, so a vomiting message blocked in one neural route can be rerouted via another. The VC responds to afferent inputs from different parts of the body by sending efferent impulses to the motor nuclei that initiate emesis.

Serotonin subtype-3 ($5HT_3$) receptors along the vagus nerve have a key role in acute N&V from chemotherapy (CINV), radiation therapy (RT) to the chest or abdomen, pharyngeal irritation, abdominal distention or obstruction, and probably other causes. Antineoplastic drugs and abdominal RT damage or otherwise stimulate enterochromaffin cells (ECs) that are distributed throughout the gastrointestinal (GI) epithelium of the stomach. Serotonin is released in response to these insults, crosses the GI tissues, and binds to 5HT receptors. This, in turn, causes a vomiting impulse that is transmitted through the CTZ or directly to the VC.[22]

The CTZ, a highly vascular area not confined within the blood–brain barrier, lies close to the VC in the area postrema in the fourth ventricle of the brain. The CTZ detects emetogens (drugs, biochemical products, toxins) in the cerebrospinal fluid and bloodstream, and has a role in N&V from chemotherapy and other causes. The CTZ may play a greater role in nausea than in vomiting, is implicated in food intake and conditioned taste aversion, and has a role in GI tract motility.

The vestibular apparatus (VA) in the inner ear is most commonly activated to cause N&V with motion sickness and labyrinthitis. The VA *may* have a minor role in CINV, and it is relevant to assess for history of motion sickness, as it is a risk factor for acute N&V.[21]

Several areas of the higher cortex modulate the experiences of N&V, ANV, and taste aversions, although the involved neural connections and transmitters are unknown. Likewise, the limbic region—the internal alarm system of the brain that results in negative emotions to distressing symptoms—is activated when the individual experiences nausea or other distressing symptoms (e.g., pain, dyspnea).

The most important neurotransmitters in the central nervous system and the periphery involved in N&V are serotonin and substance P, while dopamine and other neurotransmitters play lesser roles. Enterochromaffin cells may release serotonin after the liver detects ingested GI tract or bloodstream toxins—including emetogenic chemotherapy—to initiate emesis. The magnitude of serotonin release corresponds to the onset, severity, and duration of N&V from chemotherapy.[24]

The importance of $5HT_3$ receptor blockade in N&V is thought to diminish on post-chemotherapy days. Other emetic pathways, neurotransmitters, and receptors may become activated during delayed CINV, and antiemetics have different mechanisms or act at different receptors during acute and delayed CINV.

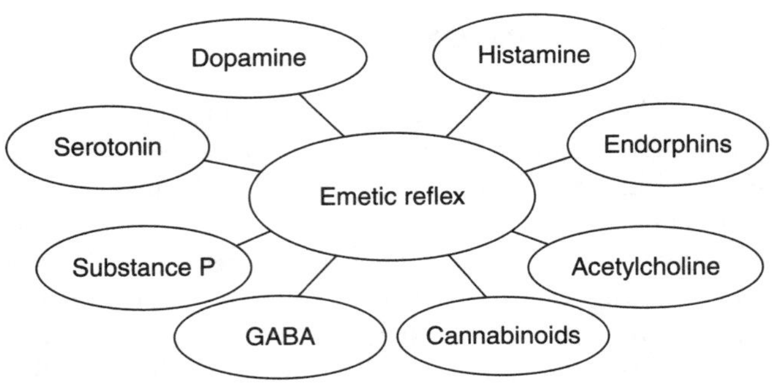

FIGURE 11-2

Neurotransmitters associated with acute and delayed chemotherapy-induced nausea and vomiting (CINV).

Abbreviation: GABA: gamma-aminobutyric acid.

Substance P (SP), a tachykinin regulatory neuropeptide found in the GI tract and near the VC, binds with several neuroreceptors to mediate several vegetative functions. The SP binding to neurokinin (NK_1) receptors occurs near the VC and is involved in N&V from a wide variety of causes. Because NK_1 binding occurs close to the final common pathway for emesis, NK receptor antagonists (NK_1-RAs) will likely have a broader range of efficacy than many other antiemetics.[24] Substance P binding at the NK_1 receptors in the medulla is more prevalent during delayed CINV.[18,24] Research has confirmed that an NK_1-RA (plus a $5HT_3$-RA and dexamethasone before moderately to highly emetogenic chemotherapy) increases control rates of acute CINV, and also significantly decreases delayed vomiting and delayed nausea. Figure 11-2 displays the multiple, common, overlapping neurotransmitters associated with acute and delayed CINV.[25] The three main groups of neurotransmitter receptors involved in this complex process are dopamine, serotonin, and substance P receptors. The dopamine receptors have more of historical interest, as the corresponding antagonists were the mainstay of antiemetic therapy in the 1980s, prior to the newer classes of agents. While histamine, acetylcholine, endorphins, gamma-aminobutyric acid (GABA), and cannabinoid receptors have a minor role in N&V, there is an overlapping involvement of these receptors for which a combination of antiemetics may have greater efficacy.[25]

SYMPTOM ASSESSMENT

A thorough baseline assessment that considers known patient history including risk factors is critical in planning the approach for nausea and vomiting prophylaxis and treatment. Key areas in the pretreatment assessment include previous cancer therapies, previous experience with N&V, comorbidities, current disease, current chemotherapy regimen, and current medications. It is also important to note any structural, metabolic, chemical, or psychological issues that may impact N&V. Physical assessment and diagnostic tests are important to preventing N&V, and ongoing assessment is equally important to promptly intervene if distressing symptoms occur, despite proactive antiemetic therapy. Oncology nurses are key healthcare providers who communicate with patients and caregivers most often, and they can best assess and document how the *patient perceives* the severity of N&V, how acceptable the antiemetic side effects are, and how both affect the patient's QOL and ADLs. Oncology nurses are also in a critical position to provide triage and education, and are essential in providing clear communication to physician colleagues.

RISK FACTORS

In terms of therapies, chemotherapy is a more frequent cause of N&V than RT or anesthesia, and the risk of N&V is augmented by individual patient and disease factors. The nurse must, therefore, consider events that can precipitate N&V, including the emetogenic potential of chemotherapy and radiation therapy, other emetogenic drugs, and possible contributing problems that are common in patients with cancer, such as constipation, intermittent bowel obstruction, hypercalcemia, infection, or uncontrolled cough. There should also be concern for patients receiving concurrent chemotherapy and radiation therapy, as the risks may be additive and significant, depending on the drug, regimen, and radiation site.

Chemotherapy-induced nausea and vomiting

The emetogenic potential of chemotherapy agents is the most important risk factor for CINV, and moderately to *highly* emetogenic agents are most likely to induce acute and delayed CINV. Time to onset and duration of CINV vary greatly, but the most emetogenic drugs (e.g., cisplatin, mechlorethamine, dacarbazine, streptozocin) tend to have the shortest time to onset of emesis (less than 1 hour to a few hours).[26–28] While this schema regarding the emetogenicity potential of chemotherapy agents was adopted in 1997[26] and modified in 2004,[27] it is still widely accepted today. Acute CINV is arbitrarily considered to occur during the first 24 hours post-chemotherapy, after which delayed CINV starts and may persist for several days. Table 11-3 displays

TABLE 11-3

Emetogenic Risk Levels for Common Chemotherapy/Biotherapy Drugs

Chemotherapy	Minimal (<10%)	Low (10%–30%)	Moderate (30%–90%)	High (>90%)
Intravenous	Bevacizumab Bleomycin Bortezomib Cetuximab Fludarabine Rituximab Vinblastine Vincristine Vinorelbine	Docetaxel Doxorubicin (liposomal) Etoposide Fluorouracil Gemcitabine Ixabepilone Lapatinib Paclitaxel Pemetrexed Topotecan Trastuzumab	Azacitadine Carboplatin Cisplatin (<50 mg/m^2) Cyclophosphamide (≤1.5 g/m^2) Cytarabine (>200 mg/m^2) Daunorubicin Doxorubicin (≤60 mg/m^2) Ifosfamide Irinotecan Oxaliplatin	AC combination (with doxorubicin or epirubicin with cyclophosphamide) Carmustine Cisplatin (>50 mg/m^2) Cyclophosphamide (>1.5 g/m^2) Dacarbazine Mechlorethamine
Oral	Chlorambucil Erlotinib Gefitinib Hydroxyurea Methotrexate Thioguanine	Capecitabine Fludarabine	Cyclophosphamide Etoposide Imatinib Temozolomide	Procarbazine

Key:
Minimal emetogenic risk: <10% of patients will experience vomiting
Low emetogenic risk: 10%–30% of patients will experience vomiting
Moderate emetogenic risk: 30%–90% of patients will experience vomiting
High emetogenic risk: >90% of patients will experience vomiting

Source: Data from Hesketh et al[28]; NCCN[29]; Basch et al[30]; Roila et al[31].

emetogenic risk for common intravenous and oral chemotherapy drugs.[26–28] The table delineates the risk categories for emesis: minimal (<10%), low (10%–30%), moderate (30%–90%), and high (>90%), with commonly used chemotherapy and biotherapy drugs.

Radiation therapy–induced nausea and vomiting

Both TBI and RT to the upper abdomen or entire abdomen are considered highly emetogenic, whereas RT to the lower hemibody, thorax, and pelvis is moderately emetogenic.[2,3,19] Large-volume fields (more than 400 cm^2) that include upper abdominal tissues pose the greatest risk for RINV, which is estimated at 90% with hemibody RT to the upper and mid-abdomen, but only 15% with lower hemibody fields. Other documented risk factors include concomitant chemotherapy and previous experience with vomiting induced by chemotherapy. It has been observed that approximately one-third of radiotherapy patients experienced nausea and vomiting, with the vast majority not receiving antiemetic prescriptions for this problem.[2,3]

Post-anesthesia nausea and vomiting

Post-anesthesia nausea and vomiting (PONV) not only increases patient discomfort, but can also lead to wound dehiscence, bleeding, dehydration, electrolyte imbalance, prolonged hospital stays and, rarely, life-threatening aspiration. Risk factors are female gender, age, history of motion sickness, nonsmoking status, history of migraine headaches, and postoperative opioid administration.[32,33] PONV, if experienced once, is likely to happen on subsequent occasions. Cancer surgeries most commonly causing PONV include craniotomy, head and neck procedures (including thyroid), mastectomy or other major breast surgery, laparotomy, or laparoscopic procedure. A few studies have begun to examine the type of anesthesia and incidence of PONV, further evaluating its risks, benefits, and financial aspects.[32,33] Higher-risk anesthetic techniques include inhalation agents, nitrous oxide, and large-dose neostigmine. Of note, one study evaluated the use of paravertebral block (PVB) and PONV on post-operative pain. While there were similar PONV and post-operative pain scores in the PVB group and those without this intervention, there may be a role for this type of anesthesia in decreasing pain medication usage, which can also induce nausea and vomiting.[34]

Nausea and vomiting related to progressive disease

Factors related to N&V during progressive cancer are often multifactorial, involving chemical, GI, CNS, and other causes, and may be mediated via different pathways.[35] Chemical causes include emetogenic drugs (e.g., chemotherapy, opioid analgesics, nonsteroidal anti-inflammatory drugs [NSAIDs], anticonvulsants, antibiotics, digoxin, and anticholinergic agents). Emetogenic mechanisms vary, so a drug could act in the CTZ, induce serotonin release, irritate the GI tract, cause gastric stasis, or do more than one of these to induce N&V. Other chemical causes of N&V include hypercalcemia, hyperglycemia, hypocortisolism, hyponatremia, and renal or hepatic failure. The causes should be identified and treated accordingly.[36] Gastrointestinal and CNS causes may be due to tumor obstruction, impacting N&V from both the GI tract and brain influences.[36]

Patient factors

Gender is an important patient-related risk factor for N&V from therapy or disease. N&V is more frequent and often poorly controlled in menstruating women than in men. This gender effect may be related to hormone status and be interrelated with age. That is, persons younger than age 55 are at greater risk for severe acute CINV and ANV than older patients are, while older men and women have similar rates of CINV.[18,37,38] In addition to age, alcohol use and other factors may influence CINV risk. There is some evidence that patients who have heavy chronic alcohol intake have less CINV than nondrinkers. Other potential patient risk factors include severe N&V with previous life events (i.e., motion sickness, hyperemesis of pregnancy).[18,37] More recently, high anxiety levels, patient expectation and perceived susceptibility of N&V before therapy, and breast cancer have been identified as risk factors.[38,39]

Table 11-4 lists common risk factors for CINV, RINV, PONV, and other causes.[2,3,18,19,35–39] As noted in Table 11-4, risk factors such as female gender and younger age are applicable to all types of N&V. Risk factors such as dose of chemotherapy, schedule, and more rapid infusion rate may increase the potential risk for CINV. For RINV, radiation site, field size, dose and frequency are specific to this type of treatment. For PONV, the type of anesthetic and surgery are major factors. The use of volatile/inhalant anesthetics, nitrous oxide, and large-dose neostigmine are noted to be PONV risk factors.[33] For other causes such as advanced cancer, the risks often relate to chemical and metabolic disturbances, as well as obstructive disease. The additive effects of patient factors and emetogenic risk of the individual drugs and combinations need to be assessed thoroughly prior to chemotherapy and the antiemetic regimens need to be carefully planned, depending on disease state. Table 11-5 highlights common chemotherapy regimens and unique considerations due to disease and other risk factors.[35–39]

TABLE 11-4

Risk Factors for Chemotherapy-Induced Nausea and Vomiting (CINV), Radiation-Induced Nausea and Vomiting (RINV), Post-Anesthesia Nausea and Vomiting (PONV), and Other Causes

CINV
- Female gender
- Younger age (<55)
- History of CINV
- History of emesis with pregnancy
- History of motion sickness
- Low alcohol intake history
- Performance status
- Anxiety
- Pretreatment expectation of nausea
- Emetogenicity of chemotherapy drugs
- Dose, schedule, route, and rate of administration

RINV
- Female gender
- Younger age (<55)
- Low alcohol intake history
- History of RINV
- Concurrent chemotherapy
- Previous history of CINV
- Radiation site
- Field size
- Radiation dose and frequency

PONV
- Female gender
- Younger age (<50 years)
- History of PONV
- Nonsmoking status
- History of motion sickness
- History of migraines
- Anxiety
- Volatile anesthetics
- Inhalation agents, nitrous oxide, large-dose neostigmine
- Prolonged anesthesia and surgery
- Type of surgery
- Intra-, peri-, or post-operative opioids

Other Causes (i.e., Advanced Cancer)
- Younger age (less common >65 years)
- Female gender
- Low alcohol intake
- Chemical: concurrent chemotherapy, opioids, antibiotics, digoxin
- Metabolic: hypercalcemia and other electrolyte imbalance
- Obstructive/advanced disease: liver or brain metastases, obstructive uropathy, ascites, bowel obstruction
- Psychological: anxiety and pain

Source: Data from Enblom et al[2]; Maranzano et al[3]; Feyer et al[17]; Schwartzberg[19]; Bakshi et al[32]; Vari et al[33]; Shoemaker et al[35]; NCCN[36]; Thompson[37]; Roscoe et al[38]; Warr et al[39].

SELF-ASSESSMENT

Preferable tools for self-assessment would include assessments of nausea, vomiting, and retching, such as the Index of Nausea, Vomiting, and Retching (INVR),[40] an instrument designed to measure the frequency, severity, and distress of CINV. The MASCC Antiemesis Tool (MAT)[40] specifically measures frequency and severity of CINV both acutely (day 1) and on a delayed basis (days 2–4). One advantage of the MAT is that it is readily available online in several languages. The numeric rating scale (NRS)[41] is part of the MAT, and a visual analog scale can also be used to measure nausea.

Of note, the time when the self-assessment is completed may be critical to better understand the nausea and vomiting events, so as to best capture the timing of the occurrence, frequency, and severity.[41,42] If seen just prior to subsequent chemotherapy visits, patients may forget or minimize their reports, as they are feeling well and have recovered from the treatment-related symptoms.

OBJECTIVE ASSESSMENT

History

In addition to risk factors, it is important to collect baseline information about associated problems that could cause or result from N&V—including use of other medications (prescription and over the counter) and fluid volume status—and to link such information with physical and laboratory findings. For instance, a bowel history that focuses on constipation is particularly important for a patient taking opioid analgesics. If N&V is a current problem, questions regarding pattern (occurring before or after eating, infrequent large volume secondary to partial or complete bowel obstruction, movement related) and accompanying symptoms (heartburn, reflux, polyuria with hypercalcemia or hyperglycemia) are important. The nurse should also ask patients about strategies (drug and other) they found helpful and unhelpful for dealing with past episodes of N&V.

Physical assessment

The physical assessment for N&V focuses on possible causes identified by the history and risk profile assessment, particularly related to the GI system. It starts with examining the mouth for oral candidiasis, herpes, or other infection. A thorough abdominal assessment includes examining the abdominal contour for distention and auscultating bowel sounds in all four quadrants to discern partial or total small bowel obstruction. Palpation is also important to detect tenderness, hepatomegaly, severe splenomegaly, ascites, masses, or large feces in the colon.

Persistent vomiting, exacerbated by persistent nausea, can lead to fluid volume deficit (FVD), hypokalemia, and

TABLE 11-5

Common Moderately and Highly Emetogenic Regimens and Specific Cancer Types and Risk Factor Challenges

Cancer type	Regimen*	Risk Factor Challenges
Breast	AC, TAC, TC, TCH	• Female gender • Younger age <55 • Expectations, anxiety • Potential history with pregnancy associated emesis
Lung	Carbo-Taxol, Cis-Taxol, Cis-Vinorelbine, Cis-Gemcitabine, Cis-Pemetrexed, Cis-Etoposide	• Concurrent chemotherapy and radiation therapy • Multi-day regimens
Colorectal/ Gastrointestinal	FOLFOX, CapeOx, Irinotecan	• Concurrent chemotherapy and radiation therapy • Absorption issues with oral medications
Ovarian/Gynecologic	Carbo-Taxol, IP Cisplatin, Cisplatin	• Female gender • Younger age <55 • Expectations, anxiety • Potential history with pregnancy associated emesis • Intraperitoneal (IP): intra-abdominal treatment
Testicular	Cisplatin-based regimens	• Multi-day regimens • Younger age
Head and neck	Cispatin or Carboplatin-based regimens	• Concurrent chemotherapy and radiation therapy • Difficulty with nutrition, mucositis, and dry mouth

*AC: Doxorubicin + Cyclophosphamide
TAC: Docetaxel + Doxorubicin + Cyclophosphamide
TC: Docetaxel + Cyclophosphamide
TCH: Docetaxel + Carboplatin + Trastuzumab
Carbo-Taxol: Carboplatin + Paclitaxel
Cis-Taxol: Cisplatin + Paclitaxel
Cis-Vinorelbine: Cisplatin + Vinorelbine
Cis-Gemcitabine: Cisplatin + Gemcitabine
Cis-Pemetrexed: Cisplatin + Pemetrexed
Cis-Etoposide: Cisplatin + Etoposide
FOLFOX: Oxaliplatin + Leucovorin + Fluorouracil
CapeOx: Capecitabine + Oxaliplatin
IP Cisplatin: Intraperitoneal Cisplatin

Source: Data from Thompson[37]; Roscoe et al[38]; Warr et al[39].

metabolic alkalosis. Actual weight should be documented at baseline and before each course of chemotherapy to evaluate changes in fluid volume status (FVS). Rapid weight loss over a few days post therapy in a vomiting patient provides more accurate information about FVD than intake and output (I&O) or skin turgor.[40] Moisture or dryness between the gingiva and buccal mucosa can differentiate dryness caused by mouth breathing from FVD.[40] Postural hypotension may also occur with FVD, so heart rate (HR) *and* blood pressure (BP) should be checked in both the supine and sitting positions.

Diagnostic evaluation

Laboratory tests augment physical findings to confirm FVD and alkalosis, or to pinpoint other factors contributing to N&V. The ratio of blood urea nitrogen (BUN) to creatinine reflects the degree of dehydration. Other serum chemistries are often useful; creatinine reflects normal renal function or insufficiency, electrolytes may confirm hyponatremia or other electrolyte imbalances associated with N&V, and liver function tests (LFTs) reflect hepatic function. A flat plate radiograph of the abdomen (KUB) is indicated if obstruction or obstipation are suspected. Other visualization studies may be useful, depending upon the patient's clinical presentation.

DEGREES OF TOXICITY

A physician or nurse generally completes the Common Terminology Criteria for Adverse Events (CTCAE), which is used in cancer chemotherapy trials to define tolerable and safe doses, to evaluate toxicities, and to make dose changes for patients who experience adverse effects, including N&V (Table 11-6).[43] However, there are no data that

TABLE 11-6

National Cancer Institute Common Terminology Criteria for Adverse Events (CTCAE): Nausea and Vomiting

	1	2	3	4	5
Nausea	Loss of appetite without alteration in eating habits	Oral intake decreased without significant weight loss, dehydration, or malnutrition	Inadequate oral caloric or fluid intake; tube feeding, total parenteral nutrition (TPN), or hospitalization indicated	—	—
Vomiting	1–2 episodes (separated by 5 minutes) in 24 hours	3–5 episodes (separated by 5 minutes) in 24 hours	≥6 episodes (separated by 5 minutes) in 24 hours; tube feeding, TPN, or hospitalization indicated	Life-threatening consequences; urgent intervention indicated	Death

Definitions:
Nausea: A disorder characterized by a queasy sensation and/or urge to vomit.
Vomiting: A disorder characterized by the reflexive act of ejecting the contents of the stomach through the mouth.
Source: Data from National Cancer Institute Common Terminology Criteria for Adverse Events (CTCAE)[43].

substantiate the reliability, sensitivity, and validity of the CTCAE—that is, to show whether this grading system accurately reflects patients' perceptions regarding the severity and impact of nausea *and* vomiting.[44] Nurses' and physicians' ratings of patients' symptom severity and the relative importance of nausea and vomiting frequently do not agree with patient ratings, so while it is necessary to estimate and document CTCAE data, this does not replace patient self-report.[40] The CTCAE may be the most familiar to practicing nurses, and is commonly used in clinical research.

SYMPTOM MANAGEMENT STRATEGIES

The goal of antiemetic management is the prevention of N&V. Antiemetic medications are the mainstay of prevention and treatment, whether N&V is related to cancer therapy, disease, or other factors. Antiemetic selection should be evidence based—when there is adequate research—and be targeted toward the probable causes of N&V; the selected agent should have few adverse effects, be practical to administer, and be affordable. A growing body of data supports the use of complementary measures, which may be useful adjuncts to pharmacotherapy.

THERAPEUTIC APPROACHES

Pharmacologic management

Antiemetics are classified as $5HT_3$ receptor antagonists, NK_1 receptor antagonists, dopamine receptor antagonists, corticosteroids, cannabinoids, benzodiazepines, and others. No antiemetic in any class controls N&V all of the time in all patients, which illustrates our incomplete understanding of N&V and complicates its management.

$5HT_3$ receptor antagonists. Ondansetron, granisetron, and dolasetron are the first-generation $5HT_3$ receptor antagonists ($5HT_3$-RAs) currently available in the United States. $5HT_3$-RAs act primarily in the GI tract, but may have a lesser role in the CTZ, to block transmission of vomiting impulses to the VC.[18,22] Oral doses, if available, are equally or more efficacious than intravenous (IV) doses because $5HT_3$-RAs act in the GI tract, and either route prevents acute CINV in the majority of adults. Many of the $5HT_3$-RAs are available in multiple forms including IV, oral tablet, oral disintegrating tablet, oral disintegrating filmstrip, liquid, and transdermal patch formulations. Many of the $5HT_3$-RAs are superior to other antiemetics in preventing RINV after TBI or RT to the abdomen or pelvis,[2,3] as well as for PONV.[32–34] $5HT_3$-RAs may have some utility in N&V from other causes (e.g., gastric irritation, obstruction or distention, neurological problems, carcinoid syndrome, or uremia), but there is little research to support their use in such cases—probably because they are expensive and often cost prohibitive in palliative care. At present, little evidence is available to establish clear guidelines in this setting.[44]

$5HT_3$-RAs are not structurally identical, so their efficacy and adverse effects may vary among patients. Palonosetron is a second-generation $5HT_3$-RA with a longer half-life (approximately 40 hours), which also has a stronger binding affinity for the serotonin receptor.[22] Current data and guidelines now support the use of palonosetron for the prevention of N&V with moderately and highly emetogenic chemotherapy regimens, and its use is preferred in some guidelines.[29,30,45] $5HT_3$-RAs are metabolized in the liver by cytochrome p450 (CYP450) enzymes. There is variability in terms of which CYP450 enzymes metabolize particular $5HT_3$-RAs, and this might explain why patients who have inadequate antiemetic control with one $5HT_3$-RA may achieve better control with a second agent.[18]

The most common adverse effects associated with $5HT_3$-RAs are headache, constipation, lightheadedness, and sedation, which are less severe than side effects of other antiemetics. Constipation is related to slowed colonic transit and is more common when $5HT_3$-RAs are taken for several days. Infrequent side effects include dizziness, diarrhea (which may be related to cisplatin), tremor, anxiety, and cardiovascular (CV) effects.[18,22]

Dolasetron's packaging includes a warning about potential electrocardiogram changes, but this agent's CV effects were not evaluated in premarketing studies of other $5HT_3$-RAs. Subsequent research has found rare patients who experience clinically nonsignificant CV effects after $5HT_3$-RA administration.[23] Recently, however, dolasetron in the IV form was removed from the market due to increased incidence of cardiac arrhythmias noted with its use. Oral dolasetron continues to be available as an alternative in national guidelines.[22,29,30] Patients with cancer might be at risk for CV events by virtue of concomitant cardiac disease, dehydration, electrolyte imbalances, malnutrition, cardiotoxic chemotherapy, or use of other drugs with CV effects. The nurse should bear in mind that $5HT_3$-RA administration *may* increase the potential for CV problems in at-risk individuals.

NK_1 receptor antagonists. Antiemetic prophylaxis with an NK_1-RA is currently supported in the literature and recommended for patients receiving moderately and highly emetogenic chemotherapy.[29,30] The NK_1-RAs are helpful in preventing both acute and delayed N&V. Aprepitant and IV fosaprepitant are currently the only NK_1-RAs available. Aprepitant's recommended dosing is 3 days (125 mg on day 1, and 80 mg on days 2 and 3); it is included as part of a multidrug regimen, along with a $5HT_3$-RA and dexamethasone.[29,30] More recently, fosaprepitant has been introduced, and allows for a single IV dose. The IV dosing of fosaprepitant was deemed equivalent to the aprepitant oral 3-day dosing.[46] A large study has demonstrated improvement in control of acute and delayed CINV, particularly in women, with the use of fosaprepitant.[47]

Dopamine receptor antagonists. The dopamine receptor antagonists are now considered older antiemetics, and are primarily used for breakthrough N&V. Prior to the advent of the $5HT_3$ and NK_1-RAs, the dopamine receptor antagonists were the best available antiemetics. Now that the pathophysiology of N&V is better understood, they are rarely used in prophylaxis due to the minor role they play in receptor blockade.[18] Phenothiazines (e.g., prochlorperazine, chlorpromazine), butyrophenones (haloperidol), and substituted benzamides (metoclopramide) bind with dopamine (D_2) receptors in the CTZ and block emetic impulse transmission to the VC. The D_2 receptor antagonists (D_2-RAs) are effective for acute CINV after mildly emetogenic chemotherapy, delayed CINV, RINV after radiation to sites other than chest or abdomen, and N&V from other causes.[2,3] Prochlorperazine, the most widely used phenothiazine, is less sedating than chlorpromazine.[29] Haloperidol is chemically similar to phenothiazines and useful for the same indications; thus it may be useful when other antiemetics fail, or in antiemetic combinations for CINV, PONV, and N&V in terminal illness.

Antiemetic efficacy must outweigh adverse effects, particularly in palliative care. The D_2-RAs are not "clean" and bind, with varying degrees, to non-dopamine receptors—an action that results in enhanced antiemetic or adverse effects. For example, metoclopramide binds to D_2 receptors in the CNS, and to $5HT_3$ and $5HT_4$ receptors in the peripheral GI tract. On the one hand, agonist activity at $5HT_4$ receptors results in prokinesis (accelerated gastric emptying and small bowel transit), thereby decreasing N&V related to stasis. On the other hand, metoclopramide may cause diarrhea. Binding at other receptors can also cause adverse effects. Alpha$_1$-adrenergic (α_1) receptor binding may cause sedation, dizziness, and orthostasis, whereas histamine (H_1) receptor binding causes sedation and anticholinergic effects (e.g., dry mouth, constipation, nasal congestion).[14]

Any D_2-RA can trigger extrapyramidal symptoms (EPS)—most commonly akithesia and infrequently dystonia. Extrapyramidal symptoms are more common in children, young adults, and women than in older individuals and men, and with high-dose D_2-RAs (e.g., metoclopramide). Akithesia (dancing legs syndrome) ranges from a feeling of inner disquiet to an inability to sit still, while dystonia presents as torticollis or spasm of the lower jaw that causes a frightening sensation of breathlessness. Akithesia is managed with a benzodiazepine (e.g., lorazepam or diazepam), and dystonia is reversed with diphenhydramine 25–50 mg PO or IV or benztropine 1–2 mg IV. Agents used to reverse EPS are sedating and have anticholinergic effects, so patient safety must be a major concern when considering the duration of drug action.[23,48]

Corticosteroids. Dexamethasone, alone or in combination, is effective for acute and delayed CINV, RINV, PONV, and N&V related to progressive disease. Dexamethasone and $5HT_3$-RAs, when used to counteract the adverse effects of moderately and highly emetogenic chemotherapy, increases complete control of acute and delayed CINV by 15% to 20%.[29,30] The mechanism by which dexamethasone works to decrease N&V has yet to be elucidated, but this agent remains a cornerstone in antiemetic therapy.

There is no established optimal dose and schedule for dexamethasone, but single or multiple doses of 8–20 mg (IV or PO) are similarly effective for emesis (higher doses may be more effective for nausea).[29,30] Corticosteroids are nonsedating, and may increase appetite and enhance a sense of well-being; on the down side, they cause hiccups, insomnia, elevated blood glucose in diabetic patients, dysphoria, and insomnia. Rapid IV administration of dexamethasone causes perineal burning, tingling, or itching; thus the medication should be administered over several minutes. Preexisting diabetes should not be a contraindication to corticosteroid use; however, increased monitoring of blood sugar levels and treatment of hyperglycemia may be necessary.

Cannabinoids. Endogenous endocannabinoids bind to cannabinoid$_1$ receptors (CB_1) in many areas of the brain to affect a wide variety of neuroregulatory roles, which may explain the antiemetic effect of dronabinol and nabilone. Dronabinol is more effective than prochlorperazine or low-dose metoclopramide for mildly to moderately emetogenic chemotherapy.[18] However, it is not used as a first-line antiemetic for N&V from any cause because other antiemetics are equally or more effective and have fewer adverse effects. However, low doses of dronabinol may be useful in some instances of refractory N&V, such as in terminally ill patients with N&V from GI metastases.[14] Distressing adverse effects of cannabinoids can include depersonalization, drowsiness, dizziness, euphoria or dysphoria, loss of coordination, dry mouth, and postural hypotension, and are more common in elderly than young patients.[47] Caution should also be exercised in patients with a history of psychiatric illness. Other disadvantages of dronabinol and nabilone are formulation and prescription. Cannabinoids are classified as Schedule II drugs, meaning they are considered to have a high potential for abuse and physical or psychological dependence. In recent years, some states have adopted legislation to legalize the use of marijuana. Despite the society-imposed stigma on marijuana and tetrahydrocannabinol (THC), there is high interest in investigating other potential uses of these cannabinoids to relieve insomnia and pain, induce muscle relaxation, and elevate mood.

Benzodiazepines. Benzodiazepines have modest antiemetic effects at best and are used as adjuncts to other antiemetics.[18] Oral or parenteral lorazepam is most commonly used to decrease anxiety associated with chemotherapy administration, which may explain its value in minimizing acute N&V.[48] Sublingual lorazepam is absorbed through the oral mucosa, resulting in a rapid effect similar to IV dosing. Intravenous administration may induce perceptual disturbances, urinary incontinence, hypotension, and sedation. Intravenous lorazepam has frequently been on the drug shortage list, and healthcare providers need to plan accordingly when planning and ordering this antiemetic regimen. Benzodiazepines can cause respiratory depression and are to be administered cautiously to elderly or debilitated patients or to patients taking other CNS depressant drugs. Patients need to be cautioned on the sedating effect, and to plan accordingly for transportation if such drugs are administered intravenously with chemotherapy.

Other drugs. Drugs that bind to other receptors exert relatively modest antiemetic effects. These medications include drugs that bind to histamine receptors, including dimenhydrinate, diphenhydramine, hydroxyzine, and promethazine; as well as drugs that bind to muscarinic cholinergic (M) receptors, such as scopolamine. Such drugs are most commonly used for N&V related to vestibular and motion/position disorders, hepatic disease, opioid administration, and GI disturbances. Antihistamines and anticholinergic agents have similar side effects that include drowsiness, dry mouth, disorientation, dizziness, ataxia, constipation, and even N&V, which may be dose limiting or otherwise require management.[18]

Some evidence also suggests that olanzapine—an atypical antipsychotic agent with antidepressant effects—may significantly reduce nausea in patients with advanced cancer and breakthrough CINV; this drug has been studied in combination with other standard antiemetics.[49,50] Interestingly, olanzapine is a potent $5HT_3$-RA and also has effects at D_2 and other receptors. Possible side effects include sedation, weight gain, hyperglycemia, and diabetes.

Commonly used antiemetic agents used for CINV are listed in Table 11-7.[48,51,52]

CINV management

Several professional groups have published antiemetic management recommendations for CINV.[29–31] These recommendations are similar because they were developed by expert consensus panels that reviewed the research and categorized available data based on their strength. There are some differences in guidelines—for example, related to the number of chemotherapy risk categories, the agents included in each risk level, and whether chemotherapy doses are considered to influence emetogenicity. Antiemetic guidelines are intended to help clinicians make reasonable antiemetic choices, but lengthy publications are not practical in clinical settings and are probably not widely used. Thus practitioners may continue to prescribe less desirable antiemetics, and over- or under-prescribe appropriate antiemetics.[53–57]

The newest guideline categorizes chemotherapy drugs by risk for CINV as high (>90% risk), moderate (30%–90% risk), low (10%–30% risk), or minimal (<10% risk); in this guideline, emetogenic risk is the basis for antiemetics on the day of chemotherapy (Figure 11-3)[48,51,52] and days following.[29,48,58] Antiemetic guidelines do not consider gender or other variable patient risks, and guideline authors stress that clinicians should consider these factors when selecting antiemetic medications. Furthermore, combination chemotherapy regimens are probably more emetogenic than each single agent, and this may need to be considered in planning antiemetic therapy.

TABLE 11-7

Commonly Used Antiemetic Agents for the Treatent of Chemotherapy-Induced Nausea and Vomiting

Class/Drugs	Dosage Forms	Issues
	$5HT_3$ Receptor Antagonists	
• Ondansetron	PO (tablet, oral disintegrating tablet, film strip, liquid), IV	• Variety of routes • Cost, some have generic formulations • Common side effects are headache and constipation
• Granisetron	PO, IV, transdermal patch	
• Dolasetron	PO	
• Palonosetron	IV	
	NK-1 Receptor Antagonists	
• Aprepitant	PO tri-pack	• Access: Cost for oral formulation • Common side effects are fatigue, hiccups, constipation, headache
• Fosaprepitant	IV	
	Corticosteroids	
• Dexamethasone	PO, IV	• Side effects are increased energy, mood swings, insomnia, heartburn, elevated blood sugar
	Dopamine Receptor Antagonists	
• Metoclopramide	IV, PO, R	• Side effects include sedation, agitation, restlessness, orthostatic hypotension, extrapyramidal symptoms
• Prochlorperazine	PO, IV, IM, R	
• Haloperidol	PO, IM	
	Benzodiazepines	
• Lorazepam	PO, IV, IM	• Side effects include sedation • Driving may be an issue

Abbreviations: PO: oral; IV: intravenous; IM: intramuscular; R: rectal.

Source: Data from Polovich et al[48]; Bragalone[51]; Wilkes and Barton-Burke[52].

Many of the available recommendations apply to single-day chemotherapy regimens, so these definitions and guidelines may not be applicable to multiday regimens. While the recommendations differ somewhat between guidelines, the challenge of managing multiday chemotherapy is being examined.[29,31,48,59] Although there is agreement regarding the use of $5HT_3$-RAs, dexamethasone, and NK_1-RAs, few data have been published regarding the use of repeating doses of palonosetron and aprepitant. The National Comprehensive Cancer Network (NCCN) Guidelines do provide additional information, recognizing the safety issues and the need for antiemetic coverage for a considerably longer period of time.[29]

Another area characterized by scant data is high-dose chemotherapy with stem cell transplantation. Many of the regimens used in stem cell transplantation are considered highly emetogenic, and the antiemetic agents recommended are a combined modality.[30,59] This is also a setting where complementary strategies are being studied.

Oral chemotherapy agents are being increasingly utilized in the oncology setting: 25%–30% of new drugs in development are oral drugs.[60] The risk of emetogenicity of the individual drug, along with assessment of other patient risk factors, should be evaluated when such agents are used. Risk stratification and antiemetic recommendations for oral chemotherapy agents have been added to the NCCN guidelines.[29] Oral chemotherapy drugs are costly, have side effects, and require adequate antiemetic therapy. Food and drug interactions may impact the effectiveness of therapy; therefore, collaboration of pharmacy and nursing personnel is important in identifying these interactions, as is education of patients/families.[61] Increased education and use of calendars may be helpful in successful administration of oral agents.

The topic of adherence to outpatient antiemetic regimens is an area of recent study. In high-risk patients receiving moderately or highly emetogenic chemotherapy, adherence to the antiemetics used for delayed N&V can

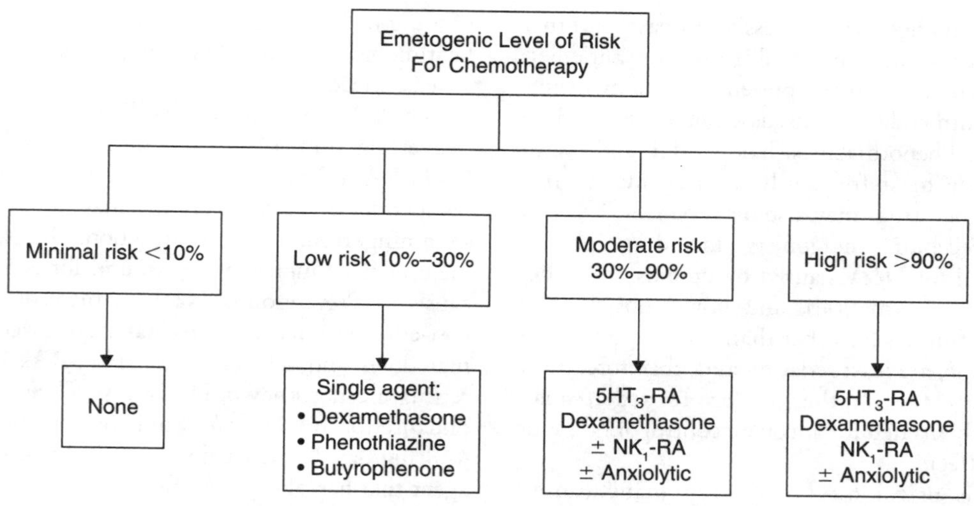

FIGURE 11-3

Antiemetic treatment options for acute chemotherapy risk.

Abbreviations: $5HT_3$ RA: Serotonin$_3$-receptor antagonist; NK_1-RA: Neurokinin 1-receptor antagonist.

Source: Data from Polovich et al[48]; Bragalone[51]; Wilkes[52].

be extremely important to minimize CINV. One study found that 42% of patients with breast cancer receiving anthracycline-based therapy were nonadherent with the dose administration of antiemetics as recommended.[62] The nonadherent behaviors were more common in patients who had higher educational levels, greater alcohol consumption, and prior exposure to other chemotherapy regimens. Further research should be done, focusing on evaluating the reasons for nonadherence to prescribed antiemetics and implementing interventions to improve adherence.[62]

Few data have been published regarding use of second-line antiemetics when first-line antiemetics, particularly a $5HT_3$-RA, are ineffective or cause distressing side effects. However, some patients achieve superior antiemetic control with a second $5HT_3$-RA, so it would seem prudent to administer this therapy before turning to other antiemetics having more adverse effects.[18,63,64] Similarly, patients who experience either poorly controlled N&V or objectionable side effects with other antiemetics should be changed to a $5HT_3$-RA regimen. There is no advantage in using $5HT_3$-RAs on an as-needed basis, when compared to older, more inexpensive drugs such as metoclopramide.[63–67] The benefits and side effects must be taken into consideration when selecting antiemetic agents for individual patients.

RINV management

The currently available guidelines recommend that patients at high risk for RINV (e.g., those patients receiving TBI, hemibody RT, or RT to the upper abdomen) receive an oral $5HT_3$-RA prophylactically, but few include specific suggestions for doses and schedules.[21,29] Alternatively, small doses of dexamethasone (2 mg PO TID) may be as effective as a $5HT_3$-RA to prevent RINV in patients at moderate to high risk, and the combination a $5HT_3$-RA and dexamethasone may represent a superior regimen.[35] The recommended antiemetics to be given before each fraction of moderately emetogenic RT (e.g., thorax, pelvis, lower hemibody) include a $5HT_3$-RA or a D_2-RA (prochlorperazine, metoclopramide, thiethylperazine). Recommended antiemetics for RINV associated with low-risk RT (e.g., head and neck, extremities, or skin) are somewhat controversial and vary in the literature.[17,27,29,31]

PONV management

Published guidelines exist for PONV, but a significant body of literature supports using single or combination antiemetics (e.g., $5HT_3$-RA, droperidol, phenothiazine, or a corticosteroid) for patients at high risk for PONV (i.e., female: male risk is 3:1, previous PONV, surgery associated with PONV, obesity, a history of motion sickness).[68–70] Furthermore, $5HT_3$-RAs and corticosteroids offer advantages relative to older antiemetics in that they cause fewer and less bothersome adverse effects, such as sedation.

Management of nausea arising from other causes

There is little research regarding N&V from other causes, and management is largely based on empirical experiences reported in the hospice and palliative care literature. Antiemetic management in these situations is often challenging because the exact causes of N&V are not clear, and interventions often must be directed toward more than one cause. In addition, there are no "standard" doses or schedules of antiemetics for progressive disease or other causes. Guidelines cannot be established for antiemetics in advanced cancer, with the present level of evidence. Many of the recommendations discussed here are based on limited literature. Phenothiazines, haloperidol, and metoclopramide are the most frequently used agents for this indication, but other drugs may also be of benefit.[71,72]

Dopamine receptor antagonists including phenothizines are useful for N&V caused by opioids and other drugs, metabolic abnormalities, and bowel obstruction. Drugs with low affinities for other than D_2 receptors, such as prochlorperazine, are least sedating and, therefore, most useful for N&V.[14,20,45] Phenothiazines are started at small doses and carefully titrated for adequate control of N&V or intolerable side effects.

Haloperidol is useful for N&V from many causes, such as opioid-induced effects, or related to other drugs or metabolic abnormalities. Haloperidol has a long half-life, and low doses are less sedating than most phenothiazines (doses greater than 5 mg may cause dose-limiting sedation or EPS).[45] Haloperidol is not excreted by the kidney and is safe for patients with renal failure, as well as for elderly individuals in whom N&V may be controlled with small doses (e.g., 1 mg PO every 12 hours).

Metoclopramide—the only currently available prokinetic agent—may be useful for N&V related to gastric stasis or irritation, incomplete or high GI obstruction, or unexplained chronic nausea.[51,52] Its oral administration is appropriate to prevent N&V, while rectal and parenteral administration are reserved for patients unable to take oral medications because of uncontrolled N&V or altered mental status. Metoclopramide accelerates gastric emptying and can increase colicky pain and should not be administered to patients with complete obstruction or obstipation.

Other antiemetics, including corticosteroids, dronabinol, and $5HT_3$-RAs, may be indicated for some instances of N&V. Olanzapine and related drugs may be effective broad-spectrum antiemetics used to concomitantly alleviate other symptoms such as sleeplessness and weight loss. Additionally, antihistamines, anticholinergic agents, octreotide, and benzodiazepines may be useful in treating increased secretions, diarrhea, and anxiety.

Varying doses of corticosteroids are recommended for N&V. Although they have some potential to irritate the stomach, the potent anti-inflammatory effect of corticosteroids means they may be useful for N&V related to increased intracranial pressure (ICP), GI obstruction, or biochemical problems (e.g., hypercalcemia, uremia).[45]

Dronabinol is infrequently used, but may be beneficial alone or with a phenothiazine to control intractable N&V from GI mucosal metastases.[14] Dronabinol may also stimulate appetite and alleviate neuropathic pain, but can lead to psychoactive side effects (i.e., euphoria in young patients and dysphoria in the elderly). This agent is started at low doses (2.5 mg or 5 mg PO every 6 hours, or before meals and at bedtime) and is carefully titrated to maximal therapeutic or adverse effect.

The $5HT_3$-RAs are not first-line antiemetics in the palliative setting, primarily because of direct drug costs. However, $5HT_3$-RAs (alone or in combination with other drugs, such haloperidol or dexamethasone) may be effective for N&V stemming from bowel obstruction, drugs, uremia, CNS metastases or injury, or sepsis, and for N&V of unknown cause.[72,73] Prevention of N&V in these instances would be cost-effective if repeated hospitalizations were avoided. Optimal doses and schedules for $5HT_3$-RAs in the palliative setting are not known, but in a small number of patients, ondansetron 16–24 mg/day did not seem more effective than 4–8 mg/day.[14] Smaller doses would be less costly (another agent that has $5HT_3$-RA effects may be a practical alternative) and less likely to induce adverse effects, particularly constipation and dizziness. Nausea and vomiting not mediated by $5HT_3$ receptor binding, such as opioid-related N&V and motion sickness, will not be controlled with a $5HT_3$-RA.[14]

Olanzapine and mirtazapine have effects at $5HT_3$ and other serotonin receptors, D_2 and other dopamine receptors, as well as $alpha_1$, histaminergic, and muscarinic cholinergic receptors. Neither of these agents causes EPS, and both may be superior alternatives to prochlorperazine and haloperidol.[36,71] Olanzapine (5 mg or 10 mg) and mirtazapine (15 mg or 30 mg) may decrease nausea and vomiting, as well as decrease other distressing symptoms associated with progressive disease (e.g., anorexia, weight loss, pain, diarrhea, mood, insomnia, depression, anxiety). These agents require further study, but may be less expensive alternatives to usual $5HT_3$-RAs.

Antihistamines and anticholinergic agents have limited usefulness for N&V related to motion, GI obstruction, and increased intracranial pressure. Antihistamines include diphenhydramine, meclizine, promethazine, and hydroxyzine; anticholinergic agents include hyoscyamine, scopolamine, and glycopyrrolate. Glycopyrrolate has little CNS penetration (and less sedation) and is occasionally used for N&V associated with colicky pain from GI obstruction. Other antihistamines and anticholinergics are used for similar situations, but are more sedating and cause anticholinergic side effects. Octreotide decreases GI secretions, N&V, and abdominal cramping from malignant bowel obstruction.[14] When a patient is close to dying, other interventions that increase N&V (IV fluids) should be discontinued, but oral fluids should be allowed to maintain patient comfort.

Benzodiazepines are not antiemetics, but lorazepam or alprazolam may decrease anxiety that exacerbates N&V. There are no clear dose recommendations for use of these medications in terminal care, but initial doses should be small (lorazepam 0.5 mg–2 mg PO or IV every 6–8 hours) and doses titrated cautiously because lorazepam may be very sedating.

Combination antiemetic regimens may be more effective than single drugs, particularly for patients with N&V secondary to malignant involvement of abdominal structures (e.g., stomach, pancreas, colon, rectum, ovary, uterus, gallbladder). For instance, the use of a combination antiemetic cocktail is effective when used as first-line therapy (metoclopramide, diphenhydramine, dexamethasone) with greatly enhanced control of N&V.[74] Furthermore, patients who took combination antiemetics did not have more adverse effects than patients who took single antiemetics.[74] Table 11-8 lists selected agents that may be used for RINV, PONV, or nausea of other causes (e.g., advanced cancer).[45,69,71,72]

Nonpharmacologic interventions

Complementary measures. Complementary measures, such as behavioral interventions, massage, music or art therapy, acupressure or acupuncture, and dietary modifications, may enhance antiemetic efficacy and should be considered as useful adjuncts to pharmacologic interventions. Some complementary measures are evidence-based, inexpensive, nontoxic, and pleasant, and can be self-administered. Nurses, physicians, social workers, psychologists, or others can teach patients relaxation techniques, such as guided imagery and passive muscle relaxation (PMR), and assist patients to gain a greater sense of self-control. These techniques are used more often than other behavioral interventions (systematic desensitization and attentional distraction) that require a trained therapist or psychologist to provide instruction. Behavioral interventions have been successful for some cases of ANV, but are ineffective for acute and delayed CINV.[48]

Needle acupuncture of the P6 (Neiguan) point is used in traditional Chinese medicine to decrease N&V. A growing body of data indicates that this therapy alleviates acute nausea, but not delayed nausea and vomiting.[75,76] This knowledge has led to the use of transcutaneous manual acupuncture and electroacupuncture, which are sometimes helpful in enhancing control of CINV (when used with antiemetics including $5HT_3$-RAs), PONV, and motion sickness.[75,76] The P6 point is located on the inner wrist about three fingerbreadths above the skin crease of the wrist, between the tendons of the palmaris longus and flexor carpi radialis. Acupressure bands are inexpensive, adjustable elastic wristbands that have a rounded stud that is positioned over the P6 point of the dominant wrist or both wrists. Data on the use of these acupressure bands have been mixed; thus the effectiveness of the intervention has not yet been established.[41,77]

General comfort measures and individualized dietary modifications may also be useful adjuncts. One strategy is to encourage patients to use interventions that were helpful for N&V with pregnancy, with illness, or during stressful periods. Altering food preparation and eating may also be helpful, such as preparing and freezing meals for later use between cycles when chemotherapy-related nausea is not a problem, or having family members cook meals. Other helpful tips include keeping the mouth clean and moist, consuming small and frequent meals, taking a glass of wine with meals, and eating cold or room-temperature foods that give off fewer odors than hot foods. Foods to avoid when N&V is anticipated include fatty foods, which delay gastric emptying, and spicy, salty, and sweet foods, which may exacerbate N&V. Many of these interventions are based on expert opinion, rather than randomized, controlled trials.[41]

Herbal remedies, most notably ginger, are sometimes used to decrease N&V. Doses of 500 mg–1000 mg (standardized doses should be used) of ginger may decrease N&V (several components of ginger are antagonists at $5HT_3$ receptors).[77–79] Ginger is most often used for motion sickness and morning sickness, but may be beneficial for patients with cancer. The data from studies on ginger for CINV have been mixed; therefore, the effectiveness of this therapy has not yet been established. While ginger produces little in the way of detrimental effects, the dosing and regulation of this substance have not been standardized.[41,77–79]

Structured education by nurses may not yet be supported by a wealth of evidence, but it is drawing attention, study, and acceptance in promoting self-care and improved patient outcomes. Due to time constraints, shorter counseling sessions with tailored information should continue in the ambulatory setting. Further research is needed to better understand the impact of the information, patient expectations, and overall symptom assessments.[80]

Many patients with cancer use complementary and alternative medicine (CAM) to enhance antitumor effects and to increase comfort and control and, therefore, may appreciate information and tips about CAM therapies that might be helpful antiemetic adjuncts. Helping patients undergoing chemotherapy to learn relaxation or distraction therapies may decrease their ANV, but may be burdensome and ineffective for patients who have progressive disease. In contrast, patients may find acupressure, ginger or other herbs, or dietary modifications to be helpful at various times throughout the cancer experience.[81–83]

NURSING IMPLICATIONS

The control of CINV and RINV has improved with optimal use of $5HT_3$-RAs, but some nurses and physicians incorrectly assume that $5HT_3$-RA regimens effectively control every individual instance of N&V and, therefore, that N&V is no longer a problem. In reality, all patients must be considered at risk for N&V—even when they receive

TABLE 11-8

Selected Antiemetic Agents for Radiation-Induced Nausea and Vomiting (RINV), Post-Anesthesia-Induced Nausea and Vomiting (PONV), and Nausea Due to Other Causes

Classification	Use	Issues
	Phenothiazines	
• Prochlorperazine	• RINV (low risk) • PONV (low risk) • Advanced cancer	May be sedating, may cause extrapyramidal symptoms (EPS)
	Butyrophenones	
• Haloperidol	• RINV • PONV • Advanced cancer	Less sedating than phenothiazines
	Benzamides	
• Metoclopramide	• RINV • PONV • Advanced cancer	May be helpful for gastrointestinal (GI) motility May cause EPS
	Corticosteroids	
• Dexamethasone	• RINV (high risk) • PONV • Advanced cancer	May increase appetite and mood, may cause insomnia Caution with rapid intravenous infusion due to perineal burning
	Antihistamines	
• Promethazine • Diphenhydramine	• PONV • Advanced cancer	Confusion, drying of mucosal membrances, sedation, urinary retention
	Serotonin Antagonists	
• Ondansetron • Granisetron	• RINV (moderate risk) • PONV (moderate risk) • Advanced cancer	Constipation and headache common Cost may be a deterrent in palliative care, not usually first line
	Cannabinoids	
• Dronabinol	• Advanced cancer	Not a first line drug, sedating
	Benzodiazepines	
• Lorazepam	• RINV • Advanced cancer	Sedating, may cause disorientation in elderly (anxiety, claustrophobia)
	Other	
• NK-1 antagonists • Olanzapine • Mirtazapine	• PONV • Advanced cancer • Advanced cancer	May increase appetite and weight gain, may cause sedation

Source: Data from Davis et al[45]; Ignoffo[69]; Hamling[71]; Laugsand et al[72]; Jimenez et al[73].

"optimal" antiemetics. Ongoing assessments are essential to making timely changes in suboptimal antiemetics. For example, when a patient is receiving any new, moderately to highly emetogenic chemotherapy regimen, the nurse should coordinate a telephone follow-up on day 2 or 3 post treatment to assess the patient for delayed CINV and antiemetic side effects. A brief diary completed for several days after chemotherapy (or during RT) is another valid way to evaluate an antiemetic regimen and captures the patient's perceptions about vomiting and nausea (intensity and duration), symptom effects on ADLs and QOL, and antiemetic acceptability.

Nursing assessment of the patient who is vomiting includes the number of emeses, ability to drink fluids, thirst, concentrated urine, and rapid weight loss. The character of the vomitus may provide clues about its etiology; stomach contents may be identifiable as food, medication, bile, or blood (coffee grounds), while distal ileum obstruction may lead to brown, fecal-smelling emesis. Telephone triage is critically important in identifying those patients who are need of more emergent care, and in intervening with those patients who can improve with education and encouragement.

CONSIDERATION OF VULNERABLE POPULATIONS

Many individuals in our aging population will develop cancer over the course of a lifetime. Increasing numbers of elderly patients are receiving treatment for cancer, and will consequently need attention to side effects of therapy. The elderly population poses additional risk factors such as increased risk for constipation, electrolyte disturbances, and anorexia.[84,85] Treatment of the elderly may also be complicated by the presence of multiple comorbidities, which may impact morbidity and tolerance of therapy. With increasing age, many patients may already be taking multiple medications. The use of multidrug regimens is made more complex by tolerance of additional medications, drug–drug interactions, understanding of new medications, and cost.[84,85] Adherence to medication regimens among the elderly can be an issue owing to the various risk factors, such as dementia, impairments in vision and dexterity, and social isolation that could come into play. Individual assessment of the elderly patient and detailed attention to the issues discussed are paramount to managing a patient on cancer treatment. The unique issues of the elderly (Table 11-9) pose a major concern for the future.[84,85]

Medically underserved groups, including low-income populations and minorities, are more likely to be undertreated for symptoms related to breast cancer treatment. One study suggested that resolution of symptoms can be improved by better patient–physician communication. In addition, perceived patient self-efficacy in communicating with physicians and physician awareness may help in resolving nausea. Increasing cultural competence and appropriate educational interventions are potential strategies to improve treatment-related symptoms and improve overall quality of life.[86] It has also been reported that patients and providers have differences of opinion regarding barriers to managing CINV, with providers noting financial and patient-related barriers as the most common, yet patients rarely noting cost as a barrier but instead endorsing the stoic philosophy and the desire to be strong and to not complain.[87] Addressing misconceptions and establishing mutually consistent goals will lead to better care.

The distressing side effect of N&V has been well documented. With improvements in pharmacologic strategies and increasing attention to complementary strategies, strides in reducing CINV have been made. One of the most recent studies on patient perceptions of the side effects of cancer therapy shows change on the horizon. Fatigue and psychosocial QOL concerns (such as effect on partner and hair loss) were predominant, compared to emesis and nausea in previous surveys.[88] While this study's findings hold promise, attention to individual patients, risk factors, and specific diagnosis-related challenges must continue. Further work is being done to develop more predictive tools to assess risk for both acute and delayed nausea and vomiting. While many risk factors have been documented, no real standardized method of assigning risk to individual patients has emerged. Current validation studies show accuracy in identifying patients at high risk of N&V, with the final task of demonstrating that risk-model antiemetic therapy improves overall nausea and vomiting control. If widely accepted, this type of tool would be relatively easy to use in the oncology setting.[89] It would also be a helpful adjunct to clinical guidelines. In addition, some data suggest that individuals may be at greater risk of developing side effects due to high absorption—a concept that relates to greater risk for anxiety, more reactive physiological reactions, and side effects such as nausea and vomiting. Identifying individuals who may be more physiologically reactive to stressful situations may lead to more effective interventions.[90] There may be differences among patients who are newly diagnosed versus those who have recurrent disease, and among those who are married versus those who are unmarried.[91] Understanding the perception of side effects and their distress among other social and emotional variables will be an ongoing assessment over time individual patients.

FUTURE RESEARCH

With progress comes a continued need for quality improvement. Upon review of the current antiemetic guidelines in 2009 by the Multinational Association for Supportive Care (MASCC), several directions for further research in antiemetic therapy were identified. Better capabilities in predicting nausea and vomiting may be achieved by

TABLE 11-9

Issues in the Management of Nausea and Vomiting in the Elderly

Elderly Issue	Further Consideration
Chemotherapy-related risk factors	Specific drug, combination regimens, often given lower doses, risk for neutropenic complications and potential need for white blood cell growth factors
Patient-related risk factors	Female gender
	Previous chemotherapy-induced nausea and vomiting (CINV)
	Alcohol intake
	Anxiety
	Expectation of nausea
	Emesis during pregnancy
	Motion sickness
	Constipation risk
	Electrolyte disturbance risk
Co-morbidities	Consideration for hypertension, heart disease, chronic obstructive pulmonary disease, arthritis, diabetes, renal and hepatic disease
Poly-pharmacy	Number of medications combined with renal and liver function decline may result in increased drug-drug interactions and side effects
	Nausea due to increased number of pills
	Complex medication schedules
	Cost of medications
Adherence and compliance with medications	With increasing number of medications prescribed, many are not taken properly
	Dementia, impaired vision, dexterity, and social isolation may be risk factors affecting adherence and compliance
Physiology in the elderly	Oral absorption of drugs may be delayed
	Liver function decline
	Renal function decline
	Diminished bone marrow reserves

Source: Data from Jakobsen et al[84].

combining algorithms based on patient prognostic factors and the chemotherapy agents. The current risk stratification does not include nausea. With further research in pharmacogenetics, the potential for the identification of genes that code for specific receptors may assist with prediction of emesis, selection of antiemetic agents, and identification of optimal dosages for individual patients. The measurement of QOL and more global assessments of well-being should be incorporated into clinical trials to balance the efficacy of the agents with the toxicity of the antiemetic medication. In the future, it may be possible to include other functional endpoints in studies, such as effective blockade of receptors as demonstrated by PET scan. In a cost-conscious society, economic endpoints should also be included in studies of new antiemetics and combinations. The therapeutic index—that is, minimal effective dosing and scheduling of antiemetics—needs to be examined in conjunction with the therapy's cost-efficacy. Other populations for whom there is still a need for evidence include patients receiving high-dose chemotherapy, those receiving multiple-day chemotherapy, pediatric populations, the elderly, and patients receiving concomitant chemotherapy and radiation therapy. While the emphasis has traditionally been on pharmacologic therapy, data on nonpharmacologic therapy are still needed to better understand its role and improvement in management of N&V. Further study of clinical guidelines, efficacy of dissemination, and implementation is needed to better realize the benefits of the guidelines in patient care. Lastly, the potential of new antiemetic agents with new and different receptors needs to be studied as our understanding of the pathophysiology of nausea and vomiting continues to improve.[92]

PATIENT SELF-CARE

An important role of the oncology nurse is to teach patients and families self-care measures for N&V. Self-care guides for CINV, RINV, and N&V from cancer or other diseases are included in Appendix 11A Self Care Guide for Nausea and Vomiting from Chemotherapy, Appendix 11B Self Care Guide for Nausea and Vomiting from Radiation Therapy, and Appendix 11C, Self Care Guide for Nausea and Vomiting from Cancer and other Causes.[93]

REFERENCES

1. Salsman JM, Grunberg SM, Beaumont JL, et al. Communicating about chemotherapy-induced nausea and vomiting: a comparison of patient and provider perspectives. *J Natl Compr Canc Netw.* 2012;10:149–157.
2. Enblom A, Bergius Axelsson B, Steineck G, et al. One third of patients with radiotherapy-induced nausea consider their antiemetic treatment insufficient. *Support Care Cancer.* 2009;17:23–32.
3. Maranzano E, De Angelis V, Pergolizzi S, et al. A prospective observational trial on emesis in radiotherapy: analysis of 1020 patients recruited in 45 Italian radiation oncology treatment centres. *Radiother Oncol.* 2009;94:36–41.
4. Kurtin SE. Chemotherapy-induced nausea and vomiting: clinical updates. *Oncol Pharmacist.* 2010;3:44–45.
5. Viale PH, Grande C, Moore S. Efficacy and cost: avoiding undertreatment of chemotherapy-induced nausea and vomiting. *Clin J Oncol Nurs.* 2012;16:E133–E141.
6. Hesketh PJ. Penny wise, dollar foolish approach to antiemetic use may compromise patient care. *J Oncol Pract.* 2009;5:221–222.
7. Herrstedt J. Antiemetics: an update and the MASCC guidelines applied in clinical practice. *Nat Clin Pract Oncol.* 2008;5:32–43.
8. Bloechi-Daum B, Deuson RR, Mavros P, et al. Delayed nausea and vomiting continue to reduce patients' quality of life after highly and moderately emetogenic chemotherapy despite antiemetic treatment. *J Clin Oncol.* 2006;24:4472–4478.
9. Farrell C, Brearley SG, Pilling M, et al. The impact of chemotherapy-related nausea on patients' nutritional status, psychological distress, and quality of life. *Support Care Cancer.* 2013;21(1):59–66.
10. Tina Shih YC, Xu Y, Elting LS. Costs of uncontrolled chemotherapy-induced nausea and vomiting among working-age cancer patients receiving highly or moderately emetogenic chemotherapy. *Cancer.* 2007;110:678–685.
11. Burke TA, Wisniewski T, Ernst FR. Resource utilization and costs associated with chemotherapy-induced nausea and vomiting (CINV) following highly or moderately emetogenic chemotherapy administered in the US outpatient hospital setting. *Support Care Cancer.* 2011;19:131–140.
12. Craver C, Gayle J, Balu S, et al. Clinical and economic burden of chemotherapy-induced nausea and vomiting among patients with cancer in a hospital outpatient setting in the United States. *J Med Econ.* 2011;14:87–98.
13. Haiderali A, Meditto L, Good M, et al. Impact on daily functioning and indirect/direct costs associated with chemotherapy-induced nausea and vomiting (CINV) in a US population. *Support Care Cancer.* 2011;19:843–851.
14. Glare P, Miller J, Nikolova T, et al. Treating nausea and vomiting in palliative care: a review. *Clin Int Aging.* 2011;6:243–259.
15. Molassiotis A, Farrell C, Bourne K, et al. An exploratory study to clarify the cluster of symptoms predictive of chemotherapy-related nausea using random forest modeling. *J Pain Symptom Manage.* 2012; 44(5):692–703.
16. Hawkins R, Grunberg S. Chemotherapy-induced nausea and vomiting: challenges and opportunities for improved patient outcomes. *Clin J Oncol Nurs.* 2009;13:54–64.
17. Feyer PC, Maranzano E, Molassiotis A, et al. Radiotherapy-induced nausea and vomiting (RINV): MASCC/ESMO guideline for antiemetics in radiotherapy: update 2009. *Support Care Cancer.* 2011;19(suppl 1):S5–S14.
18. Jordan K, Sippel C, Schmoll HJ. Guidelines for antiemetic treatment of chemotherapy-induced nausea and vomiting: past, present, and future recommendations. *Oncologist.* 2007;12:1143–1150.
19. Schwartzberg L. Chemotherapy-induced nausea and vomiting: state of the art in 2006. *J Support Oncol.* 2006;4(suppl 1):3–8.
20. Dy SM, Apostol CC. Evidence-based approaches to other symptoms in advanced cancer. *Cancer J.* 2010;16:507–513.
21. Sanger GJ, Andrews PL. Treatment of nausea and vomiting: gaps in our knowledge. *Auton Neurosci.* 2006;129:3–16.
22. Bayo J, Fonseca PJ, Hernando S, et al. Chemotherapy-induced nausea and vomiting: pathophysiology and therapeutic principles. *Clin Transl Oncol.* 2012;14:413–422.
23. Oncology Nursing Society. Proposed chemotherapy-induced nausea and vomiting (CINV) pathways. Slide from CINV Regional Oncology Nursing Society (ONS) program, Pittsburgh PA 2006.
24. Trigg ME, Higa GM. Chemotherapy-induced nausea and vomiting: antiemetic trials that impacted clinical practice. *J Oncol Pharm Pract.* 2010;16:233–244.
25. Darmani NA, Crim JL, Janoyan JJ, et al. A re-evaluation of the neurotransmitter basis of chemotherapy-induced immediate and delayed vomiting: evidence from the least shrew. *Brain Res.* 2009;1248:40–58.
26. Hesketh J, Kris MG, Grunberg SM, et al. Proposal for classifying the acute emetogenicity of cancer chemotherapy. *J Clin Oncol.* 1997;15:103–109.
27. Roila F, Hesketh PJ, Herrstedt J, et al. Prevention of chemotherapy and radio-therapy-induced emesis: results of the 2004 Perugia International Antiemetic Consensus Conference. *Ann Oncol.* 2004;17:20–28.
28. Hesketh PJ. Chemotherapy-induced nausea and vomiting. *N Engl J Med.* 2008;358:2482–2494.
29. National Comprehensive Cancer Network. Clinical practice guidelines in oncology: antiemesis [v. 1.2012]. http://www.nccn.org/professionals /physician_gls/pdf/antiemesis.pdf.
30. Basch E, Prestrud AA, Hesketh PJ, et al. Antiemetics: American Society of Clinical Oncology clinical practice guideline update. *J Clin Oncol.* 2011;29:4189–4198.
31. Roila R, Herrstedt J, Aapro M, et al. Guideline update for MASCC and ESMO in the prevention of chemotherapy and radiotherapy-induced nausea and vomiting: results of the Perugia consensus conference. *Ann Oncol.* 2010;21(suppl 5):v232–v243.
32. Bakshi SG, Jibhkate B, Sareen R, et al. Nausea and vomiting after breast cancer surgery, and relationship with hormonal status. *J Anesth.* 2011;26:187–195.
33. Vari A, Gazzanelli S, Cavallaro G, et al. Post-operative nausea and vomiting (PONV) after thyroid surgery: a prospective, randomized study comparing totally intravenous versus inhalational anesthetics. *Am Surg.* 2010;76:325–328.
34. Aufforth R, Jain J, Morreale J, et al. Paravertebral blocks in breast cancer surgery: is there a difference in postoperative pain, nausea, and vomiting: *Ann Surg Oncol.* 2011;19:548–552.
35. Shoemaker LK, Estfan B, Induru R, et al. Symptom management: an important part of cancer care. *Cleve Clin J Med.* 2011;78:25–34.
36. National Comprehensive Cancer Network. Clinical practice guidelines in oncology: palliative care [v.2.2012]. http://www.nccn.org /professionals/physician_gls/pdf/palliative.pdf.

37. Thompson N. Optimizing treatment outcomes in patients at risk for chemotherapy-induced nausea and vomiting. *Clin J Oncol Nurs.* 2012;16:309–313.
38. Roscoe JA, Morrow GR, Colagiuri B, et al. Insight in the prediction of chemotherapy-induced nausea. *Support Care Cancer.* 2010;18:869–876.
39. Warr DG, Street JC, Carides AD. Evaluation of risk factors predictive of nausea and vomiting with current standard-of-care antiemetic treatment: analysis of Phase 3 trial of aprepitant in patients receiving adriamycin-cyclophosphamide–based chemotherapy. *Support Care Cancer.* 2011;19:807–813.
40. Friend PJ, Johnston MP Chemotherapy-induced nausea and vomiting. In Eaton LH, Tipton JM, eds: *Putting Evidence into Practice: Improving Oncology Patient Outcomes.* Pittsburgh: Oncology Nursing Society; 2009: 71–83.
41. Irwin MM, Lee J, Rodgers C, et al. *Putting Evidence into Practice: Improving Oncology Patient Outcomes—Chemotherapy-Induced Nausea and Vomiting Resource.* Pittsburgh: Oncology Nursing Society; 2012.
42. Wood JM, Chapman K, Eilers J. Tools for assessing nausea, vomiting, and retching. *Cancer Nurs.* 2011;34:E14–E24.
43. U.S. Department of Health and Human Services, National Institutes of Health, National Cancer Institute. *Common Terminology Criteria for Adverse Events (CTCAE),* v.4.03. June 14, 2010.
44. Eaton LH, Tipton JM. Assessment and measurement. In Eaton LH, Tipton JM, eds, *Putting Evidence into Practice: Improving Oncology Patient Outcomes.* Pittsburgh: Oncology Nursing Society; 2009: 63–69.
45. Davis MP, Hallerberg G. A systematic review of the treatment of nausea and/or vomiting in cancer unrelated to chemotherapy or radiation. *J Pain Symptom Manage.* 2010;39:756–767.
46. Grunberg S, Chua D, Maru A, et al. Single-dose fosaprepitant for the prevention of chemotherapy-induced nausea and vomiting associated with cisplatin therapy: randomized, double-blind study protocol—EASE. *J Clin Oncol.* 2011;29:1495–1501.
47. Hesketh PJ, Aapro M, Street JC, et al. Evaluation of risk factors predictive of nausea and vomiting with current standard-of-care antiemetic treatment: analysis of two phase III trials of aprepitant in patients receiving cisplatin-based chemotherapy. *Support Care Cancer.* 2010;18:1171–1177.
48. Polovich M, Whitford JM, Olsen M. *Chemotherapy and Biotherapy Guidelines and Recommendations for Practice.* 3rd ed. Pittsburgh: Oncology Nursing Society; 2009.
49. Navari RM, Einhorn LH, Loehrer PJ, et al. A phase II trial of olanzapine, dexamethasone, and palonosetron for the prevention of chemotherapy-induced nausea and vomiting: A Hoosier Oncology Group study. *Support Care Cancer.* 2007;15:1285–1291.
50. Navari RM, Gray SE, Kerr AC. Olanzapine versus aprepitant for the prevention of chemotherapy-induced nausea and vomiting: a randomized Phase III trial. *J Support Oncol.* 2011;9:188–195.
51. Bragalone DL, ed. *Drug Information Handbook for Oncology: A Complete Guide to Combination Chemotherapy Regimens.* 9th ed. Hudson, OH: Lexicomp; 2011.
52. Wilkes GM, Barton-Burke M. *2012 Oncology Nursing Drug Handbook.* Burlington, MA: Jones & Bartlett Learning; 2012.
53. Grunberg SM. New findings regarding chemotherapy-induced nausea and vomiting in cancer patients. *Clin Adv Hematol Oncol.* 2011;9(suppl 27):3–10.
54. Todaro B. Cannabinoids in the treatment of chemotherapy-induced nausea and vomiting. *J Natl Compr Canc Netw.* 2012;10:487–492.
55. Grunberg SM. Obstacles to the implementation of antiemetic guidelines. *J Natl Compr Canc Netw.* 2009;7:601–605.
56. Roscoe JA, Morrow GR, Aapro MS, et al. Anticipatory nausea and vomiting. *Support Care Cancer.* 2011;19:1533–1538.
57. Schwartzberg LS. Incorporating chemotherapy-induced nausea and vomiting guidelines into clinical practice. *Clin Adv Hematol Oncol.* 2011;9(suppl 27):9–10.
58. Tipton JM. Side effects of chemotherapy and molecular targeted therapy. In Skeel RT,, Khleif SN, eds. *Handbook of Cancer Chemotherapy.* 8th ed. Philadelphia: Lippincott, Williams, and Wilkins; 2011, 543–565.
59. Einhorn LH, Grunberg SM, Rapoport B, et al. Antiemetic therapy for multiple-day chemotherapy and additional topics consisting of rescue antiemetics and high-dose chemotherapy with stem cell transplant: review and consensus statement. *Support Care Cancer.* 2011;19(suppl 1):S1–S4.
60. Weingart SN, Brown E, Bach PB, et al. NCCN Task Force report: oral chemotherapy. *J Natl Compr Canc Netw.* 2007;6:S1–S14.
61. Jatoi A. Cancer chemotherapy: with or without food? *Support Care Cancer.* 2010;18(suppl 2):S13–S16.
62. Chan A, Low XH, Yap KY. Assessment of the relationship between adherence with antiemetic drug therapy and control of nausea and vomiting in breast cancer patients receiving anthracycline-based chemotherapy. *J Manag Care Pharm.* 2012;18:385–394.
63. Middleton J, Lennan E. Effectively managing chemotherapy-induced nausea and vomiting. *Br J Nurs.* 2011;20(suppl):S7–S15.
64. Feyer P, Jordan K. Update and new trends in antiemetic therapy: the continuing need for novel therapies. *Ann Oncol.* 2011;22:30–38.
65. Frame DG. Best practice management of CINV in oncology patients: I. Physiology and treatment of CINV: multiple neurotransmitters and receptors and the need for combination therapeutic approaches. *Support Oncol.* 2010;8(suppl 1):5–9.
66. Wickham R. Best practice management of CINV in oncology patients: II. Antiemetic guidelines and rationale for use. *Support Oncol.* 2010;8(suppl 1):10–15.
67. Nevidjon B, Chaudhary R. Controlling emesis: evolving challenges, novel strategies. *Support Oncol.* 2010;8(suppl 2):1–10.
68. American Society of PeriAnesthesia Nurses PONV/PDNV Strategic Work Team. ASPAN's evidence-based clinical practice guideline for the prevention and/or management of PONV/PDNV. *J Perianesth Nurs.* 2006;21:230–250.
69. Ignoffo RJ. Current research on PONV/PDNV: practical implications for today's pharmacist. *Am J Health Syst Pharm.* 2009;66(1 suppl 1):S19–S24.
70. Chandrakantan A, Glass PS. Multimodal therapies for postoperative nausea and vomiting, and pain. *Br J Anaesth.* 2011;107(suppl 1):27–40.
71. Hamling K. The management of nausea and vomiting in advanced cancer. *Int J Palliat Nurs.* 2011;17:321–327.
72. Laugsand EA, Kaasa S, Klepstad P. Management of opioid-induced nausea and vomiting in cancer patients: systematic review and evidence-based recommendations. *Palliat Med.* 2011;25:442–453.
73. Jimenez A, Madero R, Alonso A, et al. Symptom clusters in advanced cancer. *J Pain Symptom Manage.* 2011;42:24–31.
74. Kumar G, Hayes KA, Clark R. Efficacy of a Schedule IV cocktail of antiemetics for the palliation of nausea and vomiting in a hospice population. *Am J Hosp Palliat Care.* 2008;25:184–189.
75. Smith ME, Bauer-Wu S. Traditional Chinese medicine for cancer-related symptoms. *Semin Oncol Nurs.* 2012;28:64–74.
76. Ezzo J, Richardson M, Vickers A, et al. Acupuncture-point stimulation for chemotherapy-induced nausea or vomiting. *Cochrane Database Syst Rev.* 2006;19:CD002285.
77. Wickham R. Evolving treatment paradigms for chemotherapy-induced nausea and vomiting. *Cancer Control.* 2012;19(suppl 2):3–9.
78. Ryan JL, Heckler CE, Roscoe JA, et al. Ginger (*Zingiber officinale*) reduces acute chemotherapy-induced nausea: a URCC CCOP study of 576 patients. *Support Care Cancer.* August 5, 2011 [Epub].
79. Zick SM, Ruffin MT, Lee J, et al. Phase II trial of encapsulated ginger as a treatment for chemotherapy-induced nausea and vomiting. *Support Care Cancer.* 2009;17:563–572.
80. Jahn P, Renz P, Stukenkemper J, et al. Reduction of chemotherapy-induced anorexia, nausea, and emesis through a structured nursing intervention: a cluster-randomized multicenter trial. *Support Care Cancer.* 2009;17:1543–1552.

81. Panahi Y, Saadat A, Sahebkar A, et al. Effect of ginger on acute and delayed chemotherapy-induced nausea and vomiting: a pilot, randomized, open-label clinical trial. *Integr Cancer Ther.* 2012;11(3):204–211.
82. Haniadka R, Popouri S, Palatty PL, et al. Medicinal plants as antiemetics in the treatment of cancer: a review. *Integr Cancer Ther.* 2012;11:18–28.
83. Lawenda BD, Johnstone PA. CAM therapies to mitigate the toxicities of cancer therapy. In Abrams DI, Weil AT, eds, *Integrative Oncology.* New York: Oxford University Press; 2009, 232–243.
84. Jakobsen JN, Herrstedt J. Prevention of chemotherapy-induced nausea and vomiting in elderly cancer patients. *Crit Rev Oncol Hematol.* 2009;71:214–221.
85. Saylor MS, Smetana RF. Potential for drug–drug interactions in treating cancer-related nausea and distress. *J Oncol Pharm Pract.* 2010;17:403–408.
86. Maly RC, Liu Y, Leake B, et al. Treatment-related symptoms among underserved women with breast cancer: the impact of physician–patient communication. *Breast Cancer Res.* 2010;119:707–716.
87. Hershman D, Calhoun E, Zapert K, et al. Patients' perceptions of physician–patient discussions and adverse events with cancer therapy. *Arch Drug Info.* 2008;1:70–78.
88. Carelle N, Piotto E, Bellanger A, et al. Changing patient perceptions of the side effects of cancer chemotherapy. *Cancer.* 2002;95:155–163.
89. Dranitsaris G, Bouganim N, Milano C, et al. Prospective validation of a prediction tool for identifying patients at high risk for chemotherapy-induced nausea and vomiting. *J Support Oncol.* 2012;20:1–7.
90. Zachariae R, Paulsen K, Mehlsen M, et al. Chemotherapy-induced nausea, vomiting, and fatigue: the role of individual differences related to sensory perception and autonomic reactivity. *Psychother Psychosom.* 2007;76:376–384.
91. Sun CC, Bodurka DC, Weaver CB, et al. Rankings and symptom assessments of side effects from chemotherapy: insights from experienced patients with ovarian cancer. *Support Care Cancer.* 2005;13:219–227.
92. Olver I, Molassiotis A, Aapro M, et al. Antiemetic research: future directions. *Support Care Cancer.* 2011;19:S49–S55.
93. Wickham R. Nausea and vomiting. In Yarbro CH, Frogge MH, Goodman M, eds. *Cancer Symptom Management.* 3rd ed. Sudbury, MA: Jones and Bartlett; 2004, 187–214.

Nausea and Vomiting from Chemotherapy

Name: ____________________

Symptom and Description

You may have nausea (feeling queasy or sick to your stomach) and/or vomiting (throwing up) from your chemotherapy. Nausea and vomiting (if they happen) often occur a few days after chemotherapy and can last for 3 or more days.

Most people will have nausea more than vomiting, and both symptoms can range from slight to more severe (where you cannot do normal activities). If nausea or vomiting occurs and lasts for more than a day, you can become dehydrated if you are not able to drink fluids. This can have an effect on your body and you will need to contact your doctor or nurse.

Prevention

We have medicine to prevent and control nausea and vomiting. Based on the type of chemotherapy, your doctor and nurse will give you one or more medicines before your treatment. If nausea and vomiting happen after the chemotherapy, you will get orders for medicines for you to take at home.

- Make sure that you get your medicine for nausea and vomiting. Let your doctor or nurse know if your drugstore does not have the medicine or if you cannot afford to pay for them.
- If you are not sure how to take the medicine for nausea and vomiting, call your doctor or nurse.
- Take the medicine for nausea and vomiting that your doctor has ordered. If you have vomiting and cannot take them, call your doctor or nurse.
- If you still have nausea or vomiting even after taking your medicine, call your doctor or nurse. You should tell your doctor or nurse if you do not get relief, because your medicine can be changed and things can be done to help.

Management

When nausea and vomiting last for more than 1 day, you may need to come to the office for fluids through a vein (IV) and to receive medications for nausea and vomiting. Sometimes your doctor may order blood tests to find out if you are low on body salts or other problems. Most of the time, your doctor and nurse will be able to control your nausea and/or vomiting so that pills can be used to control it at home.

Self-Management

There are other things that you can do to decrease nausea and vomiting. It may be helpful to try these steps:

- Eat a small amount of food before your chemotherapy treatment.
- Eat smaller, more frequent meals (about every 3 hours).
- Try to eat foods and drink fluids that have made you feel better in the past or are "comfort foods." These might be bland foods, dry crackers, ginger ale or other soda, chicken soup, and others.
- Do not eat your favorite foods when you have nausea.
- Do not eat fatty, fried, spicy, or salty foods when you have nausea.
- Reduce food odors if possible, or have someone else prepare your foods. It is helpful to plan ahead, and prepare meals that can be frozen and reheated.
- Eat foods that are room temperature or cool. The smells from hot foods can make nausea worse.
- Take your antinausea medicines as ordered, or before meals so that they are working during and after meals.
- Keep your mouth clean, brush your teeth twice a day, and rinse your mouth out with water after meals.
- Relaxation exercises or music may help you feel less anxious, and may help decrease your nausea.

Follow-Up

Call your nurse or doctor if any of these things happen:

- Your nausea and vomiting last for more than 1 day, or nausea keeps you from doing the things you enjoy.
- You vomit, and it looks like it may have blood in it.
- You cannot drink or keep down fluids.
- You cannot keep down your antinausea medicines.
- You lose 2 or more pounds in 1–2 days. This may mean you are losing water. You may be thirsty, and have a dry mouth and tongue.
- You do not urinate as much as normal, or your urine looks dark yellow.
- You feel light-headed or dizzy, faint (pass out), or become confused.

Phone Numbers

Nurse: ______________________ Phone: ______________________

Doctor: ______________________ Phone: ______________________

Evenings or Weekends: ______________________ Phone: ______________________

Other: ______________________ Phone: ______________

Comments:

Source: Tipton J. Nausea and Vomiting. In: Yarbro CH, Wujcik D, Gobel BH, eds. *Cancer Symptom Management*. 4th ed. Burlington, MA: Jones & Bartlett Learning; 2014.

Nausea and Vomiting from Radiation Therapy

Patient Name: ____

Symptom and Description

You may have nausea (feeling queasy or sick to your stomach) and/or vomiting (throwing up) from radiation therapy. These symptoms are more likely to occur if you receive radiation to your abdomen, stomach, chest, or spine. Nausea and vomiting are less common when radiation therapy is given to other parts of your body. Nausea and vomiting may start within 1–2 hours after your radiation treatment, and can last for many hours.

Most people will have nausea more than vomiting, and both symptoms can range from slight to more severe (where you cannot do normal activities). If nausea or vomiting occurs and lasts for more than a day, you can become dehydrated if you are not able to drink fluids. This can have an effect on your body and needs attention by your doctor or nurse.

Prevention

There are medicines to help control nausea and vomiting. If nausea and vomiting are likely with your radiation therapy, your doctor and nurse will order a medicine that you should take before each radiation treatment, or as needed when you are at home.

- Make sure that you get your medicine for nausea and vomiting. Let your doctor or nurse know if your drugstore does not have the medicine or if you cannot afford to pay for them.
- If you are not sure how to take the medicine for nausea and vomiting, call your doctor or nurse.
- Take the medicine for nausea and vomiting that your doctor has ordered. If you have vomiting and cannot take them, call your doctor or nurse.
- If you still have nausea or vomiting even after taking your medicine, call your doctor or nurse. You should tell your doctor or nurse if you do not get relief, because your medicine can be changed and things can be done to help.

Management

When nausea and vomiting last for more than 1 day, you may need to come to the office for fluids through a vein (IV) and to get medicine for nausea and vomiting. Sometimes your doctor may order blood tests to find out if you are low on body salts or there are other problems. Most of the time, your doctor and nurse will be able to control your nausea and/or vomiting so that pills can be used to control it at home.

Self-Management

There are other things that you can do to decrease nausea and vomiting. It may be helpful to try these steps:

- Eat a small amount of food prior to your radiation therapy.
- Eat smaller, more frequent meals (about every 3 hours).
- Try to eat foods and drink beverages that have made you feel better in the past or are "comfort foods." These might be bland foods, dry crackers, ginger ale or other soda, chicken soup, and others.
- Do not eat your favorite foods when you have nausea.
- Do not eat fatty, fried, spicy, or salty foods when you have nausea.
- Reduce food odors if possible, or have someone else prepare your foods. It is helpful to plan ahead, and prepare meals that can be frozen and reheated.
- Eat foods that are room temperature or cool. The smells from hot foods can make nausea worse.
- Take your antinausea medicines as ordered, or prior to meals so that they are working during and after meals.
- Keep your mouth clean, brush your teeth twice a day, and rinse your mouth out with water after meals.
- Relaxation exercises or music can help you feel less anxious, and may help decrease your nausea.

Follow-Up

Call your nurse or doctor if any of the following happen:

- Your nausea and vomiting last for more than 1 day, or nausea keeps you from doing things you enjoy.
- You vomit, and it looks like it may have blood in it.
- You cannot drink or keep down fluids.
- You cannot keep down your antinausea medicines.
- You lose 2 or more pounds in 1–2 days. This may mean you are losing water. You may be thirsty, and have a dry mouth and tongue.
- You do not urinate as much as normal, or your urine looks dark yellow.
- You feel light-headed or dizzy, faint (pass out), or become confused.

Phone Numbers

Nurse: ______________________________ Phone: ______________________________

Doctor: ______________________________ Phone: ______________________________

Evenings or Weekends: ________________ Phone: ______________________________

Other: ______________________________ Phone: __________________

Comments:

Source: Tipton J. Nausea and Vomiting. In: Yarbro CH, Wujcik D, Gobel BH, eds. *Cancer Symptom Management*. 4th ed. Burlington, MA: Jones & Bartlett Learning; 2014.

Nausea and Vomiting from Cancer or Other Causes

Patient Name: ______________________________

Symptom and Description

The cancer itself or other problems can cause nausea (feeling queasy or sick to your stomach) and/or vomiting (throwing up). These symptoms may be worse if you are receiving chemotherapy and/or radiation therapy. Nausea and vomiting can come on slowly or quickly. Your doctor will treat the problem causing the nausea and vomiting.

Nausea and vomiting can be unpleasant, and can range from slight to more severe (where you cannot do normal activities). If nausea or vomiting occurs and lasts for more than a day, you can become dehydrated if you are not able to drink fluids. This can have an effect on your body and needs attention by your doctor or nurse.

Prevention

There are medicines to help control nausea and vomiting. If nausea and vomiting are likely with your treatment, your doctor and nurse will order a medicine that you should take before each chemotherapy or radiation treatment, or as needed when you are at home.

- Make sure that you get your medicine(s) for nausea and vomiting. Let your doctor or nurse know if your drugstore does not have the medicines or if you cannot afford to pay for them.
- If you are not sure how to take the medicine(s) for nausea and vomiting, call your doctor or nurse.
- Take the medicine(s) for nausea and vomiting that your doctor has ordered. If you have vomiting and cannot take them, call your doctor or nurse.
- If you still have nausea or vomiting even after taking your medicine(s), call your doctor or nurse. You should tell your doctor or nurse if you do not get relief, because your medicine(s) can be changed and things can be done to help.

Management

When nausea and vomiting last for more than one day, you may need to come to the office for fluids through a vein (IV) and to receive medicine for nausea and vomiting. Sometimes your doctor may order blood tests to find out if you are low on body salts or there are other problems. Most of the time, your doctor and nurse will be able to control your nausea and/or vomiting so that pills can be used to control it at home.

Self-Management

There are other things that you can do to decrease nausea and vomiting. It may be helpful to try these steps:

- Eat a small amount of food prior to your chemotherapy or radiation therapy.
- Eat smaller, more frequent meals (about every 3 hours).
- Try to eat foods and drink fluids that have made you feel better in the past or are "comfort foods." These might be bland foods, dry crackers, ginger ale or other soda, chicken soup, and others.
- Do not eat your favorite foods when you have nausea.
- Do not eat fatty, fried, spicy, or salty foods when you have nausea.
- Reduce food odors if possible, or have someone else prepare your foods. It is helpful to plan ahead, and prepare meals that can be frozen and easily reheated.
- Eat foods that are room temperature or cool. The smells from hot foods can sometimes make nausea worse.
- Take your antinausea medicines as ordered, or before meals so that they are working during and after meals.
- Keep your mouth clean, brush your teeth twice a day, and rinse your mouth out with water after meals.
- Relaxation exercises or music can help you feel less anxious, and may help decrease your nausea.

Follow-Up

Call your nurse or doctor if any of the following happen:

- Your nausea and vomiting last for more than 1 day, or nausea keeps you from doing important or things you enjoy.
- You vomit, and it looks like it may have blood in it.
- You cannot drink or keep down fluids.
- You cannot keep down your antinausea medicine.
- You lose 2 or more pounds in 1–2 days. This may mean you are losing water. You may be thirsty, and have a dry mouth and tongue.
- You do not urinate as much as normal, or your urine looks dark yellow (concentrated).
- You feel light-headed or dizzy, faint (pass out), or become confused.

Phone Numbers

Nurse: ______________________ Phone: ______________________

Doctor: ______________________ Phone: ______________________

Evenings or Weekends: ______________________ Phone: ______________________

Other: ______________________ Phone: ______________

Comments:

Source: Tipton J. Nausea and Vomiting. In: Yarbro CH, Wujcik D, Gobel BH, eds. *Cancer Symptom Management.* 4th ed. Burlington, MA: Jones & Bartlett Learning; 2014.

Chapter 12

Malignant Ascites

Kim Slusser, RN, MSN, CHPN®

THE PROBLEM

Malignant ascites is the abnormal collection of fluid within the peritoneal cavity associated with an array of cancer diagnoses. Malignancy is the second leading cause of ascites after cirrhosis, accounting for 10% of all cases of ascites.[1–3] Malignant ascites is often an indicator of advanced disease, and it continues to be a major source of discomfort and frustration to patients and a management challenge for the healthcare team. Nearly 60% of patients with malignant ascites present with symptoms.[1] The abnormal accumulation of fluid may initially be subtle, with vague abdominal discomfort. As the fluid accumulates, it affects the respiratory and gastrointestinal systems, causing the patient's condition to deteriorate. Decreased oral intake, fatigue from efforts to perform even simple tasks, and anxiety and fear over the uncertainty about what is happening may all negatively impact the patient's quality of life. A study that explored symptom clusters in patients referred for paracentesis with symptomatic malignant ascites showed patients experienced distressing symptom clusters of (1) depression–anxiety and (2) fatigue–mobility–well-being–appetite.[4]

Oncology nurses play an active role in providing symptom management interventions and education for these patients. Increased knowledge of the pathogenesis, treatment options, and patient experience of malignant ascites enhances the nurse's response in meeting the physical, psychological, educational, and spiritual needs of these patients and their families.

INCIDENCE

At least half of all patients with cancer present with ascites at the initial diagnosis (50%–54%).[1,5,6] Females are more likely (64%–67%) to experience malignant ascites than males (33%–36%).[1,2,5] This is primarily due to ovarian cancer being the most common cancer associated with malignant ascites. Malignant ascites is seen in 29%–37% of all cases of ovarian cancer.[1,2,5] More than three-fourths of patients initially diagnosed with ovarian cancer present with ascites, and nearly all will develop ascites during tumor progression.[5,7] Other cancers associated with malignant ascites include the following:[1,2,5,8,9]

- Breast
- Colorectal
- Endometrial
- Esophageal
- Gastric
- Genitourinary
- Lung
- Lymphoma
- Pancreaticobiliary
- Primary peritoneal

Historically, the primary tumor in 20% of cases of all malignant ascites was unknown,[3,8] but recent studies citing improved diagnostic testing have demonstrated rates as low as 8%.[5,10] More than 95% of patients with malignant ascites also present with metastatic disease, including that involving the peritoneum (90%), liver (27%), bone (12%), and lung (8%).[5]

With the exception of cases seen in ovarian cancer, duration of survival is generally poor.[9] Patients with malignant ascites secondary to ovarian cancer have a significantly higher median survival rate of almost 2 years as compared to a median survival rate of 5.7 months for all other cancers.[5] Patients with gastrointestinal cancer and metastasis to the liver have the lowest survival rates.[5,6] Low levels of serum albumin and total proteins and poor performance status are also significant factors predicting low survival rates, especially in the non-ovarian cancer patient population with liver metastasis.[5,6] Regardless of the primary cancer, once patients develop intractable symptoms from their ascites, survival ranges from 1 to 4 months.[1,2]

ETIOLOGY

Malignant ascites is caused by direct invasion of the peritoneum such as peritoneal carcinomatosis, or secondarily by the local effect of tumor or vena cava compression.[1,3,9] Two-thirds of patients with malignant ascites have peritoneal carcinomatosis with evidence of cancer cells in the peritoneal fluid; the remaining one-third experience ascites due to portal hypertension or lymphatic obstruction.[9] Portal hypertension is most commonly seen in cancer patients with liver metastasis, but patients may also exhibit portal hypertension from cirrhosis, congestive heart failure, constrictive pericarditis, nephrotic syndrome, and peritoneal infections.[9,11] These conditions could be related to comorbidities or complications of previous cancer treatment. The main extra-abdominal tumors causing lymphatic obstruction originate from breast cancer, lung cancer, and lymphoma.[8]

It can be difficult to determine the cause of an individual patient's ascites, making it challenging to develop and implement preventive strategies and effective treatment plans. When ascites is the presenting symptom of cancer, a definitive diagnosis of the primary tumor is helpful, as the treatment and prognosis will vary. Therapy aimed at improved survival may be appropriate in some cases, especially for female patients with ovarian and breast cancers and patients with lymphoma.[1,2,5,6,8,9] More invasive and aggressive interventions may also be considered for those patients with a high performance status.[5,6,9] In most other cases, the goals of therapy become symptom relief, improved performance status, and enhancement of quality of life. Even in cases of palliative symptom relief, knowledge of the primary source of the ascites is helpful in identifying interventions and developing a plan of care. While many interventions have been tried and clinical investigations are ongoing, attempts to control malignant ascites still achieve varying degrees of success.

PATHOPHYSIOLOGY

The peritoneum encases the abdominal organs and covers the abdominal and pelvic space; it comprises a layer of mesothelial cells overlying layers of connective tissue. Normal physiology of the peritoneal cavity is dependent on the balance of peritoneal fluid production and drainage. In healthy individuals, there is a constant movement of fluid into (influx) and out of (efflux) the peritoneal cavity. This fluid is derived from the transudation of plasma and proteins through capillaries in the peritoneal membrane and drained by the lymphatic channels of the peritoneum. Normally, a small amount of peritoneal fluid (approximately 50–100 mL) is present and continuously circulates in the peritoneum.[8,12,13] Circulation and drainage of the fluid are driven by the movement of the diaphragm and bowel peristalsis. In a healthy individual, nearly two-thirds of the peritoneal fluid is reabsorbed by the lymphatic channels and eventually reaches the right subclavian vein and the right thoracic duct. The entire process of fluid production, drainage, and reabsorption is dependent on the stable relationship between oncotic and hydraulic pressure gradients, capillary permeability, and the surface area for filtration.[9] This relationship of net capillary filtration is described by Starling's law of capillary dynamics (see Figure 12-1).[9]

In malignant ascites, there is an imbalance of peritoneal fluid production and drainage, leading to water and sodium retention in the abdominal cavity. This condition may involve an increase in fluid production, a decrease in drainage, or a combination of both.[8,9] Factors influencing

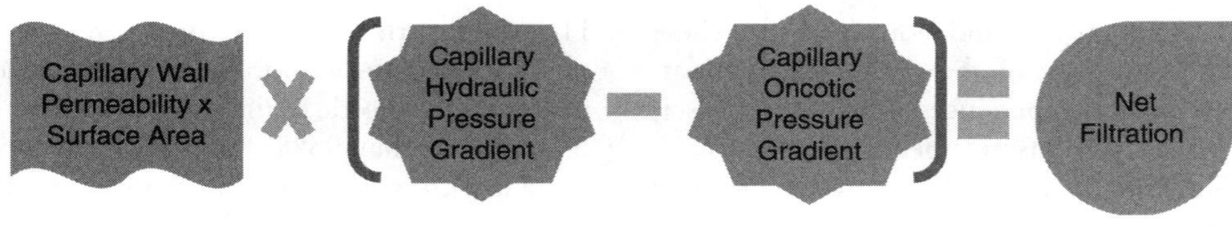

FIGURE 12-1

Starling's law of capillary hemodynamics.

Source: Data from Kammula[9].

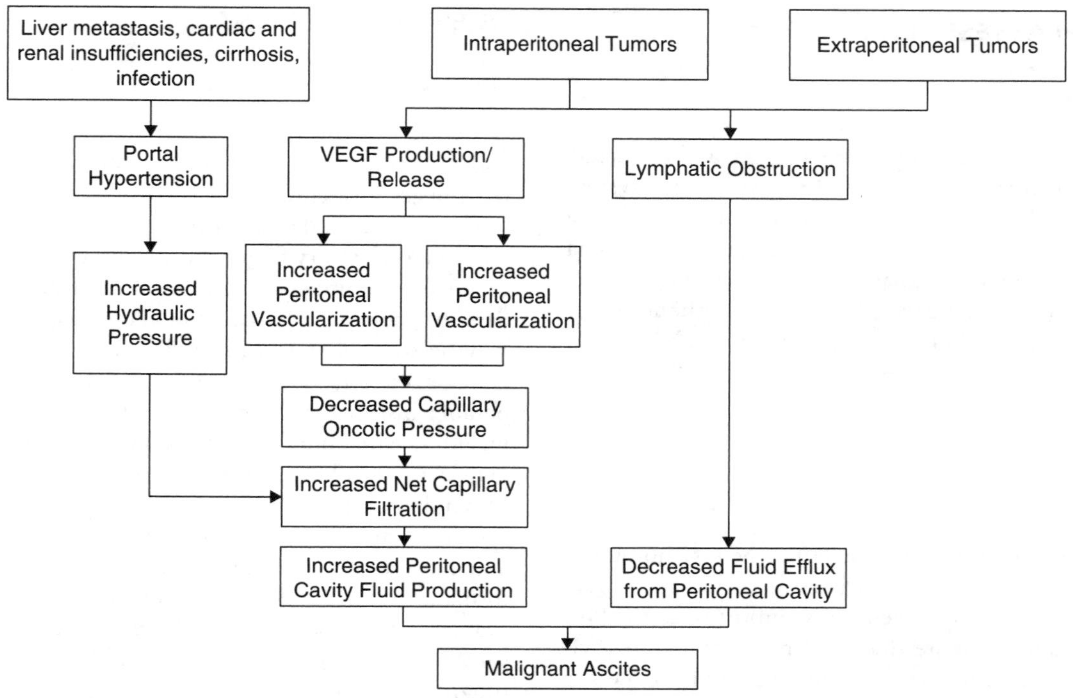

FIGURE 12-2

Causes of malignant ascites.

Abbreviation: VEGF: vascular endothelial growth factor.

Source: Data from Chung and Kozuch[1]; Cavazzoni et al[8]; Kammula[9].

the increased production and decreased drainage of peritoneal fluid include the following:[1,8,9]

1. Cytokine release from intraperitoneal tumor cells. Increased production of glycoproteins such as vascular endothelial growth factor (VEGF) and tumor necrosis factor (TNF) results in increased peritoneal neovascularization and capillary permeability. This process decreases oncotic pressure.
2. Lymphatic obstruction by intra- and extraperitoneal tumors resulting in impaired drainage of peritoneal fluid content.
3. Portal hypertension causing an increase in capillary hydraulic pressure. The increase in pressure leads to increased fluid production.

After ascites has developed, overactivation of the renin–angiotensin–aldosterone system secondary to reduced intravascular volume associated with ascites leads to sodium and water retention and reduced urinary output, increasing the ascites.

Figure 12-2 illustrates the causes of malignant ascites, and Figure 12-3 displays malignant ascites within the peritoneal cavity. The development of malignant ascites is most likely dependent on a combination of factors, with each factor playing a greater or lesser role in each individual patient.

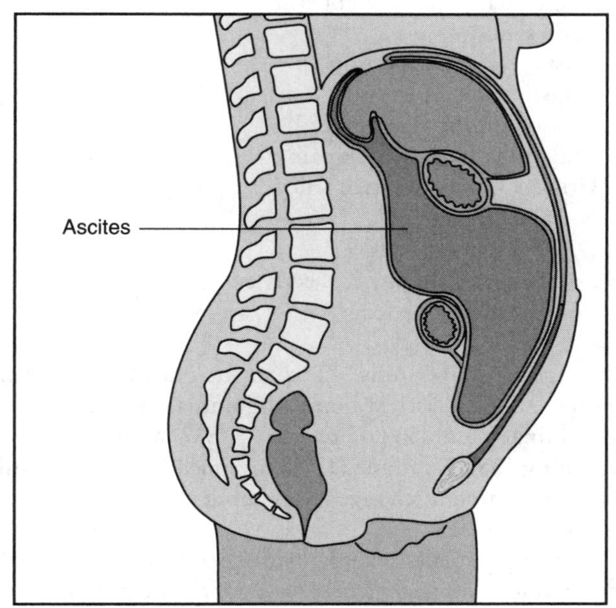

FIGURE 12-3

Ascites.

Source: Courtesy of Gardiner, P. 2012. Photo Researchers, Inc.

SYMPTOM ASSESSMENT

RISK FACTORS

Patients at risk for developing malignant ascites include those with primary tumors of the gynecologic system, gastrointestinal system, breast, liver, and lymphoma. Comorbid conditions, such as cirrhosis, cardiac and renal disorders, and previous radiation treatments, may increase a patient's risk for the development of malignant ascites. Other risk factors include hypoalbuminemia and hypoproteinemia, which are often seen in a patient with end-stage disease.[14]

SELF-ASSESSMENT

Understanding how patients describe their symptoms of ascites will facilitate a thorough assessment and appropriate plan of care. Patients experience discomfort once the fluid volume increases to more than 500 mL.[13] Symptoms will reflect the pressure of the accumulating fluid on the surrounding structures of the intestines, bladder, lungs, and back. A detailed history will reveal a variety of complaints that may have started with a vague discomfort that have progressed to any of the following:

- Recent weight gain
- Tight-fitting clothing
- Abdominal bloating
- Decrease in or lack of appetite
- Early satiety
- Dyspepsia or indigestion
- Constipation
- Nausea and/or vomiting
- Abdominal or low back pain
- Urinary urgency or frequency
- Fatigue
- Difficulty breathing
- Low tolerance to physical activity
- Lower extremity edema

In a retrospective study, 122 patients out of 209 patients with malignant ascites noted abdominal swelling (55%), abdominal pain (53%), nausea (37%), anorexia (36%), vomiting (25%), fatigue (17%), dyspnea (11%), early fullness (6%), weight change (5%), ankle swelling (3%), and heartburn (1%).[5]

Having patients record their experiences assists in the evaluation of management interventions and progression of disease. Patients should be encouraged to keep a log of their symptoms and to note how the symptoms affect their quality of life. Appendix 12A provides a self-assessment tool patients can use at the initial and subsequent clinic visits.

OBJECTIVE ASSESSMENT

History

A detailed history of the gastrointestinal, genitourinary, and respiratory systems should be obtained in addition to the impact of ascites on the patient's quality of life. This information includes frequency and consistency of bowel movements; urinary frequency; dietary intake; and presence of nausea, vomiting, and shortness of breath. Patients may describe anorexia, early satiety, and decreased intake. Weight may be stable despite decreased intake, as the ascites fluid increases but total body mass decreases. It is also important to obtain a history of previous cancer and associated treatments including radiation; liver, cardiac, and renal disease; and past and current alcohol consumption.[15] A baseline weight should be obtained, and the patient's usual weight assessed.

The Karnofsky index scoring system (Table 12-1)[16] and Eastern Cooperative Oncology Group (ECOG) performance scale (Table 12-2)[17] are well-established tools to evaluate performance status. They can be simple and easy ways for the healthcare team to evaluate the baseline and progressive effects that the presenting symptoms have on the patient's quality of life.

Physical assessment

Evaluation of the extent of ascites accumulation begins with the abdominal assessment. This will include inspection, auscultation, measurement of abdominal girth, percussion of the abdomen, and determination of a fluid wave.

TABLE 12-1

Karnofsky Performance Status Scale

100	Normal activity; no evidence of disease
90	Normal activity; minor signs/symptoms of disease
80	Normal activity with effort; some signs/symptoms of disease
70	Cares for self; unable to carry on all normal activity
60	Requires occasional assistance
50	Requires considerable assistance and frequent medical care
40	Disabled; requires special care and assistance
30	Severely disabled; hospital admission is indicated
20	Very sick; hospital admission necessary; active supportive treatment needed
10	Moribund; fatal processes progressing rapidly
0	Dead

Source: Data from Karnofsky performance status scale definitions rating (%) criteria[16].

TABLE 12-2

ECOG Performance Status*

Grade	ECOG
0	Fully active, able to carry on all pre-disease performance without restriction
1	Restricted in physically strenuous activity but ambulatory and able to carry out work of a light or sedentary nature, e.g., light house work, office work
2	Ambulatory and capable of all self care but unable to carry out any work activities. Up and about more than 50% of waking hours
3	Capable of only limited self care, confined to bed or chair more than 50% of waking hours
4	Completely disabled. Cannot carry on any self care. Totally confined to bed or chair
5	Dead

Source: * As published in Oken MM, Creech RH, Tormey DC, Horton J, Davis TE, McFadden ET, et al. *Toxicity And Response Criteria Of The Eastern Cooperative Oncology Group. Am J Clin Oncol 5:649–655, 1982.* Credit to Eastern Cooperative Oncology Group, Robert Comis M.D., Group Chair[17].

With the patient supine, inspection of the abdomen will reveal skin that is taut and shiny if ascites is present. The umbilicus may evert and the flanks may begin to bulge.[18]

Auscultation should always be performed prior to any palpation or percussion. This prevents the altering of the frequency and characteristics of the patient's bowel sounds.[19] Visually separate the abdominal area into four equal quadrants, and place the diaphragm of the stethoscope over each quadrant for 5–20 seconds.[19] Upon auscultation, bowel sounds may be high pitched, hypoactive, or absent due to ascites fluid interfering with bowel function. Measurement of the abdominal girth will provide a reference for later evaluation of regression or progression related to therapeutic measures. The umbilicus is used as the starting point with the measuring tape wrapped around the patient, documenting the measure in either centimeters or inches.

Percussion of the abdomen will reveal a shifting dullness if ascites is present. With the patient supine, fluid will gravitate to the flanks, displacing the bowel upward. This requires the presence of at least 1500 mL of fluid in the abdominal cavity; therefore early fluid accumulation in some patients may not be detected by percussion.[9,10] Percussion from the midline of the abdomen down to the side reveals a change from tympany to dullness (where the ascites fluid rests). Next, the patient rolls onto his or her side, resulting in fluid flowing to the dependent flank and the gaseous bowel being displaced upward. Percussion from the topside downward now reveals a new level of dullness at the lower flank. In an abdomen distended with gas, no change in percussion is noted.

A fluid wave test can be performed to confirm ascites. The patient or another clinician places a hand firmly along the midline of the abdomen to prevent transmission of the wave through the abdominal wall. The clinician then places his or her left hand against the patient's right side and firmly slaps the left flank with the other hand.[19] If ascites is present, a wave will be felt as a distinct sharp tap on the left hand of the examiner.

Gross distention of the abdomen caused by the peritoneal fluid accumulation will create upward pressure on the diaphragm and restrict lung expansion. Patients typically exhibit dyspnea, tachypnea, and orthopnea. As ascites continues to accumulate, it can cross through the diaphragm into the pleural space, resulting in pleural effusion. The thoracic cavity is assessed to detect the presence of pleural effusion. Upon physical exam, respirations per minute are measured and the difficulty of respirations is assessed. Auscultation of the lungs may reveal diminished breath sounds over the area of fluid, with sounds above the fluid level being hyperresonant. Percussion will reveal a dull or flat sound where fluid is located. Increased respiratory rate and effort add to the workload of the heart, resulting in tachycardia.

The patient with advanced or progressive disease often presents with a tense, distended abdomen; dyspnea; and difficulty walking. In end-stage disease, patients appear fatigued, malnourished with cachectic extremities, and ashen color.

Diagnostic evaluation

Imaging techniques including x-ray, ultrasound, computerized tomography (CT) scan, and magnetic resonance imaging (MRI) are effective in detecting small amounts of fluid in the abdomen and can provide early identification of unsuspected ascites. Ultrasound can detect as little as 5–10 mL of free peritoneal fluid.[9] Although imaging cannot distinguish between benign and malignant ascites, it can detect the presence of a solid tumor that may be the cause of ascites. Ultrasound, CT, and MRI have significant diagnostic accuracy in identifying liver metastases and other hepatic tumors, with CT and transvaginal ultrasound providing radiologic findings suspicious for ovarian tumors. Pancreatic cancer can be detected on CT scan. Radiologic imaging techniques are useful in visualizing tumors of the esophagus and gastric and colon cancers, although endoscopy is the primary diagnostic tool for gastrointestinal cancers. Radiologic confirmation of ascites in the presence of a tumor guides the clinician in the next step of differential diagnosis, including cytologic verification of a malignancy and selection of management approaches.[10]

A diagnostic paracentesis can both confirm the diagnosis and provide temporary relief of malignant ascites. Paracentesis is not recommended for women with a suspected gynecologic malignancy.[20] In this group of patients, an exploratory laparotomy, tumor debulking, or staging and cytologic evaluation will provide the diagnosis of gynecologic cancer and subsequent relief of ascites. Patients with gynecologic cancer often respond to first-line chemotherapy and have a better median survival than all other groups of patients with malignant ascites.

The color and character of the ascites fluid assist clinicians in determining the principal cause of ascites:[9,10]

- Bloody or serosanguineous fluid is usually associated with ovarian, liver, and other cancers that cause intraperitoneal dissemination.
- Chylous ascites is a milky fluid containing an elevated triglyceride concentration commonly associated with lymphoma; it is also observed with damage of lymphatics after external beam radiation.
- Serous ascites is usually associated with nonmalignant conditions, such as congestive heart failure, renal disease, or cirrhosis.
- Cloudy ascites fluid may be due to an infection.

Initial laboratory testing of peritoneal fluid focuses on the presence of infection, portal hypertension, or malignancy.[9] To rule out infection, fluid is evaluated via a white blood cell count with differential. If the neutrophil count is greater than 250/mm^3, a Gram stain and culture for bacterial, fungal, and acid-fast organisms is ordered to determine treatment options.[9]

Serum and peritoneal fluid testing of albumin levels can indicate whether portal hypertension or malignancy is the cause of the ascites.[1,3,9–11] Determining the serum to ascites albumin gradient (SAAG)—that is, serum albumin concentration minus ascitic fluid albumin concentration—is a better diagnostic test than the historical total protein-based criteria.[9–11,21] A gradient greater than or equal to 1.1 g/dL indicates portal hypertension with 97% accuracy; which is most commonly caused by cirrhosis, hepatic congestion, congestive heart failure (CHF), or portal vein thrombosis.[9–11] Twenty percent of patients with cancer will have a high SAAG.[3] A lower gradient (high protein ascites) indicates a lack of portal hypertension and more likely the presence of malignancy. High protein ascites is most commonly seen in peritoneal carcinomatosis, but can also indicate an infectious process of the peritoneum, nephrotic syndrome, or malnutrition/hypoalbuminemia.[9–11] Additional testing to distinguish between malignant and nonmalignant ascites can include determining lactate dehydrogenase (LDH) and cholesterol levels. An ascites LDH level greater than 250 μg/mL and a cholesterol level greater than 70 mg/dL are associated with malignancy.[3]

In general, when a malignant etiology is suspected, peritoneal fluid cytology will be performed. Not all tumors shed cells into the peritoneum: thus only 60% of cytology tests will be positive for cancer.[10] Patients with peritoneal carcinomatosis have positive cytology 97% of the time.[9,10] Traditional serum markers such as CA 125 and CA 19–9 can be helpful in linking the presence of ascites with an underlying primary malignancy, but testing the ascitic fluid levels of these markers has not been determined to be beneficial in choosing treatment options.[9] Improved sensitivity and specificity may be achieved in the diagnosis of malignant ascites by checking ascitic levels of sialic acids, human chorionic gonadotropin-beta, VEGF, and fibronectin levels and telomerase activity, however, there is not enough evidence to support these tests' routine clinical use.[9]

The role of laparoscopic evaluation in diagnosing ascites of unknown primary origin has been studied as a means of determining the cause of ascites.[22] The laparoscopic technique enables visualization of the peritoneal surfaces, offers the ability to obtain a tissue diagnosis, and provides relief of ascites without the trauma of open laparotomy and subsequent recovery. A study spanning more than 20 years evaluated the usefulness of laparoscopic procedures in determining the cause of ascites in patients. The study demonstrated rare complications and a definitive cause of ascites was identified in more than 90% of all cases.[22] In this study, 44%–56% of the cases were positive for peritoneal carcinimatosis.[22]

DEGREES OF TOXICITY

To evaluate the patient with ascites and provide standardized information, the National Cancer Institute has developed toxicity criteria that grade the degree of ascites on a scale of 1 to 5. Table 12-3 provides details of these grading criteria.[23]

TABLE 12-3

National Cancer Institute Common Terminology Criteria for Adverse Events (CTCAE): Ascites

Grade 1 Mild	Grade 2 Moderate	Grade 3 Severe	Grade 4 Life-threatening or disabling	Grade 5 Death
Asymptomatic, clinical or diagnostic observations only; intervention not indication	Symptomatic, medical intervention indicated	Severe symptoms, invasive intervention indicated	Life-threatening consequences, urgent operative intervention indicated	Death related to adverse event

Source: Data from National Cancer Institute Common Terminology Criteria for Adverse Events (CTCAE)[23].

TABLE 12-4

Patient Assessment for Ascites

Patient Assessment for Ascites	
Patient Self-Assessment	**Physical Findings**
Recent weight gain	Measurable weight gain
Tight-fitting clothing	Taut and shiny skin appearance of the abdomen
Abdominal bloating or "fullness"	Everted umbilicus
Decrease or lack of appetite	Bulging flanks
Early satiety	High pitched, hypoactive, or absent bowel sounds
Indigestion	Increased abdominal girth
Constipation	Percussed shifting dullness
Nausea and/or vomiting	Fluid wave of the abdomen
Abdominal or lower back pain	Dyspnea/increased respiratory rate
Urinary urgency or frequency	Diminished breath sounds
Fatigue	**Radiologic Studies**
Difficulty breathing	Flat plate of abdomen
Low tolerance to physical activity	Abdominal computerized tomography
Lower extremity edema/swelling	Ultrasound
Detailed History	Magnetic resonance imaging
Frequency and consistency of bowel movements	**Laboratory Studies**
Urinary frequency	Serum to ascites albumin gradient $<$ 1.1 g/dL
Dietary intake	Ascites fluid
Usual weight	Lactate dehydrogenase $>$ 250 μ/ml
Previous cancer and treatment	Cholesterol $>$ 70mg/dL
Liver, cardiac, or renal disease	Bloody, serosanguineous, chylous, or milky fluid
Past and current alcohol use	Positive malignant cytology
Quality of Life Assessment	Gram stain and culture
Karnofsky Performance Scale Score: less than baseline	Laproscopic evaluation
ECOG Performance Scale Score: less than baseline	

Abbreviation: ECOG: Eastern Cooperative Oncology Group.

Source: Data from Rosenberg[3]; Ayantunde and Parsons[5]; Kammula[9]; Ammouri and Prommer[10]; Scallan et al[14]; Nettina[15]; Talley and O'Connor[18]; Han et al[22]; Vogel et al[24]; Economua[25]; Murphy[26].

Progression of malignant ascites also adversely impacts the patient's quality of life. The Karnofsky index scoring system (Table 12-1) and ECOG performance status scale (Table 12-2) are helpful tools to measure this impact.

Table 12-4 summarizes the complete symptom assessment, including history, objective, and subjective assessment measures.[3,5,9,10,14,15,18,22,24–26]

SYMPTOM MANAGEMENT STRATEGIES

Malignant ascites is a complex condition, and the management of this condition is dependent on the tumor of origin. The patient with ovarian cancer or lymphoma-associated ascites will undergo a markedly different treatment regimen than the patient with a gastrointestinal malignancy. In the situation of ovarian cancer or lymphoma, the individual usually responds to primary therapy such as surgical debulking, chemotherapy, or radiation, which controls the malignancy and the ascites for an extended period of time.[27] For patients who experience malignant ascites as a result of persistent, recurrent, or advanced disease, or those who have failed standard first-, second-, or third-line treatment, the presence of ascites is a grave sign.[9] The chance for "cure" of disease and subsequent "cure" of the ascites is not a realistic goal. Life expectancy varies, but has been estimated to be in the range of 1–4 months.[5] The goal for patients in this palliative phase of care becomes symptom relief with a focus on maintaining or enhancing quality of life.

THERAPEUTIC APPROACHES

When malignant ascites becomes symptomatic, there are a variety of treatment options. There are no standard criteria of efficacy of response to treatment. Instead, a patient's expression of relief from symptoms is used as the standard for continuing a particular treatment; in cases of worsened or unrelieved symptoms, new approaches are explored.[1,8]

Diuretic therapy

Diuretic therapy can be beneficial in patients with hepatic metastases and cirrhotic ascites, in whom there is retention of sodium and water as a result of portal hypertension and the activation of the renin–angiotensin–aldosterone pathway.[8] Retrospective studies of diuretic therapy using spironolactone and a loop diuretic, such as furosemide, have shown that such therapy can provide relief of symptoms in 43% of patients with various cancers[28]; nevertheless, there is a lack of randomized and prospective studies solidifying the effectiveness of this therapy.[7–9] When using diuretics, implementation of a sodium-restricted diet can prevent additional fluid accumulation.

The ineffectiveness of diuretics is related to the pathogenesis of different malignant ascites. Patients with massive hepatic metastasis are reported to benefit most from the use of spironolactone because of their increased plasma renin and aldosterone levels secondary to increased portal pressure.[29] Dosages of spironolactone can range from 150 mg/day to 450 mg/day, and doses of furosemide can range from 40 mg/day to 80 mg/day.[7,8] The effectiveness of diuretic therapy is limited and the expected maximum ascites fluid reabsorption is 800 mL, which translates into less than 1 kg/day weight loss.[8]

Complications related to diuretic therapy for the management of malignant ascites include hypovolemia, hypotension, and hyperkalemia, which can lead to circulatory and renal failure.[7,8] In some cases, the use of diuretics can increase the hematocrit and potentially induce thromboembolic events.[7] Routine checks of electrolytes are needed to prevent complications. Clinicians should avoid using diuretics in patients with a low SAAG and evidence of ascites containing cancer cells, as such therapy will have little benefit for these patients.[1]

Paracentesis

Paracentesis is still the mainstay of treatment for malignant ascites, providing immediate, albeit temporary, relief of symptoms; improving pain and dyspnea; and increasing the patient's mobility and overall comfort.[7] It is a widely chosen intervention owing to its ability to create an immediate response in approximately 90% of patients.[2,8–10] Fluid drainage via paracentesis can range from a few liters to more than 20 liters[8]; there is no consensus on the maximum amount of fluid drainage per session without experiencing complications.[1,7,8] The amount of fluid drainage depends on the patient's ability to tolerate the procedure. Drainage is stopped when the patient is experiencing discomfort from the procedure. It is generally safe to perform "blind" paracentesis; however, ultrasound guidance is used in patients who have loculated ascites, large tumor masses, or adhesions from previous surgery or who have received chemotherapy or radiation.[30] While the procedure can be done safely and quickly in the outpatient setting, the major drawback of paracentesis treatments is that the therapeutic effects are short-lived. Serial paracentesis procedures are usually required every 10 days.[1,31]

Complications of paracentesis procedures are infrequent. They can include secondary peritonitis, perforation, hypoproteinemia, pulmonary embolism, and hypotension.[1,7] The effectiveness of concurrent volume expansion such as albumin replacement in reducing severe hypotensive complications has not been established.[1] In a systematic review, Becker et al. state that a patient can have as much as 5 liters of fluid drained without any major hemodynamic complications.[28] Blood tests of electrolytes, proteins, and renal function should be routinely monitored to prevent complications.[7] Patients may be instructed to adopt a high-protein diet to lessen the potential of low serum protein, a condition sometimes associated with frequent paracentesis.[1]

Immediately prior to the procedure, patients should empty their bladder to prevent injury.[32] Patients are seated upright to allow the intestines to float away from the tap site. After the site is prepped, the abdominal wall is punctured with a needle or trocar instrument. If cytology is desired, a drainage system with a three-way stopcock can be set up. If not, fluid is drained either by gravity or by suction.[32] The cannula can be removed after the complete aspiration of fluid or can be sutured in place to allow drainage over a period of 12–24 hours. Exceeding cannula placement beyond 24 hours increases the risk of infection.[1]

An indirect negative effect that impacts patients receiving serial paracentesis is fatigue. It arises due to frequent hospital or clinic visits or waiting until symptoms are intolerable to reduce the frequency of treatments.[3] Despite the short-term benefits, paracentesis is commonly used because most patients are not candidates for more aggressive treatment modalities.

Permanent catheter placement. When patients require paracentesis more often than every 7 days to relieve symptoms, the placement of a permanent catheter is often considered, especially in patients who have a life expectancy of more than 2–3 months.[7,8] This allows for more frequent drainage that can be done by the patient at home, eliminating the need for frequent trips to the hospital or clinic. Catheter placement can reduce the fatigue and discomfort from the paracentesis procedure and allows for increased autonomy.[10]

Tunneled catheters are preferred to nontunneled catheters due to their reduced risk of infection (2%–5% versus 12%–34%, respectively).[8,10] Tunneled catheters also have a reduced risk of occlusion.[8] The Pleurx® and Aspira© catheters are most often tunneled and are the two approved catheters by the Food and Drug Administration (FDA) for the long-term drainage of peritoneal fluid.[33] The advantages of these catheters as opposed to other options (e.g., peritoneal ports, Tenckhoff® catheters, and dialysis catheters) are that the Pleurx® and Aspira© catheters (1) have a one-way rubber valve rather than a clamp device to close the system, so that the valve remains sealed even if the cap becomes dislodged, thereby maintaining a closed system; and (2) have attachment supplies that contain a line connected to vacuum bottles to access the catheter.[3,30] Nontunneled catheters, such as pigtail catheters, are used in patients who have a life expectancy of a few weeks to a month.[3] Pigtail catheters are not an acceptable longer-term drainage option owing to their increased risk of infection, occlusion, and leakage.[30] In the majority of cases, the catheter type chosen for the patient is highly dependent upon what is available in a given healthcare setting.[3] Tunneled catheters are easily inserted under local anesthesia as an outpatient surgery.

Recommendations for drainage schedules vary depending on the patient's symptoms. The most serious complication with permanent catheters is peritonitis.[8] Antibiotic prophylaxis is recommended for catheter placement and sometimes continued throughout the first week or two of treatment.[7,8,30] Patients need to be warned of the consequences of poor catheter care, which can include infection and occlusion. If necessary, intraperitoneal antibiotics can be delivered through the catheter in an effort to avoid removing the catheter. In addition to the complications of poor catheter maintenance, malfunction of the catheter can occur from occlusion by fibrin clot formation or by blood or peritoneal fluid that becomes thickened or gelatinous. Unfortunately, areas of fluid can become loculated as the cancer progresses or adhesions form. As with any therapeutic measure for malignant ascites, the patient's physical status, peritoneal fluid characteristics, and tumor type must be considered to accurately evaluate the individual's ability to gain benefits that outweigh risks. In particular, the appropriate candidate for an external catheter is a patient who is cognitively and physically able to care for the device and has a supportive network of caregivers who can help provide care.

Peritoneovenous shunts

The use of a peritoneovenous shunt (PVS) is an alternative to repeated paracentesis. A PVS is a one-way tube connecting the peritoneum to the vena cava in which the valve opens at a specific pressure and leads the fluid into the vein.[7] The three shunts used for this purpose are the Hyde, LeVeen, and Denver® shunts. PVS has been used for treatment of peritoneal ascites since the early 1970s.[3,31] There is no evidence to support the use of one type of PVS over the others.[3,7]

Peritoneovenous shunting of ascites fluid out of the "third space" and return of this fluid to the circulatory system maintains vascular volume and reduces protein loss. Another advantage for some patients is the avoidance of external drainage devices in those persons who may be unable to maintain and manage the drainage system, and for patients who cannot cope with the self-image of external devices.[3]

PVS has been shown to be more effective in nongastrointestinal malignancies such as ovarian and breast cancers. PVS for malignant ascites related to ovarian cancers achieves palliation in more than 50% of all cases; in contrast, gastrointestinal malignancies have a relatively poor response rate, ranging from 10% to 15%.[7]

While placement of the PVS is a relatively simple procedure carried out under local anesthesia and intravenous sedation, it is used less often because of the high rates of early mortality in this patient population and shunt-associated complications.[8] Contraindications for shunt placement include congestive heart failure and renal failure due to the significant hemodilution and blood volume overload produced by the shunt, jaundice, portal hypertension, severe pleural effusion, and clotting disorders.[8] Because the PVS catheter must be tunneled from the peritoneum to the vena cava, healthcare providers have noted difficulty placing a PVS in patients with marked cachexia.[31] In addition, catheter occlusion rates range from 16% to 45%, which is much higher than the rates observed with tunneled permanent catheters.[8] Patients with hemorrhagic or chylous ascites should not undergo PVS placement due to high rates of shunt clotting and occlusion.[9] Patients with loculations would not be ideal candidates for PVS use, either, as the fluid may not be able to reach the catheter for appropriate drainage.

Identifying whether the patient's peritoneal fluid has positive cytology is important in determining PVS therapy. The median shunt survival time in patients with negative cytology is approximately 140 days, compared with 26 days in patients with positive cytology.[10] In general, post-PVS-placement complications include disseminated intravascular coagulation due to the protein- and clotting factor–rich ascites fluid, pulmonary edema, shunt occlusion resulting from increased cellular debris and protein, and infection.[9,34] Infections can be treated with antibiotics and usually necessitate shunt removal.

In summary, PVS can provide effective palliation of ascites in approximately 70% of patients.[9] However, practitioners may be reluctant to use PVS because of concerns about subjecting terminally ill patients to palliative surgery and the fear of complications. The associated risks of PVS should be weighed against the benefits when evaluating a potential candidate. Patient screening for PVS should include a thorough cardiac, respiratory, and renal evaluation to determine the patient's ability to tolerate increased fluid load.

Intraperitoneal therapy

Intraperitoneal chemotherapy. Administering chemotherapeutic agents directly into the peritoneal cavity via a temporary or permanent catheter allows direct exposure of the chemotherapeutic agent to the affected area while minimizing systemic effects. Often the intention of using chemotherapy for malignant ascites is to cause irritation to the peritoneal surface, thereby causing scarring and fibrosis, which prevent further ascites accumulation.[8] The chemotherapy may also control the primary cancer. Agents that have been used include mitoxantrone, cisplatin, and mitomycin C. Side effects of intraperitoneal chemotherapy can include nausea and vomiting, leukopenia, abdominal pain, and infection. See Table 12-5 for a review of intraperitoneal chemotherapy.

TABLE 12-5

Intraperitoneal (IP) Chemotherapy for Malignant Ascites Management

IP Chemotherapy	Side Effects
Bleomycin	Fever Hypersensitivity Infection Nausea/vomiting Noncardiac chest pain
Cisplatin	Abdominal pain Diarrhea Nausea/vomiting Neutropenia Peritonitis Systemic toxicity
Mechlorethamine	Nausea/vomiting Neutropenia Pain
Mitomycin C	Bowel leak Ileus Neutropenia Pulmonary embolism Sepsis Serous wound leak Small bowel perforation Thrombocytopenia
Mitoxantrone	Abdominal pain Anemia Infection Nausea/vomiting Neutropenia Thrombocytopenia
Thiotepa	Intesitinal obstruction

Source: Data from Chung and Kozuch[1].

A limitation of this type of treatment is the inability of the drugs to penetrate into bulky, large solid tumors, as penetration is estimated to be no more than 1–5 mm.[3,7,8] Similar to systemic chemotherapy agent decision making, agent selection should be determined based on the tumor type, patient's performance status, prior chemotherapy, and drug toxicity profile.[1] Intraperitoneal chemotherapy has demonstrated variable success ranging between 33% and 85%; ovarian cancer is the most sensitive to therapy, with ascites control being achieved in more than 65% of patients.[8] The success rate for intraperitoneal chemotherapy for ascites control of all cancer types, however, is less than 50%.[8] Cisplatin alone or in combination with other agents seems to be one of the most effective agents while demonstrating less systemic toxicity and fewer side effects.[8]

Intraperitoneal chemotherapy attempts to minimize the side effects and toxicities associated with systemic therapy, but it is not completely free of adverse effects and toxicities. In one study, 34% of patients with primary ovarian cancer had to stop treatment with cisplatin and paclitaxel due to catheter-related complications of infection, catheter blockage and leaks, and abdominal pain.[35] In 2006, the National Cancer Institute (NCI) announced after a large Phase III study by Armstrong et al. that intraperitoneal chemotherapy in conjunction with systemic treatment in optimally debulked ovarian cancer should be encouraged, but cautioned clinicians and patients that more research needed to be conducted.[36–38] Due to the limited use of intraperitoneal chemotherapy for the treatment of malignant ascites mainly in clinical trials, this option is usually offered only at major cancer centers.[2]

Other approaches to intraperitoneal chemotherapy include perioperative administration or immediate postoperative administration, as in gastric malignancies, in an effort to prevent ascites formation. Intraperitoneal hyperthermic chemotherapy (HIPEC) both alone and in combination with aggressive cytoreductive surgery has been investigated, with results revealing improved palliation and survival in nonovarian intraperitoneal disseminated malignancies.[1] The premise underlying the efficiency of this treatment is that a hyperthermic medium (40°C–43°C) enhances the cytotoxicity of some chemotherapeutic agents.[2] There have been only a handful of studies with small sample sizes examining HIPEC therapy without surgery, but one study's response rate after one month showed greater than 94% resolution of ascites and a median survival of 98 days as well as an improvement in the Karnofsky index score.[39] Studies require replication before the use of this therapy can be recommended. Complications in the handful of studies included bowel wall damage, bleeding, abdominal fluid collection and abscesses, pleural effusion, electrolyte disorders, and hypotension.[8]

Radioisotopes. Radioisotopes have also been investigated in the treatment of ascites, primarily in the 1950s and 1960s; their use for malignant ascites has not been robustly developed, however, owing to this treatment modality's significant side effect profile.[2] Use of Au-198 has been abandoned and is considered hazardous due to its toxicity, including its propensity to cause intestinal obstruction, which prohibits dose escalation.[1,2] Chromic phosphate colloid (^{32}P) has been used most often because of its ability to penetrate tissues to a depth of 8 mm and its long half-life of 14 days, but it has not been recently studied.[1] Patients with small peritoneal seedings are more likely to respond to such therapy than those with large volume of solid tumors. Response rates range from 30% to 80% but response is of short duration, requiring repeated administration of the radioisotopes.[1] Use of radioactive suspensions has fallen out of favor because of their infliction of significant bowel damage, including necrosis that can occur with poor distribution of the radioactive agent.[1]

Emerging treatments: immunotherapy and targeted agents

Although a variety of cytokines and immunotherapy agents have been the subject of research since the 1980s, the studies have generally had very small sample sizes and the generalizability of their results to standard therapy has not been determined.[8,9] The main drugs studied are tumor necrosis factor agents (TNF), interferon, and OK-432. Researchers have been interested in the efficacy of TNF due to its ability to inhibit the interaction between VEGF and its receptor.[8] A small study comparing paracentesis with TNF treatment and paracentesis alone showed no clinical advantage, although a phase I trial using intraperitoneal recombinant TNF-α in refractory malignant ascites noted a complete or partial resolution in 76% of patients with mild side effects of fever, chills, nausea, vomiting, and fatigue.[40,41] More research is needed to definitively establish the benefit of TNF treatment.

With the increase in discovery of targeted therapies, there has been some study of anti-VEGF antibodies such as bevacizumab, and the trifunctional antibody, catumaxomab. Small studies evaluating bevacizumab intraperitoneal therapy alone or in combination with taxane therapy for malignant ascites associated with gastrointestinal, gynecological, and breast cancers have demonstrated success in the treatment of malignant ascites, eliminating the necessity of serial paracentesis.[42–44] Catumaxomab is a trifunctional antibody that has been studied for intraperitoneal application in patients with ovarian cancer. Phase I and II trials have better defined the dosing parameters, as grade 3 and 4 toxicities could be reduced with a decrease in dose while maintaining a positive response rate in the majority of subjects.[45] The side effects of fever, nausea, vomiting, and abdominal pain occurred on the day of or the day after infusion and were reversible. A dose of paracetamol 1000 mg (oral or rectal) is given 30 minutes prior to the start of infusion to minimize febrile reactions and risk for anaphylaxis. To improve the agent's distribution, 500 mL of 0.9% sodium chloride solution is administered intraperitoneally 30 minutes before initiation of the catumaxomab infusion.[45] Catumaxomab has received European approval for the treatment of malignant ascites and clinical trials have been conducted in the United States, but further studies are warranted.[2,7]

These emerging therapies hold some promise as alternative approaches to management of malignant ascites. Because the majority of patients presenting with malignant ascites having advanced stages of cancer, however, the benefits, risks, and tolerance to aggressive therapy need to be assessed to offer a treatment that maximizes quality of life and symptom relief.

NURSING IMPLICATIONS

The effectiveness of a therapeutic intervention for malignant ascites must encompass parameters that assess the patient's physical and psychological response. Nursing plays a key role in (1) assessing interventions directed toward symptom relief and improvement of quality of life, (2) providing essential patient education to minimize complications and enhance therapeutic responses, and (3) implementing independent nursing symptom management strategies to relieve discomfort and improve the patient's overall well-being. Even prior to initiating treatment for malignant ascites, nurses assist patients in exploring the benefits and risks of treatment options and considering how these options relate to the patient's goals. Knowledge of the patient and family over time places the nurse in the unique position of patient advocate, teacher, and counselor.

It is critical to document the evaluation of treatments over time. Pertinent data include the patient's subjective description of improvement in comfort, oral intake, respiratory function, gastrointestinal function, and activity tolerance. Objective data include abdominal girth measurement, weight, blood count values, chemistry, and tumor markers. If the patient is receiving treatment for the cancer and a measurable tumor is being followed, this information can be included in the evaluation as well. Any adverse effects to treatment should also be recorded.

Patient assessment and evaluation of interventions can be maintained on a nursing flow sheet. This form includes information on physical assessment and measurements such as vital signs, weight, intake and output, abdominal girth, laboratory values, nutritional intake, pain control, skin integrity, toxicity grading using the NCI grading system, and performance status measurement using Karnofsy index scoring scale or ECOG performance scale measurements. The frequency of fluid drainage via paracentesis or permanent catheter drains, the amount and character of fluid, and laboratory analysis of fluid if indicated can be recorded. Consultations with support services such as social work, home health care, dieticians, palliative care, and physical therapy can be documented to provide continuity of care.

Patients can be encouraged to be independent in their self-care as much as possible. Activities can be planned around therapeutic options. Patients can conserve energy by limiting visitors, delegating tasks to others, and taking frequent rest breaks after activities.[24–26] Many patients need to be advised to accept the assistance of family members and support services such as home care or psychological counseling for themselves or their families.[24–26] As the patient's physical status and options for treatment diminish, patients and families will need reassurance that members of their healthcare team are available for questions and advice on managing end-of-life issues.[24] Advance directives, if not already discussed, should be considered.

Many patients pursue alternative methods such as acupuncture, acupressure, and therapeutic touch for palliation of symptoms. Nurses can provide insight into their availability.

Meeting the psychological and spiritual needs of the patient and family may require referral to other healthcare professionals and support services. Once curative treatment is no longer an option for the patient, nurses have a role in promoting quality of life and assisting the patient and family with the dying process. The nurse can arrange a hospice representative to meet with the patient and family in the home to provide information about the hospice philosophy and service provisions.[24,26] Patients and families can be reassured that end-of-life physical and psychological needs will be met.

Nursing specific considerations and interventions to provide supportive measures throughout the course of malignant ascites are described in Table 12-6.[24–26,46] Also, Figure 12-4 provides a symptom management algorithm.

TABLE 12-6

Nursing Guidelines for Management of Ascites

Management Goal	Intervention
Promote fluid mobilization	• Assess peripheral edema • Monitor intake and output, electrolytes, serum protein, albumin • Administer diuretics as ordered • Obtain daily weight, abdominal girth • Elevate feet/legs when sitting • Apply compression stockings, boots • Assist patient in maintaining mobility
Promote respiratory function	• Elevate head of bed • Promote activity as tolerated • Provide oxygen as needed • Administer analgesics as ordered
Promote gastrointestinal function	• Maintain adequate nutrition as tolerated: Small, frequent meals Food supplements Bland diet Calorie counts • Obtain daily weights • Assess frequency of bowel movements • Administer antacids, H_2 blockers, antiemetics, bowel regimen, as ordered • Encourage oral hygiene after meals and as needed • Provide diversional therapy • Instruct in guided imagery
Promote skin integrity	• Encourage and assist in ambulation, positioning, turning • Apply lotion to relieve pruritus and dry skin • Massage bony prominences • Provide air mattress, foam cushions on bed, chairs • Encourage nutritional intake
Promote safety	• Monitor for signs of bleeding, infection, peritonitis • Provide clutter-free environment • Minimize invasive procedures • Assist in ambulation
Promote comfort	• Assess severity and quality of pain, discomfort • Provide air mattress, foam cushions on bed, chairs • Instruct in relaxation techniques, guided imagery • Administer analgesics, antianxiety agents, diuretics, antiemetics as ordered • Assist in positioning for comfort • Provide uninterrupted rest periods • Provide psychosocial and spiritual support/counseling
Promote self-care	• Instruct patient/family in interventions for self-care at home and in follow-up appointments • Assess equipment/resources needed within the home • Provide appropriate referrals to home-care agency, hospice • Provide referral for psychosocial counseling as indicated

Source: Data from Vogel et al[24]; Economua[25]; Murphy[26]; Winkelman[46].

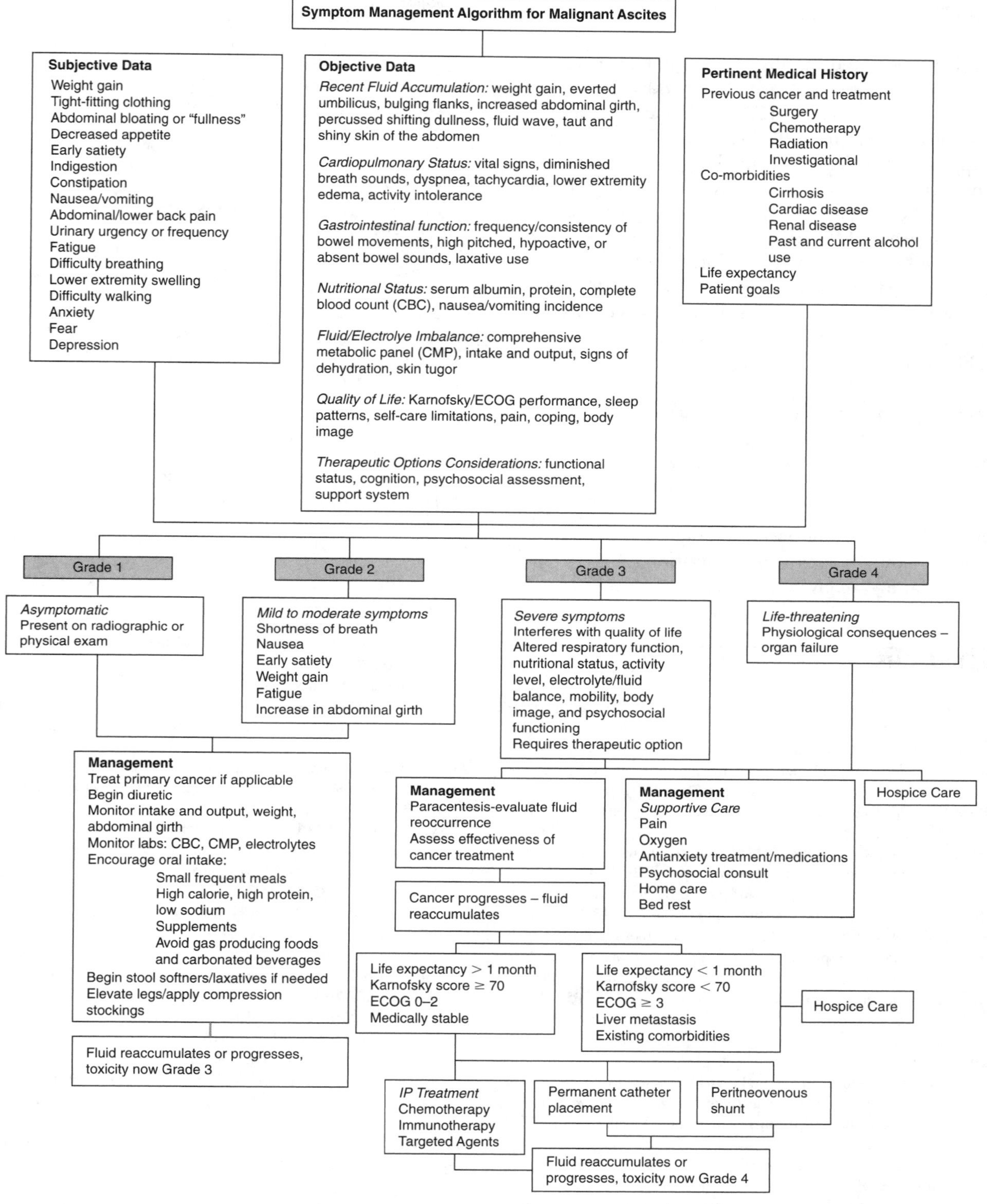

FIGURE 12-4

Symptom management algorithm for malignant ascites.

Abbreviation: ECOG: Eastern Cooperative Oncology Group.

PATIENT SELF-CARE

To assist patients and families in symptom management and self-care, written tools can be provided to reinforce verbal teaching. Appendix 12A (Malignant Ascites Self-Assessment), Appendix 12B (Self-Care Guide: Ascites), and Appendix 12E (Ascites Daily Log) can be given to all patients, whereas Appendix 12C (Removing Ascites Fluid: Paracentesis) can be given to patients undergoing paracentesis and Appendix 12D (Shunt Care) to patients with PVS.

There are several trustworthy Internet sites nurses can use to inform patients about additional self-care resources. Websites specific to the patient's disease, patient advocacy groups, and community and government resources are available, including the following:

- American Cancer Society: www.cancer.org
- Cancer Care Inc.: www.cancercare.org
- The Wellness Community: www.twcvv.org
- National Hospice and Palliative Care Organization: www.nhpco.org
- Hospice Link: www.hospiceworld.org
- National Family Caregivers Association: www.thefamilycaregiver.org

REFERENCES

1. Chung M, Kozuch P. Treatment of malignant ascites. *Cur Treat Opt Oncol.* 2008;9:215–233.
2. Barni S, Cabiddu M, Ghilardi M, Petrelli F. A novel perspective for an orphan problem: old and new drugs for the medical management of malignant ascites. *Crit Rev Oncol/Hematol.* 2011;79:144–153.
3. Rosenberg SM. Palliation of malignant ascites. *Gastroenterol Clin North Am.* 2006;35:189–199.
4. Hussain A, Bezjak A, Easson A. Malignant ascites symptom cluster in patients referred for paracentesis. *Ann Surg Oncol.* 2010;17:461–469.
5. Ayantunde AA, Parsons SL. Pattern and prognostic factors in patients with malignant ascites: a retrospective study. *Ann Oncol.* 2007;18:945–949.
6. Ayantunde AA, Parsons SL. Predictors of poor prognosis in patients with malignant ascites: a prospective study. *Clin Med Diagnost.* 2012;2(2):1–6.
7. Woopen H, Sehouli J. Current and future options in the treatment of malignant ascites in ovarian cancer. *Anticancer Res.* 2009;29:3353–3360.
8. Cavazzoni E, Bugiantella W, Graziosi L, Franceschini M, Donini A. Malignant ascites: pathophysiology and treatment. *Int J Clin Oncol.* 2013;18(1):1–9.
9. Kammula US. Malignant ascites. In: DeVita VT, Lawrence TS, Rosenberg SA, eds. *DeVita, Hellman, and Rosenberg's Cancer: Principles and Practice of Oncology.* 9th ed. Philadelphia: Lippincott Williams & Wilkins; 2011;2214–2219.
10. Ammouri L, Prommer EE. Palliative treatment of malignant ascites: profile of catumaxomab. *Biol Targets Therap.* 2010;4:103–110.
11. LeBlanc K, Arnold RM. Evaluation of malignant ascites #176. *J Palliat Med* 2010;13(8):1027.
12. Levy A. Peritoneum and mesentery. Part I: anatomy. http://www.radiologyassistant.nl/en/4a252c5303035. Accessed April 1, 2012.
13. Cope D. Malignant effusions. In: Yarbro CH, Wujcik D, Gobel BH, eds. *Cancer Nursing Principles and Practice.* 7th ed. Burlington, MA: Jones & Bartlett Learning; 2011;873–877.
14. Scallan J, Huxley VH, Korthuis RJ. Pathology of edema formation. In: *Capillary Fluid Exchange: Regulation, Functions, and Pathology.* San Rafael, CA: Morgan, Claypool, and Life Sciences; 2010. http://www.ncbi.nlm.gov/books/NBK53445/.
15. Nettina S, ed. Hepatic, biliary, and pancreatic disorders. In: *Lippincott Manual of Nursing Practice.* 9th ed. Ambler, PA: Lippincott Williams & Wilkins; 2010;712–745.
16. Karnofsky performance status scale definitions rating (%) criteria. http://www.hospicepatients.org/karnofsky.html. Accessed April 1, 2012.
17. Oken MM, Creech RH, Tormey DC, et al. Toxicity and response criteria of the Eastern Cooperative Oncology Group. *Am J Clin Oncol.* 1982;5:649–655.
18. Talley N, O'Connor S. The gastrointestinal system. In: *Clinical Examination: A Systematic Guide to Physical Diagnosis.* 6th ed. Australia: Elsevier; 2010;153–182.
19. deWit S, ed. Assessing health status. In: *Fundamental Concepts and Skills for Nurses.* 3rd ed. New York: Elsevier Science; 2008:370–393.
20. Eisenhauer E, Salani R, Copeland L. Epithelial ovarian cancer In: Disaia P, Creasman W, eds. *Clinical Gynecologic Oncology.* 8th ed. New York: Saunders, Elsevier; 2012;285–328.
21. Fleming ND, Alvarez-Secord A, Von Gruenigen V, Miller MJ, Abernethy AP. Indwelling catheters for the management of refractory malignant ascites: a systematic literature overview and retrospective chart review. *J Pain Symptom Manage.* 2009;38(3):341–349.
22. Han C, Lee C, Huang K, et al. Diagnostic laparoscopy in ascites of unknown origin. *Chang Gung Me J.* 2008;31(4):378–383.
23. National Cancer Institute Common terminology criteria for adverse events v4.0 (CTCAE). 2009. http://www.acrin.org/Portals/0/Administration/Regulatory/CTCAE_4.02_2009-09-15_QuickReference_5x7.pdf. Accessed April 1, 2012.
24. Vogel WH, Wilson MA, Melvin MS. (eds) Part I. *Advanced Practice Oncology and Palliative Care.* Philadelphia: Lippincott Williams & Wilkins; 2004.
25. Economua D. Bowel management: constipation, diarrhea, obstruction, and ascites. In: Ferrell BR, Coyle N, eds. *The Oxford Textbook of Palliative Nursing.* 3rd ed. New York: Oxford University Press; 2010:269–290.
26. Murphy D. Malignant ascites. In: Chernecky CC, Murphy-Endik C, eds. *Acute Care Oncology Nursing.* 2nd ed. St. Louis, MO: Saunders; 2009: 26–34.
27. von Gunten T. CF: Diagnosis and management of ascites. In: Berger A, Von Roenn J, Schuster J, eds. *Principles and Practice of Palliative Care and Supportive Oncology.* 3rd ed. Philadelphia, PA: Lippincott, Williams and Wilkins; 2005:185–192.
28. Becker G, Galandi D, Blum H. Malignant ascites: systematic review and guideline for treatment. *Eur J Cancer.* 2006;42:589–597.
29. Sangisetty SS, Miner TJ. Malignant ascites: a review of prognostic factors, pathophysiology, and therapeutic measures. *World J Gastrointest Surg.* 2012;4(4);87–95.
30. LeBlanc K, Arnold R. Palliative treatment of malignant ascites #177. *J Palliat Med.* 2010;13(8);1028–1029.
31. Mullard AP, Bishop JM, Jibani M. Intractable malignant ascites: an alternative management option. *J Palliat Med.* 2011;14(2):251–253.
32. Kawalak J, ed. *Lippincott's Nursing Procedures.* 5th ed. Philadelphia: Lippincott, Williams, and Wilkins; 2009.
33. 510(k) Summary 21 CFR 807.92. Aspira peritoneal drainage system. 2011. http://www.accessdata.fda.gov/cdrh_docs/pdf11/K110396.pdf. Accessed April 1, 2012.
34. Tomiyama K, Takahashi M, Fujll T, et al. Improved quality of life for malignant ascites patients by Denver peritoneovenous shunts. *Anticancer Res.* 2006;26:2393–2396.
35. Walker J, Armstrong D, Huang H, et al. Intraperitoneal catheter outcomes in a phase 3 trial of intravenous versus intraperitoneal chemotherapy in an optimal stage 3 ovarian and primary peritoneal cancer: a Gynecologic Group study. *Gynecol Oncol.* 2006;100:27–32.

36. Armstrong DK, Bundy B, Wenzel L, et al. Intraperitoneal cisplatin and paclitaxel in ovarian cancer. *New Engl J Med.* 2006;354:34–43.
37. National Cancer Institute. NCI clinical announcement: intraperitoneal chemotherapy for ovarian cancer. January 5, 2006. www.cancer.gov/newscenter/pressreleases/2006/ipchemotherapyrelease. Accessed August 5, 2012.
38. Trimble EL, Thompson S, Christian MC, Minasian L. Intraperitoneal chemotherapy for women with epithelial ovarian cancer. *Oncologist.* 2008;13(4):403–409.
39. Valle M, Van der Speeten K, Garofalo A. Laparoscopic hyperthermic intraperitoneal preoperative chemotherapy (HIPEC) in the management of refractory malignant ascites: a multi-institutional retrospective analysis in 52 patients. *Surg Oncol.* 2009;100(4):331–334.
40. Seimetz D, Lindhofer H, Bokemeyer C. Development and approval of the trifunctional antibody catumaxomab (anti-Ep_CAM x anti-CD3) as a targeted cancer immunotherapy. *Cancer Treat Rev.* 2010;36(6);458–467.
41. Heiss M, Murawa P, Koralewski P. The trifunctional antibody catumaxomab for the treatment of malignant ascites due to epithelial cancer: results of a prospective randomized phase II/III trial. *Int J Cancer.* 2010;127(9);2209–2221.
42. Pichelmayer O, Gruenberger B, Zielinski C, et al. Bevacizumab is active in malignant effusion. *Ann Oncol.* 2006;17:1853.
43. Numnum TM, Rocconi RP, Whitworth J, et al. The use of bevacizumab to palliate symptomatic ascites in patients with refractory ovarian carcinoma. *Gynecol Oncol.* 2006;102:425–428.
44. El-Shami K, Elsaid A, El-Kerm Y. Open-label safety and efficacy pilot trial of intraperitoneal bevacizumab as palliative treatment in refractory malignant ascites. *J Clin Oncol.* 2007;25(18 suppl):9043.
45. Burges A, Wimberger P, Kumper C, et al. Effective relief of malignant ascites in patients with advanced ovarian cancer by a trifunctional anti-EpCAM x anti-CD3 antibody: a phase I/II study. *Clin Cancer Res.* 2007;12(13):3899–3905.
46. Winkelman LA. Malignant ascites. In: Yarbro CH, Frogge MH, Goodman M, eds. *Cancer Symptom Management.* 3rd ed. Sudbury, MA: Jones and Bartlett; 2004;401–419.

Malignant Ascites Self-Assessment

Patient Name: ____________________

This guide will help you find any signs and symptoms of excess fluid in your belly. Picking up even small changes in your body and how you are feeling can help your healthcare team in finding excess belly fluid, so that they can work with you to develop ways to help take care of this problem.

Please answer the following questions:

Question	Yes	No
Have you had recent weight gain that you could not explain in the past 6 months? If yes, how much weight have you gained? ____________ pounds		
Are your clothes fitting tighter around the waist and upper legs?		
Do you have a feeling of belly "bloating" or "fullness"?		
Have you had a decrease in your appetite?		
Do you have frequent upset stomach or nausea?		
Do you have constipation?		
Do you have new belly or lower back pain? How would you rate the pain on a scale of 0–10 (0 = no pain, 10 = severe pain)? 0 1 2 3 4 5 6 7 8 9 10		
Do you need to urinate more often?		
Do you have urinary urgency?		
Are you more tired than usual?		
Are you short of breath?		
Do you have swelling in your lower legs or ankles?		
Medical History		
Have you had radiation therapy or chemotherapy?		
Do you have a history of liver, heart, or kidney disease? Please circle: Liver Heart Kidney		
Do you drink alcohol? If yes, how many drinks each week do you drink? ____________		

Source: Slusser K. Malignant Ascites. In: Yarbro CH, Wujcik D, Gobel BH, eds. *Cancer Symptom Management.* 4th ed. Burlington, MA: Jones & Bartlett Learning; 2014.

Ascites

Patient Name: ____

This guide will help you to know how to live with fluid that collects in your belly. It provides ways to deal with the symptoms.

What Is Ascites?

Ascites is a symptom that is seen when large amounts of fluid collect in your belly. The fluid can cause a feeling of fullness and make your clothes fit tightly. There are many ways listed in this guide that can be used to decrease the discomfort, reduce the fluid buildup or prevent it from getting worse, and prevent other problems.

Management

Diet

There are no limits to your diet. If possible, eat foods high in calories and protein and low in sodium. Because you may feel "fullness" or "bloating" in your belly, eating small, frequent meals (6 small meals per day) may be helpful.

- High-protein, low-sodium foods include unprocessed, unseasoned beef, lamb, pork, poultry, and fish; eggs and egg substitutes; dried beans and peas, unsalted nuts, and salt-free nut butters.
- To reduce sodium in your food, try to prepare fresh fruits and vegetables instead of canned or frozen ones.
- Foods you may choose to *avoid* (to reduce sodium) in your diet include cured, smoked, and salted meats (sausage, ham, hot dogs, bacon, cold cuts) and already prepared marinated meats in your grocery's meat section.
- You can also discuss the use of supplements with your healthcare team if eating causes fullness and bloating, making it hard to take in adequate nutrition.

Pain Control

You can rate your pain daily using a scale of 0–10, in which 0 equals no pain and 10 equals the worst pain you can think of. It is helpful to write your pain ratings in a diary or log and include things like whether the pain is aching, sharp, or dull. You can also include things that make your pain worse or better.

Based on your pain level, your healthcare team will discuss options with you to help with your pain. These options can include medicine, positioning, and nonmedicine methods such as distraction, meditation, and others.

Activity

There are no limits to your activity. You may find it helpful to take frequent rests or breaks between daily tasks, errands, or activities. To reduce lower leg and ankle swelling, you can put your legs up when sitting.

(continued)

Diary

Keeping a diary of how the fluid collection in your belly makes you feel can help both the healthcare team and you know if the symptoms are getting worse or better. This is important in checking the current treatment methods being used and if new methods need to be found. A sample daily log is included for your use.

Follow-Up

Call your nurse or doctor if any of the following occur:

- Weight gain where your clothes are not fitting
- Trouble breathing or shortness of breath
- Nausea and/or vomiting
- Pain greater than a 4 rating for 2 consecutive days

Phone Numbers

Doctor's name: ____

Number: ____________________

Nurse's name: ____

Number: ____________________

Other: ____

Number: ____________________

Source: Slusser K. Malignant Ascites. In: Yarbro CH, Wujcik D, Gobel BH, eds. *Cancer Symptom Management*. 4th ed. Burlington, MA: Jones & Bartlett Learning; 2014.

Removing Ascites Fluid: Paracentesis

Patient Name: ______________________________

This guide will help you to know how the procedure called paracentesis is done, what to expect, and when to call for help.

Symptom and Description

Ascites is a symptom that occurs when large amounts of fluid pool in your abdomen. The fluid can cause a sense of fullness, make your clothes fit tightly, and affect your ability to eat.

The Procedure

A paracentesis is a small incision into your abdomen to place a tube to drain the fluid. The tube is placed into a drainage bag or container. The procedure provides quick relief of pressure on your abdomen.

An ultrasound machine is used to help find the best place to put the drainage tube. Your skin will be cleaned with a special solution and a numbing medicine will be injected into your skin. You may feel a pinching and burning sensation for a few seconds. The tube will then be placed into your belly and fluid will be drained. When the fluid is drained, the tube will be removed. Pressure will be applied to the site to stop the bleeding. A gauze dressing will then be placed over the area.

You will go home as soon as you are ready. The dressing should stay on for 1 day. You will not be able to take a shower, drive, or lift heavy objects for 1 day. You may take the medicine your doctor gave you for pain. If you experience leakage, you should apply direct pressure with a clean gauze for 10 minutes.

Follow-up

You should make arrangements with your doctor for a follow-up visit to the office.

After the procedure, call your doctor if you have:

- Fever over 101°F
- Shaking, chills
- Sudden, intense abdominal pain
- Unexplained weakness
- Nausea, vomiting, diarrhea, or constipation that last more than 24 hours
- Fluid builds up again

Phone Numbers

Nurse: ______________________ Phone: ______________________

Doctor: ______________________ Phone: ______________________

Other: ______________________ Phone: ______________________

Source: Slusser K. Malignant Ascites. In: Yarbro CH, Wujcik D, Gobel BH, eds. *Cancer Symptom Management.* 4th ed. Burlington, MA: Jones & Bartlett Learning; 2014.

Shunt Care

Patient Name: ______________________________

This guide will help you to know how to live with the fluid and shunt in your abdomen. You will learn how to take care of the shunt and how to handle the effects of the shunt and fluid.

Symptom and Description

Ascites is a symptom that occurs when large amounts of fluid pool in your abdomen. The fluid can cause a sense of fullness and make your clothes fit tightly. The shunt is a tube that has been placed to reduce this fluid by draining it into your bloodstream. The excess fluid can then be removed by your kidneys into the urine. The fluid can be removed and managed with the care outlined in this guide.

Management

1. *Diet:* There are no limits to your diet. Try to eat foods high in protein and calories. Small, frequent meals (up to 6 meals a day) may be easier for you to eat.
2. *Pain control:* Rate your pain daily using a scale of 0 to 10 in which 0 equals no pain and 10 equals the worst pain that you can imagine. Select the number that best describes your level of pain.

0	1	2	3	4	5	6	7	8	9	10
no pain									worst pain	

3. *Activity:* There are no limits to your activities. You should do what you feel like doing. Rest periods may be helpful. Elevate your feet/legs when sitting. Wear an abdominal binder while up to increase pressure and enhance fluid flow.
4. *Fluid flow:* If you notice an increase in size around your abdomen, you may increase fluid flow into the bloodstream by any of the following:
   - Lying down flat on your back
   - Using the spirometer for 15 minutes 4 times a day
   - Wearing an abdominal binder while up to increase pressure and enhance fluid flow
   - If you have a Denver shunt in place, compress it as you were taught by your doctor or nurse
5. *Diary:* Keep a record of your daily pain rating, measurement around abdomen, and weight on the Patient Data Record included. Be careful to measure your abdomen in the same place each day. Bring this record with you to your next visit with your nurse or doctor.

Follow-up

Call your nurse or doctor if any of the following occurs:

- A weight gain or increase in abdominal size so that your clothes do not fit
- Trouble breathing or shortness of breath
- Nausea, vomiting
- Increase in pain rating to above 4 for 2 days in a row.
- Fever greater than 101°F

Phone Numbers

Nurse: ____________________ Phone: ____________________

Physician: ____________________ Phone: ____________________

Other: ____________________ Phone: ____________________

Source: Slusser K. Malignant Ascites. In: Yarbro CH, Wujcik D, Gobel BH, eds. *Cancer Symptom Management.* 4th ed. Burlington, MA: Jones & Bartlett Learning; 2014.

Ascites Daily Log

Patient Name: ______________________________

This log can be used to keep track of the symptoms you feel from the fluid excess in your belly. It is helpful to bring this log with you when you see your healthcare team. You can check with your healthcare team to decide how often you should weigh yourself and measure your abdominal girth; these may not need to be done daily.

Week beginning: ______________

Day	Weight	Abdominal Girth	Pain (0–10)	Appetite (Good, Fair, Poor)	Nausea or Vomiting (Y/N)	Number of Bowel Movements	Urinary Frequency (Y/N)	Urinary Urgency (Y/N)
Sun								
Mon								
Tues								
Wed								
Thurs								
Fri								
Sat								

Comments:

Source: Slusser K. Malignant Ascites. In: Yarbro CH, Wujcik D, Gobel BH, eds. *Cancer Symptom Management*. 4th ed. Burlington, MA: Jones & Bartlett Learning; 2014.

PART V

Alterations in Genitourinary Function

Chapter 13
Bladder Disturbances

Chapter 13

Bladder Disturbances

Connie Henke Yarbro, RN, MS, FAAN
Donna L. Berry, RN, PhD, AOCN® FAAN

THE PROBLEM

Disturbances of the bladder that are associated with cancer symptoms, treatment side effects, or disease sequelae can be categorized into three basic groups of human responses: pathophysiologic responses, sensory or experiential responses, and behavioral responses. Table 13-1 depicts the three groups of responses and respective symptoms. To establish clarity of terms as used in this chapter, symptom definitions are provided in Table 13-2.

A bladder disturbance in a person with cancer most likely will be composed of a set of symptoms involving more than one type of response. For example, an individual with an *Escherichia coli* infection of the bladder may experience the sensations of dysuria and urgency (sensory responses) and report urinary frequency (behavioral response). As with most cancer symptomatology, the complexity of human responses creates challenges for both self-care and management by the healthcare provider.

TABLE 13-1

Human Responses and Bladder Symptoms

Pathophysiologic	Hematuria; lower urinary tract infection; radiation or drug-induced cystitis; hemorrhagic cystitis; outflow obstruction; sphincter incompetence
Sensory/experiential	Dysuria; urgency; bladder pain
Behavioral	Frequency; voiding dysfunction

The impact of bladder disturbances on quality of life can be dramatic. The pain or discomfort of irritative bladder symptoms not only can cause personal suffering, but also can motivate an individual to withdraw from curative therapy. Voiding dysfunction may be difficult to manage and so embarrassing that the individuals may avoid social activities or become isolated by never leaving their house.

INCIDENCE

When a person with cancer presents with a disturbance of the bladder, the situation is most often related to one of the following typical scenarios.

First, an individual with carcinoma of the bladder is at risk for hematuria and irritative bladder symptoms (dysuria, urgency, frequency). *Hematuria*—that is, either gross or microscopic blood in the urine—is the hallmark manifestation of bladder cancer and is the presenting symptom in as many as 80% of individuals with superficial bladder cancer.[1–4] Irritative bladder symptoms (IBSs) are present at diagnosis in 20% to 30% of patients with bladder cancer.[2] Drug-induced cystitis associated with intravesical chemotherapy has been reported in as many as 44% of cases,[5,6] and IBSs have been reported in nearly 80% of those individuals receiving intravesical bacillus Calmette-Guérin (BCG).[2] Although the majority of patients with bladder cancer present with early-stage disease, some tumors will progress to invade the entire bladder wall. For these individuals and those who are diagnosed with muscle-invasive disease, removal of the bladder is the first-line therapy.[7]

TABLE 13-2

Bladder Disturbance Symptom Definitions

Symptom	Definition
Hematuria	Blood in the urine: can be microscopic or visible to eye alone as pink-tinged or red urine, with or without clots
Dysuria	Painful and/or burning sensations during urination
Frequency	Voiding more often than every 2 hours; daytime frequency is sometimes described as *diurnal* frequency; *nocturia* is used to describe nighttime voiding more than once if under 65 years of age and more than twice if over 65 years of age
Urgency	Compelling feeling of the need to urinate as soon as possible
Irritative bladder symptoms	A symptom index generally including dysuria, urgency, and frequency
Cystitis	Inflammation of the bladder epithelium
Hemorrhagic cystitis	An often sudden onset of hematuria combined with bladder pain and irritative bladder symptoms
Urinary outflow obstruction	An impediment near the bladder neck that can create urinary retention and overflow incontinence; usually prostate tumor in the oncology setting
Sphincter incompetence	A common complication of radical prostatectomy due to the necessary distortion of the urethrovesical junction

A second scenario involving bladder disturbances in patients with cancer is that of a *lower urinary tract infection* (UTI). The incidence of bacteriuria (defined as more than 10^5 colony-forming units/mL) is highest in the elderly, the age group also most likely to develop cancer. Bacteria typically involved in such infections include *E. coli*, *Enterobacter*, and *Streptococcus* species.[8] Immunosuppressed individuals are at additional risk for infections of the bladder, with their immunosuppression often allowing the growth of normally less virulent organisms such as *Candida*. Individuals receiving or recuperating from cancer therapy are also at risk if they are catheterized. Catheter-associated UTIs are the most common nosocomial infection worldwide.[9]

A third typical bladder disturbance scenario, manifested in men with cancer, is that of voiding dysfunction associated with *prostate cancer*. Prostate cancer accounted for nearly one-third of all malignancies diagnosed in men in 2011.[10] Most men with localized disease are asymptomatic or present with bladder outlet obstruction and bladder irritability.[11] Radical prostatectomy (RP) is one of the most common treatments for localized carcinoma of the prostate. However, one year after a prostatectomy, the majority of men will not be fully continent. Peterson and Chen[12] reviewed data from the Center for Prostate Disease Research related to 4374 patients undergoing RP between 1990 and 2007. Complete data were available for 1616 men (37%), of whom 1459 (90.3%) reported urinary incontinence more than one year after RP. When treatment for prostate cancer includes either external beam radiation therapy to the pelvic region or radioactive implants to the prostate, radiation cystitis is a common side effect, ranging from mild to severe.[11,13,14]

Fourth, urinary incontinence and voiding dysfunction have been reported in other populations. Urinary incontinence is an ongoing concern in women after treatment of rectal cancer.[15] Manchana[16] noted that voiding dysfunction and urinary incontinence are prevalent in gynecologic cancer survivors after radical hysterectomy.

Finally, functional urinary incontinence associated with *neurologic deficits,* or altered dexterity and mobility, is observed in some individuals with cancer. Cognitive dysfunction caused by metabolic derangements, chemotherapy, or radiation therapy side effects can impair toileting behaviors of the affected individual. Peripheral neuropathy—a side effect of numerous chemotherapeutic agents[17,18]—can impair both dexterity and mobility, making voiding behaviors much more difficult. Urinary incontinence, along with pain and leg weakness, are symptoms of spinal cord compression.[19]

Clearly, these scenarios are not inclusive of all individuals with bladder disturbances related to cancer; however, they are typical of the bladder disturbances frequently encountered by oncology nurses. In addition, many patients, particularly the elderly, have multiple illnesses and may have bladder disturbances unrelated to their malignant processes.

ETIOLOGY AND PATHOPHYSIOLOGY

The etiology and pathophysiology of bladder disturbances associated with cancer can be discussed either as problems of the bladder urothelium or as problems of the neuromuscular function of the bladder. The mucosal lining of the bladder consists of the urothelium (formerly called the transitional epithelium), plus five to seven layers of transitional epithelial cells (Figure 13-1).[20] The mucosa overlies the collagenous lamina propria containing blood vessels, lymphatic vessels, and nerves. Beyond that, the muscularis propria is organized in bundles of smooth muscle, and the perivesical tissue encases the bladder.[7]

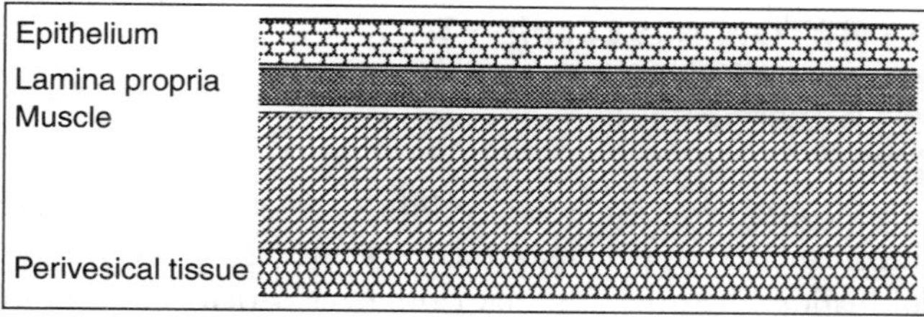

FIGURE 13-1

Graphic depiction of the tissue layers of the bladder.

BLADDER CANCER

Malignant growth confined to the transitional epithelium and the lamina propria accounts for more than 90% of all diagnosed bladder cancers.[7,21] These superficial bladder tumors and carcinoma in situ disrupt the mucosal integrity and can infiltrate the lamina propria, causing hematuria and irritation. Hematuria may fluctuate, occurring off and on over the course of weeks to months. However, if it always recurs, it is likely that the cause is due to bladder cancer.[22] The less common, invasive tumors manifest the same type of symptoms but more severe discomfort.

BLADDER INFECTION

The bladder epithelium undergoes inflammatory change when colonized with infectious agents. Polymorphonucleocytes (PMNs) infiltrate the mucosa, while edema develops within the cellular matrix and the lamina, causing irritability.[23] Muscle irritability and painful bladder spasms may result in urge incontinence, dysuria, urgency, and frequency. A very similar mechanism ensues when BCG is administered intravesically for treatment of superficial bladder cancer. Although the BCG is an attenuated form of the bacillus, the bladder epithelium reacts with an inflammatory sequence of events that ultimately leads to tumor elimination and delay of recurrence.[24] An individual receiving the treatment can experience the irritative bladder symptoms of dysuria, frequency, and urgency, along with pain localized to the lower pelvic region.[25] Treatment of the irritative sensations includes eliminating the causative agent (in the case of bladder infection) and reducing exposure of the bladder epithelium to additional irritants such as highly concentrated or acidic urine.[26]

CHEMOTHERAPY-INDUCED CYSTITIS

Hemorrhagic cystitis is a complication associated with ifosfamide and cyclophosphamide, cytotoxic alkylating agents used in a variety of malignancies. Patients will report a sudden onset of dysuria and hematuria, which less commonly is massive and intractable. The damage to the epithelium is most likely caused by the metabolic breakdown products of cyclophosphamide and includes mucosal ulcerations, vascular telangiectasia, severe edema, and hemorrhage within the lamina propria.[23] Fortunately, this drug-induced hemorrhage is less common than in the past, due to the use of mesna, an agent that, when administered with ifosfamide or cyclophosphamide, protects the urothelium.[17,27]

Other cancer agents that have been reported to cause hemorrhagic cystitis include gemcitabine,[17] dacarbazine,[28] and temozolomide.[29]

Intravesical cytotoxic chemotherapies such as mitomycin-C and valrubicin have been used for treatment of transitional cell carcinoma of the bladder. The local irritative effects of these agents are those of a chemical cystitis, similar to that of an infectious inflammation but without the evidence of bacteriuria.

RADIATION INJURY

Individuals receiving radiation therapy to the pelvic area can experience radiation cystitis that is time and dose dependent. The disturbance is manifested as acute cystitis approximately 3 to 5 weeks after initiation of treatment and usually subsides 2 to 8 weeks after completion of treatment. Late reactions also have been reported months or years after therapy and are related to bleeding, symptomatic cystitis, and contracture.[30] Histologically, the bladder epithelium becomes transiently hyperemic, followed by development of extensive vascular dilation, stromal edema, and focal ulcerations.[23] External beam radiation or implanted source radiation (brachytherapy) can damage the urethra and impair urethral blood supply, inducing fibrosis, stricture, or atrophy.[31]

VOIDING DYSFUNCTION

Various types of voiding dysfunction are possible. The following etiologies are those that may frequently be encountered by oncology nurses.

Many patients with cancer are taking opioids for pain relief. Reduced bladder muscle contractility and subsequent urinary retention can be side effects of systemic and spinal opioids.[32]

Overflow incontinence or bladder outflow obstruction can occur in men with benign prostatic hypertrophy and carcinoma of the prostate.[11] As seen in Figure 13-2, the prostate surrounds the urethra as it exits from the bladder through the bladder neck. A tumor may cause narrowing of the urethra or disruption of normal urinary sphincter

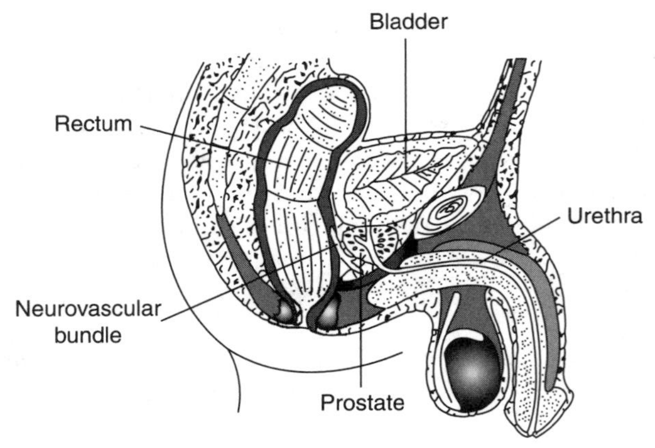

FIGURE 13-2

Anatomic relationships of the male bladder.

function. The obstruction leads to hypertrophy and instability of the detrusor muscle, which normally empties the bladder by contracting. Urinary retention occurs despite intravesical pressures that may be relatively high. The bladder then spontaneously releases urine, and the man experiences incontinence, including dribbling, frequent urination, and nocturia. Concomitant UTI is common because of the higher residual volumes and may result in sensations of dysuria and urgency.

A common postoperative complication of radical prostatectomy is urinary incontinence.[11,13,33,34] Because of the excision of the prostate plus the portion of the urethra located within the prostate, the bladder neck must be surgically repaired and reconnected to the remaining urethra during the prostatectomy procedure. Given the disruption in normal urinary anatomy and voiding function, the patient wears a urinary catheter for 2 to 3 weeks after the operation and then begins to regain urinary continence. The necessity of removing prostate tissue with tumor-free margins often results in partial resection of the tissues of the urinary sphincter mechanism and, consequently, stress incontinence.

SPINAL CORD INJURY

Injury to the spinal cord due to bony metastasis or direct tumor extension can lead to detrusor paralysis and associated sphincter weakness. The detrusor muscle, which normally contracts during bladder emptying, lies flaccid, allowing the bladder to overfill, and ultimately stress incontinence occurs. Detrusor hyperreflexia can also occur during the bladder-filling phase, limiting the storage capabilities of the bladder.[35]

SYMPTOM ASSESSMENT

SELF-ASSESSMENT

Dysuria during or after voiding, frequency, urgency, incontinence, and hematuria are some of the symptoms of bladder disturbances that can affect patients' quality of life. Patients do not always verbally describe their urinary symptoms or complications to their physician or nurse, yet will often report a higher level of symptomatology on a self-report questionnaire.[36] For this reason, it is important to provide a self-report tool at regular intervals for gathering bladder disturbance information.

In 1992, members and consultants of the American Urological Association (AUA) reported the development and validation of a symptom index for benign prostatic hyperplasia (BPH).[37] This index discriminates between male patients likely to have BPH and those without urologic problems; however, it is suitable for both men and women with urinary dysfunction. The AUA Symptom Index is recommended for use in following and monitoring urinary symptomatology before and over the course of treatment for obstruction.[38] It includes both obstructive symptom items (hesitancy, incomplete emptying, intermittency, and weak stream) and irritative symptom items (frequency, urgency, and nocturia). Dysuria is not included, however.

The Expanded Prostate Cancer Index Composite (EPIC)[39] is a validated self-report questionnaire designed for men with prostate cancer. This tool addresses irritative symptoms, and the "urinary domain" question set could be adapted for use in individuals with bladder cancer. The International Prostate Symptom Score (IPSS) has been commonly used to assess lower urinary tract symptoms but it is not as comprehensive as the Core Lower Urinary Tract Symptom Score (CLSS).[40–42]

A written record of voiding activity is helpful in the assessment and evaluation of treatment for bladder disturbances, particularly for individuals experiencing incontinence. The diary is most useful if kept simple and easy to complete. The record can be kept for a few days before a diagnostic evaluation or during certain times within a treatment period. The simplest of diaries documents only the pattern of voiding. For a more comprehensive diary, additional information can be gathered regarding fluid intake, urgency, and even dysuria. Appendix 13A provides a sample bladder diary.

OBJECTIVE ASSESSMENT

History

All diagnostic evaluations begin with a health history. After ascertaining what has brought the individual to the practice setting, focus the history interview on more specific inquiries relevant to the lower urinary system and related systems (Table 13-3).

Physical assessment

Physical examination of the lower urinary tract is indicated when there is a complaint of a bladder disturbance; it entails evaluation of the abdomen and the external genitalia. Ask the individual to empty the bladder before the examination and to recline in a comfortable supine position. The bladder can then be inspected, palpated, and percussed for signs of distention. Dull sounds on percussion and resistance to light palpation, all in the suprapubic area, are indications of a distended or retentive bladder. Urinary tract infection or a mass can also produce resistance to palpation.

Inspect the perineal skin for integrity in both men and women, noting rashes or excoriations that might be caused by urinary leakage. The penis, including the glans penis and meatus, should be inspected for inflammation. In an uncircumcised man, the glans is normally moist and pink. Inspect the perineum, vulvar area, and meatus of a woman as she reclines in a lithotomy position. The labia minora should be soft and nontender. Rashes or excoriations on the labia and vaginal opening may indicate vaginitis or UTI.

Certain aspects of a general physical examination are pertinent to evaluation of a bladder disturbance. Some physical findings significant to carcinoma of the bladder include pallor and edema of the lower extremities, indicating impaired circulation related to a possible mass. Systemic findings, such as fever and chills, anorexia, weight loss, and malaise, are important to note when identifying an infection that has colonized the kidneys or has become systemic, and when evaluating disease progression.

TABLE 13-3

Health History Questions for a Complaint of an Altered Voiding Pattern
Chief Complaint: Altered Voiding Pattern (Incontinence/Retention/Dysuria) Voiding patterns
How often does the patient urinate during the day and night?
How long can the patient wait comfortably between urinating?
How long can urination be postponed before the need to urinate is urgent?
Does involuntary loss of urine occur during coughing, sneezing, changing positions, or during physical exercise?
Is there a sense of urgency before loss of urine? Is the involuntary loss of urine continuous or intermittent, before or after urinating or both? Are pads worn, and how often do they become saturated or changed? Are any other urinary devices worn or used?
Does the patient have difficulty starting the stream of urine? Is the stream weak or involuntarily interrupted? Is there incontinence or other urinary symptoms during sexual activity?
Urologic history
Does the patient describe sensations of discomfort or burning before, during, or after urination, and where it is felt, in the bladder or urethra?
Has the patient been evaluated and treated for urinary tract infection(s)?
Were there any congenital urinary disorders?
Has the patient been evaluated and treated for kidney or bladder stones or genitourinary tumors?
Has the patient noticed any urine color or odor changes?
Related system disorders
Are there any previously diagnosed neurologic conditions such as Parkinson's disease, multiple sclerosis, spinal cord injury or malignant metastasis, diabetes, or stroke?
Does the patient have any changes in normal bowel patterns?
Are there indications of sexual dysfunction?
If a woman, is she premenopausal or postmenopausal?
Medications affecting continence
Is the patient taking any antispasmodics, antidepressants, or narcotics (agents that decrease detrusor contractility)?
Is the patient taking any cholinergics (agents that increase detrusor contractility)?
Is the patient taking any alpha-blockers or skeletal muscle relaxants (agents that reduce sphincter resistance)?
Is the patient taking any alpha-sympathomimetics (agents that increase sphincter resistance)?
Surgical history
Has the patient had any genitourinary procedures, abdominopelvic surgery, or spinal surgery?

Diagnostic evaluation

A variety of diagnostic procedures are available and indicated for the various bladder disturbances. Most common are the cystourethroscopy (also referred to as *cystoscopy*) and urodynamic testing. Table 13-4 lists several genitourinary diagnostic procedures and relevant information.

DEGREES OF TOXICITY

The severity of selected bladder disturbances has been quantified in the AUA Symptom Index (Figure 13-3). Generally, the more frequent the disturbance, the more severe the symptom and the higher the score on the tool. The Common Terminology Criteria for Adverse Events (CTCAE)[43] uses a grading system for reporting of adverse events. These criteria are not suited for patient self-report alone because they require synthesis of patient-reported sensory information and clinical assessment, such as which medications have been used for symptom relief or which type of catheterization was required for urinary obstruction. Table 13-5 provides the CTCAE grading scale for selected urinary disorders.

SYMPTOM MANAGEMENT STRATEGIES

THERAPEUTIC APPROACHES

Preventive strategies

For the individual receiving therapy for carcinoma of the bladder, prevention should focus on minimizing irritative bladder symptoms related to intravesical therapy. The goal of prevention is to minimize conditions known to enhance bladder inflammation—primarily acidic, concentrated urine. Pretreatment fluid restriction should be avoided unless the individual has difficulty retaining the intravesical treatment agent for the prescribed duration. Oral fluids should be increased as tolerated after the intravesical retention of the treatment agent. Acidic foods and fluids should be eliminated or minimized in the diet.

Prevention of lower UTIs is particularly important in those individuals with cancer who are immunocompromised. Urinary catheterization should be avoided whenever possible. When urinary catheterization is necessary, strict aseptic technique must be followed during the procedure and meticulous catheter care implemented for

TABLE 13-4

Selected Genitourinary Procedures

Procedure/Test	Selected Indications	Contraindications	Nursing Care
Intravenous pyelogram/ urogram (IVP/IVU)	Recurrent or febrile urinary tract infection (UTI) Hematuria Abdominal/pelvic mass Urinary system tumor Obstruction	Allergy to either iodine-bound contrast material or iodine-based cleansing solution Allergy to shellfish	Preparation includes catharsis and dehydration Monitor for hypersensitivity reactions. renal output
Computed tomography (CT scan)	Abdominal/pelvic mass Genitourinary tumor detection and staging	Allergy to iodine-bound contrast material	Monitor for hypersensitivity reactions
Magnetic resonance imaging (MRI)	Abdominal/pelvic mass Genitourinary tumor detection and staging	Pacemaker History of aneurysm surgery with clips	Teaching of procedure Removal of metal objects from patient
Urodynamic testing (cystometrics)	Urinary incontinence Bladder outlet obstruction Neuropathic bladder Urinary retention	Current UTI Acute, debilitating illness limiting mobility	Teaching of procedure preparation and aftercare Increase fluids and abstain from voiding 1–4 hours prior to test Prophylactic antibiotics Monitor for discomfort; treat with increased fluids and warm bath
Cystourethroscopy	Recurrent or febrile UTI Obstruction of bladder outlet Urethral or bladder fistula Incontinence Hematuria	Current UTI	Antibiotics for bacteriuria Monitor for frank bleeding/clots, signs of systemic infection

Question	Not at All	Less Than 1 Time in 5	Less than Half the Time	About Half the Time	More than Half the Time	Almost Always
1. During the last month or so, how often have you had a sensation of not emptying your bladder completely after you finished urinating?	0	1	2	3	4	5
2. During the last month or so, how often have you had to urinate again less than 2 hours after you finished urinating?	0	1	2	3	4	5
3. During the last month or so, how often have you found you stopped and started again after several times when you urinated?	0	1	2	3	4	5
4. During the last month or so, how often have you found it difficult to postpone urination?	0	1	2	3	4	5
5. During the last month or so, how often have you had a weak urinary stream?	0	1	2	3	4	5
6. During the last month or so, how often have you had to push or strain to begin urination?	0	1	2	3	4	5
7. During the last month or so, how many times did you most typically get up to urinate from the time you went to bed at night until the time you got up in the morning?	None	1 Time	2 Times	3 Times	4 Times	5 or More Times
	0	1	2	3	4	5
AUA Symptom Index = sum of questions 1 to 7.						

FIGURE 13-3

Health history questions for a complaint of an altered voiding pattern.

Source: Data from Barry MJ, Fowler FJ, O'Leary MP, et al. The American Urological Association symptom index for benig prostatic hyperplasia. *J Urol* 1992;148:1555.[37] Reprinted with permission.

TABLE 13-5

National Cancer Institute Common Terminology Criteria for Adverse Events (CTCAE)

	GRADE				
Adverse Event	**1**	**2**	**3**	**4**	**5**
Hematuria (A disorder characterized by laboratory test results that indicate blood in the urine)	Asymptomatic; clinical or diagnostic observations only; intervention not indicated	Symptomatic; urinary catheter or bladder irrigation indicated; limiting instrumental ADL	Gross hematuria; transfusion, IV medications or hospitalization indicated; elective endoscopic, radiologic or operative intervention indicated; limiting self-care ADL	Life-threatening consequences; urgent radiologic or operative intervention indicated	Death
Urinary frequency and urgency (A disorder characterized by urination at short intervals and sudden compelling urge to urinate)	Present	Limiting instrumental ADL; medical management indicated	–	–	–
Urinary incontinence (A disorder characterized by inability to control the flow of urine from the bladder)	Occasional (e.g., with coughing, sneezing, etc.) pads not indicated	Spontaneous; pads indicated; limiting instrumental ADL	Intervention indicated (e.g., clamp, collagen injections); operative interventions indicated; limiting self-care ADL	–	–

Abbrevations: ADL: activities of daily living; IV: intravenous.

Source: Data from National Cancer Institute: Common Terminology Criteria for Adverse Events (CTCAE)[43].

an indwelling catheter. Urinary retention must be minimized to reduce risk of a UTI.

Urinary voiding dysfunction in the person with cancer is often the result of the disease process or the surgical intervention and is not highly amenable to prevention. Nevertheless, preoperative teaching of pelvic floor exercises to strengthen bladder sphincter muscles may increase the chance of postoperative continence.[44] In medically induced voiding dysfunction, careful monitoring of the individual can enable early detection of a problem and prevent further complications. For example, a person receiving vincristine may begin to exhibit peripheral neuropathies in the extremities and subsequently experience urinary retention. Notation of the phenomenon and cessation of vincristine may prevent further progression of the neuropathy.

Management

Hematuria. Mild hematuria is commonly associated with carcinoma of the bladder and sometimes with drug-induced inflammation of the urothelium; however, it is generally tolerated without special treatment. Individuals receiving therapy for superficial bladder tumors should be informed that mild hematuria (pink-tinged urine) is not cause for alarm, but that any increase in the amount of blood should be reported to their nurse or doctor. More severe, gross hematuria and hemorrhagic cystitis are managed by bladder irrigation with saline and, as needed, with red cell transfusions to counteract blood loss. For refractory bleeding, surgical intervention may be required, including cystotomy and urinary diversion with cystectomy in life-threatening cases.[45]

Irritative bladder symptoms. Dysuria, daytime frequency, nocturia, and urgency are sensory and behavioral symptoms often associated with intravesical therapy of superficial bladder cancer and with lower UTIs. The goals of symptom management in IBSs are to eliminate the sensations of pain, burning, or urgency and to return altered patterns of urinary elimination to a premorbid state. One study reported intravesical instillation of sodium hyaluronate to be efficacious in relieving dysuria and pain in patients with radiation cystitis or chemical cystitis due to intravesical BCG or mitomycin C.[46]

Other medical interventions usually include analgesic medications. Phenazopyridine provides urinary-specific analgesia in some individuals. Antibiotic therapy for bacterial bladder infections is based on the result of a urine culture and sensitivity. Trimethoprim/sulfamethoxazole given orally twice a day provides cost-effective coverage for most UTIs. Comfort measures for pain relief include urinary analgesics such as phenazopyridine and warm, moist heat to the lower back or soaking in warm bath water.

Voiding dysfunction. Bladder outlet obstruction can be caused by direct prostate tumor extension and pressure. Prompt surgical resection is indicated when urinary retention is manifested as a symptom and also because of the metastatic potential of the disease. In addition, radical prostatectomy often results in urinary incontinence due to sphincter incompetence. Nursing care focuses on interventions to minimize postoperative complications and enhance continence.

A variety of therapies are available for men with unresolved postsurgical or postradiation urinary incontinence. Behavioral therapies include timed voiding, pelvic floor exercises (Kegel exercises), biofeedback, electrical stimulation, and medications.[11,14] Surgical therapies include transurethral collagen injections to the bladder neck, sling procedures, or placement of an artificial urinary sphincter to enhance urinary control.[47] The necessity for repeated collagen injections increases the cost of this therapy, and artificial sphincter placement has been found more cost effective.[48] The artificial sphincter device contains a reservoir, pump, and cuff. The cuff is implanted and surrounds the urethra so that urine is blocked when the cuff is inflated. The pump is implanted in the scrotum and activated by the patient to release the cuff pressure and initiate voiding.[47] Complications of the artificial sphincters include urethral erosion and infection. Some of these devices will require replacement or surgical revision, particularly if the man has received radiation for his prostate cancer,[31] but reimplantation can be quite successful.[49] Some men prefer the sling procedure because it avoids the use of a mechanical device.[50]

Functional urinary incontinence is managed based on the etiology of the dysfunction. For those individuals with impaired cognitive functioning due to brain tumor enlargement or metastasis, nursing interventions focus on developing and instituting a toileting program based on habitual patterns along with a behavioral modification program to encourage toileting behaviors. However, the intensity of such a patient/family teaching program must be determined by the prognosis and general functional status of the impaired individual. On some occasions, continued incontinence necessitates placement of a long-term indwelling catheter. Patients who are dependent on institutionalized care or who are experiencing serious skin care problems, patients with a short life expectancy, and those with a chronically painful condition may prefer, or may be asked to comply with, the placement of an indwelling urinary catheter. Home care focuses on maintaining the patency of the catheter and drainage system, along with minimizing bacterial colonization of the bag or catheter and subsequent UTI. Appendix 13B contains a self-care guide for urinary catheter care.

The symptom management algorithms found in Figures 13-4 and 13-5 detail treatment strategies for hematuria, IBS, and urinary incontinence. Table 13-6 is a clinical

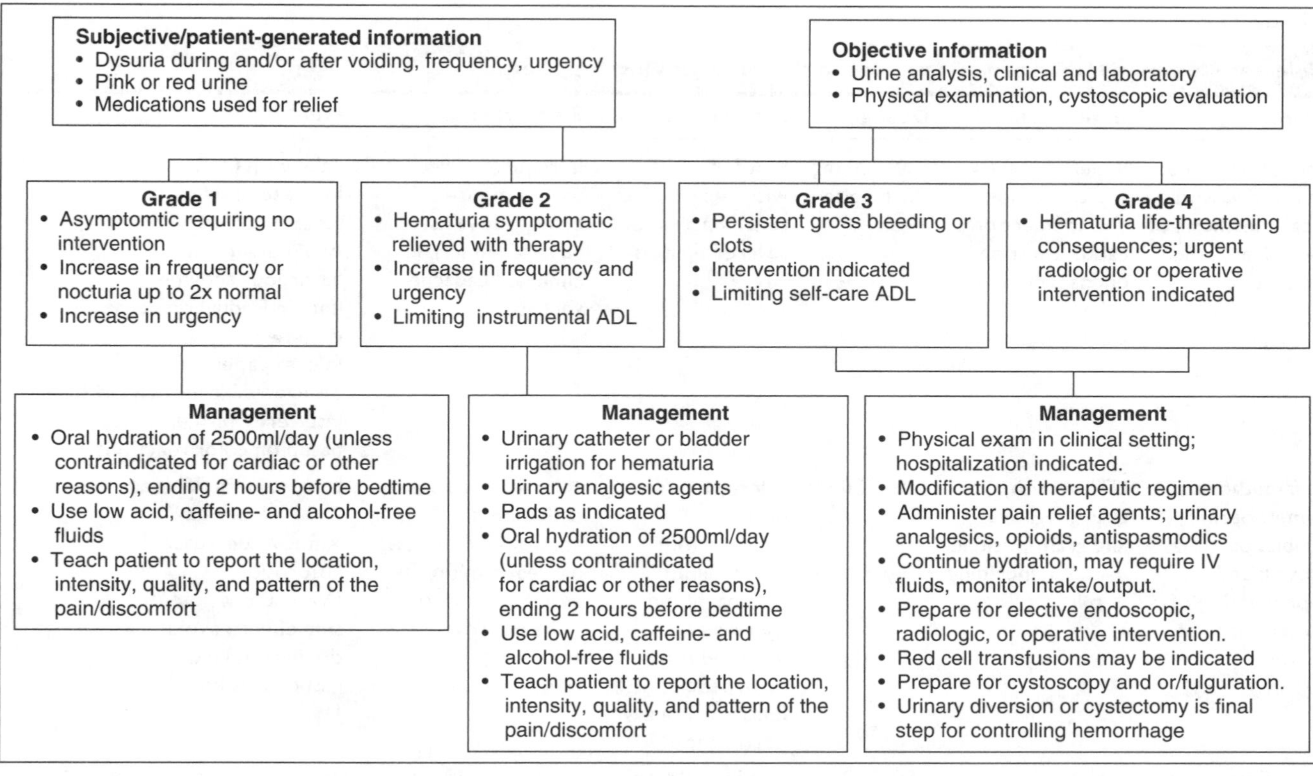

FIGURE 13-4

Treatment management strategies for hematuria and irritative bladder symptoms.

Abbreviation: ADL: activities of daily living.

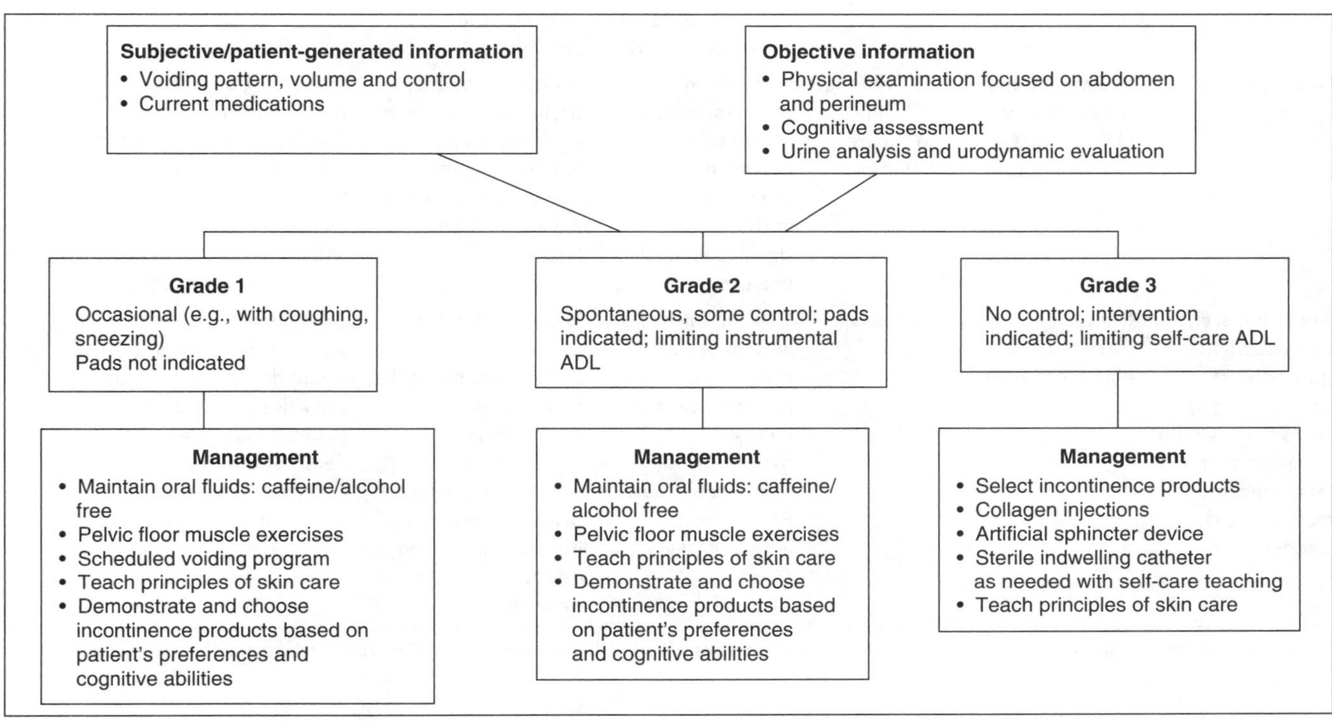

FIGURE 13-5

Management of urinary incontinence.

TABLE 13-6

Selected Common Medications Prescribed in the Urologic Oncology Setting

Agent	Indications	Dosage	Precautions	Side Effects	Nursing
Phenazopyridine: an azo dye with local anesthesia of the urinary tract mucosa	Relief of urinary tract irritation due to infection, catheterization, endoscopy, and other urinary tract procedures	100–200 mg PO tid after meals	Not for use with impaired renal function or severe hepatitis	Infrequent except with prolonged or high-dose use: nausea, hemolytic anemia, headache, vertigo	Take with food Increase oral fluids to 2500 mL per day Avoid driving or hazardous activities until individual response is known Inform patient that urine turns orange-red, can stain clothing, interferes with urine tests based on color reactions
Sulfamethoxazole/ trimethoprim: inhibits bacterial growth and reproduction of a wide range of bacteria	UTI of both gram-negative and gram-positive bacteria, including *E. coli*	160–800 mg PO q12h	Allergy to sulfa drugs Caution with concomitant asthma, blood dyscrasias, impaired renal or hepatic function, urinary obstruction	Allergic reactions, drowsiness, confusion, dizziness, nausea/vomiting, stomatitis, diarrhea, bone marrow suppression, jaundice, fever	Increase oral fluids to 2500 mL per day Antacids decrease absorption Warn about potential side effects, avoid driving until individual response is known
Ciprofloxacin: one of the quinolones, antibiotics that inhibit DNA replication causing bacterial death	UTI due to various bacteria, particularly effective against *Pseudomonas*	250–750 mg PO q 12 hours	Use by children and pregnant or nursing mothers is not recommended Caution with CNS disorders or impaired renal or hepatic function	Allergic reactions, headache, dizziness, anorexia, restlessness, hypertension, nausea/ vomiting, diarrhea, back and joint pain, hematuria, dyspnea, reduces caffeine clearance	Take on an empty stomach Do not administer with antacids or oral iron
Nitrofurantoin	Treatment and prevention of UTI	50–100 mg PO qid, for acute infection	Not safe in pregnant women at term and in newborns Do not use in those with significant renal impairment	Allergic reactions, dizziness, drowsiness, headache, peripheral neuropathy, bone marrow suppression, nausea/ vomiting, dyspnea, cough	Urine may turn dark yellow to brown Avoid concomitant antacids Take with food or milk to minimize GI disturbance Dilute oral suspension and do not crush tablets, to avoid staining teeth
Anticholinergics/ antispasmodics/ spasmolytics, e.g., oxybutynin, flavoxate; a group of agents that relax smooth muscle in the bladder	Instability incontinence, bladder spasms	Varies	Caution in those with impaired renal or hepatic function, cardiac disease, hypertension, reflux esophagitis, BPH, chronic lung disease	Allergic reactions, confusion, drowsiness, headache, nervousness, dysrhythmias, dry mouth, GI hypomotility, urinary hesitancy/ urgency, impotence, blurred vision, decreased sweating	Administer on an empty stomach 1 hour before meals Avoid driving or hazardous activities until individual response is known Teach about dry mouth and orthostatic hypotension effects; avoid overheating

Abbreviations: BPH: benign prostatic hypertrophy; CNS: central nervous system; GI: gastrointestinal; UTI: urinary tract infection.

nursing guide to be used as a quick reference to common medications prescribed in the urologic oncology setting.

NURSING IMPLICATIONS

Bladder disturbances are a major problem in certain populations of patients with cancer as a result of the disease or treatment. Few fully validated instruments are available for assessment of bladder disturbances in the oncology setting. The EPIC tool[39] may be adapted for most any bladder disturbance by using the appropriate subscales. The Common Terminology Criteria for Adverse Events address the relevant disturbances and could be used in a clinical oncology setting to monitor individuals' responses to symptom management; however, this scale is not intended for self-report or self-monitoring. The addition of patient report instruments to clinician grading of symptoms will enhance the quality and completeness of data collected for use in evaluating the efficacy of symptom management.

Nurses can play an instrumental role in the prevention, management, and follow-up care of patients with various bladder disturbances. Many patients will not openly discuss their problems with bladder disturbances, so objective assessment will provide insight into these individuals' problems. Nursing care, through patient education, advocacy, and psychosocial support, can help improve the quality of life of the patient with bladder disturbances.

TABLE 13-7

Resources for Patients with Bladder Disturbances

Professional Specialty Groups

Society of Urologic Nurses and Associates, Inc.
East Holly Avenue, Box 56
Pitman, NJ 08071–0056
888-827-7862
Website: http://www.suna.org

Wound Ostomy and Continence Nurses Society
National Office
15000 Commerce Parkway
Suite C
Mount Laurel, NJ 08054
Ph: 888-224-9626
Website: http://www.wocn.org

Educational and Support Services

American Urologic Association Foundation
1000 Corporate Boulevard
Linthicum, MD 21090
Phone: 410-689-3700 or 1-800-828-7866
Website: http://www.urologyhealth.org

Us Too: International Prostate Cancer Education and Support Network
5003 Fairview Avenue
Downers Grove, IL 60515
Phone: 630-795-1002
Website: http://www.ustoo.org/

PATIENT SELF-CARE

Self-care guides for catheter care (Appendix 13B), IBSs (Appendix 13C), and urinary incontinence (Appendix 13D) are provided to facilitate patient education efforts. A bladder diary is provided as well (Appendix 13A). Table 13-7 lists resources available to nurses who manage bladder disturbances in the oncology setting and to patients with bladder disturbance symptoms.

REFERENCES

1. Hollenbeck BK, Dunn RL, Ye Z, et al. Delays in diagnosis and bladder cancer mortality. *Cancer.* 2010;116(22):5235–5242.
2. Steinberg GD, Bladder cancer. http://emedicine.medscape.com/article/438262-overview. Accessed October 30, 2012.
3. Gorin MA, Ayyathurai R, Soloway MS. Diagnosis and treatment of bladder cancer: how can we improve? *Postgrad Med.* 2012;124(3):28–36.
4. Shephard EA, Stapley S, Neal RD, Rose P, Walter FM, Hamilton WT. Clinical features of bladder cancer in primary care. *Br J Gen Pract.* 2012;62(602):598–604.
5. Shelley MD, Wilt TJ, Court J, Coles B, Kynaston H, Mason MD. Intravesical bacillus Calmette-Guérin is superior to mitomycin C in reducing tumour recurrence in high-risk superficial bladder cancer: a meta-analysis of randomized trials. *BJU Int.* 2004;93(4):485–490.
6. Mangiarotti B, Trinchieri A, Del Nero A, Montanari E. A randomized prospective study of intravesical prophylaxis in non-muscle invasive bladder cancer at intermediate risk of recurrence: mitomycin chemotherapy vs BCG immunotherapy. *Arch Ital Urol Androl.* 2008;80(4):167–171.
7. National Comprehensive Cancer Network. NCCN guidelines version 2.2012. Bladder cancer. http://www.nccn.org/professionals/physician_gls/pdf/bladder.pdf. Accessed October 30, 2012.
8. Shelton B. Infection. In: Yarbro CH, Wujcik D, Gobel BH, eds. *Cancer Nursing: Principles and Practice.* 7th ed. Burlington, MA: Jones & Bartlett Learning: 2011:713–749.
9. Tambyah PA, Oon J. Catheter-associated urinary tract infection. *Curr Opin Infect Dis.* 2012;25(4);365–370.
10. Siegel R, Naishadham D, Jemal A. Cancer statistics 2012. *CA Cancer J Clin.* 2012;62(1):10–29.
11. Kazer MW, Harmon AS. Prostate cancer. In: Yarbro CH, Wujcik D, Gobel BH, eds. *Cancer Nursing: Principles and Practice.* 7th ed. Burlington, MA: Jones & Bartlett Learning; 2011:1609–1633.
12. Peterson AC, Chen Y. Patient reported incontinence after radical prostatectomy is more common than expected and not associated with the nerve sparing technique: results from the Center for Prostate Disease Research (CPDR) database. *Neurourol Urodyn.* 2012;31(1):60–63.
13. Dunn MW, Kazer MW. Prostate cancer overview. *Semin Oncol Nurs.* 2011;27(4):241–250.

14. Mirza M, Griebling TL, Kazer MW. Erectile dysfunction and urinary incontinence after prostate cancer treatment. *Semin Oncol Nurs.* 2011;27(4);278–289.
15. Panjari M, Bell RJ, Burney S, Bell S, McMurrick PJ, Davis SR. Sexual function, incontinence, and wellbeing in women after rectal cancer: a review of the evidence. *J Sex Med.* 2012; 9(11):2749–2758.
16. Manchana T. Long-term lower urinary tract dysfunction in gynecologic cancer survivors. *Asian Pac J Cancer Prev.* 2011;12(1);285–288.
17. Camp-Sorrell D. Chemotherapy toxicities and management. In: Yarbro CH, Wujcik D, Gobel BH, eds. *Cancer Nursing: Principles and Practice.* 7th ed. Burlington, MA: Jones & Bartlett Learning; 2011:458–503.
18. Wilkes GM. Peripheral neuropathy. In: Yarbro CH, Frogge MH, Goodman M, eds. *Cancer Nursing: Symptom Management.* 3rd ed. Sudbury, MA: Jones and Bartlett; 2004:333–357.
19. Wilkes GM. Spinal cord compression. In: Yarbro CH, Frogge MH, Goodman M, eds. *Cancer Nursing: Symptom Management.* 3rd ed. Sudbury, MA: Jones and Bartlett; 2004:359–373.
20. Chaux A. Bladder: Normal histology. 2011. http://www.pathologyoutlines.com/topic/bladderhistology.html. Accessed October 30, 2012.
21. Wood LS, Zhou M. Pathology of genitourinary malignancies implications for clinical management. *Semin Oncol Nurs.* 2012; 28(3): 143–153.
22. Tyler A. Urothelial cancers: ureter, renal pelvis, and bladder. *Semin Oncol Nurs.* 2012;28(3):154–162.
23. Petersen RO, Sesterhem IA, Davis CJ. *Urologic Pathology.* 3rd ed. Philadelphia: Lippincott; 2008.
24. Muehlbauer PM. Biotherapy. In: Yarbro CH, Wujcik D, Gobel BH, eds. *Cancer Nursing: Principles and Practice.* 7th ed. Burlington, MA: Jones & Bartlett Learning; 2011:530–560.
25. Shelton G. Bladder cancer In: Yarbro CH, Wujcik D, Gobel BH, eds. *Cancer Nursing: Principles and Practice.* 7th ed. Burlington, MA: Jones & Bartlett Learning; 2011:1080–1090.
26. Berry D. Measurement of irritative bladder symptoms. *Oncol Nurs Forum.* 1997;24:319.
27. Klastersky J. Side effects of ifosfamide. *Oncology.* 2003;65(suppl 2):7–10.
28. Mohammadianpanah M, Shirzai M, Mosalaei A, Omidvari S, Ahmadloo N. Hemorrhagic cystitis in a patient receiving conventional doses of dacarbazine for metastatic malignant melanoma: case report and review of the literature. *Clin Ther.* 2007;29(6):1161–1165.
29. Islam R, Isaacson BJ, Zickerman PM, Ratanawong C, Tipping SJ. Hemorrhagic cystitis as an unexpected adverse reaction to temozolomide: case report. *Am J Clin Oncol.* 2002;25(5):513–514.
30. Haas ML. Radiation therapy: toxicities and management. In: Yarbro CH, Wujcik D, Gobel BH, eds. *Cancer Nursing: Principles and Practice.* 7th ed. Burlington, MA: Jones & Bartlett Learning; 2011:312–351.
31. Manunta A, Guille F, Patard JJ, Lobel B. Artificial sphincter insertion after radiotherapy: is it worthwhile? *BJU Int.* 2000;85(4):490–492.
32. McMenamin E. Cancer pain management. In: Yarbro CH, Wujcik D, Gobel BH, eds. *Cancer Nursing: Principles and Practice.* 7th ed. Burlington, MA: Jones & Bartlett Learning; 2011:685–712.
33. Khoder WY, Trottmann M, Stuber A, Stief CG, Becker AJ. Early incontinence after radical prostatectomy: a community based retrospective analysis in 911 men and implications for preoperative counseling. *Urol Oncol.* 2011 epub ahead of print.
34. Martin AD, Nakamura LY, Nunez RN, Wolter CE, Humphreys MR, Castle EP. Incontinence after radical prostatectomy: a patient centered analysis and implications for preoperative counseling. *J Urol.* 2011;186(1):204–208.
35. Wein AJ, Dmochowski RR. Neuromuscular dysfunction of the lower urinary tract. In: McDougal WS, Wein AJ, Kavoussi R, et al., eds. *Campbell's Walsh Urology.* 10th ed. Philadelphia: W. B. Saunders; 2012:351–358.
36. Lee R, Penson DF. Treatment outcomes in localized prostate cancer: a patient-oriented approach. *Semin Urol Oncol.* 2002;20(1):63–73.
37. Barry MJ, Fowler FJ Jr, O'Leary MP, Bruskewitz, RC, Holtgrewe HL, Mebust WK. The American Urological Association symptom index for benign prostatic hyperplasia. The Measurement Committee of the American Urological Association. *J Urol.* 1992;148(5):1549–1557, discussion 1564.
38. Barry MJ, Fowler FJ Jr, O'Leary MP, et al. Correlation of the American Urological Association symptom index with self-administered versions of the Madsen-Iversen, Boyarsky, and Maine Medical Assessment Program symptom indexes. Measurement Committee of the American Urological Association. *J Urol.* 1992;148(5):1558–1563, discussion 1564.
39. Wei JT, Dunn RL, Litwin MS, Sandler HM, Sanda MG. Development and validation of the Expanded Prostate Cancer Index Composite (EPIC) for comprehensive assessment of health-related quality of life in men with prostate cancer. *Urology.* 2000;56(6):899–905.
40. Fujimura T, Kume H, Nishimatsu H, et al. Assessment of lower urinary tract symptoms in men by international prostate symptom score and core lower urinary tract symptom score. *BJU Int.* 2012;109(10):1512–1516.
41. Fujimura T, Kume H, Tsurumaki Y, et al. Core Lower Urinary Tract Symptom Score (CLSS) for the assessment of the female lower urinary tract symptoms: a comparative study. *Int J Urol.* 2011;18(11):778–784.
42. Homma Y, Yoshida M, Yamanishi T, Gotoh M. Core Lower Urinary Tract Symptom Score (CLSS) questionnaire: a reliable overall assessment of lower urinary tract symptoms. *Int J Urol.* 2008;15(9):816–820.
43. National Cancer Institute. Common terminology criteria for adverse events (CTCAE) version 4.0. http://evs.nci.nih.gov/ftp1/CTCAE/CTCAE_4.03_2010-06-14_QuickReference_8.5x11.pdf. Accessed October 30, 2012.
44. Sueppel C, Kreder K, See W. Improved continence outcomes with preoperative pelvic floor muscle strengthening exercises. *Urol Nurs.* 2001;21(3):201–210.
45. Russo P. Urologic emergencies in the cancer patient. *Semin Oncol.* 2000;27(3):284–298.
46. Sommariva ML, Sandri SD, Ceriani V. Efficacy of sodium hyaluronate in the management of radiation cystitis. *Minerva Urol Nefrol.* 2010;62(2):145–150.
47. Klutke JJ. Current status of urethral occlusive devices in management of urinary incontinence. *Curr Opin Obstet Gynecol.* 2000;12(5):415–419.
48. Gomes CM, Broderick GA, Sanchez-Ortiz RF, Preate D Jr., Rovner ES, Wein AJ. Artificial urinary sphincter for post-prostatectomy incontinence: impact of prior collagen injection on cost and clinical outcome. *J Urol.* 2000;163(1):87–90.
49. Frank I, Elliott DS, Barrett DM. Success of de novo reimplantation of the artificial genitourinary sphincter. *J Urol.* 2000;163(6):1702–1703.
50. Kumar A, Litt ER, Ballert KN, Nitti VW. Artificial urinary sphincter versus male sling for post-prostatectomy incontinence: what do patients choose? *J Urol.* 2009;18(1);1231–1235.

Bladder Diary

Patient Name: ______________________ Date: ______________________

Physician: ______________________ Phone: ______________________

Nurse: ______________________ Phone: ______________________

Your nurse or doctor will tell you which information is to be included on this bladder diary form and how many days to keep the diary. Write down the time of day, including AM or PM, in the column labeled *Time.* Place a checkmark in the *Urinated* column when you urinate on purpose. Place a checkmark in the *Leakage* column when you leak or pass urine by accident. Write down the approximate amount of fluid you *drink.* (Use ounces or cups or whatever measurement of volume you are most familiar with.) Do not forget to write down the time for each event—drinking, urinating, or leaking. In the *Comments* column, add symptoms that your nurse or doctor may ask you to describe or notes that will help you remember what happened. If you have questions about how to complete the diary, call your nurse or doctor.

Time	Urinated	Leakage	Fluid Amount	Taken In	Comments

Source: Yarbro CH, Berry DL. Bladder Disturbances. In: Yarbro CH, Wujcik D, Gobel BH, eds. *Cancer Symptom Management.* 4th ed. Burlington, MA: Jones & Bartlett Learning; 2014.

(continued)

Bladder Catheter Care

Name: ____

You can help the catheter work safely by preventing blockage and infection of the catheter.

Symptom and Description

An indwelling urinary catheter is a tube that drains urine from your bladder into a collection bag. Some persons need a catheter after certain surgeries. Others may have a catheter placed because it is too difficult or impossible to use the bathroom or because urine leakage cannot be controlled.

Management

Equipment

- Wash your hands with soap and water before and after handling the catheter, tubing, or bag.
- Use a leg bag during the day and the larger bedside bag at night or if you will be resting in bed more than 2 hours. Any drainage bag must be kept below the level of the bladder. Hang the larger bag on the bed or place it on a low stool. Do not lay the bag on the floor. Check the tubing for kinks that might stop the flow of urine.
- Empty the leg bag at least every 2 hours and the bedside bag at least every morning. After emptying, clean the end of the drainage tube with a cotton ball and povidone-iodine (Betadine) or 70% alcohol.
- When you change from the one type of drainage bag to the other, follow these directions to clean the bag that is not being used. If you are not using both a leg bag and a bedside bag, change or clean the drainage bag about once a week.

  1. Rinse the bag with cold water; wash it with warm, soapy water; and rinse it very well with cold, clear water.
  2. Fill the bag with a solution of one part vinegar to four parts water and soak for 30 minutes.
  3. Empty the bag and let it air dry.

- If your indwelling catheter is permanent, talk with your nurse about using bleach to disinfect the bags.
- Store any green or blue protection caps in a container of 70% alcohol.

Drinking Fluids

- It is important to keep your bladder flushed with plenty of fluids. Drink at least 2 quarts of water (64 ounces or 8 cups or about 2 liters) each day.
- Ask your doctor or nurse about drinking more or taking drinks that will make your urine more acid. If you are not at risk for irritative bladder symptoms, you may be able to avoid problems with bladder infections by drinking certain juices.

Hygiene and Washing Yourself

- You may take a shower or any kind of bath with the catheter in place. Also wash the genital area with a soapy washcloth and dry well twice a day.
- *Women* should wipe the length of the catheter with the washcloth, starting where the catheter enters the body. Then wipe the genital area from front to back, starting where the catheter enters the body, cleaning the folds around the vagina as well.
- *Men* should wipe the length of the catheter with the washcloth, starting where the catheter enters the body. Uncircumcised men should pull back the foreskin and wash the end of the penis; then wash the penis, scrotum, and groin areas.

Follow-Up

Talk to your doctor or nurse about bacteria and infections related to the catheter. People with an indwelling catheter often have some bacteria in their urine. An actual urinary tract infection occurs when enough bacteria grow to cause symptoms, such as fever or blood in the urine. Call your doctor or nurse right away if you notice any of these symptoms:

- Low back pain or stomach pain
- Cloudy, bad-smelling urine
- Material (sediment) in the urine
- Blood in the urine
- Fever or chills

Phone Numbers

Nurse: ______________________________ Phone: ______________________

Physician: ___________________________ Phone: ______________________

Other: ______________________________ Phone: ______________________

Comments

Source: Yarbro CH, Berry DL. Bladder Disturbances. In: Yarbro CH, Wujcik D, Gobel BH, eds. *Cancer Symptom Management.* 4th ed. Burlington, MA: Jones & Bartlett Learning; 2014.

Irritative Bladder Symptoms

Name: ____________________

This guide will help you prevent and manage bladder symptoms that are irritating.

Symptom and Description

Irritative bladder symptoms (IBSs) include three symptoms that often occur together:

- *Dysuria* is an unpleasant sensation of pain, discomfort, or burning that occurs during urination.
- *Urgency* is when it feels like you have to urinate right away or immediately, even sometimes if your bladder is not full.
- *Frequency* is having to urinate more frequently than what is normal for you, generally more often than every 2 hours during the day.

People who are receiving treatment for cancer, or who have certain urinary tests that require insertion of an instrument or catheter into their bladder, are sometimes at risk for IBSs and bladder infections. If you have IBSs, your doctor or nurse will want to conduct other tests to determine whether there is an infection in your bladder. People who are receiving treatment for bladder cancer through a catheter directly into their bladder are also at risk for IBSs. Such symptoms would occur after the treatments for a few hours (but can last up to several days), due to the effect of the treatment drug on the lining of the bladder. This IBS side effect usually begins after the second or third treatment.

Prevention

Although some IBSs may happen in certain people, you may be able to prevent IBSs by taking the following steps:

- Drinking plenty of liquids. Try to drink at least 2 quarts (almost 2 liters) of water every day.
- Avoiding fluids with caffeine and acid fluids (this includes most juices). Water is best!
- Not delaying if you feel the need to urinate.

Management

1. Once you have experienced IBSs, you should notify your doctor or nurse as soon as possible, describing the following details:
   - Where the discomfort is
   - How bad it is
   - What it feels like
   - How long it lasts
   - How often you feel the need to urinate

- How often you actually are urinating
- Whether your urine is pink or red

Your doctor or nurse may give you a bladder diary to record how often you urinate and how much you are drinking.

2. You must take any medication that is prescribed to treat a bladder infection or treat the discomfort.
3. Continue to drink a lot of nonacid and noncaffeinated fluids, increasing the amount to 2½ quarts (80 ounces or 10 cups) each day while the symptoms last.
4. Take warm baths in water up to your waist to reduce bladder pain, and use warm, moist heat for any low back pain you feel.

Follow-Up

Call your physician or nurse as soon as irritative bladder symptoms begin and if you have a new fever along with the IBSs. Bring with you any record of urination and fluids you have consumed when you see your doctor or nurse.

When your IBSs get better, you can return to your normal level of drinking fluids, but it should remain at least 2 quarts (almost 2 liters) per day (64 ounces or 8 cups).

Phone Numbers

Nurse: ______________________________ Phone: ______________________________

Physician: ______________________________ Phone: ______________________________

Other: ______________________________ Phone: ______________________________

Comments

Source: Yarbro CH, Berry DL. Bladder Disturbances. In: Yarbro CH, Wujcik D, Gobel BH, eds. *Cancer Symptom Management.* 4th ed. Burlington, MA: Jones & Bartlett Learning; 2014.

Urinary Incontinence

Name: ____

This guide will help you manage leakage of urine or lack of bladder control.

Symptom and Description

A person who cannot control the flow of urine has urinary incontinence. This loss of bladder control can involve a little leakage of urine when a person sneezes or coughs, or a total lack of control over urination. Urinary incontinence commonly occurs for several months after surgery, such as removal of the prostate or uterus, because of the surgery in the area of the bladder. Temporary incontinence can also occur with urinary tract infections and irritations.

Learning Needs

You can help manage incontinence when it occurs by learning to do the following:

- Keep track of the times that you urinate and/or are incontinent
- Perform certain exercises
- Take good care of your skin
- Take certain medications

Prevention

It is common to experience some loss of bladder control after surgeries such as removal of the prostate, but you can help to prevent its continuation by participating in its management.

Management

- Keep track of when you urinate by completing a "bladder diary" (included).
- Try to urinate according to a schedule. If you have been leaking or urinating every hour or more, then try to urinate only once every 60 minutes. If you have been leaking or urinating every half hour, then try to urinate only once every 30 minutes. Keep on that schedule even if you do not feel the urge to urinate.
- When you have been able to urinate on that schedule without leaking in between, then increase the time interval between attempts to urinate, by 30 minutes at a time. If you feel an urgent need to urinate in between the scheduled times, try relaxation or distraction (for instance, balance your checkbook!) and the urgency may go away for a while.
- Practice pelvic muscle exercises taught to you by your nurse or doctor.
- Keep the skin around your genital area, groin, buttocks, and upper thigh clean and as dry as possible. Wash with soap and water to remove urine. Your nurse can help you select a moisture barrier to protect your skin, if needed. Change wet clothing or bedding immediately.

Wear loose clothing. Wear adult briefs with pads or absorbent pads to help absorb urine and keep your skin dry.

- Call your nurse if your skin becomes reddened or irritated.
- Take any medications prescribed to relax your bladder muscles.

Follow-Up

Bring any record of urination and leakage with you when you see your doctor or nurse. Extending the time intervals between urination can eventually get you back to "normal" or to a point at which you are satisfied with your urinary control. Many institutions have incontinence clinics with specialists who treat urinary incontinence of all types. Your nurse or doctor may refer you to these services.

Phone Numbers

Nurse: ______________________ Phone: ______________________

Physician: ______________________ Phone: ______________________

Other: ______________________ Phone: ______________________

Comments

Source: Yarbro CH, Berry DL. Bladder Disturbances. In: Yarbro CH, Wujcik D, Gobel BH, eds. *Cancer Symptom Management.* 4th ed. Burlington, MA: Jones & Bartlett Learning; 2014.

PART VI

Alterations in Cardiopulmonary Function

CHAPTER 14

Bleeding and Thrombotic Complications

Anna Liza Rodriguez, MHA, MSN, RN, OCN®

THE PROBLEM

Bleeding and thrombotic events associated with dysregulation of the coagulation system are significant clinical complications in patients with cancer, contributing greatly to morbidity and mortality.[1] Multiple factors cause bleeding and thrombotic complications, including disease, marrow infiltration, and megakaryocyte progenitor cell death related to chemotherapy or technology such as radiation therapy. The complexity and variation in these complications demand that the clinician caring for patients with cancer be knowledgeable of normal coagulation and the various hemostatic changes that can occur in patients with cancer.

INCIDENCE

Bleeding

Thrombocytopenia is the primary hematological problem causing bleeding in patients with cancer. Thrombocytopenia is multifactorial in origin and may be due to disease, marrow infiltration, or megakaryocyte progenitor cell death related to chemotherapy or technology such as radiation therapy. Certain cytotoxic agents can also induce thrombocytopenia—particularly, platinum-based agents, cyclophosphamide, irinotecan, dactinomycin, and fludarabine.[1,2] Bleeding in patients with cancer also results from damage to local vessels, tumor invasion, and systemic processes such as disseminated intravascular coagulopathy (DIC).

The relationship between hemorrhage and low platelet level was first described by Gaydos et al.[3] in the 1960s, and it is now clearly recognized that neoplasms increase the risk for bleeding. Certain malignancies carry a higher probability for hemorrhage, including the leukemias, especially acute promyelocytic leukemia (APL). As many as 90% of patients with APL may develop a hemorrhagic complication, with the frequency of fatal hemorrhage being as high as 17.3%.[4] Gaydos et al.[3] first demonstrated that risk of hemorrhage seemed to correlate with platelet counts of less than 20,000/mm^3 in patients with hematological malignancies. Since then, there have been multiple randomized trials evaluating the risk of bleeding with thrombocytopenia in adult patients with leukemia.[5] Historical data demonstrate that the incidence of bleeding in thrombocytopenic patients with acute myelogenous leukemia (AML) (excluding APL) ranges from 20% to 32%, and from 34% to 58% in patients undergoing allogeneic stem cell transplantation (SCT).[6,7] In a multicenter retrospective study by Holler et al., a statistically significant ($p = 0.001$) higher number of bleeding events occurred in SCT patients with platelet counts of less than 13,000/mm^3.[5] Further, analysis of the relationship between the platelet count and mortality revealed a significantly ($p = 0.001$) increased risk of death in patients with a platelet count less than 15,000/mm^3.[5] The study showed that hemorrhage is the direct cause of mortality in 2.8% of SCT patients.[5]

Profound thrombocytopenia is not the only cause of bleeding in the patient with cancer. The risk of bleeding is affected not only by the level of thrombocytopenia, but also by other relevant clinical factors, including fever, sepsis, uremia, infection, medications, low albumin, low hematocrit, recent bone marrow transplant, and recent hemorrhage.[6,8]

Studies establishing the relationship between platelet count and incidence of bleeding in solid tumors are limited, and available studies have not been examined in a prospective fashion. Belt et al. demonstrated in 1978 that the incidence of hemorrhage was low in patients with solid tumors until the platelet count fell below 10,000/mm^3.[9] A retrospective review in 1984 by Dutcher and colleagues of 1274 records of patients with solid tumors treated with combination chemotherapy or experimental agents between 1972 and 1980 revealed a very low incidence of significant thrombocytopenia or bleeding.[10] These findings are supported by a study by Etling et al. indicating that the incidence of bleeding is low among solid tumor patients.[11] However, certain categories of patients may be at increased risk for bleeding—in particular, patients with poor performance status and a history of bleeding, in whom the incidence may be as high as 20%.[12] Results of a recent retrospective study by Hitron et al. revealed that clinically significant chemotherapy-induced thrombocytopenia (CIT) is commonly seen in patients following treatment with cisplatin/gemcitabine, carboplatin/gemcitabine, or cisplatin/etoposide regimens, although the relationship between CIT and bleeding was not established.[13]

Thrombosis

The relationship between cancer and thrombosis has been well established since the 1800s, following Trousseau's discovery of the association between migratory thrombophlebitis and an underlying malignant process. Tumor-associated thrombophlebitis, now referred to as Trousseau's syndrome, can be the first symptom of an undiagnosed or occult malignancy.

Cancer-associated thrombotic complications may take the form of venous thromboembolism (VTE) or DIC. VTE may present as deep vein thrombosis, pulmonary embolism, arterial thrombosis, catheter-related thrombosis, or hepatic veno-occlusive disease. Certain malignancies are associated with higher risk of VTE, including hematologic malignancies, mucin-secreting adenocarcinomas of the ovary, and pancreas, stomach, and brain tumors. Chemotherapy treatment significantly increases patient risk for developing VTE, which has an estimated annual incidence of 10.9%.[14] Thromboembolism is the second most common cause of death in patients with cancer.[15] Postmortem studies in patients with cancer indicate VTE is the second leading cause of death.[16] Fortunately, evidence is emerging that the antithrombotics, and particularly low-molecular-weight heparins, may exert an antitumor effect that could contribute to improved survival in patients with cancer when given for long-term prophylaxis.[17]

The impact of bleeding or thrombosis on the patient's quality of life depends on the acuity and the site of the bleeding or clotting. Bleeding may present as minor continuous low-volume oozing, episodic major bleeding, or acute hemorrhage. Visible bleeding can be distressing to patients with cancer, while occult bleeding may go unnoticed. Frank bleeding frequently prompts patients to seek medical attention. Bleeding can also cause increased discomfort with a relatively small amount of blood loss, as in hematuria. Low-level bleeding results in anemia, causing fatigue and weakness. Hemorrhage may be dramatic and life threatening, as in rupture of the carotid artery due to cancers of the head and neck. The location of the bleeding may be more significant in determining its severity than the volume of blood loss, such as in the case of an intracranial hemorrhage.

ETIOLOGY

Bleeding

Bleeding occurs when a blood vessel is injured and blood escapes. Therapy can damage normal tissue, as well as bone marrow, making the individual more prone to bleeding. Individuals may have one or multiple causes for altered hemostasis. Hemostasis may be altered if the platelet function or the coagulation pathways are abnormal. Multiple mechanisms alter vascular integrity, platelet function, and coagulation in the individual with cancer. Platelet dysfunction might be due to abnormal platelet counts from disease, medications, or therapy. Infection, liver disease, and high-viscosity proteins expressed by the tumor can also alter the coagulation pathway, leading to an increased risk of bleeding. Treatments such as radiation therapy or steroid treatment can lead to increased vessel fragility. Antineoplastic therapy frequently increases the risk for bleeding. Chemotherapy and radiation therapy can cause myelosuppression, including thrombocytopenia. Damaged marrow that is slow to recover or unable to fully recover after antineoplastic therapy limits the aggressiveness of further treatment for the person with cancer. Doses are diminished or eliminated because of marrow suppression. Less intensive chemotherapy may be administered in future treatments and has important implications for treatment outcomes.

The tumor itself can affect bleeding by invading surrounding structures or blood vessels or by invading and occupying the bone marrow (myelophthisis). In addition, the cancer may cause DIC by producing high-viscosity proteins. Tumors that invade local tissues or blood vessels can erode into mucous membranes, such as oropharyngeal, genitourinary, gastrointestinal, or gynecological tumors, and can cause bleeding by local tissue disruption. Tumors lying in close proximity to large blood vessels put the individual at risk for massive hemorrhage.

Leukemias and lymphomas are the most common cancers invading the bone marrow, although this effect has been seen in other cancers. With these cancers, the malignant cells are overproduced, crowding out normal hematopoietic cells, resulting in thrombocytopenia, anemia, and frequently neutropenia. The marrow's space and resources are spent making an abundance of malignant cells, causing normal cells to be underproduced. Primary bone marrow malignancies, bone marrow metastasis, cytotoxic chemotherapy, and radiation can diminish platelet production.

The degree and duration of the thrombocytopenia secondary to chemotherapy depends on the type of chemotherapy, dose, and interval between cycles. The chemotherapeutic drugs mithramycin, carmustine, and the anthracyclines are associated with abnormal platelet aggregation and other coagulopathies. Vinca alkaloids such as vincristine and vinblastine are also associated with platelet dysfunction.[1] L-Asparaginase inhibits the synthesis of clotting factors and can lead to either hemorrhage or thrombosis, especially in individuals with a history of hemostatic disorders.[18] Mitomycin can cause a thrombotic microangiopathy, manifested as hemolytic uremic syndrome (HUS),[19] as can commonly used immunosuppressive agents such as cyclosporine and tacrolimus.[20] Antiangiogenesis agents such as thalidomide have been associated with a significant increased risk of thrombosis, especially when used in combination with other chemotherapeutic drugs.[21] In the event that a systemic form of treatment, usually chemotherapy, is especially effective, the resulting tumor necrosis may cause significant bleeding, especially when the tumor involves blood vessels.

Thrombocytopenia may also be caused by destruction of platelets by immune or nonimmune mechanisms. Immune thrombocytopenia is due to antibody-mediated destruction of the platelets. Nonimmune destruction or consumption of platelets occurs in DIC, thrombotic microangiopathy (thrombus forming in the arterioles and capillaries), and platelet loss during hemorrhage. Once platelets leave the bone marrow, they are sequestered by the spleen. If the spleen is enlarged or congested, the platelets are retained within the spleen for a longer period of time. The spleen may become so congested and enlarged that the sequestration causes thrombocytopenia. The marrow tries to respond to the thrombocytopenia by increasing platelet production. Platelets continue to be sequestered in the spleen, increasing the splenomegaly.

Another important factor in the etiology of bleeding is infection or, more precisely, sepsis. The hemostatic changes occurring during sepsis range from a hypercoagulable state contributing to localized venous thromboembolism, to acute DIC causing consumption of platelets and coagulation proteins and, eventually, bleeding signs and symptoms.[22] This is due to the initiation of the coagulation cascade by complement, which is activated via the process of sepsis. The pathophysiology of sepsis-associated DIC begins with a systemic inflammatory response to an infectious agent.[23] DIC is a dangerous sequela of sepsis contributing to a high mortality rate.[24] It is most frequently seen in gram-negative sepsis due to the endotoxins released from the bacteria. Systemic disorders, such as sepsis and DIC, also put the individual at higher risk for gastritis and potential bleeding. Some viruses can cause myelosuppression or thrombocytopenia. Viral and bacterial infections may irritate or ulcerate linings of the gastrointestinal or genitourinary tracts, causing bleeding. Invasive fungal infections, especially in the lungs, can cause fatal hemorrhage.[25] Antibiotics can also be associated with increased risk of bleeding. High-dose β-lactam antibiotics, such as carbenicillin, ticarcillin, and penicillins, impair the aggregation of platelets and prolong bleeding time. Once the causative medication is stopped, platelet counts usually return to normal within a week.[26] Cephalosporins inhibit platelet function much like penicillin does, and also affect the abdominal flora, diminishing vitamin K absorption and thereby affecting coagulation. Vitamin K may be given parenterally to counter this effect. Antibiotic-related coagulation disorders can be potentiated in uremic patients. Other medications such as phenothiazines, tricyclic antidepressants, heparin, cimetidine, and thiazide diuretics may suppress platelet activity.[26,27] Corticosteroids irritate the gastric mucosa, impair wound healing, and make skin thin and fragile.

Malnourished individuals or those who have significant liver disease may have a vitamin K deficiency or coagulation defects and, are therefore, at significant risk for bleeding. The liver is the production site of all coagulation factors except factor VIII, and vitamin K is necessary for the production of some of these factors.[28] As such, vitamin K deficiencies can result in a failure to produce an adequate supply of factors needed for proper coagulation. Dietary deficiency, prolonged biliary obstruction, malabsorptive syndromes, liver disease, anticoagulation therapy, and intestinal sterilization by antibiotic therapy can all contribute to the depleted stores of vitamin K.[29] Liver impairment may result in decreased synthesis of these factors, leading to coagulation defects. Liver failure frequently is associated with altered platelet function and abnormal production of fibrinogen.[30]

Numerous drugs exert qualitative and quantitative effects on platelets. Platelet dysfunction combined with another mild hemostatic abnormality can have a cumulative effect, resulting in serious hemorrhage.[30] Aspirin is the most common medication associated with platelet dysfunction. Aspirin and other nonsteroidal anti-inflammatory drugs (NSAIDs) such as ibuprofen reduce platelet aggregation. Alteration in platelet aggregation from aspirin may last up to 4 days after ingestion, until sufficient platelet turnover occurs to replenish the system with new platelets having normal function.

Bleeding in the person with cancer may also be related to uremia. Uremic plasma inhibits normal platelet response, causing a prolonged bleeding time and impaired platelet function.[30] The most frequent presentations of bleeding in persons with uremia include petechial hemorrhages, blood blisters, ecchymoses on puncture sites, low-grade gastrointestinal bleeding, and subdural hematoma.[31] The best way to control or diminish uremic-associated hemorrhagic complications is by dialysis, which corrects or at least improves the hemostatic defect and subsequent bleeding time.[30,31] In emergencies, administration of cryoprecipitate normalizes bleeding times temporarily. Desmopressin (DDAVP) and other vasopressins are widely used hemostatic drugs that can be administered in uremia-induced platelet dysfunction and decrease the bleeding time in 50%–75% of patients.[30]

Thrombosis

Hypercoagulability, stasis, and vascular endothelial damage constitute the triad of risk factors for VTE identified by Virchow in 1856.[16,32,33] Thrombosis in patients, particularly those with acute leukemia, is related to intravascular clotting activation resulting in clotting/bleeding syndromes.[34] Thrombosis can also result from a large tumor compressing venous circulation, leading to stasis and clot formation. This is most commonly seen in superior vena cava syndrome. Thromboses in patients with cancer are found in sites other than the lower extremities. Thrombosis may be superficial or deep, migrate regularly, and may occur or recur.[35]

Non-tumor-associated risk factors for thrombosis in the patient with cancer include chemotherapy, reduced activity or immobilization, and the pervasive use of central venous catheters.[7,35,36] Cancer treatments associated with thrombosis include L-asparaginase,[7] cyclophosphamide, methotrexate, 5-fluorouracil, bevacizumab,[37] thalidomide, lenalidomide,[38] interferons, tamoxifen, medroxyprogestererone, megace,[39] and erythropoietin-stimulating agents.[7] A meta-analysis identified risk factors for catheter-related thrombosis as including a previous history of venous thrombosis, subclavian venipuncture site, improper position of the catheter tip, and peripherally inserted central catheters (PICCs).[40] Sepsis-associated thrombus formation occurs as a result of several simultaneous mechanisms following an inflammatory response: up-regulation of procoagulant pathways, down-regulation of physiological anticoagulants, and suppression of fibrinolysis, eventually causing microvascular fibrin deposition.[22]

PATHOPHYSIOLOGY

HYPERCOAGULABILITY OF MALIGNANCY

A hypercoagulable state may be an inherited or acquired disorder in which there is an increased propensity to form thrombosis. Thrombosis is a common complication of malignancy,[15] and most commonly presents as deep vein thrombosis (DVT) of the lower extremities, pulmonary embolism (PE), and venous thromboembolism (VTE). Other thrombotic complications include DIC, hemolytic uremic syndrome, and thrombotic thrombocytopenia purpura (TTP). Complex interdependent mechanisms involving tissue factor (TF), inflammatory cytokines, and platelets induce hypercoagulability. TF is the main physiologic initiator of coagulation and is expressed by malignant cells in many tumor types, including solid tumors, leukemia blast cells, tumor-associated macrophages, and endothelial cells.[15] A hypercoagulable state is induced after tumor secretion of procoagulant factors (tissue factor and cancer procoagulant).[15] Both factors can directly activate factor X, resulting in initiation of the clotting pathway. Tumors can also directly invade blood vessels, affecting the vascular endothelium and promoting clotting.[41]

THROMBOTIC COMPLICATIONS

Disseminated intravascular coagulopathy

Disseminated intravascular coagulation is the most common life-threatening hypercoagulopathy in the individual with cancer, and affects approximately 10% of patients with cancer.[42] Although DIC is not a primary disorder, with this condition normal coagulation is pathologically overactivated. It may be triggered by a number of factors, including malignancy, sepsis, hemolytic transfusion reactions, or shock. In acute DIC, there is exaggerated overstimulation of normal coagulation, and both thrombosis and hemorrhage may simultaneously occur. Activation of the clotting pathways ultimately leads to excessive fibrin production and the dissemination of fibrin thrombi, which may lodge in the microvasculature of various organs, such as the kidneys, lungs, or brain. This can result in organ damage and necrosis. This process of rapid clot formation depletes both platelets and clotting factors, thereby increasing the risk of bleeding. The excess fibrin formation also increases fibrinolysis in a compensatory attempt to break down the thrombi. Activated fibrinolysis results in high levels of circulating fibrin degradation products (FDP), which interfere with platelet aggregation and act as potent anticoagulants. As a result, DIC is a potentially fatal complication in cancer.[24]

Hemolytic uremic syndrome

Hemolytic uremic syndrome refers to a clinical syndrome characterized by microvascular thrombi composed of aggregated platelets and fibrin.[43] The pathologic trigger comprises endothelial damage and subsequent platelet aggregation, which leads to thrombocytopenia and renal, neurologic, and pulmonary dysfunction. The renal vasculature is particularly affected, often resulting in irreversible oliguria or anuric renal failure. Even though HUS is a rare clinical complication, its incidence in patients with cancer is estimated to be approximately 4%–15%.[44]

HUS is not a single disease, but rather a variety of conditions. In patients with cancer, most cases of HUS have been reported with adenocarcinoma of the breast, lung, pancreas, prostate, stomach, and lymphoma. It has also been associated with chemotherapy, mostly with mitomycin-C, 5-fluorouracil, gemcitabine, bleomycin, cisplatin, cytosine arabinoside, and daunorubicin,[45] and has also been reported after bone marrow transplant.[44,45] An association with immunosuppressive drugs such as cyclosporine and tacrolimus has been described with HUS, which may account for the higher incidence in patients receiving an allogeneic stem cell transplant.[44]

Treatment for HUS is mainly supportive and consists of plasma exchange, dialysis, and other supportive therapies. Additionally, discontinuation of the causative drug should be considered. Platelet transfusions are generally contraindicated, as they can lead to worsening of the microvascular thrombi.

Thrombotic thrombocytopenic purpura

Cancer-associated TTP is distinct from the classical form of TTP, but is generally considered to be indistinguishable from HUS. In classical TTP, patients present with a syndrome of fever, hemolytic anemia, thrombocytopenia, and renal and neurologic abnormalities due to the widespread formation of microvascular thrombi. In contrast, in patients with cancer, TTP symptoms are less pronounced. Similar vascular injury can occur, but the renal failure is found to be milder. Thrombocytopenia is believed to be due to both platelet activation and consumption at sites of endothelial injury. HUS, TTP, and microangiopathic hemolytic anemia (MAHA) are characterized by localized microvascular thrombosis or localized intravascular coagulation.

Plasma exchange is the primary treatment for TTP. Platelet transfusion is contraindicated unless given for life-threatening bleeding complications.[43]

SYMPTOM ASSESSMENT

RISK FACTORS

Assessment of bleeding and thrombosis in patients should include evaluation of risk factors. The multiple factors associated with increased risk of bleeding include fever, sepsis, uremia, infections, low hematocrit, anatomic lesions, endothelial injury, hypoalbuminemia, recent hemorrhage, thrombocytopenia, hyperleukocytosis, acquired hemophilia, anticoagulant therapy, platelet function defects, coagulation abnormalities, adverse effects of medications, and bone marrow transplantation.[6,7]

General risk factors for thrombosis include, age, gender, immobility, venous stasis, infections, and previous thrombotic history.[34] Patient-related risk factors for thrombosis include older age and female gender. African Americans are more predisposed to developing thrombosis, while Asian-Pacific Islanders have lower risk. Comorbidities such as infection, renal disease, pulmonary disease, obesity, inherited prothrombic mutations, and a prior history of VTE predispose a patient with cancer to developing thrombosis. Chemotherapy, hormone therapy, central venous access devices, and supportive therapies such as erythrocyte-stimulating agents (ESAs) are all treatment-related risk factors for thrombosis. Certain solid tumor sites are related to higher risk of thrombosis—specifically, brain, pancreas, kidney, gastric, lung, and gynecologic cancers and lymphoma.[15] The risk of thrombosis is greater at diagnosis and in patients with distant metastases or advanced stage cancer.[32] Several biomarkers are also associated with increased risk for thrombosis. For example, platelet count equal to or greater than $350{,}000/mm^3$ and leukocyte count greater than $11{,}000/mm^3$ prior to chemotherapy increase a patient's risk for thrombosis. Elevated levels of other biomarkers, including tissue factor (TF) plasma level or TF expression by tumor cells, soluble P-selectin, D-dimer, and C-reactive protein, are associated with increased risk of VTE in cancer.[15] Table 14-1 lists various risk factors for thrombosis in patients with cancer.

Lippi and Franchini cite an analysis done by Levitan and colleagues in 1999 of the Medicare Provider Analysis and Review Record (MEDPAR), showing the calculated relative risk of VTE by tumor site compared to patients with various medical comorbidities as follows: uterus (3.4), brain (2.4), leukemia (2.2), ovary (2.2), pancreas (2.1), lymphoma (1.8), stomach (1.5), kidney (1.4), colon (1.4), and rectum (1.1).[32] Clinicians should ensure that patients with a higher calculated relative risk are assessed and monitored for VTE during each clinic visit.

Recently, Khorana and colleagues developed and validated a predictive model (Table 14-2) for chemotherapy-associated thrombosis in patients with cancer based on clinical and laboratory parameters, which clinicians can use for evaluating risk for thrombosis in patients.[16,46] Points are assigned to predetermined clinical and laboratory indicators. Very high-risk tumor sites are assigned 2 points; high-risk sites are scored with 1 point. One point was assigned to each of the following biomarker/laboratory findings: pre-chemotherapy platelet count equal to or greater than $350{,}000/mm^3$; hemoglobin level less than 100 g/L; pre-chemotherapy leukocyte count greater than $11 \times 10^9/L$; use of ESAs; and body mass index (BMI) equal to or greater than 35 kg/m^2. Three risk categories based on risk scores were distinguished: low risk (0 risk score), intermediate risk (1–2 risk score), and high risk ($\geq$ 3 risk score).[46]

TABLE 14-1

Risk Factors for Thrombosis in Patients with Cancer

Patient-related factors	Older Age Female gender Race • Higher in African Americans • Lower in Asian-Pacific Islanders Comorbidities • Infection, renal disease, pulmonary disease, obesity, arterial thromboembolism • Prior history of venous thromboembolism (VTE)
Cancer-related factors	Primary site of cancer • Brain, pancreas, kidney, stomach, lung, gynecologic, lymphoma, myeloma Advanced stage of cancer (metastatic disease) Initial period after diagnosis of cancer (3–6 months after diagnosis)
Treatment-related factors	Major surgery Hospitalization Active cancer therapy: chemotherapy, hormone therapy, antiangiogenic therapy (thalidomide, lenalidomine, bevacizumab) Erythropoiesis-stimulating agents Transfusions Central venous catheters
Biomarkers	Pre-chemotherapy platelet count ≥ 350,000/mm^3 Pre-chemotherapy leukocyte count > 11,000/mm^3 Tissue factor (TF) • High TF expression by tumor cells • High TF plasma levels Soluble P-selectin D-Dimer C-reactive protein

Source: Data from Shelke and Khorana[15]; Lyman and Khorana[16].

TABLE 14-2

Risk Assessment for Chemotherapy-Associated Venous Thromboembolism (VTE)

Patient Characteristic	Risk Score
Tumor Site	
Stomach	2
Pancreas	2
Lung	1
Lymphoma	1
Gynecologic	1
Bladder	1
Testicular	1
Prechemotherapy platelet count ≥ 350 × 10^9/L	1
Hemoglobin level < 100g/L or use of ESAs	1
Prechemotherapy leukocyte count > 11 × 10^9/L	1
BMI equal to or greater than 35 kg/m^2	1

Risk Category	Total Risk Score
Low Risk	0
Intermediate Risk	1–2
High Risk	≥ 3

Abbreviation: BMI: body mass index.

Source: Data from Shelke and Khorana[15]; Khorana et al[46].

SELF-ASSESSMENT

Patients with cancer experience a broad range of symptoms throughout their treatment course. Clinicians must always provide patient instructions on which bleeding signs and symptoms to look for and report. Instructions for patient self-assessment should include definitions of bleeding events; differentiating between new and normal bleeding events (i.e., abnormal vaginal bleeding or menses); sites and duration of bleeding; amount of visible blood; and platelet levels. In addition, clinicians should explain and ensure patient understanding of basic laboratory parameters (i.e., platelet levels) in relation to observed bleeding manifestations. Emphasize that the severity of bleeding is inversely related to the platelet level.

The bleeding self-assessment checklist (Table 14-3) is a practical tool to assist patients in reporting bleeding symptoms.[47] This tool captures clinically significant bleeding events and assists clinicians in classifying severity of reported bleeding. It is important for patients to note the duration of the bleeding episode: whether the bleeding lasted only for a few minutes, for less than an hour, or for more than an hour. The patient should assess the mouth for the presence of blood blisters or active bleeding on gums or lips. When nose bleeding occurs, note whether nasal packing was required. Changes or impairment in vision as well as bloodshot eyes should be reported.

Thrombocytopenic patients should check their body daily for any new bruises or red spots, and determine if bruising or petechiae are more extensive than the day before. Painful joints or muscles should be inspected for swelling and bruising. Invasive line sites should be inspected daily for signs of bleeding. The patient should check urine and stool for visible blood, or for dark and tarry stool. Coughing up blood and bright red emesis should be reported immediately.

TABLE 14-3

Patient Self-Assessment Checklist for Bleeding

Yes	No	Sympton
☐	☐	Bleeding or blood blisters on gums or lips
☐	☐	Continuous bleeding less than 1 hour?
☐	☐	Continuous bleeding greater than 1 hour?
☐	☐	Nose bleeding (epistaxis)
☐	☐	Was packing required?
☐	☐	Continuous bleeding less than 1 hour?
☐	☐	Continuous bleeding greater than 1 hour?
☐	☐	Blood shot eyes
☐	☐	New changes/impairments in vision
☐	☐	Visible red spots or bruising on any part of body
☐	☐	More spots than day before?
☐	☐	Mild/Moderate
☐	☐	Extensive
☐	☐	Bruised swollen, and painful joints or muscles
☐	☐	Bleeding from invasive sites (for example: central venous access line)
☐	☐	Bright red blood in vomit (hematemesis)
☐	☐	Coughing up blood
☐	☐	Visible blood in urine (hematuria)
☐	☐	Vaginal bleeding
☐	☐	Is this normal menses/period?
☐	☐	Using more than 2 pads per day?
☐	☐	Bright red blood in stool (hematochezia)
☐	☐	Black tarry stool (melena)
☐	☐	Bleeding episode other than described above
Platelet Level:		**Date:**

Source: Data from Stanworth et al[47].

OBJECTIVE ASSESSMENT

History and physical assessment

A thorough assessment for alterations in hemostasis in the individual with cancer involves a complete patient and family history (Table 14-4). Because bleeding is a common disorder, close attention should be paid to any history of bleeding or clotting disorders or anything that might suggest blood loss. The history includes any bleeding tendencies such as petechiae and easy bruising, pain, headaches, nosebleeds, and changes in the color of stool or urine. Assess for prolonged bleeding following cuts, bruises, surgery, or dental extractions. If available, obtain previous laboratory tests and results to evaluate platelet and hemoglobin levels. The hemoglobin level may indicate anemia related to bleeding. An evaluation of nutritional status can identify any vitamin K deficiency or generalized malnutrition. Reviewing all medications, including over-the-counter and herbal medications, may uncover a potential interference with coagulation. Information regarding recent transfusions, possible reactions, and response to transfusions is important. Individuals with a history of prior transfusions and multiparous women are at risk of alloimmunization. As patients are exposed to antigens in donor blood products, they may develop antibodies to these specific antigens, resulting in destruction of transfused cells. With alloimmunization, patients fail to achieve the expected therapeutic increment in platelet levels. Any recent or acute episodes of infections should be determined, as infections can alter platelet production.

Physical assessment can detect early signs of bleeding. Some of these signs may be subtle, others overt. Bleeding can be internal or external, mild or life threatening, occurring anywhere in the body. The most common sites of hemorrhage include the nose, brain gingiva, bladder, gastrointestinal tract. Because bleeding frequently occurs internally, it is essential to investigate all complaints of weakness, pain, discomfort, or change in level of consciousness in the person at risk.

TABLE 14-4

Relevant History in the Assessment of Bleeding
History of bleeding and or clotting disorders
Medications including over the counter medications
Bleeding tendencies: petechiae, easy bruising. nosebleeding
Previous laboratory test results: complete blood count, coagulation tests
Previous blood product transfusions including any transfusion-related reactions and response to treatment

General performance status is evaluated and may identify the effects of the disease or presence of complications. Signs or symptoms of anemia, such as fatigue, malaise, weakness, headaches, pallor, orthostatic hypotension, or tachycardia, may be indicative of undetected chronic blood loss. Assessment for localized thrombosis should include detection of unilateral swelling of an affected extremity, positive Homan's sign, and chest pain or shortness of breath, indicative of a possible pulmonary embolus (PE).[48] The physical assessment of the patient at risk for bleeding or thrombosis must be thorough, because these complications can occur anywhere in the body (Table 14-5). A detailed head-to-toe assessment is described next.

Central nervous system. Individuals with brain cancer, leukemia, or those undergoing SCT have the highest risk of developing hemorrhage into the CNS. Alterations in level of consciousness, irritability, confusion, mental status changes, seizures, and coma may occur with impaired tissue perfusion of the brain due to bleeding or thrombosis. Intracranial hemorrhage may occur due to tumor invasion, thrombocytopenia, or coagulopathy accompanied by hypertension or increased intracranial pressure. Hemorrhages usually occur over a matter of minutes, unless the bleeding is due to anticoagulant therapy, which may develop over 24 to 48 hours. The individual may complain of a severe sudden headache. Edema around the tissue injury of the hemorrhage often leads to an increased compression and worsening clinical state. Symptoms are dependent on the location and extent of the bleed or clot. Assess the patient for signs and symptoms of neurologic deficit including widening pulse pressure, changes in pupil size and reactivity, motor strength and coordination, speech changes, and paralysis.

Eyes, ears, nose, and throat. Assess the patient for visual disturbances such as blurry vision, diplopia, alteration in visual fields, nystagmus, conjunctival hemorrhage, and periorbital edema. Inspect nares for petechiae, blood-tinged drainage, and epistaxis. The oral mucosa and gum line should be inspected for frank bleeding, blood blisters, lesions, and ulcerations.

Pulmonary. Respiratory assessment is an important measure of the anemic state of the individual who is bleeding, indicating the respiratory system's attempt or inability to compensate for a diminished blood supply. Assess the patient for cyanosis, dyspnea, tachypnea, orthopnea, and shortness of breath. Evaluate lung sounds for crackles, wheezing, or stridor. Bleeding can occur in the major airways, the pleural space, and the alveoli. Hemoptysis occurs when there is bleeding into the major airways. Malignant pleural effusions caused by cancers (lymphomas, lung cancers, and breast cancers) are frequently bloody. The severity of the symptoms is frequently associated with the rate at which the effusion fills the pleural space. Patients who are severely immunosuppressed and have a coagulopathy are most likely to bleed into the alveoli. These individuals are usually stem cell transplant recipients or have leukemia. The alveoli fill with blood, inhibiting gas exchange and leading to hypoxia. During bronchoscopy, if more bleeding occurs when washings are taken, saline is injected into the airway and aspirated; this is indicative of alveolar hemorrhage.

Cardiovascular. The hemorrhaging individual frequently shows changes in vital signs, color and temperature of extremities, and peripheral pulses. Assess the patient for tachycardia and hypotension.

Gastrointestinal. The person with cancer is prone to having hemorrhagic complications along the gastrointestinal (GI) tract. Hematemesis usually indicates bleeding proximal to the duodenum, because blood entering the GI tract below that structure cannot enter the stomach. Hematochezia indicates frank blood in stool. Melena usually indicates bleeding from the esophagus, stomach, or duodenum. One acute episode of blood loss may produce melena for as long as 3 days. Once the stool color has returned to normal, the stool may remain guaiac positive for 1 week. Blood in the GI tract is cathartic, increasing the motility with increased volume of the hemorrhage—assess the patient for bloody diarrhea. In addition, assess the patient for nausea, vomiting, fever, weakness, anorexia, and abdominal pain.

Genitourinary. Dysuria, burning, frequency, pain on urination, suprapubic pain, and cramping are also symptoms the patient can experience. Frank or gross hematuria is an indication of serious bleeding. The frequency and size of clots, as well as the number of sanitary pads used, should be noted and reported.

Musculoskeletal. Bleeding into joints is indicative of a coagulation deficit. Joints may be swollen, warm, and sore, with diminished mobility for both active and passive range of motion. It is difficult to distinguish between infection and bleeding into the joints without tapping the joint.

Diagnostic evaluation

A number of point-of-care tests are used in the assessment of bleeding. Such tests include the hemoccult tests of stools and excreta and urine dipstick to quantify microscopic hematuria. In addition, actual quantification of gauze or other material used to absorb the blood and volume measurement of melena or hematemesis constitute objective information used to assess severity of bleeding.

Scans are also used in the assessment of internal bleeding or clotting. Tests assessing internal hemorrhage or clotting

TABLE 14-5

Physical Assessment for Patients at High Risk for Bleeding or Thrombosis

Organ	Assessment
Central nervous system (CNS): Symptoms dependent on site and size of bleeding or clot	Headache, nausea/vomiting, retching, mental status changes (restlessness, confusion, lethargy, obtundation, coma), vertigo, seizures, changes in pupil size and reactivity; eye deviations, sensory or motor strength alterations, speech alterations, paralysis
Eyes	Visual disturbances—blurring, diplopia, absent or altered fields of vision, nystagmus, increased injections in sclera, conjunctival hemorrhage, periorbital edema; note if sclera are icteric
Nose	Petechiae, blood-tinged drainage, epistaxis
Mouth	Petechiae of oral mucosa, pain, dysphagia, hematemesis, bleeding gums/mucosa, blood-tinged secretions, ulcerations with frank bleeding
Upper gastrointestinal: esophagus/stomach	Dysphagia, hematemesis, blood-tinged secretions, substernal burning and pain, epigastric discomfort (burning, tenderness, or cramping), coffee ground emesis, nausea, vomiting, fever, weakness, anorexia, melena, hyperactive bowel sounds
Lower gastrointestinal: duodenum/anus	Pain (location, occurrence, duration, quality), nausea, vomiting, tarry stools, diarrhea, bowel sounds (hyper- or hypoactive), cramping, occult blood in stools, frank blood in stools (rectum or lower), blood around anus, frequency and quantity of stools, pain with bowel movements (hemorrhoids)
Lungs	Tachypnea, dyspnea, air hunger, respiration rate, depth, and exertion Crackles, rubs, wheezing, diminished breath sounds, hemoptysis (frothy BRB sputum—major airway bleeding), stridor, tickling in throat or chest with desire to cough
Cardiovascular	Tachycardia and hypotension (characteristic of anemia and acute blood loss) Changes in VS, color and temperature of extremities, peripheral pulses (present, quality), and changes in peripheral perfusion Pericardial effusions: dyspnea, cough, pain, orthopnea, venous distension, tamponade (muted heart sounds, hypotension, pulsus paradoxus, tachycardia, angina, palpitations)
Abdomen	Hepatomegaly (liver disease—possible coagulation disorder), RUQ pain, abdominal distension Splenomegaly (increased risk for bleeding): Assess for any trauma; if spleen ruptures, rapid hypovolemic shock ensues; left flank or left shoulder pain Retroperitoneal bleeding: vague abdominal complaints, ecchymoses over flank, occasional bulging flanks and tenderness; associated with hypovolemia
Genitourinary	Decreased urinary output due to massive bleeding is associated with hypovolemia and shock Hematuria: dysuria, burning, frequency, pain on urination, suprapubic pain and cramping, gross blood in urine, clots Menorrhagia: suprapubic pain and cramping, gross blood in urine, clots (may need to straight catheterize female patients to distinguish between urinary or vaginal bleeding) Frequency and size of clots, number of sanitary napkins used and color of urine are important in measuring bleeding
Musculoskeletal	Bleeding into the joints is usually associated with alterations in coagulation; swollen, warm, sore joint with decreased mobility (active and passive ROM); usually unilateral; tapping the joint's synovial fluid is frequently required to distinguish infection from bleeding Unilateral swelling of affected extremity, with or without positive Homan's sign
Skin	Petechiae, ecchymosis, purpura, hematoma; oozing from venipuncture sites, central lines, catheters, injection sites, incisional sounds, nasogastric tubes Gangrene, alterations in skin color (e.g., pallor, cyanosis), alterations in skin temperature

Abbreviations: BRB: bright red blood: VS: vital signs; RUQ: right upper quadrant; ROM: range of motion.

Source: Data from Friend and Pruett[48].

include computed tomography scans, magnetic resonance imaging, x-ray, and ultrasound. A fundoscopic examination is the initial testing undertaken in diagnosing intraocular hemorrhage. The diagnosis of the site of bleeding in the GI tract is usually done by visualization. An urgent esophagogastroduodenoscopy procedure is performed to determine the potential source of bleeding such as peptic ulcer, arteriovenous malformations, Mallory-Weiss tears, and erosive esophagitis.[49] For lower GI bleeding, diagnostic evaluation may include a colonoscopy, flexible sigmoidoscopy, or proctoscopy. A digital rectal exam can diagnose bleeding internal hemorrhoids. Occult blood is also detected by guaiac-positive stool and excreta; however, the exact location of the bleeding in the GI tract would need to be diagnosed by endoscopy.

Laboratory tests. Laboratory values are frequently the most useful information for assessing altered hemostasis and determining the potential pathophysiology. Treatments are generally based on the test results. Common screening laboratory tests, normal ranges, and the meaning of their measurements are shown in Table 14-6.

Tests used to determine platelet disorders include the platelet count, bleeding time, platelet function studies, and bone marrow aspirate. Laboratory tests used for screening coagulation disorders include the prothrombin time, partial thromboplastin time, International Normalized Ratio (INR), fibrin degradation products, fibrinogen, D-dimer, levels of specific coagulation factors, and thrombin time. Hemoglobin and hematocrit values are used to monitor blood loss. Individuals with cancer often have anemia due to multiple factors and have a tendency to run on the low side of the normal ranges. A sudden drop in hemoglobin or hematocrit, however, indicates an acute blood loss. In general, red blood cell transfusions are given to keep the hemoglobin above 7–8 g/dL and the hematocrit above 21–24 mL/dL. Cardiopulmonary compromise can occur when levels fall below this level.

TABLE 14-6

Common Screening Laboratory Tests for Assessment of Hemostasis

Laboratory Test	Normal Range	Evaluates
	Platelet evaluation	
Platelet count	150,000–400,000/mm^3	Quantification of platelets in blood
Bleeding time	2–9 minutes	Platelet plug formation
Bone marrow aspiration	Megakaryocytes present	Thrombopoiesis in bone marrow
	Coagulation evaluation	
Prothrombin time (PT)	Varies; compare with normal control (approx. 70%–130%)	Coagulation mechanism via extrinsic and common pathways
Partial thromboplastin time (PTT)	Varies; compare with normal control (approximately 21–40 seconds)	Coagulation mechanism via extrinsic and common pathways
International normalized ratio (INR)	Less than 2.0; 2.0–3.0 considered anticoagulated	Anticoagulation via manipulation of the extrinsic and common pathways
Fibrin degradation products (FDP)	Less than 10 μg/mL	Presence of FDP in serum, assessing fibrinolysis
Fibrinogen	200–400 mg/dL	Plasma concentration of fibrinogen
Specific factor assays	50%–150% activity in pooled normal plasma	Concentration of functional factors in plasma
Thrombin time	10–15 seconds	Estimated plasma fibrinogen levels
D-dimer	30–400 ng/mL	Useful in the diagnosis of disseminated intravascular coagulation, elevated levels indicate hyperfibrinolysis

Source: Data from Friend and Pruett[48].

Quantitative and qualitative measurement of platelets. The platelet count is the best indicator of the potential risk of bleeding in the person with cancer. The platelet count is the actual quantification of platelets in a blood volume. A count less than 100,000/mm^3 is indicative of thrombocytopenia. Many laboratory tests are now available to accurately diagnose conditions of platelet dysfunction.

The bleeding time provides clinicians with an idea of the integrity of vascular, platelet, and fibrin clot formation by measuring the time taken to stop bleeding from a small skin incision on a patient's forearm.[50] The bleeding time is dependent on both platelet number and function and on the normal function of blood vessels, particularly the capability of capillaries to vasoconstrict. A prolonged bleeding time can be due to alterations in any of these components and is seen with thrombocytopenia, tumor infiltration of the bone marrow, and consumption of platelets in DIC, and with the use of medications affecting platelet function. A consensus recommendation from Quality Management Program–Laboratory Services (QMP-LS) in Ontario, Canada (10 laboratories), and the North American Specialized Coagulation Laboratory Association (NASCOLA) suggested that bleeding time tests should no longer be performed to evaluate bleeding problems; nevertheless, some laboratories continue to perform such tests.[51]

A bone marrow aspirate is done to evaluate marrow function and determine the etiology of thrombocytopenia. Reduced numbers of megakaryocytes in the bone marrow indicate a primary thrombocytopenia or reduced production of platelets. If the number of megakaryocytes in the bone marrow is normal or elevated, it indicates that thrombocytopenia is a result of increased peripheral destruction of platelets or splenic sequestration. As much as 50% to 90% of the peripheral platelet pool can be sequestered in an enlarged spleen. In the absence of splenomegaly, only 30% of the platelet pool is normally found in the spleen.[52,53]

Laboratory tests may quantify specific factors or screen for efficacy of a pathway along the coagulation cascade. The prothrombin time (PT) screens for coagulation deficiency along the extrinsic and common pathways and may be prolonged due to a deficiency or inhibition of clotting factors.[50] This effect might be due to liver disease, vitamin K deficiency, obstructive biliary disease, or warfarin therapy. Activated partial thromboplastin time (aPTT) is an indicator of the integrity of the intrinsic and final common pathways of the coagulation cascade.[50] A prolonged aPTT occurs when there is a diminished quantity of any factor, except factor VII or factor XIII. This may occur due to heparin therapy, increased fibrin degradation products, and consumption of the clotting factors. If both PT and aPTT is prolonged, then the hemostatic alteration is likely found along the specific coagulation pathway. Prolongation of both PT and PTT is attributable to deficiencies in the intrinsic and extrinsic pathways along the common pathway or in all three pathways; alternatively, inhibitors may be acting on both the intrinsic and extrinsic pathways or on the common pathway.[50] Prolongation of both PTT and aPTT is related to liver diseases, vitamin K deficiency, DIC, and use of anticoagulation therapy. If both PT and PTT are within normal limits, then either the platelets or the blood vessel is defective.

Table 14-7 explains the differential diagnosis with coagulation test results.[54] The INR is a more standardized measurement, used for assessing overall anticoagulation status. An INR greater than 2.0 is considered sufficient coagulation for prophylaxis and treatment of DVT and PE.

Other measurements of coagulation (see Table 14-6) include fibrin degradation products (FDP), thrombin time, fibrinogen, and specific factor levels. The FDP measures the breakdown of fibrin and fibrinogen activity. An elevated FDP (greater than10 μg/mL) can result from surgery, obstetric complications, trauma, or DIC. A positive D-dimer test indicates fibrin degradation and thrombotic activity.[55] Positive test results are seen in individuals with DIC, pulmonary and cerebral embolism, phlebitis, thrombosis, and postoperative prothrombotic risks. Thrombin time estimates the plasma fibrinogen. It can be prolonged due to heparin, warfarin, streptokinase, or urokinase therapy; liver disease; DIC; or fibrinogen deficiency.[1] Fibrinogen may be low due to congenital or acquired hypofibrinogenemia, DIC, fibrinolysis, or severe liver disease.[56] It may be elevated in some malignant or inflammatory disorders, however. Measuring the specific factor levels in the plasma identifies individual or group factor deficiencies, aiding in the diagnosis of the bleeding or thrombotic disorder.

DEGREES OF TOXICITY

Several classification systems have been developed to grade the severity of bleeding. The most commonly used classification system is the World Health Organization (WHO) Bleeding Scale (Table 14-8), which details increasing levels in bleeding severity (grades 1 to 4).[6,7,57,58] An eight-point modified and expanded grading scale was developed by Gruppo Italiano Malattie Ematologiche Maligne dell'Adulto (GIMEMA), which includes specific sites of bleeding (Table 14-9).[6,59] The National Cancer Institute (NCI) has developed Common Terminology Criteria for Adverse Events (CTCAE; Table 14-10) to standardize reporting of treatment-related adverse events.[60] The CTCAE allows for grading of the severity of the adverse event. Toxicities, such as hemorrhage or bleeding, are graded on a scale of 0–5, and specific sites of bleeding (e.g., vaginal, gastrointestinal) are graded separately, with 0 = no bleeding; 1 = mild, no intervention needed; 2 = moderate symptoms, medical

TABLE 14-7

Differential Diagnosis for Coagulation Tests

Coagulation Test Results	Related Disorders If With Bleeding Symptoms	Related Disorders If Without Bleeding Symptoms
Increased PT Normal aPTT	Severe factor VII deficiency Warfarin Disseminated intravascular coagulation (DIC) Factor deficiency due to: • Liver disease • Vitamin K deficiency	Mild factor VII deficiency Vitamin K deficiency Use of oral anticoagulatants Sepsis
Normal PT Increased aPTT	Isolated factor deficiency: VIII, IX, XI Inhibitors of Factors VIII, IX, XI Hemophilia A and B VonWillebrand disease Heparin	Isolated factor deficiency (VIII, IX, XI, XII, contact pathway proteins) Heparin Lupus inhibitor
Increased PT Increased aPTT	Dysfibrinogenemia Severe deficiencies Factors II, V, VIII, X Factor deficiencies due to liver disease Severe vitamin K deficiency DIC Paraprotenemia Amyloidosis Heparin	Multiple coagulation factor deficiencies • Liver disease • Vitamin K deficiency Isolated factor X, V, II deficiency Factor V inhibitors Heparin therapy Warfarin therapy Low fibrinogen (< 50 mg/dL) Dilutional Lupus anticoagulants

Abbreviations: PT: prothrombin time; aPTT: activated partial thromboplastin time.

Source: Data from Rodriguez and Gobel[1]; DeLoughery[54].

intervention indicated; 3 = bleeding requiring transfusion; 4 = catastrophic bleeding requiring major intervention; and 5 = death related to bleeding. Specific bleeding events, such as DIC, can also be graded separately.

Bleeding resulting from various pathophysiology manifests differently among patients. Clinicians must carefully consider all signs and symptoms presented by the patient to appropriately prevent or manage bleeding.

SYMPTOM MANAGEMENT STRATEGIES

PREVENTIVE STRATEGIES

Preventive measures, including bleeding precautions to promote physical safety and/or guard against trauma, are critical in the care of the patient at high risk for bleeding. It is important for patients and families/caregivers to understand the risks and implications associated with the patient's platelet levels.

For the thrombocytopenic person, environmental safety, such as receiving assistance when gait is unsteady or when the person is mildly sedated or confused, is required. Strict fall precaution measures should be observed at all times for these patients in all settings to avoid potential sources of injury. Provide patients and family or caregivers instructions on fall precautions:

- Keeping floors dry
- Use of night lights
- Bed placed on lowest level possible
- Keeping the environment free from clutter
- Wheelchairs locked before the patient stands
- Patient to wear non-skid footwear when out of bed
- Assistance during ambulation, toileting, and bathing for patients with unsteady gait
- Placing items frequently used by patient (e.g., phone, TV remote, tissue, assistive devices) within reach

General bleeding precautions to initiate when the patient's platelet level is less than 20,000 cells/mm^3 include the following:[1]

- Avoid taking aspirin or other NSAIDs.
- Avoid cutting toenails and fingernails.
- Use only electric razors to prevent cuts.

TABLE 14-8

World Health Organization (WHO) Bleeding Severity Grading Scale

Grade	Description	Manifestation
0	No bleeding	
1	Minor bleeding	• Petechiae/ecchymosis • Epistaxis or oropharyngeal bleeding < 1 hour • Occult blood in stool (from trace to 1+) • Hemoglobinuria (from trace to 1+) • Retinal hemorrhage without reduction in vision • Minimal vaginal bleeding
2	Mild blood loss	• Melena, hematemesis, hematuria, hemoptysis, hematochezia, vaginal bleeding, skin bleeding that does not require transfusion or increase over routine transfusion needs • Epistaxis or oropharygeal bleeding > 1 hour • Occult blood in stool (moderate or from 2+ and greater) • Hemoglobinuria (moderate or from 2+ and greater)
3	Major bleeding	• Gross blood loss causing rapid falls in hematocrit • Melena, hematemesis, hemoptysis, hematuria, epistaxis and oropharyngeal bleeding • Abnormal vaginal bleeding that requires transfusion of one or more units of RBC • CNS bleeding detected by CAT scan without clinical consequences • Bleeding from site of venipuncture or insertion of a central venous access or catheter that requires transfusion support
4	Disabling bleeding	• Debilitating blood loss • Life threatening hemorrhage-massive bleeding causing a severe hemodynamic compromise • Bleeding into a vital organ: intracranial hemorrhage, pericardial hemorrhage, diffuse alveolar hemorrhage, cerebral hemorrhage • Retinal hemorrhage with reduction in vision • CNS hemorrhage with neurological signs and symptoms • Fatal hemorrhage regardless of site

Source: Data from Webert[6]; Kwaan and Huyck[7]; Cartoni et al[57]; Liumbruno et al[58].

TABLE 14-9

Gruppo Italiano Malattie Ematologiche Maligne dell'Adulto (GIMEMA) Bleeding Severity Grading Scale

0	No bleeding
1	Petechiae or mucosal or retinal bleeding that did not require red cell transfusion
2	Melena, hematemesis, hematuria, or hemoptysis
3	Any bleeding that required red cell transfusion
4	Retinal bleeding accompanied by visual impairment
5	Non-fatal cerebral bleeding
6	Fatal cerebral bleeding
7	Fatal non-cerebral bleeding

Source: Data from Webert et al[6].

TABLE 14-10

National Cancer Institute Common Terminology Criteria for Adverse Events (CTCAE): Bleeding

0	No bleeding
1	Mild, no intervention needed
2	Moderate symptoms, medical intervention indicated
3	Bleeding requiring transfusion
4	Catastrophic bleeding requiring major intervention
5	Death related to bleeding

Source: Data from National Cancer Institute Common Terminology Criteria for Adverse Events (CTCAE)[60].

- Use emollient lotion to keep the skin hydrated.
- Use laxatives/stool softeners if experiencing constipation.
- Apply direct pressure to puncture sites for at least 5 minutes.
- Avoid venipuncture, invasive procedure, and use of rectal thermometers or suppositories.
- Use a soft-bristled toothbrush, use only alcohol-free mouthwash, and avoid using dental floss to prevent trauma to the oral cavity.

In some instances, prophylactic blood component therapy transfusion might be indicated.[1]

Prevention of cancer-related thrombosis can involve prophylactic anticoagulation therapy in the absence of contraindications.[61,62] However, such therapy is tailored to the individual patient condition and may vary according to the clinical setting—for example, inpatient, surgery, or ambulatory/outpatient care setting.[15] A thorough history and assessment of the patient are conducted to determine the presence of any of the contraindications to anticoagulation medications listed in Table 14-11.[15] The current American Society of Clinical Oncology (ASCO) recommendations for VTE prophylaxis and treatment follow: [61]

- Anticoagulants are not currently recommended to improve survival in patients with cancer without VTE.
- Low-molecular-weight heparin (LMWH) is the preferred treatment for patients with established VTE to prevent recurrence.
- Hospitalized patients with cancer should be considered for VTE prophylaxis with anticoagulants in the absence of bleeding or other contraindications.
- Venous thromboembolism prophylaxis for patients with cancer undergoing major surgical intervention for malignant disease should be considered unless contraindicated.
- Routine VTE prophylaxis is not recommended for ambulatory patients with cancer during systemic therapy, with the exception of patients receiving thalidomide or lenalidomide with chemotherapy or dexamethasone.

TABLE 14-11

Contraindications to Anticoagulation
• Active, uncontrollable bleeding
• Active cerebrovascular hemorrhage
• Dissecting or cerebral aneurysm
• Bacterial endocarditis
• Pericarditis
• Active peptic or other gastrointestinal ulceration
• Severe, uncontrolled, or malignant hypertension
• Severe head trauma
• Pregnancy (for warfarin)
• Heparin-induced thromocytopenia
• Epidural catheter placement

Source: Data from Shelke and Khorana[15].

THERAPEUTIC APPROACHES

Thrombocytopenia

For patients undergoing multiple treatment cycles, chemotherapy dose reduction or chemotherapy dose delay is the standard preventive measure against chemotherapy-induced thrombocytopenia (CIT).[63] Prophylactic and therapeutic platelet transfusions remain the standard of care in managing CIT. Platelets transfused are either single-donor platelets derived from apheresis or pooled platelet concentrates from random donors. Both platelet products are equally efficacious, but single-donor platelets are preferred when histocompatible platelets are needed.[64] The recommended threshold for prophylactic platelet transfusion to prevent bleeding is 10,000/μL.[64,65]

A standard dose for transfusion is 300–600 $\times$ 10^9 platelets/product. A randomized controlled trial comparing standard-dose versus low-dose (150–300 $\times$ 10^9 platelets/product) platelet transfusions was conducted by Heddle et al.; the patients in the low-dose therapy arm (5.2%, $n = 58$) were observed to have grade 4 bleeds.[66] A recent study by Slichter and colleagues established that platelet dose had no significant effect on incidence of bleeding in patients with thrombocytopenia. This study further concluded that low-dose platelet transfusion is effective but requires more frequent transfusions.[67] To control platelet sequestration in the spleen, treatment with epinephrine, corticosteroids, and splenectomy may be considered. Intravenous immunoglobulin therapy (IVIG), high-dose dexamethasone, anti-D immunoglobulin, and rituximab may be indicated for patients with idiopathic thrombocytopenic purpura (ITP) to stimulate rapid platelet increases to counter platelet destruction.[1]

Thrombosis

Anticoagulants are used in treating clotting complications, and heparin is a mainstay of such therapy. Monitoring the PTT assesses the efficacy of the anticoagulation that heparin provides. Heparin does not dissolve existing clots, but rather prevents new clots from forming. It has a short half-life—1½ hours in plasma. Low-molecular-weight heparins are being used with increasing frequency (preferred to unfractionated heparin) in the initial treatment of DVT. One study suggested that enoxaparin, a LMWH, is a safe, superior, and effective alternative to heparin therapy for treating DVTs.[68] LMWHs are minimally cleared through the liver, and their clearance is not dose dependent. Such medications also have lower binding to plasma proteins, increased half-life, and a more predictable dose-response curve. LMWHs are the preferred option for both treatment and prophylaxis of thrombosis in patients with cancer, as they can be safely administered in the home and the anticoagulant effects are quite predictable, such that frequent laboratory monitoring is eliminated.[35,61]

The National Comprehensive Cancer Network's (NCCN) recommendations for inpatient thromboprophylaxis therapy for the duration of the hospital stay are as follows:[69]

- Dalteparin (LMWH): 5000 IU subcutaneously daily
- Exoxaparin (LMWH): 40 mg subcutaneously daily
- Tinzaparin (LMWH): 4400 IU subcutaneously daily
- Fondaparinux: 2.5 mg subcutaneously daily
- Unfractionated heparin: 5000 IU subcutaneously three times daily

Thromboprophylaxis significantly reduces the rate of combined symptomatic and asymptomatic VTE in patients with cancer.[50] One study demonstrated that administration of enoxaparin 40 mg daily for 4 weeks after surgery significantly reduced the frequency of postoperative venous thromboembolism, from 12% to 4.8%, in patients with cancer undergoing abdominal surgery.[70] A similar study demonstrated a significant reduction in the cumulative incidence of VTE in patients, from 16.3% with short-term prophylaxis to 7.3% when receiving dalteparin 5000 IU subcutaneously daily over an extended duration.[71]

Warfarin is an oral anticoagulant that suppresses hepatic synthesis of vitamin K-dependent clotting factors. It has no effect on platelets, and its action is cumulative and prolonged. The half-life of warfarin is 1.5–2.5 days, with steady state reached around day 4. This medication mostly affects the extrinsic pathway; therefore the PT may be monitored. Warfarin is notable for the many drug interactions that affect its efficacy. Individuals taking multiple medications need to be monitored closely when medications are added or deleted, and patient education regarding risk of bleeding is paramount.[1] A standard measurement for monitoring the effectiveness of orally administered anticoagulant is the INR, which provides a consistent ratio that can be used universally. An INR of 2.0–3.0 is generally accepted for prophylaxis and treatment of DVT and PE. Warfarin can be initiated concurrently with parenteral agent for at least 5 days and until the INR reaches or exceeds 2 for 24 hours. The INR should be monitored twice a week during the transition from concurrent to warfarin-only therapy, then weekly after the patient is on warfarin monotherapy.[69]

Central nervous system

Prevention. It is imperative to avoid activities that increase intracranial pressure, such as the Valsalva maneuver, to help prevent intracranial hemorrhage. Maintaining platelet levels greater than 10,000/mm^3, correcting coagulopathies, and controlling nausea and vomiting can decrease the risk of bleeding. Management of cough and nausea/vomiting symptoms with antitussive medications and antinausea medications should be considered to prevent forceful coughing and dry heaving.[65]

Management. The first line of treatment for intracranial bleeding is transfusion of platelets or coagulation factors. A platelet transfusion threshold to maintain platelet levels at more than 10,000/mm^3 should be established. Corticosteroids are also administered to control edema from the tissue injury, thereby preventing more elevated intracranial pressure and worse neurologic deficit. Close neurologic assessments are done, vital signs and neurologic signs are monitored, and protective measures such as strict fall precautions are instituted in the event that the patient is confused or hallucinating.

Cases involving more severe hemorrhage may require emergency burr holes or drains to release the pressure on the brain tissue, in addition to the first-line treatments just described. If inserted early enough, before pressure builds, drains could prevent more damage to brain tissue. However, because intracranial bleeds usually occur rapidly over a matter of minutes, a severe bleed is likely to result in irreversible damage. The person may become comatose and require intubation. Provision for a calm environment, explanation of actions, and pain medication for the severe headache are important to reduce anxiety.

Integumentary

Prevention. Personal hygiene is essential for maintaining maximum skin integrity. Lotions and skin emollients should be applied generously on the skin to maintain moisture and prevent dryness. Venipuncture is to be kept to a minimum, along with intramuscular and subcutaneous injections. If injections are absolutely necessary, the smallest-gauge needle possible is recommended. Paper tape is recommended rather than plastic or cloth tape to prevent trauma to the skin. Only electric razors should be used to prevent skin cuts.

Management. Direct pressure is applied to sites of bleeding from venipuncture, wound incisions, and sites of catheters. Pressure must be applied for a longer period of time than in those patients who do not have platelet or coagulation abnormalities. Cold compresses may assist in causing vasoconstriction. Hemostatic bioabsorbable dressings may be applied directly at bleeding sites. Table 14-12 lists

TABLE 14-12

Hemostatic Agents

Classification	Mechanism	Agent
Mechanical Hemostatic Agent	• Integrates an absorbable sponge, foam, pad or other material with topical hemostatic agent. • Forms a matrix at site of bleeding activating extrinsic clotting pathway	• Porcine gelatin (Gelfoam®, Gelfoam Plus®, Surgifoam®) • Cellulose (Surgicel®, Surgicel Nu-Knit®) • Bovine collagen (Avitene® sheets, Ultrafoam™ collagen sponges) • Polysaccharide spheres (Arista®)
Active Hemostatic Agent	• Topical thrombins stimulating fibrin clot formation at bleeding site	• Bovine thrombin (Thrombin-JMI®) • Recombinant thrombin (Recothrom®) • Pooled human plasma thrombin (Evithrom®)

Source: Data from Schreiber[72]; Achneck et al[73].

commonly used topical hemostatic agents.[72,73] Gelatin foams and oxidized cellulose control bleeding by providing a physical matrix for clotting initiation. Topical thrombins convert fibrinogen to fibrin to form clots. Thrombin cleaves fibrinogen to fibrin in fibrin sealants, forming a clot. Aminocaproic acid is a medication used to control acute mucocutaneous bleeds that can be given orally, topically, or intravenously (50–70 mg/kg) every 4–6 hours.[74]

Eyes

Ocular complications occur in approximately 50% of all leukemias,[75] resulting from metastases, hypercoagulopathies, and microvascular ischemias.[76] Thrombocytopenia and severe anemia are critical factors in the mechanism of intraorbital hemorrhage. Other factors affecting intraocular infarction and hemorrhage include hyperviscosity due to high blast cell counts and disease duration.[76] Bleeding in the optic fundus can result in permanent vision damage (Figure 14-1).

Prevention. For the individual with significant thrombocytopenia or altered coagulation status, transfusion of blood products may prevent or minimize the bleeding. Avoiding increased intracranial pressures also reduces the risk of bleeding.

Management. For intraocular hemorrhage, transfusion of blood products assists in controlling the bleeding. Scleral bleeding is made worse by rubbing the eyes. The eyes will feel dry and burning. Artificial tears or eye drops to moisten the eye frequently help relieve the burning and itching. If the eyes are irritated, patients should be taught to not wear contact lenses until symptoms resolve.

Nose and Mouth

Chemotherapy, radiation therapy, cancer, and oral infection all put individuals at risk for mucous membrane bleeding (Figure 14-2).

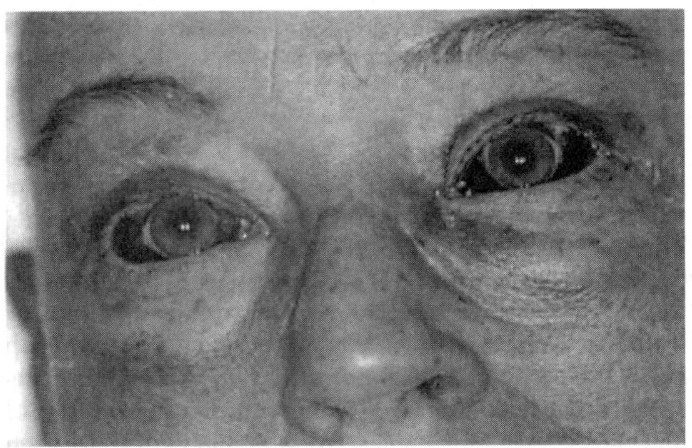

FIGURE 14-1

Scleral bleeding due to thrombocytopenia.

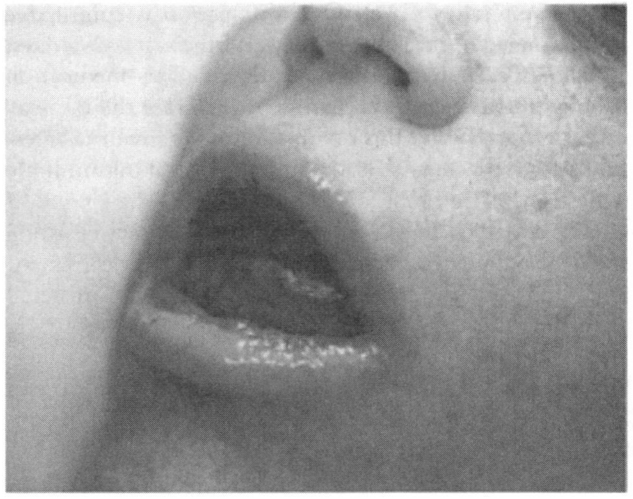

FIGURE 14-2

Drug-induced purpuric hemorrhage of lips and tongue.

Prevention. Good oral hygiene is important to ensure health and integrity of the oral mucosa. Evidence-based strategies for oral care include use of a soft toothbrush, brushing for at least 90 seconds at least twice daily, and rinsing the mouth with a bland, alcohol-free, nonirritating mouth rinse (saline, sodium bicarbonate, or saline and sodium bicarbonate mixture).[77,78] Maintaining adequate hydration and use of water-based lip moisturizers are also recommended. Dentures or dental prostheses that do not fit well should not be used when the oral membranes are irritated or while the high risk for bleeding remains. Forcefully blowing and picking one's nose should be avoided to prevent epistaxis.

Management. For epistaxis, the individual is put in high Fowler's position, with direct pressure on the nare that is bleeding. Cold compresses may help in vasoconstriction and stopping the hemorrhage. If the bleeding has not stopped with pressure in 10–15 minutes, topical thrombin may be applied to the nare to initiate hemostasis.[79,80] Nasal passages may need to be packed to stop the hemorrhage. Care must be taken not to dislodge the clot until hemostasis returns. The vessel can also be cauterized with a laser. Mechanical pressure can also be directly applied by inflating balloon catheters (balloon Foley).[81]

Bleeding oral lesions need to be kept clean; therefore meticulous and frequent mouth care is important. Diminishing infection of oral lesions decreases damage to the mucosa, allowing for more rapid healing of the ulcerations. Gentle suction may be necessary to clear out thick bloody secretions, while rinsing with cool saline helps vasoconstriction. Topical thrombin may be applied to oral lesions to help control excessive bleeding episodes. In severe bleeding from mucositis, intubation may be necessary to keep the airway open from clot formation.

Pulmonary

Management. Intrapleural bleeding may be drained to eliminate the fluid if it is causing symptoms of dyspnea. Frequent thoracentesis to relieve reaccumulation of fluid may be needed. Sclerosis may be necessary if the effusion and bleeding return too rapidly. Malignant pleural effusions are frequently managed by treating the disease with chemotherapy.

Hemoptysis related to pulmonary bleeding is usually scant and will stop spontaneously within a short period of time. Codeine or hydrocodone for cough suppression might help, as coughing is an aggravating factor for increased bleeding. For the treatment of substantial hemoptysis, the individual needs to be kept calm and on bed rest. Antianxiety medications and cough suppressants may be used. Unnecessary procedures should be eliminated. The person is placed on his or her side, with the side of hemorrhage dependent, so as not to cause asphyxiation by draining the blood in to the other lung. Suctioning and intubation are imperative to control severe hemorrhage. Arterial embolization is an effective strategy to manage hemorrhage.[82]

Alveolar hemorrhage is much more diffuse and more difficult to treat. Bleeding occurs in the alveoli, diminishing or preventing gas exchange between the alveoli and the surrounding capillaries. Respiratory support with oxygen is required. Glucocorticoids are used to control acute bleeding, but this treatment is not a long-term therapy of choice. Acute respiratory failure is associated with severe alveolar hemorrhage. Diffuse alveolar hemorrhage (DAH) occurs in approximately 5% of stem cell transplant patients and has a reported mortality rate ranging from 50% to 100%.[83] For the dying patient, oxygen and pain medications are appropriate; antianxiety medications may also be given, as anxiety increases as dyspnea becomes more acute. Placing the individual in the high Fowler's position often decreases dyspnea. Assistance is necessary due to fatigue.

Cardiovascular

Management. Severe bleeding into the pericardium can occur in patients who are thrombocytopenic or have other coagulation alterations. Due to the risk of cardiac surgery, a cardiac window is not suggested unless the pericardial hemorrhage is risking tamponade. An aspiration may be attempted but is a risky procedure. A "window" procedure may be necessary to relieve pressure and allow the heart to regain its normal functioning capacity. Heart rate, blood pressure, pulsus paradoxus, and peripheral pulses are closely monitored.

Gastrointestinal

Prevention. Antiemetics will decrease the potential for tearing of mucosa and esophagitis from vomiting. Individuals who have poor oral intake or are on corticosteroids are put on H_2 blockers or proton pump inhibitors to decrease the acid secretion in the stomach, thereby reducing the risk for upper GI bleeding. Indwelling catheters and tubes should be eliminated unless absolutely necessary. Rectal manipulation, such as digital examination and use of rectal thermometers, medications, and tubes, should be avoided in the thrombocytopenic individual. Stool softeners may be used so straining and constipation are avoided. Proper diet and exercise will also help prevent constipation.[84]

Management. Antiemetics are important to keep the gastric juices from irritating the esophagus and to prevent stress in the mucosa. Individuals with hiatal hernias and reflux esophagitis can develop significant bleeding with ulceration. This condition is especially prevalent with corticosteroid therapy or with prolonged vomiting. Antacid treatment, H_2 blockers, and dietary management usually provide sufficient control.[48]

Bleeding from esophageal varices is usually acute and massive. Vasoactive medications such as vasopressin, somatostatin, terlipressin, vapreotide, and octeotride are standard therapies used in the management of acute variceal bleeding.[85,86] Blood component therapy and fluids are administered to keep pressure stable. If bleeding continues, the varices may be repaired with endoscopic sclerosis or by balloon tamponade.[49,85]

For a Mallory-Weiss tear—a mucosal laceration at the junction of the esophagus and stomach resulting from severe retching, coughing, or vomiting—continued use of antiemetics and H_2 blockers is appropriate.[87] If bleeding is significant, gastric decompression may be necessary, as blood in the stomach can cause nausea and vomiting. Intra-arterial vasopressin may control excessive bleeding from a Mallory-Weiss tear or from a gastric ulcer.

Gastric and duodenal ulcers are initially treated with antacids, H_2 blockers, antibiotics, or coating agents such as sucralfate. A peptic ulcer causing an arteriole bleed may be stopped by endoscopic coagulation using a laser, heater probe, or electrocautery.[49] In cases of severe hemorrhage, with large ulcers unresponsive to endoscopic coagulation or bleeding tumors, surgical resection may be necessary.

Genitourinary

Prevention. Cyclophosphamide and ifosfamide are frequent causative agents of hemorrhagic cystitis. On the days of treatment, hyper-hydration, frequent (every 1–2 hours) voids, and administration of a uroprotective agent (Mesna) will reduce the risk of chemotherapy-induced hemorrhagic cystitis.[88] For high-dose cyclophosphamide or ifosfamide infusion, continuous bladder irrigation to force diuresis is used to decrease the exposure of the bladder lining to the irritant.[88]

Management. The causative agent must be determined for hemorrhagic cystitis, whether it be infection, therapy such as cyclophosphamide, or radiation therapy. If infection is the cause, antibiotics should be started. Viral infections, which are the infections most frequently seen in immunosuppressed individuals, may be more difficult to treat, as viruses do not always respond well to antiviral medications. Cytomegalovirus (CMV) infections are treated with gancyclovir or foscarnet.[89]

In chemotherapy-induced hemorrhagic cystitis, the chemotherapy should be discontinued if bleeding is severe. It is not uncommon for the urine to become heme- positive during the infusion or shortly after the infusion of chemotherapy. Increased hydration and frequent voiding, with or without diuretics, may be needed. Bleeding may become more severe later in the course for those individuals whose thrombocytopenia is severe and prolonged from the chemotherapy. Hydration and frequent voids will help clear blood and clots from the bladder. Phenazopyridine hydrochloride may decrease pain and burning, and oxybutynine chloride can help relieve spasms of the urethra and bladder.[90] Measurement of blood in the urine by urinalysis or 24-hour urine may be necessary. Platelets are transfused, if needed, and counts monitored until full recovery is seen.

Significant blood loss can occur due to hemorrhagic cystitis. A number of agents may be used to stop the hemorrhage. Continuous bladder irrigation with saline or alum may be implemented. Bed rest is recommended at this time, as the catheter may cause more irritation due to trauma. If continuous irrigation does not stop the hemorrhage, the individual may be taken to surgery for sclerosing by formalin, silver nitrate, or prostaglandins. Pain management, hydration, and assessment for continued bleeding are important interventions postoperatively. If hemorrhage continues after multiple attempts to stop it, eventually a cystectomy is recommended.

Women may have their menses suppressed with pharmacologic agents when they are experiencing or anticipating severe and prolonged thrombocytopenia, as large volumes of blood may be lost vaginally.[91] Suppression is generally accomplished with progestational medications. Sanitary napkins—not tampons—should be used to absorb the blood. A close count of pads will help measure the blood loss. If hemorrhage is severe, high-dose progestational hormonal therapy is attempted when lower doses do not inhibit the bleeding. High-dose progestational hormonal therapy, along with platelet transfusions, is usually successful. The problem with this approach is that the lining of the uterus thickens greatly with the high dose of hormones, such that when the hormones are reduced, the lining will be sloughed, leading to further blood loss. Ideally, the platelet count will have become sufficient to control the hemorrhage when hormones are reduced. If the bleeding is life threatening and unresponsive to hormonal therapy, a hysterectomy may be necessary.

Musculoskeletal

Management. Coagulation factor deficits may be corrected by administering vitamin K, improving nutrition, and administering plasma or specific coagulation factors. Physical therapy and pain medications may be necessary if the hemorrhage into the joint is substantial. Figure 14-3 provides an algorithm related to management of bleeding.

Disseminated intravascular coagulation

Prevention. Prevention of DIC may be difficult, as it has many etiologies. Infections should be treated, especially in the neutropenic person. Infection (not tumor related) is the most common initiating factor for DIC. Treating infections promptly diminishes the risk of DIC. For DIC associated with APL, the advent of treatment with all-trans retinoic acid (ATRA) has profoundly affected the management

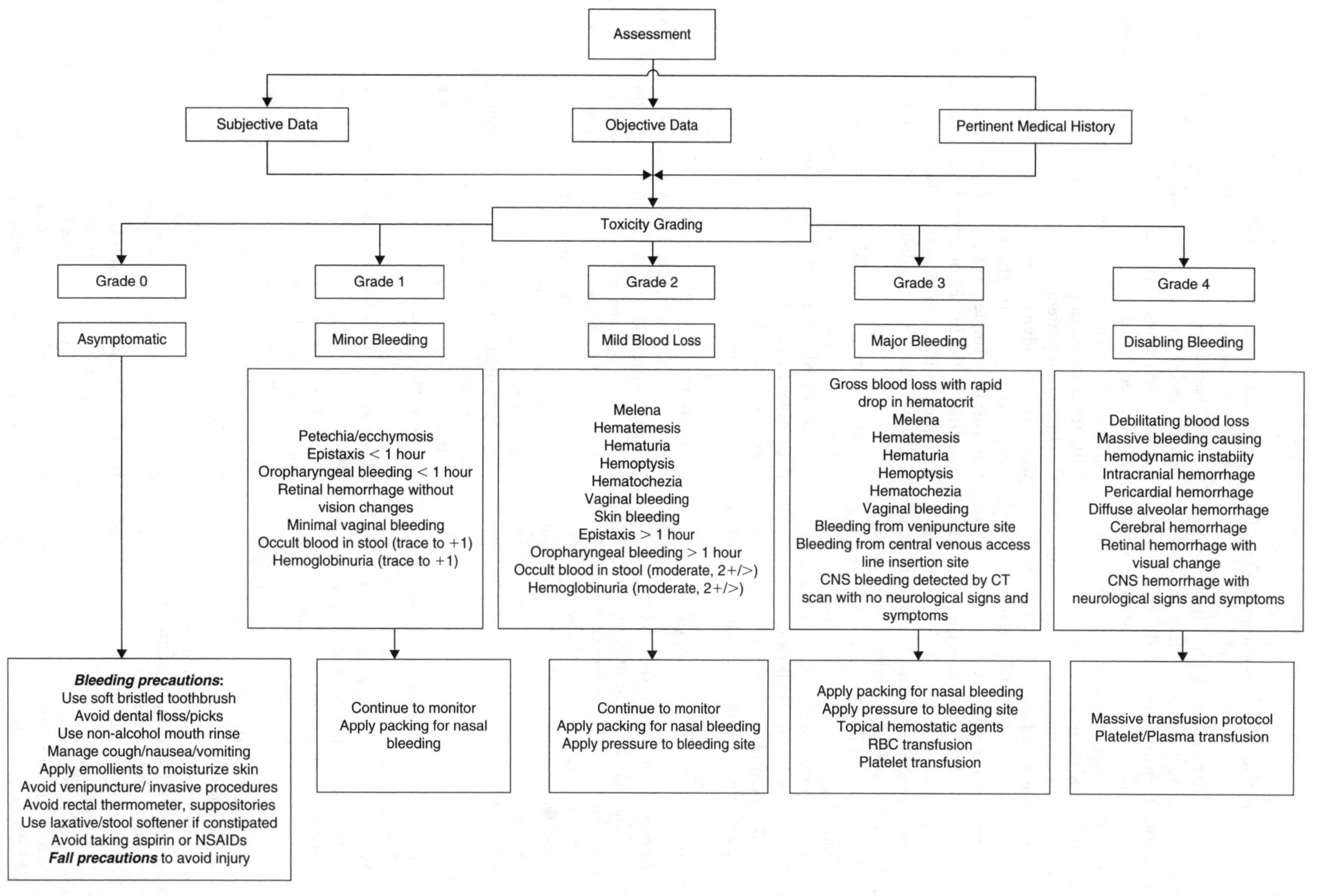

FIGURE 14-3

Management of bleeding.

Abbreviations: CNS: central nervous system; CT: computerized tomography; NSAIDs: nonsteroidal anti-inflammatory drugs; RBC: red blood cell.

of this potentially fatal coagulopathy. Indeed, the use of ATRA for remission induction of APL has produced high rates of complete remission with rapid resolution of DIC.[92]

Management. The initial treatment of DIC is to always treat the underlying cause, whether it is infection, malignancy, or another cause. Treatment is then directed at the particular bleeding or thrombotic manifestations. After treating the cause of DIC, supportive measures are similar: fluid replacement for hemodynamic support, blood support, and blood component support of vascular volume, and replenishment of coagulation factors and platelets that have been consumed. Prophylactic platelet transfusion is not considered for nonbleeding patients. In patients with DIC presenting with elevated prothrombin time and activated partial thromboplastin time, transfusion of fibrinogen-containing blood products (fresh frozen plasma, cryoprecipitate) is useful but should be implemented with caution, as fibrinogen will increase the bleeding and thrombotic complications.[93] The role of heparin in the treatment of DIC has not been established in randomized controlled clinical trials.[93] VTE prophylaxis using unfractionated heparin and low-molecular-weight heparin in critically ill patients without bleeding is recommended.[93]

Transfusion therapy

Transfusing blood components replenishes deficiencies in the individual who either has bleeding or is at significant risk for bleeding. Comprehensive and evidence-based platelet transfusion practice guidelines are available[64,94]; these guidelines are summarized in Table 14-13. Common blood components, a description of each component, and the indications are found in Table 14-14.[58]

Blood components

Whole Blood. The use of whole blood has decreased with the fractionation of the unit of whole blood into its different components. Whole blood is rarely used in the individual with cancer unless a massive bleed occurs, requiring both volume and red cell replenishment.

Red Blood Cells. The decision to replace red blood cells (RBCs) is made according to the physiologic effects of anemia. Anemia in the patient with cancer may be due to decreased bone marrow production of red blood cells or to active bleeding. Signs and symptoms of anemia include tachypnea, tachycardia, pallor, weakness, angina or palpitations, and shortness of breath with exertion. Packed red blood cells are administered for relief of symptoms. A more restrictive guideline using hemoglobin level less than 7–8 g/dL as a transfusion trigger was recently recommended by the AABB (formerly the American Association of Blood Banks).[95] The use of hemoglobin levels alone as a transfusion trigger should be avoided; instead, transfusion should be based on the individual patient's symptoms.[95] In the absence of active bleeding, the transfusion of 1 unit of packed red blood cells should increase the hematocrit by 3% and the hemoglobin by 1 g/dL.[48,96]

The Eastern Association for the Surgery of Trauma (EAST) and the Society of Critical Care Medicine (SCCM) have also developed evidence-based clinical practice guidelines for red blood cell transfusion for adult trauma and critically ill patients.[97] These recommendations include RBC transfusion for patients with evidence of hemorrhagic shock, and for patients with evidence of acute hemorrhage who are hemodynamically unstable or with inadequate oxygen delivery.[97] In the absence of acute hemorrhage, transfusion of single units of RBCs is recommended. RBC transfusion should be considered for hospitalized patients with preexisting cardiovascular disease who are symptomatic or who have a hemoglobin level of 8 g/dL or less.[95]

Platelets. Platelets are used in the prophylaxis and treatment of bleeding. Transfusion is recommended for the individual with decreased platelet production, consumption of platelets due to bleeding, and platelet dysfunction. Platelets must be stored and transfused properly for the person to acquire the appropriate transfusion increment; mishandled platelets may cause transfusion failure. Platelets should be stored at room temperature with gentle agitation; their shelf life is 5 days.

If infection or a rapidly decreasing platelet count is present, the individual should be closely monitored for bleeding. The life span of a platelet is approximately 7–10 days once released from the bone marrow. Generally, if an individual is not producing any platelets and is not bleeding, the transfusion requirement should be approximately one platelet pack every 3 days. Clinicians evaluate response to platelet transfusions by assessing increment (post-transfusion minus pre-transfusion platelet count) or percentage platelet recovery (post-transfusion increment/number of platelets transfused) corrected for blood volume.[65]

Plasma. The transfusion of plasma or specific coagulation factors found in the plasma is typically used as treatment for coagulation disorders. The amount and frequency of the transfusions depend on the severity of the deficiency, the specific factor deficiency, the risk of bleeding, and the duration of the therapy. Treatment with vitamin K can also be used if there is no active bleeding and the coagulopathy is amenable to vitamin K replacement.

Complications of Transfusion Therapy

Blood component therapy is not without risk. A variety of complications can occur due to transfusions, although many of the infectious risks (i.e., transmission of known viruses such as HIV and hepatitis C) have been eliminated due to highly sensitive methods of screening for presence of these viruses in the donated product.[97,98] The most serious complications are generally immune mediated, such

TABLE 14-13

Evidence-Based Platelet Transfusion Guidelines	
Platelet Product	Pooled random donor platelet concentrates and single donor apheresis platelets have similar qualities and can be used interchangeably. Both products are equally efficacious in post-transfusion increments, hemostatic benefit. Side-effects are similar. Both products maintain platelet viability stored up to 5 days after collection.
Platelet Processing	Leukoreduction of platelets indicated for AML patients. Clinical significance of leukoreduction: 1. Reduces platelet alloimmunization rates 2. Prevents CMV transmission by transfusion 3. Reduces febrile non-hemolytic transfusion reactions γ-Irradiation of platelets prevent transfusion related GVHD are indicated for: 1. Patients receiving allogeneic stem cell transplant 2. Patients receiving blood products from related donors 3. Patients who are severely immunocompromised (patients with Hodgkin's disease or other lymphomas) Volume reduction of platelets should only be considered when really necessary since centrifugation can damage platelets.
Prophylactic and Therapeutic Platelet Transfusion	A prophylactic platelet trigger = 10,000 platelets/μl is recommended for chronically thrombocytopenic patients. • AML – 10,000 platelets/μl • HSCT – similar to AML • Patients with chronic, stable thrombocytopenia can be observed without prophylactic transfusion[4] • Solid tumors – 20,000 platelets/μl Therapeutic platelet transfusion triggers for patients undergoing surgical procedure: • Neurosurgery – 100,000 platelets/μl • Other invasive procedures – between 50,000 – 100,000 platelets/μL • Trauma – between 50,000 – 100,000 platelets/μL
Platelet Alloimmunization	ABO-compatible platelets are recommended to achieve best post-transfusion platelet increment and to reduce alloimmune platelet refractoriness. Alloimmunized patients should be transfused only for hemorrhagic events if no available matched platelets.
Platelet Refractoriness	Obtain platelet post-transfusion count after all transfusions. Diagnosis of platelet refractoriness only after at least two ABO-compatible transfusions resulted in poor increments. Transfuse HLA-matched platelets/crossmatched platelets for refractory patients. Anecdotal data supports the following measures for persistently refractory patients: 1. Administer platelets frequently in smaller doses (3–4 platelet concentrates every 4–8 hours) 2. IVIG 3. Fibrinolytic inhibitors 4. Recombinant factor VIIa

Abbreviations: AML: acute myelogenous leukemia; CMV: cytomegalovirus; GVHD: graft versus host disease; HLA: human leukocyte antigen; HSCT: hematopoietic stem cell transplantation; IVIG: intravenous immunoglobulin.

Source: Data from Park et al[4]; Schiffer et al[64]; NCCN[69]; Slichter[94].

as acute or delayed hemolytic reactions as well as febrile nonhemolytic and allergic reactions. Other non-immune complications include metabolic disturbances, circulatory overload, and hypothermia.[97] Even though viral transmission via this means has been largely eliminated, transfusion therapy can still lead to bacterial sepsis. Bacterial contaminants in transfused blood are rare but may occur, causing sepsis and shock. Delayed complications may include alloimmunization, iron overload, and rarer complications such as transfusion-associated graft-versus-host disease (TA-GVHD) and transfusion-related acute lung injury (TRALI).[97–100] Febrile nonhemolytic and allergic reactions are the most common complications of blood component therapy. Complications and treatment of transfusion therapy reactions are summarized in Table 14-15.

TABLE 14-14

Commonly Transfused Blood Products for the Bleeding Individual

Blood Component	Indication	Nursing Considerations
	Whole blood	
Entire contents of blood	• Massive blood loss for which volume is needed along with red cell replacement—very few indications, rarely used	• Assess for fluid overload • Monitor for transfusion reactions
	Packed red blood cells (PRBCs)	
Red blood cells with most of plasma and platelets removed, 70% of hematocrit of whole blood	• Anemia • Bleeding • Replacement of red blood cells without the volume	• Transfuse over 2–4 hours • Assess for fluid overload • Monitor for transfusion reactions
	Fresh frozen plasma (FFP)	
Prepared from whole blood or collected by apheresis. Contains clotting factors, albumin, immunoglobulins	• Bleeding • Coagulation deficiencies • Volume expander	• Transfuse as rapidly as tolerated (usually less than 30 minutes) • Must not be refrozen once thawed • Must be ABO-compatible with recipient • Monitor for transfusion-related allergic reactions
	Cryoprecipitate	
10–20 mL fibrinogen, factors VIII, XIII, VonWillebrand factor	• Severe VonWillebrand disease • Hypofibrinogenemia	• Transfuse rapidly less than 30 minutes
	Random donor platelets (RDPs)	
Platelets taken from 4 + units of whole blood, approximately 200 mL	• Prophylaxis and treatment of bleeding in patients with thrombocytopenia	• Transfuse rapidly to prevent clot formation (usually 20–30 minutes) • ABO compatibility not required but preferred to give good yield • Obtain platelet count 1 hour post-transfusion • Monitor for transfusion reactions
	Single-donor platelets (SDPs)	
Platelets obtained from one donor by apheresis, approximately 200–300 mL	• Prophylaxis and treatment of bleeding in patients with thrombocytopenia	• Transfuse as for RDP
	HLA-matched platelets	
Platelets obtained by apheresis from one donor, HLA matched, approximately 300 mL	• Alloimmunized patients • Refractory to RDP and SDP alloimmunization	• Transfuse as for other platelets • Wait 2 hours to infuse amphotericin B • Consider leukodepletion to reduce: – Risk of immunization against leucocyte antigens – Refractoriness – Febrile non-hemolytic reactions • Consider irradiation to inactivate lymphocytes to prevent severe graft versus host disease (GVHD) in stem cell transplant patients

Source: Data from Friend and Pruett[48]; Liumbruno et al[58].

TABLE 14-15

Blood Transfusion Reactions

Transfusion Reaction	Mechanism	Physical Findings	Management
		Hemolytic	
Onset is usually within 15 minutes	• Ab-Ag reaction to major blood incompatibility, causing intravascular hemolysis • Ab-Ag complex activates classical complement pathway, lysing RBCs within the vasculature	• Fever, temp rise >1°C • Chills/rigors • Chest pain/back pain • Hypotension • Nausea • Flushing • Dyspnea • Diffuse bleeding • Anemia • Oliguria • Hemoglobinuria	• Stop transfusion • Notify MD • Monitor VS • Maintain BP with fluids if necessary • Obtain and send blood and urine samples • Follow transfusion reaction protocol of institution • Return product to blood center • Document occurrence
		Delayed hemolytic	
Onset occurs between 7 days to weeks after transfusion	• Ab-Ag reaction to minor RBC antigens • Extravascular hemolysis (RE system)	• Decreasing Hgb without bleeding • Low-grade fevers	• Obtain blood samples to assess for antibody against minor RBC antigens • Transfuse as needed
		Febrile nonhemolytic	
Onset is immediate to 6 hours post-transfusion (prevalent in those exposed to multiple WBCs and platelet antigens)	• Ab directed against WBC or platelet antigens previously exposed to (may be HLA specific, WBC specific, or platelet specific)	• Fever, temp rise > 1°C • Rigors • Nausea • Pallor • Flushing	• Stop transfusion • Notify MD • Follow blood transfusion reaction protocol of institution • Send unit back to blood center • Document occurrence
Allergic		**Mild:**	**Mild:**
Onset immediate to 1 hour post-transfusion (the more severe the reaction, the more immediate)	• Ab reaction to plasma proteins in the blood product	• Hives • Pruritus	• Slow transfusion • Administer antihistamines or corticosteroids • Complete transfusion
		Anaphylactic:	**Anaphylactic:**
		• Flushing • Dyspnea • Wheezing • Hypotension • Shock	• Stop transfusion • Notify MD • Administer fluids, respiratory support as required • Epinephrine may be required • Monitor VS • Follow transfusion reaction protocol of institution • Obtain and send blood and urine samples • Send unit back to blood center • Document occurrence

Abbreviations: Ab: antibody; Ag: antigen; BP: blood pressure; Hgb: hemoglobin; HLA: human leukocyte antigen; RBC: red blood cell; RE: reticuloendothelial; VS: vital signs; WBC: white blood cell.

Source: Data from Friend and Pruett[48].

Many of the immune-mediated reactions are due to the presence of leukocytes in the blood product. Many blood centers routinely perform procedures that remove leukocytes from the blood product. This depletion is achieved by passing the product through a filter. Leukodepletion can prevent or avoid the febrile reactions as well as minimize viral transmission of CMV and HIV. Red blood cells and platelets can also be washed, which depletes the plasma. Patients who are hypersensitive to plasma proteins as indicated by allergic reactions of hives or pruritus should receive washed cells.

TA-GVHD is a rare but often fatal complication of transfusion, with mortality approaching 90% with a full-blown syndrome.[101] It can occur in a severely immunocompromised individual and is caused by the immunocompetent T lymphocytes in the transfused product, which attack the body tissues of the immunosuppressed host after transfusion. The population at risk for this complication usually includes stem cell transplant patients and individuals with leukemia. Irradiating the blood product with 25 Gy makes the lymphocyte incapable of proliferating.[101] TRALI is another rare but serious complication that presents as noncardiogenic pulmonary edema.[97]

Pharmacologic interventions

Agents that enhance intrinsic hemostatic functions include corticosteroids, estrogens, desmopressin, aprotinin, tranexamic acid, and epsilon-aminocaproic acid (EACA). EACA is an antifibrinolytic agent used in controlling bleeding in non-oncology settings (i.e., surgery). A review by Kalmandi et al of 77 patient records demonstrated the efficacy of EACA in the treatment of thrombocytopenic hemorrhage, with reduced transfusion requirements for patients within 24 hours of initiation and improved hemostasis (overall response rate of 83%).[102] Tranexamic acid (TA) is another antifibrinolytic agent that is 10 times more potent than EACA; although it is used to manage bleeding, studies on its efficacy remain limited.[80]

Thrombopoietic growth factors such as recombinant human thrombopoietin (rhTPO) and pegylated recombinant human megakaryocyte growth development factor (PEG-rHuMGDF) showed preliminary success in the treatment of thrombocytopenia, but unfavorable side effects and subsequent refractory thrombocytopenia halted further investigation of these agents.[103,104] Newer thrombopoietic growth factors—AMG531 and eltrombopag—have demonstrated efficacy and safety in the treatment of immune thrombocytopenia purpura and hepatitis C virus–induced thrombocytopenia, but their clinical application in chemotherapy-induced thrombocytopenia has not been established.[103]

NURSING IMPLICATIONS

Nurses can significantly impact patient outcomes in a variety of areas.[104] Nursing-sensitive patient outcomes (NSPO) specific to cancer care include quality of life, symptom management, functional performance, social and psychological issues, patient satisfaction with care, and safety.[106] Cancer affects the patient's quality of life at all stages of the disease course, from initial diagnosis through survivorship. Disease- and treatment-related complications such as bleeding and thrombotic complications impose a significant burden on patients and families, and can be physically and psychologically distressing. Nursing-specific interventions for favorable NSPO include bleeding symptom control and management. Nurses caring for patients need to monitor for early signs and symptoms to ensure prompt diagnosis and treatment. Nursing interventions to ensure functional status and safety include modification in activities of daily living to create activities the patient can tolerate and carry out, taking into consideration any physical limitations related to bleeding and fall prevention measures. Patient and family education teaching should include these preventive measures to ensure patient safety outside the clinical setting. Prompt management and treatment of bleeding episodes can significantly reduce the psychosocial distress of the patient who is alarmed at the sight of bleeding.

PATIENT SELF-CARE

The importance of teaching patients self-care strategies cannot be overemphasized, especially when the risk of bleeding is a possibility. Individuals are frequently instructed to have their blood counts checked between treatments to determine their nadir counts and make any needed dose adjustments. It is not uncommon for patients to monitor and record their blood counts over time to see how their counts change. This involvement should be encouraged, as it promotes the ideal of self-care as patients and their families begin to understand how blood counts can change with treatment and how risk for bleeding can be determined. Appendix 14A is a self-care guide that is useful for teaching patients how to determine if they are bleeding and what to do about it.

REFERENCES

1. Rodriguez AL, Gobel BH. Bleeding. In: Yarbro CH, Wujcik D, Gobel BH, eds. *Cancer Nursing: Principles and Practice.* 7th ed. Burlington, MA: Jones & Bartlett Learning; 2011:745–771.
2. Aster RH, Bougie DW. Drug-induced thrombocytopenia. *N Engl J Med.* 2007;357(6):580–586.
3. Gaydos LA, Freireich EJ, Mantel N. The quantitative relation between platelet count and hemorrhage in patients with acute leukemia. *N Engl J Med.* 1962;266:905–909.

4. Park JH, Qiao B, Panageas KS, et al. Early death rate in acute promyelocytic leukemia remains high despite *all-trans* retinoic acid. *Blood.* 2011;118:1248–1254.
5. Holler E, Kolb HJ, Greinix H, et al. Bleeding events and mortality in SCT patients: a retrospective study of hematopoietic SCT patients with organ dysfunctions due to severe sepsis or GVHD. *Bone Marrow Transplant.* 2009;43:491–497.
6. Webert KT, Cook RJ, Sigouin CS, et al. The risk of bleeding in thrombocytopenic patients with acute myeloid leukemia. *Haematologica.* 2006; 91:1530–1537.
7. Kwaan HC, Huyck T. Thromboembolic and bleeding complications in acute leukemia. *Expert Rev Hematol.* 2010;3:719–730.
8. Nevo S, Fuller A, Hartley E, et al. Acute bleeding complications in platelets after hematopoietic stem cell transplantation with prophylactic platelet transfusion triggers of 10×10^9 and 20×10^9 per L. *Transfusion.* 2007;47:801–812.
9. Belt RJ, Leite C, Haas CD, et al. Incidence of hemorrhagic complications in patients with cancer. *JAMA.* 1978;239:2571–2574.
10. Dutcher, JP, Schiffer CA, Aisner J, et al. Incidence of thrombocytopenia and serious hemorrhage among patients with solid tumors. *Cancer.* 1984;53:557–562.
11. Etling LS, Rubenstein EB, Martin CG, et al. Incidence, cost, and outcomes of bleeding and chemotherapy dose modification among solid tumor patients with chemotherapy-induced thrombocytopenia. *J Clin Oncol.* 2001;19:1137–1146.
12. Elting LS, Martin CG, Kurtin DJ, et al. The Bleeding Risk Index: a clinical prediction rule to guide the prophylactic use of platelet transfusions in patients with lymphoma or solid tumors. *Cancer.* 2002;94:3252–3262.
13. Hitron A, Steinke D, Sutphin S, et al. Incidence and risk factors of clinically significant chemotherapy-induced thrombocytopenia in patients with solid tumors. *J Oncol Pharm Pract.* 2011;17:312–319.
14. Haddad TC, Greeno EW. Chemotherapy-induced thrombosis. *Thromb Res.* 2006;118:555–568.
15. Shelke AR, Khorana AA. Cancer-associated thrombosis: an update. *Drug Discovery Today: Disease Mechanisms.* 2011;8(1–2):e39–e45.
16. Lyman GH, Khorana AA. Cancer, clots and consensus: new understanding of an old problem. *J Clin Oncol.* 2009;27:4821–4826.
17. Robert F. The potential benefits of low-molecular-weight heparins in cancer patients. *J Hematol Oncol.* 2010;3:1–2.
18. Hunault-Berger M, Chevallier P, Delain M, et al., for the GOELAMS (Groupe Ouest-Est des Leucémies Aiguës et Maladies du Sang). Changes in antithrombin and fibrinogen levels during induction chemotherapy with L-asparaginase in adult patients with acute lymphoblastic leukemia or lymphoblastic lymphoma. Use of supportive coagulation therapy and clinical outcome: the CAPELAL study. *Haematologica.* 2008;93:1488–1494.
19. Blake-Haskins JA, Lechleider RJ, Kreitman RJ. Thrombotic microangiopathy with targeted cancer agents. *Clin Cancer Res.* 2011;17:5858–5866.
20. Moake, J. Thrombotic thrombocytopenia purpura (TTP) and other thrombotic microangiopathies. *Best Pract Res Clin Haematol.* 2009;22:567–576.
21. Goz M, Eren MN, Cakir O. Arterial thrombosis and thalidomide. *J Thrombosis Thrombolysis.* 2008;25:224–226.
22. Semeraro N, Ammollo CT, Semeraro F, et al. Sepsis, thrombosis, and organ dysfunction. *Thrombosis Res.* 2011;129:290–295.
23. Hardaway RM, Williams CH, Vasquez Y. Disseminated intravascular coagulation in sepsis. *Semin Thromb Hemost.* 2011;27:577–583.
24. Levy M, Seligsohn U. Disseminated intravascular coagulation. In: Kaushansky K, Lichtman MA, Beutler E, et al., eds. *Williams Hematology.* 8th ed. New York: McGraw-Hill Medical; 2011:2101–2120.
25. Qui L, He J, Ye X, et al. Invasive pulmonary fungal infection accompanied by severe hemoptysis in patients with hematologic diseases: a report of nine cases. *Int J Hematol.* 2009;90(1):108–112.
26. Aster RH, Bougie DW. Drug-induced immune thrombocytopenia. *N Engl J Med.* 2007;357:580–587.
27. George JN, Aster RH. Drug-induced thrombocytopenia: pathogenesis, evaluation, and management. *Hematology.* 2009;153–158.
28. Mitchell RN. Hemodynamic disorders, thromboembolic disease, and shock. In: Kumar V, Abbas AK, Fausto N, Aster JC, eds. *Robbins and Cotran Pathologic Basis of Disease.* 8th ed. Philadelphia: Saunders Elsevier; 2010:111–134.
29. Seligsohn U, Kaushanky K. Classification, clinical manifestations, and evaluation of disorders in hemostasis In: Kaushansky K, Lichtman MA, Beutler E, et al, eds. *Williams Hematology.* 8th ed. New York: McGraw-Hill Medical; 2011:1883–1889.
30. Abrams CS, Shattil SJ, Bennett JS. Acquired qualitative platelet disorders. In: Kaushansky K, Lichtman MA, Beutler E, et al, eds. *Williams Hematology.* 8th ed. New York: McGraw-Hill Medical; 2011:1971–1983.
31. Galbusera M, Remuzzi G, Boccardo P. Treatment of bleeding in dialysis patients. *Semin Dialysis.* 2009;22:279–286.
32. Lippi G, Franchini M. Pathogenesis of venous thromboembolism: when the cup runneth over. *Semin Thromb Hemost.* 2012;34:747–761.
33. Wolberg AS, Aleman MM, Leiderman K, et al. Procoagulant activity in hemostasis and thrombosis: Virchow's triad revisited. *Anesthesia Analgesia.* 2012;114:275–285.
34. Falanga A, Marchetti M. Venous thromboembolism in the hematologic malignancies. *J Clin Oncol.* 2009;27:4848–4857.
35. Gillespie TW. Nursing interventions in the management of patients with cancer-associated thrombosis. *Semin Oncol Nurs.* 2005;21:50–59.
36. Noble S, Pasi J. Epidemiology and pathophysiology of cancer associated thrombosis. *Brit J Cancer.* 2010;102:S2–S9.
37. Zangari M. Thrombotic events in patients with cancer receiving antiangiogenesis agents. *J Clin Oncol.* 2009;27:4865–4873.
38. Rajkumar SV, Blood E, Vesole D, et al. Phase III clinical trial of thalidomide plus dexamethasone compared with dexamethasone alone in newly diagnosed multiple myeloma: a clinical trial coordinated by the Eastern Cooperative Oncology Group. *J Clin Oncol.* 2006;24:431–436.
39. Viale PH. Abnormal clotting in cancer: an overview of pathophysiology and etiology. *Semin Oncol Nurs.* 2005;21:12–20.
40. Saber W, Moua T, Williams EC, et al. Risk factors for catheter related thrombosis (CRT) in cancer patients: a patient-level data (IPD) meta-analysis of clinical trials and prospective studies. *J Thrombosis Haemostasis.* 2011 9:312–319.
41. Lopez JA, Chen J. Pathophysiology of venous thrombosis. *Thrombosis Res.* 2009;123(suppl 4):S30–S34.
42. Gobel BH. Disseminated intravascular coagulation. In: Yarbro CH, Wujcik D, Gobel BH, eds. *Cancer Nursing: Principles and Practice.* 7th ed. Burlington, MA: Jones & Bartlett Learning; 2011:928–938.
43. Sadler JE, Poncz M. Antibody-mediated thrombotic disorders: thrombotic thrombocytopenic purpura and heparin-induced thrombocytopenia. In: Kaushansky K, Lichtman MA, Beutler E, et al, eds. *Williams Hematology.* 8th ed. New York: McGraw-Hill Medical; 2011:2163–2184.
44. Zakarija A. Thrombotic and microangiopathy syndromes. *Cancer Treat Res.* 2009;148:115–136.
45. Fojo AT. Metabolic emergencies. In: DeVita VT, Lawrence TS, Rosenberg SA, eds. *DeVita, Hellman, and Rosenberg's Cancer Principles and Practices of Oncology.* 9th ed. Philadelphia, PA: Lippincott Williams & Wilkins; 2011:2142–2152.
46. Khorana AA, Kuderer NM, Culakova E, et al. Development and validation of a predictive model for chemotherapy-associated thrombosis. *Blood.* 2008;111:4902–4907.
47. Stanworth SJ, Dyer C, Casbard A, et al. Feasibility and usefulness of self-assessment of bleeding in patients with haematological malignancies, and the association between platelet count and bleeding. *Vox Sanguinies.* 2006;91:63–69.

48. Friend PH, Pruett J. Bleeding and thrombotic complications. In: Yarbro CH, Frogge MH, Goodman M, eds. *Cancer Symptom Management.* 3rd ed. Sudbury, MA: Jones and Bartlett; 2004:231–251.
49. Wilkins TH, Khan N, Nabh A, Schade RR. Diagnosis and management of upper gastrointestinal bleeding. *Am Fam Physician.* 2012;85:469–476.
50. Kamal AH, Tefferi A, Pruthi RK. How to interpret and pursue an abnormal prothrombin time, activated partial thromboplastin time and bleeding time in adults. *Mayo Clin Proc.* 2007;82:864–873.
51. Hayward CPM, Moffat KA, Raby A, et al. Development of North American consensus guidelines for medical laboratories that perform and interpret platelet function testing using light transmission aggregometry. *Am J Clin Pathol.* 2010;134:955–963.
52. Aster RH. Pooling platelets in the spleen: role in the pathogenesis of hypersplenic thrombocytopenia. *J Clin Investig.* 1966;5:645–657.
53. Rinder HM, Tomer A. Platelet production, kinetics, and hemostasis. In: Simon TL, Snyder EL, Solheim BG, et al., eds. *Rossi's Principles of Transfusion Medicine.* 4th ed. Bethesda, MD: Wiley-Blackwell; 2009:149–167.
54. DeLoughery T. Management of acquired bleeding problems in cancer patients. *Emerg Med Clin North Am.* 2009;27:423–444.
55. Cunningham RS. Therapeutic options for the treatment of cancer-associated thrombosis. *Semin Oncol Nurs.* 2005;21:21–40.
56. Neerman-Artez M, deMoerloose P. Hereditary fibrinogen abnormalities. In: Kaushansky K, Lichtman MA, Beutler E, et al, eds. *Williams Hematology.* 8th ed. New York: McGraw-Hill Medical; 2011:2051–2068.
57. Cartoni C, Niscola P, Breccia M, et al. Hemorrhagic complications in patients with advanced hematological malignancies followed at home: an Italian experience. *Leukemia Lymphoma.* 2009;50:387–391.
58. Liumbruno G, Bennardello F, Lattanzio A, et al. Italian Society of Transfusion Medicine and Immunohaematology (SIMTI) Work Group: recommendations for the transfusion of plasma and platelets. *Blood Transfus.* 2009;7:132–150.
59. Koreth R, Weinert C, Weisdorf DJ, et al. Measurement of bleeding severity: a critical review. *Transfusion.* 2004;44:605–617.
60. United States Department of Health and Human Services, National Institutes of Health, National Cancer Institute (NCI). *Common Terminology Criteria for Adverse Events (CTCAE).* Version 4.03. Bethesda, MD: NCI; 2010. evs.nci.nih.gov/ftp1/CTCAE/CTCAE_4.03_2010-06-14_QuickReference_8.5x11.pdf. Accessed April 28, 2012.
61. Lyman GH, Khorana AA, Falanga A, et al. American Society of Clinical Oncology guideline: recommendations for venous thromboembolism prophylaxis and treatment in patients with cancer. *J Clin Oncol.* 2007;25:5490–5505.
62. Wagman LD. Venous thromboembolic disease. NCCN. Clinical practice guidelines in oncology. *J Natl Compr Cancer Netw.* 2008;6(8):716–753.
63. Bhatia M, Davenport V, Cairo M. The role of interleukin-11 to prevent chemotherapy-induced thrombocytopenia in patients with solid tumors, lymphoma, acute myeloid leukemia and bone marrow failure syndromes. *Leukemia Lymphoma.* 2007;48(1):9–15.
64. Schiffer CA, Anderson KC, Bennett CL, et al. Platelet transfusion for patients with cancer: clinical practice guidelines of the American Society of Clinical Oncology. *J Clin Oncol.* 2001;19:1519–1538.
65. Slichter S. New thoughts on the correct dosing of prophylactic platelet transfusions to prevent bleeding. *Curr Opin Hematol.* 2011;18:427–435.
66. Heddle NM, Cook RJ, Tinmouth A, et al. A randomized controlled trial comparing standard- and low-dose strategies for transfusion of platelets (SToP) to patients with thrombocytopenia. *Blood.* 2009;113:1564–1573.
67. Slichter SJ, Kaufman RM, Assman SF, et al. Dose of prophylactic platelet transfusions and prevention of hemorrhage. *N Engl J Med.* 2010;362:600–613.
68. Robert F. The potential benefit of low-molecular weight heparins in cancer patients. *J Hematol Oncol.* 2010;3:1–12.
69. National Comprehensive Cancer Network (NCCN). NCCN clinical practice guidelines in oncology (NCCN guidelines): venous thromboembolic disease. Version 2.2011. http://www.nccn.org/professionals/physician_gls/pdf/vte.pdf. Accessed July 17, 2012.
70. Bergqvist D, Agnelli G, Cohen AT, et al. Duration of prophylaxis against venous thromboembolism with enoxaparin after surgery. *N Engl J Med.* 2002;346:975–980.
71. Rasmussen MS, Jorgensen LN, Wille-Jorgensen P, et al. Prolonged prophylaxis with dalteparin to prevent late thromboembolic complications in patients undergoing major abdominal surgery: a multicenter randomized open label study. *J Thrombosis Haemostasis.* 2006;4:2384–2390.
72. Schreiber MA. Achieving hemostasis with topical hemostats: making clinically and economically appropriate decisions in surgical and trauma settings. *AORN J.* 2011;94(5):S1–S20.
73. Achneck H, Siloshi B, Jamiolkowsi RM, et al. A comprehensive review of topical hemostatic agents: efficacy and recommendations for use. *Ann Surg.* 2010;251:217–228.
74. Rodriguez KD, Sun GH, Pike F, Mandel EM, Casselbrant ML, Chi DH. Post-tonsillectomy bleeding in children with von Willebrand disease: a single institution experience. *Otolaryngol Head Neck Surg.* 2010;142:715–721.
75. Hua LV, Williams SK. Sudden unilateral visual loss as an initial presentation of chronic myelogenous leukemia. *Clin Optometry.* 2010;2:29–35.
76. Lin P, Mrunthyunjaya P. Retinal manifestations of oncologic and hematologic conditions. *Int Ophthamol Clin.* 2012;52(1):67–91.
77. Harris DJ, Eilers J, Harriman A, et al. Putting evidence into practice: evidence-based interventions for the management of oral mucositis. *Clin J Oncol Nurs.* 2008;12(1):141–152.
78. Eilers J, Million R. Clinical update: prevention and management of oral mucositis in patients with cancer. *Semin Oncol Nurs.* 2011;27:e1–e16.
79. Cote D, Baber R, Diamond C, Wright E. Floseal hemostatic matrix in persistent epistaxis: prospective clinical trial. *J Otolaryngol Head Neck Surg.* 2010;39:304–308.
80. Damron BH, Brant JM, Belansky HB, et al. Putting evidence into practice: prevention and management of bleeding in patients with cancer. *Clin J Oncol Nurs.* 2009;13:573–583.
81. Pope LE, Hobbs CG. Epistaxis: an update on current management. *Postgrad Med J.* 2005;81:309–314.
82. Daliri A, Probst NH, Jobst B, et al. Bronchial artery embolization in patients with hemoptysis including follow-up. *Acta Radiologica.* 2011;52:143–147.
83. Lara AR, Schwarz MI. Diffuse alveolar hemorrhage. *Chest.* 2010;137:1164–1171.
84. Woolery M, Bisanz A, Lyons HF, et al. Putting evidence into practice: evidence based interventions for the prevention and management of constipation in patients with cancer. *Clin J Oncol Nurs.* 2008;12:317–337.
85. Wells M, Chande N, Beaton M, et al. Meta-analysis: vasoactive medications for the management of acute variceal bleeds. *Aliment Pharmacol Therapeut.* 2012;35:1267–1278.
86. Abid S, Jafri W, Hamid S, et al. Terlipressin vs. octeotride in bleeding esophageal varices as an adjuvant therapy with endoscopic band ligation: a randomized double-blind placebo-controlled trial. *Am J Gastroenterol.* 2009;104:617–623.
87. Yin A, Li Y, Jiang Y, et al. Mallory-Weiss syndrome: clinical and endoscopic characteristics. *Eur J Intern Med.* 2012;23:e92–e96.
88. Ribeiro RA, Lima-Junior RCP, Leite CA, et al. Chemotherapy induced hemorrhagic cystitis: pathogenesis, pharmacological approaches, and new insights. *J Experi Integr Med.* 2012;2:95–112.
89. Boeckh M. Complications, diagnosis, management, and prevention of CMV infections. *ASH Education Book.* 2011:305–309.

90. Smit SG, Heyns CF. Management of radiation cystitis. *Nat Rev Urol.* 2010;7:206–214.
91. Bates JS, Buie LW, Woodis CB. Management of menorrhagia associated with chemotherapy-induced thrombocytopenia in women with hematologic malignancy. *Pharmacotherapy.* 2011;31:1092–1110.
92. Falanga A, Rickles FR. Management of thromhemorrhagic syndromes (THS) in hematologic malignancies. *Hematology ASH Education Book.* 2007(1):165–171.
93. Levi M, Toh CH, Thachil J, et al. Guidelines for the diagnosis and management of disseminated intravascular coagulation. British Committee for Standards in Hematology. *Brit J Haematol.* 2009;145(1):24–33.
94. Slichter SJ. Evidence-based platelet transfusion guidelines. *Hematology ASH Education Book.* 2007:172–178.
95. Carson JL, Grossman BJ, Kleinman S, et al. Red blood cell transfusion: a clinical practice guideline for the AABB. *Ann Intern Med.* 2012. http://annals.org/article.aspx? doi: 10.7326/0003-4819-156-12-201206190-00429. Accessed July 19, 2012.
96. Dicato M, Plawny L, Diederich M. Anemia in cancer. *Ann Oncol.* 2010;21(suppl 7):vii167–vii172.
97. Napolitano LN, Kurek S, Luchette FA. Clinical practice guideline: red blood cell transfusion in adult trauma and critical care. *Crit Care Med.* 2009;37:3124–3157.
98. Eder AF, Chambers LA. Non-infectious complications of blood transfusion. *Arch Pathol Lab Med.*2007;131:708–718.
99. Vamvakas EC, Blajchman MA. Transfusion related mortality: the ongoing risk of allogeneic blood transfusion and the available strategies for their prevention. *Blood.* 2009;113:3406–3417.
100. Rojkjaer LP, Rojkjaer R. Clotting stabilization for the prevention of bleeding. *Hematol Oncol Clin North Am.* 2007;21:25–32.
101. Alter HJ, Klein HG. The hazards of blood transfusion in historical perspective. *Blood.* 2008;112:2617–2626.
102. Kalmandi S, Tiu R, Lowe C, Jin T, Kalaycio M. Epsilon aminocaproic acid reduces transfusion requirements in patients with thrombocytopenic hemorrhage. *Cancer.* 2006;107(1):136–140.
103. Levy B, Arnason E, Bussel JB. The use of second-generation thrombopoietic agents for chemotherapy-induced thrombocytopenia. *Curr Opin Oncol.* 2008;20:690–696.
104. Vadhan-Raj S. Management of chemotherapy-induced thrombocytopenia: current status of thrombopoietic agents. *Semin Hematol.* 2009;46(1 suppl 2):S26–S32.
105. Gobel BH, Beck SL, O'Leary C. Nursing-sensitive patient outcomes: the development of the putting evidence into practice resources for nursing practice. *Clin J Oncol.* 2006;10:621–624.
106. Given BA, Sherwood PR. Nursing-sensitive patient outcomes: a white paper. *Oncol Nurs Forum.* 2005;32:773–784.

Bleeding

Patient Name: ______________________________

Symptom and Description

Patients with cancer may develop bleeding. Some cancer treatments such as chemotherapy and radiation therapy can cause your platelet level to drop. The platelets are cells in your blood that help stop bleeding.

Bleeding can happen in any part of your body. You can often see where you are bleeding; but sometimes, bleeding can occur inside your body. Bleeding can occur because of an injury directly to your body or a cut on your skin. It may also occur without injury, such as in a nose bleed. Bleeding can cause you to become tired, weak, dizzy, and short of breath. You may also have pain.

You should report the following signs to your doctor:

- Nose bleeds
- Black stool
- Severe headaches
- Bright red blood in stool
- Coughing up blood
- Blood in your urine
- Sudden bloodshot eyes and any changes in your vision
- Visible red spots on any part of your body
- Bruising on any part of your body
- Bleeding from your central line site
- Bright red blood in your vomit
- Abnormal vaginal bleeding (not your regular menses)
- Pain in your stomach, joints, and muscles
- Difficulty waking up or staying up
- Shortness of breath, difficulty breathing
- Bleeding on gums or lips, or if you notice blood blisters inside your mouth
- Dizziness, severe headaches, changes in your mental status

Prevention

When your platelet levels are low, you can bleed easily. It is important for you to follow these steps to prevent bleeding when your platelets are low.

1. Skin care
   a. Always keep your skin clean and dry.
   b. Use a thick lotion on your skin.

c. Protect your skin from cuts, scrapes, and sharp objects.
d. Use an electric razor.
e. Carefully trim and cut nails.

2. Mouth care
   a. Use only a soft-bristled toothbrush.
   b. Do not use dental floss or a dental pick.
   c. Use mouthwash that does not contain alcohol.
3. Digestive system
   a. Promote a normal bowel pattern and avoid constipation.
   b. Use stool softeners and laxatives.
   c. Maintain proper diet and exercise.
   d. Drink water.
   e. Avoid straining.
   f. Do not use suppositories or enemas.
   g. Do not take rectal temperature.
4. Fall prevention
   a. Keep your home free from clutter.
   b. Adjust your bed at the lowest level.
   c. Ask for help walking if you are weak or feeling dizzy.
   d. Wear non-skid shoes when you are out of bed.
   e. Use a night light.

Management

- If bleeding occurs, stay calm.
- Apply direct pressure where you are bleeding for at least 10 minutes.
- Apply an ice pack for 10–15 minutes to stop bleeding.
- Raise your arms or legs above your heart if you are bleeding from your limb.
- If you are bleeding from your nose, gently pack the bleeding side of your nose with gauze or tissue. Leave the packing in place until bleeding stops.
- If you are having abnormal vaginal bleeding, take note of how many pads you use.
- Take note of how long the event of bleeding lasts.
- Notify your nurse and/or doctor.

Phone Numbers

Nurse: ______________________________ Phone: __________________________

Physician: ___________________________ Phone: __________________________

Other: ______________________________ Phone: __________________________

Source: Rodriguez AL. Bleeding and Thrombotic Complications. In: Yarbro CH, Wujcik D, Gobel BH, eds. *Cancer Symptom Management*. 4th ed. Burlington, MA: Jones & Bartlett Learning; 2014.

Chapter 15

Dyspnea

Margaret Joyce, PhD, ANP-BC, AOCN®

THE PROBLEM

The term *dyspnea* is generally applied to the sensation of respiratory discomfort that individuals experience as an unpleasant awareness of breathing.[1] The word *breathlessness* is often used interchangeably with dyspnea, although someone who is breathless may or may not be in distress.[2] Short of breath and shortness of breath are clinical terms also used to document the symptom of dyspnea.

The American Thoracic Society (ATS) published a consensus statement in 1999 and proposed the following broader definition of dyspnea:

> A term used to characterize a subjective experience of breathing discomfort that consists of qualitatively distinct sensations that vary in intensity. The experience derives from interactions among multiple physiological, psychological, social, and environmental factors, and may induce secondary physiological and behavioral responses.[3 (p. 322)]

In a recent update to that consensus statement, the ATS gives emphasis to the subjective nature of dyspnea, noting that the symptom of dyspnea should be distinguished from signs that clinicians use as evidence of dyspnea such as tachypnea (increased respiratory rate), use of accessory muscles, or intercostal retraction during respiration. The evaluation of a patient with dyspnea continues to be dependent upon a thorough history and physical exam; however, ATS stresses that an adequate assessment of the symptom of dyspnea depends upon patient self-report.[4] Common phrases used by patients with cancer-related dyspnea to describe the experience include "out of breath," "cannot get enough air," "breathing requires work/effort," and "chest feels tight."[5] The language used to describe dyspnea may not be specific to the medical condition (e.g., cancer), but rather may reflect features of chronic respiratory impairment or the reactive component of dyspnea.[6]

INCIDENCE

The incidence of cancer-related dyspnea varies widely depending on the cancer diagnosis, stage of disease, cancer therapy and presence of other cardiopulmonary or neurological diagnoses. In one systematic review, the pooled prevalence of dyspnea from 40 studies in patients with advanced cancer was 35%.[7] In another study, more than 50% of patients with advanced lung cancer reported dyspnea.[8] The prevalence of dyspnea increased as end of life approached, with 70% of patients admitted to a hospice home care program reporting shortness of breath[9]; by comparison, the prevalence of dyspnea in ambulatory patients newly starting chemotherapy was only 13%.[10]

Symptoms commonly reported with cancer-related dyspnea and thought to constitute symptom clusters are cough and fatigue[11] and fatigue and anxiety.[12] These symptoms (cough, fatigue, and anxiety) that occur concurrently with dyspnea may or may not be related or have a common etiology but certainly can have a synergistic or collective effect on patient outcomes. Dyspnea frequently affects many aspects of patient behavior, including functional status.[3] The most severe consequences of increasing levels of chronic dyspnea are profound reductions in physical functions such as the basic activities of daily living, role functions such as work, and changes in emotional behavior.[8]

Acute dyspnea refers to rapid-onset severe dyspnea often precipitating emergency health care. In the absence of other clinical features, acute dyspnea raises concern for airway obstruction, pneumothorax, or pulmonary embolism.[13] Chronic dyspnea, in contrast, has a slow, gradual onset. Chronic dyspnea is persistent, gradually increases over time, and may have interspersed acute episodes that vary in severity from the baseline symptom.[14] This chapter primarily focuses on chronic cancer-related dyspnea.

ETIOLOGY

Dyspnea is particularly common in patients with cancer who have primary or metastatic lung tumors or pleural involvement; however, many patients with cancer without direct lung involvement also report it. Many clinical factors can converge to cause and contribute to the symptom of dyspnea, including anemia and cachexia, as well as underlying cardiopulmonary or neurological diseases. A past or present history of tobacco use or smoking often correlates with the presence of dyspnea. Table 15-1 summarizes cancer-related dyspnea risk factors and correlates.[15]

Cancer-related dyspnea can have multiple etiologies. Clinical classification of dyspnea in cancer patients falls into four categories: direct tumor effects, indirect tumor effects, treatment related causes, and unrelated causes.[16] Elaboration of possible causes of dyspnea in each of these four categories appears in Table 15-2.[16]

TABLE 15-1

Risk Factors and Correlates for Moderate-to-Severe Dyspnea in Patients with Cancer

Smoking – past or present
Chronic obstructive pulmonary disease
Cardiac disease, especially congestive heart failure
Asthma
Environmental exposures (asbestos, coal dust, cotton dust, grain dust)
Lung radiation
Lung cancer – primary or metastatic
Anxiety – either as cause or effect of dyspnea
Fatigue / tiredness
Maximal inspiratory pressure <80% predicted
Vital capacity <80%
Low Karnofsky performance score

Source: Data from Williams, Dyspnea. *Cancer J. 2006; 12(5)*:365. Reprinted with permission[15].

TABLE 15-2

Causes of Dyspnea in Patients with Cancer

Dyspnea caused directly by cancer
- Pulmonary parenchymal involvement (primary or metastatic)
- Lymphangitic carcinomatosis
- Intrinsic or extrinsic airway obstruction by tumor
- Pleural tumor
- Pleural effusion
- Pericardial effusion
- Ascites
- Hepatomegaly
- Phrenic nerve paralysis
- Multiple tumor microemboli
- Pulmonary leukostasis
- Superior vena cava syndrome

Dyspnea caused indirectly by cancer
- Cachexia
- Electrolyte abnormalities
- Anemia
- Pneumonia
- Pulmonary aspiration
- Pulmonary emboli
- Neurologic paraneoplastic syndromes

Dyspnea from cancer treatment
- Surgery
- Radiation pneumonitis or fibrosis
- Chemotherapy-induced pulmonary toxicity
- Chemotherapy-induced cardiomyopathy
- Radiation-induced pericardial disease

Dyspnea unrelated to cancer
- Chronic obstructive pulmonary disease
- Asthma
- Congestive heart failure
- Interstitial lung disease
- Pneumothorax
- Anxiety
- Chest wall deformity
- Obesity
- Neuromuscular disorders
- Pulmonary vascular disease

Source: Data from Dudgeon, Kristjanson, Sloan, Lertzman, Clement. Dyspnea in cancer patients: Prevalence and associated factors. *J Pain Symptom Manage*, 2001. *21(2)*:95–102. Reprinted with permission[16].

PATHOPHYSIOLOGY

Normal respiratory physiology is complex. Dyspnea is the perception of a mismatch between outgoing central respiratory motor activity and incoming information from both central and peripheral receptors in the airways, lungs, and chest wall structures. Specifically, the sensation of dyspnea is that the drive to breathe is not being matched by adequate pulmonary ventilation.[4]

Possible physiologic derangements that underlie dyspnea are sorted into two main categories: (1) "controller or gas exchanger problems that lead to increased ventilation" and (2) "pump problems" secondary to impaired mechanical response or inspiratory muscle weakness (or a combination of the two).[16] The goal of the respiratory controller is to satisfy the metabolic requirements of the body. Controller or gas exchange problems include hypoventilation, oxygen shunting, diffusion impairment, and ventilation–perfusion inequality. Diffusion impairment can accompany radiation fibrosis, lymphangitic disease, or pneumonectomy. Ventilation–perfusion inequality is seen in pulmonary embolus, tumor, and chronic obstructive pulmonary disease (COPD).[17] The respiratory pump can be visualized as the pressure generator for ventilation. Pump problems leading to dyspnea include normal spirometry with anemia or psychological interference, obstructive interference from asthma or airway disease, and restrictive consequences such as those seen in pleural or chest wall disease or respiratory muscle weakness.[16]

The respiratory motor system is unusual in having both automatic (brain stem) and voluntary (cerebral cortex) sources of motor command, and discharge from these separate sources may give rise to different sensations.[4] Like pain, dyspnea has an affective component. The affective component is an emotional or behavioral response to the physiologic stimulus of respiratory compromise. This component can vary greatly among persons to modulate the intensity of the symptom. Hence, the threshold perception of dyspnea and intensity of breathing discomfort varies widely among individuals and is related only moderately to the degree of pulmonary dysfunction.[3]

SYMPTOM ASSESSMENT

SELF-ASSESSMENT

Assessment of dyspnea is a clinical challenge because of the symptom's subjective nature, which is compounded by the fact that the sensation often has more than one physiologic cause. In addition, the quality and intensity of dyspnea can be episodic as it varies over time from a chronic baseline.[14] Therefore, it is important to measure the patient's perception of dyspnea. No single tool measures all of the dimensions of dyspnea,[4] but regular and consistent assessment of the presence and intensity of dyspnea is facilitated by the use of a form or tool that will document the patient's perception or rating of the symptom and change over time such as the weekly breathing log found in Appendix 15A.

The presence of dyspnea usually is noted with respect to the context in which it occurs, such as on exertion, at rest, or nocturnally. The most common method of screening for dyspnea is self-report of the activity level that causes awareness of the symptom. The Medical Research Council (MRC) dyspnea scale is part of a standardized interview guide and respiratory epidemiologic questionnaire that has been used for many years to grade the effect of dyspnea on daily activities and the extent to which breathlessness impairs mobility.[18] This scale determines whether a person gets short of breath while (1) hurrying on level ground or walking up a slight hill or (2) walking with other people at ordinary pace on level ground. If answers to those questions are negative, the MRC screening questions continues: (3) Do you have to stop for breath when walking at your own pace on level ground? The final question is (4) Are you short of breath on washing and dressing? Another version of this question is (4) Are you too breathless to leave the house or on dressing or undressing? The grade or level of dyspnea is assigned based on the number of the last question answered with a "yes," indicating the most disability experienced by the respondent.[18] Providers in clinical practice can ask these screening questions to determine and label the extent to which dyspnea interferes with daily function.

One limitation of the MRC screening questions is that it depends on the ability to exert oneself or on ambulation (questions are not applicable if a person requires a wheelchair). As dyspnea increases, patients often reduce exertion and learn to compensate for inability to perform activities that cause distress, thereby minimizing the reported intensity of the symptom.[19]

OBJECTIVE ASSESSMENT

History and physical exam

Initially patients can be grouped into two categories: those with new-onset dyspnea and those with clinical deterioration or worsening of dyspnea. A rapid initial assessment of airway, breathing, and circulation is appropriate when confronted with a report of dyspnea to exclude an emergent situation. The stability and the circumstances of the patient's condition will guide the urgency of the subsequent evaluation. One goal of triage is to place a patient into one of three categories: (1) distress with unstable vital signs, (2) distress with stable vital signs, or (3) no distress and stable vital signs.[20]

A general approach to dyspnea evaluation includes a focused history and review surrounding the symptom, such as dyspnea intensity and descriptors, temporal onset and duration, precipitating or relieving events, and response to medication or behavioral approaches.[1,4] Elements of a patient's medical history that are critical to analysis of dyspnea include current medications and an assessment of coexisting diagnoses such as cardiac or pulmonary disease, history of current or past tobacco use or exposure to secondhand or environmental tobacco smoke, and relevant work history that provides information about toxin exposure (e.g., asbestos). Elements of a patient's current cancer therapy as well as prior radiotherapy or chemotherapy also provide valuable data with which to evaluate dyspnea etiology.

Instruments or scales commonly used in practice to measure dyspnea are the numerical rating scale (NRS)[21], the visual analog scale (VAS)[22], and the Cancer Dyspnea Scale (CDS).[23] The VAS and CDS have evidence of either reliability or validity in patients with cancer.[21] The CDS is a multidimensional 12-item tool that measures sense of effort, sense of anxiety, and sense of discomfort related to dyspnea.[23] The VAS and NRS are one-dimensional instruments; that is, they measure only one dimension of dyspnea (intensity or severity). The VAS instructs a patient to put a mark on a 100-mm line indicating how much shortness of breath he or she is having right now. The score is the millimeter distance from the start of the line to the patient's mark. The NRS instructs a person to volunteer a numerical score that indicates the amount of dyspnea experienced—for example, on a scale of 0–10, with 0 being no shortness of breath and 10 being the most severe dyspnea. A clinician's purpose and reason for measuring dyspnea—such as to obtain a clinical baseline, to determine the effect of treatment, or as part of a protocol answering a specific research question—often guides the choice of instrument or tool to measure dyspnea.

A physical examination that focuses on the cardiac and respiratory systems as well as evidence of tissue oxygenation is essential for evaluating dyspnea.[1] Initial evaluation includes all vital signs (blood pressure, pulse, respiratory rate, and temperature). Evaluation of respiration mechanics includes (1) observation of the use of accessory respiratory muscles, or pursed lip breathing; (2) stethoscope auscultation for absent breath sounds or the presence of adventitious sounds such as rales, rhonchi, wheezing, or friction rub; (3) lung field percussion to assess for dullness indicating atelectasis, consolidation, or effusion; and (4) chest palpation for respiratory excursion and fremitus. Cardiovascular assessment focuses on heart sounds, palpation of central pulses, and observation of jugular venous distention. Signs of deficient tissue oxygenation include pallor; cyanosis of fingernails, lips, and mucous membranes; and clubbing of the digits (indicating chronic hypoxia). Additionally, mental status changes such as restlessness, anxiety, disorientation, and confusion may indicate cerebral hypoxia.[2]

Diagnostic evaluation

Appropriate diagnostic testing for dyspnea is guided by cancer stage, usefulness of the diagnostic information for possible therapeutic intervention, and patient choice. Basic dyspnea diagnostic testing includes noninvasive pulse oximetry at rest and with exertion, and a complete blood count (CBC). Pulse oximetry results that show oxygen saturation less than 94% almost always represents clinically significant hypoxemia.[13] A CBC may show anemia; any decrease in hemoglobin concentration from one's usual baseline hemoglobin may be attended by a reduced oxygen-carrying capacity of the blood.[4]

Additional imaging studies can provide helpful data but extensive diagnostic testing is appropriate only to determine pathophysiological causes of dyspnea that are potentially reversible with therapy. A chest radiograph may be indicated to evaluate acute problems, such as pneumothorax, pneumonia, or pleural effusion. Chest computed tomography (CT) may provide information such as tumor outline or tumor progression if sequential scans are performed for comparison. A high-resolution spiral CT scan of the chest can evaluate for a pulmonary embolus as potential cause of dyspnea. Pulmonary function tests that measure lung volumes and gas diffusion may be helpful to diagnose a reversible airway obstruction or hypoxemia that can be improved with therapy. Patient clinical status and wishes should guide testing efforts.

DEGREES OF TOXICITY

A widely accepted terminology to grade the severity of dyspnea as an adverse event in cancer therapy clinical trials is the Common Terminology Criteria for Adverse Events (CTCAE) v4.03 five-point categorization. The CTCAE grading scale evaluates not only dyspnea's precipitating circumstance (at rest or with minimal or moderate exertion), but also the limiting impact of dyspnea on activities of daily living or self-care. The more severe grades indicate life-threatening consequences or death.[24] The limit of this classification is that it relies on exertion or a decrease in functionality as a proxy assessment of dyspnea, rather than dyspnea itself. The usefulness of the CTCAE grading scale is that it can quickly rate the presence of dyspnea and limits imposed by the symptom. Table 15-3 displays the CTCAE 4.03 grading scale for dyspnea.[24]

SYMPTOM MANAGEMENT STRATEGIES

THERAPEUTIC APPROACH

Therapy that produces small alterations of physiologic and psychological variables can result in a clinically meaningful reduction in dyspnea.[3] Desirable outcomes of dyspnea therapy should focus on the patient's self-report or expression of dyspnea rather than the observed level of dyspnea as judged by physiologic signs.[1]

Two categories of dyspnea management are therapeutic and palliative. The optimal treatment of dyspnea is to

TABLE 15-3

National Cancer Institute Common Terminology Criteria for Adverse Events (CTCAE): Respiratory, Thoracic, and Mediastinal Disorders

	Grade				
Adverse Event	**1**	**2**	**3**	**4**	**5**
Dyspnea	Shortness of breath with moderate exertion	Shortness of breath with minimal exertion; limiting instrumental activities of daily living (ADL)	Shortness of breath at rest; limiting self-care	Life-threatening consequences; urgent intervention indicated	Death

Definition: A disorder characterized by an uncomfortable sensation of difficulty breathing.

Source: Data from National Cancer Institute Common Terminology Criteria for Adverse Events (CTCAE)[24].

treat reversible causes with specific therapies (therapeutic) and to use nonspecific or palliative therapy to treat irreversible causes. The National Comprehensive Cancer Network (NCCN) palliative care guidelines advise that palliative therapy be delivered concurrently with therapeutic care.[25]

The initial focus in treating dyspnea is to optimize treatment of the underlying disease.[4] Treatment options for cancer-related dyspnea can be organized according to the same categories listed in Table 15-1—that is, dyspnea directly caused by tumor, indirectly caused by tumor, or caused by cancer therapy.[16]

Dyspnea caused by tumor

If the tumor itself is the cause of dyspnea, appropriate therapy to treat the cancer with surgery, radiotherapy, chemotherapy, or biologic therapy could reduce dyspnea.[25] Even a minor response to cancer treatment can reduce breathlessness. Dyspnea from airway obstruction due to intralumenal bronchial tumor or extrinsic compression of the airway from tumor mass may potentially be relieved with high-dose corticosteroids combined with external-beam radiotherapy, brachytherapy, or airway stenting with or without laser ablation.[1,26] Respiratory compromise from pleural effusion or ascites temporarily can be relieved by thoracentesis or paracentesis. In most instances, however, the fluid reaccumulates shortly after removal.[26] If dyspnea relief is obtained with pleural fluid drainage, pleurodesis with a sclerosing agent such as talc can obliterate the pleural space and prevent further accumulation of pleural fluid. However, subsequent dyspnea described as a sense of lung restriction sometimes results from the pleurodesis procedure. Intermittent pleural drainage through the insertion of an indwelling pleural catheter with a one-way valve to prevent reintroduction of air or fluid into the pleural space is an alternative to pleurodesis. Required ongoing care of the indwelling pleural catheter and expense of supplies are potential barriers to use of this intervention.[27]

Dyspnea indirectly caused by cancer

Chronic illness as well as certain cancer therapies can predispose an individual to secondary conditions, which may result in increased respiratory effort or discomfort. Two common complications of cancer as a chronic illness that may contribute to dyspnea are pneumonia and anemia. Pneumonia—an acute inflammation of the lung—can be effectively treated with appropriate antibiotic therapy, leading to a degree of dyspnea relief.[1] Anemia—a decrease of oxygen-carrying hemoglobin from the normal baseline level—may cause an increased sense of breathing effort. If appropriate to the patient's condition, anemia can be treated with red cell transfusion or erythropoietin therapy; however, correcting the anemia may or may not lessen dyspnea. Erythropoiesis-stimulating therapy is associated with risk of cardiovascular complications and risks of tumor growth stimulation and decreased survival.[28] Malnutrition, electrolyte and mineral imbalances, and overall deconditioning also seen in chronic cancer illness may contribute to dyspnea as well. Again, depending on the patient's status, attempts to correct these clinical circumstances may improve dyspnea control.

Dyspnea due to cancer treatment

Dyspnea, and hypoxia due to either acute or chronic pneumonitis, may be a consequence of thoracic radiation therapy or some chemotherapy agents. An oral corticosteroid, usually prednisone starting at 40–60 mg daily for 1–2 weeks, followed by a slow taper, such as reducing the dose by 10 mg every 1–2 weeks, is the mainstay of therapy.[29] Supplemental oxygen and bronchodilators as indicated are administered to treat pneumonitis.[30]

Chemotherapy agents can cause pulmonary toxicity with dyspnea and hypoxia as predominant manifestations. The agents associated with pulmonary toxicity are bleomycin, nitrosureas, and mitomycin, plus combinations of several agents that individually may have only modest pneumotoxicity (e.g., gemcitabine and weekly docetaxel).[30] Biologic targeted therapy agents such as tyrosine kinase inhibitors are associated with an uncommon but sometimes severe interstitial pneumonitis. Rituximab also has been rarely implicated in pneumonopathy.[30]

PALLIATIVE APPROACH

Palliative management of cancer-related dyspnea usually is based on a combination of drug therapy, oxygen therapy, and general supportive measures.[1] Evidence derived solely from research in cancer populations for each of these modalities is scant, however. With some exceptions, evidence supporting use of specific interventions for cancer-related dyspnea is not strong because it comes from uncontrolled research conducted in small samples. Additional evidence comes from consensus opinion of experts.

A synthesis of interventions for cancer-related dyspnea is available from the Oncology Nursing Society as part of the "Putting Evidence into Practice" (PEP) initiative.[31] The evidence in the PEP synthesis is classified by the weight or strength of existing evidence and placed into categories such as what is recommended for practice, what is likely to be effective but lacks sufficient evidence to be recommended, and what is judged to be ineffective or may be harmful and, therefore, is not recommended. Typically most of the interventions for cancer-related dyspnea, with the exception of immediate-release opioids, lack sufficient evidence to be recommended and fall into the "effectiveness not established" category.

Pharmacologic therapy

Opioids. The mechanism of action by which opioids relieve dyspnea is presumably a depression of opioid receptors found in the lung, spinal cord, and central respiratory center.[1] Opioids may diminish dyspnea by reducing the central perception of the sensation, decreasing anxiety associated with dyspnea, lessening the ventilatory responses to hypoxia and hypercapnia, and improving cardiovascular function.[1]

The use of immediate-release oral or parenteral opioids for dyspnea relief is supported by several systematic reviews of randomized controlled trials that evaluated pharmacologic interventions for breathlessness in the cancer population.[32–34] The opioid most frequently administered in these studies was morphine, although some other opioids were also used. Currently and frequently used opioids such as oxycodone and fentanyl were not included in any of the oral/parenteral studies. Although the beneficial effect of systemic opioids for dyspnea relief is well accepted, an optimal drug, dose, and modality of administration cannot be recommended because of the wide variety of doses examined in the studies.[1] Nevertheless, one study determined that a supplemental opiod dose consisting of 25% of the regular dose is sufficient to decrease dyspnea during the subsequent 4 hour period.[35] In general, although the numbers of opioid-tolerant and opioid-naive patients were small when the groups were compared in the studies, no difference in dyspnea relief was seen; reported opioid adverse effects such as nausea, vomiting, constipation, dizziness, and drowsiness were more problematic in the opioid-naive patients.[34]

Nebulized therapy. The use of nebulized opioids to relieve dyspnea is not supported by evidence.[4] Several pharmacologic agents (morphine, fentanyl, hydromorphone, furosemide, lidocaine) have been administered by the nebulized route in different studies to relieve dyspnea.[34,36] Inhalation deposits a fine mist of aerosolized medication on the respiratory tract, which has the potential to modify dyspnea through local action in the lungs. With respect to opioids, a local binding to pulmonary sensory receptors in the lung is thought to deliver the pulmonary effect and minimize systemic toxicity. Although this theory is appealing, there is a lack of data to support the use of nebulized opioids in the treatment of dyspnea.[32–34,36]

Benzodiazepines. Currently there are no convincing data from controlled studies suggesting that benzodiazepines should be used as first-line therapy for dyspnea.[4,37,38] However, perhaps because dyspnea and anxiety can occur concurrently as a symptom cluster, benzodiazepines are commonly used as an adjunct to opioids in the management of cancer-related dyspnea.[1,25] The NCCN palliative care guidelines recommend a starting dose of lorazepam 0.5–1 mg orally for benzodiazepine-naive patients who are experiencing dyspnea and have a life expectancy of years to months to weeks.[25] Benzodiazepines are known for their tendency to cause increased somnolence and delirium, especially among older adults; consequently, increased caution with their use is advised.[38]

Oxygen

Established evidence supports the use of supplemental oxygen therapy for all patients who are hypoxemic. Oxygen therapy can help to relieve dyspnea in those who are hypoxemic at rest or with minimal exertion.[4,39,40] A beneficial effect of supplemental oxygen therapy to provide dyspnea relief "could be related to changes in chemoreceptor stimulation with resulting changes in breathing patterns and/or stimulation of receptors related to gas flow through the upper airway."[4 (p. 444)]

However, many patients who report dyspnea are not hypoxic (i.e., their oxygen percent saturations are in the normal range). The use of oxygen to relieve the sensation of dyspnea, and not necessarily to correct hypoxemia, is called palliative oxygen therapy. At present, no data are available to support the use of palliative oxygen therapy. Several research trials have shown that when oxygen therapy to relieve the overall sensation of dyspnea was compared to the use of medical air (78.9% nitrogen and 21.1% oxygen), oxygen was equivocal or not superior to air.[39,41–44] On average, patients improved symptomatically with both the oxygen and the air—a finding that supports the multifactorial etiology of dyspnea. The prescription of medical air is not a common therapy encountered in practice. Medicare reimbursement for oxygen therapy requires evidence of oxygen saturation equal to or less than 88%, demonstrating hypoxemia. Supplemental oxygen without a specific oxygen saturation requirement is usually provided within a hospice care program.

Ambient airflow. Patients who are short of breath often seek to sit near a fan or open window. It is thought that cold air directed across the cheek and through the nose affects sensory receptors in the distribution of the trigeminal (fifth) cranial nerve that respond to both thermal and mechanical stimuli and can alter ventilation and reduce the perception of breathlessness.[26] In one study, the use of a handheld fan reportedly provided a significant reduction in dyspnea when air was directed toward the face.[45] This low-cost, low-risk intervention can be easily tried; thus it is recommended to see if it makes the patient feel better.

Persons often find measures such as positioning, limiting exertion, and relaxation strategies helpful in coping with dyspnea. NCCN palliative care guidelines recommend stress management and relaxation therapy as a means to manage dyspnea.[25] Evidence from three nurse-led programs that included breathlessness rehabilitation techniques and emotional support showed a positive effect in terms of reduction in dyspnea scores.[46–48] The nurse-led programs examined the use of a structured weekly approach that included assessment, education, and instruction in breathing control and coping techniques.

Because the symptom of dyspnea can change rapidly or insidiously, patients and caregivers should be instructed to report changes in baseline dyspnea, particularly increasing shortness of breath, fever, pain, and change in sputum production. Patients should be taught to avoid respiratory irritants such as primary or secondary tobacco smoke and exposure to individuals with respiratory infections. Nurses can advise about the prevention benefit of immunizations (if not contraindicated) such as pneumococcal vaccine and annual influenza vaccine.

Proper administration of medications can be challenging for both patients and caregivers. Education about medication regimens for dyspnea should include the expected actions and side effects of medications and administration techniques. If inhaled medications are included in symptom management, their use requires instruction and practice in using the devices to gain confidence in their proper use. Proper and safe use of oxygen equipment is important information to be taught.

Many patients discover body positions and a variety of breathing techniques that improve their dyspnea out of trial and error. Nonetheless, reinforcement of proper technique and encouragement to use breathing techniques in times of anxiety or distress is an important teaching goal. Individualized teaching could include the following topics: (1) the leaning forward position, (2) pursed lip breathing, and (3) diaphragmatic breathing. Dyspnea positioning and breathing techniques are described in Appendix 15B.

Relaxation training is another recommended strategy that may be helpful in cancer-related dyspnea. There are many different approaches for relaxation training, including progressive muscle relaxation, visual imagery, biofeedback, and meditation. Relaxation can cause a patient to focus on sensations other than breathlessness. Encouragement and practice will help individuals to acquire the relaxation skill.

Patient and caregiver education can empower them to use self-care strategies to promote symptom reduction. Self-care education is reinforced in multiple areas of oncology care. Symptom management education is an integral component of nurses' dialog with patients and caregivers, and is an area where nurses can be an important influence in the care of patients with dyspnea.

NURSING IMPLICATIONS

Patient outcomes can relate to specific indicators such as relief of dyspnea or comfort during palliative care. Nursing-sensitive patient outcomes are outcomes amenable to nursing intervention (either accomplished by nursing alone or as part of composite multidisciplinary plan of care).[49] Because dyspnea is a subjective symptom (like pain), patient report is the gold standard with respect to determination of intensity and assessment of relief from any intervention. One clinical recommendation is that dyspnea ought to be measured with a quantitative measure such as numerical rating scale or visual analog scale or other reliable tool; nurses should employ this dyspnea measurement in a longitudinal manner so that the symptom may be monitored and addressed over time. Understanding that the symptom of dyspnea may or may not resolve despite correction of abnormal physiologic parameters such as tachypnea, use of accessory muscles, cyanosis, or oxygen percent saturation will help care providers assess symptom status. The expectation of an intervention for dyspnea is that initial attempts to correct reversible causes will be made and attempts to palliate irreversible causes will be pursued to until patients will report relief or comfort.

PATIENT SELF-CARE

Although self-care measures for persons with dyspnea can be intuitive or learned from trial and error, education and reinforcement of techniques from healthcare providers have been shown to relieve dyspnea. The main components of dyspnea education are knowledge of signs and symptoms to report to healthcare providers, understanding medication regimens, and self-care strategies that range from recognizing maneuvers that initiate dyspnea to maximizing body positions and breathing techniques to decrease breathlessness. A tool to record the daily worst breathing level and associated fatigue, anxiety, and activity level is found in Appendix 15A. This tool can help patients communicate with their healthcare providers as well as understand and manage their own care. A self-care guide that can be used to inform patients and caregivers about the problem of shortness of breath is found in Appendix 15B.

REFERENCES

1. Dalal S, Palat G, Bruera E. Management of dyspnea. In: Berger AM, Shuster JL, Von Roenn JH. eds. *Principles and Practice of Palliative Care and Supportive Oncology.* 3rd ed. Philadelphia, PA: Lippincott Williams & Wilkins; 2007:278–290.
2. Joyce M. Dyspnea. In: Brown CG, ed. *A Guide to Oncology Symptom Management.* Pittsburgh, PA: Oncology Nursing Society; 2010:199–223.
3. American Thoracic Society. Dyspnea mechanisms, assessment, and management: a consensus statement. *Am J Respir Crit Care Med.* 1999;159(1):321–340.
4. American Thoracic Society. An official American Thoracic Society statement: update on the mechanisms, assessment, and management of dyspnea. *Am J Respir Crit Care Med.* 2012;185(4):435–452.
5. Wilcock A, Crosby V, Hughes A, et al. Descriptors of breathlessness in patients with cancer and other cardiorespiratory diseases. *J Pain Symptom Manage.* 2002;23(3):182–189.
6. Garrard AK, Williams, M. The language of dyspnoea: a systematic review. *Inter J Allied Health Sci Pract.* 2008;6(1):1–14.
7. Teunissen SC, Wesker W, Kruitwagen C, deHayes H, Voest EE, deGraeff A. Symptom prevalence in patients with incurable cancer: a systematic review. *J Pain Symptom Manage.* 2007;34(1):94–104.
8. Tishelman C, Petersson L, Degner LF, Sprangers MA. Symptom prevalence, intensity, and distress in patients with inoperable lung cancer in relation to time of death. *J Clin Oncol.* 2007;25(34):5381–5389.
9. McMillan SC, Small BJ. Symptom distress and quality of life in patients with cancer newly admitted to hospice home care. *Oncol Nurs Forum.* 2002;29(10):1421–1428.
10. Yamagishi A, Morita T, Miyashita M, Kimura F. Symptom prevalence and longitudinal follow-up in cancer outpatients receiving chemotherapy. *J Pain Symptom Manage.* 2009;37(5):823–830.
11. Cheville AL, Novotny PJ, Sloan JA, et al. Fatigue, dyspnea, and cough comprise a persistent symptom cluster up to five years after diagnosis with lung cancer. *J Pain Symptom Manage.* 2011;42(2):202–212.
12. Chan CW, Richardson A, Richardson J. A study to assess the existence of the symptom cluster of breathlessness, fatigue and anxiety in patients with advanced lung cancer. *Eur J Oncol Nurs.* 2005;9(4):325–333.
13. Gonzales R, Nadler PL. Common symptoms. In: McPhee SJ, Papadakis MA, Rabow MW, eds. *Current Medical Diagnosis and Treatment 2012.* New York: McGraw-Hill; 2012:2246.
14. McCarley C. A model of chronic dyspnea. *Image J Nurs Sch.* 1999;31(3):231–236.
15. Williams CM. Dyspnea. *Cancer J.* 2006;12(5):365–373.
16. Dudgeon DJ, Kristjanson L, Sloan JA, Lertzman M, Clement K. Dyspnea in cancer patients: prevalence and associated factors. *J Pain Symptom Manage.* 2001;21(2):95–102.
17. Dyspnea in cancer patients needs more attention. *J Support Oncol.* 2006;4(2):63–64.
18. Medical Research Council's Committee on the Aetiology of Chronic Bronchitis. Standardized questionnaires on respiratory symptoms. *BMJ.* 1960;2(5213):1665.
19. Joyce MJ, Camporeale M. Symptom management. In: Houlihan N, Tyson L, eds. *Lung Cancer Site-Specific Cancer Series.* Pittsburgh, PA: Oncology Nursing Society; 2012:131–151.
20. Shiber JR, Santana J. Dyspnea. *Med Clin North Am.* 2006;90(3):453–479.
21. Dorman S, Byrne A, Edwards A. Which measurement scales should we use to measure breathlessness in palliative care? A systematic review. *Palliat Med.* 2007;21:177–191.
22. Joyce M, Beck S. Measuring oncology nursing sensitive patient outcomes: evidence based summary. http://www.ons.org/Research/PEP/media/ons/docs/research/measurement/dyspnea.pdf. Accessed June 19, 2012.
23. Tanaka K, Akechi T, Okuyama T, Nishiwaki Y, Uchitomi Y. Development and validation of the Cancer Dyspnoea Scale: a multidimensional, brief, self-rating scale. *Br J Cancer.* 2000;82(4):800–805.
24. National Cancer Institute, Common terminology criteria for adverse events (CTCAE) v4.03 http://evs.nci.nih.gov/ftp1/CTCAE/CTCAE_4.03_2010-06-14_QuickReference_5x7.pdf. Accessed June 20, 2012.
25. NCCN palliative care guidelines version 2. 2012. http://www.nccn.org/professionals/physician_gls/pdf/palliative.pdf. Accessed June 22, 2012.
26. Dudgeon DJ. Managing dyspnea and cough. *Hematol Oncol Clin North Am.* 2002;16(3):557–577.
27. Brubacher S, Gobel BH. Use of the Pleurx pleural catheter for the management of malignant pleural effusions. *Clin J Oncol Nurs.* 2003;7(1):35–38.
28. U.S. Food and Drug Administration. 2/26/2012 FDA drug safety communication: Erythropoiesis-stimulating agents (ESAs): Procrit, Epogen and Aranesp. http://www.fda.gov/Drugs/DrugSafety/PostmarketDrugSafetyInformationforPatientsandProviders/ucm200297.htm. Accessed June 22, 2012.
29. Ghafoori P, Marks LB, Vujaskovic Z, Kelsey CR. Radiation induced lung injury. *Oncology.* 2008;22(1):37–47.
30. Machtay M. Pulmonary complications of anticancer treatment. In: Abeloff MD, Armitage JO, Niederhuber JE, Kastan MB, McKenna WG, eds. *Abeloff's Clinical Oncology.* Philadelphia, PA: Churchill Livingstone Elsevier; 2008:969–981.
31. DiSalvo WM, Joyce MM, Culkin AE, Tyson LB, Mackay K, Lubejko B. Dyspnea. In: Eaton, LH, Tipton, JM, eds. *PEP: Putting Evidence into Practice.* Pittsburgh, PA: Oncology Nursing Society; 2009:141–148.
32. Ben-Aharon I, Gafter-Gvili A, Paul M, Leibovici L, Stemmer SM. Interventions for alleviating cancer-related dyspnea: a systematic review. *J Clin Oncol.* 2008;26(14):2396–2404.
33. Viola R, Kiteley C, Lloyd NS, Mackay JA, Wilson J, Wong RK. The management of dyspnea in cancer patients: a systematic review. *Support Care Cancer.* 2008;16(4):329–337.

34. Jennings AL, Davies AN, Higgins JP, Gibbs JS, Broadley KE. A systematic review of the use of opioids in the management of dyspnoea. *Thorax.* 2002;57(11):939–944.
35. Allard P, Lamontagne C, Bernard P, Tremblay C. How effective are supplementary doses of opioids for dyspnea in terminally ill cancer patients? A randomized continuous sequential clinical trial. *J Pain Symptom Manage.* 1999;17(4):256–265.
36. Charles MA, Reymond L, Israel F. Relief of incident dyspnea in palliative cancer patients: a pilot, randomized, controlled trial comparing nebulized hydromorphone, systemic hydromorphone, and nebulized saline. *J Pain Symptom Manage.* 2008;36(1):29–38.
37. Simon S, Higginson IJ, Booth S, Harding R, Bausewein C. Benzodiazepines for the relief of breathlessness in advanced malignant and non-malignant diseases in adults. *Cochrane Database Syst Rev.* 2010;20(1):CD007534.
38. McCannon J, Temel J. Comprehensive management of respiratory symptoms in patients with advanced lung cancer. *J Support Oncol.* 2012;10(1):1–9.
39. Xue D, Abernethy AP. Management of dyspnea in advanced lung cancer: recent data and emerging concepts. *Curr Opin Support Palliat Care.* 2010;4(2):85–91.
40. Bruera E, deStoutz N, Velasco-Leiva A, Schoeller T, Hanson J. Effects of oxygen on dyspnoea in hypoxaemic terminal-cancer patients. *Lancet.* 1993;342(8862):13–14.
41. Uronis HE, Currow DC, McCrory DC, Samsa GP, Abernethy AP. Oxygen for relief of dyspnoea in mildly- or non-hypoxaemic patients with cancer: a systematic review and meta-analysis. *Br J Cancer.* 2008;98(2):294–299.
42. Qaseem A, Snow V, Shekelle P, et al. Evidence based interventions to improve the palliative care of pain, dyspnea, and depression at the end of life: a clinical practice guideline from American College of Physicians. *Ann Intern Med.* 2008;148(2):141–146.
43. Simon ST, Bausewein C. Management of refractory breathlessness in patients with advanced cancer. *Wien Med Wochenschr.* 2009;159(23–24):591–598.
44. Currow DC, Smith J, Davidson PM, Newton PJ, Agar MR, Abernethy AP. Does palliative home oxygen improve dyspnoea? A consecutive cohort study. *Palliat Med.* 2009;23(4):309–316.
45. Galbraith S, Fagan P, Perkins P, Lynch A. Booth S. Does the use of a handheld fan improve chronic dyspnea? A randomized, controlled, crossover trial. *J Pain Symptom Manage.* 2010;39(5):831–838.
46. Corner J, Plant H, A'Hern R, Bailey C. Non-pharmacological intervention for breathlessness in lung cancer. *Palliat Med.* 1996;10(4):299–305.
47. Bredin M, Corner J, Krishnasamy M, Plant H, Bailey C, A'Hern R. Multicentre randomised controlled trial of nursing intervention for breathlessness in patients with lung cancer. *BMJ.* 1999;318(7188):901–904.
48. Moore S, Corner J, Haviland J, et al. Nurse led follow up and conventional medical follow up in management of patients with lung cancer: Randomised trial. *BMJ.* 2002;325(7373):1145.
49. Gobel B, Tipton J. PEP up your practice: an introduction to the Oncology Nursing Society Putting Evidence into Practice resources. In: Eaton LH, Tipton JM, eds. *Putting Evidence into Practice: Improving Oncology Patient Outcomes.* Pittsburgh, PA: Oncology Nursing Society; 2009:1–8.

APPENDIX 15A SELF-CARE DATA FORM

Weekly Breathing Log

Patient Name: ______________________________

Day 1 Date ____________
At the end of the day, score your usual and worst breathing for the day by making a mark on each line between no problems and as bad as it can be.

Usual breathing today — Worst breathing today

Shortness of breath as bad as it can be

No shortness of breath

Days 2–7
At the end of the day, draw an arrow in each box to show if the symptom is worse (↓), better (↑) or the same (–). At the bottom of this page, note things that make your breathing worse and things you are doing that help your breathing. Share this information with the doctors and nurses providing your care.

Symptoms	Day 2	Day 3	Day 4	Day 5	Day 6	Day 7
Usual breathing today						
Worst breathing problems today						
My activity level today, compared to day 1						
My fatigue level today, compared to day 1						
My anxiety level today, compared to day 1						

Things that make my breathing worse ______________________________

Things that make my breathing better ______________________________

Shortness of Breath (Dyspnea)

Patient Name: ____

This self-care guide will help you with your problem of shortness of breath.

Symptom and Description

Dyspnea, or shortness of breath, is the feeling of having trouble breathing. Most often, people have this feeling because their bodies are working hard to move air in and out of their lungs. Less often, dyspnea occurs because the body is not getting enough oxygen. Many things can contribute to dyspnea. Shortness of breath can be caused or worsened by:

- partial or complete removal of a lung
- some chemotherapy drugs
- radiation therapy to the lungs
- tumor blocking the airways or pushing on the lungs from the outside
- lung damage from smoking
- anemia (low blood count)
- lack of muscle fitness
- infection
- obesity
- seasonal allergies
- anxiety

Feeling short of breath can cause anxiety, and anxiety can worsen the feeling, creating a cycle that is hard to break. However, there are things you can do to make you feel less short of breath.

Prevention

You may be able to decrease your shortness of breath, which will help you do more and enjoy life. You will learn positioning, breathing, air flow, and relaxation techniques. Other things to try include:

- Plan your day to lessen those activities that increase your dyspnea, such as stair-climbing and bending over.
- Wear slip-on shoes. Pull socks and shoes on while sitting. Use special devices to pick up items on the floor or ground.
- Move slowly and breathe deeply.
- Remain physically active, doing mild, gentle exercises such as walking to stay fit.
- Anticipate and plan medications, rest, or other measures before and after activities that cause you to have more shortness of breath.
- Ask family and friends for help. Accept their help. Have them read the management tips below so they can help you.

(continued)

- Avoid panic when breathing is difficult. Have someone nearby help you.
- Avoid things that make your breathing worse, such as cold air, humidity, pollen, or tobacco smoke.
- Consult with your doctor or nurse to make sure your "flu shot" and pneumonia vaccination are up to date.

Management

Positioning: These positions will help your lungs expand:

- Sit upright in a chair, lean forward slightly, and rest your forearms on the arms of the chair, on another piece of furniture, or on your knees.
- Sleep with your head on several pillows or sitting up in a recliner.

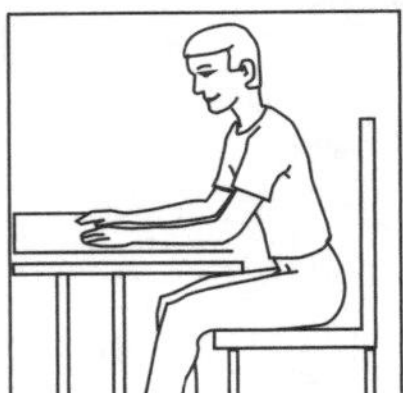
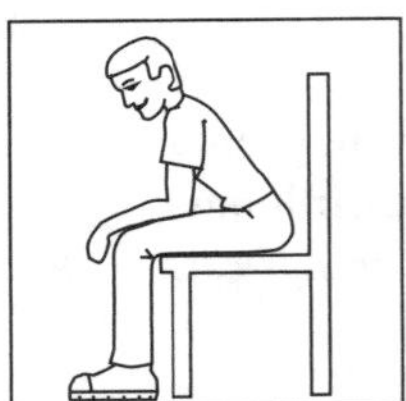
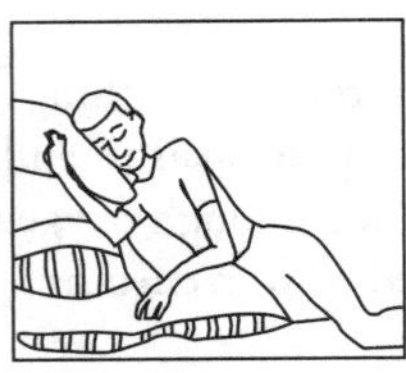
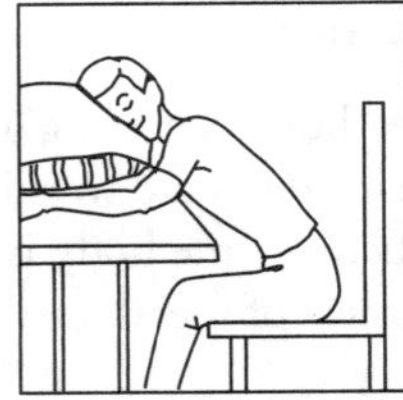
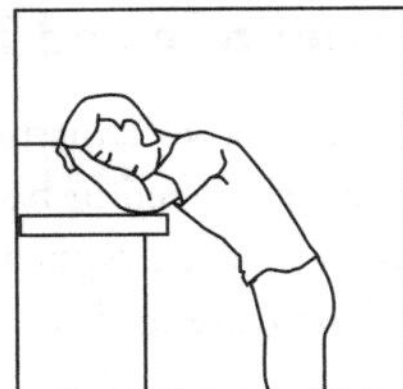

Breathing Techniques: *Pursed-lip breathing* slows the flow of air as you breathe out. This helps the smallest areas of your lungs open up. It is most helpful if you have chronic obstructive pulmonary disease (COPD).

- Breathe in through your nose, as you normally would.
- Breathe out for twice as long as you breathe in. Keep your lips tightly together, except for the very center. Blow out through this small opening.

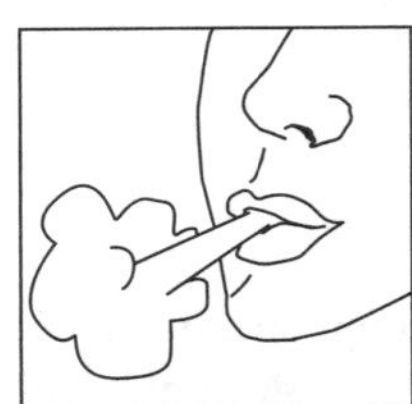

Abdominal breathing, also called diaphragmatic breathing, may lessen dyspnea by making the muscles that help you breathe more effective and stronger. If you have not been taught abdominal breathing, healthcare providers can help you learn this technique. To try it on your own:

- Find your diaphragm by placing your fingers just below your breastbone and sniffing. The muscle you feel moving is your diaphragm.
- Lie on your back as flat as is comfortable. Bend your knees and put a book on your abdomen. Breathe in deeply. As your diaphragm contracts, the book will rise. Continue to practice, with your goal being to move the book with each breath.

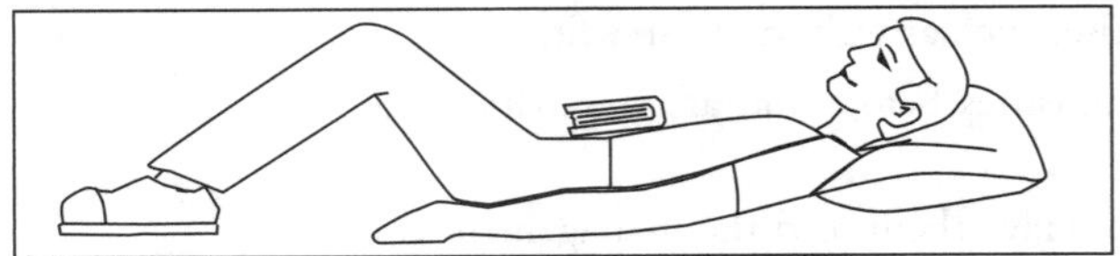

Air flow: Some people with shortness of breath feel better with oxygen treatments. Many people, however, will get the same results from cool air blowing on their cheek.

Relaxation Techniques: Dyspnea can cause anxiety. Anxiety can worsen dyspnea. It is important to learn ways to break the cycle of dyspnea and anxiety.

- Concentration: Progressive muscle relaxation is a technique you can use at home to help you relax and reduce dyspnea. While training may help you learn more quickly, audio and video taped training in progressive muscle relaxation is also helpful and can be found at many bookstores.
- Diversion: You may find activities that distract you from thinking about your breathing to be helpful. Examples are reading or listening to music.

Follow-up

There are other treatments for shortness of breath that can be tried, if your efforts aren't working well enough. Your healthcare provider may prescribe oxygen therapy or medications. In some cases, a lung or heart rehabilitation program may be suggested.

- Tell your healthcare team about the methods you are using at home and how well they are working.
- It may be helpful to keep a diary of changes in your breathing to help you report to your healthcare team.
- If you are unsure of any instructions you are given, tell your doctor or nurse.
- Be sure you understand when to call your doctor or nurse, and have both regular and emergency phone numbers handy.

Phone Numbers

Nurse: ______________________________ Phone: ________________

Physician: ______________________________ Phone: ________________

Respiratory Therapist: ______________________________ Phone: ________________

Physical Therapist: ______________________________ Phone: ________________

Pulmonary/Cardiac Rehab Program: ______________________________ Phone: ________________

Comments

Source: Joyce M. Dyspnea. In: Yarbro CH, Wujcik D, Gobel BH, eds. *Cancer Symptom Management.* 4th ed. Burlington, MA: Jones & Bartlett Learning; 2014.

Chapter 16

Effusions

Diane G. Cope, PhD, ARNP, BC, AOCNP®

THE PROBLEM

Malignant effusions, which are characterized by the excessive collection of fluid in a serous cavity, pose a significant health problem in individuals with cancer. Pleural effusions are an accumulation of fluid in the pleural cavity; pericardial effusions occur in the pericardial cavity. Effusions also create a negative impact on quality of life and a person's ability to carry out activities of daily living.

Fluid accumulation in the pleural or pericardial space can inhibit normal function of the lungs and the heart, resulting in dyspnea, fatigue, and pain.[1,2] Because malignant effusions are often late complications of progressive cancer, individuals tend to be debilitated with a low performance status and have a short life expectancy. Malignant pleural effusions are usually identified in individuals with advanced and generally incurable disease, with a 3-month mortality rate of 65% and a 6-month mortality rate of 80%.[3] Malignant pericardial effusions likewise signify a poor prognosis, with a median survival of less than 6 months.[3]

Therapeutic approaches used in the management of malignant effusions aim to maintain or improve the quality of life of the individual, yet take into consideration the clinical course of the disease. In some cases, aggressive therapy may eradicate the effusion and be appropriate in individuals with a high performance status. Comfort measures and supportive care may be preferable in individuals with advanced disease, marked pleural involvement, and low performance status.[4] In this chapter, symptom management of pleural and pericardial effusions are discussed. Maintenance or improvement of quality of life is the most important goal in treating both types of effusions, whether by medical intervention, nursing intervention, or a combination of both.

PLEURAL EFFUSIONS

INCIDENCE

A malignant effusion may be the first indication of cancer in 10% to 50% of individuals with a new cancer diagnosis, but more often it is detected in individuals with advanced metastatic disease.[3] As many as 40% of pleural effusions are caused by cancer, and 50% of patients with a cancer diagnosis are at risk for developing an effusion during their disease course.[1] It is estimated that almost 150,000 new cases of malignant pleural effusions are identified yearly in the United States.[1,3,5] Aside from primary brain neoplasms, all other neoplasms have the capability of producing malignant pleural effusions, due to lymphatic drainage through the hilar lymphatic system.[3]

ETIOLOGY

Although the majority of cancers can cause effusions, the tumor types most commonly associated with malignant pleural effusions are lung, breast, lymphoma, ovarian cancer, and gastric cancer (Figure 16-1).[3] With the rising incidence of breast and lung cancer, more than half of all malignant pleural effusions are attributed to these

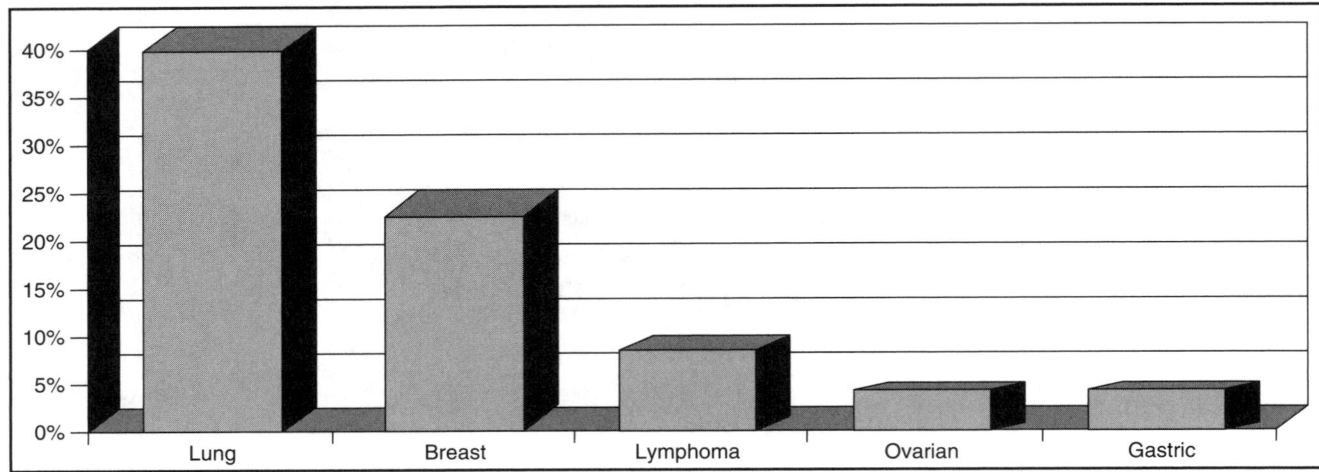

FIGURE 16-1

Tumor types associated with pleural effusions. Incidence is illustrated as a percent of all pleural effusions.

Source: Data from Kwong and Nguyen[3].

tumor types, and approximately one-third of patients will have bilateral pleural effusions.[3] Patients with a history of chest irradiation are also at risk for the development of pleural effusion.[4]

PATHOPHYSIOLOGY OF PLEURAL EFFUSIONS

NORMAL AND ABNORMAL PLEURAL FLUID FORMATION

The pleura is a thin layer of mesothelium that encases the lungs on one side (*visceral pleura*) and the thoracic cavity on the other side (*parietal pleura*). The pleural space, which is located between the visceral and parietal pleurae (Figure 16-2),[6] contains 5–15 mL of hypoproteinemic plasma at one time, although 100–200 mL of fluid moves through the space during a 24-hour period.[7] This serous fluid serves as a lubricant and is secreted by the mesothelial cells of the pleurae. Approximately 80%–90% of the fluid is reabsorbed by the lymphatic and capillary systems of the parietal pleura.[8]

Continuous pleural fluid movement is influenced by a dynamic equilibrium maintained through capillary permeability, hydrostatic and colloidal osmotic pressures, interstitial osmotic pressures, and lymphatic drainage. Changes in the balance among these parameters may result in pleural fluid accumulation, and can be caused by several neoplastic processes that include pleural implantation of cancer cells, venous obstruction, tumor cell shedding, and lymphatic obstruction.[6,9,10] Pleural implantation occurs by direct invasion of the tumor or by seeding of the primary tumor onto the serosal surface of the visceral or parietal pleura. Pleural implants lead to increased capillary permeability through inflammation of the pleural surfaces, with an increased net filtration of fluid into the pleural space. Both of these processes are common in malignant mesothelioma and lung cancer.[6,11]

Pulmonary venous obstruction causes increased hydrostatic pressure at the pleurae, thereby decreasing the pressure gradient, resulting in fluid accumulation in the pleural space. This process often occurs in lung cancer.[6]

Tumor cell suspensions, observed in lung, breast, and ovarian cancers, are malignant cells that are shed into the pleural space and change the colloid osmotic pressure. Pleural implants result in mesothelial shedding and thickening of the pleurae. It is the number of tumor cells in the pleural space that differentiates a tumor cell suspension from a pleural implant. Cytological evaluation of the pleural fluid would indicate average white cell counts greater than 3000 cells/mL in a tumor cell suspension.[12]

Lymphatic obstruction is often seen with lymphomas and metastatic breast or lung cancer. Obstruction of the lymphatic channels interferes with fluid and protein reabsorption from the pleural space, resulting in pleural effusion. The mediastinal lymph nodes are most commonly involved.[6,11]

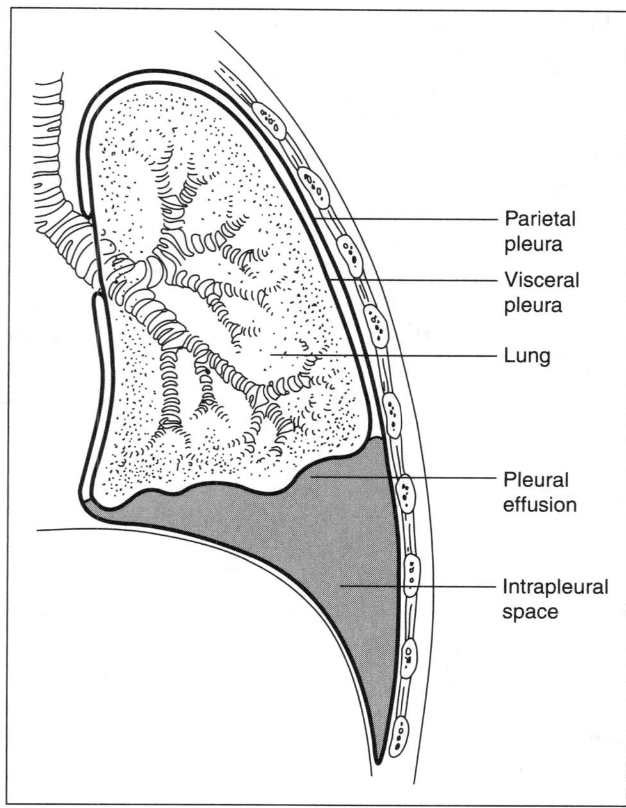

FIGURE 16-2

Structure of the lung with pleural effusion.
Source: Data from Cope[6].

SYMPTOM ASSESSMENT OF PLEURAL EFFUSIONS

RISK FACTORS

Risk factors are directly related to the underlying tumor type causing the effusion, such as breast cancer, lung cancer, lymphoma, or adenocarcinoma of unknown primary. Patients with a history of chest irradiation are at risk of developing pleural effusion due to pulmonary fibrosis.

SELF-ASSESSMENT

A patient with a pleural effusion initially will complain of shortness of breath with activity; however, this condition may progress to shortness of breath at rest when there is an increase in size of the effusion. Other symptoms that can be experienced by a patient include fatigue, dry cough, and chest discomfort or pleuritic pain.[13] These symptoms can significantly impact a patient's quality of life and will persist for the patient with cancer until therapeutic procedures are performed to remove the fluid. However, pleural effusions can recur if the cause of the effusion is not eliminated; in such a case, the patient will once again experience the same symptoms and decrease in quality of life. As a result, the patient may have increased anxiety with the dyspnea and depressed feelings related to possible progression of the cancer. For the older adult with cancer who has a pleural effusion, symptoms may be heightened because of age-related changes such as decreased respiratory function, physical decline, and presence of multiple comorbidities.

Nurses play a key role in symptom management and maximizing quality of life for patients. Dyspnea requires the same attention as pain and nausea and can be rated utilizing dyspnea assessment scales. Although several assessment scales are available,[13–15] no gold standard exists for measuring a patient's intensity or severity of breathlessness. The Numeric Rating Scale is a quick clinical assessment tool, rating dyspnea on a 0–10 scale, where 0 is no shortness of breath and 10 is shortness of breath as bad as can be.[16]

OBJECTIVE ASSESSMENT

A thorough history and physical examination are essential in the diagnosis of a malignant pleural effusion. Malignant effusions generally develop slowly over several months; nonmalignant effusions tend to have an abrupt onset. Most individuals present with complaints of dyspnea, dull aching or pleuritic chest pain, and a dry, nonproductive cough. The severity of the symptoms increases as the extent of the effusion increases. Fewer than 25% of individuals are asymptomatic.[11]

When the effusion volume reaches approximately 250 mL, physical findings may include intercostal prominence, dullness or flatness on percussion, decreased breath sounds, and decreased tactile fremitus.[3] Fever, tachypnea, labored breathing, and decreased chest wall expansion may be observed. If the effusion is large, it can cause tracheal deviation to the unaffected side.[3,4]

DIAGNOSTIC EVALUATION

Radiographic examinations

A chest radiograph will usually confirm fluid in the pleural cavity. Anterior-posterior films classically reveal a blunting of the costophrenic angle and a mediastinal shift if a large effusion is present (Figure 16-3). Lateral decubitus films are usually taken, as they can detect as little as 100 mL of pleural fluid accumulation, whereas anterior-posterior films can detect an effusion with a minimum of 200–300 mL of fluid. Ultrasound or computed tomography (CT) scan

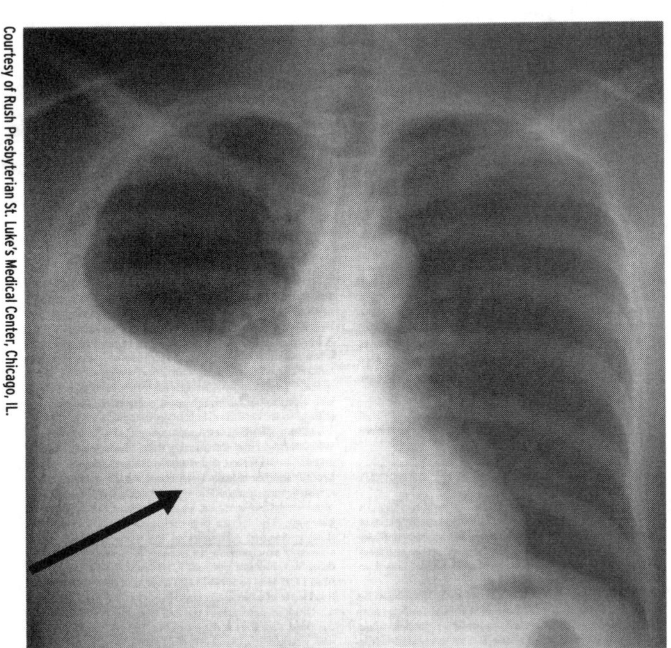

FIGURE 16-3

Chest x-ray film showing right pleural effusion.

may be useful as well, especially if the pleural effusion is the presenting symptom of a malignancy, and can identify fluid loculations, lymphadenopathy, or pleural-based masses.[1,3]

Pleural fluid evaluation

A thoracentesis is typically used in the diagnosis of pleural effusion to confirm the presence of fluid in the pleural space and allow for the evaluation of the pleural fluid. Removal of the pleural fluid often relieves the physical symptoms. A thoracentesis is performed at the bedside or in the outpatient setting under local anesthetic by inserting a needle through the posterior chest wall. The posterior axillary line and the seventh intercostal space are landmarks. A chest x-ray film should be obtained after the procedure to ensure that a pneumothorax has not occurred. Large volumes of fluid can be slowly removed, but fluid removal should not exceed 1500 mL at one time to avoid re-expansion pulmonary edema, hypotension, or circulatory collapse.[3,4,6]

At least 25–50 mL of fluid is needed as a sample to obtain an accurate diagnosis. Pleural fluids are classified as transudates or exudates. Classification of the pleural fluid distinguishes between a benign and a malignant etiology, which in turn directs treatment—either observation or medical/surgical management. A transudative pleural effusion is low in protein and occurs when systemic factors such as cirrhosis or congestive heart failure cause fluid to leak from blood vessels into the pleural space. It is watery, clear, and/or straw colored. Transudative effusions are often seen in individuals with lymphomas, although most transudates indicate a benign process.[3,4,6,17]

Most malignant effusions are classified as exudates. An exudative pleural effusion is a high-protein fluid that leaks from capillary blood vessels that have an increased permeability. Exudates are yellowish and cloudy, or bloody. The visceral and parietal pleurae are often seeded with tumor, which accounts for the typical blood-tinged or bloody fluid. The lactate dehydrogenase (LDH) level of the fluid is elevated secondary to the tissue destruction. Glucose amylase levels, protein levels, and lymphocyte counts are part of the evaluation, as is the appearance of the fluid (straw colored, bloody, turbid, or milky).[3,4,8,12,17,18]

Most malignant effusions are bloody. The chance of misclassifying an exudate is decreased when these three variables are utilized: LDH level, the ratio of pleural fluid LDH level to serum LDH level, and the ratio of pleural fluid protein to serum protein.[3,12,19,20] Studies suggest that the presence of tumor markers in pleural fluid is predictive of a poorer outcome.[21,22] Researchers are also investigating the role of complement factors and genetic analysis of pleural fluid.[11,23]

Cytology determines the cell count and composition of the fluid. This technique is diagnostic in 70%– 80% of individuals with malignant pleural effusions, but is diagnostic in fewer than 33% of patients with leukemia or lymphoma.[19] Pleural fluid pH and glucose levels may be obtained. Pleural glucose less than 28.8 mg/dL and pleural fluid pH less than 7.2 can occur with malignant neoplasms and are associated with a poor prognosis.[12,20]

Thoracoscopy

Thoracoscopy is used for diagnostic purposes when cytological evaluation is unable to confirm a benign or malignant origin for the effusion. Thoracoscopy can be performed under local anesthesia with intravenous sedation or by a video-assisted approach under general anesthesia.[24] This procedure allows visualization of approximately 75% of the visceral and parietal pleurae, and enables the healthcare practitioner to obtain biopsies. A diagnosis may be obtained by this means in nearly 100% of individuals.[1,3] Other advantages of thoracoscopy include complete drainage of pleural fluid, breakdown of loculations, and evaluation for lung entrapment.[3]

DEGREES OF TOXICITY

The toxicity grading for pleural effusions ranges from grade 1 through grade 5. The patient with a grade 1 pleural effusion is asymptomatic and requires observation only. Patients with grade 2 and grade 3 pleural effusions are symptomatic and may require diuretics, oxygen, thoracentesis, pleurectomy, sclerosis, a shunt, or radiation therapy. Grade 5 represents a toxicity-related death. (See Table 16-1.)[25]

TABLE 16-1

National Cancer Institute Common Terminology Criteria for Adverse Events (CTCAE): Non-malignant and Malignant Pleural Effusion

Degree of Toxicity	Symptoms	Treatment
Grade 1	Asymptomatic	Observation, no treatment at this time
Grade 2	Symptomatic	Requires diuretics or limited therapeutic thoracentesis
Grade 3	Symptomatic with respiratory distress	Requires surgical intervention including chest tube or pleurodesis
Grade 4	Life-threatening	Aggressive life-support, end-of-life care if aggressive measures unwarranted
Grade 5	Toxicity-related death	

Source: Data from National Cancer Institute Common Terminology Criteria for Adverse Events (CTCAE)[25].

SYMPTOM MANAGEMENT STRATEGIES FOR PLEURAL EFFUSIONS

THERAPEUTIC APPROACHES

The goal in the management of malignant pleural effusions is symptom relief while maintaining or improving the quality of life. Although some effusions occurring with diseases such as breast cancer, lymphoma, small-cell lung cancer, or ovarian cancer may respond well to chemotherapy, cure is not always possible.[2–4] The choice of medical or surgical treatment depends on several factors: an individual's age, performance status, and prognosis, as well as the site of the primary tumor. If an individual is asymptomatic with a small effusion, treatment is often postponed in favor of observation.[26] Promoting relaxation and stress reduction techniques and providing educational, emotional, and psychosocial support can help to improve the patient's sense of control and participation in care.[27]

Thoracentesis

Some individuals experience relief of symptoms after a diagnostic thoracentesis, and no additional therapy may be indicated. However, 98%–100% of patients with malignant pleural effusion will have fluid reaccumulation within 30 days.[11] In most cases, repeated thoracentesis is not recommended due to the increased risk of pneumothorax, adhesions, empyema, and pleural fluid loculations.[3] Patients who may be considered for repeated thoracentesis include those who have slow reaccumulation after each thoracentesis, have cancers that commonly respond to therapy with resolution of the effusion, have a life expectancy beyond 1–3 months, and are not able to tolerate more invasive interventional procedures such as pleurodesis.[11]

Tube thoracostomy

Chest tubes are inserted to drain pleural fluid and allow apposition of the visceral and parietal pleurae. Individuals are usually premedicated with a narcotic to decrease the discomfort of this procedure and to help relax them before chest tube insertion. Chest tubes connected to water-seal drainage, with negative pressure applied, are left in place until pleural fluid drainage is less than 100 mL/day. Tube thoracostomy alone has a 30-day success rate ranging from only 0% to 40%.[3]

Tube thoracostomy with sclerosing agent

After chest tube insertion, an attempt can be made to eliminate the pleural space by sclerosing together the visceral and parietal pleurae in a process called *chemical pleurodesis* or sclerotherapy. An irritant or sclerosing agent is instilled into the pleural space via the chest tube to induce a pleuritis and obliterate the space. Chest tube drainage should be less than 100 mL/day before sclerosing is attempted. Individuals are premedicated with a narcotic agent 15–30 minutes before sclerotherapy is initiated. The sclerosing agent is instilled in a total volume of 30–50 mL of saline via the chest tube. The chest tube is then flushed with normal saline and clamped for 1–2 hours. The individual is repositioned every 15–30 minutes to distribute the agent equally throughout the pleural cavity (prone, supine, left side, right side). The chest tube is then unclamped and placed to suction until drainage is less than 50–150 mL per 24 hours. Repositioning the individual after the instillation of the sclerosing agent may not be necessary, based on findings that, with some agents, distribution of the agent throughout the pleural cavity may be rapid and complete without repositioning.[28]

TABLE 16-2

Sclerosing Agents for Malignant Pleural Effusions

Most Commonly Used
Talc
Doxycycline
Minocycline
Less Frequently Used
Bleomycin
Cisplatin
Rarely or Never Used
Corynebacterium parvum[a]
Tetracycline[a]
Quinacrine

[a]Used in European and Asian countries.
Source: Data from Heffner[1]; Kwong and Nguyen[3].

Many agents have been used in chemical pleurodesis with varying degrees of effectiveness (Table 16-2).[3,28] The decision as to which sclerosing agent to use is often based on physician and institutional experience as well as patient-related factors. Nitrogen mustard, quinacrine, and thiotepa are no longer used, and injectable tetracycline and *Corynebacterium parvum* are no longer available in the United States.[3] Agents including tetracycline derivatives, minocycline, bleomycin, and sterilized talc are commonly used as sclerosing agents.[3,11,28,29] Doxycycline, which is similar to tetracycline but lacks the latter's toxicity, is commonly used in the treatment of pleural effusions. Bleomycin is an antineoplastic agent used for pleurodesis; it is well tolerated and associated with few side effects.[3]

Thoracoscopy with talc

Talc has been in use since the 1950s and has been consistently shown to be superior to other commonly used sclerosing agents, including doxycycline and bleomycin.[3,8,28] The talc must be sterilized and asbestos free to prevent malignant mesothelioma.[3] Talc is administered into the pleural cavity via the chest tube by insufflation or poudrage. A talc *slurry* consisting of 5–10 grams talc in 250 mL normal saline is instilled via the chest tube. The slurry is left in the pleural cavity for 2 hours. Side effects include pain, dyspnea, fever (up to 102°F, occurring in the first 12 hours and lasting up to 72 hours), and acute respiratory distress syndrome.[8] Talc can also be instilled directly onto the pleural surface via poudrage. Aerosolized talc (5–10 g) is instilled after thoracoscopy with local or general anesthesia. Flexible video-assisted thoracoscopic surgery (VATS) with local or general anesthesia makes this a viable alternative.

Talc pleurodesis is highly effective in controlling pleural effusions, with reported response rates ranging from 80% to 100%.[30,31] Thoracoscopy under general anesthesia is preferred for patient comfort due to the severe pain typically experienced upon talc insufflation. The risk of fever, dyspnea, and acute respiratory distress syndrome necessitate careful monitoring of the individual.[6]

Pleurectomy

Removal of the parietal pleura from the rib cage and mediastinum as well as abrasion of the visceral pleura are reserved for the individual who has failed other therapies and has a high performance status and long life expectancy.[8] The individual must be able to tolerate major surgery. Pleurectomy has been effective in controlling effusions 100% of the time, although postoperative bleeding, pneumonia, air leak, and empyema can occur, along with significant mortality rates.[32]

In addition, video-assisted thoracoscopy makes it possible for parietal pleurectomy without thoracotomy to be performed under general anesthesia via a 2-cm incision. Two small studies (n = 19; n = 11) showed symptomatic recurrence in 15.7% in the first group and 1 death (9%) in the second group.[24,26] This minimally invasive technique warrants further study in the palliative treatment of malignant pleural effusions and could be used in patients who fail to respond to less invasive and less expensive interventions.[1]

Pleuroperitoneal shunt

Although less frequently used, pleuroperitoneal shunting is an alternative for patients who fail sclerotherapy.[3] A silicone rubber catheter with a one-way valve provides palliation of malignant pleural effusions. Under local or general anesthesia, the pumping chamber is placed subcutaneously; the proximal end of the catheter is placed in the pleural cavity, while the distal end is placed in the peritoneum. Patients or families must then be taught to manually pump the chamber to prevent clogging. The chamber requires pumping for 5–10 minutes (more than 100 times) four times a day, limiting its use to only motivated individuals. Complications are few, however, so this procedure can be an alternative for some individuals.

Long-term indwelling pleural catheter

An option for patients requiring repeated thoracentesis or pleurodesis is the placement of a long-term indwelling pleural catheter. A small-caliber silicone rubber indwelling catheter such as the Pleurx® catheter (Surgimedics, Denver Biomaterials, Golden, Colorado) is inserted percutaneously and tunneled subcutaneously under local anesthesia. The external end of the Pleurx® catheter has a unidirectional valve for the removal of pleural fluid and the prevention of air influx into the pleural space. The patient or caregiver can be taught the drainage procedure, which can be performed at home on a daily basis. Advantages of the long-term indwelling catheter are its ease of insertion, ability to perform rapid repeated drainage of reaccumulating pleural fluid without hospitalization or invasive procedures, and maintenance of quality of life.[3] Although the long-term indwelling catheter is becoming more popular clinically, there is limited research comparing the efficacy and safety of the long-term catheter with other available treatments. Further randomized studies are needed before long-term indwelling catheters can be considered first-line therapy for recurrent pleural effusions.[33–40]

External radiation

Individuals with lung cancer or lymphoma diagnosed with an effusion secondary to hilar lymphatic obstruction may benefit from external beam irradiation. Radiation therapy may be the primary treatment modality, or it might be combined with systemic chemotherapy.[8]

Complementary therapies

Disease-related anxiety has a major impact on a patient's quality of life and is common in the patient with a malignant pleural effusion. It may be a result of difficult breathing related to chest pain or heaviness, fear of suffocation, persistent dry cough, or fear of recurrence of the effusion as well as having to repeatedly submit to painful, anxiety-producing procedures. The nurse can be instrumental in teaching anxiety-reducing techniques to the patient with pleural effusion.

Many of these techniques fall under the category of complementary medicine. Nurses are in the forefront of educating patients on the differences between complementary treatments, which are used in conjunction with conventional medicine, and alternative therapies, which are used in place of conventional medicine. A review of the literature reveals increased physician awareness of complementary medicine, the need to become more cognizant of its role in patient care, and patients' desire to explore this modality, especially patients with chronic disease.[41,42] Over the past decade, an increasing number of clinical studies have been conducted investigating complementary therapies and symptom management in the oncology patient population. Mind–body modalities, acupuncture, massage therapy, and relaxation techniques have all shown promising results in reducing anxiety and in improving mood disturbances and pain related to cancer processes and treatment.[43–51] Nurses should be aware of these techniques and share them with patients to help manage symptoms and improve quality of life. Further research in the form of randomized controlled studies investigating complementary therapies is needed to confirm their effectiveness.

DEGREES OF SYMPTOM SEVERITY

Management of the individual with a pleural effusion is a complex process and depends on the treatment modality selected, the individual's performance status, the underlying disease process, and the extent of the effusion (Figure 16-4). The nurse plays an important role in assessing the individual, providing education, and ensuring comfort through selected interventions. In patients whose options are limited to supportive care, complementary therapy offers a range of strategies to decrease anxiety related to symptoms and end-of-life issues, and to empower patients with the knowledge that their health care providers are not abandoning them.

For some individuals with end-stage cancer, end-of-life care may be all that is warranted and desired by the patient. These individuals may be in the last days or weeks of their lives and just wish to be kept comfortable. Morphine sulfate and oxygen therapy are appropriate, as well as complementary approaches. Nurses can help keep the patient comfortable with measures such as positioning and pulmonary hygiene. The aggressiveness that nurses use toward pain management must also be applied to dyspnea. Breathing techniques and exercises, such as breathing from the diaphragm and pursed-lip breathing, provide physical relief, can decrease breathlessness, and empower family members to be active in patient care.[27]

NURSING IMPLICATIONS

In light of patients receiving most care in the outpatient setting, nurses are at the forefront in the care and triage of patients with malignant pleural effusions. More than ever, nurses in ambulatory clinics require the methods and tools for accurate documentation of patient responses to treatment, protocols to address potential problems, and a variety of methods of symptom control. Patients may have a home care nurse who is able to visually assess the patient on a daily basis. A system of calling patients daily is another method to effectively monitor patients who are home after sclerotherapy or catheter/port insertion. This follow-up system is important to patients who may not have coverage for home care nursing services.

While protocols are typically institution specific, it is important that they be developed to address potential problems associated with sclerotherapy and implanted catheters. Highlights of the protocols would include the amount of fluid drainage in 24 hours from an implanted catheter, pain control, fever, signs of infection at the catheter insertion site, increasing shortness of breath and/or cough, and chest pain. A home care nurse or family member can be the contact person for this information. Nurses also need a variety of

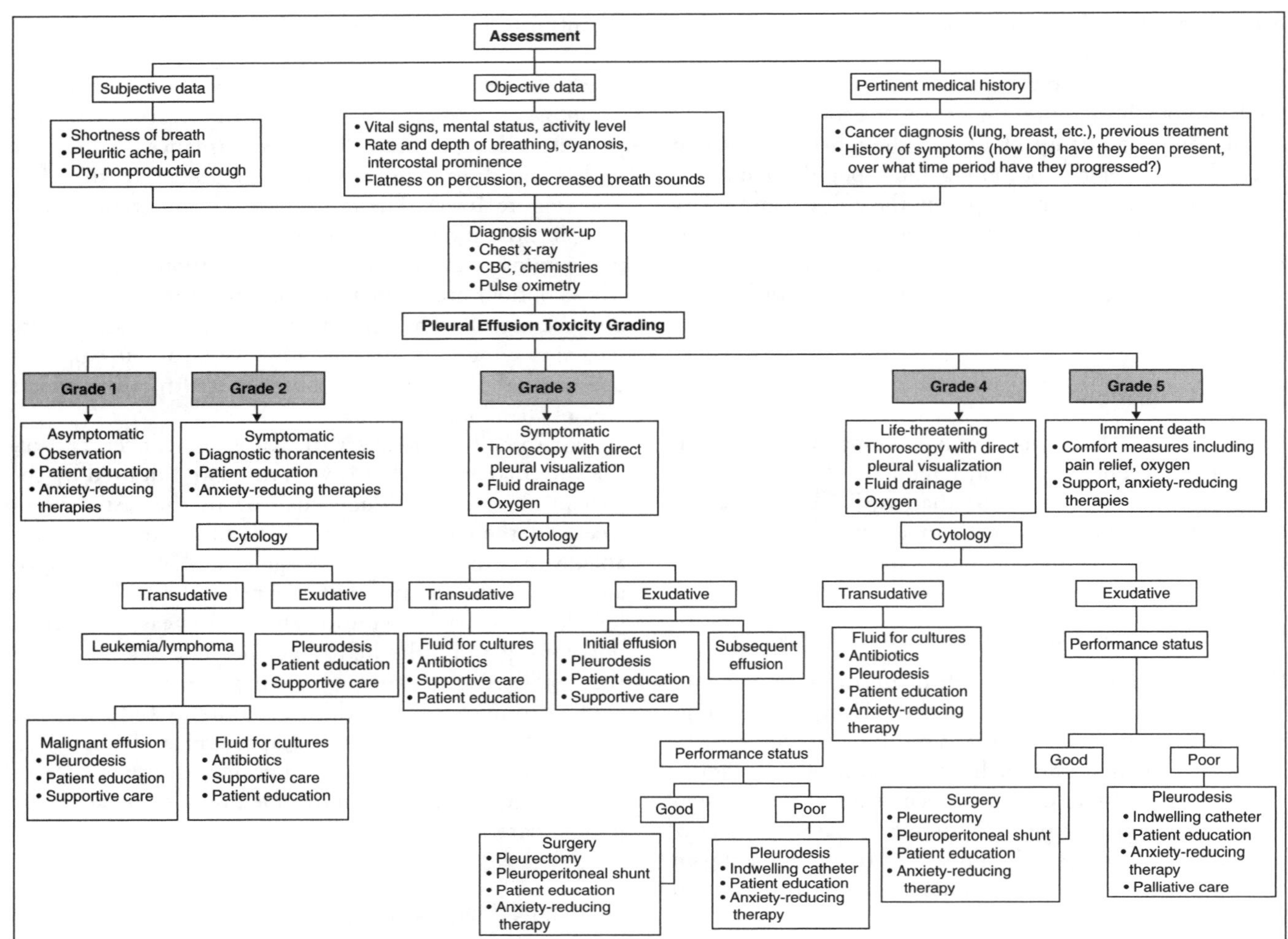

FIGURE 16-4

Nursing algorithm for the management of pleural effusions.

treatment approaches for symptom control, given that no single method is effective for all patients. These methods may include pain medications, positioning to reduce discomfort or ease breathing, energy conservation, use of oxygen, and complementary therapies to help reduce anxiety.[14,45]

PATIENT SELF-CARE FOR PLEURAL EFFUSIONS

The symptom management of malignant pleural effusion requires complex medical management. Individuals are often diagnosed with an effusion late in their disease process and are managed at home, through a hospice, or in the hospital. It is reassuring to individuals if they understand what a pleural effusion is and its symptoms. Appendix 16A includes information for individuals at risk for malignant pleural effusion. In addition, the self-care guide on shortness of breath (see the "Dyspnea" chapter) will help individuals effectively manage dyspnea.

PERICARDIAL EFFUSIONS

INCIDENCE

Pericardial effusion is the most common cardiac complication of cancer. Lung, breast, and hematologic malignancies are responsible for more than 75% of pericardial effusions (Figure 16-5).[6,52]

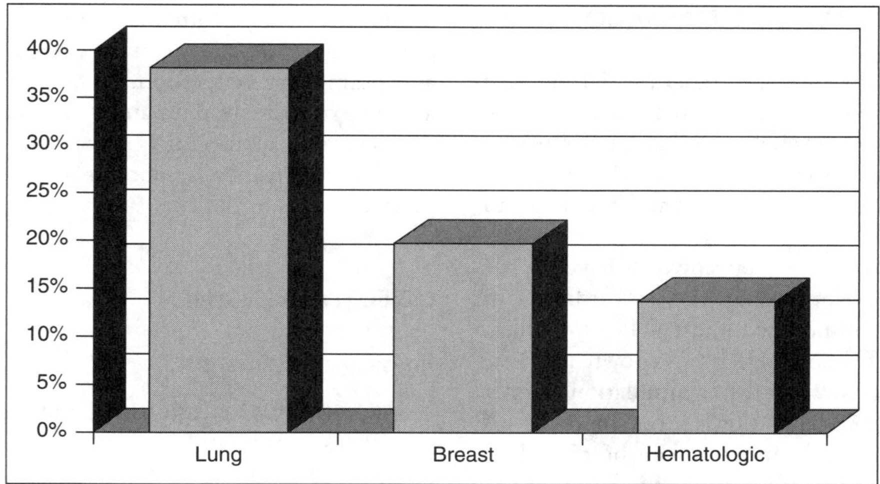

FIGURE 16-5

Tumor types associated with pericardial effusions. Incidence is illustrated as a percent of all pericardial effusions.
Source: Data from Cope[6]; Rahman and Liu[52].

ETIOLOGY

Many patients with cancer develop pericardial effusions that are not directly attributed to their primary malignancies. Although individuals treated with external radiation in doses exceeding 4000 cGy can develop pericardial effusions, the frequency of radiation-induced pericardial effusions has been greatly decreased through dose fractionation, reduced irradiation of heart volume, and modern radiation techniques.[53] Pericardial effusions also can be related to anthracycline therapy, rheumatoid arthritis and other collagen-vascular disease, infection, heart injury, cardiothoracic surgery, renal failure, hypoalbuminemia, or hypothyroidism.[54,55] Treatment of the pericardial effusion may vary depending on its etiology.

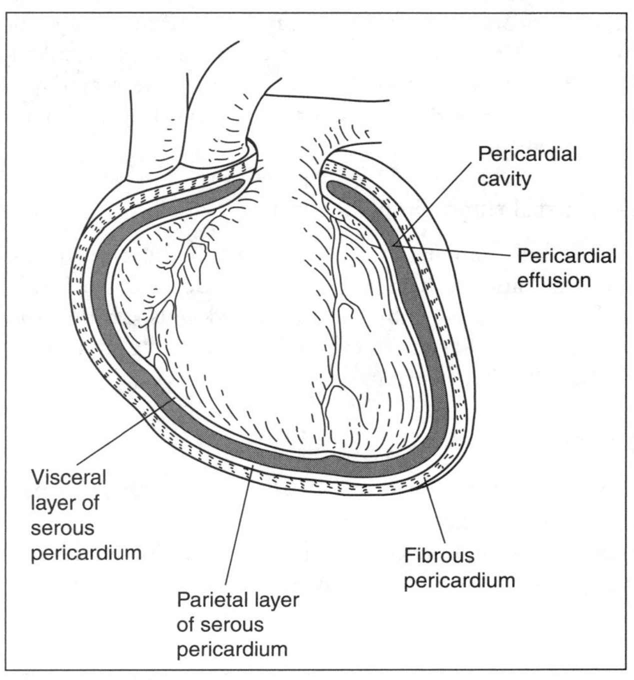

FIGURE 16-6

Structure of the pericardium with effusion present.
Source: Data from Cope[6].

PATHOPHYSIOLOGY OF PERICARDIAL EFFUSIONS

NORMAL PERICARDIAL FLUID FORMATION

The heart and a portion of the great vessels are surrounded by the double-layered pericardium. The outer fibrous layer, or *parietal pericardium*, protects the heart and holds it in position. The inner serous layer, termed the *visceral pericardium* or *epicardium*, surrounds the surface of the heart. Between these two layers is the pericardial cavity (Figure 16-6). The pericardial cavity is lubricated by 10–20 mL of fluid, averaging less than 50 mL fluid at any one time.[3,56] As with pleural effusions, Starling's hypothesis dictates that the equilibrium of pericardial fluid is maintained through four factors: capillary permeability, hydrostatic and osmotic pressures, and lymphatic drainage. Both the visceral and parietal pericardia have channels that empty into the mediastinal lymphatics.[6,56]

ABNORMAL PERICARDIAL FLUID FORMATION

As pericardial fluid accumulates, intrapericardial pressure increases, which compresses the heart. To maintain cardiac output, the body compensates by increasing heart rate and by increasing peripheral vasoconstriction. If left untreated, these compensatory mechanisms progress and are unable to maintain cardiac output.[6]

Pericardial effusions can develop slowly or have a rapid onset. If an effusion develops slowly, the pericardium can actually stretch to accommodate almost 4 liters of fluid. Rapidly developing effusions have been known to cause severe cardiac compromise with the accumulation of only 50–80 mL of fluid.[53] An alteration in the mechanisms that control pericardial fluid formation can be caused by lymphatic obstruction, pericardial tumor implantation, or direct tumor invasion of the heart.

Lymphatic obstruction

Obstruction of the mediastinal lymph nodes with tumor, as occurs in patients with lung and breast cancer, interrupts pericardial fluid flow. Capillary permeability and hydrostatic and osmotic pressures are altered, resulting in increased pericardial fluid formation. The majority of malignant pericardial effusions are the result of lymphatic and venous obstruction.[6]

Pericardial tumor implantation

Tumor cells can metastasize directly to the pericardium via lymphatic or hematogenous spread. The pericardial surfaces are irritated by the implanted cells, leading to a change in capillary permeability and resulting in a malignant pericardial effusion.[6]

Direction invasion

Mediastinal tumors can invade the heart directly. Primary tumors of the heart are uncommon; instead, the condition usually represents a variant of sarcomas, lymphoma, malignant fibrous histiocytoma, and mesothelioma of the pericardium.[53]

SYMPTOM ASSESSMENT OF PERICARDIAL EFFUSIONS

SELF-ASSESSMENT

A patient with a pericardial effusion initially may be asymptomatic until there is progression of cardiac involvement. The first symptom reported by patients is dyspnea, which can be accompanied by complaints of dull, diffuse chest pain. The experience of dyspnea can diminish quality of life and limit performance status. With additional fluid accumulation, a patient can experience fatigue, dry cough, and pulmonary congestion.[53] The patient may experience anxiety with the dyspnea and depressed feelings related to the decreased quality of life and activity limitations. For the older adult, these symptoms may be greater because of preexisting comorbidities.

OBJECTIVE ASSESSMENT

Physical assessment

Many pericardial effusions go undetected as individuals remain asymptomatic for cardiac involvement throughout the course of their disease. Physical findings often are present only when a pericardial effusion causes a decrease in cardiac output. Because individuals are increasingly being supported in the outpatient setting, nurses should be familiar with the signs and symptoms of pericardial effusions.

Pericardial effusions are usually characterized by a slow onset, but in some individuals they develop rapidly as the first sign of a malignancy. The malignancies that account for the majority of malignant pericardial effusions are lung cancer, breast cancer, and hematologic malignancies.[53] Symptoms of pericardial effusion include dyspnea, cough, chest pain, orthopnea, fever, edema, fatigue, weakness, and dizziness.[8,53] *Cardiac tamponade* is the term used to describe the severe decrease in cardiac output caused by pericardial effusion. Symptoms include a rapid progression of dyspnea with chest tightness. Individuals are anxious and often assume a forward-leaning position to obtain relief.[6,8,53,55,57]

Physical findings include tachycardia (more than 100 beats/minute), cyanosis, tachypnea, jugular venous distention, peripheral edema, and irregular heart rate.[53] Cardiac assessment may also reveal cardiac enlargement, pericardial dullness, pericardial friction rub, and distant weak heart sounds. Hepatosplenomegaly and ascites are less common. Breath sounds are usually clear. Cardiac tamponade includes hypotension and pulsus paradoxus (a large decrease in systolic pressure, more than 10 mm Hg on inspiration).[53]

Diagnostic evaluation

Many individuals with slowly developing pericardial effusions remain asymptomatic for a long time. Routine chest x-ray and electrocardiogram may reveal subtle abnormalities, increasing suspicion for pericardial effusion. Knowledge of the etiology of malignant pericardial effusions will help nurses identify those individuals at increased risk.

An anterior-posterior chest x-ray typically reveals an enlargement of the normal contour of the heart due to the increased amount of fluid in the pericardial sac. However, a normal chest x-ray does not rule out the possibility of a pericardial effusion. Therefore, due to their lack of specificity, chest x-rays are combined with other diagnostic tools in the evaluation of pericardial effusions.[2]

Some nonspecific changes noted on electrocardiogram (ECG) that are seen with pericardial effusions include sinus tachycardia, atrial and ventricular arrhythmias, and nonspecific ST-segment changes and T-wave changes.[2] Cardiac tamponade classically produces electrical alternans, a change in amplitude of the P wave and QRS complex with every other beat.[2,57]

Computerized tomography (CT) can be helpful in the diagnosis of pericardial effusions. High-density areas of fluid, pericardial thickening, and pericardial masses are visualized when viewing the heart.

Echocardiography (ECHO) is a quick, reliable, noninvasive diagnostic tool that can establish the presence of small amounts of pericardial fluid. An echocardiogram accurately demonstrates the effect of the effusion on ventricular function. It is the most commonly used diagnostic test when a pericardial effusion is suspected.

Another tool used in the diagnosis of pericardial effusion is percutaneous pericardiocentesis, used only for individuals with symptoms from large effusions or cardiac tamponade.[2,53] This invasive procedure is performed with the assistance of fluoroscopy or echocardiography to decrease the risk of cardiac puncture, ventricular tachycardia, and tension pneumothorax. Under local anesthetic, the pericardial sac is entered just to the left of the xiphoid process. The pericardial fluid aspirated is classified as a transudate or an exudate and then may be assessed for bacteria, fungi, and mycobacteria. Cytology has confirmed malignant cells in approximately 60% of patients with neoplastic pericarditis.[3]

DEGREES OF TOXICITY

Toxicity associated with pericardial effusions is divided into five grades (Table 16-3). Grade 1 is asymptomatic and requires observation only. Grade 2 also requires observation, but is associated with pericarditis. Patients with grade 3 toxicity are symptomatic and generally require oxygen, pericardiocentesis, or surgical placement of a pericardial window or catheter. A patient with grade 4 toxicity has cardiac tamponade and requires aggressive life support, or end-of-life care if aggressive measures are unwarranted. Grade 5 toxicity is toxicity-related death.

SYMPTOM MANAGEMENT STRATEGIES FOR PERICARDIAL EFFUSIONS

THERAPEUTIC APPROACHES

The goal of therapy in the treatment of malignant pericardial effusion is to completely remove the pericardial fluid and prevent reaccumulation, with minimal morbidity. The individual's primary diagnosis, stage of disease, and performance status must be considered. Some individuals may require immediate systemic treatment of cardiac tamponade to increase cardiac output before mechanical interventions can be considered. Emergency measures include intravenous plasma or colloid solutions for volume expansion and sympathomimetic agents such as isoproterenol hydrochloride.[57]

Pericardiocentesis

Therapeutic pericardiocentesis is most often utilized in the initial management of pericardial effusion. Pericardiocentesis alone has been successful in removing fluid and initially

TABLE 16-3

National Cancer Institute Common Terminology Critieria for Adverse Events (CTCAE): Nonmalignant and Malignant Pericardial Effusion

Degree of Toxicity	Symptoms	Treatment
Grade 1	Asymptomatic	Observation, no treatment at this time
Grade 2	Asymptomatic effusion small to moderate	Observation, no treatment at this time
Grade 3	Symptomatic effusion with physiologic consequenses	May require O_2, therapeutic pericardiocentesis, surgery, pericardial window, catheter
Grade 4	Life-threatening	Aggressive life-support, end-of-life care if aggressive measures unwarranted
Grade 5	Toxicity-related death	

Source: Data from National Cancer Institute Common Terminology Criteria for Adverse Events (CTCAE)[25].

alleviating symptoms, but fluid reaccumulation occurs in approximately 40%–50% of patients; thus this approach is not beneficial except in cases of life-threatening cardiac tamponade.[54]

Pericardiocentesis with sclerosing agent

Pericardiocentesis with the use of sclerosing agents is often attempted in an effort to obliterate the pericardial space when there is persistent or relapsing effusion.[54] Chemical agents are used for their antitumor activity or to induce an inflammatory response in the pericardium to achieve symphysis of the epicardium and parietal pericardium. Sclerosing agents include bleomycin, cisplatin, vinblastine, sterile talc, tetracycline, and doxycycline.[3,6] Pain, fever, and myelosuppression are reported side effects. Many of the studies that have been conducted included only small numbers of subjects, making it difficult to compare the efficacy of these sclerosing agents. Randomized controlled studies need to be conducted to confirm the effectiveness of this approach.

Radiation therapy

Radiation therapy to treat pericardial effusions has been used most successfully in radiosensitive tumors such as lymphomas, leukemias, or breast cancers. When radiation therapy was used to treat pericardial effusion in lymphomas and leukemias, the success rate was reported as 93%, whereas a success rate of 71% was reported with breast cancers.[3]

Chemotherapy

Systemic chemotherapy with or without external beam radiation has been used to treat pericardial effusions in lymphoma, breast, and solid tumors.[57,58] After initial drainage of the effusion by pericardiocentesis, chemotherapy may help prevent recurrence of pericardial fluid.

Surgery

Surgery is a treatment reserved for individuals who require repeated pericardiocentesis and can withstand the stress of surgery. Surgery may also be necessary if the diagnosis is uncertain and a biopsy is needed. Surgical interventions include indwelling pericardial catheter, subxiphoid pericardial window, thoracotomy with pleuropericardiotomy, thoracotomy with pericardiectomy, and percutaneous balloon pericardiotomy (Table 16-4).

The subxiphoid pericardiectomy (window) is performed under local anesthesia with intravenous sedation or general anesthesia; it is associated with few side effects and low morbidity.[3] Biopsies can be obtained with this procedure. An incision is made beneath the xiphoid process, and a portion of the parietal pericardium is excised, creating a "window" to allow pericardial fluid to drain into the pleural space or subcutaneous tissue. This procedure has been effective in controlling effusions 90% to 100% of the time.[3,58]

TABLE 16-4

Approaches for Prevention of Recurrent Pericardial Effusion
Subxiphoid pericardiectomy (window)
Thoracotomy with pleuropericardiotomy (window)
Percutaneous balloon pericardiotomy
Indwelling pericardial catheter
Thoracotomy with pericardiectomy

Source: Data from Kwong and Nguyen[3]; Lestuzzi[58].

A *thoracotomy* requires general anesthesia and a patient with a high performance status. This approach may not be appropriate for all patients and does not offer a reduced rate of recurrence.[3] Through a median sternotomy, the pericardium is entered, fluid is drained, and biopsies can be taken. In a *pericardiectomy*, the majority of the pericardium is excised while protecting the phrenic nerves on both sides. Chest tubes are left in place until drainage is minimal. Complications include arrhythmias (particularly atrial arrhythmias), bleeding, infection, and hemothorax. In a *pleuropericardiotomy*, a smaller portion ("window") of the pericardium is excised.

Pericardioperitoneal shunt

As for pleural effusions, implanted shunts using a Denver® catheter have been successfully used to treat patients with pericardial effusions. Under local anesthesia, one end of the catheter is placed in the pericardial sac, with the other end placed in the peritoneum to allow for continuous fluid drainage. Patients are generally discharged within 4 days. There is limited experience with this shunt method, but further studies may show it to be effective in controlling pericardial effusions with less morbidity and mortality.[3]

Percutaneous balloon pericardiotomy

A percutaneous balloon pericardiotomy is an alternative method used to prevent the reaccumulation of pericardial fluid that allows for a shorter hospital stay. Using the same approach as a pericardiocentesis, a guide is placed into the pericardial space. A balloon-dilating catheter is exchanged over the guide wire and inflated, creating a "window" in the pericardium.[3,58] A catheter is left in place to drain the effusion, and a chest x-ray is obtained to assess for pneumothorax. This procedure can be done under local anesthesia, which has a success rate of 92%, but it has a complication rate of 18%, with potential adverse effects including fever, balloon rupture, and pleural effusion requiring drainage.[58]

DEGREES OF SYMPTOM SEVERITY

Due to the possibility that fluid might develop rapidly in the pericardial space, giving rise to symptoms of cardiac tamponade, nurses must have a clear understanding of pericardial effusion and its management. Nurses play an important role in the assessment of individuals in the outpatient, home, or hospital setting. Figure 16-7 provides an algorithm for the management of pericardial effusion.[53] Initial management may require emergency interventions; further treatment of a pericardial effusion will depend on the stage of disease and performance status of the individual. Nurses need to educate, reassure, and comfort the individual as well as perform specific nursing interventions. As in the management of pleural effusions, complementary alternatives provide patients and their caregivers with strategies to reduce anxiety and provide symptom management.

NURSING IMPLICATIONS

Like their counterparts with pleural effusions, patients with pericardial effusions are receiving a greater amount of care in the outpatient setting. Nurses are generally the patient's first contact whenever there is a problem in the outpatient setting. Methods and tools for accurate documentation

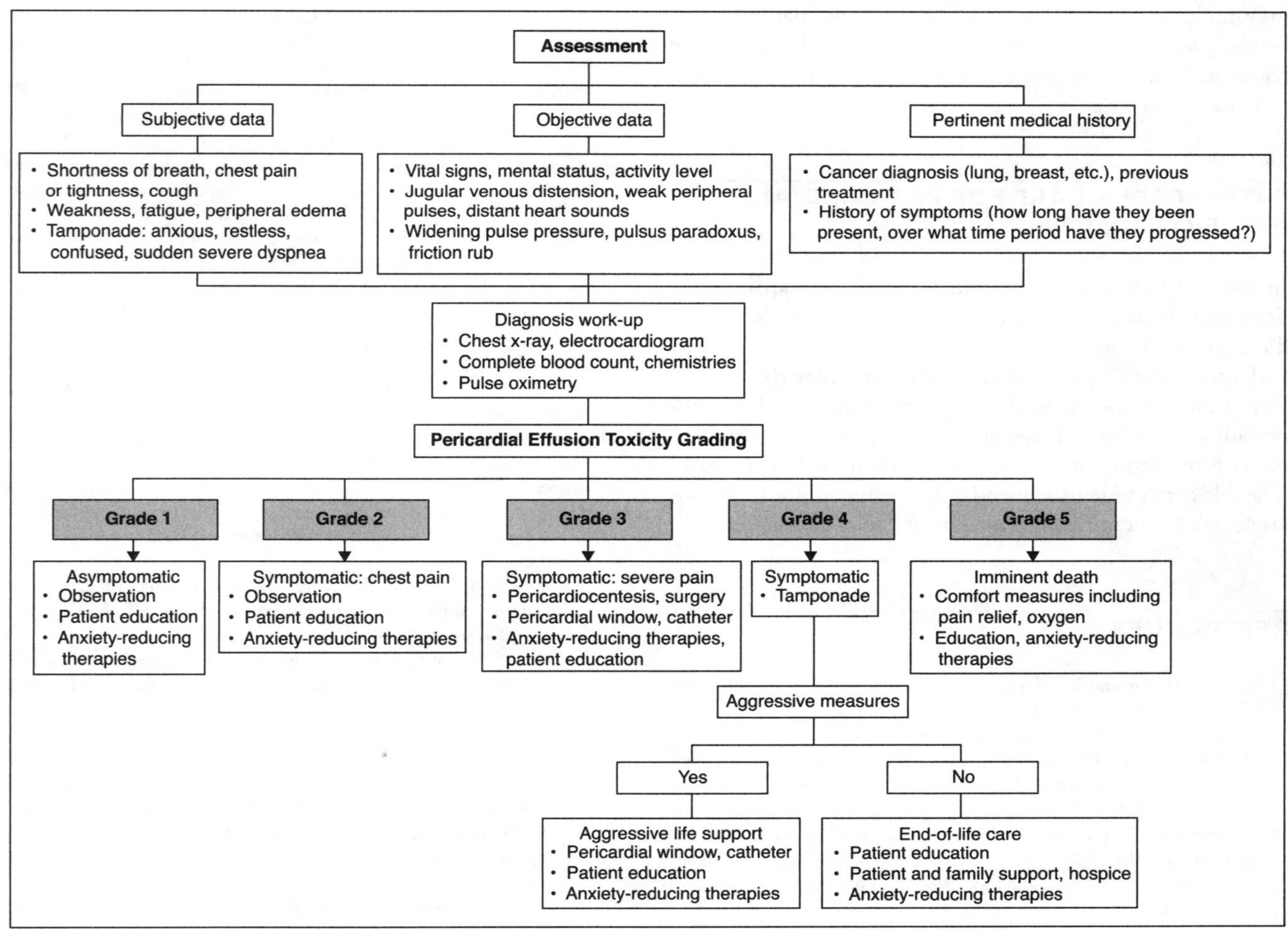

FIGURE 16-7

Algorithm for the management of pericardial effusion.

of patient responses to treatment, protocols to address potential problems, and a variety of methods of symptom control are crucial to optimize patient care. Patients being discharged from the hospital may have a home care nurse who is able to directly assess the patient on a daily basis. A system of calling patients daily is another method to effectively monitor patients who are home after having pericardial windows, balloon pericardiotomy, or placement of a pericardioperitoneal shunt.

Protocols are usually institution specific and should address potential problems associated with patients undergoing procedures to control pericardial effusions. Critical areas include the amount of fluid drainage in 24 hours from an implanted catheter, pain control, fever, signs of infection or bleeding, and signs of pleural effusion or pneumothorax. A home care nurse or family member can be the contact person for this information. Nurses also need a variety of methods for symptom control, given that no one method is effective for all patients. These methods may include a change in pain medications, patient positioning to reduce discomfort or ease breathing, energy conservation, use of oxygen, or complementary therapies to help reduce anxiety.[53,57]

PATIENT SELF-CARE FOR PERICARDIAL EFFUSIONS

In some asymptomatic individuals, small pericardial effusions may be detected on a routine chest x-ray or electrocardiogram. It is important to teach these patients the signs and symptoms of pericardial effusions so that they might alert a member of the healthcare team before cardiac tamponade occurs. Knowledge of potential problems empowers patients to become active members of their healthcare team. The self-care guide in Appendix 16B is useful for individuals at risk for pericardial effusions or their recurrence.

REFERENCES

1. Heffner JE. Diagnosis and management of malignant pleural effusions. *Respiration.* 2008;13:5–20.
2. LeWinter MM, Tischler MD. Pericardial diseases. In: Bonow RO, Mann DL, Zipes DP, Libby P. *Braunwald's Heart Disease: A Textbook of Cardiovascular Medicine.* 9th ed. St. Louis, MO: Elsevier/Saunders; 2011:1655–1660.
3. Kwong KF, Nguyen DM. Malignant effusions of the pleura and the pericardium. In: DeVita VT, Lawrence TS, Rosenberg SA. *Cancer: Principles and Practice Oncology.* 9th ed. Philadelphia: Lippincott Williams & Wilkins; 2011:2729–2744.
4. Mulley AG. Evaluation of pleural effusions. In: Gorall AH, Mulley AG. *Primary Care Medicine: Office Evaluation and Management of the Adult Patient.* 6th ed. Philadelphia: Lippincott Williams & Wilkins; 2009:361–365.
5. Held-Warmkessel J, Schiech L. Caring for the patient with malignant pleural effusion. *Nursing.* 2008;38:43–47.
6. Cope DG. Malignant effusions. In: Yarbro CH, Wujcik D, Gobel BH. *Cancer Nursing: Principles and Practice.* 7th ed. Burlington, MA: Jones & Bartlett Learning; 2011:863–878.
7. Cope DG. Pleural effusions: malignant. In: Chernecky CC, Murphy-Ende K, eds. *Acute Care Oncology Nursing.* 2nd ed. St. Louis, MO: Elsevier/Saunders; 2008:435–441.
8. Juergens RA, Spira AI, Brahmer JR. Effusions. In: Abeloff MD, Armitage JO, Niederhuber JE, et al. *Abeloff's Clinical Oncology.* 4th ed. New York: Churchill Livingston; 2008:925–944.
9. Clark JW. Approach to the patient with lung cancer. In: Goroll AH, Mulley AG. *Primary Care Medicine: Office Evaluation and Management of the Adult Patient.* 6th ed. Philadelphia: Lippincott Williams & Wilkins; 2009:433–438.
10. Lewis GM, Chai A. The cancer patient in the emergency department. In: Wolfson AB. *Harwood-Nuss' Clinical Practice of Emergency Medicine.* 5th ed. Philadelphia: Lippincott Williams & Wilkins; 2010:984–989.
11. Heffner JE, Klein JS. Recent advances in the diagnosis and management of malignant pleural effusions. *Mayo Clin Proc.* 2008:83:235–250.
12. McGrath EE, Anderson PB. Diagnosis of pleural effusion: a systematic approach. *Am J Crit Care.* 2011;20:119–128.
13. Ripamonti C, Bruera E. Dyspnea: pathophysiology and assessment. *J Pain Symptom Manage.* 1997;13:220–232.
14. Gift AG, Narsavage G. Validity of the numeric rating scale as a measure of dyspnea. *Am J Crit Care.* 1998;7:200–204.
15. Lareau SC, Carrieri-Kohlman V, Janson-Bjerklie S, Roos PJ. Development and testing of the Pulmonary Functional Status and Dyspnea Questionnaire (PFSDQ). *Heart Lung.* 1994;23:242–250.
16. Gaguski ME, Brandsema M, Gernalin L, Martinez E. Assessing dyspnea in patients with non-small cell lung cancer in the acute care setting. *Clin J Oncol Nurs.* 2010;14:509–513.
17. Reddy RM. Chest wall, pleura, mediastinum, and nonneoplastic lung disease. In: Mulholland MW, Lillemoe KD, Doherty GM, et al, eds. *Greenfield's Surgery Scientific Principles and Practice.* 5th ed. Philadelphia: Lippincott Williams & Wilkins; 2011:1391–1429.
18. Heffner J. Discriminating between transudates and exudates. *Clin Chest Med.* 2006;27:241–252.
19. Froudarakis ME. Diagnostic work-up of pleural effusions. *Respiration.* 2008;75:4–13.
20. Porcel JM, Light RW. Diagnostic approach to pleural effusion in adults. *Am Fam Physician.* 2006;73:4–13.
21. Bielsa S, Esquerda A, Salud A, et al. High levels of tumor markers in pleural fluid correlate with poor survival in patients with adenocarcinomatous or squamous malignant effusions. *Eur J Intern Med.* 2009;20:383–386.
22. Liang QL, Shi HZ, Qin XJ, Liang XD, Jiang J, Yang HB. Diagnostic accuracy of tumor markers for malignant pleural effusion: a meta-analysis. *Thorax.* 2008;63:35–41.
23. Shitrit D, Ollech JE, Ollech A, et al. Diagnostic value of complement components in pleural fluid: report of 135 cases. *Respir Med.* 2008;102:1631–1635.
24. Heffner JE. Management of the patient with a malignant pleural effusion. *Semin Respir Crit Care Med.* 2010;31:723–733.
25. National Cancer Institute Common terminology criteria for adverse events (CTCAE) http://evs.nci.nih.gov/ftp1/CTCAE/CTCAE_4.03_2010-06-14_QuickReference_5x7.pdf. Accessed 1/21/13.
26. Musani AI. Treatment options for malignant pleural effusion. *Curr Opin Pulm Med.* 2009;15:380–387.
27. DiSalvo WM, Joyce MM, Tyson LB, Tyson LB, Culkin AE, Mackay K. Putting evidence into practice: evidence-based interventions for cancer-related dyspnea. *Clin J Oncol Nurs.* 2008;12:341–352.
28. Rodriguez-Panadero F, Romero-Romero B. Management of pleural effusions. *Curr Opin Pulm Med.* 2011;17:269–273.

29. Noppen MMP. Pleurodesis for malignant pleural effusion: the optimal agent and methodology. http://www.chestnet.org/accp/pccsu/pleurodesis-malignant-pleural-effusion-optimal-agent-and-methodology. Accessed December 3, 2012.
30. Tan C, Sedrakyan A, Browne J, et al. The evidence on the effectiveness of management of malignant pleural effusion: a systematic review. *Eur J Cardiothorac Surg.* 2006;29:829–838.
31. Steger V, Mika U, Toomes H, et al. Who gains most? A 10 year experience with 611 thoracoscopic talc pleurodeses. *Ann Thorac Surg.* 2007;83:1940–1945.
32. Nakas A, Martin Ucar AE, Edwards JG, Waller DA. The role of video-assisted thoracoscopic pleurectomy/decortication in the therapeutic management of malignant pleural mesothelioma. *Eur J Cardiothorac Surg.* 2008;33:83–87.
33. Sioris T, Sihvo E, Salo J, Räsänen J, Knuuttila A. Long-term indwelling pleural catheter (Pleurx®) for malignant pleural effusion unsuitable for talc pleurodesis. *Eur J Surg Oncol.* 2008;35:546–51.
34. Tremblay A, Michaud G. Single-center experience with 250 tunnelled pleural catheter insertions for malignant pleural effusion. *Chest.* 2006;129:362–368.
35. Khaleeq G, Musani A. Emerging paradigms in the management of malignant pleural effusions. *Respir Med.* 2008;102:939–948.
36. Neragi-Miandoab S. Malignant pleural effusion, current and evolving approaches for its diagnosis and management. *Lung Cancer.* 2006;54:1–9.
37. van den Toorn LM, Schaap E, Surmont VFM, et al. Management of recurrent malignant pleural effusions with a chronic indwelling pleural catheter. *Lung Cancer.* 2005;50:123–127.
38. Tremblay A, Mason C, Michaud G. Use of tunnelled catheters for malignant pleural effusions in patients fit for pleurodesis. *Eur Respir J.* 2007;30:759–762.
39. Warren WH, Kalimi R, Khodadadian LM, Kim AW. Management of malignant pleural effusions using the Pleur(x) catheter. *Ann Thorac Surg.* 2008;85:1049–1055.
40. Van Meter ME, McKee KY, Kohlwes RJ. Efficacy and safety of tunneled pleural catheters in adults with malignant pleural effusions: a systematic review. *J Gen Intern.* 2011;26:70–76.
41. Lee RT, Hlubocky FJ, Hu JJ, Stafford RS, Daugherty CK. An international pilot study of oncology physicians' opinions and practices on complementary and alternative medicine (CAM). *Integr Cancer Ther.* 2008;7:70–75.
42. Verhoef MJ, Boon HS, Page SA. Talking to cancer patients about complementary therapies: is it the physician's responsibility? *Curr Oncol.* 2008;suppl 2:s88–93.
43. Falkensteiner M, Mantovan F, Muller I, Them C. The use of massage therapy for reducing pain, anxiety, and depression in oncological palliative care patients: a narrative review of the literature. *ISRN Nurs.* 2011; 929868.
44. Wilkinson S, Barnes K, Storey L. Massage for symptom relief in patients with cancer: systematic review. *J Adv Nurs.* 2008;63:430–439.
45. Ernst E. Massage therapy for cancer palliation and supportive care: a systematic review of randomised clinical trials. *Support Care Cancer.* 2009;17:333–337.
46. Russell NC, Sumler SS, Beinhorn CM, Frenkel MA. Role of massage therapy in cancer care. *J Altern Complement Med.* 2008;14:209–214.
47. Mansky PJ, Wallerstedt DB. Complementary medicine in palliative care and cancer symptom management. *Cancer J.* 2006;12:425–431.
48. Wilkinson S, Barnes K, Storey L. Massage for symptom relief in patients with cancer: systematic review. *J Adv Nurs.* 2008;63(5):430–439.
49. Wilkinson SM, Love SB, Westcombe AM, et al. Effectiveness of aromatherapy massage in the management of anxiety and depression in patients with cancer: a multicenter randomized controlled trial. *J Clin Oncol.* 2007;25:532–539.
50. Smith ME, Bauer-Wu S. Traditional Chinese medicine for cancer-related symptoms. *Semin Oncol Nurs.* 2012;28:64–74.
51. Dean-Clower E, Doherty-Gilman AM, Keshaviah A, et al. Acupuncture as palliative therapy for physical symptoms and quality of life for advanced cancer patients. *Integr Cancer Ther.* 2010;9:158–167.
52. Rahman A, Liu D. Pericarditis: clinical features and management. *Aus Fam Phys.* 2011;40:791–796.
53. Shelton BK. Pericarditis/pericardial effusion/pericardial tamponade. In: Camp-Sorrell D, Hawkins RA, eds. *Clinical Manual for the Advanced Oncology Nurse.* 2nd ed. Pittsburgh, PA: Oncology Nursing Press; 2006:369–383.
54. Sagrista-Sauleda J, Merce AS, Soler-Soler J. Diagnosis and management of pericardial effusion. *World J Cardiol.* 2011;3:135–143.
55. Hoit BD. Pericardial disease and pericardial tamponade. *Crit Care Med.* 2007;35(suppl):S355–S364.
56. Khandaker MH, Espinosa RE, Nishimura RA, et al. Pericardial disease: diagnosis and management. *Mayo Clin Proc.* 2010;85:572–593.
57. Shelton BK. Cardiac tamponade and pericardial effusions. In: Chernecky CC, Murphy-Ende K, eds. *Acute Care Oncology Nursing.* 2nd ed. St. Louis, MO: Saunders/Elsevier; 2009:45–58.
58. Lestuzzi C. Neoplastic pericardial disease: Old and current strategies for diagnosis and management. *World J Cardiol.* 2010;26:270–279.

Pleural Effusion (Fluid Around the Lungs)

Patient Name: ____

Symptom and Description

A pleural effusion occurs when fluid collects in the space around the lungs. Pleural effusions can occur with cancer, but can also occur in people with other illness. When this happens, the lungs cannot fully expand, and breathing may become difficult and painful. Pain, shortness of breath, and lung infections can occur if an effusion gets bigger or is not treated.

Prevention

There is no method to prevent a pleural effusion that is caused by cancer. But, you should know about the symptoms and report them to your doctor or nurse right away:

- Feve.
- A dry cough
- Shortness of breath
- The need to breathe fast
- Chest pain, which may be slight or severe. The pain may be worse when you lie on one side or the other.

Management

If you have any of these symptoms, your doctor may want to see you. The doctor will order a chest x-ray to see if there is fluid in the lungs. If fluid is seen or suspected, a test called a thoracentesis is done. This test takes off fluid from the space around the lung. Many times, people breathe easier when the fluid is taken off.

If you are short of breath or if breathing is difficult or painful, there are things you can do to help yourself breathe easier:

- Some movements allow your lungs to better expand. Sit upright, lean forward, and rest your forearms on a table.
- Sleep with the head of the bed raised or use pillows to raise your upper body. Some people feel better sleeping in a chair that reclines.
- Save your energy. Do chores early in the day (bathing, stair climbing). Take time to rest and relax.
- The doctor may order oxygen to help you breathe.
- Take your pain medication. Some medicines help to relax you and help you breathe easier.
- There is no special diet to follow. Small frequent meals (as many as 6 meals per day) might be easier for you and may tire you less.
- Drink 2–3 liters of fluids per day, unless your doctor or nurse tells you differently.

Follow-Up

The fluid is sent to the lab for more tests. The doctor will talk to you about further treatment when those results are in. Let your doctor or nurse know if the symptoms are getting worse.

Phone Numbers

Nurse: ______________________ Phone: ______________________

Physician: ______________________ Phone: ______________________

Other: ______________________ Phone: ______________________

Source: Cope DG. Effusions. In: Yarbro CH, Wujcik D, Gobel BH, eds. *Cancer Symptom Management.* 4th ed. Burlington, MA: Jones & Bartlett Learning; 2014.

Pericardial Effusion (Fluid Around the Heart)

Patient Name: ____________________

This guide will help you learn the signs of pericardial effusion.

Symptom and Description

Pericardial effusions can develop in patients with cancer. A pericardial effusion occurs when fluid collects in the space around the heart. This can happen slowly or very quickly.

You should report any of the symptoms to your doctor or your nurse:

- Cough
- Weakness
- Feeling dizzy
- Feeling restless
- Shortness of breath
- Swollen hands or feet
- Feeling tired all the time
- Chest pain or chest tightness
- A change in memory or feeling confused

Management

If you have any of these symptoms, your doctor may want to see you. The doctor will order a test to look at your heart, called an echocardiogram. A chest x-ray and electrocardiogram (EKG) may also be ordered. If fluid is seen around your heart, you will need to come to the hospital for test called a pericardiocentesis. This test will remove fluid from the space around your heart.

Follow-Up

The doctor will talk to you about any further treatment. Further treatment will try to prevent more fluid from collecting in the space around your heart.

Phone Numbers

Nurse: ____________________ Phone: ____________________

Physician: ____________________ Phone: ____________________

Other: ____________________ Phone: ____________________

Source: Cope DG. Effusions. In: Yarbro CH, Wujcik D, Gobel BH, eds. *Cancer Symptom Management.* 4th ed. Burlington, MA: Jones & Bartlett Learning; 2014.

PART VII

Alterations in Nutrition

CHAPTER 17

The Cancer Cachexia Syndrome

Regina S. Cunningham, PhD, RN, AOCN®

THE PROBLEM

Although it is a consequence of a number of serious illnesses, including chronic heart failure, infectious diseases, rheumatoid arthritis, and Alzheimer's disease, cachexia may reveal its most profound and debilitating face in patients with cancer. The term *cachexia* derives from the Greek *kakos*, meaning "bad," and *hexis*, meaning "condition." Hippocrates described patients with cachexia as having their flesh consumed, falling from their bones, or melting away, and indicated that the illness was fatal.[1] Cachexia is characterized by progressive loss of body weight, incremental tissue wasting with loss of somatic muscle, poor performance, decreased quality of life, and ultimately death.[2–5] Loss of skeletal muscle and fat are factors that distinguish this condition from starvation.[6]

Myriad definitions of cachexia can be found in the literature. Recently, an international group of experts engaged in a formal consensus process to develop a framework for the definition and classification of cachexia.[7] This group defined cancer cachexia as a multifactorial syndrome associated with an ongoing loss of skeletal muscle mass that cannot be fully reversed by traditional nutrition support interventions and leads to progressive impairment in functional status. Experts agreed that diagnostic criteria for cancer cachexia should include weight loss greater than 5%, or any significant weight loss greater than 2% in the presence of either low body mass index (BMI) or low skeletal muscle mass (sarcopenia).[7] This definition underscores the fundamental role of muscle loss in the development of frailty, decreased function, and impaired duration and quality of life in cachectic cancer patients.[8] Developing clarity on the definition of, and diagnostic criteria for, cachexia represents an important step in advancing care for patients; this work should facilitate clinical trial design, assist in the development of clinical practice guidelines, and ultimately improve the routine clinical management of this condition.[7,8]

Cachexia is typically associated with a number of other symptoms that contribute to weight loss and exacerbate the clinical picture. Anorexia, for example, so commonly clusters with cachexia that the phenomenon is frequently referred to as anorexia–cachexia syndrome. Anorexia is defined as an involuntary loss of appetite that is associated with decreased oral intake.[9] Anorexia in cancer is often associated with other symptoms that contribute to decreased consumption of calories, such as alterations in taste or smell and early satiety. Although an important component, anorexia alone is not responsible for the loss of body mass seen in cachexia. Body composition changes in anorexia are primarily related to fat loss, whereas equal losses of muscle and fat are seen in cachexia.[2,3]

Early satiety is also commonly associated with cachexia. Satiety is a feeling of satisfaction that is usually associated with the cessation of food intake. Early satiety refers to the inability to consume more than a few mouthfuls of food despite the desire to eat.[10] The sense of fullness decreases oral intake and subsequently contributes to nutritional issues and weight loss.

Other symptoms that are frequently seen in the setting of cachexia include alterations in taste or smell. These changes can be moderately severe and are often associated with decreased appetite and oral intake, contributing to or exacerbating cancer-related weight loss and cachexia.[11] Moreover, because taste and smell are associated with desirable flavors and pleasure, changes in these sensations have been associated with decreased quality of life.[12]

Commonly reported taste sensations include decreased tasting ability (hypogeusia), complete absence of taste (ageusia), or dysgeusia, which refers to a persistent bitter, metallic, or hot taste in the mouth that is related to injury to the gustatory nerve or ascending nerve pathways.[11] These changes may cause food aversions to meats such as beef and pork or other foods such as chocolate, coffee, or tomatoes. Patients may experience an increased threshold for sweets, an increased desire for salt, or an intolerance of sour foods. Taste changes can be transient and resolve after treatment completion, or they may linger.[10]

Distorted perception of smell (dysosmia) is often unpleasant, with patients describing the odor perceived as rancid. Dysosmia is categorized according to whether it is preceded by environmental stimuli (parosomia), such as the administration of chemotherapy, or occurs spontaneously (phantosmia).[10,13] In one small qualitative study investigating patient experiences with changes in smell, all subjects reported an increased sensitivity to odors that were perceived as unpleasant, such as automobile fumes, body odors, and hospital smells.[14]

Cachexia has consistently been associated with adverse outcomes, including diminished overall survival, poorer chemotherapy response rates, greater toxicity, decreased quality of life, longer length of hospital stay, diminished functional status, and higher cost of care.[1–7,15,16] Weight loss and performance status are variables often used to predict survival in the cancer population. In a classic study that included more than 3000 patients participating in Eastern Cooperative Oncology Group clinical trials, De Wys et al.[17] found a positive correlation between weight loss and performance status. Patients who experienced a weight loss of at least 5% of total body weight had shorter median survival and lower response rates to chemotherapy. Patients with specific types of malignancies who experienced no weight loss had median survival rates twice as long as their counterparts who experienced weight loss.[17]

INCIDENCE

Cachexia is common in cancer patients; recent estimates indicate that it may be present in 60% to 80% of patients with advanced cancer.[1] Incidence varies by tumor type, site, and mass, with higher rates found among patients who have aerodigestive and gastrointestinal cancers, and in those with advanced disease. Anorexia commonly accompanies cachexia and is also frequently associated with advanced disease; however, anorexia is present in approximately 50% of newly diagnosed cancer patients and may be one of the reasons why patients seek medical attention.[9] In addition, anorexia has been associated with the administration of a number of cancer treatments, and this relationship can be exacerbated when patients are receiving aggressive multimodality therapy. Myeloablative conditioning regimens are associated with anorexia and poor oral intake. In one study of patients undergoing allogeneic stem cell transplantation for hematologic malignancies, decreased oral intake was reported in 92% of subjects.[18]

Early satiety is highly correlated with anorexia, although this often goes unnoticed in clinical practice because it is frequently excluded from assessment tools and patients may not spontaneously report its presence.[9,19]

Changes in taste and smell often coexist with cachexia, but these issues are frequently overshadowed by more pressing symptoms. A recent report of patients with advanced cancer indicated that 86% of subjects experienced some type of chemosensory alteration.[13] In another investigation that included more than 500 patients, 66% experienced alterations in taste and smell; another 8% experienced changes in smell without changes in taste.[14]

Over the past few decades, the introduction of increasingly sophisticated cancer therapeutics has shifted survival rates substantially. The growing number of cancer survivors have unique health needs as a result of their disease and treatment process. Nutritional issues in the survivor population are common. Although cachexia per se has not been identified as an issue among survivors, the ability to return to pretreatment weight has been reported in subsets of the survivor population. Decline in body mass index over time has been reported in survivors of pediatric malignancies.[18] More commonly, overnutrition has been an area of focus among cancer survivors. Long-term follow-up of patients who were treated for pediatric malignancies has demonstrated increased risk for obesity among this population. The reasons for this tendency are multifactorial and not well understood, but it is thought to be related to treatment with cranial radiation at a young age.[20]

ETIOLOGY

Cachexia is classically associated with a negative protein and energy balance that stems from a combination of reduced caloric intake and abnormal metabolism. Reduced caloric intake can be related to physical, psychological, or physiologic factors associated with either the disease or treatment process or, in most cases, a combination of both.[3,4,6,8,21,22]

Physical factors

Cachexia often occurs as a result of physical and/or functional deficits that prevent the ingestion or absorption of adequate calories and nutrients. Mechanical factors such as oral ulceration related to stomatoxic chemotherapy, for example, would prevent the ingestion of adequate calories.

Severe xerostomia in a patient receiving radiation therapy to the head and neck would produce a similar effect. Any clinical situation that alters physical functioning of the gut can result in both decreased intake and changes in absorptive function. Surgical procedures to eradicate tumors in the oral cavity, esophagus, stomach, biliary tract, or bowel, for example, frequently involve the removal of portions of these anatomical structures, which often changes their function.[10] The internal lumen of the gut is lined with a mucosal layer containing microvilli at the brush border of the enterocytes. These structures maximize the surface area and are critical to the effective absorption of nutrients. Damage from chemotherapy, radiation, or infection can lead to alterations in the structure of these microvilli, reducing their efficiency. Moreover, a lack of microvilli stimulation, such as when patients are placed on nothing by mouth (NPO) status, can result in atrophy and degeneration of these structures with subsequent changes in their ability to effectively absorb proteins, carbohydrates, and fats.

Cancer and the administration of antineoplastic therapeutics are associated with the development of a broad array of symptoms; many of these conditions are associated with the physical changes that contribute to the development and progression of cachexia. Nausea and vomiting, for example, are extremely common side effects in patients receiving chemotherapy; they can result in loss of protein- and electrolyte-rich gastrointestinal contents, which leads to fluid and electrolyte imbalances. If left unchecked, dehydration and nutritional deficiencies, as well as other complications, may develop. Many cancer treatments can irritate the gastrointestinal tract and cause diarrhea. Patients receiving radiation therapy to the large or small intestine, for example, commonly develop diarrhea as a consequence of treatment. Several chemotherapeutic agents, such as irinotecan and 5-fluorouracil, are also associated with diarrhea that can quickly become severe. The development of this symptom can contribute to a lack of adequate absorption of calories and nutrients and lead to rapid weight loss. Other symptoms that commonly contribute to the development of cachexia include anorexia, early satiety, and alterations in taste and smell.[10] Eating behavior is stimulated by hunger, cravings, and hedonic sensations that are controlled by myriad physical, gastrointestinal, physiologic, and metabolic factors. The multifactorial alterations that lead to anorexia in the cancer patient may be attributable to cancer- or treatment-related factors, or both.

Physiologic factors

Physiologic alterations feature prominently in the etiology of cachexia. Current biological evidence supports theories that center on the immune effects of cancer as factors in the development of cachexia. Translational research in the area of nutritional oncology has significantly increased our understanding of the interactive relationship between and among pro-inflammatory or procachectic cytokines, neuropeptides, and neurotransmitters and the development of cancer cachexia.[23]

PATHOPHYSIOLOGY

The pathogenicity of cancer cachexia is multifactorial and results from a complex series of interrelated tumor–host interactions. Developing a clear understanding of the specific physiologic mechanisms underlying cancer cachexia is critical to the design of rational interventions directed at potentially preventing and treating this condition. Although this has been a very active area of research, current evidence suggests that many of the processes underlying cancer cachexia remain hypothetical.

THE EFFECTS OF CYTOKINES

Cytokines are soluble polypeptides, produced by a variety of immune cells, including monocytes, macrophages, lymphocytes, and endothelial cells, that are secreted in response to malignancy, trauma, or sepsis, and that exert their effects locally on target tissue receptors. Cytokines are the most frequently implicated mediators of cachexia. Tumor necrosis factor-α (TNF-α), interleukin-1 (IL-1), interleukin-6 (IL-6), interleukin-10 (IL-10), interferon-α, -β, and -γ (IFN-α, -β, and -γ) have all been identified as cytokines that contribute to the cachectic process. It appears that these substances work in concert to create cachectic effects; however, the precise mechanisms of cytokine–host interactions have not yet been fully described.[23]

Cytokines are responsible for exerting a multitude of effects that contribute to the development of cancer cachexia. Primary alterations include the development of anorexia, changes in hormonal milieu, and derangements in carbohydrate, protein, and fat metabolism. As a consequence, physical deterioration and involuntary weight loss occur, leading to diminished performance and quality of life.

ALTERATIONS IN SKELETAL MUSCLE

Marked decreases in skeletal muscle mass are associated with cancer cachexia. Microscopic examination of muscle in cachetic patients reveals increased fat infiltration between muscles and a decrease in muscle fiber diameter.[8] Muscle mass is determined by the balance of protein synthesis and degradation; in cachexia, loss of skeletal muscle results from both decreased protein synthesis and increased degredation.[24] Activation of the ubiquitin–proteosome pathway is the most significant contributor to protein degradation in cachexia, but other degradation pathways, such as the lysosomal cathepsins B, H, D, and L and activation of the calcium calpains have also been implicated in protein loss. Proteolysis has been shown to occur even in the absence of weight loss in cancer patients.[5] Apoptosis plays a role in muscle atrophy in animal models, although this finding has yet to be demonstrated in patients with cancer.[2] Other metabolic changes that deplete protein include increased whole-body turnover, changes in circulating amino acid patterns, decreased muscle amino acid uptake, and increased branched-chair amino acid turnover. These changes have been empirically linked to TNF-α, IL-6, and IL-1 activity. In addition, recent research has demonstrated that metabolic and protein turnover-related pathways appear to be suppressed in cachexia, limiting protein synthesis.[2,3]

Although muscle wasting is most typically seen in advanced disease, a number of patients with cancer demonstrate some degree of wasting at presentation. Moreover, activation of proteolysis is thought to be an early event in tumor growth and may be present long before it becomes clinically evident.[5] Loss of skeletal muscle in cachectic patients is clinically significant because of its profound effect on functional status and quality of life outcomes.[25]

ALTERATIONS IN GLUCOSE AND FAT METABOLISM

Glucose is the most essential substrate of the human body and is required to support all critical organ functions. Glucose is liberated to meet energy needs in response to hormonal stimulation. In cachexia, a number of inefficiencies in glucose metabolism occur. These changes limit the amount of glucose available for utilization by essential organs. In response to diminished supply, the liver uses gluconeogenic amino acids from skeletal muscle catabolism to produce additional glucose. In healthy individuals, this compensatory mechanism would be rapidly replaced with a process of fat conversion. In the setting of cachexia, however, continued use of protein as a source of energy occurs, further exacerbating the depletion of skeletal muscle mass.[26]

Glucose intolerance and an abnormal insulin response have also been reported in cachectic patients. In noncachectic individuals, insulin stimulates appetite and promotes fat and protein synthesis in response to elevated glucose levels. Moreover, insulin inhibits amino acid release from muscle, thereby inhibiting gluconeogenesis, reducing amino acid degradation, and conserving muscle mass. In cachexia, a slower clearance in blood glucose levels is seen due to insensitivity of insulin to tissue, which results in a lower insulin response to hyperglycemia or lack of exogenous glucose production in response to hypoglycemia. This lack of response may decrease appetite and subsequently food intake.

An increase in Cori cycle activity has been documented in cachectic individuals.[10] The Cori cycle is a process that converts glucose first to lactic acid, and then back to glucose. This cycle requires substantial energy; therefore increased activity requires additional calories. In the context of limited caloric intake, this inefficient utilization can be especially problematic.[26]

Multiple changes in fat metabolism and loss of adipose tissue have also been documented in cachectic individuals.[3] Loss of adipose tissue is largely due to lypolysis, which is driven by lipid-mobilizing factor (LMF) and tumor factor zinc-alpha-2 glycoprotein. These substances sensitize adipocytes to lipolytic stimuli and have direct lipolytic effects. Fat loss may account for most of the weight loss seen in patients with cachexia. The continued depletion of body stores causes further weakness, progressive weight loss, wasting, and perpetuation of the cachectic cycle. Cytokines have been implicated as etiological factors in this process. TNF-α, IL-1, and IFN-α, -β, and -γ have been specifically associated with decreased lipoprotein lipase activity, increased lipolysis, and increased thermogenesis.[2–5,8,10]

Figure 17-1 provides a brief overview of the factors influencing the development of cachexia.[1–10]

PATHOPHYSIOLOGY OF RELATED SYMPTOMS

Anorexia is a complex physiologic phenomenon that results from an imbalance between orexigenic and anorexigenic signals and resting energy expenditure. The release of chemicals by the tumor or the host's immune system can induce anorexia. Loss of appetite can be stimulated by the effects of hormones (e.g., leptin, ghrelin), neuropeptides, and cytokines. Many cytokines have been shown to effect appetite, including IL-1α, IL-1β, IL-6, and TNF-α. These cytokines cross the blood–brain barrier; once in the brain, they interact with lumenal surfaces of brain endothelial cells to release substances that affect appetite.[2] TNF-α and IL-1 receptors are found in the hypothalamus, a key area of the brain involved in energy homeostasis and appetite. Cytokines can also inhibit the neuropeptide-Y (NPY) pathway. NPY is one of the most potent inducers of feeding in mammals; as such, its inhibition contributes to the development of severe anorexia.[27]

Hormones, such as leptin, influence body fat stores by inhibiting food intake and energy expenditure biofeedback loops. Increased melanocortin, a neuropeptide hormone, can also induce anorexia. Increased central nervous system melanocortin signaling has been implicated in the pathogenesis of cancer anorexia.[2]

Early satiety may be related to physical obstacles or physiologic changes that influence the gastrointestinal tract.[10] Physical issues can include decreased gastric motility and emptying, decreased intestinal motility, and modification of

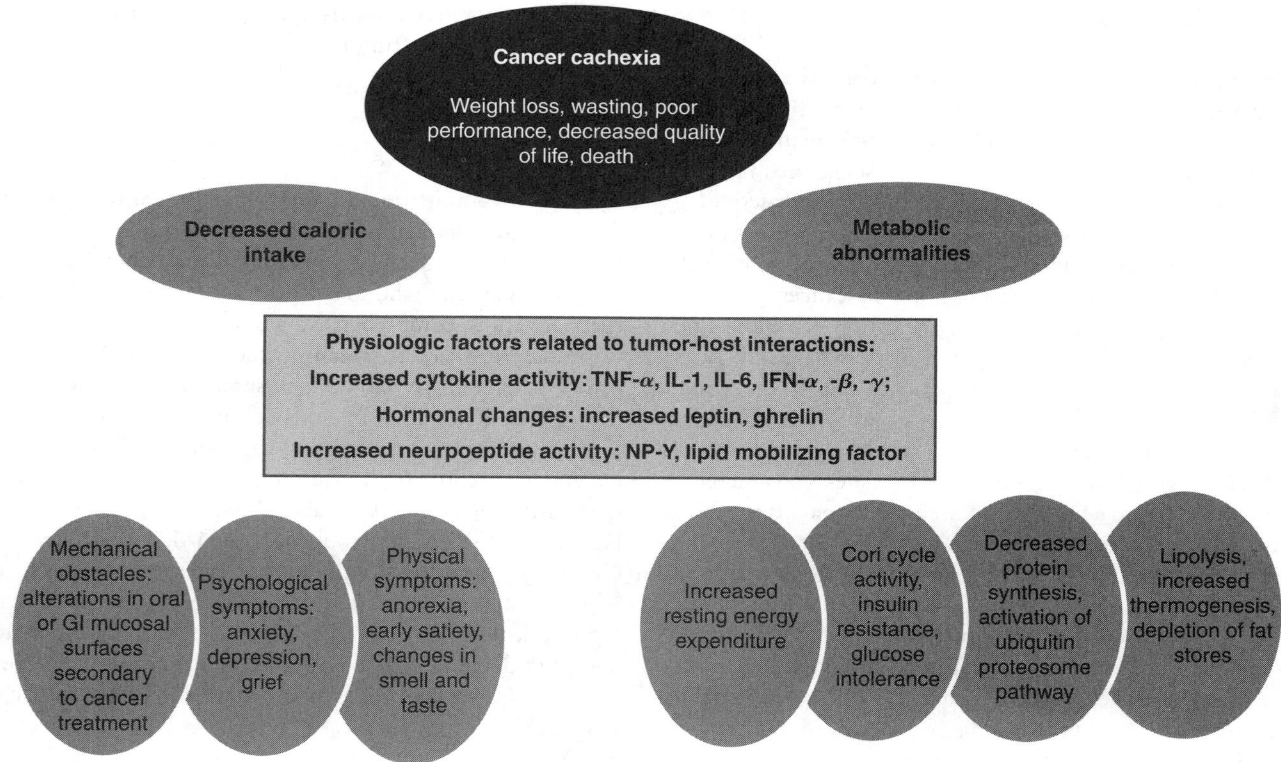

FIGURE 17-1

Factors influencing the development of cachexia.

Abbreviations: GI: gastrointestinal; IL: interleukin; NP-Y: neuropeptide-Y; TNF: tumor necrosis factor.

gastric acid secretion—all of which can inhibit the desire to eat and have been associated with cytokine activity in cancer patients. Organ enlargement, such as hepatomegaly or splenomegaly, due to progressive tumor infiltration, infection, or the extramedullary hematopoiesis seen in patients with myeloproliferative disorders, can create a profound sensation of being full. Malignant ascites has also been implicated as an etiological factor in the development of early satiety.

Alterations in taste perception may result from direct effects of the tumor, cancer-induced deficiencies of vitamins and minerals, infectious processes, therapeutic interventions including chemotherapeutic or biological agents, radiation, or surgery, and antibiotics or other pharmacologic interventions.

SYMPTOM ASSESSMENT

RISK FACTORS

Age has been identified as a risk factor in the development of cachexia, with patients at both ends of the age spectrum being at greater risk. Recent evidence suggests that genetic factors also play a role.[28] Although there is an increased incidence of cachexia within specific tumor types, there is variation among patients who develop this condition, which may be related to host genotype. Preliminary association studies in unrelated individuals have demonstrated that single-nucleotide polymorphisms in the IL-1, IL-6, and IL-10 genes that are linked to the production of these cytokines may increase susceptibility to cachexia.[8,28] Moreover, these factors have been associated with the prevalence of cachexia in both pancreatic and gastric cancers.[29,30]

Additional risk factors include conditions that have the potential to influence food intake, such as nicotine use, alterations affecting digestive or absorptive function, diseases of metabolism, and primary anorexia. Patients with cancer commonly experience other symptoms that increase their risk for the exacerbation of cachexia, such as anorexia, early satiety, or mucositis. These symptoms may be related to the disease or treatment process and may be present from the onset of disease. Each of these symptoms can contribute profoundly to increasing risk for cachexia.

SELF-ASSESSMENT

In most cultures, eating occurs in a social context and is associated with pleasure. In the cachectic patient, this connection is often lost. Encumbered by symptoms, many patients lose their desire to eat and interact in a social setting. This may lead to social withdrawal, isolation, and decreased quality of life. The accompanying weight loss often serves as an ostensible reminder of illness. Psychological symptoms, such as anxiety or depression, are common in cancer and may contribute to poor appetite, abnormal eating behaviors, and learned food aversions. Anxiety and distress have also been reported in caregivers of cachectic patients. Nutrition, eating, and food are all associated with nurturing. When caregivers are unable to effectively nurture loved ones during times of illness, feelings of hopelessness and helplessness can emerge.[22]

It is essential to ensure that patients understand the need to proactively manage symptoms and food intake early in the trajectory of illness and throughout the course of their disease. Based on their specific disease and therapeutic regimen, they should be informed about the symptoms to anticipate and the approximate time frame in which those conditions might develop. Education on preventive treatment strategies to minimize the occurrence of anticipated symptoms should be provided. These symptoms should be monitored, and patients need to understand the importance of notifying a member of the healthcare team when issues arise. Monitoring nutritional intake and weight is essential, and these parameters should also be tracked over time. Patients need to be taught that this is a real priority; they should understand that proactive interventions can help to improve outcomes. Patients who are undergoing treatment are especially vulnerable, as they may develop symptoms that decrease oral intake. It is essential that they are taught about the importance of eating and drinking, during this time.

Practical resources to guide patients, such as the National Cancer Institute publication *Eating Hints: Before, During, and After Cancer Treatment*, offer helpful information that can be readily used by patients and families.[31] Providing specific information about the right foods to consume can also be helpful. Engaging trained dietary specialists when they are available to assist with education is recommended. Tools such as food diaries or trackers can also be very helpful for patients. See Appendix 17A, Self-Care Guide: Weekly Food Diary, for more information about teaching patients.

OBJECTIVE ASSESSMENT

The importance of objective screening and assessment cannot be underestimated in optimizing the care of patients with or at risk for cancer cachexia. The early identification of changes in nutritional status during the pre-cachexia period is essential to preventing or minimizing the progression of cachexia.

Nutritional screening

The process of nutritional screening facilitates the proactive discovery of characteristics or risk factors known to be associated with dietary or nutritional problems. Screening identifies patients who are potentially at risk, earmarking them for more comprehensive assessments and early interventions. Nutritional screening tools need to have established validity and reliability and should be efficient, so that they can easily be used in a busy clinical practice setting.

One example of a screening tool with established validity and reliability in the cancer population is the Patient Generated-Subjective Global Assessment (PG-SGA; see Figure 17-2A).[33] This tool has been identified by the Oncology Practice Group of the American Academy of Nutrition and Dietetics as the standard for nutritional screening in oncology patients. The PG-SGA is a straightforward, one-page document that uses a checkbox format. The first four boxes are completed by the patient and assess history of weight change, food intake, symptoms, and functional capacity. The remainder of the form is completed by the healthcare provider. A worksheet for scoring the PG-SGA has been developed (Figure 17-2B). Each of the patient-reported responses is scored from 0 (least) to 4 (most) depending on nutritional impact. Objective data from the clinician are then combined with this score and a total value is calculated. This value indicates whether the patient is well nourished, suspected of being malnourished, or severely malnourished. An algorithm of nutritional intervention has been developed to manage each of the nutritional screening categories (Figure 17-2C).[33]

Comprehensive nutritional assessment

Patients who meet risk criteria should undergo a comprehensive nutritional assessment. Typically, this includes a careful medical and dietary history, anthropometric measurements, body composition analysis, evaluation of selected nutritional biomarkers, and an assessment for symptoms that may interfere with nutritional status. The purpose of this more comprehensive approach is to gather additional data to establish an individualized plan for nutritional support. Comprehensive nutritional assessments allow for planning of effective nutritional care; immediate issues can be addressed, short- and long-term goals established, teaching plans developed, and appropriate referrals initiated.[10]

Medical and dietary history. A comprehensive medical and dietary history is the first step in a comprehensive nutritional assessment. The history should ascertain the presence of medical issues that may interfere with effective

Scored Patient-Generated Subjective Global Assessment (PG-SGA)

Patient ID Information

History (Boxes 1–4 are designed to be completed by the patient.)

1. Weight *(See Worksheet 1)*

In summary of my current and recent weight:

I currently weigh about ________ pounds
I am about ________ feet ________ tall

One month ago I weighed about ________ pounds
Six months ago I weighed about ________ pounds

During the past two weeks my weight has:
☐ decreased$_{(1)}$ ☐ not changed$_{(0)}$ ☐ increased$_{(0)}$

Box 1 ☐

2. Food Intake: As compared to my normal intake, I would rate my food intake during the past month as:

- ☐ unchanged$_{(0)}$
- ☐ more than usual$_{(0)}$
- ☐ less than usual$_{(1)}$

I am now taking:

- ☐ *normal food* but less than normal amount$_{(1)}$
- ☐ little solid food$_{(2)}$
- ☐ only liquids$_{(3)}$
- ☐ only nutritonal supplements$_{(3)}$
- ☐ very little of anything$_{(4)}$
- ☐ only tube feedings or only nutrition by vein$_{(0)}$

Box 2 ☐

3. Symptoms: I have had the following problems that have kept me from eating enough during the past two weeks (check all that apply):

- ☐ no problems eating$_{(0)}$
- ☐ no appetite, just did not feel like eating$_{(3)}$
- ☐ nausea$_{(1)}$
- ☐ vomiting$_{(3)}$
- ☐ constipation$_{(1)}$
- ☐ diarrhea$_{(3)}$
- ☐ mouth sores$_{(2)}$
- ☐ dry mouth$_{(1)}$
- ☐ things taste funny or have no taste$_{(1)}$
- ☐ smells bother me$_{(1)}$
- ☐ problems swallowing$_{(2)}$
- ☐ feel full quickly$_{(1)}$
- ☐ pain; where?$_{(3)}$ ________
- ☐ other**$_{(1)}$ ________________

** Examples: depression, money, or dental problems

Box 3 ☐

4. Activities and Function: Over the past month, I would generally rate my activity as:

- ☐ normal with no limitations$_{(0)}$
- ☐ not my normal self, but able to be up and about with fairly normal activities$_{(1)}$
- ☐ not feeling up to most things, but in bed or chair less than half the day$_{(2)}$
- ☐ able to do little activity and spend most of the day in bed or chair$_{(3)}$
- ☐ pretty much bedridden, rarely out of bed$_{(3)}$

Box 4 ☐

Additive Score of the Boxes 1-4 ☐ A

The remainder of this form will be completed by your doctor, nurse, or therapist. Thank you.

(Optional for completion by clinicians)

5. Disease and its relation to nutritional requirements *(See Worksheet 2)*

All relevant diagnoses (specify) ________________

Primary disease stage (circle if known or appropriate) I II III IV Other ________

Age ________

Numerical score from Worksheet 2 ☐ B

6. Metabolic Demand *(See Worksheet 3)*

Numerical score from Worksheet 3 ☐ C

7. Physical *(See Worksheet 4)*

Numerical score from Worksheet 4 ☐ D

Global Assessment *(See Worksheet 5)*

- ☐ Well-nourished or anabolic (SGA-A)
- ☐ Moderate or suspected malnutrition (SGA-B)
- ☐ Severely malnourished (SGA-C)

Total PG-SGA score

(Total numerical score of A+B+C+D above) ☐

(See triage recommendations below)

Clinician Signature ________________ RD RN PA MD DO Other ___ Date ________

Nutritional Triage Recommendations: Additive score is used to define specific nutritional interventions including patient & family education, symptom management including pharmacologic intervention, and appropriate nutrient intervention (food, nutritional supplements, enteral, or parenteral triage). First line nutrition intervention includes optimal symptom management.

0–1 No intervention required at this time. Re-assessment on routine and regular basis during treatment.

2–3 Patient & family education by dietitian, nurse, or other clinician with pharmacologic intervention as indicated by symptom survey (Box 3) and laboratory values as appropriate.

4–8 Requires intervention by dietitian, in conjunction with nurse or physician as indicated by symptoms survey (Box 3).

≥9 Indicates a critical need for improved symptom management and/or nutrient intervention options.

 email: fdottery@btgc.com or noatpres1@aol.com

FIGURE 17-2A

Scored PG-SGA.

Source: Reproduced by permission of Faith D. Ottery, MD, PhD.

Worksheets for PG-SGA Scoring

Boxes 1–4 of the PG-SGA are designed to be completed by the patient. The PG-SGA numerical score is determined using 1) the parenthetical points noted in boxes 1–4 and 2) the worksheets below for items not marked with parenthetical points. Scores for boxes 1 and 3 are additive within each box and scores for boxes 2 and 4 are based on the highest scored item checked off by the patient.

Worksheet 1 - Scoring Weight (Wt) Loss

To determine score, use 1 month weight data if available. Use 6 month data only if there is no 1 month weight data. Use points below to score weight change and add one extra point if patient has lost weight during the past 2 weeks. Enter total point score in Box 1 of the PG-SGA.

Wt loss in 1 month	Points	Wt Loss in 6 months
10% or greater	4	20% or greater
5–9.9%	3	10–19.9%
3–4.9%	2	6–9.9%
2–2.9%	1	2–5.9%
0–1.9%	0	0–1.9%

Score for Worksheet 1 ☐
Record in Box 1

Worksheet 2 - Scoring Criteria for Condition

Score is derived by adding 1 point each of the conditions listed below that pertain to the patient.

Category	Points
Cancer	1
AIDS	1
Pulmonary or cardiac cachexia	1
Presence of decubitus, open wound, or fistula	1
Presence of trauma	1
Age greater than 65 years	1

Score for Worksheet 2 = ☐
Record in Box B

Worksheet 3 - Scoring Metabolic Stress

Score for metabolic stress is determined by a number of variable known to increase protein & caloric needs. The score is additive so that a patient who has a fever of >102 degrees (3 points) and is on 10 mg of prednisone chronically (2 points) would have an additive score for this section of 5 points.

Stress	none (0)	low (1)	moderate (2)	high (3)
Fever	no fever	>99 and <101	≥101 and <102	≥102
Fever duration	no fever	<72 hrs	72 hrs	>72 hrs
Corticosteroids	no corticosteroids	low dose (<10mg prednisone equivalents/day)	moderate dose (≥10 and <30mg prednisone equivalents/day)	high dose steroids (≥30mg prednisone equivalents/day)

Score for Worksheet 3 = ☐
Record in Box C

Worksheet 4 - Physical Examination

Physical exam includes a subjective evaluation of 3 aspects of body composition: fat, muscle, & fluid status. Sine this is subjective, each aspect of the exam is rated for degree of deficit. Muscle deficit impacts points score more than fat deficit. Definition of categories: 0 = no deficit, 1+ = mild deficit, 2+ = moderate deficit, 3+ = severe deficit. Rating of deficit in these categories are *not* additive but are used to clinically assess the degree of deficit (or presence of excess fluid).

Fat Stores:				
orbital fat pads	0	1+	2+	3+
triceps skin fold	0	1+	2+	3+
fat overlying lower ribs	0	1+	2+	3+
Global fat deficit rating	**0**	**1+**	**2+**	**3+**
Muscle Status:				
temples (temporalis muscle)	0	1+	2+	3+
clavicles (pectoralis & deltoids)	0	1+	2+	3+
shoulders (deltoids)	0	1+	2+	3+
interosseous muscles	0	1+	2+	3+
scapula (latissimus dorsi, trapezius, deltoids)	0	1+	2+	3+
thigh (quadriceps)	0	1+	2+	3+
calf (gastrocnemius)	0	1+	2+	3+
Global muscle status rating	**0**	**1+**	**2+**	**3+**
Fluid Status:				
ankle edema	0	1+	2+	3+
sacral edema	0	1+	2+	3+
ascites	0	1+	2+	3+
Global fluid status rating	**0**	**1+**	**2+**	**3+**

Point score for the physical exam is determined by the overall subjective rating of total body deficit.

No deficit	score = 0 points
Mild deficit	score = 1 points
Moderate deficit	score = 2 points
Severe deficit	score = 3 points

Score for Worksheet 4 = ☐
Record in Box D

Worksheet 5 - PG-SGA Global Assessment Categories

	Stage A	Stage B	Stage C
Category	Well-nourished	Moderately malnourished or suspected malnutrition	Severely malnourished
Weight	No wt loss **OR** Recent non-fluid wt gain	~5% wt loss within 1 month (or 10% in 6 months) **OR** No wt stabilization or wt gain (i.e., continued wt loss)	>5% wt loss within 1 month (or 10% in 6 months) **OR** No wt stabilization or wt gain (i.e., continued wt loss)
Nutrient Intake	No deficit **OR** Significant recent improvement	Definite decrease in intake	Severe deficit in intake
Nutrition Impact Symptoms	None **OR** Significant recent improvement allowing adequate intake	Presence of nutrition impact symptoms (Box 3 of PG-SGA)	Presence of nutrition impact symptoms (Box 3 of PG-SGA)
Functioning	No deficit **OR** Significant recent improvement	Moderate functional deficit **OR** Recent deterioration	Severe functional deficit **OR** recent significant deterioration
Physical Exam	No deficit **OR** Chronic deficit but with recent clinical improvement	Evidence of mild to moderate loss of SQ fat &/or muscle mass &/or muscle tone on palpation	Obvious signs of malnutrition (e.g., severe loss of SQ tissues, possible edema)

Global PG-SGA rating (A, B, or C) = ☐

FIGURE 17-2B

Tables for PG-SGA scoring.

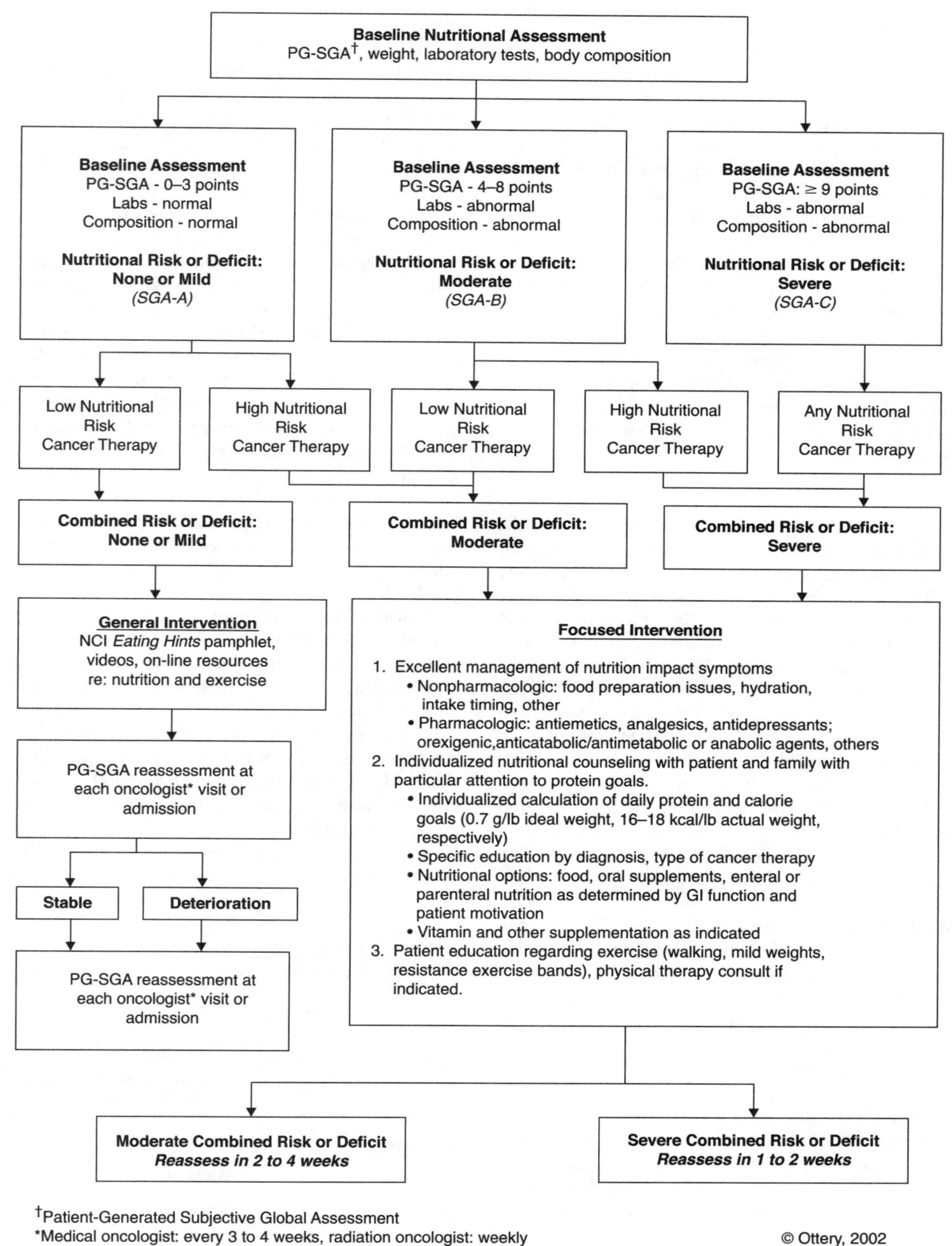

FIGURE 17-2C

Nursing algorithm for anorexia cachexia.

nutrition, such as primary anorexia, prior surgical intervention that might affect the intake or absorption of nutrients, or comorbidities that could predispose patients to or exacerbate nutritional issues. Current weight and weight changes are important to ascertain, along with specifics regarding stage of disease, treatment, accompanying symptoms, and a review of concurrent medications. An assessment of social factors, including socioeconomic, religious, cultural, or lifestyle influences that may affect food consumption, should also be completed. Other parameters of focus should include appetite; satiety level; food preferences and aversions; intolerances to foods; psychosocial or behavioral factors; family support; the ability to procure food and prepare meals; the number and size of typical meals; food groups consumed during meals; the use of nutritional supplements and vitamins, including complementary supplements; physical function; ability to work and perform other roles; and diet and nutrition educational needs. Food diaries can be used to specifically ascertain food intake history, as recall is typically unreliable.[10]

Physical examination. A physical examination of the patient should be done to assess for potential signs of malnutrition. Such an examination focuses on several key areas. The patient's general appearance is important. Body habitus, frame, and mobility provide information about general nutritional and functional status. Observe the face and assess the temporalis muscles, buccal fat pads, and zygomatic arches. Conjunctiva are observed for wrinkling and dryness (best visualized when the patient gazes laterally), which can be indicative of vitamin deficiencies. Grip strength can be assessed via a handshake. Assessments of muscle mass and tone of the forearm are made to determine if atrophy is present. Fat and muscle status can also be determined by assessing the prominence of the posterior ribs, scapula, or spine. Skin tone and turgor are examined. Scaling of the skin or a history of rashes may be indicative of vitamin (niacin) or trace element (zinc) deficiencies. Petechial and subcutaneous hemorrhages may be indicative of vitamin C and K deficiencies. Thickening of the skin may reflect inadequate amounts of vitamin A.

A gross assessment of fluid status should also be conducted. The presence of dependent ankle or sacral edema may be indicative of hypoproteinemia or problems resulting in sodium retention.

Anthropometric measurements. Anthropometrics refers to the measurement of dimensions, proportions, and ratios of the human body. Typically anthropometric measurements include height, weight, BMI, and skin fold thickness, as these measurements are noninvasive and relatively easy to assess in clinical practice. Height and weight are the measures most commonly monitored in busy oncology practices. Accuracy of these measures is especially critical in this setting because the majority of therapeutic interventions used in cancer are dosed based on body surface area (BSA), a variable that reflects a composite height and weight score.[10]

Weight alone is the outcome most relied upon to quickly assess a patient's nutritional status. Longitudinal measurement of weight from a reliable baseline is essential. Clinical practice settings should develop clear policies and procedures for the assessment of height and weight, so that personnel accountable for carrying out these activities are performing consistently. Ensuring accuracy and precision of the instruments used to assess these parameters is also critical. Using the same scale for repeated weight measurements and ensuring that periodic checks of the devices used are conducted by the manufacturer or the organization's biomedical engineering staff will help to eliminate variability. Patients should be instructed to remove heavy clothing, pocket items, and shoes. Not all patients will be able to stand for weight assessment; in these cases, chair or bed scales may be used. Height should be assessed using a stadiometer with the patient standing with feet flat on the floor or stadiometer platform. BMI can be calculated from a patient's height and weight. BMI is a measure of fat that is based on an individual's height and weight; it provides information on whether weight is within a healthy range (Table 17-1).[34]

Other anthropometric measurements include triceps and subscapular skin fold measurements. These assessments are performed to determine subcutaneous fat stores. Estimates of muscle mass and protein stores can be determined by mid-arm muscle circumference (MAMC). To obtain the MAMC, a tape measure is placed around the midpoint of the upper arm. This measurement is coupled with triceps skin fold measurements to calculate muscle mass, which gives an estimate of somatic protein stores. Comparisons of these measurements to accepted "standards" are of limited value in the cancer population, however, because "norms" are based on normal healthy subjects. In addition, variability between observers has been reported.

Nutritional biomarkers. Although a variety of laboratory tests can be used to estimate aspects of nutritional status,

TABLE 17-1

Categories of Body Mass Index

Category	Body Mass Index
Underweight	< 18.5
Normal Weight	18.5–24.9
Overweight	25–29.9
Obesity	≥30

Source: Data from National Heart, Blood and Lung Institute[34].

there is no gold standard on what or when to specifically measure. Laboratory parameters can be influenced by a multitude of other factors, and they must always be considered within the context of the patient's total clinical picture. Traditional biomarker assessments of nutritional status include the circulating proteins albumin, prealbumin, transferrin, and retinol-binding protein. C-reactive protein, total lymphocyte count, and total cholesterol have also been used for this purpose.

Albumin is the most abundant of the plasma proteins. Its concentration depends on synthesis, degradation, gastrointestinal and renal losses, volume distribution, and exchange between body compartments. Because albumin levels may be influenced by body stresses such as trauma or infection, changes in hydration status, and liver and renal disease, it is not an accurate measure of nutritional status. Serum albumin is also a negative acute-phase reactant, meaning that it can be decreased in the presence of inflammation, which occurs in many types of cancer.

Serum transferrin has also been used to assess nutritional status; however, a long (8-day) half-life limits the practicality of using this parameter. Transferrin levels can also be influenced by iron depletion or the use of hormonal agents.

Levels of electrolytes and minerals, such as calcium, potassium, phosphorus, magnesium, and zinc, are routinely assessed in cancer patients. Some of these biomarker tests can be normal even when deficiencies exist, which limits their utility in assessing nutritional status. Zinc, for example, is primarily stored in muscle and liver tissues, rather than in the serum; as such, zinc levels may appear normal even when stores are low.[10,35,36]

Body composition analysis

Body composition analysis provides a picture of nutritional intake, loss, and need over time by measuring two major body compartments: fat free (or lean body) mass and fat mass. Impairments in overall health, function, and quality of life have been associated with decreases in fat free mass.

Body composition analysis can be accomplished in a number of ways, including bioelectrical impedance analysis (BIA), dual-energy x-ray absorptiometry (DEXA), and computerized tomography (CT). BIA is based on the ability of hydrated tissues to conduct electrical energy; it measures impedance or opposition to the flow of an electrical current through body fluids contained mainly in lean and fat tissue. Impedance is proportional to the volume of body water. BIA has been validated, is relatively easy to use, and is noninvasive. Some inaccuracies may be noted in patients who have fluid losses, dehydration, or fluid retention; for these reasons, BIA is not routinely used in the cancer population.

DEXA is an accurate and reproducible method of assessing body composition; consequently, it is used as the reference method for assessment in clinical research settings. DEXA is noninvasive and provides direct measurement of three components of body composition: fat mass, fat free mass, and bone mineral mass. In the cancer population, DEXA is frequently used to assess bone mineral density, rather than to assess body composition longitudinally. Accessibility, operator skill, cost, and radiation exposure are factors contributing to its limited routine use.

CT scanning provides assessment of fat free mass through regional analysis of the third vertebra, which strongly predicts whole-body fat and fat free mass.[37] Because CT scanning is used commonly in cancer patient diagnosis and follow-up, this approach has practical benefits in that it can be integrated with routine care. Specific software is required to perform these assessments.

DEGREES OF TOXICITY

The cancer cachexia syndrome is *progressively* debilitating. Cancer cachexia should be conceptualized along a continuum that spans from pre-cachexia to cachexia to refractory cachexia. This framework can be helpful in directing interventions and resources most appropriately. Proactive and aggressive attempts to prevent weight loss and improve sarcopenia are helpful in the pre-cachectic phase, but are likely to be futile and burdensome (from a patient perspective) in the refractory phase. Patients with refractory cachexia would benefit most from symptom control and the alleviation of cachexia-induced suffering.[8]

Identifying the specific grade of toxicity for a patient with cachexia is challenging. The Common Terminology Criteria for Adverse Events (CTCAE) version 4.0 does not include a grading scheme for cachexia, and the literature does not define specific grades for this condition.[38] In clinical situations where grading criteria are not available, clinicians often use more general descriptions to denote seriousness, such as absent, mild, moderate, or severe; but perceptions of what constitutes each of these gradations vary. No descriptions denoting mild, moderate, or severe toxicity specific to cachexia could be found in the literature.

The end result of cachexia is substantial weight loss that leads to wasting, changes in performance status, and death. Weight loss is an outcome of cachexia that can be readily assessed, but always needs to be evaluated within the context of time. An involuntary weight loss of 10% or more of usual body weight over a 5-month period or 5% or more of body weight over 1 month have been used as parameters to define substantial weight loss or weight loss associated with poorer outcomes.[10] The most recent editions of the CTCAE (versions 3.0 and 4.0) include weight loss as an adverse event, although neither version makes reference to the time period over which weight change occurs (Table 17-2). The grades of toxicity associated with weight loss historically have been overly lenient, facilitating reactive versus proactive management. Weight loss

TABLE 17-2

National Cancer Institute Common Terminology Criteria for Adverse Events (CTCAE): Grading for Weight Loss, Weight Gain, and Anorexia

	Grades				
Adverse Event	**1**	**2**	**3**	**4**	**5**
Weight Loss Definition: A finding characterized by a decrease in overall body weight	5% to <10% from baseline; intervention not indicated	10% to <20% from baseline; nutrition support indicated	≥20% from baseline; tube feeding or total parenteral nutrition (TPN) indicated	___	___
Weight Gain Definition: A finding characterized by an increase in overall body weight	5% to <10% from baseline	10% to <20% from baseline	≥20% from baseline	___	___
Anorexia Definition: A disorder characterized by loss of appetite	Loss of appetite without alteration in eating habits	Oral intake altered without significant weight loss or malnutrition; oral nutritional supplements indicated	Associated with significant weight loss or malnutrition (e.g. inadequate oral caloric and/or fluid intake); tube feeding or TPN indicated	Life threatening consequences; urgent intervention indicated	Death

Source: Data from National Cancer Institute Common Terminology Criteria for Adverse Events (CTCAE)[38,39].

was not considered a grade 3 (severe or medically significant) toxicity until it reached or exceeded 20% of body weight.

Weight also needs to be contextualized within a societal framework. Obesity is an epidemic in Western society. The average body mass index of patients presenting with advanced cancer exceeds 25 kg/m^2, which is considered overweight using national Heart, Blood, and Lung Institute parameters, or a grade 2 toxicity using CTCAE criteria.[34,39] This phenomenon may lead to the underdiagnosis of cachexia and is one of the reasons why body composition analysis is an important component of patient assessment.

The degree of toxicity associated with anorexia can be determined using objective criteria; however, toxicity grading for other symptoms that frequently cluster with cachexia, such as hypogeusia, ageusia, dysosmia, and early satiety, is not found in the literature.

SYMPTOM MANAGEMENT STRATEGIES

Cancer cachexia is a complex, multifactorial syndrome that results from a whole host of intricate pathophysiologic changes that occur as a consequence of the disease (tumor–host interactions) and treatment process. The changes associated with this condition are often related to or result in a broad array of symptoms that need to be managed appropriately. Symptom management strategies may vary based on where the patient is in the disease progression trajectory. Effective management of symptoms requires a comprehensive approach and often an array of coordinated interventions. The goals of managing cachexia should be focused in five areas: 1) proactive screening and comprehensive assessment, 2) aggressive management of all symptoms that have the potential to impact nutritional status, 3) the provision of specialized nutrition support as indicated, 4) pharmacologic interventions, and 5) nutritional education for patients, caregivers, and professionals.

THERAPEUTIC APPROACHES

Cancer patients may experience symptoms concurrently or in "clusters," rather than as isolated events. This is commonly seen in the setting of cachexia, which is almost always accompanied by anorexia, taste changes, and early satiety. Although current knowledge is limited, evidence suggests that complex symptoms may act in concert to create more profound clinical effects. This concept needs to be considered in designing interventions for patients with cachexia, particularly in the setting of advanced disease, where a greater number of symptoms and more substantial symptom distress would be expected. Symptom burden refers to the combined effects of all disease- and treatment-related symptoms on a patient's ability to function.[40,41]

Strategies to effectively manage anorexia are limited (see Appendix 17B, Self-Care Guide: Anorexia–Cachexia, for more information about teaching patients). As part of the

Oncology Nursing Society's Putting Evidence into Practice (PEP) initiative, an evidence-based clinical practice resource was developed. The literature indicates that only two pharmacologic interventions—the use of corticosteroids and progestins—are recommended for clinical practice; dietary counseling is identified as likely to be effective.[9]

Evidence on the effectiveness of interventions to manage early satiety is limited. Prokinetic medications, such as metaclopromide, have been used with some effect when gastric emptying is a contributing factor.[19]

Relatively little is known about the management of taste and smell alterations in cancer. Specific patterns of taste and smell changes have not been described well in the literature. Clearly, there is a need for additional descriptive research on these symptoms. Moreover, research focused on developing an evidence base for interventions to manage alterations in smell and taste in cancer patients is also needed. Interventions for the management of dysgeusia, hypogeusia, and ageusia can be found in the literature, but these recommendations are based on the findings of specific clinical assessments, rather than on outcomes data (see Appendix 17C, Self-Care Guide: Changes in Taste and Smell, for more information about teaching patients).[11]

Nutrition support therapy

The goals of nutritional support are to ensure that patients receive an adequate amount of calories and protein, maintain weight, preserve lean body mass, minimize symptoms, and optimize function. Interventions can include dietary education and counseling, specialized nutritional support, or the use of orexigenic or pharmacologic agents. A patient's culture, ethnicity, preferences, performance status, and prognosis should all be taken into account when developing an individualized plan for nutritional support.

Nutrition support therapy should only be instituted as part of a nutrition care plan that is developed after a formal nutritional assessment is completed. The American Society of Parenteral and Enteral Nutrition (ASPEN) is a multidisciplinary organization that is dedicated to improving patient care through the advancement of the science and practice of nutrition support therapy. ASPEN has developed evidence-based guidelines outlining specific recommendations for nutrition support therapy during adult anticancer treatment and in hematopoietic cell transplantation (HCT). The ASPEN recommendations for patients receiving anticancer treatment and those for undergoing HCT are outlined in Tables 17-3 and 17-4, respectively.[42]

Dietary education and counseling

Individualized early dietary education and counseling is correlated with improved nutritional status and body weight. Dietary counseling includes the prescription of a therapeutic diet that is individualized to meet patient needs. Providing education on specific food choices, such as calorie-dense foods, and the management of symptoms so as to improve oral intake can be extremely effective.[10]

TABLE 17-3

ASPEN Clinical Guidelines: Nutrition Support Therapy During Adult Anticancer Treatment

1. Patients with cancer are nutritionally at risk and should undergo nutritional screening to identify those who require formal nutritional assessment with development of a nutrition care plan.
2. Nutrition support therapy should not be used *routinely* in patients undergoing major cancer operations.
3. Perioperative nutrition support therapy may be beneficial in moderately or severely malnourished patients if administered for 7 to 14 days preoperatively, but the potential benefits of nutrition support must be weighed against the potential risks of the nutrition support itself and of delaying the operation.
4. Nutrition support therapy should not be used *routinely* as an adjunct to chemotherapy.
5. Nutrition support therapy should not be used *routinely* in patients undergoing head and neck, abdominal, or pelvic irradiation.
6. Nutrition support therapy is appropriate in patients receiving active anticancer treatment who are malnourished and who are anticipated to be unable to ingest or absorb adequate nutrients for a prolonged period of time.
7. The palliative use of nutrition support therapy in terminally ill cancer patients is rarely indicated.
8. Omega-3 fatty acid supplementation may help stabilize weight in cancer patients on oral diets experiencing progressive unintentional weight loss.
9. Patients should not use therapeutic diets to treat cancer.
10. Immune-enhancing enteral formulas containing mixtures of arginine, nucleic acids, and essential fatty acids may be beneficial in malnourished patients undergoing major operations.

Source: Data from August and Huhmann[42].

TABLE 17-4

ASPEN Clinical Guidelines: Nutrition Support Therapy During Adult Hematopoietic Cell Transplantation

1. All patients undergoing hematopoietic stem cell transplantation (HSCT) with myeloablative conditioning regimens are at nutritional risk and should undergo nutrition screening to identify those who require formal nutritional assessment with the development of a nutritional care plan.
2. Nutrition support therapy is appropriate in patients undergoing HSCT who are malnourished and who are anticipated to be unable to ingest or absorb adequate nutrients for a prolonged period of time. When parenteral nutrition is used, it should be discontinued as soon as toxicities have been resolved after stem cell engraftment.
3. Enteral nutrition should be used in patients with a functional GI tract in whom oral intake is inadequate to meet nutritional requirements.
4. Pharmacological doses of parenteral glutamine *may benefit* patients undergoing HSCT.
5. Patients should receive dietary counseling regarding foods that may pose infectious risks and safe food handling during the period of neutropenia.
6. Nutrition support is appropriate for patients undergoing HSCT who develop moderate to severe GVHD accompanied by poor oral intake and/or significant malabsorption.

Source: Data from August and Huhmann[42].

The use of oral nutrition supplements is an intervention that is frequently suggested for cancer patients. These supplements may be of benefit in increasing caloric intake in patients who are malnourished, particularly those who have a BMI of less than 20. Moreover, in a Cochrane review, the use of supplements with energy and protein was associated with weight gain, shorter hospitalization, and improved survival.[43]

Specialized nutritional support

A variety of specialized nutritional support interventions can be utilized when patients are unable to consume adequate calories. Specialized nutrition support refers to both enteral nutrition (EN) and parenteral nutritional (PN) supplementation to bolster nutritional status. EN specifically refers to nutritional supplementation delivered through an enteral feeding device into a functioning gastrointestinal tract. PN is the administration of an admixture of nutrients systemically through the intravenous route. The use of EN is associated with improvements in nitrogen balance and consistent weight gain. PN has also been found to consistently lead to weight gain, increased body fat, and improved nitrogen balance. Neither EN nor PN has shown any ability to consistently improve levels of serum proteins.[42]

A key factor in determining the best strategy for any given patient is the functionality of the individual's gastrointestinal tract. EN is recommended in patients who have a functioning gastrointestinal tract but for whom oral intake does not adequately meet energy requirements. This approach prevents atrophy of the microvilli lining the intestinal wall and maintains normal gut flora and histology. In addition, enteral feedings prevent cholestasis by stimulating bile flow. Additional documented benefits include improvements in systemic immunity and decreased infection risk. Contraindications to EN include a malfunctioning GI tract, severe diarrhea or bleeding, GI fistulas, mechanical obstructions or malabsorption, and intractable vomiting.[42]

A variety of types of enteral feeding tubes are available. Nasoenteric tubes can be used when short-term access is required. This approach offers the advantage of exposing feedings to gastric secretions, bile acid, and pancreatic enzymes prior to the material passing into the jejunum, where most nutrient absorption takes place. Nasogastric feeding is contraindicated in patients with oral or esophageal ulcers. Further irritation of already painful ulcers can be seen when a nasogastric tube is used. In addition, these tubes can be uncomfortable for patients as well as interfere with body image.

For longer-duration (several weeks) feeding, percutaneous endoscopic gastrostomy (PEG) or jejunostomy tubes may offer patients a more comfortable option. These devices are easily inserted in the outpatient setting. PEGs are associated with a higher success and lower complication rate than other types of EN tubes, and their insertion procedures are generally easier to schedule than surgical gastrostomy. The devices are low profile and generally very well tolerated by patients. Jejunostomies access the small bowel directly; therefore, feedings are not exposed to gastric secretions and enzymes. Selection of feeding formula and schedules are prescribed to meet individual nutritional requirements and caloric needs.[44,45]

Unfortunately, feeding tubes can compromise the usual defenses against aspiration. To prevent this problem, it is recommended that continuous feedings be administered with the patient in a sitting position or with the head of the bed elevated at a 45-degree angle. Residual feeding remaining in the stomach should be checked on a 4- to 8-hour basis to determine absorption. Nursing care of the patient receiving enteral feedings focuses on preventing complications, ensuring safety, and promoting comfort. Complications associated with enteral feeding tubes include malposition, clogging, breakage, leaking, skin damage around the insertion site, and diarrhea.[44–47]

Teaching the patient and family to maintain the feeding tube and schedule is important and allows the patient to remain at home, thereby promoting the patient's self-esteem and potentially improving quality of life. Patients with gastrostomies or jejunostomies can be taught to blenderize table foods, which may cut down on expense, promote more normal digestion, and psychologically provide satiety. (See Appendix 17D, Self-Care Guide: Tube Feeding, for more information about teaching patients.)

When the enteral route cannot be used, parenteral administration provides another option for nutritional support. Parenteral formulas should include adequate amounts of hypertonic glucose, protein, fat emulsion, vitamins, electrolytes, and minerals. Parenteral nutrition is administered via a central line into a deep vein, where rapid blood flow quickly dilutes the hypertonic formula. Like EN, PN is associated with a number of complications, including fluid overload, hepatic dysfunction, subclavian vein thrombosis, delays in platelet engraftment, and catheter-related infections. PN may also diminish appetite. Specific contraindications for using the parenteral approach include a functioning GI tract, the need for nutritional support therapy for a period of less than 5 days, lack of adequate vascular access, hemodynamic instability, profound metabolic or electrolyte disturbances, anuria, and patient or caregiver preference.[42]

As with the enteral approach, PN feeding formulas and schedules are based on individual need and caloric requirements. In addition, the patient and caregiver must be evaluated for their ability to manage the complexity associated with this method of nutritional support. A home care assessment and plan should be coordinated (see Appendix 17E, Self-Care Guide: Intravenous Feeding). Oral intake should be encouraged (if not contraindicated) to ensure continued gut stimulation. In addition, food consumption may satisfy social, emotional, and psychological needs.

EN and PN can both be used in the setting of HCT to support nutritional status during the peritransplant period. ASPEN recommends the use of nutrition support therapy for patients undergoing HCT who are malnourished and who will be unable to consume or absorb adequate nutrients for a prolonged period of time, so as to minimize the complications associated with malnutrition. A span of 7 to 14 days is generally accepted as a "prolonged period," although this definition has not been clearly explicated in the literature.[42]

Complementary and alternative therapies

Cancer patients as a group are increasingly using alternative and complementary therapies. Nutrition-related alternative treatment methods are readily available, and include an assortment of nutrients, non-nutrients, and bioactive food components. Examples of nutritional alternative therapies include macrobiotic regimens, supplements, dietary macronutrients, and various vitamin regimens. Data on the use of alternative nutritional methods are extremely limited; to date, no alternative nutritional methods have demonstrated efficacy in methodologically sound clinical trials. It is important for clinicians to know whether their patients are using alternative nutritional methods; consequently, patients should be asked about this possibility during the nutrition history. Asking questions about alternative nutritional therapies opens the door to communicating about the issue. Patients often have questions about these therapies and need a reliable source of information. Clinicians should serve as a resource for patients by offering scientific evidence (if available) as well as highlighting data on potential harm that may be associated with the alternative interventions.

Pharmacologic agents

Developing pharmacologic agents to counteract the effects of cancer cachexia is a high-priority area of research. Evidence from well-designed, methodologically sound clinical trials supports the use of several pharmacologic agents in patients with anorexia or cachexia. In addition, numerous other compounds are in various stages of development for this indication. Pharmacologic agents used to treat cachexia can be grouped into three broad categories: agents that are aimed at stimulating appetite, drugs that target inflammatory cytokines, and compounds that target protein catabolism.

Appetite stimulants. Corticosteroids have been used as first-line agents in the treatment of anorexia and cachexia. In particular, dexamethasone, methylprednisolone, and prednisolone have been evaluated for this indication in randomized, double-blind, placebo-controlled clinical trials.[9] The mechanism of action by which these agents induce appetite stimulation has not been clearly explicated, but it may be related to their euphorogenic side effects. Improvements in appetite following corticosteroid use are seen within the first 1 to 3 weeks of therapy. Benefits beyond this time frame have not been reported without dose escalations.[9] Higher doses and increased duration of use place corticosteroid recipients at greater risk for the development of side effects, which often include muscle wasting or weakness (especially problematic in the cachectic population), immunosuppression, hyperglycemia that can progress to diabetes, osteoporosis, delirium, and cataract formation. Despite their negative side-effect profile, corticosteroids are frequently used on a short-term basis in the setting of cachexia.[9,10]

The progestinal agents medroxyprogesterone acetate (MPA) and megesterol acetate (MA) are synthetic derivatives of the naturally occurring hormone progesterone.[48,49] Both MPA and MA have been shown to induce appetite stimulation and weight gain in cancer patients. Other biological actions of these agents—particularly those that increase appetite, weight, and a sense of well-being—are less well understood, but are thought to be related to true appetite stimulation and anabolic effects. Recent evidence suggests that MA may also down-regulate the synthesis and release of cytokines.[2]

MA is currently used for its orexigenic effects and was granted Food and Drug Administration (FDA) approval for the treatment of AIDS-related anorexia and cachexia in 1993.[48] Multiple randomized, double-blind, placebo-controlled clinical trials evaluating the safety and efficacy of MA have been conducted in cachectic cancer patients.[2,9] Results have consistently demonstrated that patients who receive MA experience increases in appetite when compared with placebo controls. Subsequent weight gain is seen in the majority of these patients. Other benefits documented include improvements in anthropometric measures (skin fold thickness) and subjective energy levels. Progestinal agents are generally well tolerated. Side effects include mild edema, nausea, and thrombolic events.[3]

Ghrelin, a neuropeptide released from the stomach in response to fasting, has been shown to be a potent stimulator of appetite.[50] A recent study[2] demonstrated increased energy intake and meal appreciation by approximately 30% of patients with cancer and anorexia who received ghrelin, without side effects. Further studies are needed to determine if ghrelin increases lean body mass and weight. This agent needs to be administered by injection, which limits its clinical applicability. RC-1291, a ghrelin mimetic, is currently being investigated in the setting of cancer-induced anorexia. This agent has been shown to increase lean body mass and improve hand grip strength; no changes in quality of life or weight with its use have been reported to date.[3] Ghrelin-mimetic agents are an important focal area of current inquiry.

Cannabinoids are derivatives of marijuana that act via the CB_1 and CB_2 cannabinoid receptors to modulate the cytokine response of a number of immune cells. Dronabinol has been found to improve appetite and induce weight gain in phase III randomized trials[48]; however, the results were not as substantial as those induced by MA. Cannabinoids generally have a very tolerable side-effect profile. A novel inhaled formulation of dronabinol is currently in early-phase trials.[48]

Compounds targeting protein catabolism. Eicosapentaenoic acid (EPA) is an essential omega-3 fatty acid that is found in oily fish such as salmon, mackerel, or sardines. EPA has been found to decrease muscle atrophy and stimulate appetite. Moreover, evidence supports stabilization of body weight in patients with cancer, although poor compliance has been an issue with patients participating in studies involving this agent.[2] β-Hydroxy-β-methylbutyrate (HBM) is similar to EPA in that it attenuates PIF-induced protein degradation in muscle by down-regulating the ubiquitin–proteasome pathway. HBM also plays a role in protein synthesis. In placebo-controlled trials, when HBM was administered in combination with l-glutamine and l-arginine, increases body weight and lean body mass were reported; no change in fat mass was demonstrated. Additional work in this area is ongoing.[2,5]

Drugs targeting inflammatory cytokines. Melatonin is an emerging agent that has been tested in the setting of anorexia–cachexia, Melatonin is a pineal hormone that is responsible for regulating circadian rhythm. The theory supporting its mechanism of action is predicated on the assumption that cancer patients have disruptions in their circadian rhythms that stimulate the release of TNF. Melatonin may be able to treat cachexia by decreasing TNF levels. It has other biological activities, including antiproliferative actions, immunomodulatory effects on anticancer immunity, antioxidant activity, thrombopoietic activity, and psychomimetic properties that include antianxiety, antidepressant, and antiasthenic effects. Melatonin must be investigated in placebo-controlled trials before recommendations on clinical use of this agent can be made.[51]

Thalidomide is a cyclic imide that has been shown to decrease the stability of messenger RNA segments (mRNAs) coding for various pro-inflammatory cytokines, including TNF-α.[52] Thalidomide has now been investigated in several clinical trials aimed at evaluating its effectiveness in the treatment of cancer-related anorexia and cachexia. In a small preliminary study,[2] it was shown to improve symptoms, including nausea, appetite, and sensation of well-being and restedness in the morning. Another early investigation evaluating the use of an isocaloric diet in combination with thalidomide demonstrated increases in body weight and lean body mass in patients with solid tumors. In this study, thalidomide was well tolerated, with no patients developing neuropathy.[2]

Several other agents that have the ability to inhibit cytokine production have been investigated for their potential use to treat cachexia. Atractylenolide (ATR) is an agent that has been used in Chinese traditional medicine to improve gastrointestinal symptoms that include nausea, vomiting, and anorexia. Recent evidence has demonstrated its ability to markedly decrease circulating IL-1. Moreover, in a randomized, nonblinded pilot study involving a small sample of patients with cancer, ATR was shown to significantly increase body weight and arm circumference.[53] Cytokine-neutralizing agents, such as the monoclonal antibody infliximab and soluble receptors such as enteracept, both of which target TNF-α, are used to treat other chronic inflammatory pathologies and have been shown to increase weight and lean body mass in patients with rheumatoid arthritis.[54,55] Although clinical trials of these agents are under way in cancer,[56] only limited information about the use of these agents in the setting of cancer cachexia is currently available.

The use of small-molecule Janus-associated kinase 1 (JAK1) and 2 (JAK2) inhibitors in the setting of cachexia is also being investigated. A number of oral JAK2 inhibitors are currently under development for the treatment of myeloproliferative malignancies. The primary therapeutic benefit of these agents is the control of constitutional symptoms associated with these diseases. Patients participating in phase III clinical trials of these medications experienced weight gain and improvement in performance status, as well as improved quality of life.[57,58] In addition, these agents are associated with a rapid and sustained decrease in the hepatomegaly and splenomegaly that develop as a result of extramedullary hematopoiesis in this population. This factor is important because hepatomegaly and splenomegaly can lead to abdominal discomfort and pressure that often results in diminished intake of food among patients.[57–59]

While these and other molecules that block cytokine production or interfere with the proposed mechanisms of cachexia hold promise, none of them is currently available for routine use in cancer patients. Moreover, it is important to consider how agents that alter immune responses will be broadly applied in the cancer setting, particularly in patients who have hematologic malignancies.

NURSING IMPLICATIONS

Effective nutritional programs epitomize interdisciplinary care that integrates the services of trained dietary specialists, nurses, physicians, pharmacists, social workers, and specialists in pain and symptom management. Oncology nurses are in a pivotal position to provide proactive screening and assessment, as well as continuity and follow-up for cancer patients with nutritional issues. Nurses can provide quality nutritional care.

The effects of nutritional interventions need to be carefully monitored. Because the majority of cancer care is delivered in the ambulatory setting, ensuring that patients and family members are educated about potential problems and any situations that would warrant the attention of the nurse or physician is essential. Using standardized assessment tools allows patient status to be effectively monitored across the trajectory of care. At the earliest signs of deterioration, therapeutic interventions including aggressive symptom management and nutritional support should be instituted. Patients should be instructed to call with any questions or concerns and to provide updates on how interventions are working. Expected short-term outcomes of therapeutic interventions would include improvement in appetite, increased oral intake, elimination or effective control of nutrition-impact symptoms, and optimization of function. When these effects are sustained over time, normalization of laboratory values, reversal of weight loss, and repletion of lean body mass can occur.

Despite the best interventions, some patients may not respond to attempts to control cachexia. In such cases, the best supportive care should be considered.

Through screening and comprehensive patient assessment, oncology nurses can proactively identify those patients who will require nutritional interventions and education. A focus on nutritional issues at the onset of care and on a systematic basis throughout the care trajectory is essential to optimizing outcomes. Prevention of nutritional problems rather than repletion of nutritional status is preferred on the basis of risk, simplicity, and cost. Oncology nurses should ensure that processes are in place in their clinical practice settings to support systematic nutritional screening and assessment. Although tools that have been validated in the cancer population are available, they have not yet been uniformly incorporated into the practice environment. By supporting the integration of these practices, oncology nurses can contribute to driving quality and optimizing nutritional care for cancer patients.

In managing symptoms in any given patient, oncology nurses should base their interventions on the most recent evidence available. The management of symptoms is a high priority for oncology nurses; thus they have an incumbent responsibility to remain abreast of changes in practice based on new research findings. Several of the symptoms that are commonly associated with cachexia and evidence-based recommendations to manage these issues were discussed earlier in this chapter. Additional evidence is needed in many of these areas.

PATIENT SELF-CARE

Comprehensive patient and caregiver education should be incorporated into cancer programs. Resources should include printed materials, online resources, videos, and access to trained dietary specialists. Specific education, tailored to individual patient need, is also essential. Education can ensure understanding and promote compliance with the treatment plan. Patients and caregivers should be taught which symptoms to anticipate and how to monitor for and manage them. Such information should include early warning signs, self-care strategies, and instructions on when and where to contact the nurse or physician. Teaching guides that provide written instructions and "hints" can often be very useful. Several examples of self-care teaching aids are provided in the appendices for patients. (See Appendices 17D and 17E for guidance on enteral and parenteral feedings; Appendices 17B and 17C offer information on anorexia–cachexia and changes in taste and smell.)

Education for patients and caregivers should also include general information on nutrition. Many patients do not have knowledge about the fundamentals of good nutrition; consequently, they may need guidance as to which foods may be the best sources of nutritious calories and protein. Caregivers are frequently responsible for assisting with preparing meals, so they should also be included in all nutrition education efforts. Encouraging patient and family interaction and providing emotional support is helpful as well. When family members can provide the patient's favorite foods, intake usually improves and family bonds can be strengthened.

Caregivers should also be taught to monitor the patient's intake. They should be instructed on how to adequately complete food diaries and accurately report symptoms that may influence intake. The proper procedure for reporting changes in status or concerns should also be provided.

Providing nutritional education for professionals is also essential. A full range of professional educational resources should be made available to ensure that healthcare providers are up-to-date on clinical issues related to nutrition and can teach patients and families how to proactively manage nutrition. Nutritional topics should be incorporated into patient care rounds as well as other appropriate educational forums. The standard of nutritional care in cancer should include a proactive, integrated, algorithmic approach to each patient.

REFERENCES

1. von Haehling S, Anker SD. Cachexia as a major underestimated and unmet medical need: facts and numbers. *J Cachexia Sarcopenia Muscle.* 2010;1(1):1–5.
2. Tisdale MJ. Mechanisms of cancer cachexia. *Physiol Rev.* 2009;89(2):381–410.
3. Tisdale MJ. Cancer cachexia. *Curr Opin Gastroenterol.* 2010;26(2):146–151.
4. Tisdale MJ. Reversing cachexia. *Cell.* 2010;142(4):511–512.
5. Donohoe CL, Ryan AM, Reynolds JV. Cancer cachexia: mechanisms and clinical implications. *Gastroenterol Res Pract.* 2011;2011:601434.
6. Bennani-Bati N, Walsh D. What is cancer anorexia–cachexia syndrome? A historical perspective. *J R Coll Physicians Edinb.* 2009;39(3):257–262.
7. Fearon KC, Strasser F, Anker SD, et al. Definition and classification of cancer cachexia: an international consensus. *Lancet Oncol.* 2011;12(5):489–495.
8. Fearon KC. The 2011 ESPEN Arvid Wretlind lecture: cancer cachexia: the potential impact of translational research on patient-focused outcomes. *Clin Nutr.* 2012;31(5):577–582.
9. Adams LA, Shepard N, Caruso RA, Norling MJ, Belansky H, Cunningham RS. Putting evidence into practice: evidence-based interventions to prevent and manage anorexia. *Clin J Oncol Nurs.* 2009;13(1):95–102.
10. Cunningham RS, Huhman MB. Nutritional disturbances. In: Yarbro CH, Wujcik D, Gobel BH, eds. *Cancer Nursing Principles and Practice.* 7th ed. Sudbury, MA: Jones and Bartlett; 2011:818–844.
11. McLaughlin L, Mahon SM. Understanding taste dysfunction in patients with cancer. *Clin J Oncol Nurs.* 2012;16(2):171–178.
12. Epstein JB, Barasch A. Taste disorders in cancer patients: pathogenesis, and approach to assessment and management. *Oral Oncol.* 2010;46(2):77–81.
13. Hutton V, Baracos W, Wismer WV. Chemosensory dysfunction is a primary factor in the evolution of declining nutritional status and quality of life in patients with advanced cancer. *J Pain Symptom Manage.* 2007;33:156–165.
14. Bernhardson BM, Tishelman C, Rutqvist LE. Olfactory changes among patients receiving chemotherapy. *Eur J Oncol Nurs.* 2009;13:9–15.
15. Gupta D, Vashi PG, Lammersfeld CA, Braun DP. Role of nutritional status in predicting the length of stay in cancer: a systematic review of the epidemiological literature. *Ann Nutr Metab.* 2011;59(2–4):96–106.
16. Laky B, Janda M, Kondalsamy-Chennakesavan S, Cleghorn G, Obermair A. Pretreatment malnutrition and quality of life-association with prolonged length of hospital stay among patients with gynecological cancer: a cohort study. *BMC Cancer.* 2010;10:232.
17. DeWys WD, Begg C, Lavin PT, et al. Prognostic effect of weight loss prior to chemotherapy in cancer patients. *Am J Med.* 1980;69:491–497.
18. Kyle UG, Chalandon Y, Miralbell R, et al. Longitudinal follow-up of body composition in hematopoietic stem cell transplant patients. *Bone Marrow Transplant.* 2005;35(12):1171–1177.
19. Davis MP, Walsh D, Lagman R, Yavuzsen T. Early satiety in cancer patients: a common and important but underrecognized symptom. *Support Care Cancer.* 2006;14(7):693–698.
20. Green DM, Cox CL, Zhu L, et al. Risk factors for obesity in adult survivors of childhood cancer: a report from the childhood cancer survivor study. *Clin Oncol.* 2012;30(3):246–255.
21. Morley JE. Calories and cachexia. *Curr Opin Clin Nutr Metab Care.* 2009;12(6):607–610.
22. Hopkinson JB. The emotional aspects of cancer anorexia. *Curr Opin Support Palliat Care.* 2010;4(4):254–258.
23. Patra SK, Arora S. Integrative neuropeptides and cytokines in cancer anorexia–cachexia syndrome. *Clin Chim Acta.* 2012;413(13–14):1025–1034.
24. Tisdale MJ. Protein metabolism in cachexia. In: Mantovani G, Anker SD, Inui A, et al., eds. *Cachexia and Wasting: A Modern Approach.* Milan, Italy: Springer-Verlag Italia; 2006:185–190.
25. Al-Majid S, Waters H. The biological mechanisms of cancer-related skeletal muscle wasting: the role of progressive resistance exercise. *Biol Res Nurs.* 2008;10(1):7–20.
26. Maccio A, Madeddu C, Mantovanni G. Glucose metabolism. In: Mantovani G, Anker SD, Inui A, et al., eds. *Cachexia and Wasting: A Modern Approach.* Milan, Italy: Springer-Verlag Italia; 2006:477–482.
27. Yulyaningsih E, Zhang L, Herzog H, et al. NPY receptors as potential targets for anti-obesity drug development. *Br J Pharmacol.* 2011;163(6):1170–1202.
28. Dianliang Z. Probing cancer cachexia–anorexia: recent results with knockout, transgene and polymorphisms. *Curr Opin Clin Nutr Metab Care.* 2009;12(3):227–231.
29. Tan BH, Fearon KC. Cachexia: prevalence and impact in medicine. *Curr Opin Clin Nutr Metab Care.* 2008;11:400–407.
30. Tan BH, Deans DA, Skipworth RJ, Ross JA, Fearon KC. Biomarkers for cancer cachexia: is there also a genetic component to cachexia? *Support Care Cancer.* 2007;16:229–234.
31. National Cancer Institute. http://www.cancer.gov/cancertopics/coping/eatinghints. Accessed April 2, 2012.
32. Read JA, Crockett N, Volker DH, et al. Nutritional assessment in cancer: comparing the Mini-Nutritional Assessment (MNA) with the scored Patient-Generated Subjective Global Assessment (PGSGA). *Nutr Cancer.* 2005;53(1):51–56.

33. Ottery FD. Patient-generated subjective global assessment. In: McCullum PD, Polisena CG, eds. *The Clinical Guide to Oncology Nutrition.* Chicago: American Dietetic Association; 2000:11.
34. National Heart, Blood, and Lung Institute. http://www.nhlbi.nih.gov/guidelines/obesity/bmi_tbl.htm. Accessed September 12, 2012.
35. Potischman N. Biologic and methodologic issues for nutritional biomarkers. *J Nutr.* 2003;133(suppl 3):875S–880S.
36. Rzepecki P, Barzal J, Sarosiek T, Szczylik C. Biochemical indices for the assessment of nutritional status during hematopoietic stem cell transplantation: are they worth using? A single center experience. *Bone Marrow Transplant.* 2007;40(6):567–72.
37. Thibault R, Genton L, Pichard C. Body composition: why, when and for who? *Clin Nutr.* 2012: 31(4):435–447.
38. U.S. Department of Health and Human Services. Common terminology criteria for adverse events v 4.02. 2009. http://evs.nci.nih.gov/ftp1/CTCAE/CTCAE_4.03_2010-06-14_QuickReference_5x7.pdf. Accessed September 10, 2012.
39. U.S. Department of Health and Human Services. Common terminology criteria for adverse events v 2.0. 1999. http://firm-act.org/documents/appendix4.pdf. Accessed September 10, 2012.
40. Roeland E, Mitchell W, Elia G, et al. Symptom control in stem cell transplantation: a multidisciplinary palliative care team approach. Part 1: physical symptoms. *J Support Oncol.* 2010;8(3):100–116.
41. Roeland E, Mitchell W, Elia G, et al. Symptom control in stem cell transplantation: a multidisciplinary palliative care team approach. Part 2: psychosocial concerns. *J Support Oncol.* 2010;8(4):179–183.
42. August DA, Huhmann MB; American Society for Parenteral and Enteral Nutrition (A.S.P.E.N.) Board of Directors. A.S.P.E.N. clinical guidelines: nutrition support therapy during adult anticancer treatment and in hematopoietic cell transplantation. *J Parenter Enteral Nutr.* 2009;33(5):472–500.
43. Milne AC, Potter J, Avenell A. Protein and energy supplementation in elderly people at risk for malnutrition. *Cochrane Database Syst Rev.* 2005;2:CD003288.
44. Wireko BM. Enteral tube feeding. *Clin Med.* 2010;10(6):616–619.
45. Holmes S. Enteral nutrition: an overview. *Nurs Standard.* 2012;26(39):41–46.
46. Lau MT, Girard J. Ensuring safer enteral feeding. *Nurs Manage.* 2011;42(12):39–43.
47. Alivizatos V, Gavala V, Alexopoulos P, Apostolopoulos A, Bajruevic S. Feeding tube-related complications and problems in patients receiving long-term home enteral nutrition. *Indian J Palliat Care.* 2012;18(1):31–33.
48. Murphy KT, Lynch GS. Update on emerging drugs for cancer cachexia. *Expert Opin Emerg Drugs.* 2009;14(4):619–632.
49. Madeddu C, Maccio A, Panzone F, Tanca FM, Mantovani G. Medroxyprogesterone acetate in the management of cancer cachexia. *Expert Opin Pharmacother.* 2009;10(8):1359–1366.
50. DeBoer MD. Emergence of ghrelin as a treatment for cachexia syndromes. *Nutrition.* 2008;24:806–814.
51. Strasser F. Appraisal of current and experimental approaches to the treatment of cachexia. *Curr Opin Support Palliat Care.* 2007;1(4):312–316.
52. Penna F, Minero VG, Costamanga D, et al. Anti-cytokine strategies for the treatment of cancer-related anorexia and cachexia. *Expert Opin Biol Ther.* 2010;10(8):1241–1250.
53. Liu Y, Jia Z, Dong L, Wang R, Qiu G. A randomized pilot study of atractylenolide I on gastric cancer cachexia patients. *Evid Based Complement Alternat Med.* 2008;5(3):337–344.
54. Brown RA, Spina D, Butt S, Summers GC. Long-term effects of anti-tumor necrosis factor therapy on weight in patients with rheumatoid arthritis. *Clin Rheumatol.* 2012; 31(3):455–461.
55. Florin V, Cottencin AC, Delaporte E, Staumont-Salle D. Body weight increment in patients treated with infliximab for plaque psoriasis. *J Eur Acad Dermatol Venereol.* 2012 May 23.Epub ahead of print
56. Jatoi A, Ritter HL, Dueck A, et al. A placebo-controlled, double-blind study of infliximab for cancer-associated weight loss in elderly and/or poor performance non-small cell lung cancer patients (N01C9). *Lung Cancer.* 2010;686(2):234–239.
57. Santos FP, Verstovsek S. JAK2 inhibitors: are they the solution? *Clin Lymphoma Myeloma Leuk.* 2011;11(suppl 1):S28–S36.
58. Santos FP, Verstovsek S. Therapy with JAK2 inhibitors for myeloproliferative neoplasms. *Hematol Oncol Clin North Am.* 2012;26:1083–1099.
59. Harrison C, Verstovsek S, McMullin MF, Mesa R. Janus kinase inhibition and its effect upon the therapeutic landscape of myelofibrosis: from palliation to cure? *Br J Haematol.* 2012;157(4):426–437.

Weekly Food Diary

A food diary is a record of the type, amount, and time of your food intake over a 7-day period. Diaries are important because people cannot always accurately remember what or when they ate. Food diaries are helpful in understanding what you are actually eating and when. The information you record in the diary can be used to tailor nutritional planning so that it best supports your individual needs.

General Instructions for Keeping a Food Diary

- Keep a record of all foods and drinks that you consume for the next 7 days in a chart similar to the example shown here. Be sure to include all foods, drinks (including water), nutrition supplements, and any between-meal snacks.
- You should not change your food habits while keeping the diary, unless you are instructed to do so by your healthcare provider.
- It is important to write the information down immediately after you eat or drink. Do not wait until the end of the day to record this information. Keep the food diary in the kitchen or close to where you will be eating so that it is easy to accurately record the information.

Recording the Amount of Food

- Measuring the amount of food and liquid consumed is important. Use measuring spoons and cups and a small diet scale, if possible, to accurately record amounts or portion sizes. Sometimes you will have to estimate portion size. As a general rule of thumb, a 3-ounce cooked portion is approximately the size of a deck of cards. You can also estimate portions by measuring the size, such as a 3-inch by 3-inch piece of banana bread.
- Describe food as much as possible using words like "plain," "baked," "broiled," "fried," "breaded," "sweetened," "whole," "half," and "sliced."
- Remember to record all food items, including the extras like margarine, butter, sauces, gravies, cream, sugar, ketchup, mustard, pickles, and other added foods.
- Be sure to include any vitamin and mineral supplements that you take.
- Many food diaries also record activity. Include brief notes about any activities, such as walking, sitting, resting in bed, and working.

Follow-Up

Remember to bring the record back on follow-up visits!

Phone Numbers

Nurse: ______________________ Number: ______________________

Physician: ______________________ Number: ______________________

Dietitian: ______________________ Number: ______________________

7-Day Food Diary

Patient Name: ______________________________

Day 1 Date: ________________

Time	Food or Drink Consumed	Amount or Portion Size	Activity	Comments

Day 2 Date: ________________

Time	Food or Drink Consumed	Amount or Portion Size	Activity	Comments

(continued)

Day 3 Date: ______________________

Time	Food or Drink Consumed	Amount or Portion Size	Activity	Comments

Day 4 Date: ______________________

Time	Food or Drink Consumed	Amount or Portion Size	Activity	Comments

Day 5 Date: ______________

Time	Food or Drink Consumed	Amount or Portion Size	Activity	Comments

Day 6 Date: ______________

Time	Food or Drink Consumed	Amount or Portion Size	Activity	Comments

(continued)

Day 7 Date: ______________________

Time	Food or Drink Consumed	Amount or Portion Size	Activity	Comments

Source: Cunningham RS. The Cancer Cachexia Syndrome. In: Yarbro CH, Wujcik D, Gobel BH, eds. *Cancer Symptom Management*. 4th ed. Burlington, MA: Jones & Bartlett Learning; 2014.

Anorexia–Cachexia

Patient Name: ____________________

This guide is designed to help you understand and manage anorexia and weight loss. It provides practical information on how you can eat and drink enough.

Symptom and Description

Anorexia means a loss of appetite. Decreased appetite can lead to less food intake, weight loss, poor nutrition, and loss of muscle and strength. The combination of anorexia, weight loss, poor nutrition, and loss of muscle mass and strength are known as cachexia.

Anorexia is common in cancer patients and can happen because of the side effects of cancer treatment. Treatments often cause side effects such as nausea or changes in the oral mucous membranes. These problems can interfere with the ability to eat normally and usually lasts only until the side effects go away. Sometimes changes in appetite can also be related to the cancer itself. Cancers can cause changes in appetite and metabolism. The reasons why this happens are not entirely clear—it is an area of ongoing research.

Prevention

Making sure that you maintain proper nutrition is a very important part of cancer care. You should be aware of any changes in your eating habits or weight from the time of diagnosis. Be sure that you consume enough calories and maintain your weight so that you feel your best during cancer treatment. Preventing weight loss and muscle wasting are important goals that can help you to remain active. Although you are familiar with managing your own intake and weight, you may need information and tools to assist you with keeping them on track. Many people need education about what constitutes a healthy diet.

Management

Things that can help with your appetite:

- Pay attention to your appetite pattern and use it to guide your food intake. Sometimes people have a normal appetite in the morning, with anorexia worsening as the day goes on. You should eat food during the times when your appetite is best.
- Avoid large meals. Eating smaller, more manageable meals 5–6 times per day can be helpful when you do not have much of an appetite.
- It is important that you get enough calories. Selecting calorie-dense foods (foods that have a large amount of calories for their portion size) can be helpful. Examples of calorie-dense foods include pasta, rice, bread, potatoes, oils, nuts, nut butters, avocados, and bananas.

(continued)

- Make sure that your diet contains foods that are good sources of proteins, carbohydrates, and fats. Some examples of foods in each of these categories are shown in the following table:

Proteins	• Meats such as lamb, beef, chicken, turkey • Fish, water-packed tuna • Salami • Cheese • Eggs • Beans • Tofu • Greek yogurt • Protein-dense bars such as Zone Perfect, Special K® Protein, and Clif® Bars • Carnation® Instant Breakfast
Carbohydrates	• Whole grains such as oats (oatmeal), wild rice, quinoa, barley, buckwheat, amaranth, and wheatberries • Cereals • Pasta • Fruits • Starchy vegetables such as peas, potatoes, and corn • Candy, concentrated sweets
Fats	• Whole milk • Ice cream • Olives • Peanut butter • Oils

- Make an appointment with a dietitian if you have access to this resource.
- Take a multivitamin daily.
- Limit your intake of fluids with meals. Fluids can create a sense of fullness that can limit the amount of food you are able to eat. Fluids should be taken about 30 minutes before meals or between meals.
- Ask friends and family to help with preparing meals or "favorite" foods, so that you have these readily available when you want them.
- Do some form of mild exercise for 10–20 minutes each day. This helps to keep your muscles stimulated and your strength up. Taking a walk prior to meals will help stimulate appetite. Exercise following meals assists with gastric emptying.
- Eat in a pleasant space.
- There is some evidence that certain medications can help improve your appetite and help you to gain weight. Ask your doctor or nurse if such therapy might be right for you. The medicines called corticosteroids and progestins have been shown to increase appetite and weight in some groups of patients.
- A glass of wine prior to a meal can be a helpful appetite stimulant.
- Eliminate food restrictions whenever possible. For example, low-salt or restricted-calorie diets can often be eliminated. You should double-check with your physician or nurse before making such changes in your diet.
- Monitor yourself for the development of any symptoms that may interfere with your ability to eat. Examples include nausea or sores in your mouth. If symptoms develop, they should be reported to your healthcare provider, who can guide you on how to manage them. Symptoms that interfere with eating should be managed very aggressively.

Monitoring and maintaining your weight:

- It is important to monitor your weight over time.
- You should use the same scale and weigh yourself around the same time of day.

Follow-Up

You should notify your doctor or nurse if any of the following occur:

- You are unable to consume or keep down fluids or food.
- You experience symptoms that limit your intake of food/fluids.
- You experience a weight loss of 2 pounds or more over a 1-week period.

Phone Numbers

Nurse: ______________________________ Number: ________________________

Physician: ___________________________ Number: ________________________

Dietitian: ___________________________ Number: ________________________

Source: Cunningham RS. The Cancer Cachexia Syndrome. In: Yarbro CH, Wujcik D, Gobel BH, eds. *Cancer Symptom Management.* 4th ed. Burlington, MA: Jones & Bartlett Learning; 2014.

Changes in Taste and Smell

Patient Name: ____

Symptom and Description

Changes in the senses of taste and smell are often experienced by patients receiving therapy for cancer. Common types of taste changes include decreased ability to taste foods and a loss of taste. Foods may often not taste the same as they used to taste. In particular, sweet, bitter, and salty tastes can seem very different. You may crave more sweet and salty foods. Sometimes people experience a metallic taste in the mouth.

The senses of taste and smell are closely related, so patients receiving cancer treatment can also experience changes in their sense of smell. Usually, the sense of smell becomes more sensitive, particularly to odors that are unpleasant, such as body odors or hospital smells. Changes in the senses of taste and smell can lead to food dislikes, decreased intake of food, and weight loss.

Management

There has been little research on which strategies work best to manage taste changes. Most of the information available is based on assessments, rather than outcomes data. Making sure that you are able to eat properly and maintain weight during cancer treatment is very important. Being aware of issues with food intake and nutrition is important from the time you are first diagnosed. Here are a few helpful hints:

- If foods taste good, eat them. If foods no longer taste right, avoid them.
- Eliminate odors that may affect taste. This can be done by using a kitchen fan when cooking, using an outdoor barbecue grill to cook, and using boiling bags, covered pots, or microwave ovens.
- Cold foods are usually associated with fewer odors than warm or hot foods. Try deviled eggs, chicken, ham, egg salad, ice cream, milk shakes, puddings, custard, and cheese.
- If a metallic taste is present, try smooth, blended foods. Foods that are spicy with a rough texture should be avoided; alterations in taste can be influenced by texture and heat sensations.
- Chew food well and take fluid in the mouth with each bite. This can help food to get down to the taste buds.
- Chewing gum or sucking on hard candy such as Lifesavers can be helpful in minimizing a metallic taste.
- Sometimes red meats no longer taste good because of cancer treatments. If this happens, use other sources of protein, such as poultry, fish, eggs, peanut butter, cooked dried beans and peas, and dairy products.
- Marinate meat, chicken, or fish in sweet fruit juice, wine, salad dressing, or barbecue sauce to help improve the taste.
- Use herbs and spices such as oregano, rosemary, tarragon, and lemon juice to enhance the taste of foods. Aromatic herbs may enhance flavor recognition.

- Try new and attractively prepared foods to help make the meal more appetizing. It is a good idea not to try new foods before a treatment.
- Sugar can be used to tone down salty foods. Try adding sugar to grapefruit juice or tomato sauce.
- The flavor of starchy foods, such as rice or pasta, may be improved if they are not prepared with butter or margarine.
- Tart foods such as orange juice, pickles, lemonade, vinegar, and lemon juice may be helpful in improving flavor.
- Some research has focused on medications that may reduce changes in taste. The use of zinc supplements, for example, has been shown to be helpful in some patients. If changes in taste are persistent, ask your doctor of nurse if such supplements might be right for you.

Follow-Up

You should let your doctor or nurse know about the following situations:

- Changes in your sense of smell or taste prevent you from being able to maintain your intake of food or fluids.
- You experience symptoms such as nausea or vomiting that interfere with your ability to keep food or fluids down.
- You lose weight unintentionally.

Phone Numbers

Nurse: ______________________________ Number: ________________________

Physician: ___________________________ Number: ________________________

Dietitian: ____________________________ Number: ________________________

Source: Cunningham RS. The Cancer Cachexia Syndrome. In: Yarbro CH, Wujcik D, Gobel BH, eds. *Cancer Symptom Management.* 4th ed. Burlington, MA: Jones & Bartlett Learning; 2014.

Tube Feeding

Patient Name: ____

Symptom and Description

When weight loss or lack of appetite becomes severe, nutrition supplements can be given. These supplements provide calories and nutrients your body needs for energy. If you are unable to take these supplements by mouth, special tubes can be placed that allow you to receive the necessary nutrients without eating or drinking. Insertion of the tubes is relatively simple and can usually be done in the outpatient setting. There are several types of special tubes:

- **Nasogastric tube:** A tube that goes through the nose down the esophagus to the stomach. It is used to provide nutrition for a short period of time, such as a few days to a few weeks.
- **Gastrostomy tube:** A tube that is placed by the surgeon into the stomach through a small hole outside the stomach wall.
- **Jejunostomy tube:** A tube that is placed into the upper part of the intestine (jejunum), just beyond the stomach. It is placed by a surgeon through a small hole in the abdomen. Both gastrostomy and jejunostomy tubes are used to provide nutritional support for longer periods, usually several weeks.

Preventing Problems with Tubes

Many problems associated with tubes and tube feedings can be prevented with good tube care.

1. To prevent regurgitation of the feeding:
   - Sit up during feeding and for about 1 hour following feeding.
   - If your feeding is continuous, keep your head elevated on two or three pillows.
   - Before starting your feeding, check for any remaining food in your stomach. This can be done by aspirating the tube. When you aspirate, if you get back more than 2 ounces of residual food, do not take a feeding at that time. Try again in 1 hour.
   - Check placement of tube before beginning your feedings.
   - Do not begin feeding if you feel full or bloated.
2. To prevent diarrhea:
   - Allow the feeding solution to warm to room temperature before beginning the feeding.
   - Use lactose-free formulas.
   - Do not use feeding solution that has been opened and out for more than 6 to 8 hours.
   - Do not use feeding solution left open in the refrigerator for longer than 24 hours.
   - Wash your hands before handling the tube or feeding solution.
   - Keep the feeding container clean and all of your feeding equipment clean.

3. To prevent constipation:
   - Make sure you drink enough water.
   - Ask about adding fiber to your diet.
   - Consider a stool softener/laxative if you are prone to constipation.
   - Increase your physical activity as tolerated.
4. To prevent skin irritation:
   - It is important to keep the skin around tube clean and dry.
   - Check for leakage around tube and report any immediately to your caregiver.
   - Tape the tube securely to prevent pulling.
   - Change the dressing daily or as directed.
   - Apply skin protectant as needed.
5. To prevent dehydration (loss of body fluids):
   - Increase the amount of water given in the tube between feedings.
   - Observe for increased urination, which may mean that the sugar level in the urine is too high.
   - Observe for signs of thirst and fever.
   - Check with your doctor or nurse about changing the formula.
6. To prevent clogging of your feeding tube:
   - Make sure there are no kinks in the tube.
   - Flush the tube with 3 to 4 ounces of warm water after meals.
   - Dissolve all medications placed in the tube in at least 1 ounce of water.
   - Rinse your tube with warm water before and after giving medications.
   - Rinse the tube with cola or 1 part hydrogen peroxide in 3 parts water if the tube becomes sluggish.

Management

Your tube feeding will be given on a schedule that best fits your needs for care and the amount of calories required. The doctor, dietitian, or nurse will explain the schedule to you. The choices of schedules are as follows:

- **Intermittent or bolus:** Your total feeding for the day will be divided into smaller portions to be given at set times over short periods. This can be given by gravity or by a syringe.
- **Continuous tube feeding:** Your total feeding for the day will be given slowly over the 24-hour period. It is usually given by a pump to keep the rate steady.

It is very important to make sure the tube is in the right place before starting each feeding.

1. Nasogastric tube:
   - Wash your hands thoroughly using soap and warm water.
   - Draw up 10 to 20 cc of air into a syringe.
   - Insert the tip of the syringe into the end of the feeding tube.
   - Unclamp the tube.
   - Put the stethoscope into your ears and place the bell over your abdominal area.
   - Quickly push air into feeding tube. You should hear a "whoosh," a bubbling, or a quick high-pitched gurgling sound.
   - Do not give your feeding if you cannot hear this sound. Contact the doctor, nurse, or dietitian.

(continued)

2. Gastrostomy or jejunostomy tube:
   - Wash your hands thoroughly with soap and water.
   - Measure the number of inches from the stomach wall to the end of the tube.
   - If the distance is more than the recommended number of inches, do not give the feeding. Contact the doctor, nurse, or dietitian.

   Report any of the following symptoms to your doctor:
   - Tube feeding into lungs (aspiration): coughing or gagging, especially associated with fever.
   - Diarrhea: loose, watery stools, which can occur alone or be associated with other symptoms such as cramping, upset stomach, or dizziness.
   - Constipation: hard, infrequent stools.
   - Skin irritation: pain, redness, or bleeding around the tube.
   - Dehydration: thirst, weight loss, dry mouth, lack of energy, extreme tiredness.
   - Tube clogging: difficulty flushing the tube with water or air.

Follow-Up

Should any of these problems happen, call your doctor:

1. If you feel your feedings are not working well for you, check with your doctor or dietitian about changing the rate of feeding or the method of feeding.
2. If the tube becomes dislodged or falls out, apply a dressing over the opening and call your caregiver immediately.
3. Notify your caregiver if you have any of the following:
   - Temperature of 100.4°F (38°C) or more
   - Diarrhea
   - Nausea or vomiting
   - Constipation
   - Abdominal distention
   - Tube dislodgment
   - Clogging of the tube

Phone Numbers

Nurse: ______________________ Number: ______________________

Physician: ______________________ Number: ______________________

Dietitian: ______________________ Number: ______________________

Source: Cunningham RS. The Cancer Cachexia Syndrome. In: Yarbro CH, Wujcik D, Gobel BH, eds. *Cancer Symptom Management.* 4th ed. Burlington, MA: Jones & Bartlett Learning; 2014.

Intravenous Feeding

Patient Name: ______________________________

This guide will help you understand more about receiving feedings through your veins called intravenous feeding. Two schedules are commonly used to provide feedings by vein:

- Continuous: The amount of feeding for the day is given over a 24-hour period using a pump to ensure a steady rate of delivery.
- Cyclic: The amount of solution for the day is given over an 8- to 12-hour period.

Symptom and Description

When weight loss or lack of appetite becomes severe, nutrition can be given by vein. This process allows you to get the nutrients and calories your body needs for energy. The special nutrition solution can be given into an implanted port, a tunneled catheter, or any other long-term catheter placed in a large vein.

Preventing Problems

The intravenous feeding is important for giving you the nutrients your body needs to maintain its strength and health. When care is taken to give the solution safely, many problems can be avoided, including the following:

1. High blood sugar: Your blood sugar level may become high as a result of the amount of sugar in the solution. You will need to have blood tests to monitor this level as often as your doctor thinks is necessary, usually at least two to three times per week.
   - If you do develop high blood sugar, a special medication called insulin may be added at least in the beginning to your nutrition solution. The type of solution may also need to be changed.
2. Low blood sugar: Your blood sugar will become low if there is an interruption in the infusion of the nutrient solution. To avoid this problem, it is important to take the following steps:
   - Infuse the solution at the rate that you have been instructed to use.
   - Do not stop or interrupt the solution without calling your doctor first.
   - Make sure that you have your blood tests monitored as instructed.
3. Infection: Catheter infections can be prevented using evidence-based practices to manage catheter care. Clean the catheter using the method taught to you by your nurse. A few very important steps are highlighted here:
   - Use only aseptic (sterile) technique when changing the dressing of the catheter or hooking up the solution.
   - Wash hands thoroughly using soap and warm water before and after caring for the catheter.
   - Following the specific instructions provided by nurse on the products and methods to be used during catheter care.

(continued)

Management

- Have blood tests for sugar level drawn as directed.
- Should low blood sugar occur, drink one or two glasses of juice or eat several pieces of hard candy. Symptoms should resolve quickly. The symptoms of low blood sugar include sweating, nervousness, shaking of hands, hunger, weakness, irritability, numbness of tongue or lips, and headache.
- Self-administer insulin as you have been instructed or call doctor immediately if symptoms of high blood sugar occur—specifically, dry, hot flushed skin; thirst; fatigue; frequent urination; and upset stomach.
- Call the doctor for any temperature of 100.4°F (38°C) or higher.
- Do not adjust the rate of nutrition solution without talking with your doctor.

Follow-Up

1. Discuss any difficulties with the solution infusion with your doctor, nurse, or dietitian.
2. Notify your caregiver if any of the following occur:
    - Temperature of 100.4°F or higher
    - Chills
    - Tenderness or redness at the catheter site
    - Swelling of neck or arm
    - High blood sugar: dry, hot, flushed skin; thirst; fatigue; frequent urination; upset stomach
    - Low blood sugar: sweating, nervousness, shaking of hands, hunger, weakness, irritability, numbness of tongue or lips, headache

Phone Numbers

Nurse: ______________________ Number: ______________________

Physician: ______________________ Number: ______________________

Dietitian: ______________________ Number: ______________________

Source: Cunningham RS. The Cancer Cachexia Syndrome. In: Yarbro CH, Wujcik D, Gobel BH, eds. *Cancer Symptom Management*. 4th ed. Burlington, MA: Jones & Bartlett Learning; 2014.

Chapter 18

Dysphagia

Dawn Camp-Sorrell, MSN, FNP, AOCN®

THE PROBLEM

Dysphagia is a term used to describe difficulty in swallowing. It is derived from the Greek words *dys* (meaning "with difficulty") and *phagia* (meaning "to eat"). Dysphagia is best defined clinically as the sensation of delay in passage of a food bolus within 10 seconds of swallowing. The symptom indicates a delay in the passage of solids or liquids from the mouth to the stomach. To ensure adequate evaluation, dysphagia must be distinguished from odynophagia, which is discomfort or pain on swallowing.[1] Dysphagia can be described as high, affecting the pharynx and proximal esophagus, or low, affecting the esophageal body or esophagogastric junction.

Dysphagia is categorized into three major types—transfer, transit, and obstructive—according to the disruption of the normal passage of food.[1–3] Transfer dysphagia is the alteration in oral–pharyngeal bolus transfer, such as occurs with a stroke. Transit dysphagia is characterized by the absence of primary and secondary esophageal peristalsis, such as occurs with achalasia. Obstructive dysphagia is caused by mechanical stenosis in the pharynx, esophagus, or esophagogastric junction, usually from a malignancy.[4]

Malignant dysphagia describes the difficulty of swallowing due to cancer, usually resulting from a partially or completely obstructed esophageal lumen. Rarely, it can be the result of tumor invasion or esophageal innervation. The main problem with dysphagia is the person's inability to eat safely and comfortably, which leads to malnutrition and possible aspiration. Frequently patients will report, "My food sticks in my throat or my food just won't go down. I feel like I'm going to choke. I have a lump in my throat."

The incidence of dysphagia is difficult to ascertain because this symptom is the result of numerous etiologies. It has been estimated that as many as 25% of all patients with cancer have dysphagia.[5] The most common etiology of dysphagia is head and neck cancers, which account for 5% of all malignancies.[5,6] Dysphagia is the predominant symptom in most esophageal cancers.[7]

Dysphagia is a distressing symptom that indicates a difficulty in swallowing solids, semisolids, or liquids. The quality of life aspects of dysphagia and the impact it has on patients have received minimal attention in the literature. Restoration of the ability to swallow and eat normally is critical for full social rehabilitation of patients.[1,8] Inability to eat represents a barrier to fully participating in life with family and friends. Subsequently, a negative impact on the patient's quality of life can occur with the inability to return to normal eating after treatment.[6,8]

Eating is necessary to sustain life and is considered one of life's greatest pleasures. When an individual is unable to eat, the impact is tremendous.[3] To date, nurses have not studied the symptom of dysphagia as it relates to patients with cancer. Nursing research related to dysphagia needs to address all aspects of this symptom. How does dysphagia impact the patient's quality of life? Which coping mechanisms are used to overcome dysphagia? Which rehabilitative methods are beneficial to teach a patient to overcome or accommodate dysphagia? Which food consistencies are tolerated during each phase of swallowing? What is the impact of dysphagia on the overall health of the patient with cancer?

PATHOPHYSIOLOGY

Knowledge of the normal anatomy and physiology of swallowing is beneficial in understanding dysphagia and the challenges for rehabilitation. The act of swallowing is intermixed with respiration and speaking, and is coordinated with voluntary and involuntary muscle action.[3] Swallowing is a complex act that involves the coordinated activity of the mouth, tongue, pharynx, larynx, and esophagus.[4,9] Dysphagia occurs during the act of swallowing, which consists of four phases: (1) the oral preparatory phase, (2) the oral phase, (3) the pharyngeal phase, and (4) the esophageal phase (Table 18-1).[1–3,9] Once swallowing has been initiated, it takes less than 1 second for a bolus to reach the esophagus and an additional 10 to 15 seconds to complete the swallow. This process involves more than 30 muscles. Any alteration to these structures or swallowing phases, such as a mass or neurological change, can result in dysphagia.

HEAD AND NECK CANCER

Oral cavity and pharyngeal lesions tend to create worse swallowing problems than laryngeal cancer. Yet, patients with oral cavity lesions are less likely to perceive a swallowing disorder as compared with patients with tumors of the pharynx.[1] Dysphagia would be expected to accompany lesions within these areas because the structures in these regions are responsible for bolus transit and clearance. Laryngeal function during swallowing is protection of the airway.[10] As expected, patients with early-stage head and neck cancers are less likely to complain of dysphagia than those with advanced disease.

Individuals with head and neck cancer typically present with longer oral and pharyngeal transit times and residue, shorter duration of cricopharyngeal opening, and lower swallow efficiencies. After treatment, these patients have difficulties with bolus transit and bolus clearance.[10] Swallow function worsens significantly with an increase in the size of the tumor. This could be the result of disruption of the muscle function, infiltration by the tumor, ulceration related to more advanced disease, or pain.[1]

ESOPHAGEAL STRICTURE

Esophageal stricture caused by extrinsic and intrinsic tumor compression can result in dysphagia. Mechanical dysphagia can occur if the esophagus cannot distend to greater than 2.5 cm and invariably occurs when maximum distention of

TABLE 18-1

Normal Phases of Swallowing and Disorders Affecting Swallowing

Phase	Act of Swallowing	Disorders Affecting Swallowing
Oral preparatory	Processing of bolus to render to swallow	Mandibulectomy; glossectomy; palate defects; impaired tongue; xerostomia; resection of lips, anterior tongue, or floor of mouth
Oral propulsive	Propelling food from the oral cavity into the oropharynx with tongue	Impaired tongue, xerostomia, palate defects, glossectomy, mandibulectomy
Pharyngeal	Overlapping of events beginning with swallowing reflex. Structures innervated by cranial nerves IX, X, and XI Soft palate elevates hyoid bone and larynx moves upward and forward Vocal cords move to midline Epiglottis folds backward to protect airway Tongue pushes backward and downward into the pharynx to propel the bolus down Upper esophageal sphincter relaxes and pulls open, closes after food passes	Pharynx dysfunction, soft palate surgery, weak pharyngeal muscles, oropharynx surgery, pharyngolaryngectomy, laryngectomy, xerostomia, supraglottic laryngectomy, supracricoid laryngectomy, tracheotomy, palate defects, cranial nerve dysfunction or defects
Esophageal	Bolus moves downward by peristaltic wave beginning at pharynx with swallow reflex and continues in esophagus Lower esophageal sphincter relaxes and bolus is propelled into stomach	Esophageal dysfunction, cranial nerve dysfunction obstruction by tumor, tumor invasion, esophageal reconstruction

Source: Data from Raber-Dulacher et al[1]; Logemann and Larsen[2]; Logemann[3]; Lim et al[9].

the esophagus is less than 1.3 cm. Mechanical dysphagia can be caused by a large food bolus, intrinsic narrowing, or extrinsic compression.[1,11] Extrinsic compression of the esophagus can result from adenopathy in the mediastinum with lung cancer.[1,11] A benign condition, Barrett's esophagus, can cause esophageal stricture and dysphagia. Barrett's esophagus is a result of long-standing acid reflux that causes the esophageal epithelium to undergo metaplasia. The risk of developing an esophageal adenocarcinoma is increased 80-fold in individuals with Barrett's esophagus.[12]

POST-TREATMENT DYSPHAGIA

Difficult and painful swallowing can develop due to radiation therapy to the head and neck. Radiation can cause long-term xerostomia, recurrent fungal infection, tissue fibrosis, or chronic inflammation of the mucous membranes. Xerostomia can occur from the direct effect of radiation on the salivary glands. Xerostomia makes it difficult to manipulate and propel a bolus and initiate a pharyngeal swallow, and can eventually lead to dysphagia.[13] Post-radiation fibrosis of the pharyngeal muscle can impair pharyngeal motility, resulting in retention of food within the pharynx and increasing the potential risk for aspiration. Short-term side effects from chemotherapy can include stomatitis, taste changes, esophagitis, or cranial nerve neuropathy, all of which can lead to dysphagia.

Surgical resection of the oral cavity, pharynx, larynx, and esophagus can also cause varying degrees of dysphagia.[14] The type and severity of dysphagia depend on the amount of anatomic structure removed and the reconstruction procedures. Supraglottic laryngectomy and supracricoid laryngectomy are surgical procedures that usually compromise swallowing function and increase the risk for aspiration.[10,14] Supraglottic laryngectomy typically results in problems with aspiration before the swallow (delayed reflex) and during swallow because of a decrease in the vocal-fold adduction. After the swallow, pharyngeal peristalsis and laryngeal elevation both decrease, leading to dysphagia.[10,13] Esophagectomy for tumor resection can also cause postoperative anastomotic strictures leading to dysphagia.

Supracricoid partial laryngectomy increases the risk for aspiration during swallowing because it can result in premature spillage of food, pooling of secretions, insufficient clearance of the bolus, and varying degrees of laryngeal penetration.[15] Patients who have undergone a partial or total glossectomy will experience difficulty transporting and controlling a bolus of food or liquid to the oropharynx. Generally, if the tongue resection is less than 50%, the oral preparatory phase will be functional. If more than 50% of the tongue is resected, lingual peristalsis and control of the food can be reduced.[16,17] Mandibular reconstruction can cause scarring, muscle contracture, and temporomandibular joint pain that can interfere with chewing. Presence of a tracheotomy tube contributes to dysphagia because the tube impedes laryngeal elevation and results in poor clearance of the larynx.[10]

Dysphagia can also occur from cranial nerve dysfunction that arises from a cerebral or brain stem lesion. Dysphagia occurs in only a small percentage of patients with lung cancer with underlying mediastinal disease, cervical lymphadenopathy, brain stem lesions, and gastrointestinal tract metastasis.[11]

SYMPTOM ASSESSMENT

RISK FACTORS

Several factors can place a patient at risk for dysphagia. Table 18-2 describes these risk factors occurring from the cancer itself, cancer treatment, or infection. Numerous comorbidities can increase the risk of dysphagia, such as stroke, poor dentition, achalasia, and esophageal stenosis.

SELF-ASSESSMENT

Normal speech and swallowing require precise coordination of a series of rapid and complex neuromuscular actions. The impact of losing the ability to speak and swallow permanently affects the patient for a lifetime.[6] Head and neck cancer and its treatment often have devastating effects on a patient's nutritional status, dramatically altering the individual's eating habits for life.

Each type of cancer treatment, which often includes multimodality interventions, significantly hinders the patient's ability to maintain adequate intake of calories, protein, and fluid.[6] As a result, a significant decrease in quality of life occurs that affects the individual's food

TABLE 18-2

Risk Factors for Dysphagia

- Tumor invasion of oral cavity, pharynx, larynx, or esophagus
- Tumor obstruction of oral cavity, pharynx, larynx, or esophagus
- Radiation to salivary gland causing xerostomia
- Infection: viral, bacterial, fungal
- Cranial nerve neuropathy from tumor or chemotherapy
- Tracheotomy
- Odynophagia
- Past medical history: stroke, poor dentition, achalasia, esophageal stenosis

choices and intake. Changes in the ability to eat and drink in a socially acceptable fashion often pose challenges for patients with dysphagia. Treatment often exacerbates swallowing difficulties that are typically persistent and enduring long after treatment is complete.[8]

Dysphagia has a profound and multidimensional impact on the lives of patients and their families. They may avoid eating in public because of the need for extra time to eat or because of oral leakage. Patients with dysphagia may experience feelings of social isolation, altered social interaction, or embarrassment.[8] The attitude and preferences of the patient and the support of family and friends are essential components of treatment acceptance and compliance in the rehabilitation process.

OBJECTIVE ASSESSMENT

History

The history begins by ascertaining the patient's risk factors for dysphagia (see Table 18-2). The most important historical features include the duration and progression of symptoms, relation of symptoms to solids and liquids, impact of cold on swallowing, and response to swallowing a bolus.[1,2] Inquiry into these aspects can differentiate a motor disorder from a mechanical obstruction. Mechanical obstruction is characterized by a rapid onset and progressive course, more difficulty with solids than with liquids, no aggravation with cold food, and regurgitation on trying to swallow a bolus. It is usually related to a cancer process. A patient with pharyngeal dysphagia from any cause complains of symptoms immediately upon swallowing; in contrast, the onset of symptoms after swallowing is delayed in patients with esophageal dysphagia.[1]

Various signs and symptoms can indicate the degree of dysphagia and the source of the problem (Table 18-3). As part of the history, it is important to determine which types of food the patient is unable to tolerate and whether the patient is experiencing regurgitation. Undigested food and accumulated saliva occur most commonly in the recumbent position and can awaken the patient from sleep because of choking or coughing. Regurgitation becomes a major problem with disease progression. A history of dry mouth may indicate inadequate salivary production as a result of radiation or medications such as anticholinergics or antihistamines.[1]

Physical assessment

Assess the patient's weight to determine the amount of weight loss. Serial weight measurements are the single most important indicator of nutritional status.[6,11] Physical examination begins with visual assessment of the lips, oral cavity, tongue, and jaw. Observe the lips for protrusion, retraction, ulceration, and the ability to close. Inspect the oral cavity for mucosal integrity, inflammatory lesions, and masses. Observe the position and symmetry of the hard and soft palate. Inspect the dentition for secretions within the oral cavity. Evaluate the range of motion of the tongue by checking for lateralization, protrusion, elevation, and strength. Determine the ability of the jaw to close and to produce rotary movement.[11] Strength and symmetry of the jaw and facial muscles are evaluated by palpating the lower facial area while the individual clenches the jaw. Cranial nerves V, VII, IX, X, XI, and XII can be evaluated by asking the patient to frown, smile, pucker, raise the eyebrows, wrinkle the forehead, and tightly close the eyes (Table 18-4).

It is important to assess cough and gag reflexes, because these reflexes prevent food or fluid from entering the upper respiratory tract. Ask the patient to cough at least twice in rapid succession. Observe the patient for the amount of coughing and choking elicited to estimate the patient's ability to protect the airway. Presence of the gag reflex can be elicited by tickling the back of the throat with a cotton swab.

Observe the individual during eating for choking, drooling, regurgitation of fluid in the nose, and retention of food in the oral cavity.[1] Palpate the head and neck for masses

TABLE 18-3

Symptoms of Dysphagia

Phase of Swallowing	Symptoms
Oral or pharyngeal	Coughing or choking with swallowing Difficulty initiating swallow Poor bolus control Pooling of secretions Pocketing of food in lateral and anterior sulci Complaints of food sticking in throat Drooling Trismus
Esophageal	Complaints of food sticking in the chest Regurgitation Heartburn or indigestion Increase in belching
Any phase	Weight loss Change in dietary habits Recurrent pneumonia Decrease in sensation of temperature in swallowing Decrease in sensation of pain with swallowing Pain

Source: Data from Raber-Dulacher et al[1]; Logemann and Larsen[2]; Rogers[11].

TABLE 18-4

Neural Control of Swallowing

Neural Area	Assessment Technique
Efferent motor fibers of cranial nerves	Evaluate movement of the facial features and jaw.
Afferent sensory fibers of cranial nerves	Evaluate sensation of the head and neck.
Cerebral and midbrain fibers that synapse with brain stem swallowing center	Evaluate ability to swallow.
Paired swallowing centers in brain stem glossopharyngeal and vagal nerves (IX and X)	Evaluate ability to swallow.
Cervical nerves I and II with extrinsic tongue muscle control	Evaluate strength of tongue.
Cranial nerve V (trigeminal): soft palate; mouth; anterior tongue; nasopharynx; controls muscles of mastication and sensation of face, teeth, gums, and tongue	Inspect face for muscle atrophy and tremors. Palpate jaw for strength with jaw clenched. Test for superficial pain and touch sensation with patient's eyes closed.
Cranial nerve VII (facial): anterior 2/3 tongue (sense of test), controls facial muscles	Inspect symmetry of facial features: smiles, wrinkles forehead, shows teeth, closes eyes. Test ability to identify salt and sweet taste.
Cranial nerve IX (glossopharyngeal): posterior 1/2 tongue and oral hypopharynx, influences production of saliva and swallowing	Test ability to identify sour and bitter tastes. Test gag reflex.
Cranial nerves X and XI (vagus and spinal accessory): tongue base, interior larynx, controls ability to swallow	Inspect palate and uvula for symmetry with speech. Test gag reflex. Evaluate speech quality. Test trapezius and sternocleidomastoid muscle.
Cranial nerve XII (hypoglossal): tongue muscles	Inspect tongue for symmetry, tremors, and atrophy. Inspect tongue movement. Test tongue strength.

and lymphadenopathy. Evaluate the patient's palms and soles for hyperkeratosis, which is a rare symptom of esophageal cancer.[11] Auscultate the lungs for decreased breath sounds; they may indicate consolidation, such as occurs in aspiration pneumonia.

Persons with dysphagia are at great risk for compromised nutrition. A comprehensive nutritional assessment will provide necessary baseline measures (Figure 18-l). Patients who have pronounced dysphagia with long-standing malnutrition need immediate and ongoing assistance with their diet.[18] Initially ask the patient to create a written record of his or her nutritional intake for 24 hours. Review this record and calculate the amounts of protein, fat, and carbohydrate intake and total calories. Anthropometric measurements can be made at baseline and at monthly intervals to assess the patient's nutritional status. These measures include the weight, height, and skin fold thickness. Weight combined with height measurement is an indirect indicator of body composition.[18] Skin fold measurements, usually performed by a dietitian, are useful to assess the fat and muscle compartments.

Although not specific for malnutrition, certain laboratory tests can be obtained to assess nutritional status.[11] A complete blood count is used to evaluate folate and vitamin B_{12} deficiency, as indicated by macrocytosis of the red blood cells. Iron deficiency is indicated by microcytosis of the red blood cells. Total lymphocyte count is an indirect indicator of nutritional status, with low levels suggesting malnutrition. Transferrin is an indicator of visceral protein status. A low serum albumin level is also an indicator of malnutrition.

Diagnostic evaluation

Evaluation for dysphagia has three purposes: (1) to determine whether dysphagia is present, (2) to identify its cause, and (3) to develop recommendations for rehabilitation strategies. Endoscopy is usually the best diagnostic method to determine the cause of dysphagia because of its high degree of accuracy and the opportunity to take biopsies for analysis or to proceed with immediate dilatation.[11] Videofluorographic swallowing study (VFSS) is the standard diagnostic tool used to study swallowing. With this modality, the patient eats and drinks a substance mixed with barium while radiographic images are observed on a fluoroscope video monitor. Such a study allows the clinician to look closely at the anatomic structures and motion of these structures. Critical information for rehabilitation can be obtained during the study, such as the type of bolus consistencies tolerated, head positions, and swallowing techniques needed.[1,2] A barium swallow may be useful in identifying anatomic abnormalities associated with dysphagia and document the presence of aspiration.

NUTRITION ASSESSMENT

Patient Name ____________________

Date ____________________ Weight ____________________

Albumin ____________________ Protein ____________________

Symptoms (describe degree)

Pain ____________________

Cough ____________________

Choking ____________________

Nasal regurgitation ____________________

Other ____________________

Other ____________________

Nutrition

Soft diet ____________________

Supplement PO ____________________

Tube feeding ____________________

Other ____________________

Food Intake

Adequate ____________________

Good ____________________

Poor ____________________

Other ____________________

Swallowing Therapy: Yes __________ No __________

Comments:

FIGURE 18-1

Nutrition/dysphagia assessment.

DEGREES OF TOXICITY

Dysphagia can be a significant and distressful symptom that has a marked impact on the patient's quality of life. Grading of dysphagia is important in assessing the severity of the symptom and in evaluating the therapeutic interventions (Table 18-5). Use of specific parameters and operational definitions helps clinicians define the degree of dysphagia and ensures consistency in reporting this symptom.[19]

SYMPTOM MANAGEMENT STRATEGIES

THERAPEUTIC APPROACHES

Prevention of dysphagia is difficult because this symptom usually results from cancer or cancer treatment. Awareness and counseling can be beneficial to prepare the patient for the possibility that this complication might occur. Anticipation of potential nutritional deficits with dysphagia

TABLE 18-5

National Cancer Institute Common Terminology Criteria for Adverse Events (CTCAE): Dysphagia

Adverse Event	Grade				
	1	2	3	4	5
Dysphagia: a disorder characterized by difficulty swallowing	Symptomatic, able to eat regular food	Symptomatic and altered eating/ swallowing	Severely altered eating/swallowing; tube feeding or TPN or hospitalization indicated	Life-threatening consequences; urgent intervention indicated	Death

Source: Data from National Cancer Institute Common Terminology Criteria for Adverse Events (CTCAE)[19].

will facilitate the early implementation of supplemental or alternative feeding methods.[18] Patient resources should be explored to assess financial means to purchase food or nutritional supplements, food preparation facilities, and social and community supports. Xerostomia, which can lead to dysphagia, can be somewhat prevented by shielding the salivary glands during radiation therapy.[1]

The goal of therapy for dysphagia is to decrease the risk of aspiration, improve the ability to swallow, and optimize nutrition. Therapeutic intervention for this challenging symptom requires a team approach. The physician recommends when oral or alternative feedings should begin following surgery or dilatation. The dietitian recommends and monitors maintenance of adequate nutritional intake. The speech-language pathologist determines the diet consistency and attempts to reestablish adequate oral feeding. The nurse provides support to the patient and recommends available resources.

Types of food consistencies tolerated will depend on the patient's ability to handle various consistencies, such as thin and thick liquids, puree, soft and moist solids, hard and dry solids[3] (Table 18-6).[20,21] Xerostomia can be treated with artificial saliva or pilocarpine hydrochloride. Infections can be treated with appropriate antibiotic, antifungal, or antiviral agents. Routine pretreatment dental evaluation is critical for all patients regardless of the treatment modality. Rehabilitation of both speech and swallowing may be compromised by unplanned dental extractions, possible oral prosthesis, or dental caries.

Surgical intervention

Esophageal stricture causing dysphagia can be relieved by endoscopic dilatation. Endoscopic dilatation is achieved by using balloons or rigid dilators, which are typically effective for a short duration.[5,22] Repeat dilatation is usually required within two weeks; thus this procedure provides only short-term relief. Self-expanding metal stents composed of wire coils or wire mesh that expand up to 20 mm in diameter can be placed within the esophagus to open the stricture. These stents are placed using an endoscope or under radioscopic guidance.[5,22]

Laser therapy is also used to treat strictures through the direct application of a laser beam to burn and vaporize tissue at the site of the stricture. Laser therapy is most effective for exophytic lesions, short-segment discrete strictures, and proximal lesions for which other therapies, such as stenting, are not feasible.[13] Treatment is performed every other day and usually requires three to four sessions to be effective.

Injected under endoscopic guidance, 100% alcohol causes tissue fixation, ulceration, and necrosis. Like laser therapy, alcohol injection is best suited for treating exophytic bulky lesions at all levels of the esophagus. This treatment provides relief for approximately one month.

Photodynamic therapy is a nonthermal ablative technique that uses photosensitive agents. These agents are absorbed in the malignant tissue but remain inactive until exposed to specific light wavelengths. After a few days, the patient undergoes an endoscopic procedure in which a low-powered laser initiates a photochemical reaction resulting in tumor necrosis. Dysphagia is relieved for approximately two months.[23]

Brachytherapy has been used to relieve dysphagia. A sealed radiation source is placed close to or inside the esophageal tumor for approximately 1½ days. Dysphagia may worsen for about one week because of tissue edema. Once relief is achieved, the effect is longer than that noted with self-expanding metal stents.[1]

Swallowing rehabilitation

Patient motivation and the amount of individualized rehabilitation impact the rate of swallowing recovery.[24] Restoration of swallowing is the prime objective for patients with dysphagia. The most important information needed for swallowing therapy comprises the exact structures removed and the reconstruction techniques used.[1,2,14] Swallowing therapy both prior to and after

TABLE 18-6

Food Consistencies*

Consistency	Examples
Semisolid, traditionally prepared foods that are cohesive	Baked egg dishes (e.g., souffles, quiches, custards) Salads with mayonnaise or other binding agents (e.g., egg, tuna, macaroni, or meat salad) Cheese that is soft (cream cheese) or melted Pasta or rice casseroles with thick binders (eggs) Aspic, pudding, cheesecake, mousse, and gelatin
Soft foods that tend to fall apart or separate and may be difficult to control	Whole-grain breads Foods that separate into liquid and pulp (e.g., thin pureed fruits and vegetables) Dry cottage cheese Plain rice, ground meats Thin hot cereals Foods of two or more consistencies (e.g., canned fruits in juice or syrup, soups with whole vegetables, pasta, or grains)
Dense foods that are sticky and bulky	Moist white bread Peanut butter Plain mashed potatoes Bananas Refried beans
Thin liquids** (all unthickened beverages and supplements)	Fruit juices Broth and thin cream soups Coffee, tea, and milk Frozen pops, fruit ices, yogurt Water, soda, and alcohol Any food that will liquefy in the mouth within a few seconds such as watermelon Most 1.0 kcal/mL oral supplements
Thin to medium liquids (Nectar)	Vegetable juice; fruit nectars Apricot or tomato juice consistency Chocolate milk Buttermilk Thin milkshakes Cream soups
Thick liquids (Honey)	Blenderized or cream soups Eggnog Ice cream, sherbet Milk shakes, malts, and yogurt shakes Liquids thickened to honey consistency Most 1.5–2.0 kcal/mL oral supplements
Spoon-thick liquids	Thickened to pudding consistency Pudding, custard Hot cereal

*No nationally recognized standards are available for thickened liquids. A wide variety of commercially prepared thickened beverages is available and may not include the viscosity. Dry starch thickeners added to thin liquids can result in different viscosity.

**Unstable liquids (e.g., milk shakes, ice cream, sherbets, ice slushes, and frozen pops) separate into a combination to thin liquid and food mass or melt completely when allowed to stand at room temperature or when placed in the mouth. For a patient with delayed swallow, these foods should be stabilized with thickening agents.

Source: Data from Academy Nutrition care manual[20]; DMR Health Standard #07-1 Guidelines for identification and management of dysphagia and swallowing risks[21].

surgery is important in rehabilitating the patient. Several techniques can be used, including compensatory (postural maneuvers), indirect (exercises to strengthen swallowing muscles), and direct (exercises to perform while swallowing) techniques. After most surgical procedures for head and neck cancer, swallowing rehabilitation with a speech-language pathologist is essential to ensure adequate swallowing and nutrition.[18] Oromotor exercises are required to improve muscle control for swallowing.[6,24] Exercises can begin simultaneously with radiation therapy or approximately 14 days postoperatively when wound healing is complete. Areas to exercise include the lips, tongue, jaw, and palate.

Coordination of tongue movements may be improved through manipulation of objects, such as a licorice tied to a string and placed in the mouth. The licorice is grasped between the tongue and palate, then moved side to side and front to back. When the patient masters this technique, the motion is replaced with a circular movement from the middle of the mouth to the teeth and back again, as if chewing (see Appendix 18A).

Once the ability to manipulate material in the mouth has been established, the focus of exercises shifts to holding and moving a bolus.[24] A small amount of paste-consistency bolus is placed in the mouth and moved with the tongue. Once the exercise is complete, the bolus is expectorated. Practicing backward propulsion of the bolus may be accomplished by instructing the patient to squeeze juice from a long, thin cloth placed in the mouth. The amount of juice in the cloth is varied according to the individual's ability to swallow. These exercises are designed to increase the strength and range of motion of the structures of the oral and pharyngeal cavities.[14]

Indirect strategies that do not use a food bolus are also used. The indirect strategy exercises are focused on improving range of motion and strength of the swallowing mechanism from lip closure to airway protection.[3] Devices such as oral and oropharyngeal prostheses can be used to achieve successful swallowing by assisting with optimal bolus placement, manipulation, and transit in the oral cavity.

Patients who experience continued drooling may benefit from repeated attempts to close the lips and change the head position to encourage posterior movement of saliva. Atropine or antihistamines can be used to decrease secretions. Holding gauze in the mouth to absorb secretions is another option.

Stringent oral care is necessary to manage odor. The teeth or dentures and tongue should be brushed with fluoridated toothpaste and a soft toothbrush approximately four to six times per day. Rinsing the mouth several times a day with a cleansing solution will also help. Cleansing solutions with alcohol or glycerin should be avoided because they have a drying effect.

Posture and positioning

Patients gradually learn to live with dysphagia by using various maneuvers, including lifting the neck to help empty the esophagus.[3] Tilting the chin backward can facilitate oral movement or decrease oral transmit time. For patients with delayed pharyngeal swallow, the head can be tilted forward to widen the space in the larynx and reduce the chance of aspiration. This posture assists the epiglottis in protecting the airway during the swallow. For patients with unilateral vocal-cord paralysis, turning the head to the weaker pharynx side improves vocal-cord adduction by using the stronger pharyngeal wall. For patients with posterior oral cavity resections, the head can be tilted toward the stronger side of the oral cavity and pharynx to allow gravity to keep food on the stronger side.

Dietary modifications

Usually a patient can achieve adequate oral hydration with thin or thick liquids (Appendix 18B). If there is difficulty propelling food to the posterior tongue, it may help to use a long-handled spoon or syringe to place food on the posterior of the tongue. Food consistencies should match the specific physiology of each patient's swallow.[3,6] Most patients with dysphagia cannot tolerate meats or tough foods safely and, therefore, require a mechanical soft or pureed diet. Placement of a percutaneous endoscopic gastrostomy (PEG) tube may be necessary for long-term enteral nutrition (see Appendix 18C).

If the videoesophagram indicates moderate to severe swallowing dysfunction, the individual may require tube feeding.[1] Selection of nutritional products involves consideration of multiple characteristics such as osmolality, viscosity, nutritional value, cost, and convenience. The method of formula administration can be bolus or cyclic. Bolus feeding involves the rapid administration by gravity or pump infusion several times per day. Cyclic feeding can be done over an 8- to 10-hour period, usually at night.

Persons with a tracheotomy tube may eat, although swallowing is challenging.[25] The inflated tube cuff prevents aspiration but makes it difficult to swallow. When eating is complete, mouth and throat secretions should be suctioned before deflating the cuff. If food appears in or around the tracheotomy tube, feeding should be stopped.

COMPLICATIONS OF DYSPHAGIA

Consequences of dysphagia include dehydration, weight loss, weakness, starvation, fistula formation, airway obstruction, and aspiration pneumonia.[1,2,11] Aspiration has been found to be the most frequent major complication from dysphagia, especially after surgical resection (see Appendix 18D).[26] If the potential for aspiration exists, suction equipment should be readily available. The patient should maintain an upright position for 30 minutes after eating to minimize regurgitation that could result in aspiration.

NURSING IMPLICATIONS

Dysphagia usually does not resolve easily and results in a progressive, undesirable outcome. Dysphagia related to cancer usually is not relieved and sometimes can worsen after surgical resection. Ongoing assessment must be performed by the patient and/or caregivers to evaluate the degree of dysphagia. Simple techniques such as asking the individual to speak after swallowing can be used to evaluate dysphagia. If the voice is wet and gurgles, request a cough to clear the oropharynx. Inspect the oral cavity for residual food or saliva.

The main problem with dysphagia is the patient's inability to eat safely and comfortably, which may lead to malnutrition and possible aspiration. Supplemental or alternative feeding methods may be necessary to maintain adequate nutrition. The oncology nurse can assist the patient by identifying food consistencies, positions, and procedures that facilitate safe eating to minimize the risk of aspiration. The nurse, physician, dietitian, and speech-language pathologist should work together to design an individualized treatment plan and follow-up care.

Rehabilitation is a proven means of minimizing dysphagia. The patient must remain motivated to participate in rehabilitative exercises. Rehabilitation has physical, psychological, and social aspects that can improve the individual's quality of life.[8]

PATIENT SELF-CARE

Dysphagia is a frustrating symptom that is not easily relieved and not often resolved. The patient will benefit from additional resources that provide further information:

- www.dysphagiaonline.com, sponsored by Nestle Health Science, provides information on dysphagia and other websites related to dysphagia.
- www.nidcd.nih.gov, sponsored by the National Institute on Deafness and other Communication Disorders, provides useful information on dysphagia.
- www.asha.org, sponsored by the American Speech-Language-Hearing Association, provides information on swallowing exercises.
- Symptoms. WebMD.com gives an overview of dysphagia in general, causes, diagnostic studies, and potential treatments.
- www.hormelhealthlabs.com provides information on thickened beverages and other foods beneficial in the diet of the patient with dysphagia.

The self-care guide on difficulty with swallowing (Appendix 18A) provides tongue exercises that can be employed to assist with swallowing. Food consistencies must be matched with the patient's ability to swallow. Most patients with dysphagia require the ingestion of mechanical soft or pureed food (see Appendix 18B). If the dysphagia stems from an origin that prevents oral intake, tube feeding may be required; tube feeding instructions are presented in Appendix 18C. Aspiration has been found to be the most frequent major complication from dysphagia, especially after surgical resection. A self-care guide for aspiration precautions is presented in Appendix 18D.

REFERENCES

1. Raber-Durlacher JE, Brennan MT, Verdonck-deLeeus IM, Gibson RJ, Eilers JG, Waltimo T, et al. Swallowing dysfunction in cancer patients. *Support Care Cancer.* 2012;20:433–443.
2. Logemann JA, Larsen K. Oropharyngeal dysphagia: pathophysiology and diagnosis for the anniversary issue of *Diseases of the Esophagus. Dis Esophagus.* 2012:25:299–304.
3. Logemann JA. Dysphagia/speech rehabilitation. In: Berger AM, Shuster JL, Von Roenn JH, eds. *Principles and Practice of Supportive Oncology.* Philadelphia: Lippincott; 2007:131–138.
4. Morikawa S, Suzuki A, Nakase K, Yasuda K. Palliation of malignant upper gastrointestinal obstruction with self-expandable metal stent. *Korean J Radiol.* 2012;13(suppl 1):S98–S103.
5. Martinez JC, Puc MM, Quiros RM. Esophageal stenting in the setting of malignancy. *ISRN Gastroenterol.* 2011;719575:1–9 [Epub].
6. Hayward MC, Shea AM. Nutritional needs of patents with malignancies of the head and neck. *Semin Oncol Nurs.* 2009;25:203–211.
7. Hanna WC, Sudarshan M, Roberge D, David M, Waschle KA, Maryland S, et al. What is the optimal management of dysphagia in metastatic esophageal cancer? *Curr Oncol.* 2012;19:60–66.
8. Penner JL. Psychosocial care of patients with head and neck cancer. *Semin Oncol Nurs.* 2009;25:231–241.
9. Lim I, Kim Y, Oommen E, Kim H, Ko MH. The effects of bolus consistency in pharyngeal transit duration during normal swallowing. *Ann Rehabil Med.* 2012;36:220–225.
10. Scarpa R. Surgical management of head and neck carcinoma. *Semin Oncol Nurs.* 2009;25:172–182.
11. Rogers M. Dysphagia. In: Camp-Sorrell D, Hawkins R, eds. *Clinical Manual for the Oncology Advanced Practice Nurse.* 3rd ed. Pittsburgh: ONS Press; 2013 (in press).
12. Bhardwaj A, McGarrity TJ, Staris DB, Mani H. Barrett's esophagus: emerging knowledge and management strategies. *Pathol Res Int.* 2012;2012:814146 [Epub May 30, 2012].
13. Massey S. Esophageal cancer and palliation of dysphagia. *Clin J Oncol Nurs.* 2011;15:327–329.
14. Ahlberg A, Engstrom T, Nikolaidis P, Gunnarsson K, Johansson A, Sharp L, et al. Early self-care rehabilitation of head and neck cancer patients. *Oto-Laryngologicia.* 2011;131:552–561.
15. Benito J, Holsinger FC, Perez-Martin A, Garcia D, Weinstein GS, Laccourreye O. Aspiration after supracricoid partial laryngectomy: incidence, risk factors, management, and outcomes. *Head Neck.* 2011;33:679–685.

16. Hartl DV, Dauchy S, Escande C, Bretange E, Janot F, Kolb F. Quality of life after free-flap tongue reconstruction. *J Laryngol Otol.* 2009;123:550–554.
17. Chien CY, Su CY, Hwang CF, Chuang HC, Jeng SF, Chen YC. Ablation of advanced tongue or base of tongue cancer and reconstruction with free flap: functional outcomes. *Eur J Surg Oncol.* 2006;32:353–357.
18. Cunningham R. Nutritional disturbances. In: Yarbro CH, Wujcik D, Gobel BH, eds. *Cancer Nursing Principles and Practice.* 7th ed. Burlington, MA: Jones & Bartlett Learning; 2011:818–844.
19. U. S. Department of Health and Human Services, National Institutes of Health, National Cancer Institute. *Common Terminology Criteria for Adverse Events (CTCAE) Version 4.0 (v4.03).* June 14, 2010.
20. Academy Nutrition care manual, http://nutritioncaremanual.org
21. DMR Health Standard #07-1. Guidelines for identification and management of dysphagia and swallowing risks. http://www.ct.gov/dds/lib/dds/health/attachf_guidelines_consistency_mod_foodsliquids.pdf
22. Diamantis G, Scarpa M, Bocus P, Realdon S, Castoro C, Ancona E, et al. Quality of life in patients with esophageal stenting for the palliation of malignant dysphagia. *World J Gastroenterol.* 2011;17:144–150.
23. Davila ML Photodynamic therapy. *Gastrointest Endosc Clin North Am.* 2011;21:67–79.
24. Longemann JA. Treatment of oral and pharyngeal dysphagia. *Phys Med Rehabil Clin North Am.* 2008;19:803–816.
25. Coscarelli S, Verrecchia L, Le Saec O, Coscarelli A, Santoro R, de Campora E. Rehabilitation protocol of dysphagia after subtotal reconstructive laryngectomy. *Acta Otorhinolaryngol Ital.* 2007;27:286–289.
26. Jung SJ, Kim DY, Joo, SY. Risk factors associated with aspiration in patients with head and neck cancer. *Ann Rehabil Med.* 2011;35:781–790.

Difficulty Swallowing: Exercises for the Tongue

Patient Name: ______________________________

This guide will help you learn to exercise your tongue.

Symptom and Description

Your surgery or treatment may make it difficult for you to swallow or to control food in your mouth. These exercises will improve your ability to move your tongue well. Your tongue is important for eating, speaking, and swallowing.

Prevention

It is not likely you can prevent this problem from occurring, but these techniques can make it easier for you to swallow:

- Do these exercises 5 to 10 times per day.
- Keep a record of the exercises.
- Note any changes you feel while eating or swallowing.
- Call your doctor or nurse if it becomes more difficult to swallow or eat.

Management Procedure

1. General exercises: Do these 5 to 10 times per day.
    - Open the mouth as wide as possible.
    - Lift the tongue as high as possible; hold 1 second; repeat five times.
    - Lift the back of the tongue as far as possible; hold 1 second; repeat five times.
2. Tongue exercises (Figure 18A-1). Do these 5 to 10 times per day.
    - Push the tongue forward against a tongue blade or your fingers; hold for 1 second.
    - Then push the tongue to one side and forward again.
    - Then push the tongue to the other side and forward again; hold for 1 second.
    - Repeat these exercises five times.
3. Measure progress.
    - Keep a chart of exercises done and the response (such as more movement and strength).
    - These exercises will become easier to perform.
    - It will become easier to move foods in your mouth.
    - Share this information with your nurse and swallowing therapist.
    - Talk with your nurse and swallowing therapist if you believe that the exercises are not helping your tongue strength.

Log of Tongue Exercises

Patient Name: ______________________________

Date	Times Done	Response (How Is Tongue Working?)

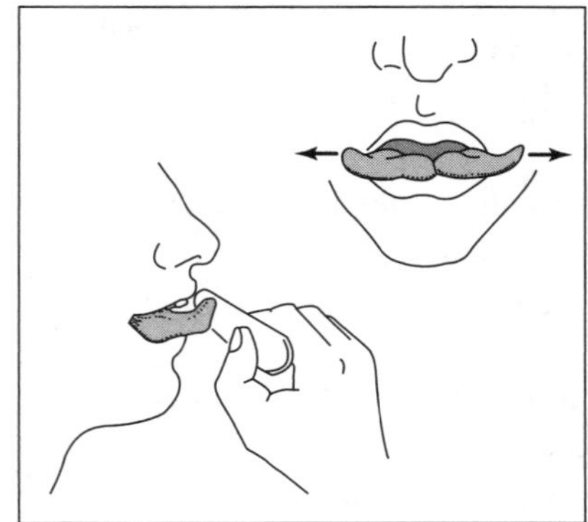

Phone Numbers

Physician: ______________________________

Other: ______________________________

Comments

Source: Camp-Sorrell, D. Dysphagia. In: Yarbro CH, Wujcik D, Gobel BH, eds. *Cancer Symptom Management.* 4th ed. Burlington, MA: Jones & Bartlett Learning; 2014.

Food Suggestions for the Person with Difficulty Swallowing

Patient Name: ______________________________

This guide will provide you with food suggestions.

Symptom and Description

Your surgery or treatments may make it difficult for you to swallow. Certain foods are easier to swallow. It is important to eat enough calories and have a balanced diet.

Management

- *Eat small meals or snacks.* It is sometimes easier to eat a small amount of food at one time. Remember to eat many times a day to get enough calories and protein.
- *Add calories to your food.* Gravies, sauces, and protein shakes can add calories. Sauces and gravies can also make the food easier to swallow.
- *Choose high-protein foods.* These include cheese, poultry, meat, fish, and beans. You may need to cut, blend, or shred the food to make it easier to swallow. Gravies and sauces may help.
- *Try milkshakes or puddings.* These are easy to swallow. The cool, smooth texture can be soothing.
- *Try cold foods or bland foods.* Cold or cool foods are soothing. Spicy foods may need to be avoided.
- *Freeze nutritional shakes.* The texture and taste of this is like ice cream, but it is more nutritious.

Follow-Up

Call your doctor or nurse if you have any of the following:

- More difficulty swallowing
- A feeling of choking
- Coughing while swallowing or drinking
- A decrease in your weight

Phone Numbers

Physician: ______________________________

Other: ______________________________

Comments

Source: Camp-Sorrell, D. Dysphagia. In: Yarbro CH, Wujcik D, Gobel BH, eds. *Cancer Symptom Management.* 4th ed. Burlington, MA: Jones & Bartlett Learning; 2014.

Tube Feeding

Patient Name: ____

This guide will help you understand tube feeding.

Symptom and Description

Tube feedings are given if you have difficulty swallowing. The difficulty swallowing is usually caused by your cancer treatment. The tube feeding is needed to prevent weight loss and to provide calories and nutrition.

Management

A feeding tube will be inserted into your nose or stomach to deliver liquid food, water, and medication (Figures 18C-1 and 18C-2).

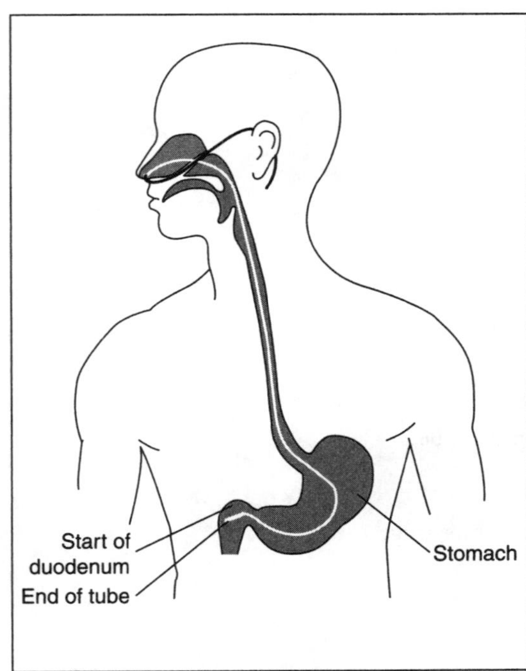

Nasal feeding tube is placed through nose into stomach. (Artist: Camille Rea.)

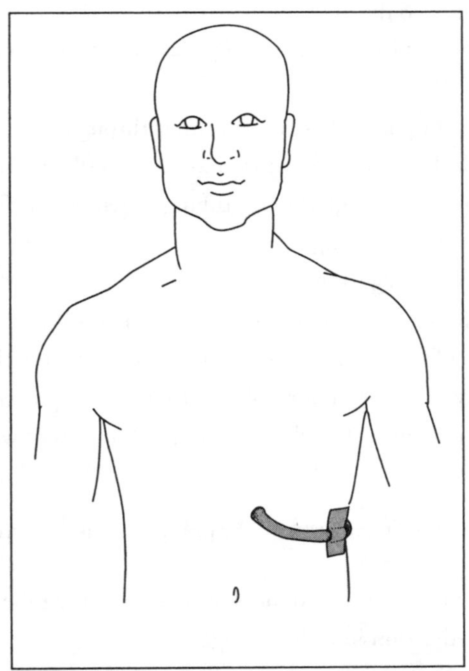

Gastrostomy feeding tube is placed through skin into stomach. (Artist: Camille Rea)

To get ready to feed yourself:

1. Follow the doctor's order for the type, amount, and time of feeding.
2. Wash hands to prevent infection.

(continued)

3. Gather the supplies. Formula may be given by syringe or feeding bag:
    - Feeding bag or large (60-cc) syringe
    - Small (10-cc) syringe
    - Two ounces of water
    - Tube feeding formula (type and amount):
    - Disposable gloves, if desired
    - Optional: a feeding pump (a pump can control flow of liquid)

To begin feeding:

1. Sit upright (45- to 90-degree angle).
2. Remove the clamp, and pinch the tubing at the end away from the nose or abdomen. This prevents leakage.
3. Using the small (10-cc) syringe, push 10 cc of air into the tube. If no choking, coughing, or pain occurs, please proceed. If choking, coughing, or pain occurs, stop now and clamp the tube. Call your doctor or nurse for advice.
4. For syringe feeding:
    - Attach the syringe to the end of the tube. Raise the syringe 18 inches above the head (if the tube is through the nose) or 18 inches above the stomach (if the tube is through the stomach).
    - Fill the large syringe with 2 ounces of water and run it through the tubing.
    - Fill the syringe with formula; allow the flow to empty gradually. Slower feeding will prevent cramping and diarrhea.
    - Refill the syringe and feed until the proper amount of feeding formula has been given.
5. For feeding bag:
    - Fill the bag with 2 ounces of water and run it through the tubing.
    - Fill the bag with the feeding formula amount prescribed.
    - Let the formula flow through the bag tubing to remove air from the tube.
    - Clamp the tube of the feeding bag.
    - Connect the feeding bag to the feeding tube.
    - Raise the bag 18 inches above the head or abdomen to start the flow of formula.
    - Change the rate of feeding flow by loosening or tightening the clamp.
    - Feeding will flow in within hours. Slower feeding will prevent cramping.
6. At the end of feeding, clear the tube by running 2 ounces of water through the tube.

To give medicine:

1. Use the large (60-cc) syringe. Remove the plunger from the syringe. Connect the syringe to the tube.
2. Clear the tube by first pushing 2 ounces of water into the tube.
3. Pour the liquid medication into the syringe.
4. If tablets are to be given:
    - Crush the tablet with the back of a spoon.
    - Put the crushed tablet into 1 ounce of water.
    - Pour the water and tablet into the syringe.
5. Push the syringe plunger to advance the medication into the feeding tube.
6. Keep rinsing medication from the cup with water until all medicine is given.
7. Finally, rinse the tube by giving 2 ounces of water.

8. Clamp the feeding tube and disconnect the syringe.
9. Call the nurse if the tube is clogged.
10. Record how much feeding is given and how much water is taken.

Call medical personnel if any of the following occur:

- Coughing or choking
- Feeding coming from tracheotomy (if present), mouth, or nose
- Nausea, vomiting, diarrhea, or stomach cramps
- Continued weight loss
- Tube becomes clogged

To be sure that the tube feeding procedure is correct, you and/or a family member will be asked to perform the tube feeding procedure for your nurse.

Follow-Up

- Keep a daily record of your weight.
- Record the amount of feeding taken each time.
- Bring the record of your feedings and your weights to your next appointment.
- The physician, nurse, and dietitian may be able to see where more help is needed.
- Call your doctor or nurse if you experience any of the following: diarrhea, constipation, continued weight loss, or indigestion.
- If you are unsure of any of the instructions, be sure to ask for help.
- Be sure you understand what to expect, what to do about it, and when to call your doctor or nurse.
- Have emergency phone numbers available.

Log of Tube Feedings

Patient Name: ______________________________

	Weight	Bowel Movement	Amount of Water	Amount of Feeding	Comments

Phone Numbers

Physician: ______________________________

Other: ______________________________

Comments

Source: Camp-Sorrell, D. Dysphagia. In: Yarbro CH, Wujcik D, Gobel BH, eds. *Cancer Symptom Management.* 4th ed. Burlington, MA: Jones & Bartlett Learning; 2014.

Difficulty Swallowing: Precautions

Patient Name: ______________________________

Symptom and Description

When you have trouble swallowing, you may swallow the wrong way. This is called aspiration. The following measures will help you to avoid aspiration.

Prevention

The following measures can help you avoid swallowing the wrong way:

- Keep your head elevated while you are eating.
- Eat your food in small bites.
- Swallow completely before taking another bite.
- Clear your throat or swallow several times to clear the food.
- Remain upright after meals for at least 30 minutes.

Management

- Only eat solids or liquids that you are able to swallow.
- Have a suction machine available if you begin to choke.
- Go to the emergency room if you feel like food has become stuck in your esophagus.

Follow-Up

- Call the office if you are unable to eat or drink.
- If you have an elevated temperature, call your physician.

Phone Numbers

Physician: ______________________________
Other: ______________________________

Comments

Source: Camp-Sorrell, D. Dysphagia. In: Yarbro CH, Wujcik D, Gobel BH, eds. *Cancer Symptom Management.* 4th ed. Burlington, MA: Jones & Bartlett Learning; 2014.

Chapter 19

Mucositis

Debra Wujcik, PhD, RN, FAAN

THE PROBLEM

The digestive tract is lined with epithelial cells from the mouth to the anus that are commonly injured as a side effect of many cytotoxic cancer therapy regimens. The mucosa acts as a protective physical and chemical barrier against pathogens that can enter the gastrointestinal system via the mouth or breaks in the mucosal integrity. The treatment of cancer with chemotherapy, radiation, and hematopoietic cell transplantation (HCT), whether alone or in combination, causes serious and life-threatening side effects in many patients. Oral mucositis is among those side effects; it is associated with pain, infection, nutritional alterations and diminished quality of life.

The terms *mucositis* and *stomatitis* have been used interchangeably to define the inflammation of the mucosa.[1,2] Mucositis is an inflammatory process that is visually seen in the mucous membranes of the oral cavity and can be present throughout the gastrointestinal tract. Inflammatory diseases of the mouth that include the mucosa and the dentition, periapces, and periodentum are collectively referred to as stomatitis.[3,4] Mucositis in both the mouth and the alimentary tract is known as alimentary tract mucositis.[1,5,6]

The oral mucosa is the most accessible part of the digestive mucosa and is examined to evaluate possible inflammation of the entire tract. Mucositis can begin with erythema and progress to confluent ulceration of the oral mucosa, including gingiva and the tongue, with the ensuing damage ranging from mild to severe.[7–9] Disruption in the integrity of the oral mucosa can have significant effects on the course of treatment such as dose delays and reductions. Many cancer patients report mucositis to be the most distressing side effect of their treatment, especially during radiation or chemotherapy for head and neck cancer.[8]

Intact oral mucosa serves as a protective barrier. Mucositis breaks that barrier, allowing for the development of local infection that can progress to life-threatening sepsis.[2,7,10] The ability to take in adequate nutrition may be compromised by excessive dryness (xerostomia), oral discomfort and pain, and alterations in taste affecting the ability and desire to eat.[10,11] The patient's quality of life may be altered when mucositis interferes with the ability to communicate and decreases oral sensation and pleasure. There are also financial implications for oral mucositis in terms of increased hospitalization, clinic visits, procedures, and medication costs.

In the past two decades, improved antiemetic therapy and use of growth factors to prevent and minimize bone marrow depression have allowed for continued dose escalation of chemotherapy agents. In turn, severe mucositis that cannot be effectively prevented or minimized has evolved into a dose-limiting side effect.[12] Along with experiencing dose reductions and dosing delays, patients who are immunocompromised can become infected and require hospitalization. Subsequently, patients with severe mucositis have higher healthcare costs[13,14] and poorer quality of life.[15–17] Oncology nurses can assist patients to manage mucositis so they can receive adequate treatment for their cancer.[18]

INCIDENCE

The National Cancer Institute[3] estimates that 10% of patients receiving adjunctive chemotherapy and 40% of those receiving primary chemotherapy experience mucositis.

It is also estimated that half of the patients with mucositis have treatment delays and one-third discontinue treatment altogether because of this side effect.[19] With mucositis, the risk of dose reduction doubles.[14] Moreover, there is increased risk of hospitalization and increased costs of care because of the need for antibiotics, parenteral nutrition, and pain management.[19] Because clinicians routinely underreport the incidence of mucositis compared to what patients report, the actual cost of mucositis in healthcare dollars is unknown.[20]

In a meta-analysis of 99 published clinical trials, Keefe et al. reviewed the toxicity data from patients treated for non-Hodgkin's lymphoma or breast, lung, or colorectal cancer (CRC).[6] They reported incidence of grade 3 and 4 (World Health Organization [WHO] grading) mucositis to be less than 10%. This figure stands in sharp contrast to a higher incidence when mucositis is the study endpoint being evaluated. For example, when Rosen et al. evaluated patients with CRC being treated with 5-fluorouracil (5FU) and leucovorin, the placebo group had a 50% greater incidence of severe mucositis than the treatment group receiving palifermin to prevent mucositis.[21]

The incidence of mucositis is higher in patients with cancers of the oral cavity, oropharynx, and nasopharynx than in patients with other cancers.[22] Nearly 100% of patients receiving radiation therapy to the head and neck have some grade of oral mucositis, and 75% to 80% of patients undergoing HCT develop significant mucositis.[7,22] Treatment combinations that include both chemotherapy and radiation are also associated with higher incidence of this side effect than either therapy alone, with the most severe grade of mucositis occurring in patients treated with chemotherapy and radiation therapy to the oral cavity.[22,23] These patients have severe oral mucositis resulting in the inability to eat solid foods and often require enteral support.[23]

ETIOLOGY

Mucositis is a common side effect of anticancer therapy and can be attributed to specific chemotherapeutic and targeted agents as well as radiation to the head and neck. Concomitant chemotherapy and radiation to the head and neck increases the incidence and severity of mucositis. Patients undergoing HCT with high-dose chemotherapy and total-body irradiation often experience severe oral and alimentary mucositis (Table 19-1).

TABLE 19-1

Chemotherapeutic Agents with a High Potential to Cause Stomatitis

Class	Agents
Alkylating agents	Busulfan Carboplatin Cisplatin Cyclophosphamide Melphalan Procarbazine Thiotepa
Antimetabolites	Cytarabine 5-Fluorouracil Floxuridine Hydroxyurea 6-Mercaptopurine Methotrexate 6-Thioguanine
DNA-interactive agents	Actinomycin D Amsacrine Bleomycin sulfate Daunomycin Doxorubicin Etoposide Idarubicin Mithramycin Mitomycin C Mitoxantrone Procarbazine hydrochloride
mTOR inhibitors	Everolimus Temsirolimus
Topoisomerase inhibitors	Etoposide Topotecan Irinotecan Teniposide
Tubulin-interactive agents	Docetaxel Paclitaxel Vinblastine sulfate Vincristine sulfate Vinorelbine

PATHOPHYSIOLOGY

Oral mucositis results from a complex interaction of local tissue damage and patient-related factors such as the local oral environment, the level of myelosuppression, and intrinsic genetic predisposition (e.g., single-nucleotide polymorphisms) to develop oral mucositis. Sonis and colleagues have expanded our understanding of the pathophysiology of mucositis from its perception as an interruption in the life cycle of epithelial cells to recognition of it as a multiphase process involving many biologic interactions.[24] The current model of the pathophysiology of mucositis includes five phases: (1) initiation; (2) up-regulation and message generation; (3) amplification and signaling; (4) ulceration; and (5) healing[19,25,26] (Figure 19-1).

Initiation begins quickly after the start of chemotherapy administration and radiation therapy. Oxygen free radicals

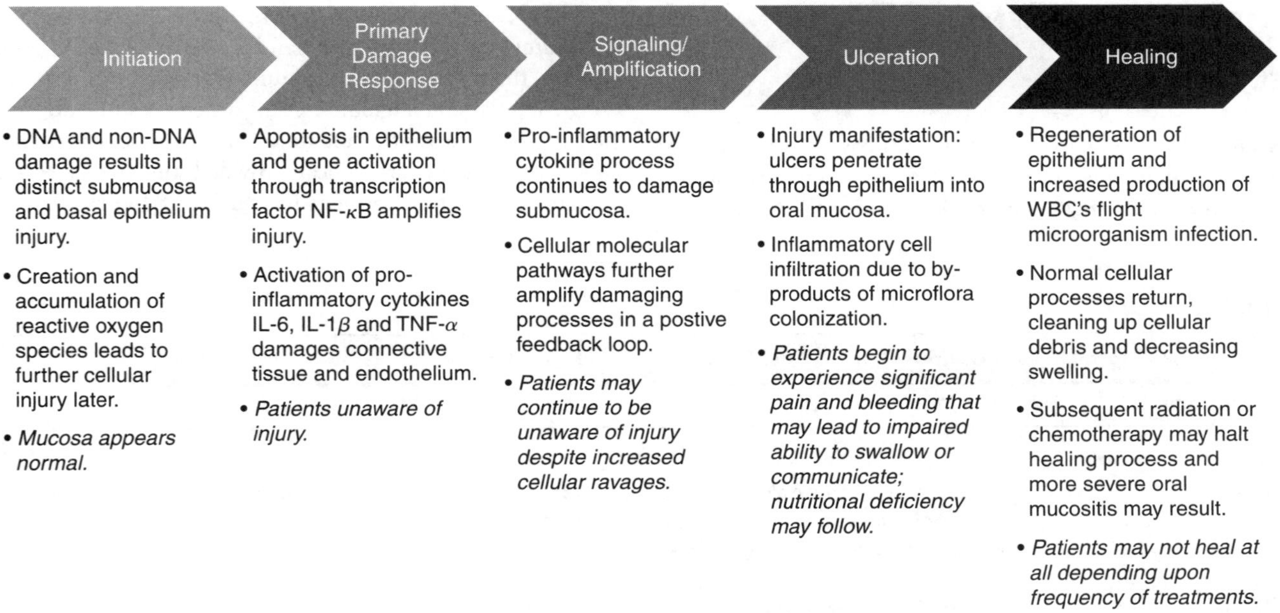

Initiation	Primary Damage Response	Signaling/ Amplification	Ulceration	Healing
• DNA and non-DNA damage results in distinct submucosa and basal epithelium injury. • Creation and accumulation of reactive oxygen species leads to further cellular injury later. • *Mucosa appears normal.*	• Apoptosis in epithelium and gene activation through transcription factor NF-κB amplifies injury. • Activation of pro-inflammatory cytokines IL-6, IL-1β and TNF-α damages connective tissue and endothelium. • *Patients unaware of injury.*	• Pro-inflammatory cytokine process continues to damage submucosa. • Cellular molecular pathways further amplify damaging processes in a postive feedback loop. • *Patients may continue to be unaware of injury despite increased cellular ravages.*	• Injury manifestation: ulcers penetrate through epithelium into oral mucosa. • Inflammatory cell infiltration due to by-products of microflora colonization. • *Patients begin to experience significant pain and bleeding that may lead to impaired ability to swallow or communicate; nutritional deficiency may follow.*	• Regeneration of epithelium and increased production of WBC's flight microorganism infection. • Normal cellular processes return, cleaning up cellular debris and decreasing swelling. • Subsequent radiation or chemotherapy may halt healing process and more severe oral mucositis may result. • *Patients may not heal at all depending upon frequency of treatments.*

FIGURE 19-1

The five biological phases of mucositis.

Source: Data from Brown[25].

are generated as a result of these treatments that cause direct cellular damage to the basal and epithelial cells in the submucosa. A cascade of biologic responses is initiated and although the mucosa still look normal, the damage has already started.[26]

The second phase comprises up-regulation and message generation. In this phase, transcription factors such as nuclear factor kappa B (NF-κB) are activated either by the reactive oxygen species released during phase 1 or by direct cytotoxicity of chemotherapy and/or radiation. Research has shown that NF-κB controls nearly 200 genes connected with mucositis.[19] A number of pro-inflammatory cytokines, such as interleukin-1 beta (IL-1β) and tumor necrosis factor alpha (TNF-α), are activated by NF-κB. IL-1β mediates inflammation and dilates vessels, potentially increasing the concentration of chemotherapeutic agents at the site. TNF-α causes tissue damage, perhaps in an escalating fashion. During the initiation and up-regulation/message generation phases, the altered pathways continue to influence one another, altering the muscosal environment. The result is erythema from increased vascularity and epithelial atrophy beginning 4 to 5 days after the initiation of chemotherapy. Microtrauma from day-to-day activities, such as speech, swallowing, and mastication, leads to ulceration.

Sonis[24] has added to his original work, proposing that the expansion of elements in the initiation phase contributes to the manifestations of mucositis seen in later stages. He postulates that the cells damaged by chemotherapy and radiation release molecules that become attached to receptors associated with epithelial and endothelial cells and fibroblasts that later serve as the "on switch" for manifestations of mucositis, including ulcers or ulceration.

Ulceration, the fourth stage in the mucositis pathophysiology model, causes the most symptoms for the patient, especially given that this period is when neutropenia is common. Ulcerations formed in the mucosa are covered with fibrinous exudates and bacteria are collected. This accumulation sets the stage for invasion of microorganisms with bacteremia and sepsis. The patient experiences pain, difficulty swallowing, and possibly bleeding from the lesions.

The final phase, healing, occurs once cancer treatment is completed. Signals from the extracellular matrix induce epithelial cells to migrate underneath the pseudomembrane (fibrin clot) of the ulcer. The epithelium then proliferates so that the thickness of the mucosa returns to normal. Although the epithelium is regenerated, it is important to understand that complete healing may not occur between cycles of treatment. In fact, the patient may experience more severe mucositis in future cycles. The direct relationship between the white blood cell count and oral mucositis is uncertain, and not all patients with mucositis demonstrate hematologic toxicity.[27,28]

SYMPTOM ASSESSMENT

RISK FACTORS

Research identifying risk factors for mucositis is limited by measurement inconsistency, use of tools without valid and reliable measures, small sample sizes, and lack of adequate controls. Confounding variables that limit the interpretation of findings include age and gender associated with specific cancers, the disease-related immunosuppression for solid versus hematologic malignancies, and differences in side effects of the various chemotherapeutic agents. In spite of these limitations, risk factors are typically divided into two categories: patient-related and treatment-related[29–33] (Table 19-2).

TABLE 19-2

Factors That Increase the Risk for Oral Mucositis in Individuals with Cancer

Risk Factor	Mechanism of Action	Prevention Strategies
Age		
Children	• Increased prevalence not well understood but may be due to immature immune response, increased cellular proliferation, and higher prevalence of hematologic malignancies	• Careful and frequent oral hygiene
Elderly	• Degenerative changes: decreased salivary flow, diminished keratinization of mucosa, and increased prevalence of gingivitis	• Careful and frequent oral hygiene • Adequate hydration • Mouth moisturizers • Avoid trauma • Dental treatment of gingivitis
Exposure to alcohol and tobacco		• Avoid or limit consumption of alcoholic beverages and tobacco products, especially during treatment
Poor oral hygiene	• Increased debris breeds infection • Lack of stimulation to enhance circulation	• Careful and frequent oral hygiene, including brushing tongue and gums
Oxygen therapy	• Moisture drawn from mucosa into oxygen, causing a drying of the mucosal lining	• Humidify oxygen • Mouth moisturizers • Adequate hydration
Oral or nasogastric suctioning	• Catheter and suctioning process cause traumatic breaks in mucosal integrity	• Minimize suctioning frequency and duration
Changes in breathing patterns	• Tachypnea and mouth breathing dry the mucosa	• Careful and frequent oral hygiene • Room humidifier
Certain drugs		
Anticholinergics and antihistamines	• Decrease salivary flow	• Careful and frequent oral hygiene
Phenytoin	• Gingival hyperplasia	• Avoid these drugs if possible
Steroids	• Fungal overgrowth	
Ill-fitting dentures	• Movement irritates mucosa and breaks integrity	• Reline dentures • Remove dentures at night and use only for eating until healing occurs
Hot, acidic, or spicy foods	• Thermal and chemical irritants inflame and traumatize mucosa	• Bland, soft foods • Avoid acidic, peppery, and spicy foods • Let hot food cool before eating it
Poor nutritional status	• Refined sugars increase dental decay • Protein/calorie malnutrition delays healing • Vitamin deficiencies cause oral complications	• Minimize intake of refined sugars • Well-balanced daily diet including fruits, vegetables, grains, and sources of protein • Daily vitamin supplement
Dehydration	• Dryness and cracking result when fluid is drawn from mucosa and lips as a protective mechanism	• Daily fluid intake of at least 2000 mL

Source: Data from Beck[33].

Patient-related risk factors

Patient-related factors contributing to the risk of mucositis include age, gender, oral health and hygiene, salivary secretory function, genetic factors, body mass index, renal function, smoking, and previous cancer treatment.

In the crisis of a cancer diagnosis and start of treatment, the patient may adjust priorities and change oral routines, especially those involved with preventive care. Due to the demands of the treatment schedule, regular dental appointments and cleanings may be delayed or missed.[10] Because the oral mucosa serves as the first line of defense against bacterial infection in the mouth, routine basic oral hygiene, including daily brushing and flossing, as well as preventive dental services to promote strong teeth and healthy gums, is necessary. Periodontal disease, caries, and overall poor oral hygiene are associated with development of mucositis. There remains a lack of randomized controlled trials to support specific oral hygiene protocols but generally providers accept the need for good oral hygiene as a way to prevent oral complications from therapy.[29,30]

Older patients and children tend to have more severe mucositis and a longer duration of mucositis.[34,35] Patients older than 50 years of age are at greater risk for mucositis likely due to decreased renal function that obstructs drug excretion.[36] The elderly also generally have lower metabolic reserves and often experience altered metabolism of chemotherapeutic agents.[37] Pediatric and adolescent patients may be at a higher risk for mucositis because a larger fraction of their basal mucosal cells are proliferating or turning over at any given time as compared to adults, whereas older adults have slower proliferation leading to slower healing.[35,38]

Some genetic factors may affect susceptibility to mucositis, including female gender and circadian variables that relate to the intrinsic endocrine system, which can affect the metabolism of certain chemotherapy-metabolizing enzymes and the mucosal response to chemotherapy or radiation.[6,10,39] The incidence of mucositis is higher in females than males.[32] Smoking and drinking alcohol while undergoing cancer treatment can increase the risk for mucositis due to damage to the epithelium of the oral cavity and alimentary canal.[40]

The incidence of mucositis is higher in patients with cancers of the oral cavity, oropharynx, and nasopharynx than in patients with other cancers, because patients with the former cancers often present with more advanced disease, necessitating multimodal and aggressive therapy.[22] In addition, prior chemotherapy or radiation to the oral cavity is associated with increased incidence and severity of mucositis.[22]

Treatment-related risk factors

The occurrence of mucositis in patients treated with chemotherapy is related to the chemotherapeutic agent, route of delivery, intensity of dose, and modality of the agent(s) used (Table 19-1). Chemotherapy affects the basal cell layer of the oral epithelium by inhibiting cellular proliferation and cell-cycle progression leading to cell death (apoptosis), which is most affected due to the high rate of mitosis in the mucosa of the oral cavity and complete alimentary canal.

Not all chemotherapy agents cause mucositis, however, and certain agents have higher potential to cause mucositis.[33] Specific groups of chemotherapeutic agents such as antimetabolites, antitumor antibiotics, and alkylating agents are known to cause mucositis. In addition, the dose and schedule of administration for certain agents promote development of mucositis. For example, mucositis is more severe with bolus 5-FU versus continuous infusion, and low-dose melphalan is less toxic than the same high-dose agent. Newer anticancer agents such as those that inhibit the mTOR pathway have been shown to cause mucositis. For example, a retrospective case-record review of 17 cancer patients who received treatment with a regimen that included an mTOR inhibitor found that all patients developed some grade of oral mucositis, with a medial pain score of 7 (range: 0–10), and 13 patients required discontinuation of therapy.[11]

The effects of combination therapies, such as the chemotherapy/radiation pairing, and high-dose chemotherapy, given either alone or as part of HCT, increase the severity of mucositis. Therapy for head and neck cancer routinely includes a combination of chemotherapy and radiation therapy. These treatments cause mucositis in 15% to 90% of patients with this type of cancer. The severity is highest when chemotherapy and radiation are given concomitantly (from 60% to 100% of patients).[41,42] Mucositis is also more severe if the radiation dose exceeds 5000 centigray (cGy) and in those patients who receive more than one treatment per day.[22] The oral mucosa becomes erythematous around the second week (when the total dose reaches approximately 2000 cGy) and worsens over the continued weeks of treatment. It does not resolve until treatment is complete.

Severe mucositis has been noted to occur in 98% of patients undergoing HCT.[40,43,44] Patients undergoing allogeneic stem cell transplantation have more severe and longer duration of mucositis than those undergoing autologous transplantation, although the mucositis in these cases is related to the intensity of the conditioning regimen. These patients receive concurrent whole-body irradiation, which produces grade 3 and 4 mucositis in more than 60% of these individuals.[19]

SELF-ASSESSMENT

Patients can be taught to assess their oral cavity for any erythema, edema, white lesions, bleeding or feelings of pain, soreness, or anything that feels different. The self-assessment should be done daily. Patients should be taught to initiate various levels of self-care and should understand when to report abnormalities to the medical team.[18]

OBJECTIVE ASSESSMENT

History

During treatment for cancer, patients may report changes in oral sensation and taste, difficulty talking and swallowing, the presence of mouth sores, and sometimes dryness (xerostomia) and difficulty eating. Bleeding, infection, and ulceration may be present.[9] The nurse should prompt the patient to reports these symptoms by asking, "Are you having any problems with your mouth?" Affirmative responses should lead to a more thorough assessment. The history should also include a pretreatment assessment of the patient's usual oral hygiene practices, ability to continue oral care, and ability to understand and perform oral care during treatment.

Physical exam

The physical assessment begins with a systematic assessment of the oral cavity (Table 19-3).[33] In a setting with good natural light, the nurse prepares for the exam by assembling nonsterile gloves, a tongue blade, a dental mirror, and gauze. The visual inspection begins with the outer lips, teeth, gums, tongue, inside cheek area, and hard and soft palates. Using the gauze to wrap the tongue will allow movement of the tongue to inspect the floor of the oral cavity. Gently pulling the upper and lower cheeks away from the gums will aid further inspection.

A healthy mouth is moist, clean, with pink, nonulcerated, intact mucosa. The patient with mucositis may have changes in color (erythema, pallor, or white patches), changes in moisture (dryness and decreased saliva), accumulation of debris or odor, changes in integrity (ulcers, cracks, lesions), and changes in perception (hoarseness, difficulty swallowing, pain).[33]

A variety of tools for assessment of mucositis have been developed and tested in the past two decades. The Oral Assessment Guide (OAG) has been widely used in research and is recommended as a comprehensive tool that is easy to use in practice.[45] The OAG is used to assess voice, swallow, lips, tongue, saliva, mucous membranes, gingiva, and teeth (or dentures); it rates the oral cavity components as 1 if normal and as 2 or 3 if abnormal changes are apparent (Table 19-4). WHO's Oral Toxicity Scale is also well known and easy to use.[46] Other assessment tools include the Oral Mucosa Rating Scale (OMRS),[47] Oral Mucositis Index,[48,49] Oral Mucositis Assessment Scale (OMAS),[50] and the Western Consortium for Cancer Nursing Research tool.[51]

TABLE 19-3

Clinical Guide: Performing an Oral Assessment

1. Gather equipment.
   - Good source of light
   - Nonsterile gloves
   - Gauze
   - Tongue blade
   - Dental mirror (optional)
2. Wash hands.
3. Apply nonsterile gloves.
4. Remove all dental appliances. Inquire regarding the fit of dentures and any sore or painful areas.
5. Inquire regarding any changes in voice, taste, ability to eat or swallow, and comfort.
6. Systematically perform each of the following, using directed light to observe for moisture, color, integrity, and cleanliness:
   a. Observe the outer lips.
   b. Pull down lower lip and raise upper lip to observe the teeth and mucosal lining of the outer vestibule. (Note: Check teeth for color, shine, debris, and caries.)
   c. Instruct the person to open the mouth so you can observe the hard and soft palates.
   d. Use a finger to displace and examine the mucosa of the inner cheeks.
   e. Note the amount and quality of the saliva. (Note: Normal saliva is thin and watery.)
   f. Examine the top of the tongue. Then ask the person to curl the tongue up to the roof of the mouth so you can observe the underside of the tongue.
   g. Use the gauze to displace the tongue to each side to observe the lateral sides of the tongue.
   h. Ask the person to take a deep breath so you can observe the oropharynx, posterior tongue, and uvula. If this technique does not allow adequate visualization, use the tongue blade to gently depress the tongue and use the dental mirror for improved visualization.
7. Based on the results of this assessment, score each category on the assessment tool.

Source: Data from Beck[33].

Diagnostic evaluation

The diagnosis of mucositis is based on the oral assessment of the practitioner and the presence of changes in the lips, tongue, saliva, mucous membranes, and gingiva and the patient's subjective complaints of pain or discomfort. The concurrent presence of infection may be proven by positive oral cultures.

DEGREES OF TOXICITY

The degree of severity of mucositis ranges from mild sensations to multiple ulcerations and bleeding lesions. These changes are often found in the mouth and throughout

TABLE 19-4

Oral Assessment Guide

Item	1	2	3
Voice	Normal	Deeper or raspy	Difficulty talking or painful
Swallow	Normal swallow	Some pain on swallowing	Unable to swallow
Lips	Smooth and pink and moist	Dry or cracked	Ulcerated bleeding
Tongue	Pink and moist and papillae present	Coated or loss of papillae with a shiny appearance with or without redness	Blistered or cracked
Saliva	Watery	Thick or ropy	Absent
Mucous membrane (buccal, mucosa, palate)	Pink and moist	Reddened or coated (increased whiteness) without ulceration	Ulceration with or without bleeding
Gingiva	Pink and stippled and firm	Edematous with or without redness	Spontaneous bleeding or bleeding with pressure
Teeth or dentures	Clean and no debris	Plaque or debris in localized area (between teeth if present)	Plaque or debris generalized along gum line or denture-bearing area

Source: Data from Eilers J, Berger AM, Peterson MD. Development, testing, and application of the oral assessment guide. *Oncol Nurs Forum*. 1988;15:325–330[45]. Reprinted with permission.

the gastrointestinal tract. The National Cancer Institute's Common Terminology Criteria for Adverse Event (CTCAE) scale is used to grade the condition of the oral cavity—specifically, dry mouth, dysphagia, oral dyesthesia, and oral pain[52] (Table 19-5).

SYMPTOM MANAGEMENT STRATEGIES

THERAPEUTIC APPROACHES

Despite ongoing research, there is not one intervention that is effective with all cancer diagnoses and treatments.[10,22,53] A number of practice guidelines have been published in the past decade. In 2004, the Mucositis Study Group of the Multinational Association of Supportive Care in Cancer (MASCC) and the International Society for Oral Oncology (ISOO) published evidence-based clinical guidelines for the prevention and treatment of mucositis.[4] These guidelines were updated in 2007.[6]

In addition, four Cochrane reviews have focused on the treatment and prevention of mucositis. The first Cochrane review, performed in 2004, found evidence to support three treatment interventions: allopurinol, immunoglobulin, and human placental extract.[55] The 2006 review focused on prevention of mucositis and recommended ten therapeutic interventions: amifostine, Chinese medicine, and hydrolytic enzymes were found to be of benefit in more than one study each, and antibiotic pastille or paste, benzydamine, calcium phosphate, honey, hydrolytic enzymes, oral care, povidone, and zinc sulfate were each supported by just one study.[56] These recommendations were again updated in 2011.[57] The 2010 guideline found low-level laser treatment to be the only intervention to effectively treat severe mucositis, and morphine was recommended for the treatment of mucositis pain.[58]

The Oncology Nursing Society's (ONS's) Putting Evidence into Practice (PEP) initiative is a source of evidence-based practice recommendations for nurses.[58,59] The ONS model uses five levels of recommendation: (1) recommended for practice; (2) likely to be effective; (3) effectiveness not established; (4) effectiveness unlikely; and (5) not recommended for practice. The PEP guidelines recommend an oral care protocol that includes patient education and guidelines for patients receiving HCT, radiation, and standard-dose chemotherapy. The prevention and treatment options described in this section are consistent with the practice guidelines of MASCC and ONS (Table 19-6).[4,58,60] Eilers and Milton recommend ongoing critical evaluation of the published evidence and frequent checking of the websites of the specific organizations.[10]

Prevention

The goal of oral hygiene is to reduce the colonization of microbes in the oral cavity and decrease the risk of oral infection by pathogens. This is especially true for patients who are immunosuppressed as the result of their cancer or cancer treatment. Patients should undergo complete oral and dental examinations, including cleaning and treatment of caries and extractions, prior to initiation of chemotherapy or radiotherapy.[40,59]

TABLE 19-5

National Cancer Institute Common Terminology Criteria for Adverse Events (CTCAE): Dry Mouth, Dysphagia, Oral Dysesthesia, Oral Hemorrhage, Oral Mucositis, and Oral Pain

	1	2	3	4	5
Dry mouth Definition: a disorder characterized by reduced salivary flow in the oral cavity	Symptomatic (e.g., dry or thick saliva) without significant dietary alteration; unstimulated saliva flow > 0.2 mL/min	Moderate symptoms; oral intake alterations (e.g., copious water, other lubricants, diet limited to purees and/or soft, moist foods); unstimulated saliva 0.1–0.2 mL/min	Inability to adequately aliment orally; tube feeding or total parenteral nutrition indicated; unstimulated saliva < 0.1 mL/min		
Dysphagia Definition: a disorder characterized by difficulty in swallowing	Symptomatic, able to eat regular diet	Symptomatic and altered eating/swallowing	Severely altered eating/swallowing; tube feeding or total parenteral nutrition or hospitalization indicated	Life-threatening consequences; urgent intervention indicated	Death
Oral dysesthesia Definition: a disorder characterized by burning or tingling sensation on the lips, tongue, or entire mouth	Mild discomfort; not interfering with oral intake	Moderate pain; interfering with oral intake	Disabling pain; tube feeding or total parenteral nutrition indicated		
Oral hemorrhage Definition: a disorder characterized by bleeding from the mouth	Mild; intervention not indicated	Moderate symptoms; medical intervention or minor cauterization indicated	Transfusion, radiologic, endoscopic, or elective operative intervention indicated	Life-threatening consequences; urgent intervention indicated	Death
Oral mucositis Definition: a disorder characterized by inflammation of the oral mucosa	Asymptomatic or mild symptoms; intervention not indicated	Moderate pain; not interfering with oral intake; modified diet indicated	Severe pain; interfering with oral intake	Life-threatening consequences; urgent intervention indicated	Death
Oral pain Definition: a disorder characterized by a sensation of marked discomfort in the mouth, tongue, or lips	Mild pain	Moderated pain limiting instrumental activities of daily living	Severe pain limiting self-care activities of daily living		

Source: Data from National Cancer Institute Common Terminology Criteria for Adverse Events (CTCAE)[52].

TABLE 19-6

Mucositis Intervention Guidelines

Treatment	Recommended	Not Recommended
Standard-dose chemotherapy	5-Fluorouracil bolus: 30-minute oral cryotherapy Edatrexate bolus: 20- to 30-minute oral cryotherapy	Chlorhexidine should not be used Acyclovir and other antivirals should not be used routinely
Radiation therapy to head and neck	Midline radiation blocks and 3D radiation treatment Benzydamine oral rinse for prevention	Sucralfate Antimicrobial lozenges
Hematopoietic cell transplantation	Patient-controlled analgesic morphine for pain Low-level laser therapy (only at centers with trained staff) Karatinocyte growth factor-1 (palifermin) intravenously High-dose melphalan: cryotherapy	Pentoxifylline Granulocyte-macrophage colony-stimulating factor mouthwashes

Sources: Data from Rubenstein et al[4]; Oncology Nursing Society[58]; Multinational Association of Supportive Care in Cancer/International Society for Oral Oncology[60].

Basic oral hygiene includes routine brushing, flossing, rinsing, and moisturizing the mouth and lips. Oral care protocols should include the routine brushing of the teeth with a soft toothbrush, flossing, and rinsing. Although flossing removes plaque and the bacteria responsible for the plaque, it is not recommended for patients who have not routinely flossed prior to the start of treatment. Frequent rinsing may effectively remove bacteria away from ulcerations. It is recommended that toothbrushes should be changed frequently (every month). All surfaces of the teeth must be brushed, and the tongue should be gently brushed to help remove debris and bacteria. Patients should brush for at least 90 seconds twice daily. Flossing should occur at least daily.[59]

Oral rinses are recommended to remove loose debris and increase oral hydration. Sodium bicarbonate reduces the acidity of oral fluids and decreases the viscosity of mucus that accumulates in the oral cavity and throat.[10,59] Patients can be instructed to rinse with a solution of ½ tsp baking soda and/or ¼ tsp table salt in 1 cup warm water several times daily to cleanse and lubricate the oral cavity.[22] All oral rinses and mouthwashes must be alcohol free, because alcohol can lead to dehydration of the mucosa and amplified irritation.[2] Patients can be encouraged to increase water consumption and ice chips as tolerated, use artificial saliva, and chew sugarless gum or suck on sugarless candy.

Treatment

Pain management should proceed in a stepwise fashion, beginning with the use of topical anesthetics and analgesics before systematic analgesics are administered. Nonsteroidal anti-inflammatory analgesics may be added next, followed by opioids (oral, transdermal, or parenteral) if the pain becomes severe. The MASCC/ISOO guidelines recommend patient-controlled analgesia with opioids for patients undergoing HCT.[60]

Patients with thrombocytopenia due to chemotherapy may experience mucosal bleeding due to ulcerative mucositis; this bleeding can be controlled with topical hemostatic agents. This side effect is of concern when the patient's platelet count falls below 20,000/mm^3 or the patient experiences spontaneous bleeding. Use of toothettes may be indicated when the platelet counts are low, and patients may require transfusions to prevent spontaneous bleeding.

Nutritional support plays a crucial role, because the patient's nutritional status can be compromised by mucositis. Patients with mucositis may begin to have taste changes that may lead to anorexia. Severe grade 3 or 4 mucositis can impair or prevent oral intake, leading to malnutrition and the need for gastrostomy tube placement when the patient is unable to maintain nutritional status and body weight. A dietician should be consulted regularly to instruct patients and providers on food options that will provide adequate caloric intake for patients.[33]

Prevention of infection is most effective when good oral hygiene is maintained. Prophylactic use of antimicrobial lozenges is not recommended for radiation-induced mucositis.[6] Although chlorhexidine is useful as an antimicrobial agent and can be effective in controlling early periodontal infection, it is not recommended for use in the prevention of mucositis.[61]

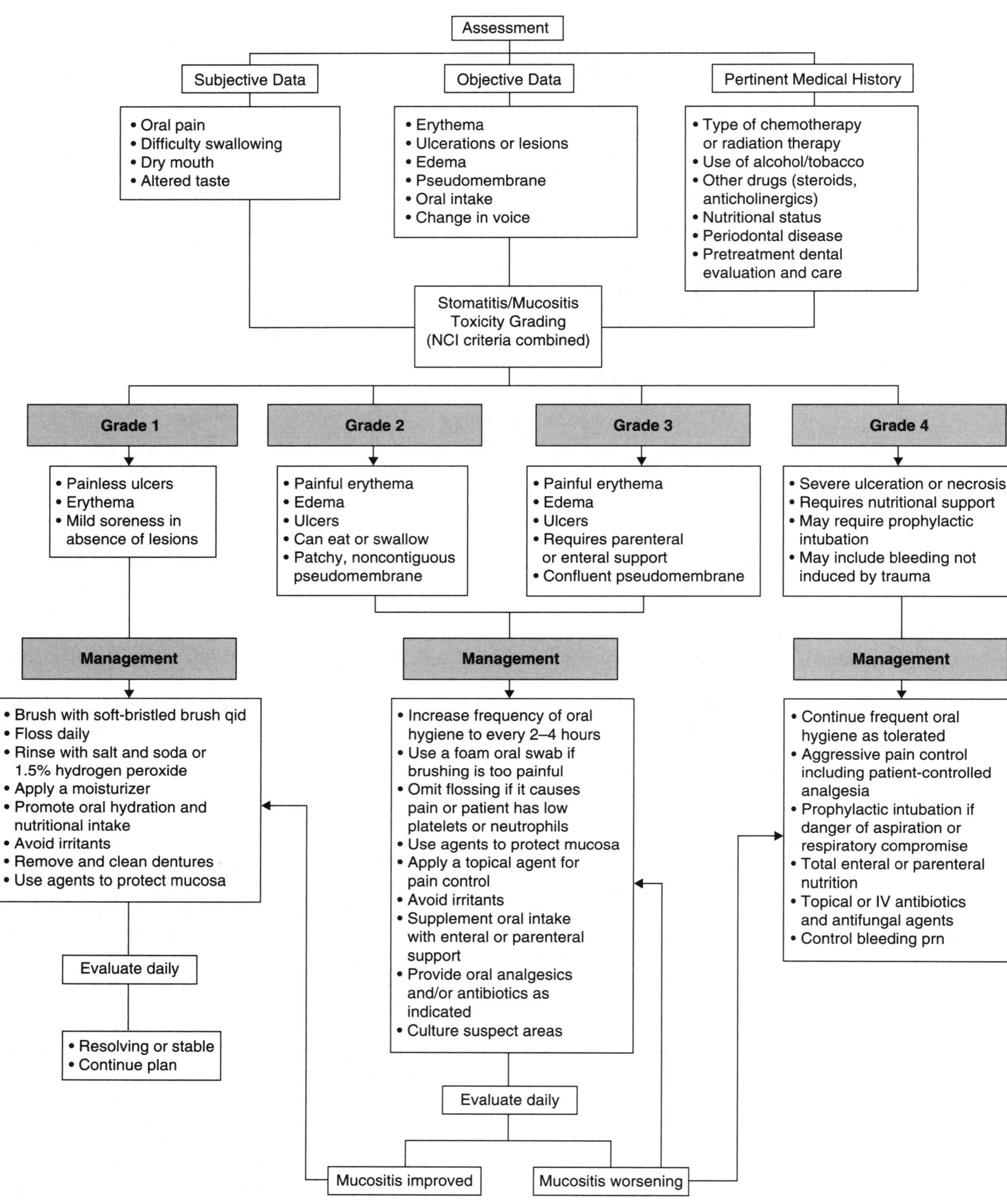

FIGURE 19-2

Oral assessment and care.

Source: Data from Beck[33].

Patients undergoing radiation therapy to the head and neck should be treated using midline radiation blocks and three-dimensional radiation treatment.[58] Benzydamine is used to prevent radiation-induced mucositis in many countries, but is not approved for use in the United States.[57]

Cryotherapy—the use of ice chips during chemotherapy administration to prevent mucositis—is hypothesized to cause local vasoconstriction and reduce blood flow to the oral tissues, resulting in decreased delivery of chemotherapy to the area.[22] Some evidence indicates that cryotherapy is effective in decreasing the severity of mucositis in patients who receive bolus doses of certain chemotherapy agents, such as fluorouracil or melphalan. Patients are instructed to hold ice or ice-cold water in their mouth for 5 minutes before and 30 minutes after infusion of these agents.

Palifermin is a recombinant human keratinocyte growth factor that stimulates epithelial cells of the oral mucosa. It is the only FDA-approved medication to prevent mucositis. Palifermin has been shown to reduce the severity and duration of mucositis in patients receiving high-dose chemotherapy and total-body irradiation with autologous stem cell transplantation.[39,40,62] The dose of this agent is 60 mcg/kg/day IV for three days prior to beginning the conditioning regimen and then for three days after the transplantation to prevent mucositis. Side effects observed with palifermin include mild rash and taste changes.

The use of acyclovir, sucrafate, and antimicrobial lozenges for prevention of mucositis is not recommended.[1,2]

NURSING IMPLICATIONS

Nurses should teach patients to self-assess and perform self-care to allow patients to participate in their own care and potentially decrease the severity of mucositis.[18] Using NCI toxicity grading and guideline-supported care, nurses can provide tailored education and care[33] (Figure 19-2). Patients should be taught to avoid tobacco products, alcohol, and certain foods and liquids (spicy, acidic, rough, or hot) that may exacerbate mucositis.[18]

PATIENT SELF-CARE

As part of self-care to prevent mucositis, patients are instructed to initiate and/or continue an oral health regimen (Appendix 19A). They are taught to brush all tooth surfaces for at least 90 seconds twice daily using a soft toothbrush; floss at least once daily or as advised by the clinician; rinse the mouth four times daily with a bland mouth rinse such as normal saline; avoid tobacco, alcohol, and irritating foods; use a water-based moisturizer to protect the lips; and maintain adequate hydration.[59]

Once the patient begins to notice the early signs of mucositis, the oral care plan is adjusted[10,25,58] (Appendix 19B). A sponge or "toothette" may be used if the patient cannot tolerate a toothbrush due to pain or bleeding. Patients can even clean the teeth with a piece of gauze wrapped around their finger. Toothbrushes are preferred to sponges for cleaning the tooth enamel, but sponges and even gauze are preferred to no cleansing. Patients should floss their teeth once daily or as advised by a clinician. They should rinse their mouth four times a day with a bland mouth rinse such as normal saline, sodium bicarbonate, or a saline and sodium bicarbonate mixture. This rinsing is thought help remove loose debris as well as moisturize the oral cavity. Many over-the-counter mouthwashes should be avoided because they contain alcohol, which can irritate the oral cavity or lesions if they are present. The patient should moisturize the lips with a water-based product.

REFERENCES

1. Peterson DE, Keefe DM, Hutchins RD, et al. Alimentary tract mucositis in cancer patients: impact of terminology and assessment on research and clinical practice. *Support Care Cancer.* 2006;14:499–504.
2. Epstein JB, Thariat J, Bensadoun J, et al. Oral complications of cancer and cancer therapy: from cancer treatment to survivorship. *CA Cancer J Clin.* 2012;62(6):400–422.
3. National Cancer Institute. Oral complications of chemotherapy and head/neck radiation. Available at: http://nci.nih.gov/cancertopics/pdq/supportivecare/oralcomplications/Health Professional. Accessed December 1, 2012.
4. Rubenstein EB, Peterson DE, Schubert M, et al. Clinical practice guidelines for the prevention and treatment of cancer therapy-induced oral and gastrointestinal mucositis. *Cancer.* 2004;100(suppl):2026–2046.
5. Keefe DM, Peterson DE, Schubert MM. Developing evidence-based guidelines for management of alimentary mucositis: process and pitfalls. *Support Care Cancer.* 2006;14:492–498.
6. Keefe DM, Schubert MM, Elting LS, et al. Updated clinical practice guidelines for the prevention and treatment of mucositis. *Cancer.* 2007; 109:820–831.
7. Fall-Dickson JM, Ramsay ES Castro, et al. Oral mucositis-related oropharyngeal pain and correlative tumor necrosis factor-alpha expression in adult oncology patients undergoing hematopoietic stem cell transplantation. *Clin Ther.* 2007;29 (suppl):2547–2561.
8. Bhide SA, Gulliford S, Schick U, et al. Dose–response analysis of acute oral mucositis and pharyngeal dysphagia in patients receiving induction chemotherapy followed by concomitant chemo-IMRT for head and neck cancer. *Radiother Oncol.* 2012;103(1):88–91.
9. Caplinger J, Royse M, Martens J. Implementation of an oral care protocol to promote early detection and management of stomatitis. *Clin J Oncol Nurs.* 2010;14(6):799–802.
10. Eilers J, Million R. Clinical update: prevention and management of oral mucositis in patients with cancer. *Semin Oncol Nurs.* 2011;27(4):1–16.

11. De Oliveira MA, Martins E, Martins F, et al. Clinical presentation and management of mTOR inhibitor-associated stomatitis. *Oral Oncol.* 2011;47(10):998–1003.
12. Arvitscher EB, Cooksley CD, Elting LS. Scope and epidemiology of cancer therapy-induced oral and gastrointestinal mucositis. *Semin Oncol Nurs.* 2004;20(1):3–10.
13. Nonzee NJ, Dandade NA, Patel U, et al. Evaluating the supportive care costs of severe radiochemotherapy-induced mucositis and pharyngitis: results from a Northwestern University costs of cancer program pilot study with head and neck and non-small cell lung cancer patients who received care at a county hospital, a Veterans Administration hospital, or a comprehensive cancer care center. *Cancer.* 2008;113(6):1446–1452.
14. Elting L, Cooksley C, Chambers M, et al. The burdens of cancer therapy: clinical and economic outcomes of chemotherapy-induced mucositis. *Cancer.* 2003;98(7):1531–1539.
15. Armstrong JA, McCaffrey R. The effects of mucositis on quality of life in patients with head and neck cancer. *Clin J Oncol Nurs.* 2006;10(1):53–56.
16. Duncan GG, Epstein JB, Tu D, et al. Quality of life, mucositis, and xerostomia from radiotherapy for head and neck cancers: a report from the NCIC CTG HN2 randomized trial of an antimicrobial lozenge to prevent mucositis. *Head Neck.* 2005;27(5):421–428.
17. Dodd MJ, Dibble S, Miaskowski C, et al. A comparison of the affective state and quality of life of chemotherapy patients who do and do not develop chemotherapy-induced oral mucositis. *J Pain Symptom Manage.* 2001;21(6):498–505.
18. Brown CG. Mucositis. In: *A Guide to Oncology Symptom Management.* Pittsburgh, PA: Oncology Nursing Society; 2010:333–346.
19. Sonis ST. Pathology of mucositis. *Semin Oncol Nurs.* 2004;20(1):11–15.
20. Sonis ST. Oral mucositis in cancer therapy. *J Support Oncol.* 2004; 2(suppl 3):3–8.
21. Rosen LS, Abdi E, Davis ID, et al. Palifermin reduces the incidence of oral mucositis in patients with metastatic colorectal cancer treated with fluorouracil-based chemotherapy. *J Clin Oncol.* 2006; 24(33):5194–200.
22. Lalla RV, Sonis ST, Peterson DE. Management of oral mucositis in patients who have cancer. *Dent Clin North Am.* 2008;52(1):61–77.
23. Treister, N and Sonis S. Mucositis: biology and management. *Curr Opin Otolaryngol Head Neck Surg.* 2007;15(2):123–129.
24. Sonis S. The quest for effective treatments of mucositis. *J Support Oncol.* 2011;9(5):170–171.
25. Brown CG. Oral mucositis. In: Yarbro CH, Wujcik D, Gobel BH, eds. *Cancer Nursing: Principles and Practice.* 7th ed. Sudbury, MA: Jones and Bartlett; 2011:807–817.
26. Denham JW, Hauer-Jensen M. The radiotherapeutic injury: a complex "wound." *Radiother Oncol.* 2002;53(2):129–145.
27. Sonis S. New trends in the management of oral mucositis. *J Natl Compr Cancer Netw.* 2005;3(suppl 1):S54–S56.
28. Sonis ST. New thoughts on the initiation of mucositis. *Oral Dis.* 2010;16(7):597–600.
29. McGuire DB. Mucosal tissue injury in cancer therapy: more than mucositis and mouthwash. *Cancer Pract.* 2002;10(4):179–191.
30. Barasch A, Peterson DE. Risk factors for ulcerative oral mucositis in cancer patients: unanswered questions. *Oral Oncol.* 2003;39(2):91–100.
31. Porock D, Nikoletti S, Cameron F. The relationship between factors that impair wound healing and the severity of acute radiation skin and mucosal toxicities in head and neck cancer. *Cancer Nurs.* 2004;27(1): 71–78.
32. Vokurka S, Bystricka E, Koza V, et al. Higher incidence of chemotherapy induced oral mucositis in females: a supplement of multivariate analysis to a randomized multicenter study. *Support Care Cancer.* 2006;14(9):974–976.
33. Beck SL. Mucositis. In: Yarbro CH, Frogge MH, Goodman M, eds. *Cancer Symptom Management.* 3rd ed. Sudbury, MA: Jones and Bartlett; 2004:276–291.
34. Raber-Durlacher JE, Weijl HI, Abu Saris M, et al. Oral mucositis in patients treated with chemotherapy for solid tumors: a retrospective analysis of 150 cases. *Support Care Cancer.* 2000;8(5)366–371.
35. Cheng KK, Lee V, Li CH, et al. Incidence and risk factors of oral mucositis in paediatric and adolescent patients undergoing chemotherapy. *Oral Oncol.* 2011;47(3):153–162.
36. Klotz U. Pharmacokinetics and drug metabolism in the elderly. *Drug Metab Rev.* 2009;41(2):67–76.
37. Epstein JB. Mucositis in the cancer patient and immunosuppressed host. *Infect Dis Clin North Am.* 2007;21(2):503–522.
38. Gibson RJ, Bowen JM, Keefe DM. Technological advances in mucositis research: new insights and new issues. *Cancer Treat Rev.* 2008;34(5):476–482.
39. Ayago Flores D, Ferriols Lisart R. Effectiveness of palifermin in the prevention of oral mucositis in patients with haematological cancers. *Farm Hosp (Engl Ed).* 2010;34(4):163–169.
40. Rodríguez-Caballero A, Torres-Lagares D, Robles-Garcia M, et al. Cancer treatment-induced oral mucositis: a critical review. *Int J Oral Maxillofac Surg.* 2012;41(2):225–238.
41. Shih A, Miaskowski C, Dodd MJ, et al. Mechanisms for radiation induced oral mucositis and the consequences. *Cancer Nurs.* 2003;26(3):223–229.
42. Peterson DE, Cariello A. Mucosal damage: a major risk factor for severe complications after cytotoxic therapy. *Semin Oncol.* 2004;31(suppl 8): 35–44.
43. Ganzer H, Touger-Decker R, Parrott JS, et al. Symptom burden in head and neck cancer: impact upon oral energy and protein intake. *Support Care Cancer.* July 24, 2012 [Epub ahead of print].
44. Beaven AW, Shea TC. The effect of palifermin on chemotherapyand radiation therapy-induced mucositis: a review of the current literature. *Support Cancer Ther.* 2007;4(4):188–197.
45. Eilers J, Berger AM, Petersen MC. Development, testing and application of the oral assessment guide. *Oncol Nurs Forum.* 1988;15(3):325–330.
46. World Health Organization. *WHO Handbook for Report Results from Cancer Treatment.* Geneva, Switzerland: WHO; 1979:15–22.
47. Kolbinson DA, Schubert MM, Flournoy N. Early oral changes following bone marrow transplantation. *Oral Surg.* 1988;66(1):130–138.
48. Schubert MM, Williams BB, Lloid ME, et al. Clinical assessment scale for the rating of oral mucosal changes associated with bone marrow transplantation: development of an oral mucositis index. *Cancer.* 1992;69(10):2469–2477.
49. McGuire DB, Peterson DE, Muller S, et al. The 20 item oral mucositis index: reliability and validity in bone marrow and stem cell transplant patients. *Cancer Invest.* 2002;20(7):893–903.
50. Sonis ST, Eilers JG, Epstein JB, et al. Validation of a new scoring system for the assessment of clinical trial research of oral mucositis induced by radiation or chemotherapy. Mucositis Study Group. *Cancer.* 1999;85(10):2103–2113.
51. Western Consortium for Nursing Research. Priorities for cancer nursing research: a Canadian replication. *Cancer Nurs.* 1987;10(6):319–326.
52. NCI. Common terminology criteria for adverse events (CTCAE) v.4.0. 2009. Available at: http://ctep.cancer.gov/protocolDevelopment /electronic_applications/ctc.htm#ctc_40. Accessed December 2, 2012.
53. Lalla RV, Peterson DE. Treatment of mucositis, including new medications. *Cancer J.* 2006;12(5):348–354.
54. Worthington HV, Clarkson JE, Eden OB. Interventions for treating oral mucositis for patients with cancer receiving treatment. *Cochrane Database Syst Rev.* 2004;2:CD001973.
55. Worthington HV, Clarkson JE, Eden OB. Interventions for preventing oral mucositis for patients with cancer receiving treatment. *Cochrane Database Syst Rev.* 2004;2:CD000978.pub2.
56. Worthington HV, Clarkson JE, Bryan G, et al. Interventions for preventing oral mucositis for patients with cancer receiving treatment. *Cochrane Database Syst Rev.* 2011;4:CD000978.pub5.

57. Clarkson JE, Worthington HV, Furness S, et al. Interventions for treating oral mucositis for patients with cancer receiving treatment. *Cochrane Database Syst Rev.* 2010;8:CD001973.pub4.
58. Oncology Nursing Society. Evidence based practice resources area. Available at: http://www.ons.org/Research/PEP/Mucositis. Accessed December 1, 2012.
59. Harris DJ, Eilers JG, Harriman A, Cashavelly BJ, Maxwell C. Putting evidence into practice: evidence based interventions for the management of oral mucositis. *Clin J Oncol Nurs.* 2008;12(1):141–142.
60. Multinational Association of Supportive Care in Cancer/International Society for Oral Oncology. Updated clinical guidelines for the prevention and treatment of oral mucositis. Available at: http://www.mascc.org/mucositis-guidelines. Accessed November 30, 2012.
61. Hensley ML, Hagerty KL, Kewalramani T, et al. American Society of Clinical Oncology 2008 clinical practice guideline update: use of chemotherapy and radiation therapy protectants. *J Clin Oncol.* 2009;27(1):127–145.
62. Spielberger R, Stiff P, Bensinger W, et al. Palifermin for oral mucositis after intensive therapy for hematologic cancers. *New Engl J Med.* 2004;351(25):2590–2598.

A Healthy Mouth

Patient Name: ____________________

This guide will help you learn how to keep your mouth clean, what to avoid, and when to see your dentist.

Symptom and Description

Your mouth has an important role to play in keeping you healthy. Cancer and cancer treatment can sometimes cause a sore mouth. There are things you can do now to keep your mouth healthy.

Prevention

How to keep your mouth clean and moist:

1. Brush your teeth within 30 minutes after eating and at bedtime.
    - Use a soft-bristle, narrow nylon toothbrush and a sodium bicarbonate (baking soda) toothpaste with fluoride added.
    - Dip the bristles in very warm water to make them softer.
    - Place the brush at a 45-degree angle to the junction of the gums and teeth.
    - Brush all of the outside surfaces of the teeth using short back-and-forth or circular strokes. Brush the inside surfaces using only the tip of the brush. Brush the chewing surfaces with a back-and-forth motion.
    - Gently brush your gums, tongue, and top of mouth.
2. If you wear dentures, remove and brush them as described above.
    - Soak the dentures for several minutes in an effervescent denture cleanser (the kind that bubbles) or flavored 1.5% hydrogen peroxide.
    - Rinse well.
    - Do not wear dentures that do not fit well. Contact your dentist to have them adjusted or relined.
    - Do not wear your dentures at night.
3. Floss your teeth at least once daily after brushing.
    - Cut a piece of dental floss 18 inches long.
    - Wrap the ends loosely around your middle fingers, leaving a few inches of floss exposed between those fingers.
    - Guide the floss with the thumbs of both hands to clean the upper teeth and with the index (first) fingers to clean the lower teeth.
    - Gently force the floss between the teeth—from your gum line to the top of each tooth.
    - Floss both sides of each tooth using a gentle up-and-down motion.

4. Rinse your mouth after brushing and flossing.
   - Use tap water, salt solution (half teaspoon of salt in 8 ounces of water), a mouthwash containing less than 6% alcohol, or flavored 1.5% hydrogen peroxide (Peroxamint) or 1 part hydrogen peroxide to 3 parts water.
   - Use your cheeks to swish the solution all around your mouth for 1 to 2 minutes.
5. Keep your lips moist.
   - Use cocoa butter, petroleum jelly, lipstick balm or lipstick, or a water-based mouth moisturizer.
   - Apply plenty of moisturizer to your lips and mouth frequently.

What to avoid that may be irritating:

- Lemon and glycerine swabs
- Mouthwashes that contain more than 6% alcohol
- Foods and drinks that are hot, spicy, or acidic
- Smoking or chewing tobacco
- Excessive alcohol

When to see the dentist:

- Visit your dentist at least every year to have a check-up and teeth cleaning.
- Make an appointment to see your dentist before you start cancer treatment or for any tooth pain.

Management

Please see the Self-Care Guide to Mucositis: A Sore Mouth.

Follow-up

Report the following to your doctor or nurse:

- Redness
- Soreness or pain
- Cracks, ulcers, blisters, or white patches
- Temperature greater than 101.3°F

Phone Numbers

Nurse: ______________________________ Phone: ____________

Physician: ______________________________ Phone: ____________

Other: ______________________________ Phone: ____________

Source: Wujcik D. Mucositis. In: Yarbro CH, Wujcik D, Gobel BH, eds. *Cancer Symptom Management.* 4th ed. Burlington, MA: Jones & Bartlett Learning; 2014.

Mucositis: A Sore Mouth

Patient Name: ______________________________

This guide will help you manage your sore mouth.

Symptom and Description

Your mouth has an important role to play in keeping you healthy. Cancer and cancer treatment can sometimes cause mucositis, a sore mouth. There are things you can do to help your mouth heal and to make it feel better.

Prevention

Please see the Self-Care Guide: A Healthy Mouth, to learn more about how you can keep your mouth healthy.

Management

1. Examine your mouth at least once daily and report changes.
    - Use a flashlight and look in your mouth while standing in front of a mirror.
    - Look for any ulcers, pimples, sores, red areas, or patches.
    - Report these changes and any mouth pain to your doctor or nurse.
2. Keep your mouth clean and moist.
    - Clean your teeth even though your mouth is sore. If it hurts to use a soft brush, use an oral swab—that is, a cleaning stick with a soft sponge tip.
    - Hold the swab with the grooves at a 90-degree angle to the gum line so the sponge can reach in between the teeth.
    - Gently massage your gums, tongue, and top of your mouth.
    - Do not floss when your platelet count is low or if it causes pain or bleeding.
    - Keep your dentures in only during meals.
    - Rinse your mouth with a salt solution (half teaspoon of salt in 8 ounces of water) or a 1.5% hydrogen peroxide solution (1 part hydrogen peroxide to 3 parts water, or flavored 1.5% hydrogen peroxide [Peroxamint]) every 2 hours for 1 to 2 minutes. If your mouth is very sore, rinse every hour. The peroxide will foam as it cleans your mouth. This should be followed by rinsing with water.
    - Keep your lips and the inside of your mouth coated with a water-based mouth moisturizer.
    - If your mouth is very dry, drink water and other fluids frequently throughout the day. Chew sugarless gum or suck on sugarless hard candy to moisten your mouth. Use a cool mist humidifier at night while sleeping. Artificial saliva is also available; apply it frequently.
3. Avoid irritating foods, alcohol, and tobacco.
    - Do not chew tobacco or smoke cigarettes, cigars, or pipes.
    - Do not drink alcoholic beverages (beer, wine, or liquor).

4. Work with your doctor and nurse to control pain, bleeding, and infection.
   - Ask your doctor to prescribe a medication for your sore mouth.
   - Before meals and as needed for comfort, apply an anesthetic (a numbing agent), such as benzocaine (Xylocaine), to sore areas of your mouth, using an oral swab or cotton-tipped applicator. Benzocaine can also be swished around the entire mouth. This will numb your mouth and make eating easier. However, be careful that foods are not too hot, because your sense of feeling may be changed so that you could burn yourself without realizing it.
   - Take a pain medicine 1.5 to 2 hours before meals. If your mouth is constantly hurting, take the medicine at regular times around the clock (for example, every 4 hours). Liquid acetaminophen can be swished around in the mouth and then swallowed. Avoid the use of aspirin products.
   - If pain is not relieved, ask your doctor about taking something stronger. Acetaminophen (Tylenol) with or without codeine is usually helpful. If pain is severe, morphine may be needed until healing occurs.
   - If bleeding occurs, apply pressure to the site of bleeding using a piece of clean gauze dipped in ice water or a wet tea bag that has been partially frozen (the tannin in the tea will help stop the bleeding). Rinsing your mouth with ice water may also be helpful.
   - If you develop an infection in your mouth, antibiotics may be needed. Some are applied directly to the mouth; others are swallowed. Follow your doctor's instructions.
5. Eat well.
   - Eat a well-balanced diet. Be sure to include foods that are high in protein (dairy products, poultry, meats, and fish).
   - Take a vitamin/mineral supplement daily.
   - If your mouth is sore, certain foods may burn and eating may become difficult. Eat frequently and in small amounts.
   - Drink at least 3 quarts (liters) of fluid a day unless you are on a fluid restriction.
   - Avoid any food that is hot, rough, or coarse; highly spiced or acidic; or any other food that bothers you.

Follow-up

Report the following to your doctor or nurse:

- Redness or extreme dryness
- Soreness or pain
- Cracks, ulcers, blisters, or white patches
- Temperature greater than 100°F
- Bleeding from your mouth
- Difficulty swallowing

Phone Numbers

Nurse: ______________________________ Phone: ______________

Physician: ___________________________ Phone: ______________

Other: ______________________________ Phone: ______________

Source: Wujcik D. Mucositis. In: Yarbro CH, Wujcik D, Gobel BH, eds. *Cancer Symptom Management.* 4th ed. Burlington, MA: Jones & Bartlett Learning; 2014.

Chapter 20

Xerostomia

Kerri A. Dalton, RN, MSN, OCN®
Tracy K. Gosselin, RN, PhD, AOCN®

THE PROBLEM

Saliva plays an important role in the maintenance of the oral cavity through lubrication, antimicrobial breakdown, acid neutralization, and cleansing of the oral cavity. Saliva also facilitates taste perceptions, chewing, swallowing, speaking, and lubrication of the upper and lower esophageal mucosa.[1,2] Xerostomia, commonly referred to as "dry mouth," is a subjective sensation of abnormal oral dryness. The sensation of oral dryness may be related to salivary gland hypofunction where there is a reduction in saliva production or a change in saliva composition, but may also be present without salivary gland injury.[3]

Xerostomia can negatively impact quality of life. In patients receiving conventional radiotherapy, a systematic review found that xerostomia negatively affects overall quality of life by interfering with speech, sleep, eating, and swallowing; creates a barrier for social contact with eating, possibly leading to decreased oral intake requiring nutritional supplements;[1,4] and increases the risk of dental problems. Quality of life studies show that the impact on quality of life is not related solely to salivary flow rates, but also reflects the subjective sensation and experience of xerostomia.[1,5]

Xerostomia often causes difficulty when eating dry or thick foods. Meals need to be interrupted by frequent sips of fluids to aid in chewing and swallowing. Patients may avoid eating in the presence of others because of embarrassment. Saliva is important for the retention, stability, and comfort of dentures, and denture instability results in difficulty with chewing. Saliva plays a role in taste perception, and xerostomia impacts the ability to taste foods; this relationship is more pronounced in individuals with radiation exposure to the taste receptors.[4]

Acute or lifelong modifications may be necessary depending on the severity of restrictions or modifications needed to perform oral activities of daily living, such as chewing or swallowing. As a result, patients with xerostomia may become depressed or emotionally distressed due to their diminished functional capacity and suffer a subsequent negative impact on overall quality of life.[3]

INCIDENCE

Most people with cancer will experience some degree of temporary or permanent xerostomia during their treatment trajectory. Overall prevalence of xerostomia for patients undergoing chemotherapy may reach as high as 50%.[1] The most profound, and almost universally irreversible, cause of xerostomia in patients with cancer is surgical excision or radiation therapy to the salivary glands, which produces a prevalence of xerostomia as much as 90%.[1] In the palliative care setting, xerostomia has been reported as a very distressing symptom in as many as 82% of patients with advanced cancer.[6,7]

ETIOLOGY

The etiologies of xerostomia are varied and complex (Table 20-1). In the cancer population, *radiation therapy* is the most common cause of irreversible damage to the

TABLE 20-1

Etiology of Xerostomia
Cancer Treatment Related
• Surgical removal of salivary glands
• Chemotherapy and biotherapy
• Radiation therapy to the head and neck region
• Iodine-131
• Total-body irradiation
Immune Disorders
• HIV/AIDS
• Sjögren's syndrome
• Graft-versus-host disease
Other disease states and conditions
• Diabetes
• End of life
• Thyroid disease
• Nerve damage
• Late stage liver disease
• Poor fluid intake, i.e., dehydration
Pharmacotherapy
• Anxiolytics
• Antibiotics
• Anticholinergics
• Antidepressants
• Antihistamines
• Antihypertensives
• Diuretics
• Opiates
• Steroids
• Proton pump inhibitors

Source: Data from Jensen et al[1]; Davies et al[6]; Davies et al[7].

major and minor salivary glands. The severity of salivary gland hypofunction is dependent on the cumulative radiation dose and the amount of salivary tissue irradiated.[1,8] For example, therapeutic radiation to treat head and neck cancers will result in some degree of permanent xerostomia. Total-body irradiation (TBI) in the transplant population as well as use of iodine-131 and surgical removal of the salivary gland will result in temporary xerostomia.[1,9]

Certain *chemotherapy* agents have been reported to cause transient xerostomia. Such agents include 5-Fluorouracil (5-FU), cisplatin, bleomycin, methotrexate, cytarabine, epirubicin, doxorubicin, cyclophosphamide, and vinblastine.[1,2] Although it has long been thought that combined chemotherapy, biotherapy, and radiation would enhance the risk for xerostomia, the data are unclear and a conclusion cannot be drawn as to whether there is an additive risk when combining therapies.[1]

Medications that inhibit cholinergic signaling pathways in salivary tissues will result in decreased salivary output.[3] Medications with anticholinergic effects are commonly used in oncology care. Although medication-induced xerostomia is reversible, the reason for the medication use is often related to chronic conditions. Drug classes that can result in xerostomia include opioids, antianxiety agents, antidepressants, steroids, antibiotics, antihypertensives, proton pump inhibitors, diuretics, and antihistamines.[3] Complaints of dry mouth in the geriatric population are often related to medications. Salivary flow tends to decrease as the number of daily medications taken increases, and elders (persons older than age 65 years) are more likely to suffer from conditions that require concomitant use of drugs that cause xerostomia.[10]

Comorbid conditions may contribute to xerostomia, such as Sjögren's syndrome, hepatitis C, poorly controlled diabetes, and renal failure treated with dialysis. Sjögren's syndrome can cause severe hypofunction of the salivary glands as well as xeroophthalmia.[3] Some individuals infected with HIV/AIDS may experience salivary gland enlargement and xerostomia.[3] Dehydration secondary to diabetes, nausea, vomiting, and diarrhea will exacerbate xerostomia.

Graft-versus-host disease may result in xerostomia when the donor lymphocytes proliferate and infiltrate the recipient tissues, including salivary glands, resulting in a Sjögren's syndrome pattern.[11] *Smoking tobacco* can cause xerostomia; although nicotine initially stimulates salivary flow, excess smoking can reduce salivary secretions and it is recommended to avoid this irritant.[3] *Alcohol*, either ingested or as an oral rinse (as in mouth rinses), contributes to dryness of oral tissues and should be avoided.

PATHOPHYSIOLOGY

SALIVARY GLANDS

The major salivary glands consist of three well-defined entities—the parotid, submandibular, sublingual glands—plus many minor salivary glands (Figure 20-1).[8] The minor salivary glands are variable from person to person and are distributed throughout the oral cavity and pharynx. A typical salivary gland is a composite of numerous functional units: secretory end pieces known as acini, collecting ducts, and a framework of myoepithelial cells and connective tissue. Two types of acinar cells exist: mucous and serous. Secretions from each acini travel through a series of interconnected ducts and end in the duct emptying in to the oral cavity.[8,12]

The normal flow rate of saliva is approximately 1 to 1.5 liters per day during times of rest and stimulation.[4] The major glands produce nearly 90% of saliva. The parotid glands produce 60% to 65% of the total salivary volume, the submandibular glands 20% to 30%, and the sublingual glands 2% to 5%.[1,4] Secretion from the parotids is purely serous, watery, and albuminous. In contrast, the submandibular and sublingual salivary gland fluid is composed of serous and mucous acini that produce thick, sticky

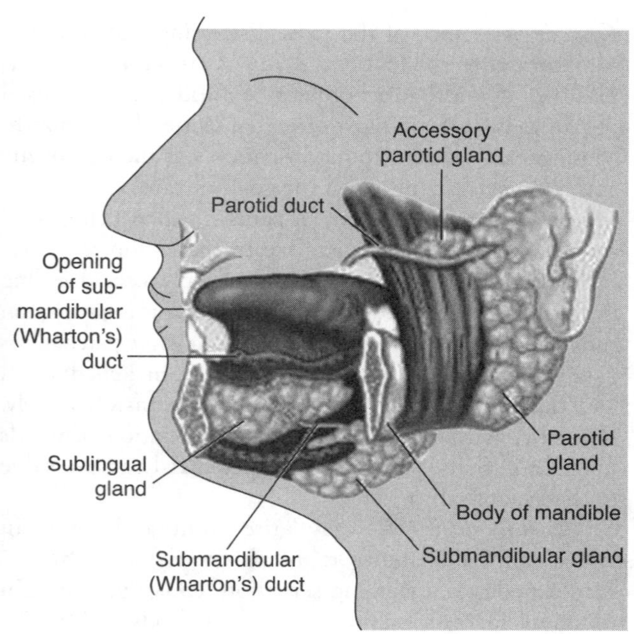

FIGURE 20-1

Salivary gland anatomy.

secretions.[8,12] The submandibular glands are also responsible for producing saliva in a resting or unstimulated state. The secretory function of the salivary glands is stimulated by taste, smell, chewing, and psychological factors, as well as by stimulation from other organs such as the esophagus and stomach.

SALIVA

The general term *saliva* refers to the fluid that surrounds all oral tissues. Saliva is composed primarily of water, but also contains antimicrobial factors, electrolytes, and enzymes that assist in the promotion of oral health and minimization of the risk of tooth decay. Saliva in normal quantity and composition exerts antimicrobial, digestive, antacid, lubricating, and homeostatic properties. The flow of saliva aids in the function of speaking by providing lubrication to the oral cavity, by assisting with the ingestion and mastication of food (chewing, food breakdown, tasting, swallowing), and by cleansing the oral cavity of food debris and residue. Long-term diminished salivary flow rate is known to be a significant risk factor for the development of dental caries due to changes in the saliva composition that impact pH and buffering capacity.[13] The maintenance of esophageal health is, to a large degree, dependent on saliva for the neutralizing effect of salivary bicarbonate on the acid that that is produced in the stomach.

RADIATION THERAPY: IMPACT ON SALIVARY GLAND FUNCTION

Radiation-induced salivary gland damage is a complex process that is not fully understood. The parotid glands are radiosensitive organs. However, parotid cells have a low mitotic rate, which would suggest that the parotid should not be radiosensitive.[4] Studies over the past several decades have led to many theories, none of which fully explains this phenomenon. The relatively low mitotic activity of the salivary glands coupled with the rapid acute response suggests something other than reproductive death as a possible explanation.[4]

The major treatment-related factors contributing to salivary gland dysfunction following irradiation are the volume of the salivary glands included in the radiation fields and the total dose of radiation administered.[1,7] Salivary cells are thought to be affected by two main mechanisms. First, cellular function is affected by selective membrane damage that inhibits water-excreting signaling pathways. Second, classical cell killing of progenitor and stem cells occurs, inhibiting cell renewal and damaging the cellular environment.[8,13] Xerostomia reflects progressive radiation-induced acinar cell inflammation, fibrosis, and degeneration that result in reduced quantity and quality of saliva.[12]

SYMPTOM ASSESSMENT

RISK FACTORS

Risk factors for xerostomia include the patient's current medication regimen; comorbid diseases, conditions, or syndromes; and cancer treatments that have been shown to contribute to oral dryness.[14] There are hundreds of medications that have the potential to contribute to a dry mouth.[15,16] Many of these medications are commonly used, including members of the antihypertensive, antidepressant, and antihistamine drug classes. Additionally, the use of chemotherapy, radiation therapy, or surgery to the head and neck region may place a patient at risk for this symptom.

SELF-ASSESSMENT

Teaching the patient and caregiver how to perform a self-assessment of the oral cavity is a key opportunity to promote oral health awareness. This assessment may be done daily while the patient is undergoing active treatment for cancer. Patients will want to use a mirror as well as a light source to examine the oral cavity. A small flashlight can also be used by the caregiver to provide light for the exam. When inspecting the oral cavity area, attention should be paid to the lips, gums, and teeth as well as the tongue, cheeks, and hard and soft palates. Patients and caregivers may choose to wear gloves, as the tongue and cheeks may need to be gently manipulated so all areas can be visualized.

The Oral Assessment Guide (OAG) has demonstrated reliability and validity and can be used by the patient or caregiver to document the status of the oral cavity as well as serve as a prompt for which areas to inspect.[17,18] The OAG has eight categories and uses a scale of 1–3 to rate severity of findings, with 1 being normal findings and 3 being severe findings. The eight assessment categories include the patient's gingiva, lips, mucous membranes, saliva, swallowing, teeth or dentures, tongue, and voice.

Other self-assessment tools that can be used to assess and measure the impact of xerostomia include the Xerostomia Inventory,[19] the Xerostomia Questionnaire,[20] and the University of Washington Quality of Life instrument.[21] These tools may be used alone or in conjunction with other symptom inventories as well as quality of life (global or disease-specific) instruments to understand all dimensions of the symptom experience and its impact on health and function. The Xerostomia Inventory is an 11-item instrument whose values are summed to give a total score and that has demonstrated validity.[19] The Xerostomia Questionnaire is an 8-item patient-reported instrument that was developed with patients who had a diagnosis of head and neck cancer.[20] The University of Washington Quality of Life instrument ranges from 10 to 12 items depending upon the version.[21] Items on this instrument were developed to address the needs of head and neck cancer patients.

A variety of functional and physical alterations of the mouth may arise due to the dryness that the patient experiences. Patients may report the following findings as well as other issues based upon their assessment:

- *Chelitis* is an inflammation of the lips that may appear as fissures and ulceration. Patients may also report dry, chapped lips and swelling.
- *Dental manifestations* can include a variety of changes in regard to acute and late effects. Patients may report changes related to dentition and periodontal disease resulting from the loss of salivary dental protection.[2,4]
- *Glossodynia* is the burning or tingling of the mouth and tongue. The tongue may appear to be depapillated and fissured, and the dorsal epithelium is atrophic or eroded and erythematous. Itching of the tongue can accompany glossodynia. Symptoms can be triggered by spicy or acidic foods as well as by toothpastes that contain sodium lauryl sulfate (SLS), which can cause irritation.[22,23] Biotene and BioXtra are SLS-free products that may be substituted for products that contain sodium lauryl sulfate.
- *Halitosis* can arise from food remnants, concurrent drug therapy, poor dentition, or the patient's inability to perform self-care due to mucositis and pain.
- *Oral dryness* is one of the most distressing and common symptoms affecting patients dying of cancer. Drug therapies (i.e., opioids, anticholinergics, antidepressants) used in palliative care are most often the cause of dry mouth. Management of xerostomia in patients at the end of life can often be difficult given the goals of care.
- *Oral infections* are common in patients experiencing xerostomia and receiving cancer treatment. Symptoms may include burning pain, taste changes, and a coated feeling in the mouth and back of throat. Candidiasis is a common fungal infection and may appear as small white patches.[13]
- *Speech difficulties* may arise due to the thickened saliva and the patient's inability to clear secretions effectively. Difficulty with conversations and enunciation of words may occur. Some patients may experience hoarseness due to the lack of saliva.
- *Swallowing difficulties* may arise from a decrease in saliva and the inability to break down food. Patients may experience a gagging sensation, choking, and pain (odynophagia) or inability to swallow foods and liquids of varying consistencies.
- *Taste alterations (dysgeusia)* including a loss of taste during radiation therapy, are expected with cancer treatment, given the role of saliva as a mediator of taste. Taste acuity is partially restored within 60 days, and is almost completely restored by 2 to 3 months post radiation. Some patients, however, are left with a degree of residual long-term or permanent hypogeusia.[24]

OBJECTIVE ASSESSMENT

It is critical for the patient to have a thorough examination of the oral cavity before, during, and after cancer treatment. This will assist the patient and provider with determining appropriate interventions to manage both the acute and late effects of treatment. This examination may be deferred or not performed as frequently in the patient who is receiving end-of-life care based on the goals of care.

History

It is important to obtain an accurate history from the patient and caregiver to understand what is directly and indirectly affecting the current symptomatology as well as what alleviates and aggravates the problem of xerostomia. Knowing a patient's past medical and surgical history as related to dry mouth is important, as is knowledge of whether the patient has received prior radiation therapy (external beam or iodine-131). An accurate list of current medications (both prescription and over-the-counter) should be reviewed as well. Asking the patient if he or she has any areas of discomfort, has loose or missing teeth, or wears dentures is important. Ascertaining when the last visit to a dentist occurred is important so care coordination can take place. Understanding the patient's current oral care habits is critical in planning interventions to promote a healthy oral cavity.

Physical assessment

The physical assessment for xerostomia includes a close inspection of the oral cavity, which includes the lips, tongue, gums, cheeks, teeth, and hard and soft palate. Visual inspection with a tongue blade and light source should be completed before any type of oral exam is undertaken. The areas should be assessed for dryness, inflammation, fissures, and any odor or plaques that might be visible. If the patient wears dentures, they should be removed for the visual inspection.

The oral mucosa may appear dry on inspection. During radiation therapy to the head and neck area, oral secretions will be copious, thick, and sticky. In addition, patients will have moderate to severe mucositis. Given the change in oral pH and microflora secondary to xerostomia, infection is common. *Candida albicans* infection may present as erythematous patches on the hard or soft palate and dorsal surface of the tongue (erythematous candidiasis), and/or with visible, removable white plaques (pseudomembranous candidiasis), which is usually diagnosed based on clinical exam. Angular chelitis—that is, cracking or fissuring of the commissures of the mouth—may be due to infection with *Candida albicans* or *Staphylococcus aureus*.[25,26]

Acute xerostomia presents symptomatically as dry mouth and some degree of functional deficit due to a decrease in saliva (mastication, speech, swallowing). Symptoms are usually temporary and can be relieved by decreasing or eliminating the causative agent(s). Acute xerostomia secondary to radiation for head and neck cancer will initially present with a dry mouth and rapidly progress to overflowing, thick, and seemingly unmanageable oral secretions. If the agent (e.g., medication, radiation therapy) contributing to or causing the xerostomia is not stopped, the decrease in saliva will persist, which leads to chronic/late xerostomia.[3]

Due to the chronic nature of xerostomia, ongoing assessment is critical both during and post treatment. Patients will be at risk for oral infections, atrophy of the oral epithelium, and ulceration. Dental caries may also arise due to changes in the composition of the saliva. The enamel becomes desiccated and weak, leading to progressive tooth wear and incisal chipping. Care coordination among oncology and dental professionals is critical to ensure optimal care. Patients should continue to be followed closely by their dentist and by the oncology team at least twice a year.[7]

Diagnostic evaluation

A diagnostic evaluation is often not warranted if an accurate history and physical assessment are completed. Salivary flow measurement (sialometry) can be conducted to determine the level of salivary function before and after radiotherapy. Stimulated and unstimulated flow rates have been quantified using different measurement techniques.[27] Measurement should be conducted using standard procedures. In patients undergoing radiation therapy, this should be done before radiation therapy is initiated and at defined intervals by the treatment team. Saliva is typically first collected in an unstimulated (resting) state, and then collected in a stimulated state. The latter collection is performed using gum, candy, or thin sheets of paraffin wax. Once the saliva is collected, it is weighed and a salivary flow rate is determined. The salivary flow rate is calculated based on the following equation[27]:

$$\text{Salivary flow rate} = \frac{\text{post-weight measure} - \text{pre-weight measure}}{\text{Collection period (time)}} = \_\_\_\_\_\_ \text{ g/min}$$

Sialography and scintigraphy (imaging studies) as well as biopsy are diagnostic methods that may also be used, but are not commonly employed for diagnosis of xerostomia in patients receiving radiation therapy for head and neck cancer. Sialography requires the patient to undergo the placement of a small catheter into the salivary duct. Contrast is then injected into the duct and appears on the x-ray. Scintigraphy is a nuclear medicine test whereby the patient receives a contrast injection and uptake is then monitored in the salivary glands.

DEGREES OF TOXICITY

The tools most commonly used in practice to objectively measure xerostomia are the Radiation Therapy Oncology Group (RTOG) Morbidity Scoring Criteria for the Salivary Gland (Table 20-2)[28,29] and the National Cancer Institute Cancer Therapy Evaluation Program, Common Terminology Criteria for Adverse Events (CTCAE) (Table 20-3).[30] The RTOG criteria cover both acute and late morbidity, whereas the CTCAE has only one criterion for morbidity, but offers subjective measurement in the form of saliva measurement.

SYMPTOM MANAGEMENT STRATEGIES

A variety of preventive approaches exist to support the patient with xerostomia. By having an accurate assessment and understanding of the severity (grade) and interventions, the nurse can serve as an advocate for care and treatment as well as

TABLE 20-2

Radiation Therapy Oncology Group - Morbidity Scoring Criteria: Salivary Gland					
	0	1	2	3	4
Acute Morbidity	No change over baseline	Mild mouth dryness/ slightly thickened saliva/may have slightly altered taste such as metallic taste/these changes not reflected in alteration in baseline feeding behavior, such as increased use of liquids with meals	Moderate to complete dryness/ thick, sticky saliva/ markedly altered taste	(Not used)	Acute salivary gland necrosis
Late Morbidity	None	Slight dryness of mouth/good response on stimulation	Moderate dryness of mouth/ poor response on stimulation	Complete dryness of mouth/no response on stimulation	Fibrosis

Source: Data from Radiation Therapy Oncology Group[28,29].

TABLE 20-3

National Cancer Institute Common Terminology Criteria for Adverse Events (CTCAE): Dry Mouth					
	1	2	3	4	5
Dry mouth	Symptomatic (e.g., dry or thick saliva) without significant dietary alteration; unstimulated saliva flow >0.2 ml/min	Moderate symptoms; oral intake alterations (e.g., copious water, other lubricants, diet limited to purees and/ or soft, moist foods); unstimulated saliva 0.1 to 0.2 ml/min	Inability to adequately aliment orally; tube feeding or TPN indicated; unstimulated saliva <0.1 ml/min	-	-

Source: Data from National Cancer Institute Common Terminology Criteria for Adverse Events (CTCAE)[30].

educate the patient on self-care measures. Table 20-4 reviews prevention and management strategies for xerostomia.[1,4,31–34]

THERAPEUTIC APPROACHES

Amifostine

Amifostine is a free radical scavenger and radioprotectant. In the pivotal study for FDA approval of amifostine, Brizel and colleagues demonstrated a decrease in the rate of both acute xerostomia grade 2 or higher, from 78% to 51% ($p < .0001$), and chronic xerostomia grade 2 or higher, from 57% to 34% ($p = .002$).[35] Other studies have also demonstrated a significant benefit with amifostine in decreasing acute and late xerostomia during radiotherapy with or without chemotherapy.[36,37]

The recommended intravenous (IV) dose of amifostine for patients receiving radiotherapy to the head and neck is 200 mg/m^2. Initial data indicated that amifostine had a short half-life; consequently, it is given IV 20–30 minutes prior to each daily radiation treatment. Further pharmacokinetic study of amifostine administered subcutaneously (SQ) demonstrated that significant concentrations of the drug reach the circulation via the SQ route. A recent phase III study with SQ amifostine demonstrated similar acute xerostomia results when compared with the IV amifostine results of the Brizel study.[36] Toxicities associated with amifostine include nausea, vomiting, hypotension, and allergic reaction. Generalized cutaneous reactions are more common when the drug is administered via the SQ route.[36] The SQ administration of amifostine is not FDA approved for use in the United States.

Patients receiving amifostine need to maintain adequate hydration during treatment. They are instructed to drink at least 2 quarts of fluid per day. Fluids can be given per gastrostomy tube or IV if the patient is unable to take oral fluids.

TABLE 20-4

Prevention and Symptom Management Strategies for Xerostomia

Prevention and Symptom Management	HCP* or SC*	Intervention	Level of Evidence
Amifostine	HCP and SC	A radioprotectant medication that is administered daily, prior to the treatment. The medicine is given either intravenously or subcutaneously during the course of radiation therapy.	Level II, grade C
Gustatory and masticatory stimulation	SC	Oral aids such as chewing gum and hard candies that provide a transient impact. These products should be sugar free.	Level III, grade D
Intensity modulated radiation therapy (IMRT)	HCP	An approach to radiation therapy whereby the dose within the field can be higher or lower (intensity) to certain areas. This allows for a decreased dose (sparing) to the salivary glands.	Level II, grade A
Muscarinic agonist stimulation	HCP and SC	An oral medication that promotes stimulation of the cholinergic receptors. Taken orally while the patient is undergoing therapy.	Level II, grade C
Oral care	HCP and SC	Includes rinsing, brushing, and flossing of the oral cavity.	Level III, grade C
Oral lubricants and saliva substitutes	SC	Offer temporary, short-term relief of xerostomia.	Level II, grade B
Salivary gland transfer	HCP	A surgical approach whereby the submandibular gland is transferred out of the radiation field. This is done in patients who received postoperative radiation.	Level IV, grade B
Symptom Management	**HCP or SC**	**Intervention**	**Level of Evidence**
Acupuncture	HCP	An approach using small needles to stimulate residual salivary gland function to secrete saliva.	Level II, grade C
Hyperbaric oxygen treatment	HCP	Typically used for the treatment of osteoradionecrosis. Not used for primary treatment of xerostomia.	Level IV, grade D

**Abbreviations*: HCP: healthcare provider; SC: self-care.

Source: Data from Jensen et al[1]; Dirix et al[4]; Vissink et al[31].

Levels of Evidence – Grading Key

Level	Definition
I	Meta-analysis of multiple well designed studies. Randomized controlled trials with high power.
II	One well designed randomized controlled trial. Randomized controlled trials with low power.
III	Well designed, quasi experimental studies. Nonrandomized, cohort, or pre/post design.
IV	Well designed, non-experimental studies. Correlational or comparative studies.
V	Case reports.
VI	Descriptive or qualitative study.
VII	Expert opinion.

Source: Data from Hadorn et al[32]; Melnyk et al[33].

(continued)

TABLE 20-4

Prevention and Symptom Management Strategies for Xerostomia (*Continued*)

Grades of Evidence – Grading Key

Grade	Definition
A	The United States Preventative Services Task Force (USPSTF) recommends the service. There is high certainty that the net benefit is substantial.
B	The USPSTF recommends the service. There is high certainty that the net benefit is moderate or there is moderate certainty that the net benefit is moderate to substantial.
C	Clinicians may provide the service to selected patients depending on individual circumstances. However, for most individuals without signs or symptoms there is likely to be only a small benefit from this service.
D	The USPSTF recommends against this service. There is moderate or high certainty that the service has no benefit of that the harms outweigh the benefits.

Source: Data from U.S. Preventative Services Task Force[34].

Premedication with an oral antiemetic is given 1–2 hours prior to amifostine therapy, and an antihistamine may be given as well if amifostine is delivered subcutaneously.[38] Subcutaneous injections are rotated to the stomach, upper leg, and upper arm. Hypotension is monitored and blood pressure is taken prior to the injection as well as 15 minutes after the injection is administered.[36]

Gustatory and mastication stimulation

Gustative substances include sugar-free gum and candy. These products provide temporary relief from xerostomia. Acidic sugar-free drinks can assist in stimulating saliva flow, but may cause demineralization and dental caries.[7,31] Mastication will stimulate salivary flow if there is some degree of functional salivary tissue. Eating foods that require vigorous chewing (e.g., carrots and celery) several times a day can be helpful.[39]

Intensity-modulated radiation therapy

Intensity-modulated radiation therapy (IMRT) allows for sparing of some or all of the salivary glands based upon dose distribution of radiation within the treatment field. With IMRT, each individual field has multiple beams with different levels of intensity within it, allowing for dose escalation or avoidance of critical anatomical structures. For patients receiving radiation therapy to the head and neck area, IMRT allows the physician to minimize or spare the glands, treating one or both of the parotid glands depending upon the location the tumor. This is done during treatment planning in which the optimal beam array is selected based upon dose distribution. In managing patient outcomes related to xerostomia, IMRT is considered to have advantages over conventional external-beam treatment.[40] Studies have found improvement in salivary recovery, decreased incidence of xerostomia, and improvement in quality of life related to IMRT in the management of head and neck cancer.[41–43]

Muscarinic agonist stimulation

Pilocarpine is a parasympathomimetic drug that acts as a muscarinic-cholinergic agonist. Pilocarpine is known to stimulate secretions from the salivary glands as well as lacrimal, gastric, intestinal, respiratory, and pancreatic secretions. It has limited efficacy in the prevention setting, but further study is needed to see if efficacy can be improved with IMRT and other salivary gland-sparing options.[3,44]

The usual dose of pilocarpine is 5–10 mg by mouth 3 times per day, starting on day 1 of radiation therapy. The most common side effect is excessive sweating, which is typically related to the dose. Other side effects include nausea, rhinitis, and increased lacrimation.[44]

In the post-treatment setting, the use of pilocarpine has been well documented. In two randomized, double-blind, placebo-controlled studies of pilocarpine as a treatment for xerostomia, researchers found that this agent increased salivary production and provided clinically significant benefits for the treatment of post-radiation–induced xerostomia. The pilocarpine dose that was most well tolerated was 5 mg.[43,44] The primary toxicity in both studies was sweating, which occurred in 21% and 27% of patients, respectively, and was described as mild to moderate.[43,45]

Oral care

Optimal oral care is critical to patients who may experience salivary gland hypofunction and xerostomia. Although research exists on oral care regimens, the best product for a particular patient is often difficult to determine.[4] The following principles are used to guide optimal patient self-care.

Patients should perform oral care at a minimum of 4 times per day and more frequently as needed (e.g., after meals, after consumption of sugary foods and drinks, before going to bed).[24,39] A soft-headed toothbrush should be used with a fluoride toothpaste. If there is pain with brushing, a soft-headed oral sponge can be substituted. Flossing should be performed daily unless the patient experiences pain, bleeding, or mucositis. A dentist may prescribe fluoride gel trays for the patient; these devices are commonly used at bedtime to minimize the risk of dental caries due to the composition changes in the saliva.[24]

Oral rinses are commonly recommended to patients and include a mixture of salt and baking soda.[24] One popular regimen is ½ teaspoon of salt and ½ teaspoon of baking soda in 1 cup of warm water. This solution should be mixed fresh each day and used 4 to 6 times per day to cleanse and buffer the oral mucosa.[24] Oral rinses that include alcohol should be avoided, as they have the potential to cause burning and pain as well as dryness. For patients who are also experiencing mucositis, a gentle lavage of the oral cavity will help clear secretions and loosen debris. A water pick device is helpful, but the patient may not tolerate the water pressure secondary to mucositis. A low-cost alternative is an enema bag and tubing that delivers water at lower pressure.

Biotene® and Oral Balance® products are commonly used for oral care in patients who are experiencing dry mouth. They include chewing gum, toothpaste, an oral rinse, and mouthwashes. These products contain components that are naturally occurring in saliva and have demonstrated a positive improvement in patients who have used them.[46–48] Patients who are experiencing mucositis concomitantly with xerostomia should also perform meticulous oral care.

Continued reinforcement of brushing, flossing, and rinsing is critical, as is the use of fluoride trays. Likewise, ongoing care and treatment by a dentist is critical. Patients should be counseled to avoid alcohol, caffeine, and tobacco, as these substances will further dry oral mucosa. If the patient also has mucositis, alcohol and tobacco will further irritate these areas.

Salivary gland transfer

Salivary gland transfer is the surgical transplantation of the submandibular gland outside of the radiation field prior to the initiation of radiation therapy. This surgical technique has shown promise in small studies.[49–51] In a prospective study of 70 patients, of whom 36 had their salivary gland transferred and shielded, the patients who received the treatment were found to have better saliva production functions, heavier mean weight of saliva, and lower grade of xerostomia.[51] This advance in care is important, as the submandibular gland is responsible for approximately 65% of unstimulated saliva, which has the potential to improve speech and symptoms of dryness.[8]

Acupuncture

Acupuncture is one of several types of alternative medicine options that patients may use in managing symptoms of disease and treatment. An ancient Chinese therapy, historically used for the treatment of pain and postoperative nausea, acupuncture is gaining ground in the area of xerostomia symptom management. Treatment is accomplished through the insertion of small needles into specified zones to unblock energy.

In a randomized trial of patients who were undergoing radiation therapy for nasopharyngeal cancer, researchers found that those who received acupuncture had greater improvement in salivary flow rate and quality of life.[52] In another small study of 12 patients with radiation-induced xerostomia, those who received real acupuncture versus a sham method were found to have increased unstimulated salivary flow rates and improved scores for dry mouth.[53] In a systematic review, limited evidence and methodological limitations were noted; thus patients who are seeking this treatment should be referred to credible practitioners of acupuncture.[54]

Hyperbaric oxygen treatment

The use of hyperbaric oxygen (HBO) is not a primary treatment modality in patients with xerostomia due to lack of clinical evidence. In patients who have required HBO for osteoradionecrosis, xerostomia has sometimes been a secondary endpoint of evaluation.[55] In a pilot study, post-radiation patients who received 30 sessions of HBO experienced significant decreases in xerostomia as well as slight increases in unstimulated and stimulated saliva.[56] A recent review of the literature noted that more clinical and experimental studies are needed before making a judgment of HBO's usefulness in managing xerostomia.[55]

Oral lubricants and saliva substitutes

Treatment of xerostomia with oral lubricants and saliva substitutes is done primarily to treat the symptom and minimize the dryness. Many of these products provide short-term relief for a long-term problem. Artificial saliva is formulated to mimic the chemical and physical characteristics of saliva. More than 99% of saliva is water; it also contains buffering agents and enzymes that play a crucial role in maintaining a healthy oral environment. Patients may find benefit in oral lubricants and saliva substitutes as well as in taking frequent sips of water. Patients with xerostomia use water frequently as a saliva substitute. Frequent intake of water or application of water aerosol is roughly half as effective as artificial saliva with regard to duration of relief of dryness.[7] Adequate oral hydration (8–10 glasses water/day) is essential.[39]

Artificial saliva contains a mixture of ions, buffering agents, cellulose derivatives (to increase viscosity and lubricate), and flavoring agents. Several commercially prepared oral lubricants are available. Cellulose-based (carboxymethylcelluose [CMC]) products are the most common, and are available as a spray or gel. Such CMC-based products tend to be viscous.

Artificial saliva is available in a variety of forms, including sprays, lozenges, gels, and swab sticks. Glycerine and lemon swabs are not recommended, due to their drying effect on the oral mucosa.[54] A recent Cochrane review of topical therapies to manage dry mouth reported there to be no strong evidence that any topical therapy is effective in relieving the symptom of dry mouth.[3]

Treatment of oral infections

Treatment of oral candidiasis involves topical or systemic antifungal medications. Troches and oral rinses, such as nystatin, are not routinely used, as each of these products has its own patient adherence issues related to dosing and timing and each must be systemically absorbed through the gastrointestinal tract.[13,58] Systemic medications include fluconazole and ketoconazole. The length of treatment varies from 7 to 14 days or longer. Liquid preparations of these antifungals are available. Chlorhexidine has shown mixed results in the prevention of oral infections in patients with xerostomia and is known to cause changes in taste as well as tooth staining.[59] Topical antifungal cream or ointment is helpful in treating angular chelitis. Dentures should be appropriately cleaned and monitored for fit.

Dental care and surveillance

Damage of the teeth is an indirect effect of radiation-induced salivary gland damage, which results in a pronounced shift toward a highly acidogenic, highly cariogenic oral microflora.[8,20] For this reason, lifelong oral care and dental surveillance is critical.[24] Teaching and reinforcing self-care practices are important before, during, and after irradiation.

Nutrition

Maintaining adequate hydration and nutrition can be a major task for individuals with xerostomia. Patients receiving radiation therapy for head and neck cancer may experience a myriad of acute and late effects from treatment that impact lubrication, mastication, and swallowing—all critical elements to maintaining oral intake. Patients often lose interest in food, and eating becomes a painful and less than pleasant experience and has the potential to impact socialization. Reduced fluid and caloric intake results in weight loss, which is an independent prognostic indicator for survival and quality of life.

Diet modification includes elimination or reduction in sugar intake. Certain foods are known to have an irritating effect on the dry oral mucosa, such as dry, acidic or spicy foods, and highly flavored foods.[24] A consultation with a dietician familiar with xerostomia can be helpful. Because swallowing may be difficult, patients are fearful of choking. A speech or swallowing therapy consultation is advised.

Experimental treatments

A variety of treatments are being explored to help with the prevention and management of xerostomia. The first of these experimental treatments is stem cell therapy, an approach based on the premise that stem cells can differentiate into salivary cells and restore salivary function.[31,60] The second area of investigation is gene therapy, in which a vector (usually a virus) is used to introduce DNA or RNA into surviving cells that help them secrete water.[43] At this time, both stem cell and gene therapy studies are primarily being conducted in animal models, but preclinical studies demonstrate that they may have the potential to work in humans as well.[31,60]

Two medications that have been studied in relation to managing xerostomia are cevilimine and palifermin. A newer sialogogue, cevilimine is approved for treating xerostomia in Sjögren's syndrome.[61] It has not been approved for use in radiation-induced xerostomia, however. Palifermin was studied in patients receiving concurrent chemoradiation. Benefits related to xerostomia were present in those who received hyperfractionated radiation, compared to standard treatment.[62] The researchers note that further studies should investigate higher doses. Dermatologic symptoms as well as fever were reported side effects with palifermin therapy.[62]

The final area of study related to the management of xerostomia is a phase II Radiation Therapy Oncology Group study that investigated the use of transcutaneous electrical nerve stimulation versus pilocarpine.[63] Patients who were 3 to 24 months post radiation therapy with or without chemotherapy, and who met study criteria, received twice-weekly acupuncture-like transcutaneous electrical nerve stimulation. Patients continued these sessions for 12 weeks and had multiple electrodes placed during each treatment. Thirty patients out of 35 at the time of evaluation had a positive treatment response, with 42.9% improvement in dry mouth symptoms as well as improved salivary flow rates.

NURSING IMPLICATIONS

Nursing-sensitive patient outcomes take into account the care and interventions that nursing provides. Such care may often be provided in collaboration with other disciplines, as is often the case in managing xerostomia. The oncology nurse is integral in the assessment, intervention, and education of patients experiencing xerostomia, as this symptom often affects patients' quality of life across the care continuum. (See Figure 20-2 for assessment and management of xerostomia.)

In addressing cancer-related xerostomia, nurses have evaluated oral care products, performed medication reviews, refined administration of radioprotectants, and developed self-care guidelines. By understanding the levels of evidence associated with interventions, nurses can further promote interventional research that can improve care.[32–34] Patient and caregiver education is essential when it comes to care and nutritional modification across the care continuum. Nursing collaboration with multidisciplinary colleagues assists in the formulation of a comprehensive

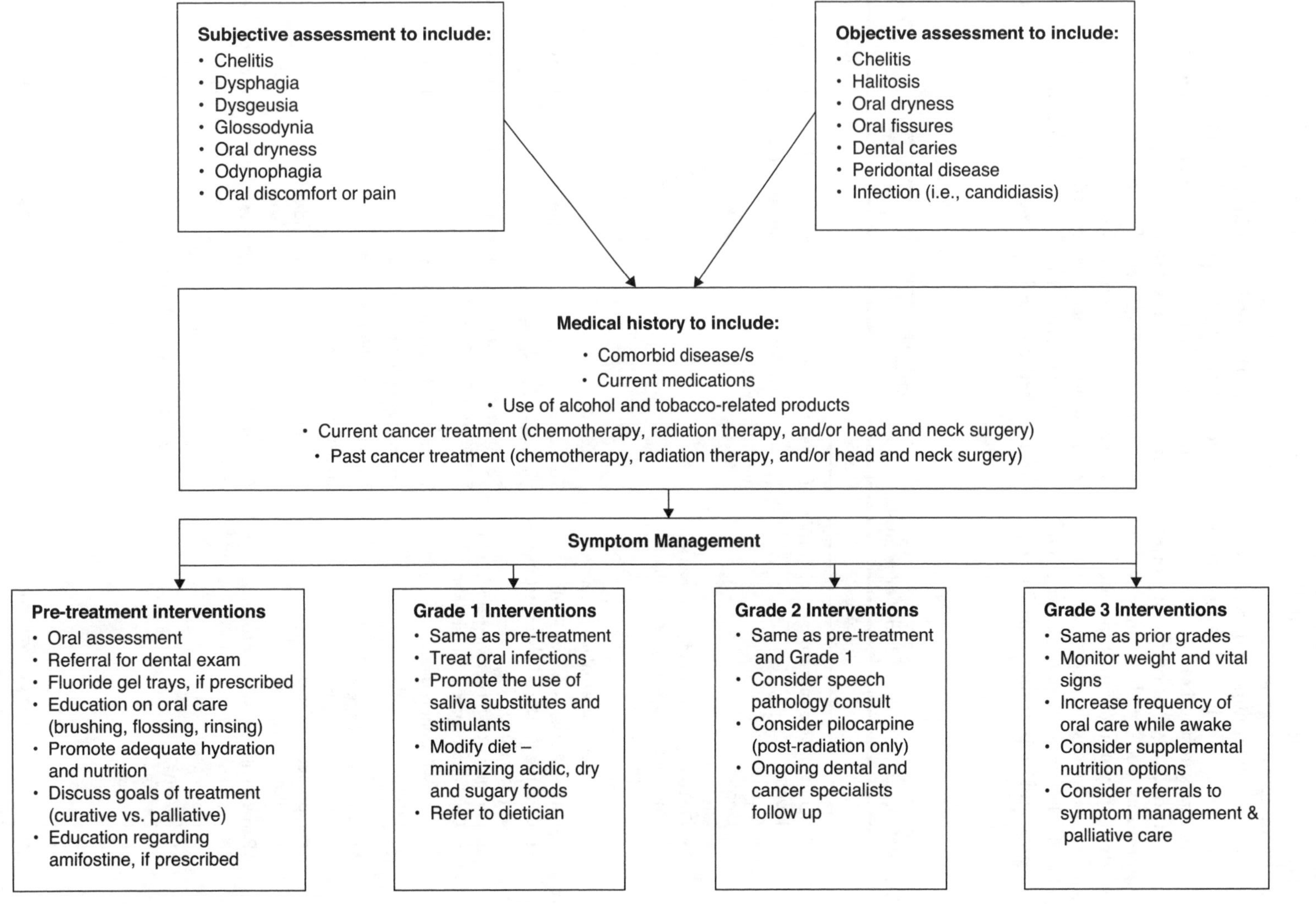

FIGURE 20-2

Xerostomia symptom assessment and management.

Source: Data from Berk et al[8]; NCI[24]; Vissink et al[31]; BC Cancer Agency[39]; Smink et al[64].

care plan that can maximize the patient's ability for self-care and minimize acute and late effects. Patient-reported outcomes play a pivotal role in understanding the patient experience and symptomatology as well as providing longitudinal data over time about nursing interventions and patient adherence to them. (Table 20-5 summarizes nursing implications related to xerostomia.)

Patients with xerostomia due to radiation therapy often experience other symptoms as well. In the acute phase of treatment, these concomitant symptoms may include dysphagia, odynophagia, fatigue, mucositis, sleep disturbance, and a decreased appetite. This constellation of symptoms requires ongoing education and support for the patient and caregiver as well as teaching tools that support practice.[64] The nurse will need to reinforce the need for good oral care (brushing, flossing, rinsing, fluoride trays) and consider how it might need to be modified as treatment progresses, along with the need to avoid irritants such as alcohol and tobacco. Early on, the patient should be referred to a dietician to learn about necessary dietary changes to avoid xerostomia. The nurse should encourage the patient to drink 8- to 10 ounce glasses of fluid per day, to use artificial saliva or to take frequent sips of water, and to adhere to any medication regimens prescribed. As the patient transitions from active treatment to follow-up care, he or she needs to be educated on the late effects that may arise, including

TABLE 20-5

Nurse Sensitive Patient Outcomes Related to Xerostomia

Intervention		Desired Outcome	Timing
Care coordination and referrals*	Patient will be evaluated by: • Nurse • Counselor • Dentist • Dietician • Oncology team (medical, radiation and surgical oncology specialists) • Speech pathology • Social worker • Supportive care/palliative care	To maintain current level of function To have proactive or early intervention to minimize symptomatology	Pretreatment During treatment Post-treatment
Medication adherence	Patient will take as prescribed: • Oral medications for xerostomia as prescribed • Antiemetics, if receiving amifostine • Oral antifungals as prescribed	To maintain functional performance To improve symptom management To minimize need for higher level symptom intervention	Pretreatment During treatment Post-treatment
Patient education	Patient will understand: • Oral assessment • Oral care • Dietary management • Hydration needs • Contact numbers • Follow-up care needs	To maintain functional performance To improve symptom management To maintain oral health To maintain weight To minimize need for hospital admission	Pretreatment During treatment Post-treatment
Symptom reporting	Patient will report symptoms related to: • Decreased oral intake • Dizziness • Dry mouth • Fatigue • Fever • Mucositis • Pain • Painful chewing or swallowing • Sleep	To identify and report symptoms for early intervention To minimize risk of potential clinic, emergency room and/or admission to the hospital	Pretreatment During treatment Post-treatment

*based upon Scope of Practice

Source: Data from Jensen et al[1]; National Cancer Institute[30]; BC Cancer Agency[39].

ongoing xerostomia and ongoing risk for dental cavities and periodontal disease. Continual reinforcement of oral care is essential, as is ensuring the patient is taking medications as prescribed. By providing education, promoting self-care, and collaborating early on with other disciplines, the oncology nurse can impact symptom burden and ultimately influence survivorship and quality of life.

PATIENT SELF-CARE

The patient self-care guide (Appendix 20A) can be used to guide patients through the care they need to perform to minimize the symptom of dry mouth due to disease, treatment, or both. As the healthcare team is an integral component of patients' care, it is essential that all patients be provided with resources that promote self-care as well as optimal outcomes.

For further information on xerostomia, patients can visit the following websites:

- http://www.cancer.net/patient/All+About+Cancer/Treating+Cancer/Managing+Side+Effects/Dry+Mouth+or+Xerostomia
- www.nidcr.nih.gov/oralhealth/topics/drymouth/
- http://www.cancer.org/Treatment/TreatmentsandSideEffects/PhysicalSideEffects/DealingwithSymptomsatHome/caring-for-the-patient-with-cancer-at-home-mouth-dryness
- http://www.cancer.gov/cancertopics/pdq/supportivecare/oralcomplications/Patient

REFERENCES

1. Jensen SB, Pederson AML, Vissink A, et al. A systematic review of salivary gland hypofunction and xerostomia induced by cancer therapies: prevalence, severity and impact on quality of life. *Support Care Cancer.* 2010;18:1039–1060.
2. Jensen S, Mouridsen H, Reibel J, Brunner N, Nauntofte B. Adjuvant chemotherapy in breast cancer patients induces temporary salivary hypofunction. *Oral Oncol.* 2008;44:162–173.
3. Furness S, Worthington HV, Bryan G, Birchenough S, McMillan R. Interventions for the management of dry mouth: topical therapies (review). *Cochrane Database Syst Rev.* 2011;7:CD008934.
4. Dirix P, Nuyts S, Van den Bogaert W. Radiation-induced xerostomia in patients with and neck cancer: a literature review. *Cancer.* 2006;107:2525–2534.
5. Kakoei S, Haghdoost A, Rad M, et al. Xerostomia after radiotherapy and its effect on quality of life in head and neck cancer patients. *Arch Iran Med.* 2012;15:214–218.
6. Davies A, Bagg J, Laverty D, et al. Salivary gland dysfunction ("dry mouth") in patients with cancer: a consensus statement. *Eur J Cancer Care.* 2009;19:172–177.
7. Davies A, Hall S. Salivary gland dysfunction (dry mouth) in patients with advanced cancer. *Int J Palliat Nurs.* 2011;17:477–482.
8. Berk L, Shivnani A, Small W. Pathophysiology and management of radiation-induced xerostomia. *J Support Oncol.* 2005;3:191–200.
9. Sugiura Y, Soga Y, Nishide S, et al. Evaluation of xerostomia in hematopoietic cell transplantation by a simple capacitance method device. *Support Care Cancer.* 2008;16:1197–1200.
10. Ram S, Kumar S, Navazesh M. Management of xerostomia and salivary gland hypofunction. *J Calif Dent Assoc.* 2011;39:656–659.
11. Johannes K, Meier H, Wolff D, et al. Oral chronic graft-versus-host disease: report from the International Consensus Conference on clinical practice in cGVHD. *Clin Oral Investig.* 2010;15:127–139.
12. Bhide SA, Miah AB, Harrington KJ, Newbold KL, Nutting CM. Radiation-induced xerostomia: pathophysiology, prevention, and treatment. *Clin Oncol.* 2009;21:737–744.
13. Kumar S, Ram S, Navazesh M. Salivary gland and associated complications in head and neck cancer therapy. *J Calif Dent Assoc.* 2011;39:639–647.
14. Jensen SB, Pedersen AML, Vissink A, et al. A systematic review of salivary gland hypofunction and xerostomia induced by cancer therapies: management strategies and economic impact. *Support Care Cancer.* 2010;18:1061–1079.
15. Daly CF. Xerostomia and cytoprotection. In: Haas ML, McBride DL, eds. *Managing the Oral Effects of Cancer Treatment: Diagnosis to Survivorship.* Pittsburgh, PA: Oncology Nursing Society; 2011:103–123.
16. Navaresh M. Saliva in health and disease. *J Calif Dent Assoc.* 2011;39:627–628.
17. Eilers J, Epstein J. Assessment and measurement of oral mucositis. *Semin Oncol Nurs.* 2004;20:22–29.
18. Knöös M, Östman M. Oral assessment guide: test of reliability and validity for patients receiving radiotherapy to the head and neck region. *Eur J Cancer Care.* 2009;19:53–60.
19. Thoman WM, Chalmers JM, Spencer AJ, Williams SM. The xerostomia inventory: a multi-item approach to measuring dry mouth. *Community Dent Health.* 1999;16:12–17.
20. Eisbruch A, Kim HM, Terrell JE, Marsh LH, Dawson LA, Ship JA. Xerostomia and its predictors following parotid-sparing irradiation of the head-and-neck cancer. *Int J Radiat Oncol Biol Phys.* 2001;50:695–704.
21. Weymuller EA, Alsarraf R, Yueh B, Deleyiannis FW, Coltrera MD. Analysis of the performance characteristics of the University of Washington Quality of Life instrument and its modification (UW-QOL-R). *Arch Otolaryngol Head Neck Surg.* 2001;127:489–493.
22. Fakhry-Smith S, Din C, Nathoo SA, Gaffar A. Clearance of sodium lauryl sulphate from the oral cavity. *J Clin Periodontol.* 1997;24:313–317.
23. Rantanen I, Tenovuo J, Pienihäkkinen K, Soderling E. Effects of a betaine-containing toothpaste on subjective symptoms of dry mouth: a randomized clinical trial. *J Contemp Dent Pract.* 2003;15;4:11–23.
24. National Cancer Institute. Oral complications of chemotherapy and head/neck radiation (PDQ). May 17, 2012. http://www.cancer.gov/cancertopics/pdq/supportivecare/oralcomplications/HealthProfessional/page1. Accessed June 16, 2012.
25. Gonsalves WC, Chi AC, Neville BW. Common oral lesions: Part I. Superficial mucosal lesions. *Am Fam Physician.* 2007;75:501–506.
26. Park KK, Brodell RT, Helms SE. Angular cheilitis, part 1: local etiologies. *Cutis.* 2011;7:289–95.
27. Navaresh M, Kumar SKS. Measuring salivary flow: challenges and opportunities. *J Am Dent Assoc.* 2008;139(5 suppl):35S–40S.
28. Radiation Therapy Oncology Group. Acute radiation morbidity scoring schema website. http://www.rtog.org/ResearchAssociates/AdverseEventReporting/AcuteRadiationMorbidityScoringCriteria.aspx. Accessed July 12, 2012.
29. Radiation Therapy Oncology Group. Late radiation morbidity scoring schema website. http://www.rtog.org/ResearchAssociates/AdverseEventReporting/RTOGEORTCLateRadiationMorbidityScoringSchema.aspx. Accessed July 12, 2012.
30. Cancer Therapy Evaluation Program. Common terminology criteria for adverse events, version 3.0. August 9, 2006. http://ctep.cancer.gov/protocolDevelopment/electronic_applications/docs/ctcaev3.pdf. Accessed July 12, 2012.

31. Vissink A, Mitchell JB, Baum BJ, et al. Clinical management of salivary gland hypofunction and xerostomia in head-and-neck cancer patients: successes and barriers. *Int J Radiat Oncol Biol Phys.* 2010;78:983–991.
32. Hadorn BC, Baker D, Hodges JS, Hicks N. Rating the quality of evidence for clinical practice guidelines. *J Clin Epidemiol.* 1996;49:749–754.
33. Melynk BM, Fineout-Overholt E. *Evidence-Based Practice in Nursing and Healthcare: A Guide to Best Practice.* Philadelphia: Lippincott, Williams & Wilkins; 2011.
34. U.S. Preventative Services Task Force. Grade definitions. http://www.uspreventativeservicestaskforce.org/uspstf/grades.htm. Accessed August 14, 2012.
35. Brizel DM, Wasserman TH, Henke M, et al. Phase III randomized trial of amifostine as a radioprotector in head and neck cancer. *J Clin Oncol.* 2000;18:3339–3345.
36. Bardet E, Martin L, Calais G, et al. Subcutaneous compared with intravenous administration of amifostine in patients with head and neck cancer receiving radiotherapy: final results of the GORTEC 2000–02 phase III randomized trial. *J Clin Oncol.* 2011;29:127–133.
37. Büntzel J, Glatzel M, Mücke R, Micke O, Bruns F. Influence of amifostine on late radiation-toxicity in head and neck cancer: a follow up study. *Anticancer Res.* 2007;27:1953–1956.
38. Law A, Kennedy T, Pellitteri P, Wood C, Christie D, Yumen O. Efficacy and safety of subcutaneous amifostine in minimizing radiation-induced toxicities in patients receiving combined-modality treatment for squamous cell carcinoma of the head and neck. *Int J Radiat Oncol Phys.* 2007;69:1361–1368.
39. BC Cancer Agency. Professional practice standard nursing standards: symptom management guidelines: xerostomia. January 2010. http://www.bccancer.bc.ca/NR/rdonlyres/5D986439-3614-4F17-9E50-7FECC73C45D1/50150/Xerostomia1.pdf. Accessed June 12, 2012.
40. O'Sullivan B, Rumble RB, Warde P, Members of the IMRT Indications Expert Panel. Intensity-modulated radiotherapy in the treatment of head and neck cancer. *Clin Oncol.* 2012;24:474–487.
41. Little M, Schipper M, Feng FY, et al. Reducing xerostomia after chemo-IMRT for head-and-neck cancer: beyond sparing the parotid gland. *Int J Radiat Oncol Biol Phys.* 2012;83:1007–1014.
42. Nutting CM, Morden JP, Harrington KJ, et al. Parotid-sparing intensity modulated versus conventional radiotherapy in head and neck cancer (PARSPORT): a phase 3 multicentre randomized controlled trial. *Lancet.* 2011;12:127–136.
43. Eisbruch A. Radiotherapy: IMRT reduces xerostomia and potentially improves QOL. *Nat Rev Clin Oncol.* 2009;6:567–568.
44. Scarantino C, LeVequw F, Swann RS, et al. Effect of pilocarpine during radiation therapy: results of RTOG 97-09, a phase III randomized study in head and neck cancer patients. *J Support Oncol.* 2006;4:252–258.
45. LeVeque FG, Montgomery M, Potter D, et al. A multicenter, randomized, double-blind, placebo-controlled, dose-titration study of oral pilocarpine for treatment of radiation-induced xerostomia in head and neck cancer patients. *J Clin Oncol.* 1993;6:1124–1131.
46. Givens E. Update on xerostomia: current treatment modalities and future trends. *Gen Dent.* 2006;54:99–101.
47. Epstein JB, Emerton S, Le ND, Stevenson-Moore, P. A double-blind crossover trial of Oral Balance gel and Biotene® toothpaste versus placebo in patients with xerostomia following radiation therapy. *Oral Oncol.* 1999;35:132–137.
48. Warde P, Kroll B, O'Sullivan B, et al. A phase II study of Biotene in the treatment of postradiation xerostomia in patients with head and neck cancer. *Support Care Cancer.* 2000;8:203–208.
49. Al-Qahtani K, Hier MP, Sultanum K, Black MJ. The role of submandibular salivary gland transfer in preventing xerostomia in the chemoradiotherapy patient. *Oral Surg Oral Med Oral Pathol Oral Radiol Endod.* 2006;101:753–756.
50. Jha N, Harris J, Seikaly H, et al. A phase II study of submandibular gland transfer prior to radiation for prevention of radiation-induced xerostomia in head-and-neck cancer (RTOG 0244). *Int J Radiat Oncol Biol Phys.* 2012. doi: 10.1016/j.ijrobp.2012.02.034.
51. Liu KK, Su Y, Jha N, et al. Submandibular salivary gland transfer for the prevention of radiation-induced xerostomia in patients with nasopharyngeal carcinoma: 5-year outcomes. *Head Neck.* 2011;33:389–395.
52. Meng Z, Garcia MK, Hu C, et al. Randomized controlled trial of acupuncture for prevention of radiation-induced xerostomia among patients with nasopharyngeal carcinoma. *Cancer.* 2012;118:3337–3344.
53. Cho JH, Chung WK, Kang W, Choi SM, Cho CK, Son CG. Manual acupuncture improved quality of life in cancer patients with radiation-induced xerostomia. *J Altern Complement Med.* 2008;14:523–526.
54. O'Sullivan EM, Higginson IJ. Clinical effectiveness and safety of acupuncture in the treatment of irradiation-induced xerostomia in head and neck cancer patients: a systematic review. *Acupunct Med.* 2010;28:191–199.
55. Spiegelberg L, Djasim UM, van Neck HW, Wolvius EB, van der Wal KG. Hyperbaric oxygen in the management of radiation-induced injury in the head and neck region: a review of the literature. *J Oral Maxillofac Surg.* 2010;68:1732–1739.
56. Forner L, Hyldegaard O, von Brockdorff AS, et al. Does hyperbaric oxygen treatment have the potential to increase salivary flow rate and reduce xerostomia in previously irradiated head and neck cancer patients? A pilot study. *Oral Oncol.* 2011;47:546–551.
57. Meurman JH, Odont D, Sorvari R. Hospital mouth-cleaning aids may cause dental erosion. *Spec Care Dentist.* 1996;16:247–250.
58. Worthington HV, Clarkson JE, Khalid T, et al. Interventions for treating oral candidiasis for patients with cancer receiving treatment (review). *Cochrane Database Syst Rev.* 2010;7(7):CD004152.
59. Su N, Marek CL, Ching V, Grushka M. Caries prevention for patients with dry mouth. *J Can Dent Assoc.* 2011;77:b85.
60. Coppes RP, Stokman MA. Stem cells and the repair of radiation-induced salivary gland damage. *Oral Dis.* 2011;17:143–153.
61. Petrone D, Condemi JJ, Fife R, Gluck O, Cohen S, Dalgin P. A double-blind, randomized, placebo-controlled study of cevimeline in Sjögren's syndrome patients with xerostomia and keratoconjunctivitis sicca. *Arthritis Rheumat.* 2002;46:748–754.
62. Brizel DM, Murphy BA, Rosenthal DI, et al. Phase II of palifermin and concurrent chemoradiation in head and neck squamous cell carcinoma. *J Clin Oncol.* 2008;26:2489–2496.
63. Wong RK, James JL, Sagar S, et al. Phase 2 results from Radiation Therapy Oncology Group Study 0537: a phase 2/3 study comparing acupuncture-like transcutaneous electrical nerve stimulation versus pilocarpine in treating early radiation-induced xerostomia. *Cancer.* 2012;118(17):4244–4254.
64. Smink KA, Gosselin-Acomb TK. Evaluation of an educational tool to enhance outcomes for patients with head and neck cancer. *Clin J Oncol Nurs.* 2004;8:490–494.

Dry Mouth (Xerostomia)

Patient Name: ______________________________

Symptom and Description

Dry mouth or "xerostomia" is the feeling of oral dryness that can be the result of some cancer treatments or medicines. Some medicines can cause your mouth to feel dry. Radiation therapy to your head and neck area will cause some dry mouth that may be permanent.

Dry mouth can cause problems with eating (chewing and swallowing), talking, and sleeping. Also, your mouth may feel sore, and your tongue may feel like it is "burning." Dry mouth will increase your risk of oral infection and dental decay.

Prevention

It is not likely that dry mouth can be prevented due to the medicines and/or treatments used for cancer. We will try to decrease radiation to your organs that make saliva during your treatment if possible, and you may receive medicines to help you to produce saliva while you are going through your cancer treatment.

Management

There are many things that may help your mouth feel better and keep your teeth healthy. Talk with your doctor, nurse, and dentist and ask them for ideas.

- **Oral care:** Keep your mouth clean by using oral rinses, brushing, flossing, and using fluoride trays as prescribed. You can ask for a mouth rinse "recipe." It is important for you to take care of your teeth. Brush your teeth and rinse your mouth after every meal. Avoid using alcohol-based mouth rinses.
- **Chewing:** Some people find that chewing sugar-free gum and sucking on sugar-free hard candies can help increase saliva in the mouth.
- **Moisture:** Water can help moisturize your mouth. You should drink at least 2 quarts of water per day. Many saliva substitutes and mouth lubricants are also available; you may select from sprays, gels, and rinses. For dry mouth at night, keep a glass of water and these products within reach.
- **Acupuncture:** Some people find that treatment with acupuncture helps to increase saliva in the mouth. Discuss this treatment with your healthcare team to see if it is an option for you.
- **Medicines:** Your doctor or nurse may prescribe medicines during your cancer treatment that may help increase saliva.
- **Diet changes:** Meeting with a dietician may help you to see what foods to avoid. Soft, moist (those with sauces and gravies) foods are easiest to chew and swallow. Try to avoid dry, hard foods (e.g., crackers, bread) as well as acidic and spicy foods.

(continued)

Follow-Up

Report the following to your doctor or nurse:

- Soreness or pain
- Difficulty swallowing
- Dry mouth that affects your normal activities
- Problems taking in food or liquid because of your dry mouth
- Redness, cracks, ulcers, or white patches on your lips, gums, tongue, or mucous membranes

Phone Numbers

Nurse: ______________________________

Doctor: ______________________________

Dentist: ______________________________

Other: ______________________________

Questions for your care team:

Source: Dalton KA, Gosselin TK. Xerostomia. In: Yarbro CH, Wujcik D, Gobel BH, eds. *Cancer Symptom Management.* 4th ed. Burlington, MA: Jones & Bartlett Learning; 2014.

PART VIII

Alterations in Neurological Function

Chapter 21
Increased Intracranial Pressure

Chapter 22
Peripheral Neuropathy

Chapter 21

Increased Intracranial Pressure

Margaret M. Fields, RN, MSN, ACNP-BC, AOCNP®

THE PROBLEM

Intracranial pressure (ICP) is the sum of the pressures exerted against the skull by the intracranial contents. The three intracranial components are brain tissue, blood, and cerebral spinal fluid (CSF). The skull is a rigid container of fixed size, so an increase in one or more of these components can lead to an increase in ICP. Brain tissue makes up 80% of the volume of intracerebral components, while blood and cerebral spinal fluid account for 10% each.[1]

Elevated ICP can result in potentially devastating complications and death. Prolonged elevation of ICP decreases cerebral perfusion, resulting in tissue hypoxia, edema, and tissue death, which further increases ICP. Therefore, it is essential to make this diagnosis quickly and intervene early and aggressively to restore equilibrium to the central nervous system. ICP is measured in millimeters (mm) of mercury (Hg). Normal ICP is 7–15 mm Hg.[2,3]

INCIDENCE

The incidence of elevated ICP in the oncology population is difficult to estimate, as this symptom may occur in the patient with cancer for a variety of reasons and may often go undetected. The most common reason for increased ICP in the oncology population is brain metastases. It is difficult to identify the number of individuals affected by brain metastases on an annual basis, as these data are not generally available. Estimates as high as 200,000 cases per year have been reported.[4] In a retrospective review of patients in Detroit who developed brain metastases from 1973 to 2001, Barnholtz-Sloan et al.[5] noted a lower overall incidence of brain metastases—10%. The patients reviewed in their analysis were diagnosed with primary lung, melanoma, breast, renal, or colorectal cancer. The highest incidence, 20%, was noted in patients with lung cancer. The most common cancers to metastasize to the brain are lung, breast, and melanoma.[6] Primary brain tumors are much less common and make up only 1.5% of total cancers diagnosed annually, or roughly 23,000 cases.[7]

Other causes of increased ICP are difficult to track in reference to the oncology population, but include intracranial bleeding, infection, heart failure, superior vena cava syndrome, and ischemic–anoxic states.[8]

ETIOLOGY

The major causes of increased ICP are as follows:

- Space-occupying lesions such as primary brain tumors, brain metastases, abscess, or hematoma;
- Cerebral edema, which can occur with hypoxic brain injury, large infarction (stroke), severe infection (meningitis), radiation injury, or traumatic brain injury resulting in alteration of the blood–brain barrier, which disrupts the flow of water and sodium and increases fluid retention;
- Increased production of CSF, which occurs with certain tumors of the choroid plexus;
- Decreased CSF absorption, which can occur with adhesions formed after bacterial meningitis or large intracerebral hemorrhage, or with tumor compressing and impeding the CSF pathway.

Decreased absorption of CSF results in accumulation of fluid and distention of the ventricles. The central nervous system normally contains approximately 150 mL of CSF at any point in time. Daily CSF production is 450–500 mL; a decrease in absorption of CSF can lead to hydrocephalus in a few days to weeks.[8] Obstructive venous outflow can occur with thrombus in venous sinus, jugular vein compression, or neck surgery.[8]

PATHOPHYSIOLOGY

The brain is divided into the right and left hemispheres, with the right side of the brain controlling the left side of the body, and the left side of the brain controlling the right side of the body. The cerebrum consists of four lobes on each side: the frontal, temporal, parietal, and occipital. The remainder of the brain is composed of the cerebellum, the midbrain, and the brain stem (Figure 21-1).[9]

The functions of the areas of the brain are delineated as follows. The frontal lobe is responsible for personality and mood, strategic and abstract thinking, judgment, speech, and voluntary motor control. The temporal lobe is responsible for auditory perception, short-term memory, sensory processing and ability to identify body position, and language and memory interpretation. The parietal lobe is responsible for logic, mathematics, ability to identify objects by touch, ability to write, taste, and ability to feel vibrations, temperature, pain, and pressure. The occipital lobe is responsible for visual processing and interpretation. The cerebellum is responsible for the integration of sensory perception, coordination, and motor control. The midbrain is responsible for relaying sensory information and motor signals between the cerebral cortex and the body, and for regulation of consciousness, sleep, and alertness. The brain stem is responsible for regulation of cardiac and respiratory function.[10]

The Monro Kellie doctrine, a hypothesis put forth by Alexander Monro more than two centuries ago, states that an increase in volume of one of the intracellular components—brain tissue, blood, or CSF—must come at the expense of the other two. Initially, when one component increases, the body attempts to maintain homeostasis by compensatory mechanisms. These mechanisms include displacement of CSF into the thecal sac, and decrease in the volume of cerebral venous blood via venoconstriction and extracranial drainage. The goal is for ICP to be maintained within normal parameters of less than 15 mm Hg. However, as compliance decreases over time, additional small volume changes can result in a dramatic increase in ICP. Changes that occur gradually produce less of an effect initially, as the body has time to adjust to them. Rapid changes, by comparison, produce a more dramatic effect.[3,11]

The brain tissue is less compliant, but may adjust by decreasing the space between gyri (rounded ridges of the brain) and by compressing the brain tissue. The ability of the brain to accommodate increased pressure is limited.

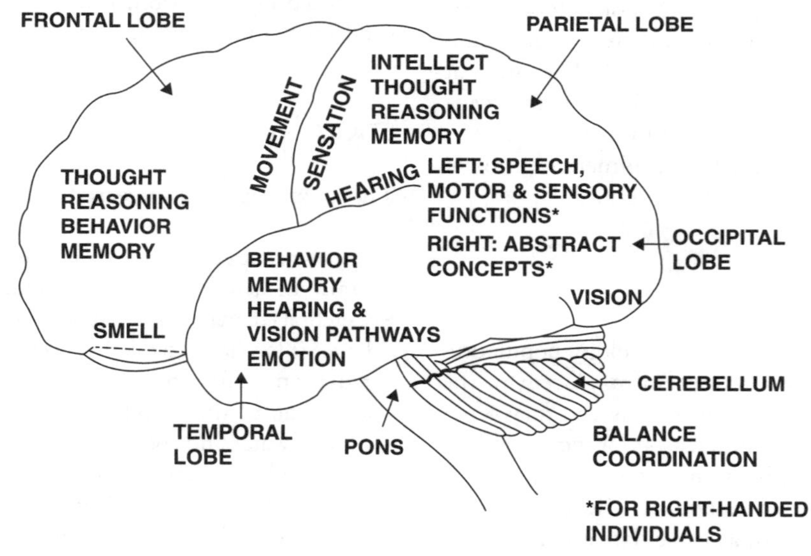

FIGURE 21-1

Areas of the brain and functions.

Source: Reprinted with permission from the American Brain Tumor Association[9].

When too much pressure is placed on a given area, the brain may herniate; herniation is the displacement of tissue across an abnormal opening (Figure 21-2).

Several types of herniation may occur in the brain. In *cingulate herniation*, a lesion compresses one side of the brain, forcing the cingulate gyrus from that side under the falx cerebri (the major fold of the dura at the top of the brain that separates the left and right hemispheres of the cerebrum) to the other side of the brain. Midline shift will be visible on imaging (Figure 21-3). *Uncal herniation* occurs when the midbrain is compressed such that the cerebral peduncle is forced against the tentorium (the major dural fold that separates the cerebrum from the cerebellum). *Central herniation* results when there is downward force on the tentorium and the brain stem is displaced through the foramen magnum. In *cerebellar herniation*, the lower portion of the cerebellum (the cerebellar tonsil) is displaced downward through the foramen magnum.[2,13]

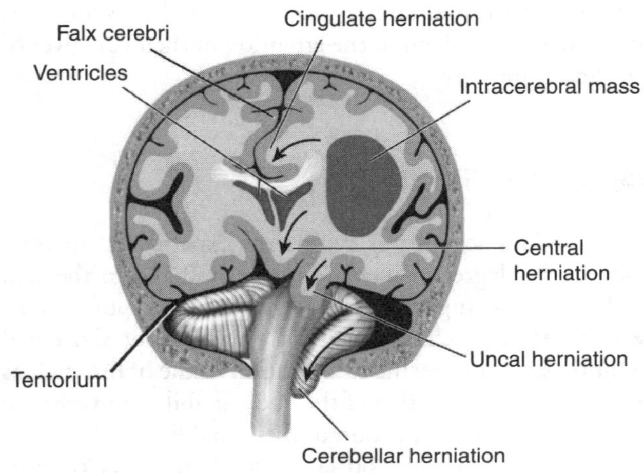

FIGURE 21-2

Cerebral herniation.
Source: Courtesy of HFS Imaging, Merion Station, PA.

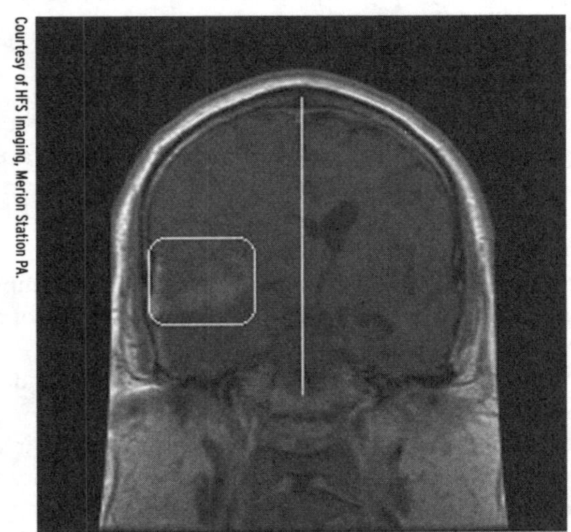

FIGURE 21-3

Coronal image of brain with midline shift and compression of lateral ventricle due to tumor. Right heterogeneous temporal tumor enclosed in box.

The earliest signs of increased ICP are headache and a decreased level of consciousness. As ICP continues to increase, more symptoms emerge—namely, diplopia, and nausea. Symptoms then progress to dilation of the ipsilateral pupil and cranial nerve III palsy (characterized by ptosis, diplopia, and limited eye movements, often with the eye deviated downward and out). Subsequent symptoms include decerebrate posturing, with progression to hemiparesis. Later, symptoms progress to the contralateral side with dilation of the opposite pupil. The final stages of increased ICP are manifested by Cushing's triad—a cluster of symptoms consisting of increased systolic blood pressure, bradycardia, and irregular breathing.[3,13] Table 21-1 details symptom progression in herniation syndromes.

The ability of the third intracerebral component, blood, to decrease so as to accommodate increased ICP is limited. A large decrease in intracerebral blood volume will ultimately worsen increased ICP. As the blood volume in the brain shrinks, cerebral perfusion is decreased, which results in hypoxia. This leads to an increase in cerebral edema, which in turn further increases ICP. Cerebral perfusion pressure (CPP) is related to the mean arterial

TABLE 21-1

Clinical Progression of Signs and Symptoms of Cerebral Herniation

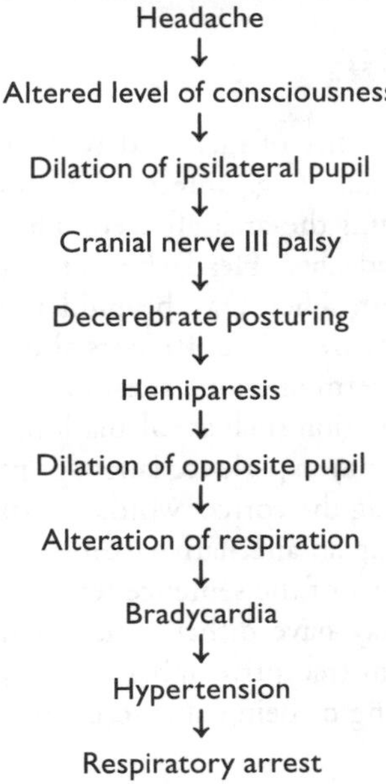
Headache
↓
Altered level of consciousness
↓
Dilation of ipsilateral pupil
↓
Cranial nerve III palsy
↓
Decerebrate posturing
↓
Hemiparesis
↓
Dilation of opposite pupil
↓
Alteration of respiration
↓
Bradycardia
↓
Hypertension
↓
Respiratory arrest

TABLE 21-2

Intracranial Blood Flow and Pressure Relationships

CPP = MAP − (ICP + CVP)

- CPP = Cerebral Perfusion Pressure : Goal is to keep >60 mm Hg.
- MAP = Mean Arterial Blood Pressure : Goal is to keep between 60–150 mm Hg.
- ICP = Intracranial Pressure: Goal is to keep <20 mm Hg.
- CVP = Central Venous Pressure

Source: Data from Hickey and Olson[13]; Ravi and Morgan[14].

pressure (MAP) and ICP. The relationship of cerebral perfusion to MAP and ICP is expressed by an equation: CPP is equal to MAP minus the combined sum of ICP and central venous pressure (CVP) (Table 21-2).[13,14] The therapeutic goal is to maintain CPP greater than 60 mm Hg, MAP between 60 and 150 mm Hg, and ICP at less than 20 mm Hg.[13–15]

SYMPTOM ASSESSMENT

RISK FACTORS

Any patient with cancer is at risk for increased ICP via several mechanisms. These pathways include infection (meningitis) due to immune suppression, intracranial hemorrhage due to thrombocytopenia, venous failure due to heart failure or superior vena cava syndrome, and space-occupying metastases in the brain.[11]

SELF-ASSESSMENT

The patient experience of increased ICP will vary depending on the root cause (e.g., infection, hemorrhage, tumor) of the problem and the area affected. The most common symptom is headache. Headaches are typically persistent and recurrent. They may be mild initially, but then increase in severity over time. Patients also often describe a decrease in short-term memory, attention span, or difficulty with executive function such as calculations or organization of tasks. Patients may experience language problems such as difficulty in finding the correct words to express themselves or incorrectly using an alternative word that does not make sense in the context of the sentence (expressive aphasia). In addition, they may have difficulty understanding what is being said to them (receptive aphasia). They may have difficulty with reading or being able to express their thoughts in writing. Some patients experience weakness resulting in inability to walk or perform self-care activities.[13] As these symptoms do not lend themselves to the patient being able to consistently and reliably record them, it may be necessary to rely on family members or caregivers to provide details of day-to-day functioning and problems the patient is experiencing.

The patient experience of increased ICP can be very distressing. Patients initially often do not know the cause of their symptoms and may question whether they are experiencing dementia or a stroke. Sometimes patients may be embarrassed and try to cover for their symptoms rather than bring them to the attention of their caregiver or healthcare provider.

OBJECTIVE ASSESSMENT

The type and severity of symptoms experienced directly relate to the degree of increase in the ICP and to the area of the brain being affected.[3] Signs and symptoms may be nonspecific, such as headache, vomiting, or shortened attention span; or specific to a location in the brain, such as inability to move one side of the body, inability to verbalize thoughts, or loss of a portion of the visual field.[11,13]

Symptoms may develop either gradually over time or suddenly, depending on the rate of increase in pressure. Symptoms can be very distressing to patients and family members, as they may result in personality changes or functional debility related to weakness or sensory loss. Patients may develop deficits that result in them requiring assistance with basic functions such as bathing or toileting. In severe cases, patients may be unresponsive or comatose and suffer permanent disability or death.[3,11]

History

Taking a comprehensive history of any symptom is facilitated with the use of the mnemonic "OLD CART":

O: onset. When did the symptom first begin?
L: location. Where is the symptom located? For example, if it is evidenced by headache, is it frontal, occipital, or all over?
D: duration. When the symptom occurs, how long does it last?
C: characteristics. Is it constant or intermittent? Is it severe or mild. Does it impact quality of life or ability to perform activities of daily living (ADLs)?
A: aggravating/associated factors. Does anything make it worse or accompany the symptom (e.g., time of day, certain positions, cough, straining with stool, nausea with headache)?

R: relieving factors. Does anything make it better (e.g., lying down in the dark; sitting up in a quiet room, leaning forward)?
T: treatments. What has the patient or family tried so far and how effective or ineffective have therapies been? Be sure to include both pharmacologic and nonpharmacologic interventions.[16]

Routinely utilizing this mnemonic when taking the history of a symptom helps to ensure that all aspects of the symptom are addressed.

Physical assessment

Neurologic assessment provides the nurse with the ability to detect changes in status that may be related to an increase in intracranial pressure. A complete neurologic assessment includes general observations, cranial nerve assessment, motor assessment, testing of reflexes, coordination, and gait assessment.

General. Neurologic assessment of the patient begins with general observation. This part of the neurologic assessment includes aspects of appearance and behavior, mood, facial expression, speech, vocabulary, thought processes, reasoning, memory, and abstract reasoning.[17] Concerning symptoms for increased ICP would be lethargy, confusion, and impaired reasoning. Table 21-3 identifies specific assessment questions and techniques used in general assessment.[18]

Cranial nerves. See Table 21-4 for cranial nerve functions and assessment.

- Cranial nerve I: This nerve is often not assessed, but can be tested by asking the patient to identify a scented substance such as coffee or spice.
- Cranial nerve II: Assess for pupil size and reactivity to light (pupil should constrict in the eye into which the light is directed *and* the contralateral eye). In early increased pressure, the pupil on the affected side will remain dilated when light is shined into it; in more advanced increased ICP, both pupils will remain dilated. Assess for intactness of peripheral vision fields by standing directly in front of the patient a few feet away. Have the patient cover one eye and focus their gaze straight ahead (e.g., on the examiner's nose). Then holding your hand to the side, display a different number of fingers on your left and right hands about 8 inches lateral to your face at about the level of your forehead, nose, and neck on your left and right sides. Ask patient to tell you how

TABLE 21-3

Neurological Assessment: General Observations

Quality/Function	Questions to Ask
Appearance and behavior	Is the person well groomed or disheveled? Does the person appear anxious or depressed? What is the person's posture like? Has there been a change from baseline?
Mood, facial expression, attitude	Does the person appear angry, depressed? Is the behavior appropriate? Has the patient or family noted a change from baseline?
Flow of speech, thought processes and perceptions, thought content	What is the pace and spontaneity of speech? Has the patient experienced any delusions, hallucinations, new phobias?
Orientation	Is the person oriented to person, place, and time?
Level of consciousness	Is the person alert or somnolent? Is this a change?
Attention and concentration	Can the patient count backward from 100 subtracting serial 7s with few errors?
Memory (remote)	Can the patient recall birthplace, age, history of illness, current events in last 5 years?
Memory (recent)	Can the patient recall arrival at the hospital/office?
Memory: retention and immediate recall	Can the patient recall list of objects or dates when asked to repeat the list in 3 to 5 minutes?
Calculations	Can the person do simple multiplication or addition?
Vocabulary	Can the patient define words such as orange, metaphor, flourish?
Abstract reasoning	Can the patient explain a simple proverb?
Similarities	Can the patient describe how a cat and a mouse are alike?
Judgment	Can the patient provide a reasonable answer to a question such as "What would you do if there was a fire on your stove?"

Source: Data from Wilkes[18].

TABLE 21-4

Cranial Nerves: Function and Examination

Number	Name	Function	Examination
I	Olfactory	Smell	Detect scented substance such as coffee or spice
II	Optic	Vision	Test for pupillary response to light and optic disk assessment for papilledema
III	Oculomotor	Most eye muscles	Move eyes to follow finger in an "H" pattern
IV	Trochlear	Superior oblique	Look down and inward (toward the nose)
VI	Abducens	Lateral rectus	Move eyes laterally to look to the side
V	Trigeminal	Facial sensation, mastication	Check for numbness along the forehead, cheek, and chin on both sides of the face (V1-V3), clench teeth
VII	Facial	Facial expression, taste	Smile, raise eyebrows, taste
VIII	Auditory (vestibulocochlear)	Hearing, balance	Finger rub, whisper, tuning fork
IX	Glossopharyngeal	Pharynx sensation, taste	Movement of palate, uvula midline
X	Vagus	Muscles pharynx, larynx, Parasympathetic innervation of the heart	Open wide and say Ahh, check for symmetric movement of uvula
XI	Spinal accessory	Controls trapezius, sternocleidomastoid	Raise shoulders, turn head: check for symmetry of strength
XII	Hypoglossal	Tongue movement	Stick out tongue; check to see if it is midline or deviates to one side; assess ability to move to sides

Source: Data from Bickley[16].

many fingers you have displayed. Using an ophthalmoscope, assess the fundus or interior surface of the eye, which includes the retina, optic disc, macula and fovea, and posterior pole. Papilledema (swelling of the optic disc) is a cardinal sign of increased intracranial pressure.

- Cranial nerves III, IV, and VI: These three cranial nerves are evaluated together by testing eye movement. Assess for full eye movements in all directional gazes (up, down, lateral, and medial) by asking patient to follow your finger while moving it in an "H" pattern. Figure 21-4 illustrates how to test extraocular movements. In increased ICP, the patient may report diplopia or you may note ptosis or difficulty in performing eye movements on the affected side. The remainder of the cranial nerves are generally not affected by increased ICP, with the exception of cranial nerve X. Loss of gag reflex is a late sign of increased ICP.
- Cranial nerve V: Assess for symmetry of facial sensation on the left and right at the level of the forehead, cheek, and chin. Ask the patient to clench the teeth, and check for symmetry of contracted jaw muscles.
- Cranial nerve VII: Assess facial symmetry by asking the patient to raise the eyebrows, close the eyes tightly, and smile broadly.

1. Ask the patient to visually follow your finger as you move it through the six cardinal gazes.
2. Draw an "H" shape in the air with your finger, moving slowly as you change direction.
3. Pause during upward and lateral gazes to identify nystagmus.

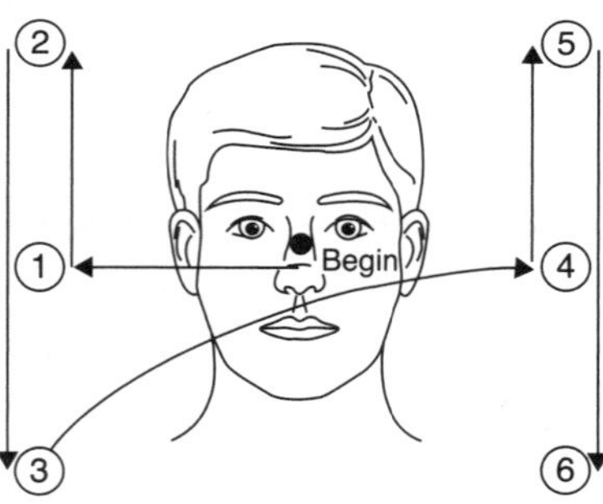

4. Normally, eyes should be conjugate (move together in the same direction). An individual may have slight nystagmus (fine, rhythmic oscillation) normally with extreme lateral gaze.

FIGURE 21-4

Testing extra ocular movement.

- Cranial nerve VIII: Hearing can be assessed by whispering into both ears or gently rubbing your fingers 3–4 inches away from the patient's ears.
- Cranial nerve IX and X: Assess for symmetry of elevation of the soft palate and uvula when patient says, "Ahh."
- Cranial nerve XI: Assess for symmetry of strength of muscles for turning the head (sternocleidomastoid) and shrugging the shoulders (trapezius).
- Cranial nerve XII: Have the patient stick out the tongue and move it from side to side. Assess whether the tongue is midline and is able to be moved freely.[12] Deviation from normal findings may indicate compression of brain tissue in the area of the affected cranial nerve, which may be an indication of an increase in intracranial pressure.[3]

Motor function. Assess for muscle bulk and tone (normal, flaccid, or spastic). Assess the strength of the muscles of the upper and lower extremities by checking for the patient's ability to move against resistance exerted by the examiner. Grading of muscle strength is on a scale of 0 to 5 (Table 21-5).[19] In patients with increased ICP in an advanced stage, you may see a decrease in strength on the side of the body opposite from the brain lesion.

Coordination. Assess for smoothness of movements and fine motor coordination. Can the patient pick up a small object such as a coin or key from a flat surface? Are rapid finger-tapping movements smooth and rhythmic? Can the patient slide the heel of one foot up and down the opposite shin from heel to knee?[16]

Reflexes. Are reflexes symmetric? Are they normal, hyperreflexive, or absent? Reflexes that are asymmetric are abnormal. Reflexes that are hyperreflexive may be a normal variant, particularly if symmetric; if asymmetric, however, they may indicate pathology in the brain. Absent reflexes may indicate pathology in the spinal cord. Reflexes are graded on a scale of 0 to 4, ranging from absent to hyperactive (Table 21-6).[16]

TABLE 21-5

Grading of Muscle Strength

0	No movement
1	Able to twitch, but no meaningful movement
2	Able to move laterally, but not against gravity
3	Able to move against gravity but unable to hold against minimal resistance
4	Able to move against gravity and resistance, but without full strength
5	Full strength

Source: Data from O'Brien[19].

Gait. Assess for stance (wide, normal, narrow based) and arm swing (present, absent, both arms). Is the gait smooth, shuffling, or a lurching movement? Assess turning for smooth pivot or en bloc turning. Assess for steadiness of gait and balance. Can the patient walk on the heels, tiptoes, and in tandem? Does the patient use any aids for ambulation such as a cane?[12]

Diagnostic evaluation

The initial assessment for elevated intracranial pressure begins with radiologic imaging to assess for a mass, intracerebral hemorrhage, or hydrocephalus. If radiologic findings support a diagnosis of increased intracranial pressure, the physician may wish to continually monitor the degree of pressure. The gold standard for ICP measurement is invasive monitoring via use of a probe inserted into the intraventricular space.[14] This method allows for continuous monitoring of ICP and rapid adjustments in therapy.

There is controversy over whether ongoing monitoring of ICP improves outcomes in the traumatic brain injury population. Early studies had shown significantly better outcomes (mortality of 12% in a monitored group versus 53% in an unmonitored group).[20] However, later studies were not able to replicate a significant survival advantage. At this time, invasive monitoring is indicated only in selected patients following traumatic brain injury: age greater than 40, unilateral or bilateral motor posturing, systolic blood pressure less than 90 mm Hg, abnormal computed tomography (CT) findings such as hemorrhage or hydrocephalus, or Glasgow Coma Scale scores in the range of 3–8.[21] The Glasgow Coma Scale assigns an overall rating based on assessment of the patient's eye response, verbal response, and motor function (Table 21-7).[22,23]

Several other measures are used to assess signs or causes of increased ICP. Noninvasive measures include fundoscopic examination of the inner eye using an ophthalmoscope to assess for papilledema, which indicates increased ICP. CT scan and magnetic resonance imaging (MRI) can be obtained to assess for space-occupying brain lesions (primary or metastatic) or hemorrhage. Newer methods to assess for elevated ICP include ocular sonography

TABLE 21-6

Grading of Deep Tendon Reflexes

0	Reflex is absent
1	Reflex is diminished
2	Normal reflex
3	Hyperactive or brisk reflex
4	Clonus (continuous rhythmic reflex present after single tap with reflex hammer)

Source: Data from Bickley[16].

TABLE 21-7

Glasgow Coma Scale

Eyes:	Opens eyes spontaneously	4 points
	Opens eyes to verbal command	3 points
	Opens eyes in response to pain	2 points
	Does not open eyes	1 point
Verbal:	Oriented	5 points
	Confused, disoriented conversation	4 points
	Inappropriate responses, words understandable	3 points
	Incomprehensible speech; sounds	2 points
	None	1 point
Motor:	Follows commands regarding movement	6 points
	Localizes painful stimuli	5 points
	Withdraws from pain	4 points
	Abnormal flexion to painful stimuli (decorticate posture)	3 points
	Extension to painful stimuli (decerebrate posture)	2 points
	No movements	1 point

The Glasgow Coma Scale (GCS) comprises three tests of response: ***eye, verbal***, and ***motor***. The sum of the three comprises the score. The lowest possible GCS is 3 (deep coma or death), while the highest GCS is 15 (fully awake, alert person).

Source: Data from Kornbluth and Bardway[23].

(checks optic nerve sheath diameter), optic tonometer to assess intraocular pressure, transcranial Doppler ultrasound to assess for cerebral vasospasm or hyperemia, and tissue resonance analysis (TRA) to assess for cerebral edema. TRA uses an ultrasound probe placed on the forehead of the patient; it emits an ultrasound wave that passes through and is reflected off the skull and soft tissue. A complex calculation is applied to a portion of the ultrasound wave to assess the speed of the wave and compare it to a constant to evaluate for tissue edema.[24,25]

Figure 21-5 illustrates an algorithm for assessment, interventions, and treatment of increased ICP.

DEGREES OF TOXICITY

Several measures are used to evaluate the impact of neurologic disease on functioning, including the common terminology criteria for adverse events (Table 21-8) established by the National Cancer Institute;[26] the Karnofsky performance scale, which is a measure of overall functioning; and the Glasgow Coma Scale, which is a measure of neurologic function. These are all validated measurement tools that are commonly known, and by which one can easily communicate the functional status of a patient.

SYMPTOM MANAGEMENT STRATEGIES

THERAPEUTIC APPROACHES

In emergent cases of increased ICP, the immediate goals are to assess the airway, breathing, and circulation. It is imperative that any deficits be corrected immediately, as hypoxia and hypotension will result in cerebral edema, further elevating ICP.[3,14]

Proper positioning of the patient should be implemented immediately. The head of the bed should be elevated at least 30 degrees, and the neck must be kept in a neutral midline position. This positioning prevents compression of the jugular veins and maximizes cerebral venous return. It is important to avoid crossing limbs or extreme hip flexion, as these maneuvers also increase ICP.[3,11,12,27]

Previously, prophylactic hyperventilation had been employed to cause cerebral vasoconstriction and reduce ICP. More recently, this technique has been shown to have a paradoxical effect. The vasoconstriction caused by hyperventilation results in reduced cerebral blood flow and hypoxia, which in turn causes edema and worsens increased ICP. This intervention is now indicated only in true emergencies to prevent herniation and death.[28–30]

Careful use of analgesics will prevent increases in ICP, which can be caused by pain or agitation. Analgesics must be cautiously titrated to achieve symptom relief without impairing neurologic monitoring, as analgesic agents may cause sedation or hypotension, resulting in impaired cerebral perfusion.[3,13,27]

Seizures increase ICP by increasing cerebral blood flow and metabolic rate; therefore, early intervention for seizure treatment is important in preventing secondary injury. Prophylaxis may be used early in the course of therapy, but prophylactic anticonvulsants are not recommended after seven days in patients with no prior seizure history.[31]

It is essential to avoid hyperthermia, as cerebral metabolic demand is increased 5% to 7% for each degree Celsius that the body temperature is elevated. The increased metabolic demand can result in relative tissue hypoxia, further increasing ICP. Fever must be aggressively treated. Because hyperthermia is known to be deleterious, there has been interest in potential benefit from hypothermia. At this point, the use of hypothermia is not clearly defined. Some studies[32,33] appeared to show benefit from this technique in patients with traumatic brain injury, while other

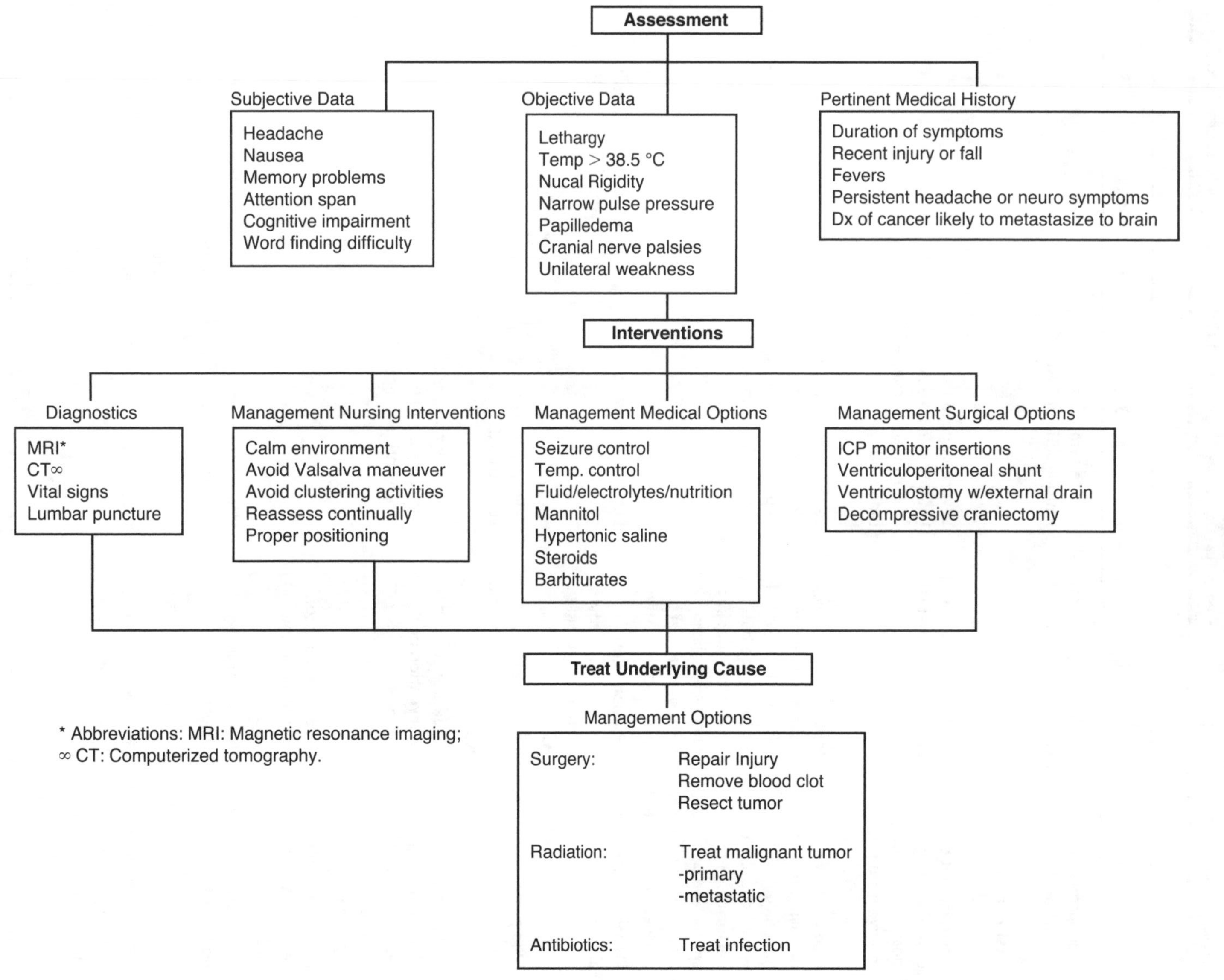

FIGURE 21-5

Algorithm for assessment and treatment of Increased intracranial pressure (ICP).

TABLE 21-8

National Cancer Institute Common Terminology Criteria for Adverse Events (CTCAE): Nervous System Toxicity

	Grade				
Adverse Event	**1**	**2**	**3**	**4**	**5**
Cranial nerve disorder	Asymptomatic; clinical or diagnostic observations only; intervention not indicated	Moderate symptoms; limiting instrumental activities of daily living (ADL)	Severe symptoms; limiting self-care ADL		
Ataxia	Asymptomatic; clinical or diagnostic observations only; intervention not indicated	Moderate symptoms; limiting instrumental ADL	Severe symptoms; limiting self-care ADL; mechanical assistance indicated		
Cognitive disturbance	Mild cognitive disability; not interfering with work/school/life performance; specialized educational services/ devices not indicated	Moderate cognitive disability; interfering with work/school/life performance but capable of independent living; specialized resources on part-time basis indicated	Severe cognitive disability; significant impairment of work/ school/life performance		
Depressed level of consciousness	Decreased level of alertness	Sedation; slow response to stimuli; limiting instrumental ADL	Difficult to arouse	Life-threatening consequences	Death
Headache	Mild pain	Moderate pain; limiting instrumental ADL	Severe pain; limiting self-care ADL		
Hydrocephalus	Asymptomatic; clinical or diagnostic observations only; intervention not indicated	Moderate symptoms; intervention not indicated	Severe symptoms or neurological deficit; intervention indicated	Life-threatening consequences urgent intervention indicated	Death
Lethargy	Mild symptoms; reduced alertness and awareness	Moderate symptoms; limiting instrumental ADL			
Seizure	Brief partial seizure; no loss of consciousness	Brief generalized seizure	Multiple seizures despite medical intervention	Life-threatening; prolonged repetitive seizures	Death
Somnolence	Mild but more than usual drowsiness or sleepiness	Moderate sedation; limiting instrumental ADL	Obtundation or stupor	Life-threatening consequences; urgent intervention indicated	Death

Source: Data from National Cancer Institute Common Terminology Criteria for Adverse Events (CTCAE)[26].

studies[34–36] have failed to note any improvement in cerebral perfusion pressure. Several approaches have been tried including use of intravenous cooling devices and cooling blankets. It is critical to avoid shivering in the patient being treated with hypothermia, as this reaction will increase metabolic demand and ICP.[3,13,27]

A euvolemic, normoglycemic state and prevention of hyponatremia are essential, as imbalances in any of these factors will exacerbate elevations in ICP. A euvolemic state is crucial because dehydration and hypotension can result in hypoxia and further increase ICP. Conversely, fluid overload increases vascular volume, which then further increases ICP. The IV hydration fluid of choice is normal saline, as dextrose solutions can increase cerebral edema. Maintaining normal glucose levels helps to prevent secondary brain injury. Hypoglycemia impairs the energy supply to damaged neurons in the brain, whereas hyperglycemia increases oxidative stress and has been associated with poor outcomes. Hyponatremia results in intracellular expansion, further increasing ICP. Maintaining a normal serum sodium level minimizes fluctuations in ICP and cerebral edema.[3,13,27]

Medications

The mainstay of drug therapy for treatment of increased ICP is medication to reduce cerebral edema and manage symptoms.

Mannitol. Mannitol is an osmotic diuretic. It is given in doses ranging from 0.25 to 1 g IV every 6 to 8 hours to maintain serum osmolality at less than 320 mOsm/kg and ICP at less than 20 mm Hg.[37] Mannitol is a vesicant, so care must be taken to avoid extravasation. The solution should be administered via a filter, as crystals may form. If crystals are noted, the solution should be warmed to remove them. In patients being treated for cerebral edema, mannitol may accumulate in the brain if it circulates for long periods of time, such as occurs with continuous infusion; therefore, intermittent boluses are preferred.[38] Each dose should be given over 20 to 30 minutes. Reduction in ICP occurs in 15 to 30 minutes, and the duration of action is 1.5 to 6 hours.

Mannitol is hypothesized to reduce ICP by reducing blood viscosity, which then briefly increases cerebral blood flow and oxygen transport. This, in turn, reduces cerebral blood volume and ICP. Furthermore, mannitol reduces ICP by withdrawing water from the brain parenchyma and excreting the excess water in the urine.[38,39]

Hypertonic saline. Hypertonic saline solutions, with concentrations ranging from 3% to 23.4%, are being used more often in the setting of increased ICP. This treatment approach has been shown to be a safe and effective option for rapidly decreasing ICP. Hypertonic saline works by creating an osmotic force that pulls water into the intravascular space. This action increases CSF absorption, increases cardiac output, and expands the intravascular volume. Collectively, it results in a positive inotropic effect that improves cerebral perfusion pressure.[2,39]

Three percent saline infusions have been effective at reducing cerebral edema when given at 0.1–2 mL/kg/hr titrated to keep serum sodium between 145 and 155 mEq/L. However, no clear guidelines or specific targets for optimal sodium concentrations have been established. Hypertonic saline has been shown to be effective in temporarily reversing transtentorial herniation when given in bolus dose of 300 mL of 3% saline, 250 mL of 7.5% saline, 75 mL of 10% saline, or 30 mL of 23.4% saline. Hypertonic saline is given over 30 minutes. It has at least equivalent efficacy to—if not greater efficacy than—mannitol when given in a bolus dose, and can even reduce ICP in patients in whom mannitol has failed.[38–40]

Potential complications of hypertonic saline infusion include shifts in electrolyte balance with increases in serum sodium and in serum creatinine, and decrease in serum potassium. Care must be taken to monitor electrolytes and renal function closely and to correct them appropriately. In patients who are hyponatremic prior to hypertonic saline infusion, there is a theoretical risk of central pontine mylinolysis due to rapid correction of this state. This outcome has not been reported in the setting of induced hypernatremia in normonatremic patients for the treatment of increased ICP.[40] An additional risk includes thrombophlebitis with infusions given peripherally; therefore, delivery of infusions via a central line is recommended.[38,40]

Steroids. The use of glucocorticoids in the setting of increased ICP is dependent upon the root cause of elevated ICP. In the setting of cerebral infarction, intracranial hemorrhage, or traumatic head injury, steroids have no role; indeed, they may be deleterious in the cases of head injury.[41] Dexamethasone, however, may be beneficial in cases of elevated ICP caused by brain tumors or infection.[42] The recommended dose is 10 mg IV initially, followed by 4 mg every 6 hours for 5 to 7 days. The drug should not be abruptly discontinued, but rather should be tapered to avoid risk of adrenal insufficiency. Side effects include elevation of blood sugar, emotional lability, fluid retention, immunosuppression, gastritis, and insomnia.[43]

Barbiturate coma. Barbiturate coma is considered a second-tier therapy and is used only in cases of refractory elevations of ICP. A barbiturate coma decreases cerebral metabolic demands, cerebral blood flow, and ICP. Care must be taken to monitor blood pressure and ensure that the patient does not become hypotensive, which will decrease cerebral perfusion, resulting in hypoxia and increased ICP. Barbiturate coma impairs neurologic examination, so monitoring of ICP measurement, mean arterial pressure, and electroencephalogram (EEG) is required to guide therapy.

The most commonly used barbiturate in this setting is pentobarbital. It is generally given in a loading dose of 10 mg/kg over 1 to 2 hours, followed by a continuous infusion rate of 1–2 mg/kg/hr titrated up to maximum of 4 mg/kg/hr. At the maximum dose, continuous EEG monitoring is recommended to assess brain function, as it is not possible to perform a neurologic examination on a comatose patient. Secondary to respiratory suppression, these patients also require mechanical ventilation. Potential complications include hypotension, hypokalemia, infections, hepatic, and renal dysfunction.[2,3,39]

Table 21-9 provides an overview of medications used to treat increased ICP.

Surgical interventions

Ventriculoperitoneal shunt. In cases of elevated ICP caused by hydrocephalus, a ventriculoperitoneal (VP) shunt to divert excess CSF from the ventricles to the peritoneal cavity is able to maintain normal ICP (Figure 21-6). Placement of such a shunt is performed for long-term management of excess CSF related to decreased absorption, which results in excess CSF leading to increased ICP. Shunting may be required in conjunction with alteration of the lining of the ventricles due to adhesions from prior infection, radiotherapy, or tumor. Insertion of a shunt delivers the excess CSF to the peritoneal cavity where it is absorbed.[8]

TABLE 21-9

Medication Overview

	Dose	Onset	Duration	Mechanism of Action	Caveats
Mannitol	0.25 - 1gm IV q 6–8 hrs over 20–30 min[37]	15–30 min	1.5–6 hrs	↓ blood viscosity which ↑ cerebral blood flow and O_2 transport. Pulls H_2O from brain tissue and excretes excess H_2O in urine[38,39]	Solution is a vesicant. Crystals may form in solution; filter must be used. If crystals present, warm solution to remove them. Electrolyte abnormalities may occur - must monitor K^+, Na^+[38]
Hypertonic saline	300ml of 3% saline 250ml of 7.5% saline 75ml of 10% saline 30ml of 10% saline Infuse each IV over 30 min[38–40]	10–20 min	3–5 hours	↑ CSF absorption, ↑ cardiac output and expands intravascular volume, which improves CPP[2,39]	Electrolyte abnormalities may occur - must monitor K^+, Na^+, BUN, creatine. Can cause thrombophlebitis, central line recommended. Contraindicated if serum Na > 150mEq/L[38,40]
Dexamethasone	10mg/kg over 1–2 hours then continuous infusion 1–2 mg/kg/hour[43]	10–15 minutes	72 hours	Suppresses inflammation, interferes with mediators of inflammatory response[41]	↑ blood sugar; Risk of gastritis; must give concomitant gastric protection (H_2 blocker or PPI). Causes immunosuppression. Do not discontinue abruptly; should be tapered to ↓ risk of adrenal insufficiency[42]
Pentobarbital	10mg/kg over 1–2 hours then continuous infusion 1–2 mg/kg/hour[39]	10–15 minutes	Variable	↓ brain metabolism and cerebral blood flow[39]	Cannot monitor neurologic exam on comatose patient. Requires monitoring of ICP; EEG; CPP. Can cause respiratory suppression; requires ventilatory support. Monitor for hypotension, ↓K^+, hepatic or renal dysfunction[2,3,39]

Abbreviations: BUN: blood urea nitrogen; CPP: cerebral perfusions pressure; CSF: cerebral spinal fluid; EEG: electroencephalography; ICP: increased intracranial pressure; PPI: proton pump inhibitor.

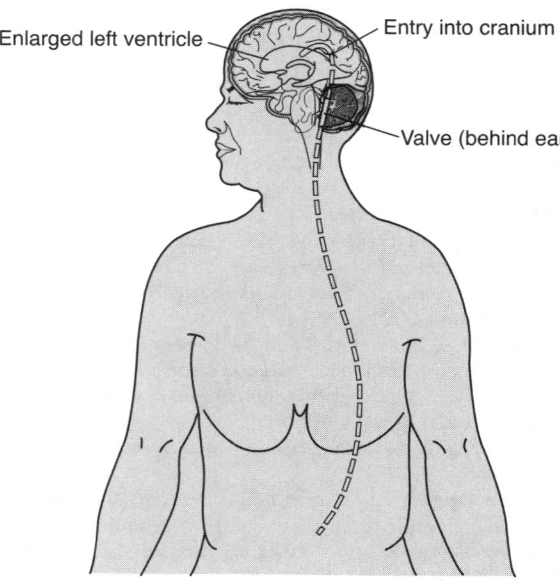

FIGURE 21-6

Ventriculoperitoneal shunt.

Source: Illustration copyright © 2012 HFS Imaging.

External ventricular drain. If urgent removal of CSF for a limited period is needed, an external ventriculostomy drain may be placed. These devices are sometimes left in place postoperatively or inserted in cases of subarachnoid hemorrhage to provide a means of rapid ICP reduction.[12]

Decompressive craniectomy. If emergent removal of material (blood clot, tumor, or abscess) is required to alleviate elevated ICP, a decompressive craniectomy may be performed. Postoperatively, the bone flap may be left off to allow for continued expansion of brain tissue from swelling until the crisis interval has passed. The goal of this procedure is to remove the primary cause of ICP elevation and prevent further brain injury related to decreased perfusion, hypoxia, or compression.[3]

NURSING IMPLICATIONS

The nurse can employ any of several interventions to minimize ICP and promote homeostasis in the affected patient (Table 21-10). Numerous authors[13,44,45] have cited the importance of maintaining a calm environment to avoid overstimulation of the patient. This approach includes applying interventions such as dim lights, avoidance of noise, and avoidance of sudden jarring of the bed, painful procedures, or emotional distress surrounding the patient.

TABLE 21-10

Nursing Interventions to Decrease ICP

Maintain proper positioning

- Head of bed elevated 30″
- Neck in neutral position
- Avoid extreme hip flexion
- Log roll when turning

Calm environment

- Avoid loud noise
- Avoid bright overhead lights
- Avoid sudden jarring of the bed
- Do not cluster noxious activities

Treat/prevent symptoms that can increase ICP

- Vomiting
- Constipation
- Coughing
- Shivering

Avoid activities that increase ICP

- Patients pushing themselves up in bed using their feet
- Patients pulling against restraints
- Patients pushing against footboard

Proper positioning of the patient (elevating the head of the bed 30 degrees and keeping the neck in a neutral, midline position) should be maintained by the nursing staff at all times. This strategy prevents compression of the jugular veins and maximizes cerebral venous return. It is important to avoid crossing limbs and extreme hip flexion, as these maneuvers also increase ICP.[3,11,13,27] Maintaining proper positioning requires the use of the log rolling position for turning when needed.

Clustering of noxious activities (suctioning or turning) that increase ICP should be avoided because this practice may cause a cumulative effect, resulting in spikes of ICP that can produce ischemia.[13,45] The Valsalva maneuver causes increased intra-abdominal and intrathoracic pressure that results in increased ICP; it occurs with coughing, vomiting, and straining with stool. Nursing staff should be mindful of the need to promptly treat symptoms with cough suppressants, antiemetic therapy, and implementation of a bowel regimen to prevent this occurrence in affected patients.[12,13]

PATIENT SELF-CARE

Caring for a patient with increased ICP and his or her family members can be challenging for even a seasoned nurse. Elevated ICP is a complex issue that can involve rapid condition changes and can be very distressing to family members. To aid in the care of the patient with increased ICP, Table 21-11 offers information regarding patient resources. A patient self-care guide dealing with pressure in the brain appears in Appendix 21A.

TABLE 21-11

Patient Resources

National Brain Tumor Society
124 Watertown Street, Suite 2D
Watertown, MA 02472
Phone: 800-770-8287
617-924-9997 Fax: 617-924-9998
http://www.braintumor.org

- Information about brain tumors
- Patient and family support groups
- Patient/family telephone network
- Brain tumor support group sites
- Resource material

American Brain Tumor Association
8550 W. Bryn Mawr Ave. Ste 550
Chicago, IL 60631
Phone: 773-577-8750
Fax: 773-577-8738
CareLine: 800-886-2282
E-mail: abtacares@abta.org
http://www.abta.org

- Information about brain tumors
- Patient and family support groups
- Patient/family telephone network
- Brain tumor support group sites
- Resource material

Brain Tumour Foundation of Canada
620 Colborne St., Suite 301
London, Ontario, Canada N6B 3R9
Phone: 800-265-5106
519-642-7755 Fax: 519-642-7192
http://www.braintumour.ca

American Cancer Society
250 Williams Street NW
Atlanta, Georgia, 30303
Phone: 800-227-2345
http://www.cancer.org

- Patient education
- Community support and resources

National Cancer Institute
NCI Office of Communications and Education
Public Inquiries Office
6116 Executive Boulevard
Suite 300
Bethesda, MD 20892-8322
Phone: 800-422-6237
http://www.cancer.gov

- Patient education
- Information on clinical trials

REFERENCES

1. Allen D. Disorders of the nervous system. In: Alexander MF, Fawcett JN, Runciman PJ, eds. *Nursing Practice: Hospital and Home.* 3rd ed. Edinburgh: Churchill Livingstone; 2006:395–442
2. Ramesh Kumar R, Singhi SC, Singhi P. Raised intracranial pressure (ICP): management in emergency department. *Indian J Pediatr.* 2012;79:518–524.
3. Pitfield AF, Carroll AB, Kissoon N. Emergency management of increased intracranial pressure. *Pediatr Emerg Care.* 2012;28:200–203.
4. Gavrilovic IT, Posner JB. Brain metastases: epidemiology and pathophysiology. *J Neurooncol.* 2005;75:5–14.
5. Barnholtz Sloan JS, Sloan AE, Davis FG, Vigneau FD, Lai P, Sawaya RE. Incidence proportions of brain metastases in patients diagnosed (1973 to 2001) in the metropolitan Detroit cancer surveillance system. *J Clin Oncol.* 2004;22(14):2865–2872.
6. Eichler AF, Loeffler JS. Multidisciplinary management of brain metastases. *Oncologist.* 2007;12:884–898.
7. American Cancer Society. Cancer facts and figures, 2012. 2012. http://www.cancer.org/acs/groups/content/@epidemiologysurveillance/documents/docurrent/acspc-031941.pdf. Accessed March 10, 2012.
8. Ropper AH, Adams RD, Brown R. Disturbances of cerebrospinal fluid and its circulation. In: Ropper AH, Brown RH, eds. *Adams and Victor's Principles of Neurology.* 8th ed. New York: McGraw-Hill; 2005:529–545.
9. American Brain Tumor Association. Brain tumors: a primer for patients and caregivers. Chicago;page 84 http://www.abta.org/secure/about-brain-tumors-a-primer.pdf, Accessed 1/31/13.
10. Arzbaecher JM. Anatomy and physiology of the brain and spine. In: Allen DH, Rice L, eds. *Central Nervous System Cancers.* Pittsburgh, PA: ONS Publications Department; 2011:5–15.
11. Lee ET, Armstrong TS. Increased intracranial pressure. *Clin J Oncol Nurs.* 2008;12:37–41.
12. Hickey JV. Comprehensive neurological examination. In: Hickey JV, ed. *The Clinical Practice of Neurological and Neurosurgical Nursing.* 6th ed. Philadelphia, PA: Lippincott Williams & Wilkins; 2009:111–153.
13. Hickey JV, Olson DM. Intracranial hypertension: theory and management of increased intracranial pressure. In: Hickey JV, ed. *The Clinical Practice of Neurological and Neurosurgical Nursing.* 6th ed. Philadelphia, PA: Lippincott Williams & Wilkins; 2009:270–304.
14. Ravi R, Morgan RJ. Intracranial pressure monitoring. *Curr Anaesthes Crit Care.* 2003; 14:229–235.
15. Stein DM, Hu PF, Brenner M, et al. Brief episodes of intracranial hypertension and cerebral hypoperfusion are associated with poor functional outcome after severe traumatic brain injury. *J Trauma Injury Infect Crit Care.* 2011;71:364–374.
16. Bickley LS. The nervous system. In: Bickley LS, Szilagyi PS, eds. *Bates' Guide to Physical Examination and History Taking.* 10th ed. Philadelphia, PA: Wolters Kluwer/Lippincott, Williams & Wilkins; 2008:655–735.
17. Lee ET, Westcarth LJ. Patient assessment. In: Allen DH, Rice LL, eds. *Central Nervous System Cancers.* Pittsburgh, PA: ONS Publications Department; 2011:17–34
18. Wilkes GM. Increased intracranial pressure. In: Yarbro CH, Frogge MH, Goodman M, eds. *Cancer Symptom Management.* 3rd ed. 2004:374–388. Sudbury, MA: Jones & Bartlett Learning.
19. O'Brien MD. Motor testing. In: Guarantors of Brain, ed. *Aids to the Examination of the Peripheral Nervous System.* 5th ed. London: Saunders Elsevier; 2010:1–3.
20. Ghajar J. Traumatic brain injury. *Lancet.* 2000;356:923–929.
21. Rao GS, Durga P. Changing trends in monitoring brain ischemia: from intracranial pressure to cerebral oximetry. *Curr Opin Anesthesiol.* 2011;24:487–494.
22. Frattalone AR, Stevens RD. Intracranial pressure and its surrogates. *Intens Care Med.* 2011;37:1051–1053.
23. Kornbluth J, Bhardway A. Evaluation of coma: a critical appraisal of popular scoring systems. *Neurocritical Care.* 2011;14:134–143.

24. Roque PJ, Wu TS, Barth L, et al. Optic nerve ultrasound for the detection of elevated intracranial pressure in the hypertensive patient. *Am J Emerg Med.* 2011. doi:10.1016/j.ajem.2011.09.025.
25. Rosenberg JB, Shiloh AL, Savel RH, Eisen LA. Non-invasive methods of estimating intracranial pressure. *Neurocritical Care.* 2011;15:599–608.
26. National Institutes of Health, National Cancer Institute. Common terminology criteria for adverse events (CTCAE) version 4.0. http://evs.nci.nih.gov/ftp1/CTCAE_4.03_2010-06-14_QuickReference_5x7.pdf. Accessed July 7, 2012.
27. Marcoux KK. Management of increased intracranial pressure in the critically ill child with an acute neurological injury. *AACN Clin Issues.* 2005;16:212–231.
28. Muizelaar JP, Mamarou A, Ward JD, et al. Adverse effects of prolonged hyperventilation in patients with severe head injury: a randomized clinical trial. *J Neurosurg.* 1991;75:731–739.
29. Schneider GH, von Helden A, Lanksch WR, Unterberg, A. Continuous monitoring of jugular bulb oxygen saturation in comatose patients: therapeutic implications. *Acta Neurochir.* 1995;134:71–75.
30. von Helden A, Schneider GH, Unterberg A, Lanksch, WR. Monitoring of jugular venous oxygen saturation in comatose patients with subarachnoid haemorrhage and intracerebral hematomas. *Acta Neurochir.* 1993;59:102–106.
31. Brain Trauma Foundation, American Association of Neurological Surgeons, Congress of Neurological Surgeons, et al. Guidelines for the management of severe traumatic brain injury. VII. Intracranial pressure monitoring technology. *J Neurotrauma.* 2007;24(suppl 1):S45.
32. Marion DW, Penrod LE, Kelsey SF, et al. Treatment of traumatic brain injury with moderate hypothermia. *N Engl J Med.* 1997;336:540–546.
33. Polderman KH, Hoe RTT, Peerdeman SM, Vandertop WP, Girbes AR. Effects of therapeutic hypothermia on intracranial pressure and outcome in patients with severe head injury. *Intens Care Med.* 2002;28:1563–1573.
34. Shiozaki T, Hayakata T, Taneda M, et al. A multicenter prospective randomized trial of the efficacy of mild hypothermia for severely head injured patients with low intracranial pressure. *J Neurosurg.* 2001;94:50–54.
35. Clifton GL, Miller ER, Choi SC, et al. Lack of effect of induction of hypothermia after acute brain injury. *N Engl J Med.* 2001;334:556–563.
36. Metz C, Holzschuh M, Bein T, et al. Moderate hypothermia in patients with severe head injury: cerebral and extracerebral effects. *J Neurosurg.* 1996;85:533–541.
37. Rabinstein AA. Treatment of cerebral edema. *Neurologist.* 2006;12:59–73.
38. Bratton SL, Chestnut RM, Ghajar J, et al. Guidelines for the management of severe traumatic brain injury. II. Hyperosmolar therapy. *J Neurotrauma.* 2007;24(suppl 1):S14–S20.
39. Ennis KM, Brophy GM. Management of intracranial hypertension: focus on pharmacologic strategies. *AACN Adv Crit Care.* 2011;22:177–182.
40. Torre-Healy A, Marko NF, Weil RJ. Hyperosmolar therapy for intracranial hypertension. *Neurocrit Care.* 2012;17:117–130.
41. Edwards P, Arango M, Balica L, et al. Final results of MRC CRASH, a randomized placebo-controlled trial of intravenous corticosteroid in adults with head injury-outcomes at 6 months. *Lancet.* 2005;365:1957–1959.
42. Batchelor TT, Byrne TN. Neurological complications of primary brain tumors. In: Schiff D, Kesari S, Wen P, eds. *Cancer Neurology in Clinical Practice: Neurologic Complications of Cancer and Its Treatment (Current Clinical Oncology).* Totowa, NJ: Humana Press; 2008:381–396.
43. Vallerand AH, Sanoski CA, Hopfer-Deglin J. Dexamethasone. In: *Davis's Drug Guide for Nurses.* 12th ed. Philadelphia, PA: FA Davis; 2011:350.
44. Tume LN, Baines PB, Lisboa PJG. The effect of nursing interventions on the intracranial pressure in paediatric traumatic brain injury. *Brit Assoc Crit Care Nurs.* 2011;16:77–84.
45. Suadoni MT. Raised intracranial pressure: nursing observations and interventions. *Nurs Stand.* 2009;23:35–40.

Increased Pressure in the Brain

Patient Name: ______________________________

Symptom and Description

This guide will help you and your family to know signs of increased pressure in your brain and understand what you can do to prevent the problem from getting worse.

Increased pressure in your brain can occur from the following causes:

- Infection or bleeding in the brain
- Injury to the head from a fall or accident
- Spread of cancer to your brain

Signs you should look for include these conditions:

- Frequent headache that worsens over days to weeks
- Decreased attention span and concentration
- Weakness on one side of the body

Management

If you have these symptoms, you need to tell your doctor or nurse. If you have already been diagnosed with this problem, the following tips will help you to minimize the seriousness of the symptom.

- Avoid activities that increase the pressure in the abdomen or chest, such as coughing, vomiting, and straining with bowel movements, lifting heavy objects, or bending at the waist.
- Take medicines such as antinausea pills, cough suppressants, and stool softeners to prevent vomiting, coughing, or constipation.
- Keep your head elevated with pillows at night and your neck straight (avoid turning the neck sharply to the side or bending the neck forward or backward).
- Keep a calm environment with low stress and tension levels.

Follow-Up

The best treatment for this problem is to eliminate its cause with the correct therapy. The cause may be infection, bleeding, or tumor. The treatment may include surgery, radiation therapy, or antibiotics. It will be important for you and your family to report any changes that may be a sign of the problem getting worse, such as more severe headache, development of nausea related to headache, weakness in one body area, or changes in vision, hearing, or other senses.

You will likely have follow-up clinic appointments scheduled during this time, but any rapid worsening of symptoms requires an urgent call to your healthcare provider.

Phone Numbers:

Doctor: ________________________________ Phone: ________________

Nurse: ________________________________ Phone: ________________

Other: ________________________________ Phone: ________________

Comments:

____

____

____

____

Source: Fields MM. Increased Intracranial Pressure. In: Yarbro CH, Wujcik D, Gobel BH, eds. *Cancer Symptom Management.* 4th ed. Burlington, MA: Jones & Bartlett Learning; 2014.

Chapter 22

Peripheral Neuropathy

Gail M. Wilkes, RNC, MS, AOCN®

THE PROBLEM

Peripheral neuropathy (PN)—a condition caused by inflammation, injury, or degeneration of one or more peripheral nerve fibers—often occurs in patients with cancer.[1] Chemotherapy-induced peripheral neuropathy (CIPN) is related to injury to the peripheral nerves from neurotoxic chemotherapy. Its mechanism of injury, incidence, and severity are related to the drug, dose, duration, and any other neurotoxic drugs coadministered. Symptoms of peripheral neuropathy relate to the specific nerve injury and depend on whether sensory, motor, autonomic, or cranial nerve dysfunction is involved. Symptoms can range from paresthesias alone to severe and disabling sensorimotor pain and muscle weakness.

The cost of peripheral neuropathy can be very expensive, in terms of both money and quality of life. In 1999, the estimated treatment cost for a patient with CIPN was approximately $5507.[2] In 2012, average costs for patients who developed CIPN within 9 months of treatment were $17,344 higher than those for controls without CIPN, largely due to outpatient costs of $8092.[3] Patients with CIPN had an average of 12 more outpatient visits than controls, as well as more extensive hospital stays.

More importantly, peripheral neuropathy can greatly diminish quality of life (QOL). This was documented in 1988 for patients receiving high-dose cisplatin who developed CIPN.[4] Patients with symptomatic CIPN had an increased likelihood of fatigue, malaise, and psychological distress, and one year post treatment, they also had significantly decreased satisfaction with life, sense of well-being, and ability to work or perform activities of daily living (ADLs). More recently, Cachia et al. studied 32 patients who had pain and peripheral neuropathy, and found physical functioning scores on QOL measures correlated with pain, QOL, and fatigue (all $p = 0.001$).[5] Tofthagen described patient perceptions associated with CIPN: pain or discomfort, loss of sensation in upper and lower extremities, and frustration as symptoms interfered with ADLs.[6] In addition, these researchers have described injuries related to numbness, muscle weakness, and loss of balance. Further, patient risk for falls increases with each chemotherapy cycle, and patients receiving taxanes may be at greater risk for falls than patients receiving platinum-based drugs.[7] Thus, the nurse should assess patients for muscle weakness, loss of balance, or patient perception that symptoms interfere with walking or driving, as affected patients may be at a higher risk for falls.[7] Other research has shown that patients with CIPN have diverse symptom patterns, and degrees of symptom distress ranging from mild to severe emotional distress, changes in functional ability, and impairment of social role.[8]

Personal independence is greatly threatened by the various manifestations of peripheral neuropathy, such as severe, painful paresthesias, footdrop, and wristdrop. Individuals who work with their hands and who lose fine motor control may be unable to work to support their families.

Nurses are key in identifying neuropathic changes early, teaching self-care measures, and, if peripheral neuropathy develops, ensuring that patients find rehabilitation services and learn measures to reduce disability. In addition, if the patient is responding to the chemotherapy drug, early identification of PN is critical, as the drug dose may be modified so the patient can continue on therapy, or a change can be made in the treatment plan to minimize worsening of PN. Throughout care, emotional support to prevent loss of self-esteem is very important as well.

INCIDENCE

While it is estimated that 10% to 20% of patients with cancer will develop PN,[9] Teravainen and Larsen found that 48% of patients with lung cancer had peripheral neuropathy before beginning chemotherapy.[10] Further, diabetes mellitus affects 8% to 18% of patients with cancer, and approximately 37% to 59% of patients with diabetes will develop PN.[11] The incidence of CIPN is estimated at 20% to 40% of patients.[12] Studies have explored the incidence related to type of chemotherapy. One study of more than 65,000 elderly patients with breast, ovarian, and lung cancer found that patients receiving taxanes alone were twice as likely to develop CIPN, while those receiving platinum–taxane combinations were three times as likely to develop this problem, compared to patients who did not receive chemotherapy.[13] However, it is generally accepted that the incidence of PN is underreported.[14] Reasons for underreporting include patient-related (e.g., reluctance to report symptoms due to fear of meaning/cancer recurrence, lack of knowledge), provider-related (e.g., underdiagnosed due to knowledge and skill deficits, lack of standardized PN assessment), and science-related (e.g., limited research findings related to standardized measurement tools) factors[15]; lack of reliable and valid diagnostic instruments to document and grade CIPN; and reported low incidences of severe PN in smaller, earlier clinical trials, which are found to be higher in larger-powered studies.[16]

Peripheral neuropathy is a significant national health problem, and it has catalyzed the formation of a number of working groups such as the National Comprehensive Cancer Network (NCCN) task force on neuropathy in cancer, which has led to a prospective surveillance model for physical rehabilitation for women with breast cancer.[17] The incidences of CIPN related to specific agents, as reported by the NCCN task force, are shown in Table 22-1.

TABLE 22-1

Incidence of Chemotherapy-Induced Peripheral Neuropathy (CIPN) Related to Specific Chemotherapy Agents

Drug	Incidence of CIPN
Paclitaxel	57%–83% overall, 2%–33% severe
Docetaxel	11%–64% overall, 3%–14% severe
Albumin-bound paclitaxel	73% overall, 10%–15% severe
Vinca Alkaloids	30%–47% overall
Cisplatin	28%–100% overall
Carboplatin	6%–42% overall
Oxaliplatin	Acute 85%–95% overall, persistent 10%–18%
Bortezomib	31%–55% overall, 9%–22% severe
Thalidomide	25%–83% overall, 15%–28% severe
Lenalidomide	10%–23% overall, 1%–3% severe
Carboplatin + paclitaxel	67% overall, 4%–9% severe
Capecitabine + ixabepilone	67%, with 21% severe

Source: Data from Stubblefield et al[18].

ETIOLOGY

Patients may have existing PN or be at increased risk for developing PN, and this relationship is aggravated by cancer or its treatment—specifically, neurotoxic chemotherapy. Risk factors are numerous and discussed in the section on symptom assessment. Cancer itself as well as the disease's treatment—most commonly chemotherapy, but also radiation therapy, surgery, and biological therapy—may cause PN. The most common chemotherapeutic agents that cause or worsen preexisting PN are shown in Table 22-2.[16,19–25]

Higher doses of neurotoxic chemotherapy or drugs given in combination with overlapping neurotoxicity increase the risk of CIPN. Research is ongoing to identify whether gene polymorphisms increase the risk of developing CIPN with various neurotoxic chemotherapy drugs.[26]

As patients with cancer survive longer due to effective multimodality treatment, the incidence of PN will likely increase. Less common causes of cancer-related peripheral neuropathy are tumor infiltration and compression of spinal nerves, and rarely paraneoplastic sensorimotor neuropathy with axonal degeneration or segmental demyelination.[16]

The focus of this chapter is on chemotherapy-induced peripheral neuropathy.

PATHOPHYSIOLOGY

The exact pathophysiology of CIPN is unknown but is thought to relate to damage to the mitochondria (energy storehouse) in the nerve cell.[27,28] To better understand the underlying process, a review of the peripheral nerves is helpful.

The central nervous system (CNS) is composed of the brain and spinal cord, and the peripheral nerves bring information from the body/periphery to the CNS, and messages from the CNS back out to the periphery. The peripheral nerves in general are sensory, motor, cranial, and autonomic fibers. They can be subdivided into large

TABLE 22-2

Drugs Associated with Peripheral Neurotoxicity (PN)

Chemotherapy	Primarily Sensory	Sensorimotor	Primarily Motor	Autonomic Nervous System	Cranial Nerves	Comments
Arsenic		√				33% incidence of paresthesias; partially reversible
Bortezomib	√; primarily small fiber sensory nerves of lower limbs	Rare		√; less common: diarrhea, constipation, nausea, vomiting, urinary or sexual dysfunction, orthostatic hypotension		Incidence 33%–66% in patients with multiple myeloma; dose dependent; reversible, unlike investigational analogues carfilzomib and marizomib
Carboplatin	√; sensory			√	√	Uncommon as single agent unless high dose, cumulative dose >400 mg/m^2; risk up to 74% when combined with paclitaxel; coasting* may occur
Carmustine				√	√ (intra-arterial)	
Cisplatin	√; primarily sensory (large) fibers			√; orthostatic hypotension	√; decreased hearing common, altered vision rare	Cumulative dose >300–500mg/m^2; increased risk when combined with paclitaxel; coasting often occurs
Cytarabine		√		√		Rare; from pure sensory to sensorimotor; cerebellar dysfunction with ataxia at high doses
Docetaxel		√; Predominantly sensory, large fibers> small or unmyelinated fibers		√		Increased risk with dose 100 mg/m^2 or cumulative dose of > 600 mg/m^2; dose-limiting toxicity; coasting may occur
Erubulin mesylate		√				Low incidence; in clinical trials, 5% of patients had CIPN >1 year
5-fluorouracil (5-FU)		√				Rare; increased risk in patients who lack the enzyme dihydropyridimidine dehydrogenase; rare cerebellar ataxia; also PN exacerbation reported after topical 5-FU treatment

(continued)

TABLE 22-2

Drugs Associated with Peripheral Neurotoxicity (PN)

Chemotherapy	Primarily Sensory	Sensorimotor	Primarily Motor	Autonomic Nervous System	Cranial Nerves	Comments
Hexamethylmelamine		√				Increased risk if preexisting cisplatin PN
Ixabepilone		√; sensory > motor				Increased risk dose >40mg/m²; severe from 4th cycle; reversible
Lenalidomide	√					CIPN significantly lower in incidence and severity than thalidomide
Methotrexate	√				√	Rare; increased risk with high-dose methotrexate, which crosses the blood-brain barrier
Oxaliplatin	√ (persistent, chronic) √ (acute)	Rare motor				Risk cumulative dose >750 mg/m²; reversible in most cases; acute pharyngolaryngeal dysestheia may occur but can be prevented with avoidance of exposure to cold; coasting may occur
Paclitaxel (all formulations)		√; large sensory fibers > small or unmyelinated fibers		√; paralytic ileus, orthostatic hypotension,	√; rare optic nerve dysfunction	Increased risk with dose >175/m² q 3 weeks, >100 mg/m² q week, or cumulative dose >500 mg/m²; dose-limiting toxicity; usually reversible
Procarbazine		√		√; orthostatic hypotension		Incidence 20% unless combined with vincristine, which increases risk
Thalidomide	√	√; sensory > motor				Reflexes usually preserved; irreversible
Vinblastine		√		√	√	
Vincristine		√		√; ileus, constipation, jaw pain	√; ptosis	Dose-limiting; extensor muscle weakness upper, lower extremities; begins early (e.g., 2 weeks); coasting may occur; reversible in up to 2 years
Vindesine		√		√	√	
Vinorelbine		√; sensory > motor		√	√	Increased PN when combined with paclitaxel

*Coasting: chemotherapy induced peripheral neuropathy (CIPN) worsens after drug is discontinued.

Source: Data from Hausheer[16]; Amato and Baron[19]; Berkowitz and Walker[20]; Renbarger et al[21]; Richardson et al[22]; Richards[23]; Saif et al[24]; Velasco et al[25].

myelinated, small myelinated, and small unmyelinated nerves. Sensory fibers can be large myelinated fibers that conduct proprioception (knowing where body parts are in relation to the body) and vibration impulses to the brain rapidly, or the small myelinated and unmyelinated fibers that conduct pain and temperature.[29] Motor axons are usually large myelinated fibers.

The peripheral nerves originate from the spinal cord and are composed of 43 pairs of nerves: 12 pairs of cranial nerves and 31 pairs that enter the spinal cord and become the spinal nerves.[30] All nerve fibers are enclosed within a Schwann cell, but some are more tightly wrapped in Schwann cell layers, forming a myelin sheath. This enhances the speed of conduction of the nerve impulse. The cranial nerves have motor or sensory function, and four have parasympathetic function, controlling involuntary body functions such as digestion and elimination. Each pair of spinal nerves has sensory afferent and motor efferent fibers that receive and give information about a specific area or distribution of the body called a *dermatome* (Figure 22-1). In the spinal cord, each spinal nerve separates into two roots: ventral and dorsal. The ventral root is made up of motor fibers that carry (efferent) impulses from the CNS to the muscles and glands of the body telling that body part what to do (e.g., voluntary movement, muscle tone, coordination). The cell body of the motor neuron lies within the spinal cord with the axon in the periphery. If a motor neuron is damaged or injured, the muscle that it innervates can weaken and atrophy over time. When injured, the surviving axon grows new branches to innervate muscle areas that have lost innervation due to injury.[30]

The dorsal root contains sensory fibers that bring (afferent) sensory messages of touch, pain, temperature, vibration, and body position from the skin, muscles, and joints to the spinal cord and up to higher brain centers. The long axon and cell body of these fibers are outside the CNS, so they are exposed to blood carrying neurotoxic chemotherapy. This may explain why sensory PN is more common than motor PN, but with continued therapy, injury may progress to become sensorimotor PN.[16]

Similar to the *somatic* nervous system, which was just described, the *autonomic* nervous system is also part of the peripheral nervous system and has sensory and motor nerve fibers that bring sensory information, such as blood pressure and level of oxygenation, from the blood vessels and internal and endocrine organs to the spinal cord. Autonomic peripheral nerves are responsible for controlling involuntary movement and intestinal motility. Motor fibers carry the CNS instructions, such as blood vessel constriction or intestinal muscle contraction, to the blood vessels and organs. The autonomic neuron has its cell body in a ganglion outside the cord where it can be exposed to blood containing neurotoxic chemotherapy.

Together with the neurofilaments that support the nerve axon, the microtubules in the sensory and motor axons form a conveyor belt-like pathway between the synapse and cell body so that key enzymes, neurotransmitters, and other proteins travel down the network of microtubules, while other organelles such as mitochondria and actin move by intermediate or slow axonal transport.[16] Motor proteins attached to microtubules are responsible for helping the message pass from the periphery to the CNS and back again, and also transport substances back and forth from the synapse or sensory nerve endings. The axon cannot function without healthy axonal microtubules, which are constantly undergoing assembly and disassembly and can be damaged by chemotherapy.

While not completely understood, CIPN is generally classified as distal *axonopathy* since it disrupts peripheral nerve function and results in degeneration of primarily terminal sensory axons and less commonly motor axons; rarely it may involve *neuronopathy* (resulting from direct damage to the dorsal root ganglia neuronal cell bodies, and destruction of axons).[16]

Distal axonopathy occurs from most neurotoxic chemotherapy and involves a progressive onset of symptoms after a number of treatment cycles. Symptoms arise first from the longest axons going to the toes, then to the fingertips. Symptom constellation involves distal symmetric paresthesias, dysesthesia, burning, pain, or numbness initially in the lower extremities, then the upper extremities, in a stocking–glove distribution. Severe symptoms may involve loss of deep tendon reflexes and ataxia.[16] Symptoms may "wax and wane" between treatment cycles, but with continued treatment, they become persistent and damage is cumulative.[16] Symptoms may continue to progress and become more severe after therapy (e.g., cisplatin) is stopped, a phenomenon called "coasting."[31] While CIPN is primarily neurosensory, motor neuropathy may also occur, characterized by distal muscle weakness and atrophy that may or may not interfere with function or ability to do ADLs.

In contrast, the less common CIPN neuronopathy (damage to the neuron) is associated with high-dose neurotoxic chemotherapy (e.g., taxanes or cisplatin), and is characterized by the rapid onset of symmetric distal sensory neuropathy of both upper and lower extremities as well as cranial nerves, and a rapid loss of deep tendon reflexes.[16] Symptoms occur rapidly (within hours to days) and are persistent.[16]

It is no surprise that chemotherapeutic agents that target the microtubules and neurofilaments of malignant cells damage normal nerve cells, causing interruption in axonal transport, degeneration of the distal axon, and damage to the sensory nerve cell bodies in the dorsal root ganglia. The incidence and severity of CIPN are related to the drug(s) (e.g., single neurotoxic drug or combination therapy), dose (e.g., dose dense versus standard dose, cumulative dose),

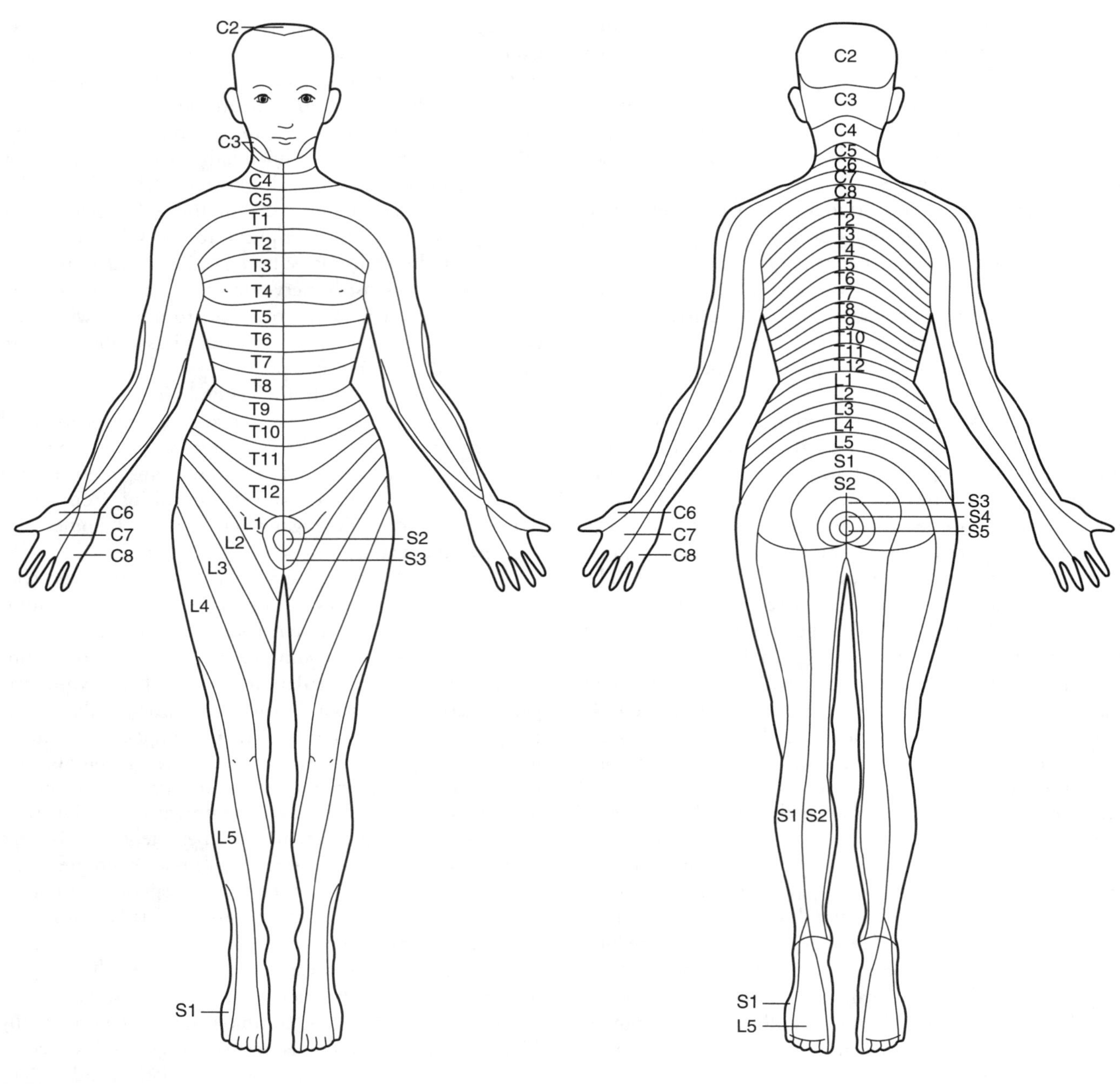

FIGURE 22-1

Dermatomes of the body.

schedule (e.g., weekly versus every 2–3 weeks), and duration of neurotoxic therapy (cumulative dose), as well as the patient's history of coexisting PN or risk for PN.[16] The sensory and/or motor axons are injured by chemotherapy, as are the Schwann cells and, if involved, the myelin sheath (depending on the drug). Sensory axons can be either large fibers or small fibers. Large fibers carry vibration and position information, and are important in proprioception. Small fibers carry touch, pain, and temperature messages. Initially, symptoms arise from damage to the longest sensory axons that stretch from the spinal cord to the toes/feet, then the fingers/hands, a pattern commonly referred to as "stocking–glove" distribution; this sort of damage affects the fine sensory nerve endings in the skin that transmit to the dorsal horn ganglia at the level of the spinal cord.[16] Demyelination reduces nerve conduction velocity, leading to loss of deep tendon reflexes. Deep tendon reflex loss is greater in the ankles than in the knees and arms.[9] Injury to the unmyelinated autonomic nerve fiber microtubules can result in bowel or bladder dysfunction, such as constipation, paralytic ileus, and bladder atony, or loss of blood pressure stability with severe orthostatic hypotension. Cranial nerve injury can result in dysfunction depending on the cranial nerve damaged—for example, impaired hearing (ototoxicity), facial nerve palsy, or vocal cord paralysis (laryngeal nerve paralysis). Individuals at greatest risk are those with preexisting PN. It is possible that genetic factors play a role in the incidence and severity of CIPN, such as single-nucleotide polymorphonucleotide polymorphisms (SNPs) related to vincristine or thalidomide in patients with multiple myeloma.[32]

Chemotherapy-induced peripheral neuropathy is a risk factor for developing neuropathic pain. In one study of patients with breast cancer who previously had received paclitaxel, and who had grade 2 or greater CIPN, patients had a three times greater likelihood of developing neuropathic pain at a mean follow-up of 9.5 years.[33] Wolf et al. showed in a prospective study that patients with severe symptoms of sensory CIPN do not all have severe neuropathic pain.[34] Neuropathic pain is challenging, and research suggests that it involves cytokines that are activated, leading to an inflammatory cascade, which leads to axonal injury, and later to CIPN-induced pain.[35] Animal studies have shown that after chemotherapy is given, two substances are likely culprits leading to neuropathic pain: peroxynitrite, an oxidant that is now overproduced and enters nerve cells, damaging or destroying the mitochondria; and sphingolipids, which also damage nerve cells.[36] By blocking these two chemicals, the researchers were able both to prevent paclitaxel-induced CIPN and to reverse it. Interestingly, peroxynitrite appears to reduce or neutralize the analgesic effects of morphine.[36]

The chemotherapy drugs most likely to cause CIPN are discussed here in terms of their pathophysiology, clinical manifestations, and recovery. Onset, rate of progression, severity, pattern, and reversibility vary by drug, dose, cumulative dose, infusion time, and schedule.

CHEMOTHERAPEUTIC AGENTS LIKELY TO CAUSE PERIPHERAL NEUROPATHY

Vinca alkaloids

Vinca alkaloids are effective anticancer drugs that destroy cells through microtubular destabilization.[37,38] Unfortunately, the microtubules in the axon transport system are inhibited as well, resulting in axonal degeneration. Vincristine binds directly to the microtubules and destroys them (depolymerizes tubulin), causing axonal sensorimotor neuropathy. Nerve studies show decreased amplitude of sensory nerve action potentials, resembling axonal degeneration.[18] Damage occurs to small sensory fibers (pain/temperature) to a greater degree than to the large fibers (vibratory/position), but both are affected. Initial symptoms are sequential and symmetric, beginning with paresthesias in the fingertips and toes, as well as decreased Achilles deep tendon reflex, which occurs in almost all patients. This progresses to myalgia, painful paresthesias of the fingers and then hands and feet, sensitivity to light touch and temperature, and absent ankle reflexes. Continued drug administration often leads to motor weakness in the wrist (extensors) and foot (dorsiflexors), resulting in wristdrop and footdrop, respectively. Vibration, position, pinprick senses, and two-point discrimination often remain intact.[18] Neuropathy is bilateral and worse in the lower extremities, so that further motor weakness creates a broad-based stance with a slapping gait. Drug discontinuance when paresthesias first appear will result in brisk resolution, whereas motor weakness may take months and sensory loss years to resolve.[18] In cases of severe CIPN, vincristine may cause a syndrome called coasting, which entails a worsening of signs and symptoms after treatment is stopped.[39]

Damage to the autonomic fibers can also occur. Dizziness (orthostatic hypotension), constipation (slowed peristalsis), abdominal colicky pain, ileus, impotence, and urinary retention are possible outcomes. Cranial nerve injury can result in bilateral palsies (bilateral ptosis, diplopia), recurrent laryngeal nerve damage (vocal cord paresis and hoarseness), trigeminal nerve inflammation (jaw pain), photophobia, and transient cortical blindness.[9] Rarely, reversible optic neuropathy has been described.[38]

Although the other vinca alkaloids may also cause neurotoxicity, they are listed here in order of decreasing risk: vincristine > vindesine > vinblastine > vinorelbine.[16] Vinorelbine causes primarily sensory CIPN that is mild to moderate and reversible when treatment ends.[37] Efforts to develop a less neurotoxic but more active vinca alkaloid led to the development of vinflunine, an investigational third-generation, bifluorinated, semisynthetic vinca alkaloid derived from vinorelbine.[40] Factors that increase risk of neurotoxicity with vincristine are (1) frequent drug administration, such as weekly; (2) dose greater than 2 mg; (3) age greater than 60 years; (4) concomitant isoniazid, teniposide, or etoposide therapy; (5) severe liver dysfunction, as the drug undergoes hepatic metabolism and clearance,[14] (6) coadministration of azole antifungals, such as itraconazole,[41] and (7) polymorphisms in CYP3A5 expression.[21]

Taxanes

In contrast to the vinca alkaloids, which cause microtubular destabilization, the taxanes and epothilones cause microtubular stabilization.[37] Paclitaxel promotes the assembly of microtubules and prevents depolymerization, thereby preventing the microtubules from reorganizing during mitosis (cell division), so the cell dies. This agent causes abnormal bundles of microtubules to form throughout the cell cycle; in the peripheral nerve, this effect leads to axonal degeneration and demyelination.[42] Risk of neurotoxicity is increased with dose per treatment cycle, the concomitant administration of neurotoxic drugs such as cisplatin, high doses (more than 200 mg/m^2), high cumulative doses, and preexisting diabetes or alcoholism. The finding that the rate of taxane-associated PN is related to dose per treatment cycle—for example, the incidence of grade 3/4 CIPN (higher toxicity grade) at a dose of 175 mg/m^2 was found to be 2% to 12%, compared to 12% to 32% with a dose of 250 mg/m^2—has led to lower taxane dosing.[37] Similarly, weekly paclitaxel with higher dose intensity resulted in higher grade 3 sensory neuropathy (23%) compared to a dosing schedule of every three weeks (12%).[43] Finally, with dose-dense paclitaxel given weekly over 1 hour, doses greater than 100 mg/m^2 may cause severe neurotoxicity.[43] Initially, patients may experience an acute pain episode described as "arthralgia" and "myalgia" that develops 1 to 3 days following treatment, which may be severe. Loprinzi et al. defined the natural history of this syndrome in a prospective North Central Cancer Treatment Group (NCCTG) cohort study (N08C1) and concluded that it represented nerve pathology rather than arthralgia and myalgia.[44]

Taxane CIPN is primarily sensory, beginning with paresthesias of the feet and hands (burning, tingling, numbness) in a "stocking–glove" distribution. Alterations in proprioception and vibration sense often result in difficulty climbing stairs.[42] Loss of deep tendon reflexes, leg muscle weakness, and loss of fine motor movement (e.g., difficulty buttoning clothing) may occur as well. In many patients, this CIPN is reversible. Survivors of breast cancer who developed CIPN related to paclitaxel may develop a post-treatment neuropathic pain syndrome, which in one study had an incidence of 27% at 9 years post treatment.[45]

Docetaxel also promotes microtubule formation, but prevents disassembly so that the elements cannot come apart, thereby halting cell division. Nerve damage results in axonal degeneration and demyelination. The CIPN resulting from docetaxel use is primarily sensory neuropathy, and less commonly motor neuropathy. Incidence is related to dose, ranging from 19% at 60 mg/m^2 to 49% at 100 mg/m^2 and to a cumulative dosage of 400 mg/m^2 or greater.[27] Combined therapy with another neurotoxic agent, such as cisplatin, oxaliplatin, or vinorelbine, also increases risk. Common symptoms of docetaxel-related CIPN include paresthesia, dysesthesia, and pain. Motor neuropathy, if it occurs, is characterized by distal extremity weakness. Discontinuation of therapy usually results in slow resolution over a period ranging from 0 to 106 weeks, with a median of 9 weeks.[46]

Cabazitaxel, a taxane microtubule inhibitor, has activity in docetaxel-resistant tumors. It is associated with a low incidence of CIPN (14%), 1% of which is classified as grade 3/4.[47]

Nab-paclitaxel (albumin-bound paclitaxel) was developed in an effort to permit increased doses of paclitaxel, which are otherwise limited by its solvent cremaphor EL, and to reduce toxicity, including CIPN. The drug, encased in albumin, acts as a Trojan horse, releasing paclitaxel into the tumor cells. Doses of paclitaxel delivered through this vehicle are significantly higher (e.g., 260 mg/m^2) than standard paclitaxel (175 mg/m^2) administered in a cremaphor EL solvent every 3 weeks. The incidence of CIPN is understandably higher than with paclitaxel, but demonstrates a fairly rapid reversibility.[48] Gradishar et al. reported the incidence of sensory neuropathy as well as the reversibility of *nab*-paclitaxel CIPN to be 71% (10% grade 3), compared to 56% (2% grades 3/4) for paclitaxel when given every 3 weeks. More than half of the *nab*-paclitaxel patients had reversal of CIPN after a median of 22 days post treatment interruption.[49] *Nab*-paclitaxel weekly (100 mg/m^2 or 150 mg/m^2 weekly) and every 3 weeks (300 mg/m^2) were compared to docetaxel (100 mg/m^2) given every 3 weeks as first-line treatment of metastatic breast cancer. The frequency and grade of CIPN were similar in all groups. Median time to improvement in CIPN was 16 days in the *nab*-paclitaxel every-3-weeks dosing group, 22 days in the lower-dose weekly group, and 23 days in the higher *nab*-paclitaxel dose given weekly, compared to 41 days in the docetaxel group. The overall response rate (ORR) was significantly higher and the time to progression (TTP) longer in both of the weekly *nab*-paclitaxel groups compared to the group who received docetaxel given every 3 weeks.[50] Rarely, cranial nerve palsies, vocal cord paresis, and paralytic ileus (autonomic neuropathy) have been described in patients receiving *nab*-paclitaxel.[51]

Epothilones

Epothilones are another group of microtubule-stabilizing agents, of which ixabepilone is FDA approved and others are under investigation. Ixabepilone binds to specific subunits of the microtubules, stabilizing them so they cannot interact during cell division, and causing cell death. It also avoids drug resistance pathways.[52] In initial clinical trials, the incidence of sensory neuropathy related to ixabepilone was 62% (14% grade 3/4) and the incidence of motor neuropathy was 10% (1% grade 3) when ixabepilone was given as a single agent. When this agent was combined with capecitabine in the treatment of metastatic breast cancer, the incidence of sensory neuropathy was 64% (20% grade 3) and the incidence of motor neuropathy was 16% (5% grade 4); 80% of patients had improvement to grade 1 or baseline, or no worsening of PN with dose reduction.[53] Reduced incidence and severity of CIPN was found with a lower dose (6 mg/m^2/day) given on days 1–5 of a 3-week cycle compared to a 40 mg/m^2 IV dose given every 3 weeks.[54]

In a study comparing it with erubulin mesylate, ixabepilone caused 15% more CIPN, and the onset of first symptoms was earlier (11.6 weeks in the ixabepilone arm versus 35.6 weeks in the erubulin mesylate arm).[55] Eribulin mesylate is a non-taxane, microtubule dynamics inhibitor that binds to one end of the microtubules so that they cannot grow (polymerize); the microtubules then clump together, preventing mitosis and causing cell death. The incidence of all grades of CIPN reported was 35%, with 8% of cases being grade 3/4. Twenty percent of patients in the reported study had baseline PN (grades 1/2). Twenty-two percent of patients had developed a new/worsened PN that did not recover after an average of 269 days after dose reduction/interruption. CIPN lasted for more than 1 year in 5% of patients.[55] CIPN was primarily sensory in nature, but motor neuropathy can also occur.[56,57]

Platinols

Cisplatin is a heavy metal that damages the dorsal root ganglia and causes axonal degeneration and secondary segmental demyelination of the large-fiber (vibration/proprioception) sensory nerves.[19] The extent of injury is dose related, and, as cumulative doses exceed 300 mg/m^2 and approach 500 mg/m^2, almost 100% of patients will experience some degree of sensorimotor neuropathy.[1]

Sensory deficits predominate with cisplatin use, and the earliest sign is decreased vibratory sense.[58] Other cisplatin-induced sensory losses involve proprioception (position) and light touch. There may be hypersensitivity to pain (hyperalgesia). Sensory losses are bilateral and follow a "stocking–glove" distribution, with paresthesias of the toes an early symptom. Paresthesias of the fingers can lead to difficulty with fine motor movement such as writing or buttoning a shirt. As injury to the large myelinated sensory fibers progresses, reflexes are lost. Decreased ankle reflexes may progress to absent reflexes with footdrop, causing a slapping gait. Motor symptoms include weakness of distal muscles and leg cramping. The patient may develop L'hermitte's sign, a sudden electric shock-like sensation as the neck is flexed. As neuropathy progresses, neuropathic pain may develop. With severe neuropathy, the individual has a broad-based stance, and as position sense becomes impaired, sensory ataxia and loss of balance result.[18] Recovery is usually partial, with symptoms progressing after treatment has stopped (coasting).[18]

Cranial nerve injury related to cisplatin therapy involves auditory and visual changes. Hearing loss begins with asymptomatic loss of high-frequency pure tone sounds that is manifested on an audiogram, emerging with cisplatin doses greater than 60 mg/m^2.[59] Tinnitus is the first symptom to appear and affects 60% to 70% of patients. If the drug is stopped at this point, tinnitus will resolve. With continued drug use, however, symptomatic loss of medium-frequency sounds occurs and may be permanent. Damage to the retina also may occur after high-dose cisplatin and can cause blurred vision and impaired color vision.[60] In a patient survey, Holden and Felde demonstrated that this loss of precise color vision was extremely distressing.[61]

Although less neurotoxic than cisplatin, the analogue carboplatin causes injury to the sensory axons with less effect on motor and autonomic fibers. Paresthesias occur in approximately 5% of patients at usual doses. Signs and symptoms of sensory CIPN increase with high-dose therapy, with higher cumulative doses greater than 400 mg/m^2, or when carboplatin is used in combination with other neurotoxic drugs such as paclitaxel.[16,18]

The third-generation platinum analogue, oxaliplatin, causes frequent peripheral neuropathy. Two distinct sensory neuropathies are observed: acute PN and cumulative, persistent PN. *Acute PN* occurs within hours to 1–3 days of drug administration, is transient and often precipitated by exposure to cold, may involve unusual symptoms such as pharyngolaryngeal dysesthesia, and usually regresses between treatments (within 2 weeks) but often recurs. *Cumulative, persistent PN*, which lasts longer than 14 days, persists between treatment cycles, with symptom severity increasing with successive cycles of treatment and increased cumulative dose. Cumulative CIPN is a dose-limiting complication.

Acute PN is thought to be related to rapid chelation of calcium by oxaliplatin-released oxalate, which affects the sodium channels in the nerve membrane and synapse (ion channelopathy). This effect stands in contrast to the cumulative, persistent PN that appears to be related to gradual drug damage to the peripheral axon and/or dorsal root ganglia.[62]

Paresthesias of the fingers or muscle cramps in the hand or forearm may occur in acute PN. Cold-induced dysesthesias occur in about 68% of patients, and pharyngolaryngeal dysesthesia in about 1% to 2% of patients (grade 3/4).[63] These effects are often precipitated by exposure to cold, such as reaching into the freezer or drinking an ice-cold beverage. The reactions, although frightening to the patient, resolve quickly and can be prevented by teaching patients strategies to avoid cold exposure during or after chemotherapy administration. Chronic sensory CIPN occurs in about 10% to 15% of patients who have received a cumulative dose of 780–850 mg/m^2, but the incidence increases with increased cumulative drug dose.[62] Paresthesias of the toes and fingertips begin first and move proximally up the limbs. If symptoms worsen and are allowed to progress, motor neuropathy may develop with resulting weakness and disability. Paresthesias appear to be reversible, with median time to recovery from grade 3 toxicity of 13 weeks.[16]

Proteasome inhibitors

Bortezomib, a proteasome inhibitor, causes primarily a sensory PN, but motor neuropathy has been reported.[64] Bortezomib inhibits nuclear factor-kappa B (NF-kB), leading to cell-cycle arrest, apoptosis, and inhibition of angiogenesis, with resulting cell death; it also blocks the transcription of nerve growth factor–mediated neuron survival.[31] This may help to explain the frequent, primarily small-fiber, axonal sensory distal neuropathy that bortezomib may cause. CIPN is a dose-limiting outcome, with symptoms beginning soon after initial treatment and reaching a plateau at cycle 5.[65] Patients with symptomatic PN at baseline are more likely to develop worsening of their symptoms.[64]

Subcutaneous (SQ) administration of bortezomib reduces the risk of CIPN in patients with multiple myeloma compared to administration via the intravenous route (IV) (24% versus 41%), as well as the incidence of grade 3 or higher (6% versus 16%).[66–68] Moreau et al. showed that SQ administration of bortezomib was noninferior to IV administration.[66] There was improvement or resolution of CIPN when the drug was discontinued for grade 2 CIPN (51%–73%),[64] and improvement or resolution occurs in most patients within 3 months after drug discontinuance, with a median duration of 47 days.[67]

Chadhry et al. studied patients who received two neurotoxic drugs together—bortezomib and thalidomide—and found that 96% of patients developed CIPN. These authors reported that CIPN (1) is not related to cumulative dose, (2) is mild to moderate and generally reversible, and (3) predominately involves axonal large fibers rather than small fibers.[69] However, a subset of patients developed a more severe demyelinating CIPN.[69]

Thalidomide analogues

Thalidomide and its analogs are immunomodulatory agents that inhibit angiogenesis.[65] Thalidomide causes a sensory/sensorimotor axonal neuropathy of both small and large sensory fibers, with symptoms beginning with tingling or painful distal paresthesias, sensory loss in lower extremities, and, if motor fibers are involved, muscle weakness and tremor.[69] The incidence of CIPN (all grades) was 96% in one study.[69] CIPN related to thalidomide is largely irreversible—a fact that led to the development of its analogue lenalidomide, which causes significantly less CIPN, an effect that is reversible (overall 8%–10%, with 2%–3% grade 3/4).[23] The investigational third-generation analogue pomalidomide is reported to be more active than thalidomide in multiple myeloma treatment, and to cause less CIPN.[70]

Chemotherapy-induced peripheral neuropathy can lead to the development of neuropathic pain. Normally, peripheral nociceptor neurons detect a painful stimulus and the nociceptive (pain) impulse is sent to the spinal cord by either C-fiber (slow, unmyelinated) or A-delta (fast, myelinated) axons. Sensitized or inflamed nociceptors fire spontaneously, causing constant pain. If C-fiber neurons are made to fire continuously, glutamine, a principal excitatory neurotransmitter, is released, which binds to *N*-methyl-D-aspartate (NMDA) receptors in the spinal cord and activates the NMDA receptor. It is thought that activation of the NMDA receptor brings about central sensitization, with increased sensitivity to all messages coming into the spinal cord.[71,72] The overexcitation results in pain without a painful stimulus and increases the intensity of the neuropathic pain impulse. Various substances are then recruited to the area, such as substance P, alpha agonists and antagonists, gamma-amino butyric acid (GABA) agonists, and free radicals. GABA and sodium-channel activity appear to down-regulate the NMDA receptor and quiet things down. It is also thought that the binding of glutamate to the NMDA receptor triggers hyperalgesia (increased perception of pain from a noxious stimulus that normally is not intense) and allodynia (pain caused by a stimulus that normally is not painful), which are both classic properties of neuropathic pain.[73]

SYMPTOM ASSESSMENT

RISK FACTORS

Risk factors for the development of CIPN include the following:

- *History of PN* or high risk of developing it, due to conditions such as concurrent diabetes mellitus, longstanding alcohol abuse, atherosclerosis/ischemic disease, vitamin B_{12} deficiency, cancer cachexia, vitamin B/folate deficiencies, Charcot-Marie Tooth disease (hereditary disease causing neuropathic joints), infection (e.g., Lyme disease, HIV, varicella-zoster, Epstein-Barr, hepatitis C), metabolic disorders (e.g., subclinical hypothyroidism, amyloidosis), or autoimmune diseases (e.g., rheumatoid arthritis, lupus)
- *Concurrent neurotoxic medicines*: isoniazid, ethambutol, gentamycin, metronidazole HCl, ciprofloxacin, phenytoin, antiretroviral drugs; or prior or concurrent administration of cisplatin, oxaliplatin, paclitaxel, docetaxel, thalidomide, lenalidomide, or bortezomib
- *High-dose chemotherapy or high cumulative doses of neurotoxic drugs*
- *Dose, schedule, and frequency of neurotoxic chemotherapy drugs*
- *Increased age* (in one study of patients receiving bortezomib, the incidence of grades 3/4 CIPN was 14% for patients younger than age 75, and 25% in patients 75 years or older[74]
- *Malignancy* (e.g., multiple myeloma, paraneoplastic neuropathy)

SELF-ASSESSMENT

Patients initially complain of a "pins and needles" sensation beginning in the tips of the toes, then the tips of the fingers. It may be intermittent at first, and may not be bothersome. As treatment continues, it becomes a more persistent sensation, to the point that the patient may describe unexpected uncomfortable sensations, such as the weight of the sheet on the toes when going to sleep (dysesthesia). Patients may be unable to distinguish hot and cold temperatures in their bathwater. Patients who develop changes in proprioception may tell the nurse that they could not find the brake pedal with their foot and now are "afraid to drive." They may tell the nurse they now wear sneakers all the time, and the nurse may notice that patients hug the wall as they enter the treatment room to avoid losing balance. Also, with changes in proprioception, patients may report how difficult it is to climb stairs and that they trip frequently. Patients with changes in fine motor movement may have difficulty with ADLs, such as buttoning clothes or preparing meals. This can lead to dependence on a family member to assist with dressing, bathing, meal preparation, and housecleaning. Patients may develop neuropathic pain, which is often described as electric, shock-like jolts on a background of pain that prevents them from sleep, comfort, and safe ambulation.

While patients receive close follow-up during treatment, for some patients sequelae of CIPN persist for more than 1 to 2 years, and may involve major disability such as decreased mobility, especially in the elderly. Elderly patients may choose not to undergo treatment with neurotoxic drugs so as to preserve their mobility.

Some patients enjoy journaling their cancer treatment experience; for them, documentation describes their symptom experience. As the validity and need for patient-reported outcomes (PRO) is recognized, patients will be asked to verbalize and document their symptoms and the effect on their ability to live as they wish. Other patients may prefer a structured diary with check-off columns of the potential symptoms they may experience given their particular neurotoxic chemotherapy drug, such as paclitaxel, which would prompt self-assessment of the impact of paresthesias and dysesthesias; sensation of temperature (hot/cold); difficulty walking, climbing steps, or driving the car (proprioception); and pain.[75]

The CIPN Assessment Tool (CIPNAT) has reported validity and reliability as a patient self-report tool that would be useful in these circumstances.[76] For example, in the authors' study of patients receiving oxaliplatin, patients reported cold sensitivity, tingling in the hands, and numbness in the hands and toes, while the most severe symptoms were cold sensitivity, nerve pain, and trouble with balance. The most distressing symptoms were trouble with balance, muscle or joint aches, and neuropathic pain. Patients reported that these symptoms interfered with many activities.

The EORTC-QlQ-CIPN20 is being tested in Europe; it is a 20-item quality of life questionnaire developed to identify patients' perceptions of symptoms and functional limitations relating to CIPN.[77] The three subscales are sensory, motor, and autonomic CIPN, and the tool is being field tested.

OBJECTIVE ASSESSMENT

Clinical nursing parameters to be assessed in the patient at risk for CIPN include sensory, motor, autonomic, and cranial nerve functions. Assessment should include the following points in the history and physical exam.

History

- Assess risk for development of CIPN: Does the patient have risk factor(s)?
- Assess medication profile: Is the patient taking any neurotoxic medications such as isoniazid? Is the patient receiving concomitant neurotoxic chemotherapy drugs (e.g., vincristine, cisplatin, paclitaxel, docetaxel)?
- What is the dose and schedule of chemotherapy? Is it high-dose, dose dense, or weekly versus every three weeks?
- Symptom analysis: Which symptoms does the patient have? When did symptom(s) begin? Intensity? Location(s)? Are the symptoms symmetrical on both sides of body? If paresthesias are not symmetrical, then CIPN is unlikely. Is the distribution distal in a stocking–glove manner or in a dermatome? Intermittent versus constant? Waxing and waning? Quality (radicular, burning, pins and needles, electric shock)? Alleviating and aggravating factors? Any accompanying symptoms? Impact on function and ability to do ADLs such as bathing, dressing, eating, walking, climbing stairs, and driving? If ability to do ADLs is affected, is it sometimes, most of the time, or all of the time? Dropping things? Tripping over feet? Tending to hug walls when walking?

Sensory symptoms may include numbness and tingling, burning, change/loss of sensation, difficulty distinguishing hot and cold, difficulty buttoning a shirt, difficulty walking and placing feet, tripping and falling, and pain. *Sensory signs* may include paresthesias, dysesthesias, hypoesthesia or hyperesthesia, hyporeflexia or areflexia; diminished or absent proprioception, vibratory sensation, cutaneous sensation, and discrimination between sharp and dull; diminished or absent deep tendon reflex.[1,11,16]

Motor symptoms may include muscle weakness, cramping, spasm, or tripping; difficulty lifting up the foot/toes, holding objects, or closing buttons; shaky handwriting; and arms and legs feeling "heavy." *Motor signs* may include difficulty with fine motor movement, decreased muscle strength, atrophy, and gait abnormalities.[1,11,16]

Cranial symptoms may include hoarseness or ringing in the ears; *cranial signs* may include decreased vision and hearing. *Autonomic symptoms* may include dizziness when standing, constipation, difficulty voiding, and impotence; *autonomic signs* may include orthostatic hypotension, urinary retention, diaphoresis, or anhydrosis (no sweating).[1,11,16]

Review of systems

- Head, eyes, ears, nose, throat: Usual vision? Any blurring of vision? Any changes in visual acuity or color perception? Any difficulty seeing traffic lights? Usual hearing? Any tinnitus? Decreased hearing? Any dizziness when changing position?
- Gastrointestinal: Usual bowel elimination pattern? Any changes? Constipation? Colicky abdominal pain?
- Genitourinary: Usual bladder pattern? Any difficulty voiding? Changes? Retention?
- Musculoskeletal: Any muscle weakness, cramping, stumbling, abnormal gait, or falls?
- Neurologic: Numbness or tingling of fingers/toes, hands/feet, or around the mouth? Any change in ability to write name, button clothes, or pick up a dime? Any loss of sensation (e.g., to temperature, vibration, touch, pain, or proprioception [knowing where body parts are in relation to the body])? Any weakness or paralysis? Any pain? Location, intensity, and character of pain?

Physical exam

- Vital signs: Assess for orthostatic changes in blood pressure and heart rate.
- Cranial nerve assessment: Table 22-3 depicts a complete examination of the cranial nerves. Vincristine may damage cranial nerve V (CN-V), causing acute jaw pain, which usually resolves within a few days and may not recur. Cisplatin may cause damage to CN-VIII, resulting in tinnitus, loss of hearing, nystagmus, and vertigo; damage to CN-IX may result in altered taste or dysphagia. Injury to CN-X may appear as hoarseness or dysphagia; to CN-XI, as neck and shoulder weakness; and to CN-XII, as asymmetry or fasciculations of the tongue.[78]
- Motor function assessment: Examine skeletal muscles for size, tone, strength (extensor/flexor), any involuntary movements, and gait. Motor CIPN can appear as muscle weakness, atrophy, or ataxia. Compare both sides of the body for symmetry and equality of motor strength, starting distally and working proximally. A few simple tests should be sufficient. Key techniques are shown in Table 22-4.[1,11,78]
- Muscle stretch reflexes (deep tendon reflexes): Assess reflexes as shown in Table 22-5. Patients with early motor neuropathy may be asymptomatic and show only decreased Achilles tendon reflexes; other reflexes become diminished with continued chemotherapy, and disappear, resulting in muscle weakness of the hands and feet (wristdrop and footdrop). Vincristine is known for causing loss of deep tendon reflexes (DTRs), although recovery of sensation and DTRs occurs in more than half of patients.[79] Assess the biceps, triceps, quadriceps, and Achilles tendon. Observe the briskness of response. If the reflex is not elicited, have the person perform isometric exercises (e.g., cup two hands together and try to pull them apart).[11,78]
- Sensory function assessment: Sensory function is evaluated to identify areas of damage in the sensory cortex or pathways. Table 22-6 describes techniques to assess sensory function.[1,11,78] The exam begins distally, and moves proximally, comparing one side of the body to the other, while the patient keeps his or her eyes closed. The senses of pain, light touch, position, and vibration are tested, followed by fine discrimination and temperature. The location of the sensory loss helps to pinpoint the site of sensory damage. Damage to large sensory nerve fibers results in impairment of vibration and proprioception, whereas damage to small sensory nerve fiber impairs recognition of hot and cold, and pain sensation may be abnormal.[11] Table 22-7 identifies terms used to describe neuropathic pain.

  Deficits are described in terms of the *dermatomal* distribution. A dermatome is the area of skin innervated by the sensory nerve root of a spinal segment, as shown in Figure 22-1.

  Vibration is often the first sensation lost in peripheral neuropathy. Patients with small sensory nerve damage may develop a diminished response to temperature and touch in addition to the numbness and tingling commonly experienced. In addition, proprioceptive losses in the lower extremities can lead to ataxia if the person has also lost reflexes.
- Autonomic assessment: Dysfunction is related to involuntary physiologic functions such as bowel and bladder function and maintenance of blood pressure during movement. Difficulty initiating urination can progress to urinary retention, overflow, or incontinence. Bowel dysfunction can be manifested by loss of rectal sensation, constipation, or paralytic ileus. Orthostatic hypotension can increase risk of falls.[7]

TABLE 22-3

Physical Examination of the Cranial Nerves

Cranial Nerve	Test
CN-I: Olfactory	• This is tested by recognition of a common odor, such as coffee or cinnamon, with the eyes closed. Each nostril is tested separately.
CN-II: Optic	• To test for visual acuity, ask the patient to hold a newspaper 15–18 inches away, close one eye, and read a few sentences. Repeat with the other eye, then with both eyes open. For more accuracy, use a Snellen eye chart from 20 feet away or a hand-held chart that is comparable. • To test for peripheral vision, face the person so that your eyes are at the same level. Have the person cover the right eye while you cover your left eye, and have the person stare into your eye; then, extend your right arm out to the side and down ("5 o'clock"), point your finger, and slowly raise it into the field of vision. Ask the person to let you know when your finger is seen. Repeat with your arm extended straight out to the side ("3 o'clock") and up toward the ceiling ("1 o'clock"). Now, ask the person to cover the other eye while you do the same, and repeat your arm movements with the left arm. • The last part of the exam is done using the ophthalmoscope, which will not be discussed here.
CN-III: Oculomotor CN-IV: Trochlear CN-VI: Abducens	• These three cranial nerves are evaluated together by testing the muscle movements that rotate the eyeball. Ask the person to keep the head in one position facing you. Hold your forefinger about 12–18 inches from the person's eyes, and ask the person to follow with eyes only as you move your finger through the six cardinal gazes. When the person's eyes have followed as far as possible, stop, hold your finger, and observe for nystagmus. Throughout, you must observe both eyes to see if they move together; disconjugate gaze suggests dysfunction in the extraocular muscles. • Observe the pupils for ptosis (CN-III controls the muscles elevating the eyelid) and for equal size and shape. • Finally, observe for pupillary light responses. Darken the room if possible. For direct response, cover one of the person's eyes and shine a penlight into the pupil in the other eye. The pupil should constrict. Repeat with the other eye. For consensual light reflex, ask the person to keep both eyes open. Shine the penlight into the right pupil from the side, and observe the left pupil constricting (both pupils should constrict); repeat in the other pupil.
CN-V: Trigeminal	• To test the motor strength of the temporal and masseter muscles, which are innervated by this nerve, place your fingers on the person's temples and ask the person to clench the teeth; then repeat with your fingers on the person's jaws. • To test the sensory tract, ask the person to close the eyes, and gently touch the skin on the forehead, cheek, and jaw bilaterally with a wisp of cotton.
CN-VII: Facial	• This nerve innervates taste buds (not usually tested) and facial muscles, which are tested for motor strength. Ask the person to frown, puff out the cheeks, smile showing the teeth, and tightly close the eyes and resist as you try to gently open the person's eyes.
CN-VIII: Vestibulocochlear (Acoustic)	• The nerve has two branches, one for hearing (cochlear) and the other for balance (vestibular). Hearing is tested by standing about 2 feet behind the person and lightly whispering a two-digit number, then asking the person to repeat it. A ticking watch can also be used and brought from a distance to just outside the ear. Ask the person to let you know when the ticking is heard. • If there is a hearing abnormality, use the Weber's (tests air and bone conduction using a vibrating tuning fork on forehead, looking for lateralization or the sound being louder in one ear or the other) and Rinne's (compares bone to air conduction using tuning fork on mastoid eminence below the ear, and ask when stops hearing vibration) tests. Normally the sound is heard in the center of the head, or both ears equally (Weber), and air conduction is greater than bone conduction (Rinne) which help to assess lateralization and bone versus air conduction. The use of the otoscope will not be discussed.
CN-IX: Glossopharyngeal CN-X: Vagus	• Both these nerves help regulate gag and palatal reflexes. To test motor strength, place your hand on the person's throat and ask the person to swallow. • To test the gag reflex, gently touch the back of the person's throat with a tongue depressor.
CN-XI: Spinal Accessory	• This nerve innervates the sternocleidomastoid and trapezius muscles. Test for motor strength by placing your hands on the person's right cheek and asking the person to turn the cheek against your hand as you resist. Repeat on the other cheek. Then, place your hands on the person's shoulders, and ask the person to shrug the shoulders up against the resistance of your hands.
CN-XII: Hypoglossal	• This nerve innervates the tongue. To test, ask the person to stick out the tongue, and note whether it moves in the midline and whether there is any involuntary movement or atrophy. Also note whether the uvula is midline or deviated.

Source: Data from Bickley[78].

TABLE 22-4

Assessment of Motor Function

Function and Assessment Technique	
Gait:	• Ask the person to walk back and forth in a room, and note the posture, body movements, and step. For example, is the step a steppage gait in which the foot is lifted high with knees flexed then dropped to the floor with a slapping sound; or is the gait staggering, unsteady, and wide-based as with cerebellar ataxia? • Ask the person to walk heel-to-toe along an imaginary line to test cerebellar function.
Muscles:	• Starting with the upper limbs, provide fixed resistance by pushing against the extremity and ask the person to oppose it by pushing back as forcefully as possible. Grade the strength as follows: 5/5 can raise and hold limb against active resistance (push) 4/5 can raise and hold limb, but not against active resistance (push) 3/5 can raise limb, but cannot hold it against active resistance (touch) 2/5 moves limb, but cannot raise or lift limb to overcome gravity 1/5 slight contraction visible (patient tries to move limb but no movement) 0/5 no movement • Test plantar flexion and dorsiflexion at the ankle by asking the person to push down against your hand and then to pull the foot away as you cup your hand around the foot. • Test for drift of the arms and legs. Have the person close the eyes and extend arms with palms facing upward for 10 seconds; ask the person to sit on the edge of a chair or bed, close the eyes, and hold both legs out in front, holding this position for 30 seconds. You should observe for any upward or downward drift of the arms or legs, wrist pronation, or curled fingers.
Involuntary movements:	• Are tremors, spasms, or other involuntary movements observed?
Coordination:	• Test the integrity of the cerebellum, which is responsible for balance and coordination. Ask the person to sit down and then to touch the nose with a finger, first with eyes open then closed. Next, ask the person to touch your finger as you move it in different directions. This point-to-point action helps to identify intention tremors. • Then ask the person to alternately tap the right and left hands against the knee as quickly as possible and to alternately pronate and supinate hands and forearms. • Ask the person to move one foot down the shin of the other leg, and repeat this with the other leg. • Finally, ask the person to stand up with feet together and arms at the sides, first with eyes open then closed. A person maintains balance by proprioception, vestibular function (knowing the head position in space), and hearing. The person can have a proprioception problem but can use vision and vestibular function to maintain balance. If the person loses balance with eyes closed, this is a positive Romberg sign. This helps to find out the cause of loss of motor coordination (ataxia)

Source: Data from Armstrong et al[1]; Visovsky et al[11]; Bickley[78].

TABLE 22-5

Examination of the Muscle Stretch Reflexes (Deep Tendon Reflexes)

Reflex	Examination
General	Help the person become comfortable sitting on the edge of the bed or examining table. Use the end of the reflex hammer to gently strike the tendon. Response is graded on a 0 to 4+ scale: 4+ Very brisk, hyperactive, and abnormal; with clonus 3+ Brisk, but excessive 2+ Normal 1+ Slightly diminished (sluggish), but may be normal 0 Absent, often abnormal
Achilles reflex	Foot should plantar flex. If there is abnormality, it may reflect a problem at nerves S-1 and S-2 of the spinal cord.
Quadriceps reflex	Elicits knee jerk, which should extend the leg. Tests nerves L-3, L-4.
Biceps reflex	Elbow should flex. Tests nerves C-5, C-6.
Triceps reflex	Elbow should extend. Tests nerves C-7, C-8.

Source: Data from Visovsky et al[11]; Bickley[78].

TABLE 22-6

Sensory Examination

Dimension	Examination
General	To begin, ask the person to keep *his/her eyes closed during* the exam. It is important to compare one side with the other throughout the exam. Identify areas where there is decreased sensation using a washable marker.
Pain	If the sensation of pain is intact, touch and temperature should be intact. Use a sterile 22-gauge needle or a safety pin cleansed with alcohol and, starting at the shoulders, gently touch the metal to the skin, asking the person to tell you when it is felt. Touch one side, then the other, and move down to the distal aspects of the arms and legs.
Light Touch	Using a wisp of cotton, touch the areas assessed under pain, and ask the person to tell you when the cotton is felt.
Position	Grasping the person's index finger (at the last joint) from the side, move the joint up or down and ask the person whether the finger is pointing up or down. Repeat this on the opposite side as well as with each of the big toes. If position sense is impaired, move on to the next proximal joint (e.g., wrist or ankle).
Vibration	Test both sides of the body for vibratory sense using a tuning fork. Tap the tuning fork on the heel of the hand to begin vibration, then place the rounded end on the interphalangeal joint of the middle finger. Ask the patient to tell you what is felt. If pressure, then ask the patient to tell you when the sensation stops and touch the fork to stop the vibration. Repeat on the other hand. Then test the feet, placing the tuning fork on the bony joint of each great toe. If the patient has no sense of vibration, move proximally, placing the vibrating fork on the bony prominence of the wrists and the medial malleoli of the ankle joints. If still no vibration is felt, move to the elbow and knee.
Fine discrimination	Place a common object, e.g., coin, in the patient's hand, and ask patient to identify it; test other hand with a different object (e.g., key). This ability is called *stereognosis.*

Source: Data from Armstrong et al[1]; Visovsky et al[11]; Bickley[78].

TABLE 22-7

Neuropathic Pain Vocabulary

Term	Definition
Allodynia	Pain sensation caused by a stimulus that normally is not painful
Analgesia	Absence of pain sensation
Deafferentiation pain	Electric shock-like pain superimposed on a background of burning sensation; caused by interruption of an afferent nerve pathway (loss of sensory input into the central nervous system [CNS]) and release of pain message from other neural tissue
Dysesthesia	Unpleasant abnormal sensation resulting from activities that normally do not cause pain
Hyperalgesia	Increased perception of pain from a noxious stimulus that normally is not this intense
Hyperpathia	Exaggerated reaction to a painful stimulus; may occur with allodynia, hyperesthesia, hyperalgesia, and/or dysesthesia
Hyperesthesia	Excessive sensitivity to touch
Hyposthesia	Decreased sensitivity to touch
Neuropathic pain	Complex chronic pain state following injury to the nervous system (CNS or brain and spinal cord, or peripheral nerves outside the brain and spinal column)
Paresthesia	Spontaneous sensation of numbness, tingling, burning, or "pins and needles" without stimulation
Paroxysmal	Occurring intermittently with a sudden onset, typical of neuropathic pain
Phantom Limb Syndrome	Perceived sensations, including pain, in an area where a limb has been amputated.

Diagnostic evaluation

Patients who will be receiving potentially neurotoxic chemotherapy should have a comprehensive baseline history and physical exam. If the patient has PN prior to starting chemotherapy, then further neurological evaluation is often performed by a neurologist or rehabilitation specialist, together with neurodiagnostic testing to determine the etiology. This is specifically recommended for patients with breast cancer using a rehabilitation model.[17] This model can be applied to all patients.[79]

Neurodiagnostic testing for PN includes nerve conduction velocity and electromyography (EMG) testing. Nerve conduction velocity studies can help identify the severity and location of peripheral neuropathy, and identify whether the damage (degeneration) involves the myelin sheath or the axon. A nerve is stimulated, which then sends an electrical response along the axon. The speed is measured, and if it is slow or demonstrates any blockage of the impulse, it is likely due to damage to the myelin sheath, while a decrease in the strength of the impulse suggests degeneration of the axon. Testing is combined with EMG to identify early axonal degeneration (normal conduction velocity but abnormal EMG) and demyelination (reduced conduction velocity and normal EMG). Other available testing includes skin biopsy to evaluate the nerve fiber endings and determination of the vibration perception threshold. The value of nerve conduction studies in objectively assessing CIPN has been questioned except when the etiology of the PN is unknown or during clinical trials.[80] As there are no data showing that these quantitative studies reliably (1) diagnose, quantify, or monitor response to CIPN treatment, (2) correlate with clinical symptoms,[81] or (3) correlate with patients' subjective reports of CIPN,[18] these tests are not commonly used.

Audiometry assesses pure tone hearing and high- and low-frequency hearing; it includes speech audiometry, tone decay testing, and acoustic reflex testing. Baseline testing is useful for comparison with serial audiograms for patients receiving cisplatin chemotherapy. This is especially recommended for patients with preexisting hearing loss. For this test, the patient sits in a small, soundproof testing room and wears headphones to listen to varying frequencies. The test lasts 40 to 60 minutes.

DEGREES OF TOXICITY

Grading scales for quantifying the degree of CIPN toxicity exist, but the challenge remains to identify a simple yet comprehensive, clinically useful, and clinimetrically sound CIPN-specific measurement tool.[82] This has made it very difficult to evaluate interventions aimed at prevention, minimization, and reversal of CIPN.[82] The most commonly used tools are the National Cancer Institute's Common Terminology Criteria for Adverse Events (NCI-CTCAE),[83] the Total Neuropathy Score (TNS) and its derivatives (reduced [TNSr], reduced short form [TNSr-SF], modified [mTNS], and clinical [TNSc]), and the Eastern Cooperative Oncology Group's Common Toxicity Criteria (ECOG).[84–88] Separate tools must be used to assess neuropathic pain, such as the Neuropathic Pain Scale for CIPN (NPS-CIN).[81]

When using the NCI-CTCAE v4.03, grade 1 CIPN symptoms would be classified as mild, and require no special treatment as symptoms will resolve over time. Grade 2 symptoms are moderate and interfere with instrumental ADLs such as meal preparation, with assistance being required to accomplish this activity; often the neurotoxic chemotherapy drug will be dose reduced. Patients will need rehabilitative intervention to restore function if possible.[17] Grade 3 symptoms are severe, and interfere with ability to do basic ADLs; the patient requires assistance and rehabilitation,[17] and the neurotoxic drug is held. If pain is present, that issue also requires immediate intervention. Most of the assessment/grading tools have not been tested for validity and reliability in the CIPN patient population.

The ideal evaluation tool is one that combines the patient's subjective assessment with a physical assessment. Griffith et al. conducted a systematic review of psychometric properties of CIPN measures.[85] Of the 15 studies that met their criteria (e.g., reliability, validity, responsiveness), two measures emerged as potentially useful: the TNS versions that included both subjective measures of CIPN-related quality of life and objective examinations of nerve function; and the Functional Assessment of Cancer from the Gynecologic Oncology Group, dealing with neurotoxicity (FACT/GOG-Ntx).[89] The FACT/GOG-Ntx is often used in clinical trials. While it assesses patient outcomes, it was validated against the NCI-CTCAE and Karnofsky Performance Scale, which are unable to capture the dimensions of CIPN.[90]

More recently, Smith et al. established the validity of the TNSr, TNSrSF, tendon reflex item, NPS-CIN, and NCI-CTC sensory grading scale, and the reliability of the TNSr and NPS-CIN scales when measuring taxane- and platinum-induced PN.[84,86] Tofthagen et al. developed and tested a patient self-assessment and report tool to measure CIPN called the CIPN Assessment Tool (CIPNAT).[87] The tool was found to be valid and reliable when tested in patients receiving paclitaxel, docetaxel, cisplatin, and oxaliplatin. Selected grading scales are shown in Table 22-8.[82,83,88]

As CIPN is a problem for patients across boundaries, a group of international oncologists (U.S. and European) are undertaking a collaborative study entitled the Chemotherapy-Induced Peripheral Neuropathy Outcome Measures Standardization (CI-Perinoms) Study to formally determine validity and reliability of the different assessment tools in a CIPN patient population.[90]

TABLE 22-8

Selected Grading Scales for Chemotherapy Induced Peripheral Neuropathy (CIPN)

Name of Scale	Grade I	Grade 2	Grade 3	Grade 4	Comments
NCI-CTCAE[83]	**CTCAE**				**Grade 5 Death omitted**
Peripheral motor neuropathy	Asymptomatic; clinical or diagnostic observations only; intervention not indicated	Moderate symptoms; limiting instrumental ADL[A]	Severe symptoms; limiting self-care ADL;[B] assistive device indicated	Life-threatening consequences; urgent intervention indicated	Validity and reliability not established in CIPN population
Peripheral sensory neuropathy	Asymptomatic; loss of DTRs[C] or paresthesia	Moderate symptoms; limiting instrumental ADLs	Severe symptoms; limiting self-care ADLs	Life-threatening consequences; urgent intervention indicated	Validity not established in CIPN
Paresthesia	Mild symptoms	Moderate symptoms, limiting instrumental ADLs	Severe symptoms, limiting instrumental ADLs	—	Validity and reliability not established in CIPN population
Neuralgia[D]	Mild pain	Moderate pain; limiting instrumental ADLs	Severe symptoms, limiting instrumental ADLs	—	Validity and reliability not established in CIPN population
Other, non-specified, e.g., autonomic neuropathy, cranial neuropathy	Asymptomatic or mild symptoms; clinical or diagnostic observations only; intervention not indicated	Moderate; minimal, local or noninvasive intervention indicated; limiting age-appropriate instrumental ADL	Severe or medically significant but not immediately life-threatening; hospitalization or prolongation of existing hospitalization indicated; disabling; limiting self-care ADL	Life-threatening consequences; urgent intervention indicated	Validity and reliability not established in CIPN population
ECOG[88]					
Neuro motor	Subjective weakness, no objective findings	Mild objective weakness without significant impairment of function	Objective weakness with impairment of function	Paralysis	Validity and reliability not established in CIPN population
Neuro a) sensory	Mild paresthesias; loss of DTRs	Mild or moderate objective sensory loss; moderate paresthesias	Severe objective sensory losss or paresthesias that interfere with function	—	Validity and reliability not established in CIPN population
b) hearing	—	—	Hearing loss interfering with function but correctable with hearing aid	Deafness, not correctable	Validity and reliability not established in CIPN population
c) constipation	Mild	Moderate	Severe	Ileus >96 hours	Validity and reliability not established in CIPN population

(continued)

TABLE 22-8

Selected Grading Scales for Chemotherapy Induced Peripheral Neuropathy (CIPN) (*Continued*)					
Name of Scale	**Grade 1**	**Grade 2**	**Grade 3**	**Grade 4**	**Comments**
TNS: Total Neuropathy Score[82]					
					Measures subjective, and objective; validity and reliability established in CIPN for the TNS-reduced (TNSr), TNSr-Short Form (SF)[84,85] Modified version omits nerve conduction tests
Motor symptoms	Slight difficulty	Moderate difficulty	Requires assistance	Functionally disabled	Scores range from 0–36 (original was 44), higher scores denote more severe PN[82]
Sensory symptoms	Limited to fingers or toes	Extension to ankle or wrist	Extension to knee or elbow	Extension to above the knee or elbow, functionally disabling	Psychometric properties supported but limited evidence[83,85]
Pin sensibility	Reduced in fingers and toes	Reduced to ankle	Reduced to elbow or knee	Reduced above elbow or knee	Too burdensome for use by oncology nurses
Vibration sensibility	Reduced in fingers and toes	Reduced to ankle	Reduced to elbow or knee	Reduced above elbow or knee	Simplified versions being tested for psychometrics
Reflexes	Reduced ankle reflex	Absent ankle reflex	All reflexes reduced	All reflexes absent	
Strength	Mild weakness	Moderate weakness	Severe weakness	Paralysis	
Vibration and thermal thresholds percentile	95–96 percentile (Normal is <95 percentile)	97 percentile	98 percentile	>99 percentile	
[F]Nerve conduction:sural amplitude score	76%–95% LLN[E] (Normal or reduced <5%)	76%–95% LLN	51%–75% LLN	26%–50% LLN	0%–25% LLN
[F]Nerve conduction: Peroneal amplitude score	76%–95% LLN (Normal or reduced <10%)	76%–95% LLN	51%–75% LLN	26%–50% LLN	0%–25% LLN

Abbreviations: NCI: National Cancer Institute; CTCAE: common terminology criteria for adverse events; ECOG: Eastern Cooperative Oncology Group; TNS: Total Neuropathy Score; Instrumental ADLs: necessary activities beyond basic self-care, such as driving, performing a job, cooking, cleaning; Self-care ADLs: basic self-care activities such as bathing, grooming, eating; DTRs: deep tendon reflex or stretch reflex; Neuralgia: disorder characterized by intense painful sensation along a nerve or group of nerves; LLN: lower limit of normal; Sural and peroneal nerve amplitude.

Source: Data from Smith et al[82]; National Cancer Institute Common Terminology Criteria for Adverse Events (CTCAE)[83]; Smith et al[84]; Griffith et al[85]; Smith et al[86]; Eastern Cooperative Oncology Group Common Toxicity Criteria[88].

SYMPTOM MANAGEMENT STRATEGIES

THERAPEUTIC APPROACHES

Generally, primary prevention of peripheral neuropathy is not possible. Given that reliable and valid clinical assessment tools in a CIPN population are only now being identified, and otherwise standardized assessments are not being performed across all clinical groups, some potentially effective measures to prevent, minimize, or reverse established CIPN are not yet fully known.[85] The most commonly used measures for the prevention of CIPN are (1) reducing risk factors, such as using an alternative dose or schedule (e.g., SQ instead of IV dosing of bortezomib,[66] oxaliplatin dosing with "stop and go" intermittent schedules[91] discussed in the next paragraph); (2) assessment to identify early signs and symptoms of CIPN; and (3) dose reduction, dose interruption, or drug discontinuance to prevent CIPN from progressing to more severe symptoms. This strategy is not effective for drugs that are associated with the coasting phenomenon, as the process of PN continues after the drug has been stopped. Drug administration route, dose, schedule, and cumulative dose may be modified.

Paclitaxel CIPN can be reduced by modifying the dose and administration schedule.[42] The single dose of paclitaxel used, like the cumulative dose, relates to the severity of subsequent CIPN. The cumulative dose of paclitaxel resulting in toxicity of grade 2 or higher was 715 mg/m^2, and the rate of development is directly related to the paclitaxel dose per treatment cycle.[37] Weekly paclitaxel in adjuvant breast cancer treatment resulted in improved disease control and overall survival, but the rate of grades 2–4 CIPN was higher in the once-weekly dosing arm compared to the every-3-weeks dosing arm (27% versus 20%).[91]

Intermittent dosing of oxaliplatin can decrease the incidence of CIPN during therapy using the FOLFOX regimens.[92,93] FOLFOX stands for folinic acid (FOL), fluorouracil (F), and oxaliplatin (OX); the FOLFOX4 dose of oxaliplatin is 85 mg/m^2, while that of FOLFOX7 is 130 mg/m^2. Treatment is given in 2-week cycles. The OPTIMOX1 trial was a randomized, controlled, prospective trial that compared (1) patients receiving FOLFOX4 every 2 weeks until disease progression to (2) patients in the experimental arm, who received FOLFOX7 for 6 cycles, then maintenance 5-FU/leucovorin chemotherapy without oxaliplatin every 2 weeks for 12 cycles, followed by FOLFOX7. The "stop and go" label given to this approach refers to the intermittent oxaliplatin therapy delivered in the experimental arm. The study results showed that the incidence of CIPN was equivalent in cycles 1–6, but in subsequent cycles 7–18, those patients in the experimental arm had significantly less grades 3/4 CIPN (grade 3: 17.9% for FOLFOX4 recipients versus 13.3% for the experimental arm). However, the overall rate of grade 3 CIPN was not significantly different between groups. Planned reintroduction of oxaliplatin after cycle 18 occurred in 40% of intermittent-therapy recipients, but the response rate (RR), progression-free survival (PFS), and overall survival (OS) were similar between groups.

Taberno et al. used a similar strategy with an oxaliplatin/capecitabine combination (XELOX) plus bevacizumab for 6 cycles, followed by maintenance XELOX-bevacizumab or bevacizumab alone. There was a reduction in grades 3/4 CIPN in the bevacizumab-only arm (7%) compared to the continuous XELOX-bevacizumab arm (24%), with no differences in RR, PFS, or OS.[93] Finally, withholding the dose or dose reduction can stop the progression of CIPN, except when the neurotoxic drug has a coasting phenomenon.[93]

Table 22-9 lists agents that have been or are being studied to prevent or ameliorate CIPN.[18,92,94–128]

Many of the studies that documented promising neuroprotective agents require further validation. While early studies showed preliminary evidence that amifostine was neuroprotective for patients receiving cisplatin and paclitaxel, all of the studies did not have CIPN as an endpoint, and not all studies agreed in terms of their results.[42,129–131] Xaliproden was studied in a large, double-blind, randomized, controlled trial (RCT) in patients receiving oxliplatin.[111] The group receiving xaliproden had a reduction in grade 3 CIPN, with a corresponding increase in grade 2 CIPN, as compared to placebo recipients, but the overall incidence of all grades CIPN was the same in both arms (73%).[111]

Calcium and magnesium infusions for patients receiving oxaliplatin also appear promising, with their effectiveness assumed to be due to their action of increasing extracellular calcium.[132] Generally, the infusions are given 30 minutes prior to and after the oxaliplatin. Initially, this approach was being studied in a large cooperative trial, called the CONcePT trial (Combined Oxaliplatin Neurotoxicity Prevention Trial), which was stopped early due to an apparent lower tumor response in the calcium/magnesium group.[97] Later evaluation, correction, and final results of the CONcePT trial showed no evidence of inferiority in tumor control between groups, as well as a significant decrease in grade 2 or higher CIPN and a decrease in muscle spasms, but no significant effect on cold-induced effects of oxaliplatin in the calcium/magnesium group.[98,133]

Knijn et al. reported on the results of the CAIRO (Capecitabine, Irinotecan, and Oxaliplatin in Advanced Colorectal Cancer) randomized clinical trial (n = 755), which evaluated adding cetuximab to oxaliplatin/capecitabine (CAPOX) and bevacizumab, as well as calcium and magnesium infusions prior to oxaliplatin administration.[100] Retrospectively, the authors found that while the incidence of all grades of neurotoxicity was significantly lower in the calcium/magnesium group compared to the control group (85% versus 92%, p = 0.02), there was no difference in the incidence of grade 2 or higher CIPN. There was also no difference in PFS, OS, or RR.

Greater success has been achieved with validating neuropathic pain relief interventions. The sympathetic stress

TABLE 22-9

Chemotherapy Induced Peripheral Neuropathy (CIPN): Prevention and Treatment

Drug/Action	Mechanism of Action	Study Results	Citation
PREVENTION			
Drug interruption	[A]OPTIMOX1 study of continuous [B]FOLFOX 4 versus intermittent [C]FOLFOX7 then maintenance 5-FU	Significant decrease in CIPN cycles 7-18, but overall grade 3 CIPN similar in both groups	92
Acetyl-l-carnitine	CIPN may be related to mitochondrial injury; agent protects mitochondria	[D]REASON study, phase II, RCT (sagopilone) showed no difference between placebo and acetyl groups; ovarian patients had less high-grade PN	94 Studies continue [NCT00775645, NCT01492920]
Alpha-lipoic acid (aka thioctic acid)	Natural lipophilic antioxidant	No benefit in CIPN but poor patient adherence was identified as a possible reason for lack of benefit	95 Effective in DM-related PN; NCT00705029 clinical trial
Amifostine	Chemotherapy detoxifier, facilitates DNA repair	Conflicting results in studies	18,96
Calcium (Ca) and magnesium (Mg) infusions	With oxaliplatin, thought to bind to oxalate and reduce its effect on voltage-gated sodium channels	[E]CONcePT trial: reduced grade 3 CIPN in intermittent chemotherapy arm, stopped early	97
		N04C7-prospective, grade ≥ 2 significantly less in Ca/Mg group by NCI CTCAE (phase III RCT)	98
		[F]NEUROXA trial: RCT, positive early findings of reduced grade 3 CIPN (5% in Ca/Mg arm versus 24% in control); found Ca/Mg does not affect tumor response; unfinished study.	99
		[G]CAIRO2- retrospective, no benefit	100
		Choo study using nerve conduction to evaluate effectiveness; no significant difference between groups but Ca/Mg increased rate of abnormal nerve conduction	101
		Many positive trials, but no standardization in trial design or evaluation; NCI large prospective clinical trial planned	98
Gabapentin	Anticonvulsant, appears to affect the release of gamma-aminobutyric acid (GABA)	Not effective in CIPN.	102
Glutamine	May upregulate Nerve Growth Factor	Reduced incidence oxaliplatin CIPN; reduced CIPN with glutamine given 4 days prior to paclitaxel then 24 hrs after (reduced moderate to severe dysesthesias and distal paresthesias, and reduced interference with ADLs). Larger, prospective studies needed.	103 104
Glutathione	Antioxidant that attracts heavy metals, helps prevent platinum adducts (accumulation) in dorsal root ganglia	Reduced incidence/trend of CIPN	105

N-acetyl cysteine	Antioxidant, increases whole blood levels of glutathione	Decreased grades 2–4 CIPN	106
Oxacarbazepine	Ion channel modulation, inhibits high-frequency firing of nerves	Effective in reducing oxaliplatin-induced CIPN compared to placebo	107
Recombinant human leukemia inhibitory factor	Neuroprotective cytokine	Not effective	108
Vitamin E	Nerve health	Prior small studies showing benefit; CIPN lower in vitamin E group (5.9%) compared to placebo (41.7%), ($p < 0.01$)[109] No benefit, RCT, n = 207[110]	109,110
Vitamin B_{12}/B6	Nerve cell essential vitamins	Clinical trial ongoing	NCT00659269 (ClinicalTrials.gov)
Xaliproden	$5HT_{1a}$ serotonin receptor agonist; neurotrophic and neuroprotective effects	Patients receiving xaliproden had less grade 3, but more grade 2 CIPN, but there was no difference in overall incidence of CIPN between groups	111
TREATMENT			
Acupuncture	Relieves ^{H}Qi channels, releases endogenous opioids, activates myelinated and unmyelinated nerves	Study of the effectiveness of acupuncture on refractory CIPN in acute care hospital patients in the UK; 82% (n = 17) reported improvement; no standardized assessment, uncontrolled trial	112 NCT00891618
		Randomized trial suggests benefit but needs replication	113
		Series of 5 patient cases showed significant improvement in CIPN (pain, numbness, tingling)	114
		Well-designed, randomized trials needed	115
Baclofen/amitriptyline/ and ketamine (BAK-PLO)	Topical gel absorbed for systemic effects	Prospective trial (N = 208) showed trend for improvement over placebo, with greatest improvements in tingling, cramping, and shooting/burning pain symptoms, needs further study	116
Capsaicin	Binds to sensory nociceptors in skin, increases painful stimuli, followed by desensitization and reduced pain perception	General peripheral neuropathy, not CIPN Some relief of painful neuropathy experienced by 41% vs 26% placebo	117
Cutaneous electrostimulation device (MC5-A)	Nerve stimulation reduces pain impulse	Pilot shows dramatic reduction in pain in refractory CIPN patients (59% decrease in pain score over 10 days); requires additional study	118
Duloxetine	Serotonin-norepinephrine reuptake inhibitor increases pain-inhibiting neurochemicals in the brain	30% or greater reduction in pain scores versus CALGB cooperative phase III trial (N = 231): Decreased pain: 59% study arm, 39% placebo; no change (30% vs 33%), and increased pain (11% study arm, 28% placebo); significant decrease in interference scores in duloxetine group; 1st study to show significant benefit of any drug on CIPN-related pain	119

(continued)

TABLE 22-9

Chemotherapy Induced Peripheral Neuropathy (CIPN): Prevention and Treatment *(Continued)*

Drug/Action	Mechanism of Action	Study results	Citation
Gabapentin	Anticonvulsant, appears to affect the release of gamma-aminobutyric acid (GABA)	No benefit to treat CIPN symptoms, N=115	120
High-frequency external muscle stimulation	Increase afferent impulses to spinal cord, unknown mechanism	Patients with painful diabetic neuropathy symptoms; trial uncontrolled; 73% had marked improvement in symptoms	121
		Significant reduction in pain compared to transcutaneous electric nerve stimulation (TENS) group	122
Lamotrigine	Blocks sodium channels	No reduction in oxaliplatin CIPN	123
Physical activity/ exercise	Developing strength and stamina	Strengthening exercises moderately improve muscle strength in CIPN; aerobic exercise shown to prevent the onset or modify natural history of diabetic neuropathy	124 125
Pulsed infrared light therapy (Anodyne)	Unknown, may increase circulation that decreases pain	Anodyne light therapy no more effective than placebo therapy	126
Spinal cord stimulation	Spinal impulses block pain impulses entering the spinal cord	Evidence is case report only. A review of 707 cases showed 70 used for PN without mention of CIPN.	127
Transcutaneous electrical nerve stimulation (TENS)	Unclear, may be due to increased muscle oxidative capacity due to electrotherapy	Beneficial effect, sometimes lasting $>$ 1 year with continued use	128
Venlafaxine	Serotonin-norepinephrine reuptake inhibitor increases pain-inhibiting neurochemicals in the brain	[I]EFFOX RCT showed 31.3% relief of acute sensory symptoms of oxaliplatin compared to 5.3% with placebo ($p = 0.03$)	105

Abbreviations: RCT: randomized controlled trial. [A]OPTIMOX1 trial: oxaliplatin was given intermittently, e.g., at a higher dose (FOLFOX7) for 6 cycles, then removed for 12 cycles (5FU/ leucovorin only), then oxaliplatin was reintroduced (FOLFOX7; FOLFOX (Folinic acid, 5-fluorouracil (5-FU), oxaliplatin), [B]FOLFOX4 has oxaliplatin 85mg/m^2 and [C]FOLFOX7 has oxaliplatin dose of 130 mg/m^2. This was compared to the standard FOLFOX4 given every 2 weeks continuously. [D]REASON: Randomized phase II trial evaluating safety and efficacy of acetyl-L-carnitine in the prevention of sagopilone-induced peripheral neuropathy; [E]CONcePT(Combined Oxaliplatin Neurotoxicity Prevention Trial) trial: prospective trial to evaluate efficacy of calcium/ magnesium to reduce oxaliplatin-sensory PN; [F]NEUROXA trial: French study evaluating effect of Ca/Mg on tumor response and grade 3 CIPN; [G]CAIRO2 RCT phase 3 study comparing patients with advanced colorectal cancer receiving capecitabine, oxaliplatin, with or without bevacizumab in first-line setting; [H]Qi (energy) channels are used in acupuncture; there are 12 primary Qi channels; [I]EFFOX trial: French RCT evaluating the efficacy of venlafaxine in preventing or relieving oxaliplatin-induced acute neurotoxicity.

Source: Data from Stubblefield et al[18]; Tournigand et al[92]; Lhomme et al[94]; Guo et al[95]; Beijers et al[96]; Hochster et al[97]; Grothey et al[98]; Gamelin et al[99]; Knijn et al[100]; Choo et al[101]; Wong et al[102]; Wang et al[103]; Stubblefield et al[104]; Weickhardt et al[105]; Lin Lin et al[106]; Argyriou et al[107]; Davis et al[108]; Pace et al[109]; Kottschade et al[110]; Cassidy et al[111]; Donald et al[112]; Xu et al[113]; Wong et al[114]; Visovsky et al[115]; Barton et al[116]; Derry et al[117]; Smith et al[118]; Smith et al[119]; Rao et al[120]; Humpert et al[121]; Reichstein et al[122]; Rao et al[123]; White et al[124]; Balducci et al[125]; Lavery et al[126]; Mekhail et al[127]; Pieber et al[128].

response is involved in intensifying the pain impulse via the release of norepinephrine from sympathetic nerve endings. A nurse-led Cancer and Leukemia Group B (CALGB) prospective clinical trial (170701) has established that duloxetine has effectiveness in the treatment of CIPN.[119] Duloxetine is a selective serotonin and norepinephrine reuptake inhibitor (SSNRI). In this study, 231 patients who reported severe pain from CIPN (related to cisplatin or taxane therapy) were randomized to receive duloxetine followed by placebo, or placebo followed by duloxetine. CIPN-related pain decreased in 59% of patients taking duloxetine compared to 39% taking placebo. Another SNRI, venlafaxine has also shown significant activity. In a smaller, randomized study of 48 patients, 31.1% of patients obtained full relief from oxaliplatin CIPN pain, compared to 5.3% in the placebo arm ($p = 0.03$).[134] These drugs are also believed to block sodium channels, thereby reducing the intensity of the pain impulse.

While neuropathic pain has often been managed by gabapentin, evidence for efficacy is found in the treatment of diabetic NP and herpes zoster, not in CIPN.[120] The antiepileptic drug lamotrigine was studied in CIPN, but found to be ineffective.[123] Small studies or case reports suggest a benefit for acupuncture, but well-designed, randomized clinical trials are needed to confirm this effect.[115]

Pregabalin, an anticonvulsant, blocks certain calcium channels on neuronal membranes, and is thought to decrease pronociceptive neurotransmitters in the spinal cord, thereby reducing neuropathic pain. It is indicated for the relief of neuropathic pain in patients with diabetic PN and postherpetic neuralgia. A systematic review showed that a minority of patients will realize substantial benefit and more will have moderate benefit, when the drug is used for relief of diabetic and central neuropathic pain, postherpetic neuralgia, and fibromyalgia.[135] Vondracek et al. studied pregabalin in pediatric oncology patients with CIPN and found that significant and long-lasting relief was found in 86% of patients ($n = 28$) at daily doses of 150–300 mg for 8 weeks.[136] Saif et al. studied pregabalin in the treatment of grades 2–3 oxaliplatin-induced CIPN ($n = 23$).[137] The target dose of 150 mg three times a day provided the best benefit, with onset of relief in 2–6 weeks. In most (48%) patients, sensory neuropathy improved by one to two grades.[137] The rationale for other drugs that appear to reduce neuropathic pain but that do not have strong evidence supporting their use in CIPN is described below.

Some drugs that decrease neuropathic pain work by interfering with or down-regulating NMDA receptors. NMDA receptor antagonists such as ketamine decrease sensitization of the dorsal horn of the spinal cord. Another glutamate receptor near NMDA on the neuronal membrane is sensitive to sodium-channel opening, and increases transmission of the painful impulse if the channel is open. Drugs that stabilize the sodium channels include carbamazepine, divalproex sodium, phenytoin, and mexilitine.[138] Nonsteroidal anti-inflammatory drugs (NSAIDs) and corticosteroids may have membrane-stabilizing effects and act centrally as well as peripherally, reducing the intensity of the pain impulse. However, overall NSAIDs and opioids have limited effectiveness in the management of neuropathic pain and may be effective for only a small subpopulation of patients.[138] Evidence suggests that the NMDA receptor is responsible for opioid tolerance, and blockade of the receptor reverses tolerance.[139] Other sources suggest that initially the receptor is not sensitive and cannot be blocked by opioids. Once the receptor has been blocked by an NMDA antagonist, both the NMDA receptor antagonist and an opioid are needed to obtain full analgesia.[140] Finally, the topical anesthetics lidocaine in a transcutaneous patch and lidocaine and prilocaine cream prevent sodium channels from opening, thereby reducing the intensity of the pain impulse.

Collaboration between pharmacists, nurses, and podiatrists has resulted in the formulation of topical creams for the management of CIPN. Barton et al. conducted a double-blind, placebo-controlled trial of baclofen 10 mg, amitriptyline HCl 40 mg, and ketamine 20 mg in a gel (BAK-PLO) compared to placebo to treat CIPN ($n = 208$).[116] They found a trend toward improvement in both sensory ($p = 0.053$) and motor ($p = 0.21$) subscales, with greatest improvement in tingling, cramping, and shooting/burning pain in hands and in difficulty holding a pen.[116]

While they have not been studied in conjunction with CIPN, a number of other topical agents have been studied in diabetic neuropathy or postherpetic neuralgia. A 5% lidocaine plaster, which is indicated for the relief of postherpetic neuralgia, was compared to systemic pregabalin in patients with postherpetic neuralgia and diabetic polyneuropathy. Patients were found to have similar levels of analgesia, but fewer side effects in the topical lidocaine group.[141] Capsaicin is a derivative of hot chili peppers and is thought to deplete substance P from sensory nerves, thereby reducing the transmission of the pain impulse from the periphery to the CNS.[142] While it is FDA indicated for arthritis and musculoskeletal pain, capsaicin is used to relieve the pain from postherpetic neuralgia, arthritis, psoriasis, and diabetic neuropathy.[143] A combination lotion of capsaicin, lidocaine, menthol, and methyl salicylate has been used to treat diabetic neuropathic pain but has not been studied in CIPN.[144] Other agents currently being studied include amitriptyline and ketamine cream.[145]

Clinical studies regarding medication management for CIPN are difficult to evaluate and compare, as they tend to use different measurement tools for CIPN. The strength of evidence for efficacy is limited by lack of standardized, valid, and reliable measures for CIPN across groups; lack of sound trial designs; underpowered studies; retrospective as well as prospective studies with some blinded and others not; and evaluation of nonhomogenous patients (adjuvant versus palliative).[85]

The Oncology Nursing Society's CIPN-related Putting Evidence into Practice (PEP) resources do not make any recommendations, as effectiveness has not been established, in the following scenarios:

- Prevention: acetyl-L-carnitine, alpha-lipoic acid, amifostine, calcium and magnesium, gabapentin, glutamine, glutathione, nortriptyline, vitamin E, and recombinant human leukemia inhibitory factor
- Intervention; carbamazepine, lamotrigine, acupuncture, capsaicin, physical activity/exercise, spinal cord stimulation, pulsed infrared light therapy, external high-frequency external muscle stimulation[146,147]

NURSING IMPLICATIONS

The symptom constellations related to CIPN are amenable to nursing care.[148,149] Oncology nurses should ensure that they take the following steps:[25]

- Routinely perform subjective and objective assessments related to CIPN and related factors for all patients receiving neurotoxic chemotherapy
- Teach patients strategies for adapting to changes in physical functioning and managing the risk of injury related to CIPN
- Teach patients to report motor, sensory, and autonomic neurologic signs and symptoms
- Continue research efforts to understand the CIPN trajectory relative to single agents, combination agents, and dosing schedules to develop evidence-based guidelines for assessment

Visovsky states that the only interventions that are associated with a high level of evidence and can be recommended for nursing practice are education and support to preserve patient safety.[148] Clearly, research opportunities exist to identify and measure the impact of nursing care on patient outcomes in terms of nurse assessment to identify early signs and symptoms of CIPN, patient education to involve patients in self-assessment, early intervention, prevention of falls and injury, and the development of strategies to permit self-care and maximize independent functioning.

Peripheral neuropathy occurs over time, and assessment by the nurse is crucial to early identification of toxicity and to ongoing monitoring of progression so that timely decisions can be made. In fact, in one study, neurological monitoring reduced the incidence of bortezomib-induced CIPN in multiple myeloma patients.[25] Clinicians used the TNSc (clinical version) assessment tool, which was a good predictor of CIPN. In addition, nurses can teach patients and their families self-care measures so that injury can be prevented and make referrals to physical and occupational therapy to maintain and improve function as needed; such education can include (1) signs and symptoms of PN, and when to report them; (2) strategies for personal safety; (3) principles of foot care; (4) risks of ischemic and thermal injuries; and (5) ways to manage symptoms of autonomic neuropathy.[148] Table 22-10 presents a standardized nursing care plan.

Therapeutic approaches depend on the stage of the patient's treatment, or whether treatment is completed. Ideally, prior to treatment, the nurse will ensure that any potentially neurotoxic drugs are discussed with the physician/midlevel provider so as to eliminate or substitute any concurrent medications that are also neurotoxic, such as replacing colchicine with another anti-gout medication, and to avoid other potentially neurotoxic drugs, such as metronidazole.[150] Prior to the initiation of chemotherapy, the nurse begins a systematic assessment of risk for CIPN, signs and symptoms of PN, pain, and functional impairments at baseline, and then reassesses the patient on these points prior to each treatment. Accurate documentation is essential so that worsening PN can be identified early. Rehabilitation strategies for CIPN should start upon the initiation of potentially neurotoxic chemotherapy, as suggested for women with breast cancer.[17] The physical exam should document the patient's baseline strength, sensation, reflexes, and gait.[150] The nurse is the catalyst to ensure that the healthcare team provides ongoing monitoring and documentation of signs and symptoms, deficits, and any progression.

Treatment of peripheral neuropathy is symptomatic and requires input from the multidisciplinary team. Care is directed toward relief of pain, disability, and emotional distress; maximization of independence through the use of drugs, rehabilitation, and psychosocial support; and prevention of injury and permanent dysfunction.

Studies are beginning to describe the CIPN symptom experience for patients with specific chemotherapy-related CIPN. For example, Speck et al. reported their findings from a descriptive, exploratory study showing that paclitaxel-induced CIPN affected breast cancer patients' routine activities, functions, and behaviors.[151] Fortunately, the study also revealed that these patients developed management strategies to reduce the impact, such as exercise, mindfulness, use of occupational therapy, and environmental planning. Patient-reported outcome self-reports help to identify the patient's subjective experience of the symptoms associated with CIPN, but better, more concise, and more comprehensive instruments need to be developed.[152]

Sensory deficits place the patient at risk for injury; thus safety is a primary concern. For example, the patient with loss of temperature sensation should be instructed in how to assess water temperature (bath, dish) and how to minimize injury, such as by turning down the temperature of the home hot-water heater. Numbness and reduced sensation in the feet can lead to gait and balance problems.[153] This issue is compounded if a patient develops motor deficits, such as decreased distal muscle strength, or autonomic involvement, such as orthostatic hypotension, which further increases the risk

TABLE 22-10

Standardized Nursing Care Plan for Management of Peripheral Neuropathy

Nursing Diagnosis	Nursing Plan	Expected Outcomes
Knowledge deficit related to peripheral neuropathy or possible progression of peripheral neuropathy	Teach patient about peripheral neuropathy as a potential side effect of specific drug and to report any symptoms. 1. Oxaliplatin: pins-and-needles sensation in hands or feet, or choking sensation in throat when exposed to cold. 2. Numbness and tingling in hands or feet during or after therapy 3. Change in gait, such as tripping or stumbling. 4. Weakness in muscles. 5. Inability to perform fine motor movement, such as buttoning a shirt or picking up a coin from a flat surface. 6. Change in sexual functioning. 7. Assess need for and introduce rehabilitation interventions early.	• Patient will describe potential neurotoxic side effects. • Patient identifies signs and symptoms to report to health provider.
Potential for injury related to peripheral neuropathy (decreased sensitivity to temperature, gait disturbance, decreased proprioception)	Determine patient risk by assessing integrity of sensory function, especially proprioception and vibration, but also temperature and pain. 1. Sensory perception to light touch, pin prick, vibration, positioning, temperature. 2. Patient's ability to tolerate light touch, cold or hot water, presence of numbness and/or tingling, presence of painful sensations. 3. Proprioception testing of sense of position (station), gait, deep tendon reflexes, muscle weakness or atrophy, and balance. 4. Ability to sense placement of body parts, ability to write, evidence of muscle weakness. 5. Effect of any symptoms or changes on ability to do activities of daily living (ADLs), other activities important to patient, or comfort. a) Assess patient's ability to perform ADLs such as holding a fork, cutting food, hygiene, dressing, walking, and handwriting, cooking. b) Discuss referral to Physical Therapist and/or Occupational Therapist as needed. c) Involve family members in care planning as permitted by patient. d) Involve resources as needed, visiting nurse, homemaker, Home Health Assistants. 6. Teach self-care measures to prevent injury, including report of symptoms, and measures to improve home safety. 7. Prevent further damage: If patient has signs/symptoms of peripheral neuropathy, discuss grade and plan with physician/mid-level provider regarding any necessary modifications.	• Patient will be without injury. • Patient will report changes in tactile and proprioceptive function. • Patient will develop self-care measures that assure safety.
Knowledge deficit related to self-care measures required for safety	Teach patient self-care measures for changes related to neuropathy to remain safe, including making home safe. 1. Numbness/tingling of hands and feet: a) *Altered sensation with decreased tactile sense*: stay focused on task at hand, taking time to complete task; avoid temperature extremes; protect hands and feet with gloves/shoes, inspect toes/feet, fingers/hands for pressure sores, cuts, abrasions, burns; use zipper pulls, shoe horns, velcro attachments, large grip pens and pencils, large grip utensils when cooking; Use light-weight, plastic glasses, utensils and plates when making/serving and eating meals.	• Patient will describe self-care measures to maximize safety at home.

(continued)

TABLE 22-10

Standardized Nursing Care Plan for Management of Peripheral Neuropathy *(Continued)*

Nursing Diagnosis	Nursing Plan	Expected Outcomes
	b) *Decreased temperature sense*: Use unbreakable thermometer to test bath or shower water and water for dishwashing (should be < 110°F or 43.3°C), turn down water heater temperature; wear waterproof gloves when washing dishes; wear warm gloves when going outside in winter; use thick pot holders and plastic dishes and utensils when cooking. 2. Decreased proprioception: use shower chair, non-skid tub mat to prevent falling in the shower; remove scatter rugs and clutter from home hallways; ensure adequate home lighting; use night light if needed; wear high-top sneakers if difficulty climbing steps or feeling feet on floor; avoid driving if unsure where feet are on control pedals. 3. Motor weakness: a) *Gait changes* with stumbling, tripping: keep rooms, hallways, stairs well illuminated; secure handrails and non-slip surfaces on stairs; remove all clutter and loose rugs, furniture on wheels from living area; install safety features in bathroom: avoid use of heavy motorized equipment such as lawn mower; b) *Loss of fine motor movement:* use zipperpull, buttoner tool to assist in buttoning shirts, wear clothes with elastic waist and pullover tops; wear shoes with Velcro closures; evaluate ability to do fine motor movements to feed self, cook, and consider family meeting to reorganize home tasks.	
Impaired mobility related to peripheral neuropathy: decreased proprioception, muscle weakness	Assess patient's level of activity, muscle strength, and level of mobility baseline prior to chemotherapy, prior to each treatment, and at each visit once therapy is completed. 1. Encourage patient to use visual cues to determine position of body parts if proprioception is impaired. 2. Teach measures to prevent injury. 3. Refer for physical or occupational therapy for assistive devices as needed.	• Patient will ambulate safely.
Alterations in autonomic functioning related to peripheral neuropathy, potential	Assess autonomic functions and patient coping with changes as needed. 1. Constipation: High-fiber diet, drink 3 quarts of fluid a day, stool softeners, laxatives, try to move bowels same time each day; notify RN/MD if abdominal pain, distention, or if no bowel movement in 2–3 days. 2. Urinary retention/incontinence: Try to empty bladder at same times each day, bladder training exercises, do not drink fluids after 6 PM at night. 3. Orthostatic dizziness: Change position very slowly and hold onto secure surface when getting up, drink 2–3 quarts of water each day, thigh-high TEDS, and medications as ordered; call RN/MD right away if symptoms worsening, falls. 4. Impotence (see below).	Patient will have normal function or strategies to ensure adequate function.

Potential for sexual dysfunction related to peripheral neuropathy: altered tactile sensation, muscle weakness, changes in role	Discuss with patient the impact of treatment-related dysfunction on ability to give/receive affection, sexuality, social role, and self-esteem 1. Discuss appropriate alternative means of sexual expression and provide emotional support 2. Refer for specific sexual counseling as needed	• Patient and significant other will identify effects on sexual expression • Patient and significant other will identify alternative methods of sexual expression
Altered comfort level related to painful paresthesias	Assess comfort level and presence of severe tingling, numbness, burning, or other sensations Assess quality, intensity, and frequency of discomfort Identify precipitating factors such as warm or cold stimulation and help patient develop realistic plan to avoid triggers 1. Teach patient to recognize patterns, avoid triggers 2. Discuss with MD/midlevel provider evidence supported interventions: duloxetine, venlafaxine, or pregabalin 3. Discuss interventions where evidence requires further validation: consider topical plaster/ointment such as 5% lidocaine, EMLA (Eutechtic Mixture of Local Anesthetics) cream, massage, acupuncture, TENS if acceptable and available	• Patient will have decreased pain • Patient will have increased comfort
Potential for role change (self-concept, self-esteem, social function, occupational role) related to peripheral neuropathy disability	Assess impact of sensory/perceptual dysfunction on social and work roles; ability to meet role expectations of self and family 1. Discuss modifications in job and role, as appropriate and available 2. Refer to occupational/physical therapist for evaluation concerning assistive devices to promote rehabilitation 3. Encourage independence where possible and provide positive reinforcement for accomplishments; encourage patient to accept assistance from family and friends in areas where dependent 4. Provide emotional support during grief reaction and assess need for support or counseling 5. Provide information about support groups and other resources to promote effective coping	• Patient and family will demonstrate effective coping strategies
Oxaliplatin only: Potential for sensory perceptual alterations related to pharyngolaryngeal dysesthesia	1. Teach patient that pharyngolaryngeal dysesthesia may occur 2. Teach patient preventive measures, such as avoidance of cold before chemotherapy, during, and for 1–3 days following 3. If symptom develops, teach patient relaxation exercises	• Pharyngolaryngeal dysesthesia will be prevented • If pharyngolaryngeal dysesthesia occurs, patient will tolerate experience safely

Source: Data from Armstrong et al[1]; Visovsky et al[11]; Visovsky et al[147]; Wickham[150]; Hile et al[153].

for falls. Mobility is a priority for most patients; in fact, older adults may prefer maintenance of mobility over therapy that may lengthen survival.[154] Assessment of impairments as well as mobility-related function should occur first at baseline, and then regularly during treatment.[153] Patients commonly report tingling, burning, and allodynia, which can lead to decreased hand grip and function.[150] Involvement of physical therapists (PTs) and occupational therapists (OTs) is very important in assessment of functional disability and development of rehabilitative interventions.[155] For example, if the patient has difficulty with hand grips, an OT can evaluate the patient and recommend an appropriate assistive device.

Certain exercise therapies may increase circulation and sensory perception (skin stimulation). Pain is often a major concern. Although crampy pain may be relieved by short-acting opioids, neuropathic (dysesthetic) pain is often unrelieved by opioids and requires treatment with other agents such as duloxetine, venlafaxine, or pregabalin. Topical gels or plasters may be appropriate and deserve consideration.

A review of rehabilitation guidelines for patients with breast cancer led panelists to recommend that patients who had CIPN that interferes with functioning be referred to a physical or occupational therapist.[124] Benefits of this approach include not only therapeutic intervention, but also education and practical advice that can help patients cope more effectively with the challenges of CIPN to daily living. Physical therapy may help patients with motor deficits strengthen weakened muscles. Usual exercises focus on range of motion, stretching, and massage. In addition, the PT can make recommendations for assistive devices such as orthotic braces, canes, and appropriate splints. High-top tennis shoes may help the patient with footdrop and gait disturbances.[150] Loss of fine motor movement may have a significant impact on quality of life, so attention to self-esteem and life satisfaction is very important. Using a rehabilitation focus, occupational therapists can provide helpful tips on self-care and living with limitations.[17] The data showing that manual therapy (massage) significantly decreases sensory distress (pain, numbness, tingling) are limited to case studies,[156] although a feasibility study is under way, and instructions by an oncology massage expert are available via the Internet.[157,] Armstrong et al. caution that patients with allodynia or hyperalgesia may not be able to tolerate massage.[1]

Patient self-assessment for autonomic dysfunction (bowel, bladder, and sexual) is very important, along with specific self-care measures. For example, during chemotherapy with vincristine, constipation can be prevented through the use of bowel regimens. Patients should be instructed to eat a high-fiber diet, have a fluid intake of 2 to 3 liters per day, and exercise regularly. Constipation should be prevented, so patients should be taught self-care strategies, including the administration of laxative suppositories or cathartics if needed.[158]

Cranial nerve deficits include loss of hearing and visual changes. Patients at high risk for hearing loss should have audiograms performed prior to and during therapy to identify such losses.[159] If significant abnormalities appear, discussion of risk versus benefit of continued therapy should occur between the healthcare team and the patient. Patients should be instructed to report early changes in hearing such as tinnitus; this will also prompt early risk-versus-benefit discussions between patient and provider.

For patients receiving oxaliplatin, it is important to teach the patient before cycle 1 to avoid cold during and for 3 days after treatment. If it is winter and very cold outside, the patient should wear warm clothes, a scarf, hat, and mittens and cover his or her mouth when talking to prevent inhalation of cold air. The car should be warmed prior to the patient getting into the vehicle. Prior to, during, and after the treatment, the patient should avoid drinking cold beverages. If it is necessary to drink cool beverages, advise the patient to drink through a straw. Inside the house, when in the kitchen, the patient should wear gloves when reaching into the refrigerator or freezer. This will minimize or prevent acute pharyngolaryngeal dysesthesia, as well as cramping of the fingers and hands.[150]

If a patient has begun to develop peripheral neuropathy, it is critical to rigorously assess the patient at each encounter for signs and symptoms of progressive neuropathy using a scale that is consistent at each visit, as well as to ascertain their effect on ADLs. Patients should be advised to report signs and symptoms during intervals between treatments as well, and journaling or some form of documentation may be helpful in this regard. Symptom management revolves around the particular symptoms. The nurse assesses for risk factors for injury; ability to perform self-care such as ADLs, food preparation, and house cleaning; ability to ambulate; bowel elimination pattern; and alterations in sexuality. The nurse, together with the patient and family, develop a plan of care focusing on symptom management and injury prevention (e.g., having someone else test water temperature using an unbreakable thermometer if the patient has decreased sensitivity to temperature changes). While prospective, randomized clinical trials to document evidence of efficacy remain to be conducted, most nonpharmacologic interventions are not harmful. These include exercise (especially in water), massage, hydrotherapy, acupuncture, and TENS.[17] In terms of pharmacologic management of neuropathic pain, the goal is to interrupt or modulate the painful impulse so that the pain is less intense or absent.

PATIENT SELF-CARE

Table 22-11 provides a list of resources for patients with CIPN and their families. Appendix 22A provides a self-care guide for patients with peripheral neuropathy.

TABLE 22-11

Patient and Family Resources
Organizations
American Chronic Pain Association (ACPA) P.O. Box 850 Rocklin, CA 95677–0850 ACPA@theacpa.org http://www.theacpa.org Phone: 916–632–0922, 1-800-533-3231 Fax: 916–652-8190
Foundation for Peripheral Neuropathy 485 Half Day Road, Suite 200 Buffalo Grove, IL 60089 info@tffpn.org http://www.foundationforpn.org Phone: 877-883-9942 Fax: 847-883-9960
National Foundation for the Treatment of Pain P.O. Box 70045 Houston, TX 77270 NFTPain@cwo.com http://www.paincare.org Phone: 713-862-9332 Fax: 713-862-9346
Neuropathy Action Foundation Administration Office 1950 Old Tustin Ave Santa Ana, CA 92705 Arizona office 18650 N. Thompson Peak Parkway #1021 Scottsdale, AZ 85255 Phone: 877-512-7262 info@neuropathyaction.org http://www.neuropathyaction.org/index.htm
Neuropathy Association 60 East 42nd Street Suite 942 New York, NY 10165·0999 info@neuropathy.org http://www.neuropathy.org Phone: 888-PN-FACTS (888-763-2287) Fax: 212–692–0668
Websites American Cancer Society. www.cancer.org
American Society of Clinical Oncologists (ASCO) Cancer.net
CancerCare www.cancercare.org
Canadian Neuropathy Association http://canadianneuropathyassociation.healthunlocked.com/
Oncology Nursing Society, Ons.org
National Institute of Neurological Disorders and Stroke: NINDS Peripheral Neuropathy Information Page http://www.ninds.nih.gov/disorders/peripheralneuropathy/peripheralneuropathy.htm
Neuropathy Trust (UK) http://neurocentre.com/community/

REFERENCES

1. Armstrong T, Almadrones L, Gilbert MR. Chemotherapy-induced peripheral neuropathy. *Oncol Nurs Forum.* 2005;32:305–311.
2. Calhoun EA, Fishman DA, Roland PY, et al. Total cost of chemotherapy-induced hematologic and neurologic toxicity. *Proc Am Soc Clin Oncol.* 1999;18A:1606(abstr. 886).
3. Pike CT, Birnbaum HG, Muehlenbein CE, Pohl GM, Natale RB. Healthcare costs and workloss burden of patients with chemotherapy-associated peripheral neuropathy in breast, ovarian, head and neck, and nonsmall cell lung cancer. *Chemother Res Pract.* 2012. doi: 10.1155/2012/913848.
4. Ostchega Y, Monohoe M, Fox N. High dose cisplatin-related peripheral neuropathy. *Cancer Nurs.* 1988; 11:23–32.
5. Cachia E, Eiser C, Ezaydi Y, et al. A study of pain, peripheral neuropathy and psychosocial late effects in multiple myeloma patients. *BMJ Support Palliat Care.* 2012;2:A3. doi: 10.1136/bmjspcare-2012-000196.8.
6. Tofthagen C. Patient perceptions associated with chemotherapy-induced peripheral neuropathy *Clin J Oncol Nurs.* 2010;14:E22–E28.
7. Tofthagen C, Overcash J, Kip K. Falls in persons with chemotherapy-induced peripheral neuropathy. *Support Care Cancer.* 2012;20:583–589.
8. Bakitas MA. Background noise: the experience of chemotherapy-induced peripheral neuropathy *Nurs Res.* 2007;56:323–31.
9. Lee EL, Westcarth L. Neurotoxicity associated with cancer therapy. *Adv Pract.* 2012;3:11–21.
10. Teravainen H, Larsen A. Some features of the neuromuscular complications of pulmonary cancer. *Ann Neurol.* 1977;2:495–502.
11. Visovsky C, Meyer RR, Roller J, Poppas M. Evaluation and management of peripheral neuropathy in diabetic patients with cancer. *Clin J Oncol Nurs.* 2007;12:243–247.
12. Wolf S, Barton D, Kottschade L, Grothey A, Loprinzi C. Chemotherapy-induced peripheral neuropathy: prevention and treatment strategies. *Eur J Cancer.* 2008;44:1507–1515.
13. Zhannat N, Xia R, Liu C-C, et al. Risk of chemotherapy-induced peripheral neuropathy in large population-based cohorts of elderly patients with breast, ovarian and lung cancer. *Am J Therapeutics.* 2010;17:148–158.
14. Markman M. Chemotherapy-induced peripheral neuropathy: underreported and underappreciated. *Curr Pain Headache Rep.* 2006;10:275–278.
15. Polomano RC, Farrar JT. Pain and neuropathy in cancer survivors. *Cancer Nurs.* 2006;29(2 suppl):39–47.
16. Hausheer FH. Chemotherapy-induced peripheral neuropathy. In: Perry MC, ed. *The Chemotherapy Source Book.* 4th ed. Philadelphia: Lippincott Williams and Wilkins; 2008:234–244.
17. Stubblefield MD, McNeely ML, Alfano CM, Mayer DK. A prospective surveillance model for physical rehabilitation of women with breast cancer. *Cancer.* 2012;118(suppl 8):2250–2260.
18. Stubblefield MD, Burstein HJ, Burton AW, et al. NCCN task force report: management of neuropathy in cancer. *J Natl Compr Cancer Ntwk.* 2009;7(suppl 5):S1–S26.
19. Amato AA, Baron RJ. Peripheral neuropathy. In: Longo DL, Fauci AS, Kasper DL, Hauser JL, Jameson J, Loscalzo, eds. *Harrison's Principles of Internal Medicine.* 18th ed. New York: McGraw-Hill; 2012:3448–3473.
20. Berkowitz A, Walker S. Bortezomib-induced peripheral neuropathy in patients with multiple myeloma. *Clin J Oncol Nurs.* 2012;16:86–89.
21. Renbarger JL, McCammack KC, Rouse CE, Hall SD. Effect of race on vincristine related neurotoxicity. *Pediatr Blood Cancer.* 2008;50:769–771.
22. Richardson PG, Delforge M, Beksac M, et al. Management of treatment-emergent peripheral neuropathy in multiple myeloma. *Leukemia.* 2011;26:595–608.
23. Richards T. Managing the side effects of lenalidomide and bortezomib. *Comm Oncol.* 2009;6:56–58.
24. Saif MW, Hashmi S, Mattison L, Donovan WB, Diasio RB. Peripheral neuropathy exacerbation associated with topical 5-fluorouracil. *Anti-Cancer Drugs.* 2006;17:1095–1098.

25. Velasco R, Petit J, Clapes V, Verdu E, Navarro X, Bruna J. Neurological monitoring reduces the incidence of bortezomib-induced peripheral neuropathy in multiple myeloma patients. *J Peripher Nerv Syst.* 2010;15(1):17–25.
26. Corthals SL, Kulper R, Johnson DC, et al. Genetic factors underlying the risk of bortezomib induced peripheral neuropathy in multiple myeloma patients. *Haematologica.* 2011;96(11):1728–1732.
27. Podratz JL, Knight AM, Ta LE, et al. Cisplatin induced mitochondrial DNA damage in dorsal root ganglion neurons. *Neurobiol Dis.* 2010;41:661–668.
28. Bennett, G, Flatters S. Studies of peripheral sensory nerves in paclitaxel-induced painful peripheral neuropathy: evidence for mitochondrial dysfunction. *Pain.* 2006;122:245–257.
29. Pascuzzi RM. Peripheral neuropathy. *Med Clin North Am.* 2009;93:317–342.
30. Hall JE. The nervous system: motor and integrative neurophysiology. In: *Guyton and Hall Textbook of Medical Physiology.* 12th ed. Philadelphia: Saunders Elsevier; 2011:655–665.
31. Windebank AJ, Grisold W. Chemotherapy-induced neuropathy. *J Peripher Nerv Syst.* 2008;13:27–46.
32. Becker PS. Genetic predisposition for chemotherapy-induced neuropathy in multiple myeloma. *J Clin Oncol.* 2011;29:783–785.
33. Reyes-Gibby CC, Morrow P. Chemotherapy-induced peripheral neuropathy as a predictor of neuropathic pain in breast cancer patients previously treated with paclitaxel. *J Clin Oncol.* 2009;27(suppl): abstr e20505.
34. Wolf SL, Barton DL, Qin R, et al. The relationship between numbness, tingling, and shooting/burning pain in patients with chemotherapy-induced peripheral neuropathy (CIPN) as measured by the EORTC QLQ-CIPN-20 instrument, N06CA. *Support Care Cancer.* 2012;20:625–632.
35. Wang XM, Lehky TJ, Brell JM, Dorsey SG. Discovering cytokines as targets for chemotherapy-induced painful peripheral neuropathy. *Cytokine.* 2012;59:3–9.
36. Doyle T, Chen Z, Muscoli C, et al. Targeting the overproduction of peroxynitrite for the prevention and reversal of paclitaxel-induced neuropathic pain. *J Neurosci.* 2012;32:6149–6160.
37. Swain SM, Arezzo JC. Neuropathy associated with microtubule inhibitors: diagnosis, incidence, and management. *Clin Adv Hematol Oncol.* 2008;6:455–467.
38. Weisfeld-Adams JD, Dutton GN, Murphy DM. Vincristine sulfate as a possible cause of optic neuropathy. *Pediatr Blood Cancer.* 2007;48:238–240.
39. Versrappen CC, Koeppen S, Heimans JJ, et al. Dose-related vincristine-induced peripheral neuropathy with unexpected off-therapy worsening *Neurology.* 2005;64:1076–1077.
40. Delord J-P, Bennouna J, Mourey L, Bougaret J, Brandely-Talbot M, Ferre P. Vinflunine oral pharmacokinetics and absolute bioavailability of soft and hard gelatin capsules: results of two Phase 1 trials. *Clin Pharmacokin* 2012;51:357–364.
41. Moriyam B, Henning SA, Leung J, et al. Adverse interactions between antifungal azoles and vincristine: review and analysis of cases. *Mycoses.* 2012;55(4):290–297.
42. Scripture CD, Figg WD, Sparreboom A. Peripheral neuropathy induced by paclitaxel: recent insights and future perspectives. *Curr Neuropharmacol.* 2006;4:165–172.
43. Mielke S, Spareboom A, Mross K. Peripheral neuropathy: a persisting challenge in paclitaxel-based regimes. *Eur J Cancer.* 2006;42:24–30.
44. Loprinzi CL, Reeves BN, Dakhil SR, et al. Natural history of paclitaxel-associated acute pain syndrome: prospective cohort study NCCTG N08C1. *J Clin Oncol.* 2011;29:1472–1478.
45. Reyes-Gibby CC, Morrow PK, Buzdar A, Shete S. Chemotherapy induced peripheral neuropathy as a predictor of neuropathic pain in breast cancer patients previously treated with paclitaxel. *J Pain.* 2009;10:1146–1150.
46. Sanofi-aventis US LLC. Taxotere prescribing information. Bridgewater, NJ: September 2011.
47. Paller CJ, Antonarakis ES. Cabazitaxel: a novel second-line treatment for metastatic castration-resistant prostate cancer *Drug Des Devel Ther.* 2011;5:117–124.
48. Scheff RJ. Breast cancer and the new taxanes: focus on *nab*-paclitaxel. *Comm Oncol.* 2008;5(suppl 8):7–13.
49. Gradishar WJ, Tjulandin S, Davidson N, et al. Phase III trial of nanoparticle albumin-bound paclitaxel compared with polyethylated castor-oil based paclitaxel in women with breast cancer *J Clin Oncol.* 2005;23:7794–7803.
50. Gradishar WJ, Krasnojon D, Cheporov S, et al. Significantly longer progression-free survival with *nab*-paclitaxel compared with docetaxel as first-line therapy for metastatic breast cancer. *J Clin Oncol.* 2009;27:3611–3619.
51. Celgene Corporation. Abraxane package insert. Summit, NJ: January 2012.
52. Bristol Myers Squibb. Ixempra prescribing information. Princeton, NJ: October 2011.
53. Thomas E, Gomez HL, Li RK, et al. Ixabepilone plus capecitabine for metastatic breast cancer progressing after anthracycline and taxane treatment. *J Clin Oncol.* 2007;25:5210–5217.
54. Low JA, Wedam SB, Lee JJ, et al. Phase II clinical trial of ixabepilone (BMS-247550), an epothilone B analog, in metastatic and locally advanced breast cancer. *J Clin Oncol.* 2005;23:2726–2734.
55. Vahdat L, Gopalakrishna P, Garcia AA, et al. Comparison of the incidence of peripheral neuropathy with eribulin mesylate versus ixabepilone in metastatic breast cancer patients: a randomized phase II study. Presented at CTRC-AACR San Antonio Breast Cancer Symposium, San Antonio, TX. December 6–10, 2011. Abstr P5-19-02.
56. Eisai, Inc. Halaven package insert. Woodcliff Lake, NJ: February 2012.
57. Twelves C, Loesch D, Blum JL, et al. A phase III study (EMBRACE) of eribulin mesylate versus treatment of physician's choice in patients with locally recurrent or metastatic breast cancer previously treated with an anthracycline and a taxane. *J Clin Oncol.* 2010;28 (suppl):18s (abstr CRA 1004).
58. Weiss RB. Miscellaneous toxicity: neurotoxicity. In: DeVita VT, Hellman S, Roseberg SA, eds. *Cancer: Principles and Practice of Oncology.* 6th ed. Philadelphia: Lippincott Williams &Wilkins; 2005:2924–2936.
59. Rademaker-Lakhai JM, Crul M, Zuur L, et al. Relationship between cisplatin administration and the development of ototoxicity. *J Clin Oncol.* 2006;24:918–924.
60. Omoti AE, Omoti CE. Ocular toxicity of systemic anticancer chemotherapy. *Pharmacy Pract.* 2006;4:55–59.
61. Holden S, Felde G. Nursing care of patients experiencing cisplatin-related peripheral neuropathies. *Oncol Nurs Forum.* 1987;14:13–19.
62. Saif MW, Reardon J. Management of oxaliplatin-induced peripheral neuropathy. *Ther Clin Risk Manag.* 2005;1:249–258.
63. Sanofi-aventis US LLC. Eloxatin prescribing information. Bridgewater, NJ: December 2011.
64. Millennium Pharmaceuticals Inc. Velcade prescribing information. Cambridge, MA: January 2012.
65. Argyriou AA, Iconomou G, Kalofonos HP. Bortezomib-induced peripheral neuropathy in multiple myeloma: a comprehensive review of the literature. *Blood.* 2008;112:1593–1598.
66. Moreau P, Pylypenko H, Grosicki S, et al. Subcutaneous versus intravenous administration of bortezomib in patients with relapsed multiple myeloma: a randomized, Phase 3, non-inferiority study. *Lancet Oncol.* 2011;12:431–440.
67. Richardson PG, Briemberg H, Jagannath S, et al. Frequency, characteristics, and reversibility of peripheral neuropathy during treatment of advanced multiple myeloma with bortezomib *J Clin Oncol.* 2006;24:3113–3120.
68. Jagannath S. Current standards for first-line therapy of multiple myeloma. *Clin Lymphoma Myeloma.* 2007;7:S207–S214.
69. Chaudhry V, Cornblath DR, Polydefkis M, Ferguson A, Borrello I. Characteristics of bortezomib- and thalidomide-induced peripheral neuropathy. *J Peripher Nerv Syst.* 2008;13:275–282.
70. Mikhael J, Rajkumar V, Roy V, et al. Efficacy of pomalidomide plus low-dose dexamethasone in multiple myeloma patients despite previous use of lenalidomide [abstract]. *J Clin Oncol.* 2011;29(suppl 15): [Abstr] 8067.

71. Bennett GJ: Update on the neurophysiology of pain transmission and modulation: focus on the NMDA-receptor. *J Pain Symptom Manage.* 2000;19(1 suppl):S2–S6.
72. Wu LJ, Zhuo M. Targeting the NMDA receptor subunit NR2B for the treatment of neuropathic pain. *Neurotherapeutics.* 2009;6:693–702.
73. Callin S, Bennett MI. Assessment of neuropathic pain. *Contin Educ Anesthesia Crit Care Pain.* 2008;8:210–213.
74. Mateos, MV, Hernandez IM, Hernandez MT, et al. Bortezomib plus melphalan and prednisone in elderly untreated patients with multiple myeloma: results of a multicenter phase 1/2 study. *Blood.* 2006;108:2165–2171.
75. Hile ES, Fitzgerald GK, Studenski SA. Persistent mobility disability after neurotoxic chemotherapy. *Phys Ther.* 2010;90:1649–1657.
76. Tofthagen CS, McMillan SC, Kip KE. Development and psychometric evaluation of the chemotherapy-induced peripheral neuropathy assessment tool. *Cancer Nurs.* 2011;34:E10–E20.
77. Postma TJ, Aaronson NK, Heimans JJ, et al. The development of an EORTC quality of life questionnaire to assess chemotherapy-induced peripheral neuropathy: the QLQ-CIPN20. EORTC module for CIPN. http://groups.eortc.be/qol/qolg_projects.htm#neuropathy. Accessed June 10, 2012.
78. Bickley LS. The nervous system. In: *Bates' Guide to Physical Examination and History Taking.* 10th ed. Philadelphia: Wolters Kluwer/Lippincott Williams & Wilkins; 2009:672–678, 663–671, 690–696.
79. Legha SS. Vincristine neurotoxicity: pathophysiology and management. *Med Toxicol.* 1986;1:421–427.
80. Argyiou AA, Polychronopoulos P, Chroni E. The usefulness of nerve conduction studies in objectively assessing oxaliplatin-induced peripheral neuropathy. *Oncologist.* 2007;12:1371–1372.
81. Cleeland CS, Farrar JT, Hausheer FH. Assessment of cancer-related neuropathy and neuropathic pain. *Oncologist.* 2010;15(suppl 2):13–18.
82. Smith EM, Beck SL, Cohen J. The total neuropathy score: a tool for measuring chemotherapy-induced peripheral neuropathy *Oncol Nurs Forum.* 2008;35:96–102.
83. National Cancer Institute Cancer Therapy Evaluation Program. Common Terminology for Adverse Events[v.4.03]. 2010. http://evs.nci.nih.gov/ftp1/CTCAE/CTCAE_4.03_2010-06-4_QuickReference_8.5x11.pdf). Accessed June 3, 2012.
84. Smith EM, Cohen JA, Pett MA, Beck SL. The reliability and validity of a modified total neuropathy score-reduced and neuropathic pain severity items when used to measure chemotherapy-induced peripheral neuropathy in patients receiving taxanes and platinums. *Cancer Nurs.* 2010;33:173–183.
85. Griffith KA, Merkies IS, Hill EE, Cornblath DR. Measures of chemotherapy-induced peripheral neuropathy: a systematic review of psychometric properties. *J Peripher Nerv Syst.* 2010;15:314–25.
86. Smith EM, Cohen JA, Pett MA, Beck SL. The validity of neuropathy and neuropathic pain measures in patients with cancer receiving taxanes and platinums. *Oncol Nurs Forum.* 2011;38:133–142.
87. Tofthagen C, McAllister RD, McMillan SC. Peripheral neuropathy in patients with colorectal cancer receiving oxaliplatin. *Clin J Oncol Nurs.* 2011;15:1182–1189.
88. Eastern Cooperative Oncology Group. Common toxicity criteria. http://ecog.dfci.harvard.edu/general/common_tox.html. Accessed June 3, 2012.
89. Huang HQ, Brady MF, Cella D, Fleming G. Validation and reduction of FACT/GOG-Ntx subscale for platinum/paclitaxel-induced neurologic symptoms: a gynecologic oncology group study. *Int J Gynecol Cancer.* 2007;17:387–393.
90. Cavaletti G. The chemotherapy-induced peripheral neuropathy outcome measures standardization (CI-Perinoms) study: an answer to the unsettled questions of drug-related neuropathy assessment in cancer patients. *Eur Assoc Neurooncol Mag.* 2012;2:37–40.
91. Sparano JA, Wang M, Martino S, et al. Weekly paclitaxel in the adjuvant treatment of breast cancer *N Engl J Med.* 2008;358:1663–1671.
92. Tournigand C, Cervantes A, Figer A, et al. OPTIMOX1: a randomized study of FOLFOX4 or FOLFOX7 with oxaliplatin in a stop-and-go fashion in advanced colorectal cancer: a GERCOR study. *J Clin Oncol.* 2006;24:394–400.
93. Tabernero J, Aranda E, Gomez A, et al. Phase III study of first-line XELOX plus bevacizumab (BEV) for 6 cycles followed by XELOX plus BEV or single-agent (s/a) BEV as maintenance therapy in patients (pts) with metastatic colorectal cancer (mCRC): the MACRO trial (Spanish Cooperative Group for the Treatment of Digestive Tumors [TTD]). *J Clin Oncol.* 2010;28(15 suppl):3501.
94. Lhomme C, Berton-Rigaud D, Joly F, et al. Results from a randomized Phase II study to evaluate the safety and efficacy of acetyl-L-carnitine in the prevention of sagopilone-induced peripheral neuropathy (REASON). *J Clin Oncol.* 2011;29(suppl): abstr 9116.
95. Guo Y, Palmer JL, Forman SR, et al. A randomized, double-blinded, placebo-controlled trial of oral alpha lipoic acid to prevent platinum-induced polyneuropathy *J Clin Oncol.* 2011;29(suppl): abstr 9010.
96. Beijers AJM, Jongen JLM, Vreugdenhil G. Chemotherapy-induced neurotoxicity: the value of neuroprotective strategies. *Netherlands J Med.* 2012;70(1):18–25.
97. Hochster HS, Grothey A, Childs BH. Use of calcium and magnesium salts to reduce oxaliplatin-related neurotoxicity *J Clin Oncol.* 2007;225:4028–4029.
98. Grothey A, Nikcevich DA, Sloan JA, et al. Intravenous calcium and magnesium for oxaliplatin-induced sensory neurotoxicity in adjuvant colon cancer: NCCTG N04C7. *J Clin Oncol.* 2011;29:421–427.
99. Gamelin L, Boisdron-Celle M, Morel A, et al. Oxaliplatin related neurotoxicity: interest of calcium magnesium infusion and no impact on its efficacy. *J Clin Oncol.* 2008;26:1188–1189.
100. Knijn N, Tol J, Koopman M, et al. The effect of prophylactic calcium and magnesium infusions on the incidence of neurotoxicity and clinical outcome of oxaliplatin-based systemic treatment in advanced colorectal cancer patients. *Eur J Cancer.* 2011;47:369–374.
101. Choo S, Tan H, Lo YL, et al. Use of intravenous calcium and magnesium infusion in preventing oxaliplatin-induced sensory neuropathy. *Asian Pac J Clin Oncol.* 2010;61(4):270–277.
102. Wong GY, Michalak JC, Sloan JA, et al. A Phase III double blinded, placebo controlled, randomized trial of gabapentin in patients with chemotherapy-induced peripheral neuropathy: a North Central Cancer Treatment Group Study. *Proc Am Soc Clin Oncol.* Orlando, FL: May 14–17, 2005: 8001.
103. Wang WS, Lin JK, Lin TC, et al. Oral glutamine is effective for preventing oxaliplatin-induced neuropathy in colorectal cancer. *Oncologist.* 2007;12:312–319.
104. Stubblefield MD, Vahdat LT, Balmaceda CM, et al. Glutamine as a neuroprotective agent in high dose paclitaxel-induced peripheral neuropathy: a clinical and electrophysiologic study. *J Clin Oncol.* 2005;17:271–276.
105. Weickhardt A, Wells K, Messersmith W. Oxaliplatin-induced neuropathy in colorectal cancer. *J Oncology.* 2011:201593 [Epub December 12, 2011]. doi: 10.1155/2011/201593.
106. Lin PC, Lee MY, Wang WS, et al. *N*-acetylcysteine has neuroprotective effects against oxaliplatin-based adjuvant chemotherapy in colon cancer patients: preliminary data. *Support Care Cancer.* 2006;14:484–487.
107. Argyriou AA, Chroni E, Polychronopoulos P, et al. Efficacy of oxcarbazepine for prophylaxis against cumulative oxaliplatin-induced neuropathy. *Neurology.* 2006;67:2253–2255.
108. Davis ID, Kiers L, MacGregor L, et al. A randomized, double-blinded placebo-controlled Phase II trial of recombinant human leukemia inhibitory factor (rhuLIF, emfilermin, AM242) to prevent chemotherapy-induced peripheral neuropathy. *Clin Cancer Res.* 2005;11:1890–1898.
109. Pace A, Giannarelli D, Galie E, et al. Vitamin E neuroprotection for cisplatin neuropathy: a randomized placebo-controlled trial. *Neurology.* 2010;74:762–766.

110. Kottschade LA, Sloan JA, Mazurczak MA, et al. The use of vitamin E for the prevention of chemotherapy-induced peripheral neuropathy: results of a randomized Phase III clinical trial. *Support Care Cancer.* 2011;19:1769–1777.
111. Cassidy J, Bjarnason G, Hickish T, et al. Randomized double blind (DB) placebo (Plcb) controlled Phase III study assessing the efficacy of xaliproden (X) in reducing the cumulative peripheral sensory neuropathy (PSN) induced by the oxaliplatin (Ox) and 5-FU/LV combination (FOLFOX4) in first line treatment of patients (pts) with metastatic colorectal cancer (MCRC). *J Clin Oncol.* 2006;24(suppl 18S):3507, abstr 229.
112. Donald GK, Tobin I, Stringer J. Evaluation of acupuncture in the management of chemotherapy-induced peripheral neuropathy. *Acupunct Med.* 2011;29:230–233.
113. Xu WR, Hua BJ, Hou W, Bao YJ. Clinical randomized controlled study on acupuncture for treatment of peripheral neuropathy induced by chemotherapeutic drugs. *Zhongguo Zhen Jiu.* 2010;300:457–460.
114. Wong R, Sagar S. Acupuncture treatment for chemotherapy-induced peripheral neuropathy: a case series. *Acupunct Med.* 2006;24:87–91.
115. Visovsky C. Acupuncture for the management of chemotherapy-induced peripheral neuropathy *J Adv Pract Oncol.* 2012;3:178–1181.
116. Barton DL, Wos EJ, Qin R, et al. A double-blind, placebo-controlled trial of a topical treatment for chemotherapy-induced peripheral neuropathy: NCCTG trial N06CA. *Support Care Cancer.* 2011;19: 833–841.
117. Derry S, Lloyd R, Moore RA, McQuay HJ. Topical capsaicin for chronic neuropathic pain in adults (review). *Cochrane Database Sys Rev.* April 2009; 4. doi: 10.1002/14651858.CD07393. Accessed June 12, 2012.
118. Smith TJ, Coyne PJ, Parker GL, Dodson P, Ramakrishnan V. Pilot trial of a patient-specific cutaneous electrostimulation device (MC5-A Calmare) for chemotherapy-induced peripheral neuropathy *J Pain Symptom Manage.* 2010;40:883–891.
119. Smith EML, Pang H, Cirrincione C, et al. CALGB 170601: A Phase III double blind trial of duloxetine to treat painful chemotherapy-induced peripheral neuropathy (CIPN). *J Clin Oncol.* 2012;30(suppl): abstr CRA9013.
120. Rao RD, Michalak JC, Sloan JA, et al. Efficacy of gabapentin in the management of chemotherapy-induced peripheral neuropathy: a Phase 3 randomized, double-blind, placebo controlled, crossover trial (N00C3). *Cancer.* 2007;110:2119–2118.
121. Humpert PM, Morcos M, Oikonomou D, et al. External electric muscle stimulation improves burning sensations and sleeping disturbances in patients with type 2 diabetes and symptomatic neuropathy. *Pain Med.* 2009;10:413–419.
122. Reichstein L, Labrenz S, Ziegler D, Martin S. Effective treatment of symptomatic diabetic polyneuropathy by high-frequency external muscle stimulation. *Diabetologia.* 2005;48:824–828.
123. Rao RD, Flynn PJ, Sloan JA, et al. Efficacy of lamotrigine in the management of chemotherapy-induced peripheral neuropathy: a Phase 3 randomized, double-blind, placebo-controlled trial, N01C3. *Cancer.* 2008;112:2802–2808.
124. White CM, Pritchard J, Turner-Stokes L. Exercise for people with peripheral neuropathy. *Cochrane Database Syst Rev.* 2004; 18(4):CD003904.
125. Balducci S, Iacobellis G, Parisi L, et al. Exercise training can modify the natural history of diabetic peripheral neuropathy. *J Diab Complic.* 2006;20:216–223.
126. Lavery LA, Murdoch DP, Williams J, Lavery DC. Does anodyne light therapy improve peripheral neuropathy in diabetes? A double-blind, sham-controlled, randomized trial to evaluate monochromatic infrared photoenergy. *Diab Care.* 2008;31:316–321.
127. Mekhail NA, Mathews M, Nageeb F, Guirguis M, Mekhail MN, Cheng J. Retrospective review of 707 cases of spinal cord stimulation: indications and complications. *Pain Pract.* 2010;11:148–153.
128. Pieber K, Herceg M, Paternostro-Sluga T. Electrotherapy for the treatment of painful, diabetic peripheral neuropathy: a review. *J Rehab Med.* 2010;42:289–295.
129. Hilpert F, Stahle A, Tome O, et al. Neuroprotection with amifostine in the first-line treatment of advanced ovarian cancer with carboplatin/paclitaxel-based chemotherapy: a double blind, placebo-controlled, randomized phase II study from the Arbeitsgemeinschaft Gynakologische Onkologoie (AGO) Ovarian Cancer Study Group. *Support Care Cancer.* 2005;13:797–805.
130. Moore D, Donnelly J, McGuire WP, et al. Limited access trial using amifostine for protection against cisplatin and three hour paclitaxel-induced neurotoxicity: a phase II study of the Gynecologic Oncology Group. *J Clin Oncol.* 2003;21:4207–4213.
131. Openshaw H, Beamon K, Synod TW, et al. Neurophysiological study of peripheral neuropathy after high-dose paclitaxel: lack of neuroprotective effect of amifostine. *Clin Cancer Res.* 2004;10:461–467.
132. Khattack MA. Calcium and magnesium prophylaxis for oxaliplatin-related neurotoxicity: is it a trade-off between drug efficacy and toxicity. *Oncologist.* 2011;16:1780–1783.
133. Grothey A, Hart LL, Rowland KM, et al. Intermittent oxaliplatin administration and time-to-treatment failure in metastatic colorectal cancer: final results of the Phase III CONCEPT trial. *J Clin Oncol.* 2008;26(suppl 15S; abstr 4010),180s.
134. Durand JP, Deplanque G, Montheil V, et al. Efficacy of venlafaxine for the prevention and relief of oxaliplatin-induced acute neurotoxicity: results of EFFOX, a randomized, double-blind, placebo-controlled Phase III trial. *Ann Oncol.* 2011;23:200–205.
135. Moore RA, Straube S, Wiffen PJ, Derry S, McQuay HJ. Pregabalin for acute and chronic pain in adults. *Cochrane Database Syst Rev.* 2009;3:CD007076.
136. Vondracek P, Oslejskova H, Kepak T, et al. Efficacy of pregabalin in neuropathic pain in paediatric oncological patients. *Eur J Paediatr Neurol.* 2009;13:332–336.
137. Saif MW, Syrigos K, Kaley K, Isufi I. Role of pregabalin in treatment of oxaliplatin-induced sensory neuropathy. *Anticancer Res.* 2010;30:2927–2933.
138. Rosenquist RW. Practice guidelines for chronic pain management. *Anesthesiology.* 2010;112:1–24.
139. Barr GA, McPhie-Lalmansingh A, Perez J, Riley M. Changing mechanisms of opiate tolerance and withdrawal during early development: animal models of human experience. *ILAR.* 2011;52:329–341.
140. Ebert B, Thorkildsen C, Andersen S, Christrup LL, Hjeds H. Opioid analgesics as noncompetitive *N*-methyl-D-aspartate (NMDA) antagonists. *Biochem Pharmacol.* 1998;56:553–559.
141. Baron R, Mayoral V, Leijon G, Binder A, Steigerwald I, Serpell M. Efficacy and safety of 5% lidocaine (lignocaine) medicated plaster in comparison with pregabalin in patients with postherpetic neuralgia and diabetic polyneuropathy: interim analysis from an open-label, two-stage, adaptive, randomized, controlled trial. *Clin Drug Investig.* 2009;29:231–241.
142. Gallagher RM. Management of neuropathic pain: translating mechanistic advances and evidence-based research into clinical practice. *Clin J Pain.* 2006;22(suppl 1):S2–S8.
143. Saljoughian M. Capsaicin: risks and benefits. *US Pharmacist.* 2009;34:HS-17–HS-18.
144. Dunteman E. Targeted peripheral analgesics in chronic pain syndromes. *Practical Pain Manage.* July/August 2005: 14–25.
145. Granato J. Fast-track designation: AmiKet (EpiCept). *Formulary.* May 1, 2012. http://formularyjournal.modernmedicine.com/formulary/article/articleDetail.jsp?id=774125. Accessed July 21, 2012.
146. Oncology Nursing Society. Putting evidence into practice: peripheral neuropathy. Review completed as of May 2008. http://ons.org/Research/PEP/media/ons/docs/research/outcomes/peripheral/quickview.pdf. Accessed June 15, 2012.

147. Visovsky C, Collins M, Abbott L, Aschenbrenner J, Hart C. Putting evidence into practice: evidence based interventions for chemotherapy-induced peripheral neuropathy. *Clin J Oncol Nurs.* 2007;11:901–913.
148. Visovsky C. Measuring oncology nursing sensitive patient outcomes: evidence based summary. http://www.ons.org/Research/NursingSensitive/Summaries/media/ons/docs/research/summaries/peripheral/overview.pdf. Accessed June 10, 2012.
149. Given B, Sherwood P. Nursing sensitive patient outcomes: a white paper. *Oncol Nurs Forum.* 2005;32:773–784.
150. Wickham R. Chemotherapy induced peripheral neuropathy: a review and implications for oncology nursing practice. *Clin J Oncol Nurs.* 2007;11:361–376.
151. Speck RM, Demichele A, Farrar JT, et al. Scope of symptoms and self-management strategies for chemotherapy-induced peripheral neuropathy in breast cancer patients. *Support Care Cancer.* 2012;20(10): 2433–2440.
152. National Cancer Institute Symptom Management and Quality of Life Steering Committee. Chemotherapy-induced peripheral neuropathy. Clinical Trials Planning Meeting, Executive Summary. http://transformingtrials.cancer.gov/files/CIPN_CTPM_Final_Executive_Summary_for_CCCT_Aug_2010.pdf. Accessed July 20, 2012.
153. Hile ES, Fitzgerald GK, Studenski SA. Persistent mobility disability after neurotoxic chemotherapy. *Phys Ther.* 2010;90:1657–1659.
154. Mendelblatt JS, Sheppard VB, Hurria A, et al. Breast cancer adjuvant chemotherapy decisions in older women: the role of patient preference and interactions with physicians. *J Clin Oncol.* 2010;28:3146–3153.
155. Harris SR, Schmitz KH, Campbell KL, McNeely ML Clinical practice guidelines for breast cancer rehabilitation: synthesis of guideline recommendations and qualitative appraisals. *Cancer.* 2012;118(suppl 8):2312–2324.
156. Cunningham JE, Kelechi T, Sterba K, Barthelemy N, Falkowski P, Chin SH. Case report of a patient with chemotherapy-induced peripheral neuropathy treated with manual therapy (massage). *Support Care Cancer.* 2011;19:1473–1476.
157. Woods RD. Step-by-step massage therapy protocols for common conditions: CIPN. *Massage Today.* February 12, 2012. http://www.massagetoday.com/mpacms/mt/article.php?id=14537. Accessed June 13, 2012.
158. Wilkes GM, Barton-Burke M. *Oncology Nursing Drug Handbook.* Burlington, MA: Jones & Bartlett Learning; 2012:331–334.
159. Chang KW. Clinically accurate assessment and grading of ototoxicity. *Laryngoscope.* 2011;121:2649–2657.

Peripheral Neuropathy

Patient Name: ____

This guide will help you learn about peripheral neuropathy and how to take care of yourself.

Symptom and Description

Chemotherapy may cause damage to one or more nerves in your body. If you already have peripheral neuropathy, it may increase the risk of it getting worse. Which symptoms you feel depend on the chemotherapy drug. You may feel or have any of the symptoms in the list:

- "Pins and needles," numbness, tingling, or burning in your toes/feet and fingers/hands
- Trouble telling the difference between hot or cold
- Trouble being able to pick up a small object like a coin, or button your shirt, or dropping things
- Trouble feeling the shape of a coin in your hand
- Trouble knowing where your hands and feet are, such as where your foot is when you start to climb stairs; this may cause you to trip
- Pain along the nerve, such as in your toes/feet or fingers/hands
- Less strength in your muscles or weakness

Less common symptoms include:

- Constipation or other changes in your bowel or bladder function
- Feeling dizzy when standing

Prevention

While it is not possible to prevent peripheral neuropathy, there are things you can do to prevent it from getting worse. You should tell your nurse or doctor if you have any of these symptoms, and if it is hard to do your daily care, such as brushing your teeth and getting dressed. There may be other ways of giving your chemotherapy that lessen the risk of peripheral neuropathy, or your dose may be changed. Your doctor or nurse will also review your other medicines to make sure that any of them that cause peripheral neuropathy are changed.

If your chemotherapy is vincristine or vinblastine, you should try to keep your bowel movements regular. These tips may help prevent constipation:

- Drink 2 to 3 quarts of fluid each day.
- Eat a high-fiber diet (fruit, veggies, beans, bran, prunes).
- Try to do light exercise.
- Take a laxative as directed by your nurse or doctor if you have not moved your bowels in 1 to 2 days.

If your chemotherapy is oxaliplatin, you should avoid being cold for the first few days of treatment.

- Do not drink cold drinks, as this can make your throat feel like it is closing.
- Wear a glove when you put your hand in the freezer.
- Stay warm.

Management

Tell your doctor or nurse if you have any symptoms, and how they affect your life, such as during sleep, eating, cooking, or getting dressed.

One or more of these symptoms may put you at risk for getting hurt, such as falling, or burning yourself if you cannot feel how hot something is. These tips are helpful to keep you safe and to ease any problems:

- Stay as active as you can, walking and doing light to moderate exercise to keep your muscles toned.
- Protect your hands and feet by wearing gloves when washing dishes, working in the garden, or doing chores.
- Check your feet daily for any sores or cuts, as your shoes may be too tight and you may not feel it.
- If cooking, use thick pot holders and think about using plastic plates and utensils.
- If you have trouble feeling hot and cold, turn down the temperature of your hot water heater to prevent burning yourself. Ask someone else to test the water (bath, dish) for you.
- Use a non-skid tub mat and shower chair in the bath; use a tub rail to hold on to.
- Make sure halls and rooms are well lit and clutter free so you do not trip or fall.
- Make sure stairs are well lit, and use the stair railings for support when climbing them.
- If your fingers have trouble with zippers or buttons, wear pants with an elastic waistband or use a zipper pull or buttoner (from the occupational therapist).
- If you have trouble knowing where your feet are, avoid driving, as you may not be able to use the brakes when needed. Watch where you put your feet, and walk with one foot ahead of the other so you do not trip.
- Talk with family members about ways they can help you, such as by cooking, cleaning, and keeping the home safe.
- Talk with your nurse or doctor about trouble you are having. Physical and occupational therapists are part of the healthcare team, and they can offer helpful tips and devices.
- Ways to manage discomfort:
    - Talk with your doctor or nurse about medicines that can help relieve the pain, numbness, and tingling.
    - Talk with your nurse about nonmedicine treatment that may make you feel better, such as massage, exercise, acupuncture, and topical creams. There is some evidence that these treatments can decrease the discomfort of peripheral neuropathy.

Follow-Up

There is much that can be done to help you if you feel symptoms of peripheral neuropathy. It is important that you know what the symptoms are and are willing to report them. Ask your doctor or nurse if you have questions. Also, make sure you know when your next appointment is.

(continued)

Phone Numbers

Physician: ______________________________ Phone: ____________

Nurse: ______________________________ Phone: ____________

Home Health Nurse: ______________________________ Phone: ____________

OT/PT: ______________________________ Phone: ____________

Notes: ______________________________

Source: Wilkes GM. Peripheral Neuropathy. In: Yarbro CH, Wujcik D, Gobel BH, eds. *Cancer Symptom Management.* 4th ed. Burlington, MA: Jones & Bartlett Learning; 2014.

PART IX

Anatomical and Surgical Alterations

Chapter 23

Alopecia

Mary Callaghan, RN, MN, AOCNS®
Abby Cooper, RN, MSN, OCN®

THE PROBLEM

The impact of hair loss as a result of cancer therapy has been described in the medical literature for more than 40 years. Many references and studies state that hair loss, also known as alopecia, negatively impacts cancer patients' perception of their physical appearance, body image, sexuality, and self-esteem. In the anthropological literature, hair is an important symbol of the individual and the individual's relationship to his or her culture.[1] The way we look and the image we project says a great deal about the ways in which we value ourselves; when those values include portions of our physical appearance that are altered by therapy, anxiety ensues.

Wagner and Bye published one of the first studies to measure the impact of drug-induced alopecia on body image in patients with cancer in 1979.[2] The subjects of their study—one group with signs of chemotherapy-induced alopecia and the other group without alopecia—completed a body image and social activity questionnaire. The results revealed that subjects with alopecia decreased their social activities more than those without obvious hair loss, but body image and social activity scores between the groups showed no statistically significant difference. This study has prompted continued research in the area throughout the ensuing decades.

More recent reviews of the literature regarding cancer treatment-related alopecia indicate that alopecia continues to be a distressing side effect that negatively affects various elements of quality of life including body image and social engagement.[3,4] A number of studies have examined self-esteem, self-image, sexual problems, body image, and self-confidence in patients with chemotherapy-induced alopecia.[5–8] In the literature related to breast cancer, hair loss is just as traumatizing to some patients as losing their breast.[4]

The experience of hair loss related to their cancer therapy not only influences patients' self-image but also informs them and others of the seriousness of their illness. A phenomenological study of young adults indicated that patients discovered that hair loss was difficult to hide and was a conspicuous sign to others of their illness.[9] Even when patients felt physically well while undergoing chemotherapy, their hair loss served as a signal of their disease to others, who then treated them differently.

The media, consumer education movements, and the increased availability of medical information have sensitized the public to the many side effects of cancer therapy. Ironically, this sensitivity has made it more difficult for some patients to hide evidence of their cancer treatments. Yet society's willingness to openly discuss the difficulties that patients with cancer face has led to the creation of a myriad of resources and support services. An environment that empowers the patient to be productive and active throughout cancer therapy and beyond should be the goal of both the healthcare and the lay communities.

INCIDENCE

Alopecia is a common side effect related to radiation therapy to the head and many chemotherapeutic and biologic agents. Chemotherapy-related alopecia is estimated to occur in 65% of patients with cancer.[10] Descriptions of hair loss associated with single agents such as busulfan began to appear in the medical literature in the late 1950s.[11] By the 1960s, reports of therapy-related hair loss increased as chemotherapy was prescribed for more patients. Within the four classes of chemotherapeutic agents, the frequency of alopecia is estimated at 80% for antimicrotubule agents such as paclitaxel; 60% to 100% for antitumor antibiotic agents such as doxorubicin; more than 60% for alkylators such as cyclophosphamide; and 10% to 50% for antimetabolites such as 5-flourouracil.[10] The trend toward combining two or more agents with differing mechanisms of action (combination therapy), coupled with increased drug doses to maximize cell kill, has increased the likelihood of alopecia.

Radiation-induced hair loss is more variable, depending on the area to be radiated and the dose of radiation. Whole-brain irradiation is associated with 100% hair loss.[12] Hair loss related to directed radiation therapy to the brain occurs only over the area of the scalp included in the radiation port. Temporary alopecia occurs approximately 2 to 3 weeks after radiation exposure and resolves within 2 to 3 months of completion of radiation.[12] This point must be clearly articulated so that individuals receiving radiation to areas other than the scalp need not fear losing scalp hair. Doses of 200–500 centigray (cGy) to the scalp can produce some hair loss depending on how many treatments are required. Higher doses yield more profound alopecia and retarded patterns of regrowth.[12]

Permanent alopecia—defined as absence of or incomplete hair growth 6 months beyond completion of therapy is correlated significantly with the radiation dose administered.[12] Doses reported to cause permanent hair loss vary widely. One study reported the rate of permanent hair loss to be in the range of 0% to 80%, with a median incidence of 5% in patients receiving 36 gray (Gy) of radiation (2 Gy/fraction, 5 days/week).[13] Lawenda et al.[12] conducted a study to develop a dose-response relationship for the occurrence of permanent alopecia after cranial irradiation. The follicle dose at which 50% of the patients developed permanent alopecia in this study was estimated to be 43 Gy. The median dose for minimal alopecia (Grade 1 or 2) was 32.9 Gy (range, 10.7-54 Gy). The median dose in which moderate to severe alopecia occurred (Grade 3 and 4) was 48.4 Gy (range: 15.9–73.6 Gy).[12] This study provided a better understanding of the relationship between radiation dose and the development of alopecia.

Targeted biologic agents have recently been identified as a key therapy in cancer, but few reports in the literature have addressed alopecia as a result of the use of these agents. Small-molecule inhibitors and monoclonal antibodies targeting the epidermal growth factor receptor (EGFR) are recognized as causes of a variety of cutaneous side effects, including alopecia.[14–16] The EGFR inhibitors have been linked to alopecia and a number of hair changes, including changes in texture, slower growth of scalp hair, trichomegaly of eyelashes, and hypertrichosis of facial hair.[17] Cetuximab, a monoclonal antibody targeting EGFR, has been reported to induce alopecia in 4% of patients receiving this therapy.[18]

Multitargeted receptor tyrosine kinase inhibitors have been associated with reversible hair depigmentation and, in some cases, with mild alopecia. Sorafenib and sunitinib, both oral tyrosine kinase inhibitors, have been reported to induce alopecia in as many as 50% of patients.[17,18] The alopecia described with these agents is described as diffuse and reversible.

ETIOLOGY

Normal hair growth patterns

A single human hair comprises a hair bulb that contains a proliferating pool of undifferentiated cells, the hair root, and the hair shaft. At the base of every hair follicle is the padilla, which consists of the rapidly dividing matrix cells. Active division of matrix cells occurs in the lower portion of the bulb, which pushes the hair up from the root and projects it through the surface of the scalp. A strand of scalp (or terminal) hair is composed of rows of tightly compacted, keratinized cells. Approximately 100,000 such strands cover the human scalp, with most individuals experiencing an average loss of 100 to 150 of these hairs daily.[19]

Phases of hair growth and rest normally vary with age and body region; they can also be affected by physiological and psychological events. Normal hair growth phases are tricyclic and are not synchronized. At any single point in time, 85% to 90% of human scalp hair is in the growing (anagen) phase and 12% is in the transitional (catagen) and resting (telogen) phases. Anagen lasts from 2 to 5 years, producing hair growth at a rate of 0.35 mm/day. As hairs approach catagen (which lasts up to 2 weeks), the hair root separates from within the hair bulb and is pushed out of the bulb. During the resting phase (telogen), there is no obvious hair growth for approximately 3 to 5 months; this is a period of intense metabolic and proliferation preparation for ensuing growth.[20] Events that initiate catagen and the resultant telogen are not clear. As telogen ends, there is a repeated increase in RNA synthesis as follicles reenter anagen.

Treatment-related mechanisms of action on hair follicles

Chemotherapy, radiation therapy, and many biologic agents make no distinction between cancer and normal cells. With chemotherapeutic agents, all sites of energetic mitotic activity are prone to their chemical insult. The bone marrow, gastrointestinal tract, and rapidly proliferating cells of the hair and skin surfaces are particularly vulnerable to these effects. Not all drugs within a single pharmacologic classification produce equal degrees of alopecia; the reason that some agents and not others produce alopecia is unclear.

Many agents can produce alopecia (Table 23-1). Although some agents are more often noted to cause hair loss due to their frequent appearance in the medical literature (e.g., doxorubicin and cyclophosphamide), the degree of hair loss produced by any particular agent is influenced by the dose delivered, the schedule, and the rate and the route of administration.[20,21] Agents typically associated with alopecia include anthracyclines, antibiotics, antimetabolites, vinca alkaloids, and taxanes.[21,22] Unfortunately, the incidence of alopecia with common chemotherapeutic regimens is difficult to predict because these data are inconsistently documented in the literature. High-dose chemotherapy regimens used in stem cell transplantation are associated with complete hair loss in a short period of time.[23] The use of cyclic combination chemotherapy regimens such as cyclophosphamide, 5-fluorouracil, methotrexate (CMF) and doxorubicin and cyclophosphamide (AC) is associated with gradual hair loss over several weeks.[20,21] Low-dose therapy, oral administration, and weekly regimens are less likely to cause complete alopecia.[22]

Radiation therapy-induced hair loss is a result of the direct effect of radiation-induced damage to DNA replication and cellular replication. As described earlier, the amount of radiation dose to the hair follicle within the radiation field is an important factor influencing hair loss.[12,13]

The etiology of targeted therapy-related hair loss continues to be investigated. Indeed, hair loss in patients receiving targeted therapies has yet to be fully described. The hair changes associated with EGFR inhibitors are thought to result from the inhibitory effects on normal hair growth.[15,24] Activation of EGFR appears to be important in normal hair growth; thus inhibition of this growth factor during the anagen phase will cause hair loss.

In a recent study investigating the adequacy of common grading tools for measuring dermatologic toxicities related to oral tyrosine kinase inhibitors (TKIs), 24% of patients receiving an oral TKI experienced some degree of hair loss.[25] Hair loss occurred by the third week following initiation of therapy in 56% of patients. The National Cancer Institute Commom Terminology Criteria for Adverse Events (CTCAE) grade 1 and grade 2 toxicity occurred in 79% and 21% of patients, respectively. Additional studies are needed to adequately describe the incidence and severity of alopecia associated with the new targeted therapies.

TABLE 23-1

Cancer Therapy Agents Associated with Alopecia*
Agents that Usually Produce Alopecia
Cyclophosphamide
Daunorubicin
Docetaxel
Doxorubicin (>50 mg)
Etoposide
Ifosfamide
Irinotecan
Paclitaxel
Taxotere
Topotecan
Vindesine
Vinorelbine
Agents that Sometimes Produce Alopecia
5-Fluorouracil
Amsacrine
Bleomycin
Busulfan
Cetuximab
Cytarabine
Dactinomycin
Epirubicin
Gemcitabine
Idarubicin
Mechlorethamine
Melphalan
Mithramycin
Mitomycin
Mitoxantrone
Sorafenib
Sunitinib
Thiotepa
Vinblastine
Vincristine
Low to No Potential to Produce Alopecia
Carboplatin
Capecitabine
Carmustine
Cisplatin
Chlorambucil
Dacarbazine
Fludarabine
Hydroxyurea
Imatinib
Interleukin-2
L-Asparaginase
Lomustine
6-Mercaptopurine
Methotrexate
Procarbazine
Suramin
Teniposide
6-Thioguanine

**Note*: The degree, onset, and duration of alopecia result from a combination of treatment factors, including agent dosage, delivery schedule, route of administration, and the combination of agents and treatment modalities.

PATHOPHYSIOLOGY

Most hair follicle injury is caused by anagen arrest. Because the matrix in the hair bulbs of the follicles on the scalp is highly proliferative, hair follicles are vulnerable to cytotoxic drugs and direct damage from radiation therapy.[26] When a dose of an alopecia-causing drug is given, the cells of the hair bulbs absorb a proportion of the drug. Cellular division and protein synthesis can be suppressed or halted. If cellular activity is completely halted, the hair enters telogen (resting phase) prematurely. The hair is free to be shed, and regrowth occurs in approximately 3 to 5 months, the normal length of telogen. This sequence of events can explain the hair regrowth that some patients experience even while continuing to receive chemotherapy; it is the normal hair cycle that was precipitously interrupted by a dose of chemotherapy; the cycle resumes if there is no further insult by additional doses of drug.[20,26] Patients should be made aware that the regrowth of hair during a chemotherapy cycle is not an indication that the therapy is not working.

If a dose of drug is not sufficient to halt anagen, inhibition of mitosis in the hair bulb may occur instead, causing narrowing or constriction of the hair shaft; these narrow sections can be viewed as the follicle grows. Additional doses of drug can cause repeated areas of stricture, reflecting each exposure to the causative agent. These structural abnormalities are weakened sites and become points of breakage during normal activities such as shampooing or brushing the hair.[26,27]

Alopecia connotes a diffuse shedding of hair. To be noticeable, at least 50% of the hair must be lost.[27] Although most discussions about this toxicity of many cancer drugs focus on the loss of scalp hair, loss of hair effects can include the axillary, pubic, body, and facial hair, including the eyebrows and eyelashes. Agents that cause alopecia differ in their ability to do so through a variety of routes, doses, and schedules. High peak blood levels produced by intermittent administration of drugs on schedules such as every 2 or 3 weeks (pulse drug doses) may cause great disruption in the mitotic activity of anagenic hair cells, whereas continuous infusions of lower daily doses of drug can increase the cell's length of exposure to the causative agent. One agent classically linked to alopecia, doxorubicin, causes significantly more hair loss at doses of 50 mg/m^2 or greater.[22] Many early reported interventions to reduce alopecia focused on doxorubicin, due to the high frequency of its use and the nearly total reported occurrence of alopecia extending to the eyebrows and eyelashes.

Hair loss typically begins to appear days to weeks after the first exposure to drug, with continued loss over the next 3 to 4 weeks, but there can be dramatic exceptions to this guideline.[22,27] Typically hair on the crown and the sides of the head above the ears disappears first, possibly due to mechanical friction, as these areas come into contact with bed linens, pillows, and head coverings. Patients may complain that their scalp hurts, itches, or has heightened sensitivity just prior to major hair loss.[26]

Exposed scalp can be sensitive, so it must be protected. Regrowth may be seen in 3 months as cells move prematurely into telogen to recover and reenter anagen. As hair repopulates the scalp, it may be damaged again by additional drug doses, or it may continue to grow slowly. An early report on 14 patients with cancer who received a single infusion of busulfan noted that alopecia appeared in 6 of the 14 individuals, with slow regrowth of hair. The researchers also noted that alopecia was unrelated to clinical response. No alopecia was seen at lower doses of the drug that were also therapeutically effective.[11] Hair loss is nearly always temporary when caused by cancer drugs. Recent reviews have reported permanent hair loss after high-dose chemotherapy and stem cell transplantation with busulfan as the likely drug causing the hair loss.[22,23] Another report cited numerous changes in new hair growth, ranging from color to texture alterations; for example, straight hair can regrow waved or curly, and consistency can change from thick to fine. These changes have been reported in as many as 60% of patients.[22] Generally hair returns without interruption once all systemic therapy has been halted.[22,26]

SYMPTOM ASSESSMENT

RISK FACTORS

The primary risk factor for the development of alopecia is the specific agent used for treatment. The routes, doses, and schedules all influence the degree of alopecia.[21,22] Although most estimations of degree of alopecia are reported as case reports or anecdotal descriptions with few high-level evidence-based studies, Table 23-1 provides a general list of agents that are associated with cancer therapy-related alopecia.

OBJECTIVE ASSESSMENT

The ability to measure a phenomenon such as drug-induced alopecia is critical for three reasons:

1. To precisely describe alopecia in terms of severity, onset, duration, and recovery
2. To standardize descriptors of alopecia so that information from multiple studies and settings can be compared and contrasted
3. To evaluate responsiveness to therapeutic measures

Physical assessment

Patients who have alopecia or who receive alopecia-causing treatment are examined at serial time points to document patterns of hair loss, especially if they are enrolled in a clinical trial. The physical exam must include the following components:

- Description of patterns of hair loss on the scalp and over the entire body
- Density of remaining hair
- Shape of the front hairline
- Length, texture, and curl/wave of hair
- Color and shine
- Condition of the scalp

Additionally, hair can be gently pulled to test for excessive loss (the pull test), and subjected to a daily count and a wash test to measure amount of hair loss.[27] The patient should be questioned about finding hair on pillows or bed linens to determine timing and severity of alopecia so as to provide education and supportive care. Fine regrowth of hair may be noted between treatments or approximately 3 months after the initiation of alopecia-causing therapy. Precise documentation of the patterns of hair loss and recovery is vital and often overlooked, especially in a clinical trial setting. The global description "alopecia" on each patient visit is not sufficient, as it ignores important patient information about hair loss patterns that could be definitive for a new cancer drug or drug combination. Diaries or other patient recording devices may allow patients the chance to track daily observations and may provide the healthcare professional with precise data both for the clinical trial and for future research studies.

DEGREES OF TOXICITY

WHO toxicity grading criteria

The World Health Organization (WHO) convened meetings in 1978 and 1979 attended by representatives from 13 nations. The purpose of the meetings was to standardize reporting criteria for cancer clinical trials, especially those focused on the reporting of toxicities. WHO criteria related to alopecia that were derived from the meetings and adapted to the trials of the European Organization for Research on Treatment in Cancer (EORTC) are listed in Table 23-2.[28] The WHO criteria are often used in European clinical trials to describe toxicity, and in trials measuring prevention of alopecia.

TABLE 23-2

World Health Organization Grading for Alopecia

Grade 0	Grade I	Grade 2	Grade 3	Grade 4
No change	Minimal loss	Moderate, patchy loss	Complete alopecia but reversible	Nonreversible loss

Source: Data from World Health Organization[28].

ECOG grading criteria

The WHO grading criteria for the measurement of toxicity have not been widely used by U.S. clinical trials groups. Instead, a number of cancer cooperative group tools to assess therapy side effects have been developed. One commonly used tool is a grading scale from the Eastern Cooperative Oncology Group (ECOG), listed in Table 23-3.[29] The ECOG grading system for alopecia is simplistic, and allows for interrater scoring differences.

TABLE 23-3

Eastern Cooperative Oncology Group (ECOG) Alopecia Grading

Grade 0	Grade I	Grade 2	Grade 3	Grade 4
None	Alopecia (mild) <49%	Alopecia (severe) >50%	—	—

Source: Data from ECOG[29].

Common terminology criteria for adverse events

The Cancer Therapy Evaluation Program (CTEP) of the National Cancer Institute (NCI) developed Common Toxicity Criteria (CTC) in 1988 to provide a set of repetitive measures of commonly experienced side effects of clinical trials that could be used for all U.S. cooperative groups. The guidelines, now referred to as Common Terminology Criteria for Adverse Events (CTCAE), have been revised over the years to expand the categories, more precisely define clinical phenomena, and remove the subjectivity of measures whenever possible.[30] The resulting alopecia scale is seen in Table 23-4. In both the ECOG and CTCAE scales, the maximum score for alopecia severity is grade 2.

SYMPTOM MANAGEMENT STRATEGIES

THERAPEUTIC APPROACHES

Preventive strategies

The controversy over the preventability of therapy-induced alopecia has persisted since 1966, when report of scalp tourniquet use appeared in the medical literature.[31] Since those

TABLE 23-4

National Cancer Institute Common Terminology Criteria for Adverse Events (CTCAE): Alopecia				
Grade 0	**Grade 1**	**Grade 2**	**Grade 3**	**Grade 4**
Normal	Hair loss up to 50% of normal that is not obvious from a distance but only on close inspection; does not require wig or hair piece to camouflage	Hair loss of >50% normal that is readily apparent to others; a wig or hair piece is necessary, desire to completely camouflage the hair loss	—	—

Source: Data from National Cancer Institute Common Terminology Criteria for Adverse Events (CTCAE)[30].

first publications, interventions to prevent or minimize the loss of hair during therapy have been of three major types: scalp tourniquets, scalp hypothermia or cooling, and use of pharmacologic agents.

Scalp tourniquets or pressure to retard hair loss is accompanied by risks, however, and is not a recommended practice.[26] The use of scalp tourniquets has been abandoned and there are no reports in the current literature regarding its use.

Scalp hypothermia or cooling applies the concept of creating a drug-free area through the use of ice or temperature-controlled devices to decrease drug uptake to the scalp. Scalp cooling may also alter the metabolism of agents in the cells. Numerous reports have shown varying degrees of success in using hypothermia to retard hair loss.[21,32–38] Published reports are often difficult to analyze and compare, however, for the following reasons:

- They are frequently nonrandomized studies, with no control group.
- They use vague or unreported scales by which to measure success.
- They do not adequately define assessment periods and criteria to judge success.
- They group together patients receiving different drugs on different schedules.
- They have not reported follow-up on patients once alopecia occurs.
- They report small patient numbers.
- They use different methods to cool the scalp.

In recent reviews of literature, there has been an increased interest in scalp cooling to prevent chemotherapy-induced alopecia.[3,33–35] A recent review of nonpharmacologic methods for dealing with chemotherapy side effects concluded that based on the published literature, a tentative recommendation could be made for the prevention of chemotherapy-induced alopecia using scalp hypothermia.[35]

The success of scalp cooling may be linked to the following factors:

- *Ability to cool the scalp sufficiently.* Thus the fit, temperature, and length of application are important.
- *The drugs and doses administered.* High doses of agents deemed more likely to produce alopecia are more difficult to protect against through scalp cooling.
- *Concerns related to patient safety.* Although reports of latent scalp metastases following scalp hypothermia or cooling put the prevalence of this complication at less than 1%, the possibility of placing a patient at risk for later, perhaps resistant, sites of disease recurrence may make this intervention untenable for some healthcare professionals.[34]

Scalp hypothermia is described as uncomfortable by some patients. In addition, its benefits usually become less obvious over time for patients who use it for repeated chemotherapy treatments. In a study of female breast cancer patients, those who attempted scalp cooling with unsuccessful results report a lower health-related quality of life and body self-image than those who did not attempt to inhibit hair loss.[36] The intervention also requires time expenditure by the staff, who must apply and maintain these devices.

In the United States, the broad application of scalp hypothermia to reduce treatment-related alopecia was curtailed in the early 1980s.[3] The Food and Drug Administration (FDA) took the scalp cooling apparatus off the market based on reports of scalp metastasis occurring after scalp cooling.[34] The interest in scalp cooling has been resurrected by the American public as evidenced by an article describing scalp hypothermia.[37] The European literature indicates that researchers in Europe continue to study and use scalp hypothermia.[32–36]

Pharmacologic agents represent an area of intervention that has raised some hope among professionals who are frustrated by the risks and failure rates associated with scalp hypothermia. A review of the literature by Wang et al. summarized trials using pharmacologic agents to prevent or minimize alopecia.[38] Several agents, including minoxidil, AS 101 (a tellurium compound), ammonium tricholor (dioxoethylen-O,O-), and vitamin D were reviewed.[38]

Minoxidil is an orally active peripheral vasodilator used to treat severe hypertension, which produces a side effect of enhanced hair growth. It has been tested for its ability to retard hair loss during chemotherapy treatment and to accelerate the regrowth of lost hair. The drug offered good protection against hair loss induced by cytosine arabinoside but not against cyclophosphamide-induced alopecia in rat models.[38] Both a randomized-controlled trial and a prospective trial failed to find any benefits from the prophylactic use of 2% topical minoxidil during chemotherapy.[38] Unfortunately, the investigation of minoxidil has shown mixed responses in other trials and its use had not been advocated in practice.[38]

Vitamin D (calcitriol) has also been investigated as a prevention agent because of its ability to inhibit DNA synthesis and to arrest the cell cycle at the Gap 0/Gap 1 interphase in keratinocytes.[38] A single trial investigated the use of topical vitamin D at 0.00025% and 0.005% doses. This intervention failed to show any protection from chemotherapy-induced alopecia in women receiving 5-fluorouracil, nonliposomal doxorubicin, and cyclophosphamide.[38]

The literature reveals recent experience with a number of agents to protect and recover hair. In 2006, Wang et al. published an expert review on many pharmacologic agents studied to decrease hair loss related to cancer therapy.[38] The immunomodulator AS 101 was found to show chemotherapy and radiation hair-loss protective effects in patients with lung cancer receiving combination chemotherapy.[38] Many other agents under investigation have proved disappointing in terms of their ability to prevent alopecia related to chemotherapy.[22,38]

In summary, a variety of interventions aimed at chemotherapy-related alopecia reported since 1966 have shown a range of results. Scalp hypothermia or cooling using gel packs, ice caps, or a variety of commercially available devices remains the most commonly used scalp hair preservation intervention reported in the literature, although this practice is observed primarily in Europe. There are no clear prescriptive guidelines as to which patient groups would clearly benefit from hair loss prevention throughout treatment. Instead, a number of considerations are proposed for the healthcare professional's evaluation.

1. Currently, scalp cooling is contraindicated for those patients with hematological malignancies, and its use is controversial in patients with nonhematological malignancies who undergo curative chemotherapy.[10]
2. Scalp hypothermia cannot be predicted to be successful. Patients who may benefit the most are those who receive doxorubicin in doses of less than 50 mg/m^2 or drugs with low to moderate potential for producing alopecia.[10]
3. Scalp hypothermia appliances must fit snugly and be maintained at a uniformly low temperature. Some institutions report that wetting the hair before applying a scalp device gives a tight seal and a uniform cooling pattern. Patients must be assessed frequently throughout the cooling process for their comfort.[34,36]
4. Scalp tourniquet is a historic and not-recommended practice that has been largely replaced by hypothermia units.[26]
5. Pharmacologic approaches are relatively new, and results stemming from their use are now appearing in the medical literature with increasing frequency. Their ability to retard or prevent hair loss remains unproven.[38]

Management strategies

Patients should be advised to purchase a wig or head coverings early in their treatment schedule, while enough hair is present to allow a good match of color and style. Patients may request a prescription for a wig, or cranial prosthesis, as insurance may cover all or part of the cost.[22,39,40] Some stylists specialize in wigs for medically related hair loss. Artificial eyebrows and eyelashes are also commercially available; patients should be advised to use caution when applying them to sensitive skin, as skin irritation may occur.

Unprotected scalp and body areas are extremely sensitive.[22] Patients should be advised to use sun protection factor (SPF) products of at least SPF 15 when exposed to sunshine for more than brief periods of time. Use of a soft scarf or hat is advised to protect the scalp and reduce patients' sensitivity to temperature. Gentle massage and pain medication such as a nonsteroidal anti-inflammatory agent might be helpful in alleviating discomfort including itching and pain.[22]

Patients who experience an uneven pattern of hair loss may express the desire to shave or cut the remaining hair. This action can enhance a person's physical and emotional well-being, as a more symmetrical and acceptable body image is produced. Caregivers should alert the patient to avoid cuts or nicks to the scalp when sections of hair are cut; use of an electric razor can reduce the risk of nicking the scalp. Symptomatic relief may also be obtained by using lotions, massage, and other locally soothing approaches. Patients may also be given information regarding application of permanent make-up for eyebrows to enhance their appearance. Although the medical literature offers no guide to these practices, patients may gain relief from them, provided their safety is not jeopardized. Reassuring patients that their hair will return when systemic therapy is halted may redirect some of their anxiety toward adaptation and recovery. Hair regrowth averages 0.25 inch per month.

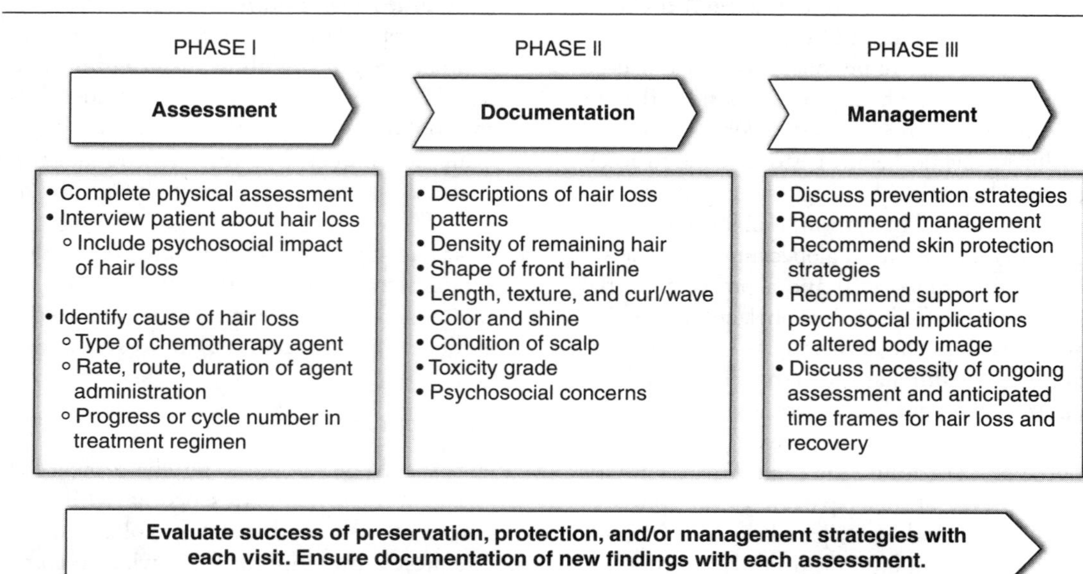

FIGURE 23-1

Nursing assessment and management guide for therapy-related alopecia.

NURSING IMPLICATIONS

Use of nursing diagnoses, often including grieving and disturbed body image, allows nurses to implement nursing interventions appropriate to a patient's experience.[39] Employing techniques such as active listening and support system enhancement can help support patients throughout the experience of this unavoidable side effect in many patients who receive chemotherapy treatment.[40]

Patients need to be prepared by their healthcare providers for the onset and transient nature of this side effect.[40–42] The appearance of hair on bed linens typically begins 2 weeks after the initiation of chemotherapy, but the onset can occur sooner, especially with high-dose regimens. Loss can be rapid and complete, resulting in a totally defoliated scalp within 3 to 4 weeks from the beginning of treatment. Figure 23-1 provides an assessment and management guide for therapy-related alopecia.

PATIENT SELF-CARE

Patients who experience alopecia as a side effect of their chemotherapy regimens do not necessarily have problems with treatment compliance.[3] Those who have difficulty with the altered self-image that alopecia imposes, however, may suffer. Healthcare professionals should be alert to patient and family reports of interference with activities because of symptoms such as alopecia, loss of appetite, withdrawal from family and significant others with verbalized feelings of loss of libido and attractiveness, depression, fatigue, and sadness. Classes such as "Look Good, Feel Better"—a series sponsored by the American Cancer Society—can help patients accept a different, perhaps transient, view of themselves until they recover from this obvious effect of their therapy program.[41] Appendix 23A provides a self-care guide for individuals experiencing alopecia.

REFERENCES

1. Hansen H. Hair loss induced by chemotherapy: an anthropological study of women, cancer, and rehabilitation. *Anthropol Med.* 2007;14:15–26.
2. Wagner L, Bye M. Body image and patients experiencing alopecia as a result of cancer chemotherapy. *Cancer Nurs.* 1979;5:365–369.
3. Trueb RM. Chemotherapy-induced alopecia. *Curr Opin Support Palliat Care.* 2010;4(4):281–284.
4. Lemieux J, Maunsell E, Provencher L. Chemotherapy-induced alopecia and effects on quality of life among women with breast cancer: a literature review. *Psychooncology.* 2008;17:317–328.
5. Zannini L, Verderame R, Cucchiara G, et al. "My wig has been my journey's companion": perceived effects of an aesthetic care programme for Italian women suffering from chemotherapy-induced alopecia. *Eur J Cancer Care.* 2012;21:650–660.
6. Roe H. Chemotherapy-induced alopecia: advice and support for hair loss. *Br J Nurs.* 2011;20:S4–S11.
7. Koszalinski RS, Williams C. Embodying identity in chemotherapy-induced alopecia. *Perspect Psychiatr Care.* 2012;48:116–121.
8. Fobair P, Stewart SL, Chang S, et al. Body image and sexual problems in young women with breast cancer. *Psychooncology.* 2006;15:579–594.

9. Snobolm C, Friedrichsen M, Heiwe S. Experiencing one's body after a diagnosis of cancer: a phenomenological study of young adults. *Psychooncology*. 2010;19:863–869.
10. Trueb R. Chemotherapy-induce alopecia. *Semin Cutan Med Surg*. 2009;28:11–14.
11. Bierman HR, Kelly KH, Knudson AG Jr, et al. The influence of 1,4-dimethyl sulfonoxy-l,4-dimethylbutane (CB 2348, Dimethyl Myleran) in neoplastic disease. *Ann NY Acad Sci*. 1958;68:1211–1222.
12. Lawenda BD, Gagne HM, Gierga DP, et al. Permanent alopecia after cranial irradiation: dose-response relationship. *Int J Radiat Oncol Biol Phys*. 2004;60:879–887.
13. Shakespeare TP, Dwyer M, Mukherjee R, et al. Estimating risks of radiotherapy complications as part of informed consent: the high degree of variability between radiation oncologists may be related to experience. *Int J Radiat Oncol Biol Phys*. 2002;54:647–653.
14. Donavan JC, Ghazarian DM, Shaw JC. Scarring alopecia associated with use of epidermal growth factor receptor inhibitor gefitinib. *Arch Dematol*. 2008;144:1524–1525.
15. Graves JE, Jones BF, Lind AC, et al. Nonscarring inflammatory alopecia associated with the epidermal growth factor receptor inhibitor erlotinib. *J Am Acad Dermatol*. 2006;55:349–353.
16. Wnorowski AM, de Souza A, Chachoua A, et al. The management of EGFR inhibitor adverse events: a case series and treatment paradigm. *Int J Dermatol*. 2012;51;223–232.
17. Widakowich C, de Castro G, de Azambuja E, et al. Review: side effects of approved molecular targeted therapies in solid cancers. *Oncologist*. 2007:12:1443–1445.
18. Hammond-Thelin LA. Cutaneous reactions related to systemic immunomodulators and targeted therapies. *Dermatol Clin*. 2008;26:121–159.
19. Elder D, Elenitsas R, Johnson BL, Murphy GF, eds. *Levery's Histopathology of the Skin*. 10th ed. Philadelphia, PA: Lippincott Williams and Wilkins; 2008.
20. Trueb RM. Chemotherapy-induced hair loss. *Skin Therapy Lett*. 2010;15:5–7.
21. Yeager CE, Olsen EA. Treatment of chemotherapy-induced alopecia. *Dermatol Ther*. 2011;24:432–442.
22. Chon SY, Champion RW, Geddes ER, et al. Chemotherapy-induced alopecia. *J Am Acad Dermatol*. 2012;67:e37–e47.
23. Tallon B, Blanchard E, Goldberg LJ. Permanent chemotherapy-induced alopecia: case report and review of the literature. *J Am Acad Dermatol*. 2010;63:333–338.
24. Balagula Y, Lacouture ME, Cotliar JA. Dermatologic toxicities of targeted anticancer therapies. *J Support Oncol*. 2010;8:149–161.
25. Chan A, Tan EH. How well does the MESTT correlate with CTCAE scale for grading of dermatological toxicities associated with oral tyrosine kinase inhibitors? *Support Care Cancer*. 2011;19:1667–1674.
26. Breed WP, Van den Hurk CJ, Peerbooms M. Presentation, impact and prevention of chemotherapy-induced hair loss. *Expert Rev Dermatol*. 2011;6:109–125.
27. Hillman K, Blume-Peytavi U. Diagnosis of hair disorders. *Semin Cutan Med Surg*. 2009;28:33–38.
28. World Health Organization. *Handbook for Reporting Results of Cancer Treatment*. Geneva, Switzerland: WHO; 1979.
29. Eastern Cooperative Group common toxicity criteria. http://ecog.dfci.harvard.edu/general/common_tox.html. Accessed April 14, 2012.
30. National Cancer Institute common terminology for adverse events (CTCAE), v. 4.0. http://evs.nci.nih.gov/ftp1/CTCAE/CTCAE_4.03_2010-06-14_QuickRefernece_5x7.pdf. Accessed April 14, 2012.
31. Simister JM. Alopecia and cytotoxic drugs. *BMJ*. 1966;2:1138.
32. Kargar M, Sarvestani, RS, Khojasteh HN, et al. Efficacy of penguin cap as scalp cooling system for prevention of alopecia in patients undergoing chemotherapy. *J Adv Nurs*. 2011;67:2473–2477.
33. Mols F, van den Hurk CJ, Vingerhoets AJ, Breed WP. Scalp cooling to prevent chemotherapy-induced hair loss: practical and clinical considerations. *Support Care Cancer*. 2009;17:181–189.
34. Grevelman EG, Breed WP. Prevention of chemotherapy-induced hair loss by scalp cooling. *Ann Oncol*. 2006;16:352–358.
35. Lofti-Jam K, Carey M, Jefford M, et al. Nonpharmacologic strategies for managing common chemotherapy adverse effects: a systematic review. *J Clin Oncol*. 2008;26:5618–5629.
36. van den Hurk CJ, Mols F, Vingerhoets A, et al. Impact of alopecia and scalp cooling on the well-being of breast cancer patients. *Psychooncology*. 2010;19:701–709.
37. Weiss S. Sub-zero therapy lets a chemo patient keep her hair. *Washington Post*. January 11, 2011; E1–E5.
38. Wang J, Lu Z, Au JL. Protection against chemotherapy-induced alopecia. *Pharm Res*. 2006;23:2505–2514.
39. Dougherty L. Using nursing diagnoses in prevention and management of chemotherapy-induced alopecia in the cancer patient. *Int J Nurs Terminol Classif*. 2007;18:142–149.
40. Borsellino M, Young M. Anticipatory coping. *Clin J Oncol Nurs*. 2011;15(3):311–315.
41. American Cancer Society. Hair loss. Updated November 12, 2009. http://www.cancer.org/treatment/treatmentsandsideeffects/dealingwithsymptomsathome/care-for-the-patient-with-cancer-at-home-hair-loss. Accessed February 12, 2011.
42. McGarvey E, Leon-Verdin M, Baum LD, et al. An evaluation of a computer-imaging program to prepare women for chemotherapy-related alopecia. *Psychooncology*. 2010;19:756–766.

Cancer Treatment-Related Hair Loss

Name: ____

Hair loss occurs with some cancer treatments. It can begin 10 to 21 days after these drugs are started, with total loss of hair in 1 to 2 months. Most of the time the hair on your head is lost first, but hair over the whole body can be lost. If you want to wear a wig during this time, it is a good idea to be fitted for one right away. Hair regrowth may begin while you are still getting cancer treatment, but it will be slow. Full regrowth of your hair will occur when your cancer treatment is done.

Stopping Hair Loss

Stopping hair loss may not be possible. Your doctor or nurse may be able to tell you some ways that can slow or lessen the loss of hair. These do not always work, and they may be used less often with some drugs that have a good chance of causing hair loss. Prevention of hair loss may be hard because of the way cancer treatments work. They are meant to reach your body by way of the blood. When this occurs, we cannot stop them from reaching hair cells, because hair cells get nourishment through your blood.

What You Should Know

Hair loss is a *temporary* side effect of cancer treatment. You need to protect your scalp and skin with head covers and skin protection factor (SPF) products while your hair is thin or missing. You will need to learn when to expect hair loss, how it may happen, and where to go to find a wig or other head covering (such as a hat). If you are getting radiation therapy, not chemotherapy, you may lose some hair only in areas of direct radiation and permanent hair loss may occur. Discuss your hair loss with your radiation therapy doctor or nurse. Think about getting a wig, hat, or scarf early in your treatments, *before* you lose your hair. Hair loss may change the way you feel about yourself. If your feelings are stopping you from doing important things, share them with your doctor or nurse. Avoid perming, dying, straightening or using other chemicals on your hair during chemotherapy as they may cause skin and scalp irritation. Use of a gentle shampoo and other gentle hair care products may help to decrease skin and scalp irritation. Increase the amount of time in between hair washing may also reduce the risk of scalp irritation.

Follow-Up

Discuss with your doctor or nurse at each treatment how you are coping with hair loss. The American Cancer Society offers Look Good, Feel Better® classes for people who have hair loss during cancer treatment. There are a lot of resources to help you to cope during this time in your life.

Phone Numbers

Nurse: ______________________________

Physician: ______________________________

Wig Vendors: ______________________________

Other: ______________________________

Comments

Patient's Signature: ____________________ Date: ____________________

Nurse's Signature: ____________________ Date: ____________________

Source: Callaghan M, Cooper A. Alopecia. In: Yarbro CH, Wujcik D, Gobel BH, eds. *Cancer Symptom Management*. 4th ed. Burlington, MA: Jones & Bartlett Learning; 2014.

Chapter 24

Altered Body Image and Sexual Health

Linda U. Krebs, PhD, RN, AOCN®, FAAN

THE PROBLEM

Alterations in sexuality and body image are recognized consequences of having and receiving treatment for cancer. They can occur at diagnosis, during treatment, both immediately after treatment or as a late effect of treatment, and throughout all stages of disease recurrence and progression.[1] However, despite being well discussed in the medical and patient advocacy literature, alterations in body image and sexual health following cancer diagnosis and treatment are frequently considered topics that are "nice for the patient to know about" rather than being perceived as necessary topics to be covered as part of quality cancer care.[2–8] Unfortunately, healthcare providers often have underrated these side effects due to lack of knowledge about how to discuss and manage sexual issues, believing others are better suited to discuss these topics or not recognizing their significance for the patient and family. Additionally, patients often do not discuss concerns about sexuality, and to a lesser extent body image, because they are embarrassed to bring up the topic or are fearful that they are raising frivolous concerns, at least in the eyes of the provider.

It is well recognized that sexual health is a component of overall health. It is equally well understood that providing information about potential sexual side effects at the time of diagnosis or initiation of treatment decreases patients' concerns and better prepares them for any complications that may arise.[2–10] Whether the effects are temporary or long term, being aware of potential sexual dysfunctions or body image changes can prepare the patient and family for sexual health consequences related to cancer and its associated treatments and, in some cases, may mitigate a specific side effect or its impact. As noted by Krebs, "without appropriate education, counseling, and support, it may be difficult for the patient and family to adapt to the alterations that cancer can produce."[2(p880)]

Multiple definitions for sexuality and sexual health exist in the popular and medical literature. Popular literature tends to focus on acts of a sexual nature such as intercourse, or on intimacy, relationships, and communication, whereas medical literature more often focuses on physical function and physical actions, body image, and fertility and reproduction. The World Health Organization (WHO) provides a global definition of sexual health, noting that "sexual health is a state of physical, mental and social well-being in relation to sexuality. It requires a positive and respectful approach to sexuality and sexual relationships."[11] In addition, WHO has identified 13 core competencies for effectively providing high-quality sexual and reproductive health care. Among them are (1) creating an environment in which sexual health can be effectively provided (Competencies 1–3); (2) providing sexual and reproductive education and counseling (Competencies 4 and 5); and (3) effectively assessing and referring individuals for sexual health concerns (Competency 6).[12] While designed for the primary care provider, these competencies are appropriate for the oncology team, and especially the oncology nurse, who should provide high-quality care that recognizes sexual health as encompassing more than intercourse, and as including intimacy, communication, body image, giving and receiving affection, and many other relationship and pleasurable attributes.[3]

According to Hatzichristou et al.,[13] sexual dysfunction is classified as follows: (1) type I: psychogenic (without biological findings); (2) type II: organic (having vascular, neurogenic, pharmacologic, hormonal, or anatomic causes); or (3) type III: mixed (having both biological findings and cognitive or emotional distress).[13] Anxiety may be present in all types. In those persons with cancer, disease, treatment, psychosocial issues, cultural factors, and economic concerns all may play a role in causing alterations in sexual health, affecting sexual function and body image.[13]

INCIDENCE

While no current statistics are available on the exact percentages of cancer survivors who experience sexual health alterations, previous data have suggested that from 30% to 100% of patients will experience some level of alteration, including decreased intimacy, decreased sexual desire and arousal, dyspareunia, and erectile dysfunction.[2–5,8,14,15] For many individuals, these alterations are brief and, while a source of discomfort, disappointments, and even anguish, do not continue to affect the patient's life once treatment is completed and side effects have subsided. For many others, however, long-term alterations will affect many aspects of life and life choices, ranging from body image alterations, to inability to have intercourse, to infertility.

When reviewing common sexual alterations in the general U.S. population, Lara et al. noted that approximately 43% of women aged 18 to 59 self-identify as having some type of sexual dysfunction.[16] Between 20% and 25% of U.S. women complain of decreased desire, with difficulties attaining orgasm, dyspareunia, vaginismus, and problems with arousal also frequently reported. Decreased sexual desire was most common in those experiencing surgical menopause. In women with gynecologic malignancies, approximately 74% report decreased desire, while dyspareunia is seen in 40%.[16] In addition, coital pain, feelings of shame, fear of bleeding, and decreases in foreplay, sexual fantasies, and masturbation are common in the women with these types of cancer.[14–18]

For all U.S. men, the incidence of erectile dysfunction (ED) generally ranges from 40% to 80%, with the incidence increasing with aging and comorbidities.[19,20] Additionally, the finding of higher incidence depends on the study population and the manner in which the question about ED was posed. In the Prostate Cancer Prevention Trial—a clinical research study for men 55 years of age and older—approximately half of the placebo group had ED at time of enrollment. Of those who did not, 57% reported ED at five years into the study, with 65% reporting ED at seven years.[21] Rapid ejaculation is the most common dysfunction in U.S. men, with incidence ranging from 14% to 30%, followed by low sexual desire and inability to reach orgasm.[22]

Statistics on alterations in intimacy, decreased communication, changes to relationships, and other nonsexual aspects of cancer are less well known and researched. Patients report that as a result of a cancer diagnosis, they experience changes in relationships that affect quality of life, communication, and sexual function. Fear of death, depression, fatigue, effects of comorbid illnesses, realities of treatment, and other aspects of life in general impact the patient, caregiver, partner, family, or any significant other and can further affect sexual health. Poor communication, inadequate coping, and prior strained relationships do not generally improve following a cancer diagnosis without some form of intervention. Such interventions may be formal or informal, brief or intense, and provided by a sex therapist or trained counselor or member of the oncology team. Assessment for sexual health alterations will guide the nature of the intervention and determine who best can provide the assistance, resources, and education needed by the patient and significant others.[2–6]

ETIOLOGY

Common causes of sexual dysfunction may be related to age, health status, comorbid conditions, and medication use, while surgical scars, presence of a colostomy or urostomy, hysterectomy, orchiectomy, weight changes, and incontinence frequently impact body image and self-perception.[23] Increasing age may be associated with decreased desire and arousal in women and difficulty attaining or maintaining an erection in men. These changes vary among individuals, however, with many older adults enjoying a satisfying sex life and being very concerned about the potential sexual side effects of disease and treatment as they age. Health status includes both illness type (e.g., cancer, diabetes, multiple sclerosis, clinical depression, obesity) and illness duration and severity (the longer one has a disease or the more severe, the more likely the dysfunction). Sexual side effects, again, vary, but are common with chronic health conditions. The most common medication categories to affect sexual health include antihypertensives, anticonvulsants, antidepressants, H_2 blockers, and psychiatric and antinausea medications, with some agents in each category causing more alterations than others.[22] In addition, for those persons with cancer, the biology of the disease, treatments and treatment-related side effects, and psychosocial issues such as culture, religion, family dynamics, and coping strategies may both cause and affect sexual alterations. These changes may, in turn, influence perceptions of body image and psychological concerns of sexual identity, self-esteem, abandonment, feelings of anger or sadness, and worries for self and others.

Tierney[6] identified three dimensions of sexuality—physiologic, psychological, and social—and described alterations in relation to each dimension. Physiologic alterations reflect changes in the hormonal milieu or neurovascular changes to the genitalia caused by cancer treatment, management of treatment side effects, or the cancer itself. Psychological alterations relate to distress such as depression, anxiety, body image changes, and fears of changing relationships, relapse, and death. Finally, alterations in the social dimension include concerns such as changing relationships and roles, lack (or perceived lack) of social support, poor communication between partners, emotional and other types of distress in the partner, and poor or unsatisfying sexual (and other) relationships prior to diagnosis and treatment. Each dimension interacts with the others, compounding or ameliorating alterations to sexual health.

Surgery

Cancer surgery has the potential to affect sexual health through removal of tissues and body parts, damage to nerves and vascular supply, and psychological ramifications of scarring and changes to the body and one's body image. Side effects of surgical treatment can include the creation of ostomies, loss of sensation, and adhesions causing pain or discomfort. While ostomies are less common today than they were 10 to 20 years ago, those individuals with an ostomy often fear leakage and odor and suffer from body image changes due to ostomy placement and management. Incontinence and erectile dysfunction are common following prostate surgery, and ejaculatory dysfunction may be seen in young men following surgery for testicular cancer. Nerve-sparing retroperitoneal lymph node dissection decreases the incidence of incontinence and ejaculatory dysfunction, but this option is not available or used in all patients.[2–5,8,24–26]

Because other forms of cancer treatment often are coupled with surgery, it may be difficult to adequately assess the exact impact of a particular surgical intervention on sexual health. Some surgeries, such as total abdominal hysterectomy and oophorectomy, vulvectomy, prostatectomy, and orchiectomy, directly remove genital body parts and are expected to cause some level of sexual dysfunction. Other abdominal surgeries, such as colectomy, cystectomy, and rectal surgery, can have a profound effect on sexual health through creation of new body orifices, alterations in enervation, damage to neurovascular tissues, and body image alterations.[21,22,27–33]

Patients with breast and uterine cancer often experience body image alterations even though others may not readily recognize the changes to the person's body. Removal of the breast can lead to body image alterations, loss of sensation, and feelings of being "less than a woman," altering sexual function and intimacy.[2–5,8]

Those persons with visually identifiable disfigurements, such as from treatment for head and neck cancer, thyroid cancer, or a cancer requiring amputation, may suffer body image alterations coupled with the stigma of having cancer or some sort of disfiguring disease. All of these individuals may also experience trouble with sexual expression and intimacy due to surgical scarring, disfigurement, and changes in sensations, including touch, smell, and taste (being unable to taste or smell may affect the desire to enjoy an intimate meal; decreased sensation in a breast may effect sexual pleasure and intimacy).[2,8,34–42]

Radiation therapy

Radiation therapy (RT) may cause sexual health alterations through primary organ failure (e.g., testicular aplasia or ovarian failure), changes in how the organ functions (e.g., erectile dysfunction or decreased vaginal lubrication), and temporary or permanent nonreproductive effects of therapy (e.g., fatigue or nausea). The treatment site, total dose, length of treatment, prior fertility status, and patient's age determine whether these treatment effects are permanent or temporary.[2,8,28,36,42,43]

RT to the pelvis affects the sexual health of men and women differently; however, women experience an increased number of direct effects to sexual function. Increasing risks to sexual health depend on the type of RT delivered, the treatment location, the length of treatment, and the overall treatment dose. Additional concomitant physiologic conditions, such as obesity or diabetes, may exacerbate RT side effects, increasing the chance for sexual dysfunction and body image changes.[2,43,44]

Men receiving RT to the pelvis experience fibrosis of blood vessels and the nerves needed for erection, leading to increased risks of ED over time that may be either temporary or permanent (the risk is approximately the same as for surgery at 5 years post RT). They also may experience decreased frequency of ejaculation, urinary incontinence, diarrhea, or rectal bleeding that may further compromise sexual function and cause body image alterations. Inability to lubricate or reach orgasm and decreased sexual pleasure are frequently reported, and infertility and sterility are common following pelvic/abdominal RT.[45–48] Irradiation to the whole pelvis is likely to result in severe side effects,[45] whereas interstitial therapy causes less ED, but still leads to bowel and bladder dysfunction or some level of ED in 6% to 90% of patients.[43,44,47] The use of newer radiation delivery methods and smaller RT ports has decreased the incidence of ED, although adding hormone therapy may negate these benefits.[49]

Women are more likely to experience direct side effects from RT leading to alterations in sexual health and causing sexual dysfunction. Menopause can be induced with radiation doses as low 600 to 1200 cGy. Generally, younger women do not experience permanent sterility until they receive a dose of 2000 cGy or greater, whereas a dose of

600 cGy often causes menopause and the associated menopausal symptoms of amenorrhea, hot flashes, loss of libido, vaginal atrophy, and dyspareunia in women older than age 40.[50] Vaginal fibrosis and stenosis, inflammation of the mucosal lining of the vagina and anus, decreased lubrication and sensation, and alterations in fertility are other common side effects of RT to the pelvis. Decreased enjoyment, inability to reach orgasm, and decreased frequency of intercourse and sexual dreams also have been reported by women with gynecologic and other malignancies receiving pelvic RT.[2,51–53] Any of these side effects may affect sexual function, self-esteem, and body image. Additionally, the psychological impact of actual or potential infertility and sterility can be profound, particularly in young adults who have yet to start a family or in those still planning for future pregnancies.[54,55]

Regardless of the site of RT, fatigue may have a major effect on sexual function, with as many as 80% of both men and women who receive such treatment experiencing mild to severe fatigue.[56] Cancer-related fatigue causes profound tiredness leading to decreased desire, decreased ability to maintain pleasurable or routine sexual positions, and inability to sustain intercourse long enough to reach orgasm. Patients may be too fatigued to consider any type of sexual activity or may substitute cuddling, hugging, or other forms of intimacy for intercourse or activities that require expending energy they do not have. Decreased range of motion, inflammation, and pain may limit or make sexual activities impossible, while diarrhea, nausea, vomiting, fear, anxiety, and stress can decrease energy, alter body image and self-esteem, and decrease feelings of desire or being desirable, further limiting sexual activity and intimacy.[2,3,8,57]

Chemotherapy

Sexual dysfunction caused by chemotherapy is related to the type of chemotherapeutic agents used, the dose of each individual agent, the treatment protocol (e.g., length, timing, and number of medications given concomitantly and singly), and the patient's age and gender. Women closer to the age of normal menopause are more likely to experience premature menopause and infertility/sterility than younger women are; men frequently will regain fertility regardless of age, but time and potential for regaining fertility depend on the drug type and dose. Chemotherapy causes sexual dysfunction through direct effects on tissues such as the lungs or nerve endings, as well as through treatment side effects such as nausea and vomiting, fatigue, mucosal changes, and diarrhea leading to decreased desire and arousal. Additionally, chemotherapy can cause vaginal atrophy, and hair loss, making intercourse painful, altering body image and self-esteem, and decreasing desire and arousal. Infertility is common with the alkylating agents and in those receiving higher-dose or longer-duration therapy.[3,58–63]

Hormonal manipulation and treatment. Men receiving androgen-ablative therapy experience reduced ability to attain or maintain an erection and decreased interest in sexual intercourse.[64,65] Decreased arousal and the ability to achieve orgasm and gynecomastia also may occur.[58] Women receiving antiestrogens, aromatase inhibitors, or similar drugs commonly experience sexual side effects. Depending on the specific drug, these changes can include decreased interest in sex, mood disturbances, dyspareunia, weight gain, hot flashes/flushes, menopausal symptoms, and altered body image.[58,66,67]

Targeted therapies. The sexual side effects of the novel, molecularly targeted agents, such as the epidermal growth factor tyrosine kinase inhibitors, fusion proteins, and antiangiogenic agents, are currently unknown. The use of these agents, which target molecular pathways responsible for tumor growth, is increasing. Over time, increased information will undoubtedly emerge regarding all side effects of these medications, including those related to sexual health. Common side effects of rash, fatigue, and diarrhea affect sexual function specifically in the areas of desire and arousal and influence one's interest in or willingness to initiate any form of sexual activity. The cardiotoxicity of some of these agents also can affect sexual function. The potential for fetal malformation is documented for some of these agents,[68] with thalidomide requiring two forms of contraception to minimize the possibility of birth defects. Because of lack of information, these novel agents are contraindicated in pregnancy and for those wishing to breastfeed.[58,68]

Biologic response modifiers. Most sexual health effects occurring in those persons receiving biologic response modifiers (BRMs) are associated with alterations in body image as well as known side effects such as fatigue, mucous membrane changes, and flulike symptoms. Decreased libido, amenorrhea, pelvic pain, uterine bleeding, and erectile dysfunction also occur and affect interest in sexual activities and the ability to have intercourse. Additionally, changes in communication, psychological distress, and treatment-related side effects seen with BRM use may affect intimacy.[3,58,59]

Medications

Medications to manage treatment side effects or concomitant illnesses also affect sexual function. Potential drug-related dysfunctions include ED, menopausal symptoms, problems with ejaculation, and decreased desire, arousal, or the ability to reach orgasm. Medications most commonly associated with sexual dysfunction (for those persons with cancer and with noncancer chronic illness such as diabetes or cardiac disease) include the antihypertensives,[69] antiemetics, narcotics, antidepressants, antianxiety medications, and sedatives. Additionally, alcohol abuse or the use of illicit drugs influence sexual function, alter sexual responsiveness, and may lead to potentially harmful sexual practices such as unprotected sex and exposure to sexually transmitted diseases that may be particularly harmful to the immunocompromised patient. Medications designed to alter the hormonal milieu, such as antiestrogens, aromatase inhibitors, and estrogens given to men or androgens given to women, can cause vasomotor symptoms and hair loss or growth in men and women and vaginal discharge, vaginal dryness, and dyspareunia in women.[3,8,58,66]

Psychological alterations

The patient's (and frequently the family's or significant other's) psychological status can influence sexual health even when cancer or its treatments do not directly alter sexual function or body image. Psychological ramifications of cancer are common and affect all patients whether single or partnered, heterosexual or homosexual. Anxiety, depression, fear, anger, or any other emotion can affect communication, intimacy, interest in sexual activity, or ability to have intercourse or otherwise pleasure one's self or partner. Questions frequently asked by singles include when to tell potential partners about the cancer diagnosis and treatment, what to tell, and how to cope with reactions from potential partners and others. Additionally, the showing of scars and sharing of feelings and concerns about cancer, treatment, and the future can affect new and mature relationships, alter communication, and impact sexual functioning.[3,70,71]

PATHOPHYSIOLOGY

To evaluate sexual health comprehensively, both the pathophysiology of gonadal function and alterations to the human sexual response cycle are evaluated. Cancer and its treatment can alter gonadal function, causing infertility and sterility, early menopause, and a multitude of side effects and symptoms that can interfere with all aspects of sexual function. Cancer and its treatments also can affect the sexual response cycle through changes to the hormonal milieu, alterations that affect vasocongestion or muscle contractions in sexual organs, or concomitant psychosocial effects or concerns (e.g., fears, depression, anxiety) leading to alterations in desire, arousal, and the ability to attain orgasm.

PHYSIOLOGICAL ALTERATIONS IN GONADAL FUNCTION

Gonadal function is regulated by the hypothalamus and the anterior pituitary gland.[73–75] The hypothalamus secretes gonadotropin-releasing hormone (GnRH), stimulating the anterior pituitary to produce both follicle-stimulating hormone (FSH) and luteinizing hormone (LH). These hormones stimulate the ovary to produce estrogen and progesterone and the testes to produce testosterone. Anterior pituitary hormone secretions are affected by a negative feedback loop; thus, when blood levels of LH and FSH are adequate, secretions cease.[72–74]

In men, GnRH is secreted by the hypothalamus, causing the anterior pituitary to secrete LH and FSH. The secretion of LH causes interstitial Leydig cells in the testes to produce testosterone, while FSH, along with testosterone, stimulates the Sertoli cells to convert spermatogonia to spermatocytes that further divide and mature into sperm. Spermatogenesis is maintained at a constant rate through a negative feedback loop in which the Sertoli cells secrete the hormone inhibin to decrease FSH production.[72–74]

In women, the initial process is the same as in men, with GnRH secreted from the hypothalamus, in turn causing secretion of LH and FSH from the anterior pituitary. FSH causes growth of ovarian follicles. Secretion of estrogen leads to a surge in LH, and a mature ovum is extruded from the ovary during ovulation. With stimulation from LH, the ruptured ovarian follicle becomes the corpus luteum and produces estrogen, which thickens the lining of the uterus, and progesterone, which prepares the lining for implantation of an embryo. As levels of these hormones increase, FSH and LH secretions decrease. If implantation does not occur, the corpus luteum degenerates, LH and FSH levels rise, a new ovarian cycle begins, and menstruation occurs.[72–74]

In the person with cancer, alterations in gonadal function may occur for a variety of reasons, including those related to the type of cancer and associated therapy, overall health and nutrition status, age, stress, comorbid conditions and their treatments, psychological issues and concerns, or, more likely, a combination of these factors. Damage can be direct, through surgical removal of the testes, ovaries, or other structures, or it may occur as a side effect of cancer therapy that leads to alterations in hormone production with resultant changes to normal ovarian or testicular function.[2,72,73]

ALTERATIONS IN THE SEXUAL RESPONSE CYCLE

In 1966, Drs. William Masters and Virginia Johnson[76] developed a four-stage model to describe the sexual response cycle. These four stages—excitement, plateau, orgasm, and resolution—correspond to episodes of muscle contraction and vasocongestion.[6,8,75,76] As identified by Masters and Johnson and others, the excitement phase can last from minutes to hours. During excitement, there is an increase in heart rate, breathing, muscle tension, and blood flow to sex organs, and nipples become hardened or erect.

In women, the clitoris swells, breasts become fuller, and vaginal lubrication begins. For men, the penis becomes erect, the scrotum tightens, the testicles swell, and the tip of the penis begins to secrete lubricating fluid. Plateau lasts until the brink of orgasm and includes continuation and enhancement of the excitement phase. Additionally, the clitoris swells and can become extremely sensitive. Orgasm is the climax of the sexual response cycle and is generally pleasurable for most individuals. It involves involuntary muscle contraction and a release of sexual tension. The vaginal walls contract, and rhythmic contractions at the base of the penis lead to emission and ejaculation. During the resolution phase, the body returns to its normal state, breathing and heart rate decrease, the penis becomes flaccid, and there may be a general sense of fatigue and an increased feeling of intimacy. Men have a refractory period during which erection and orgasm are not reattained; this refractory period varies in length and increases with age. Some women may be able to attain orgasm more rapidly with sexual stimulation, leading to multiple orgasms.[6,8,75,76]

Multiple modifications of this model have occurred since the initial development of Masters and Johnson's four-stage model. In a 1974 revision, Kaplan[77] identified desire as important to sexual response and noted that excitement can occur without desire. Kaplan omitted the resolution phase; however, Robinson[78] restored it in his 1976 revision, but maintained Kaplan's initial phase of desire. Leif[79] added a fifth phase that includes satisfaction, while Zilbergeld and Ellison[80] modified the model to include both physiological and psychological components.

Finally, in the early 2000s, Basson[81] specifically evaluated the model for women's sexual response, noting that in women the sexual response cycle is not linear, but rather circular. She stated that many women enter into the sexual response cycle from a place of sexual neutrality and then, if receptive to sexual stimuli, may become aroused. This arousal may or may not lead to orgasm, but generally is pleasurable or leads to increased intimacy. This consideration may be particularly important for those women who have problems of decreased desire, as they may still be able to participate in sexual activities and find pleasure and even reach orgasm if the person is at least willing to be receptive to the idea of sexual activity. Levin critically appraised the revisions to the model, noting that changes allowed for greater understanding of sexual dysfunctions.[82]

SYMPTOM ASSESSMENT

Southard and Keller[83] investigated the importance of assessing sexuality in 6 adult men and 46 adult women. Of the 52 participants, 42% felt being able to discuss issues of a sexual nature with their nurse was important, and identified sexual activity, emotional changes, body image, and fertility concerns as being areas that nurses should be able to competently discuss. Fewer than 25% reported that a nurse or physician had discussed sexual issues during or following treatment. The authors note that sexuality is a sensitive topic that should be broached with patients in an individualized manner before, during, and following therapy.

For a sexual assessment to be meaningful, it must include evaluation of not only the patient's physical condition, but also the patient's psychosocial, psychosexual, and mental health status. For those individuals with cancer, a comprehensive evaluation must include the patient's diagnosis, treatment plan, status of treatment (e.g., ongoing, completed), current comorbid conditions and medications, relationship status, gender orientation, and current views of self/self-esteem.[2–5,8,71,84,85] The nursing intake history should include simple, unobtrusive questions related to sexuality and sexual function for all patients. This is particularly imperative for those persons with gynecologic or genitourinary cancers, those receiving RT or surgery to the abdomen or pelvis, those receiving chemotherapy known or likely to cause any type of sexual dysfunction, and those receiving medications for nausea, pain, hypertension, or any other condition in which treatment is known to caused sexual side effects.[2–5,8,71,84,85]

RISK FACTORS

Risk factors for alterations in body image and sexual health include the patient's cancer diagnosis, stage of disease, and treatment plan, with some diagnoses and treatments being more likely to alter sexual health than others. In addition, older age, comorbidities and their treatments, certain medications (e.g., antiemetics, antihypertensives), poor coping styles and communication patterns, and psychological concerns (e.g., low self-esteem, body image alterations, and anxiety) also play a role. Most patients will have more than one risk factor, and some risk factors may have a greater impact on sexual health than other factors. Taken collectively, the impact of the various factors can be significant even when a single risk factor might cause only minimal dysfunction.[2–5,8,71]

SELF-ASSESSMENT

The medical and nursing literature support the contention that patients are more likely than providers to bring up sexual concerns, even though patients would prefer that providers discuss sexuality, fertility, and intimacy issues with them without prompting.[2–8] In general, patients want healthcare providers to ask about their sexual functioning and the impact of cancer and cancer treatment on relationships, but often fear that their providers will be uninterested or not have the time to discuss such topics. Relationships with providers, which are often tied to short clinical visits focused on specific treatment-related problems, may not allow for building sufficient trust and comfort to allow sexual health discussions. Additionally, patients' lack of knowledge about potential sexual side effects or cultural influences on their views of cancer and sexuality also may preclude any discussion.

Providers also face barriers to discussing sexual health with their patients.[2–8,71,83–87] Park et al.[88] note that barriers for providers are threefold: healthcare system barriers, patient characteristics, and provider education, knowledge, traits, and actions. System barriers include lack of time and resources, while providers' lack of education, training, knowledge, and experience may interfere with the provider's confidence in discussing intimacy and sexual issues.[88] Providers also are often reluctant to raise sexual health issues due to personal embarrassment, lack of knowledge, and fear of bridging a topic for which the provider has little experience in evaluation, diagnosis, and management.[2–5,8,71] Finally, providers may make assumptions about patients based on sexual orientation, age, gender, partner status, and overall prognosis and limit information based on false or unclear assumptions. The self-care guide for intimacy located in Appendix 24A may be helpful in assisting patients to regain comfort, intimacy and pleasure following cancer therapy.

OBJECTIVE ASSESSMENT

The objective sexual health assessment consists of four interwoven components: the medical history, the physical examination, diagnostic studies, and a sexual function and activities appraisal. These components allow providers to discriminate between sexual issues that may be simply concerns or difficulties, and thus more easily addressed, and true dysfunctions or disorders that may require more focused or intense interventions.[89,90] Some components of the assessment are accomplished easily by the oncology nurse, whereas others may require the expertise of an advanced practice nurse or physician. Each component provides a piece of the overall sexual health assessment and is integral to creating a fully integrated plan of care that will meet the patient's (and partner's, if included in the assessment) current and future needs. If alterations to sexual health are identified, assessment focuses on the context of the dysfunction for the patient (and partner), the association of the dysfunction with any comorbidity or risk factor (such as a medication), and the level of distress felt by the patient (and partner) because of the dysfunction.[90]

History

Medical assessment for sexual health includes gathering data on the patient's age, gender, current and past health and health conditions (both acute and chronic conditions, including cancer type and stage of disease), and past surgeries or other treatments (i.e., RT or treatment for depression). Questions also should be asked about current medications, including prescribed medications such as chemotherapy and side-effect management medications, oral contraceptives, and medications for erectile dysfunction, as well as herbal products and over-the-counter medications. Additionally, immunizations, allergies, past hospitalizations, body image beliefs and self-assessment, sexual orientation, and pre-illness and current relationships (including sexual relationships) are included in the comprehensive medical history. The sexual assessment component of the medical history includes questions about ED, premature ejaculation, vaginal lubrication, and dyspareunia (in both women and men).[2–6,8,25,26,71,74,91–96] The provider also should evaluate functional patterns of health, including areas such as roles and relationships, and self-perception and self-concept as outlined in Table 24-1.[74]

Physical assessment

Physical assessment for sexual health includes a genital exam for men and a genital and breast exam for women. An examination of the rectal area also is included. In general, while the external physical exam for both women and men can be accomplished by the registered nurse, the advanced practice nurse or medical practitioner more commonly conducts both the internal and external physical exams of all patients.

Female exam. To conduct the female pelvic examination, the woman is placed in the dorsolithotomy position with her feet in the stirrups. The perineal area, including the external genitalia (the labia, clitoris, urethra, vaginal orifice, and mucous membranes), and the anal triangle are inspected for lesions, swelling, inflammation, discharge, bleeding, fissures, hemorrhoids, and hair distribution or loss. The area is palpated for masses. Using a speculum, the vagina is spread and the walls inspected for lesions, swelling, inflammation, discharge, bleeding, adhesions, and stenosis. Following the speculum exam, a bimanual exam is completed. Well-lubricated and gloved index fingers are inserted into the vagina, and the cervix, if in place, or the apex of the vagina, if the cervix has been removed, is palpated for masses. Vaginal tone and length are assessed and the strength of the pubococcygeal muscle, which has a crucial role in intercourse and orgasm, is assessed by having the woman squeeze down on the fingers. Spreading the fingers laterally can break any adhesions. A gloved finger into the rectum assesses sphincter tone and palpates for masses. To complete the exam, the external hand is pressed down on the abdomen just below the umbilicus to palpate the uterus and ovaries, if present, for masses and assess for size, shape, and mobility.[74]

TABLE 24-1

Functional Health Pattern Assessment Specific to Sexual Health

Pattern	Assessment
Health perception-health management	Perception of overall health; lifestyle choices (e.g., alcohol, caffeine, smoking); strategies used to maintain health (screenings and self-exams); family history of disease
Nutrition-metabolic	Weight changes; routine diet; use of nutritional supplements; evaluation for anemia, calcium, Vitamin D and other nutrition-related deficiencies; eating disorders
Elimination	Problems with urination/elimination; vaginal infections/drainage; urinary stress incontinence; benign prostatic hypertrophy
Activity-exercise	Energy levels; amount and type of activity; routine exercise/exercise patterns
Sleep-rest	Normal sleep pattern; naps (time, duration); fatigue; insomnia; frequent urination; hot flashes/flushes; if feels rested after sleep
Cognitive-perceptual	Ability to read, write, understand instructions; languages spoken/read; memory; attention; dizziness; dyspareunia (makes it difficult to take part in sexual activities)
Self-perception-self-concept	Personal description of self; body image changes; nonphysical problems that may affect sexual function
Role-relationship	Relationships; family structure; occupation; role in family; changes to roles; living arrangements
Sexuality-reproduction	Menstrual and obstetrical history; sexual preferences; sexual orientation; acceptable and usual types of sex (e.g., vaginal, oral, anal); current sexual activities, preferences and beliefs; impact of culture, religion, etc. on sexual practices; understanding and practice of safe sex; contraceptive practices and beliefs; general satisfaction with current sexual status and function
Coping-stress tolerance	Current life stresses; methods of coping/dealing with stress; success of current methods; major life changes in past few years
Values-beliefs	Cultural, religious, moral and ethical beliefs; beliefs about sex and sexual health; beliefs about health and illness; current practices, beliefs that may impact sexual health

Source: Data from Dirksen[74].

Male exam. Conduct the male genital examination with the man in the standing position. Inspect the pubis for hair pattern distribution and examine the underlying skin for rashes or lesions. Inspect the entire penile shaft for lesions, inflammation, color changes, scars, and swelling and palpate for masses. If present, retract the foreskin. Examine the glans and urethral meatus for signs of infection or other lesions, and compress them to evaluate for discharge. Inspect the scrotum for symmetry and presence of the testicles. Palpate the scrotum and testicles for consistency, swelling, tenderness, and the presence of a mass. Palpate the inguinal region and spermatic cord, and evaluate the inguinal lymph node. The anal region is inspected for swelling, fissures, and hemorrhoids. Assess sphincter tone and the presence of masses by inserting a well-lubricated, gloved finger into the rectum. As appropriate, a prostate exam also is included in the male genital exam.[19,25,26,74,96]

Diagnostic evaluation

The third component of a sexual health evaluation includes laboratory and other diagnostic studies to assure the patient is in optimal health, to address identified abnormalities, and to assess sexual health. Basic laboratory and diagnostic evaluations specific to the cancer diagnosis and treatment/survivorship status are drawn and evaluated. These evaluations include standard blood studies (e.g., hemoglobin, white blood cell [WBC] count, liver function tests [LFTs]) as well as tumor markers and cancer screening tests such as the Pap test, digital rectal exam, or mammography.[74,96,97]

To evaluate sexual and reproductive health, a variety of tests can be conducted. Laboratory tests to evaluate sexual and reproductive dysfunction include urine studies for human chorionic gonadotropin (hCG), total and free testosterone, and FSH; common blood studies for sexual health include prolactin levels (to evaluate pituitary dysfunction), prostate-specific antigen, hCG, testosterone, progesterone, estradiol, TSH, and FSH. Additionally, studies to evaluate endocrine dysfunction or underlying chronic illnesses such as diabetes or heart disease (e.g., glucose, lipids) should be included in the assessment. Evaluations also may include computed tomography (CT) scan, magnetic resonance imaging (MRI), or sonography to assess vascular or neurologic changes to pelvic and other organs. In those individuals suspected of having a sexually transmitted disease, a test for syphilis and cultures and smears for *Chlamydia*, *Trichomonas*, and gonorrhea also may be done.

For men with erectile dysfunction, diagnostic tests may include studies of penile tumescence, measurements of penile brachial blood pressure, a RigiScan to evaluate nocturnal erections, and test injections of intercavernous alprostadil to evaluate the ability of the penis to become erect.[97] Premature ejaculation is difficult to diagnose; the sexual history may provide the best evidence.[19]

If future childbearing is desired, fertility studies including semen analysis, basal body temperature assessment, a Huhner (or Sims-Huhner) test to assess whether cervical mucus supports transport of sperm into the uterus, and endometrial biopsy may be undertaken. Additional evaluation with invasive tests such as hysteroscopy, hysterosalpingogram, and laparoscopy can further assess fertility in women.[74]

Sexual function and activities appraisal

Conducting an effective sexual function and activities appraisal includes using a variety of evaluation tools, questions, and models to assess the current and potential levels of sexual dysfunction. Assessments may be either brief or intensive, depending on factors such as the patient's needs and desires, the patient's medical condition, the status of the nurse–patient relationship, and the environment where the assessment takes place. Current relationships and level of intimacy, previous sexual activities and relationships, self-perceived body image, coping styles, cultural and religious beliefs, and communication patterns may be topics for assessment and discussion. Additional areas for assessment may include fertility and childbearing, contraception beliefs and practices, emotional or cognitive dysfunction, current levels of social and economic support, and any history of substance abuse or domestic violence, rape or abuse.[2–6,8,71,74,98–102]

Prior to beginning the sexual evaluation and appraisal, it is essential for nurses to understand their own personal beliefs about sex and sexuality, be comfortable with their own sexuality, and attempt to minimize any biases or beliefs that could affect the assessment. It is important to be aware of potential cultural and religious beliefs that may impact assessment, and to recognize the sensitive nature of questions about sexuality for the patient.

During the assessment, the nurse should act in a professional manner and attempt to build trust. Questions should be gender and sexual orientation neutral, move from less sensitive to more sensitive topics, not make assumptions or stereotype, avoid medical or value-oriented terminology, and be asked in a matter-of-fact manner that conveys a nonprying, interested, and "need to know for quality care" attitude. Questions should flow logically from one topic to the next, and time should be allowed between questions for the patient to provide answers without feeling rushed or otherwise constrained. Patients should feel they have permission to answer or not answer any question; responses should be regarded as important and normal. Verbal and nonverbal communication should be evaluated and clarifying questions posed as needed. If possible, it is best for the nurse to sit rather than stand to conduct the sexual health assessment conversations and to maintain eye contact, if culturally appropriate. The patient's partner, if there is one, should be included in the assessment and discussion only with permission from the patient.[2–6,8,71,74]

Essential to assessment and intervention is ensuring privacy, maintaining confidentiality, and focusing on the patient's goals.[102] Upon completion of the assessment, the patient and the nurse develop a plan of care that addresses current and future sexual needs and concerns, including plans for follow-up, accessing resources, and referral.[2–6,8,71,74] Table 24-2 identifies the types of questions to ask as part of a sexual function and activities appraisal.[2–5,6,8,71,74]

Sexual function assessment tools. A variety of generic and cancer-specific questionnaires and surveys are available to evaluate sexual function in both men and women.[103,104] Some of these instruments focus on a specific aspect of sexuality such as body image, specific areas of physical functioning such as erectile dysfunction, sexual orientation, or

TABLE 24-2

Sample Questions to Ask during a Sexual Assessment

Questions Specific to Both Men and Women
Are you currently in a sexual relationship? If yes, with whom and what is the length of your relationship?
Are you satisfied with your current relationship?
Has your sex life changed in the last 6–12 months? If yes, how?
Do you prefer sexual relationships with men, women, both?
How many sexual partners have you had in the last 12 months?
Do you have any cultural or religious beliefs that may affect your sex life/sexual activity?
Do you use sexual aids or participate in oral or anal sex?
Do you have a previous history of STDs? Sexual abuse/trauma? substance abuse?
Are you currently using birth control?
Do you have feelings of sexual excitement/arousal? Are you able to reach orgasm?

Questions Specific to Women
Have you been through menopause? Do you have hot flashes, mood swings?
Do you have sufficient vaginal lubrication for intercourse?
Do you have pain or bleeding with intercourse?

Questions Specific to Men
Have you ever had a problem attaining an erection?
Do you awaken with an erection?
Do you have voluntary erections? What is the quality? How firm? How long does it last?
Do you have problems with premature ejaculation?
Do you have pain with intercourse?

Source: Data from Krebs[2–5]; Tierney[6]; Katz[8,71]; Dirksen[74].

relationships; others are more comprehensive, evaluating overall sexual function. Generic instruments address specific aspects of sexuality regardless of underlying illness or disease status. Among them are (1) the International Index of Erectile Function Questionnaire[105] and IIEF-5, a five-item abridged version;[106] (2) the Female Sexual Function Index (FSFI)[107] and a six-item abridged version;[108] (3) the Derogatis Interview for Sexual Function (DISF);[109] and (4) the Changes in Sexual Functioning Questionnaire (CSFQ).[110] In addition, sexual health questions from the Patient-Reported Outcomes Measurement System (PROMIS) have been evaluated as a single sexual dysfunction instrument as well as being incorporated in global questionnaires. The tools developed through PROMIS can be administered in multiple formats and allow for comparisons across domains and diseases; while frequently used for research, they are simple enough to be used by the nurse in clinical practice.[111] The most commonly used cancer-specific instrument is the Sexual Adjustment Questionnaire (SAQ).[112]

All of the previously mentioned questionnaires and the PROMIS questions have been found to be reliable and valid measurement tools that can facilitate assessment of sexual dysfunction and can be used for both research and clinical practice purposes. In particular, the IIEF-5,[106] the short form of the FSFI,[108] and the SAQ[112] can be used by the practicing nurse.

Assessment models. Sexual assessment models assist practitioners to both assess sexual dysfunction and intervene in sexual health matters. These models generally are classified into three categories: (1) those that specifically *assess* sexual health (ALARM[113]); (2) those that *intervene* to manage sexual concerns (PLISSIT[114]); and (3) *combination* models that both assess and intervene (BETTER[115] and BLISS[116]). In addition, behavioral health counseling models have been adapted to both assess and intervene (the adapted 5A model for sexual assessment). While the majority of sexual assessment models are appropriate for use with all individuals, the ALARM, BETTER and BLISS models are specific to those persons with cancer and are designed for use by oncology nurses and other oncology providers.

The assessment models, such as ALARM,[113] tend to be medically oriented and generally are too limited for the oncology nurse whose focus is on providing support and assessing concerns.[2] The intervention models identify and address sexual dysfunctions while making the assumption that a sexual assessment has already been completed; they do not provide a comprehensive approach to evaluating sexual health.[5] The PLISSIT[114] model is the most well known of these models. The combination models such as BETTER[115] and BLISSS[116] assess both sexual health concerns and provide intervention strategies. The BLISSS model is unique in that it encourages active listening and communication and generally includes both the patient and the patient's partner. These models assume that each patient is a sexual being with sexual concerns that may need to be addressed. All include individualized methods to manage identified sexual issues and allow oncology nurses to intervene more efficiently and effectively with each patient. They generally are easier for the less experienced nurse to use. Park et al.[88] adapted the 5A model from behavioral health counseling to facilitate and enhance sexual health communication. They suggest a multidisciplinary approach, with different members of the healthcare team designated to carry out different components, and indicate that the oncology nurse could be the coordinator to ensure that all aspects are incorporated into the patient's comprehensive sexual assessment. Table 24-3 outlines the components of the ALARM, PLISSIT, BETTER, BLISSS, and 5A Sexual Health Adaptation models.

TABLE 24-3

Sexual Assessment and Management Models

ALARM[113]	PLISSIT[114]	BETTER[115]	BLISSS[116]	5A Sexual Health Adaptation[88]
A - Activity (Sexual) ***L*** - Libido/desire ***A*** - Arousal/orgasm ***R*** - Resolution/release ***M*** - Medical data	***P*** - Permission ***LI*** - Limited Information ***SS*** - Specific Suggestions ***IT*** - Intensive Therapy	***Bring*** up sexuality/sexual health ***Explain*** importance of sexuality to QOL ***Tell*** about/identify resources ***Timing*** is critical to discussions ***Educate*** patient/ partner about sexual health ***Record*** discussions in health record	***Bring*** up sexuality ***Listen*** to ***Individual's*** experience ***Support*** patient and partner ***Stimulate*** partner communication ***Supply*** individualized information and suggestions; refer as appropriate	***Ask*** about sexuality, intimacy, and body image ***Advise*** about value/ importance of discussing sexual health ***Assess*** for sexual dysfunction and concerns ***Assist*** with referrals and to find reputable resources ***Arrange*** follow-up

Source: Data from Park et al[88]; Andersen and Lamb[113]; Annon[114]; Mick et al[115]; deVocht et al[116].

DEGREES OF TOXICITY

Degrees of toxicity can be assessed with National Cancer Institute's (NCI's) most recent Common Terminology Criteria for Adverse Events (CTCAE, version 4.03).[117] Recommendations for management based on CTCAE symptom severity are shown here in the form of three algorithms: assessment of decreased sexual interest (Figure 24-1); assessment of vaginal dryness/dyspareunia (Figure 24-2); and assessment of erectile dysfunction (Figure 24-3).

SYMPTOM MANAGEMENT STRATEGIES

THERAPEUTIC APPROACHES

To provide an individualized sexual health intervention, the nurse must be comfortable assessing and discussing sexual health issues and must have the necessary knowledge and skills to carry out the assessment and ensuing discussions. Essential to these competencies are an in-depth understanding of the patient's cancer diagnosis, disease status, treatment strategies, and follow-up plan, as well as the skills and knowledge to discuss the impact of disease and treatment on sexual health.[2–5] Feeling comfortable and not embarrassed when discussing sexual concerns, being knowledgeable about the types of sexual health issues common to cancer patients and the local resources available to address them, and being able to communicate effectively without causing discomfort or embarrassment are key elements for discussing sexual health concerns.[118] Mick suggests that it is essential that the nurse encourage patient questions and discussions about sexual health, listen objectively, and personalize the discussions using the nurse's own knowledge and skills in communicating with patients about difficult topics.[119] Nurses who are not comfortable providing an assessment can refer the patient to a nurse colleague, other team member, or other healthcare professional who can provide the needed assessment and interventions.

Sexual health discussions should be incorporated into normal care before, during, and following cancer treatment and include factual information based on the patient's

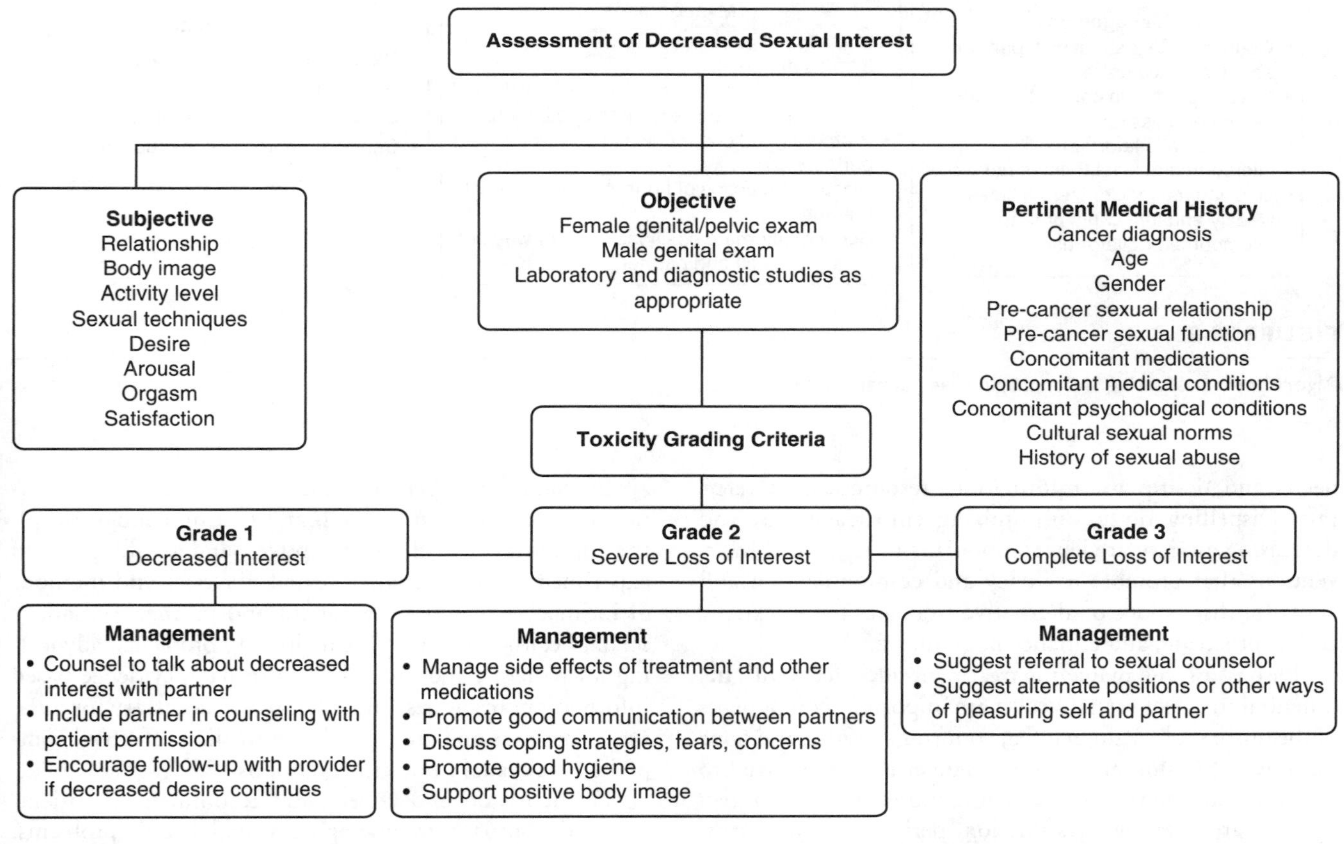

FIGURE 24-1

Algorithm for assessing decreased sexual interest.

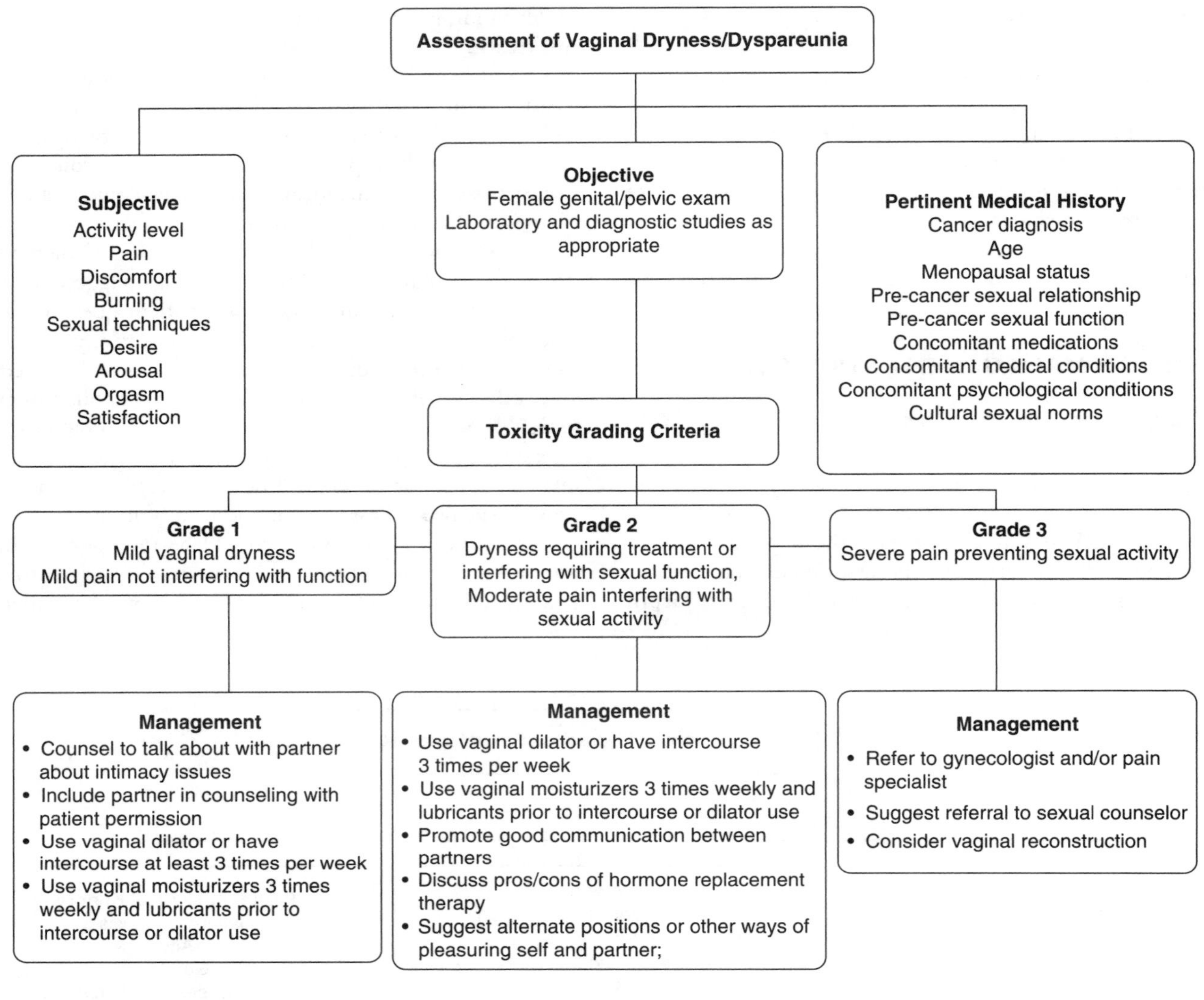

FIGURE 24-2

Algorithm for assessing and managing vaginal pain and dryness.

needs and desires for information, resources, and referrals. Dispelling myths, minimizing embarrassment, and decreasing anxiety are key components to successful interventions that promote intimacy and communication and allow for discussions of alternative strategies to be sexually active, procreate, and enhance body image.[2–5]

Discussing and managing treatment side effects with the potential to affect sexual health are important components of the nurse's role. Pain, nausea, vomiting, fatigue, and bone marrow depression are common side effects recognized to affect sexual function, body image, and intimacy. Less recognized are cognitive dysfunction, peripheral neuropathy, incontinence, stomatitis, hand–foot syndrome, and malnutrition, each of which can influence sexual desire, the ability to be sexually active, self-esteem, and body image.[2–5,58]

Encouraging open communication, healthy activities (e.g., exercise, eating well, and getting enough sleep), the appropriate use of contraceptives, and a willingness to experiment with alternative sexual practices and methods of intimacy will assist the patient and partner to manage sexual health concerns.[2–5] Anticipating problems, advocating for patients, and providing up-to-date, evidence-based information, resources, and referrals are necessary for quality cancer care and are crucial to providing effective, comprehensive sexual health interventions.[2–5,25,28]

Hatzichristou and colleagues[14] recommend a patient-centered approach to managing sexual health problems. Additionally, they recommend use of a unified and individualized management approach when assessing and treating a patient and suggest that any prescribed treatment be

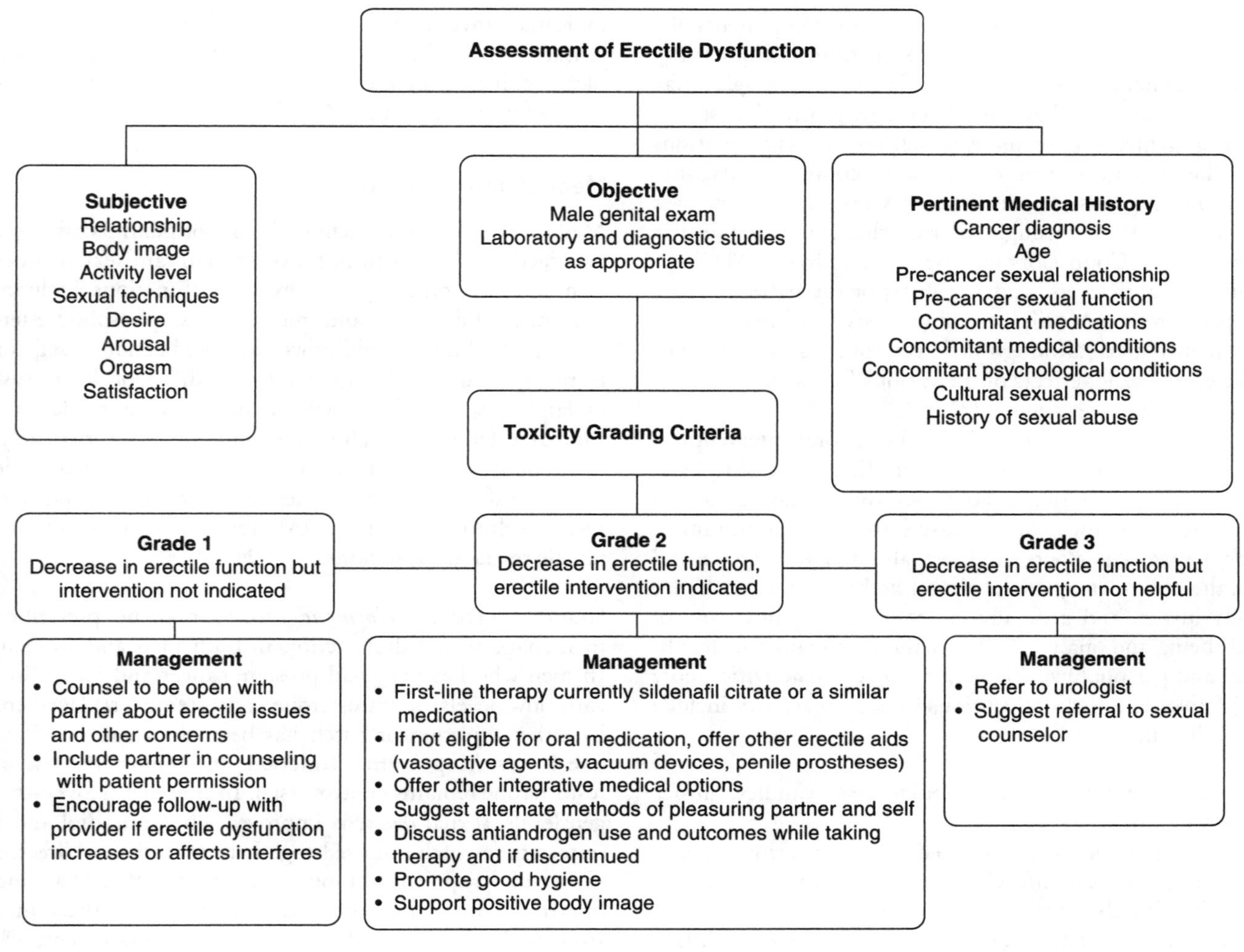

FIGURE 24-3

Algorithm for assessing and managing erectile dysfunction.

based on reproducible scientific evidence. Unfortunately, while discussed for multiple years, many current practices to manage sexual health problems have not received rigorous study and may or may not be of benefit to all or even most patients.

Psychological and behavioral interventions

The diagnosis of cancer causes anxiety, fears, concerns for the future, and a myriad of other psychoemotional feelings that can affect sexual health. Coupled with current family dynamics, past experiences, religious and cultural influences, and personal attitudes and beliefs, the addition of a cancer diagnosis and associated cancer treatment can alter relationships, communication patterns, intimacy, and sexual function. Self-esteem and body image may be affected by treatment, beliefs about illness, and side effects associated with treatment. Psychological issues play a role in multiple aspects of sexual dysfunction including ED, premature ejaculation, sexual arousal, and the ability to reach orgasm.

Brotto et al.[41] note that psychological interventions target the whole person and not just a specific organ system or region of the body. In general, the focus of psychotherapy for sexual dysfunction includes assessing for mental health and mood disorders (including depression), evaluating communication styles and patterns, assessing coping styles and skills, and investigating specific issues such as decreased libido or body image insecurities. Understanding the meaning of illness, dispelling myths, and recognizing fears and anxieties related to the cancer diagnosis, treatment, and sexuality, intimacy, sexual practices, and body image also are components of a psychological intervention for sexual health. Counseling may be general in nature or specific to sex therapy. It may include education, behavioral therapy, motivation strategies, and methods to increase self-esteem. Interventions may be through one-on-one sessions, couples counseling, or group sessions, and may be presented in person, over the telephone, or through Internet chat rooms (or similar modalities). Counselors may be nurses, physicians, chaplains, social workers, sex therapists, or the patient's peers or peer groups. Multiple combinations of counseling are frequently used, although little rigorous research is available on the exact effects of the various forms and methods of counseling over time.[2,4,5,8,14,41,70,71]

Therapy may include specific behavioral interventions such as increasing health behaviors (i.e., increasing exercise, getting more sleep, eating well, or decreasing alcohol use), or it may focus on increasing intimacy, communication between partners, and sexual activity. Exercise and weight control may make sexual activity easier, enhance body image, and generally increase the patient's sense of well-being and quality of life; methods to maintain cleanliness and personal hygiene may make sexual activities more enjoyable. Specific interventions for sexual activity include the following:

- Setting the stage for sexual activity (e.g., candles, music, sexy clothing)
- Taking pain or antinausea medications in a timely manner to promote comfort during sexual activities without undue side effects such as drowsiness
- Exploring alternative methods of intimacy such as kissing, hugging, and nongenital touching/caressing
- Using energy conservation techniques to minimize fatigue
- Using alternative positions such as lying side-by-side with the man behind, having the woman on top, or elevating the head of the bed

Creating a safe and private place to be sexually active, encouraging communication (both verbal and nonverbal) about what is pleasurable and what is not, and minimizing interruptions and distractions will enhance the sexual experience regardless of whether intercourse is the final outcome.[2,4,5,8,10,14,33,41,71,92]

A commonly prescribed intervention to enhance sexual contact is sensate focus.[71] Identified by Masters and Johnson, the goal of the sensate focus touching technique is to focus on intimacy and sensual contact rather than on genital contact and intercourse. Partners take turns touching each other, progressing from less intimate areas (nonsexual touching) to areas that are more intimate (direct genital stimulation or intercourse) over time. The goal is to take the pressure off intercourse while understanding how each partner likes to touch or be touched. As noted by Katz,[71] anyone, regardless of sexual orientation, can use sensate focus techniques to explore new ways of providing pleasure, increasing intimacy, and facilitating communication between the partners.[8,10,14,33,41,71]

Medical interventions

Medical interventions include the use of pharmacotherapy and medical devices to improve or maintain sexual function. Pharmacotherapy for sexual dysfunctions includes hormones, lubricants and moisturizers, phosphodiesterase type 5 (PDE-5) inhibitors, and medications used for intracorporeal injection (papaverine hydrochloride or prostaglandin E_1). Medical devices include vacuum devices, vaginal dilators, and clitoral stimulators. Unfortunately, while numerous options for medical management of male sexual dysfunctions exist, there is no current Food and Drug Administration (FDA)–approved treatment for female sexual dysfunctions.[14,19,20,25,41,71,92,120,121]

Pharmacotherapy. *Hormone therapy* may be prescribed to manage sexual dysfunction in both men and women. In men who have not had prostate cancer and have clinically low levels of testosterone, testosterone replacement by either injection or patch has been shown to be effective in restoring normal function. In women, the use of testosterone remains controversial. In those with low estrogen levels, sexual desire is improved when estradiol and a testosterone patch are used together; desire is not affected if estradiol supplementation is not used.[33] Van Skaa and Sprafka[122] found no increased risk of breast cancer in a study of 2100 women taking testosterone replacement; 3% of study sample had a history of cancer. However, the effectiveness of this therapy in cancer patients—in particular, those with estrogen-dependent tumors—is unclear, and the safety of its long-term use is unknown, even when supplemental estradiol is omitted.[14,33,121,122] Currently, the testosterone patch is not FDA-approved for this indication in the United States.

In women with cervical, vaginal, and vulvar cancer, estrogen replacement therapy is indicated; progesterone is added if the uterus remains intact and functional. Estrogen replacement therapy (ERT) decreases vaginal atrophy and dyspareunia and maintains vaginal integrity and moisture. If not contraindicated, local, low-dose, topical estrogen can be used to decrease vaginal atrophy and persistent vaginal dryness interfering with quality of life. ERT is available in multiple forms and in a variety of dosages, including oral, topical, and transdermal options. A low-dose, estradiol-releasing vaginal ring decreases urogenital symptoms, while estradiol vaginal tablets (i.e., local estrogen replacement tablets) relieve atrophic vaginitis. Controversy exists about the use of ERT in women with adenocarcinoma of the cervix. Current guidelines for the use of estrogen replacement therapy should be followed and are discussed in depth in the "Menopausal Symptoms" chapter.[33,121]

Tibolone is a synthetic steroid sex hormone with estrogenic, androgenic, and progestogenic effects. It is currently available in the European Union (EU) for use in postmenopausal women, but not in the United States due to concerns about increased risk for breast cancer recurrence and unknown effects in other types of cancer. Clinical trials in the EU have shown tibolone to be safe and of benefit in early-stage endometrial cancer, although further research is needed to evaluate the risks and benefits of this drug.[98,121]

Moisturizers and lubricants are essential for restoring vaginal health in women with dyspareunia, vaginal dryness, vaginal atrophy, or decreased lubrication.[14]

Moisturizers provide additional moisture to the vagina, but are not designed to provide lubrication and, therefore, are not intended for use during sexual activity. These products generally are used two to three times a week and are placed in the vagina using a special applicator. Two of the most common brands are Replens and K-Y Liquibeads. Vitamin E oil, available in capsule form, is also an effective moisturizer. The capsule is punctured, the oil is squeezed out of the capsule onto the finger, and then the oil is applied to the labia and into the vagina.[71]

Lubricants are designed for use during sexual activity to make sexual intercourse more comfortable. They have been shown to decrease dyspareunia and improve orgasmic function without raising long-term safety concerns.[92] Common products include K-Y Jelly and Astroglide; some women also use plant-based oils such as olive or coconut oil. K-Y Jelly is a water-based product that is used just before intercourse; it may dry out or become sticky. Astroglide is a glycerin-based product; it generally does not dry out or become sticky. In general, the water-based products are preferred; petroleum-based products such as Vaseline should not be used for intercourse. Products should be warmed before use and may be placed on a heating pad or in a glass of warm water for easy access during sexual activity. Newer products contain warming agents; these should be use cautiously if there is any sign of vaginal irritation. Incorporating the use of a lubricant into foreplay and other sexual activities decreases interruptions and may enhance intimacy.[71,92] The self-care guide addressing management of vaginal dryness may be of benefit; see Appendix 24B.

Erectile dysfunction is common after radical prostatectomy and RT to the prostate or pelvis and can be seen in those patients who have surgery for bladder, rectal, and testicular cancer, particularly if nerve-sparing procedures are not used. Magazine and television advertisements abound for *PDE-5 inhibitors*, touting their use in the management of ED and their effect on quality of life.[19–21,25,26,33] Sildenafil, vardenafil, and tadalafil—all PDE-5 inhibitors—have been shown to be effective in reversing or improving ED in men who underwent rectal excision for either cancer or inflammatory bowel disease, and in men who have had radical prostatectomy.[123,124] Healing following prostate surgery can take from 3 to 6 months, with full recovery occurring in approximately 1 year. Maintaining adequate blood flow to the penis and continuing to have erections is important, and early use of products that facilitate erections increases the quality and quantity of erections over time.[25,33]

The half-life for sildenafil and vardenafil is 4.5 to 6 hours, while the half-life for tadalafil is 16 to 18 hours. Nightly doses, as opposed to intermittent doses, of sildenafil and vardenafil appear to improve erectile function, promote healing of the surgical incision, and reduce scar tissue formation.[124–126] For routine sexual activity, sildenafil and vardenafil are taken approximately 1 hour prior to sexual activity. Sexual stimulation facilitates an erection that generally lasts for about 1 hour. Tadalafil can be taken daily or in a 36-hour dose, allowing for more frequent or "on demand" erections. The concomitant use of nitrate medications is contraindicated at any time. Each drug has its own particular risks and benefits that should be discussed with the patient prior to prescribing it.[25,28,120,124–127]

Sildenafil also has been tested in women experiencing decreased desire, arousal, and orgasm. Desire and arousal were not affected by sildenafil use, but orgasm dysfunction showed some improvement. Clinical trials have been small and the results not reproducible. The PDE-5 inhibitors currently are not FDA approved for use in women.[14]

Intracorporeal (intracavernosal) injections of papaverine hydrochloride, prostaglandin E_1, phentolamine, and atropine sulfate can be used to increase blood flow to the penis, leading to an erection firm enough for penetration. The choice of medication is individualized for each man and may consist of one or more agents. Medications are injected into the lateral aspect of the shaft of the penis using a 30-gauge x ½-inch needle. Following injection, erections develop in 5 to 15 minutes and generally last from 30 to 90 minutes. Foreplay often helps to achieve erection. The initial injection is done in the healthcare provider's office or clinic and the level of erection is assessed. Medication doses may be titrated and other medications added to the regimen until a firm erection is attained and can be maintained. The patient is taught to self-inject the medications, which often is difficult. Discomfort with the self-injection procedure may decrease use over time, leading to discontinuation of an otherwise effective intervention. Side effects of intracavernosal injections may include prolonged erection (priapism), bleeding or bruising, penile pain, swelling at the injection site, and fibrosis leading to erection deformities. The patient needs to be educated about frequency of medication use and potential side effects, particularly for priapism, and monitored closely for any adverse events. If an erection lasts longer than 4 hours, the patient should call his healthcare provider or go directly to the emergency department of the local hospital. The self-care guide for this procedure may be helpful and is located in Appendix 24C.[127–131]

Devices. For some patients, the use of a *vacuum constriction/erection device* to attain an erection may be the simplest and best choice. Such a device is noninvasive, requiring neither oral nor injectable medications, is relatively inexpensive, and is generally easy to use. It consists of a clear plastic tube, open at one end, with a pump at the other end, and a constriction band. The cylinder is placed over the penis (Figure 24-4).[131] The tube and pump are used to create a vacuum that helps the penis become erect. Once the penis is erect, a constriction band is placed at the base of the penis to maintain the erection. At that point, the tube is removed. The device is used either alone or in combination with oral or intracorporeal medications. Side effects are rare, but may include bruising or petechial hemorrhage of the penis. While a vacuum constriction/erection device is easy to use, many find the mechanical aspects of the procedure disconcerting and complain that it leads to decreased spontaneity. Additionally, the band can be left in place for only 30 minutes, decreasing the length of time available for sexual activity. Education is essential for safe and effective use of the device.[127,132,133]

Vaginal dilators can be helpful in managing vaginal stenosis and adhesions leading to dyspareunia. They are particularly useful in women who have received RT to the pelvis. The dilators are plastic or silicone tubes that come in a variety of sizes. They are used to mechanically stretch vaginal tissues, keeping the vagina open and pliable. Over time, the size of the dilator is increased. When these devices are combined with relaxation techniques and Kegel exercises to relax the pubococcygeus muscles, dyspareunia should lessen, making sexual intercourse and speculum exams of the vagina easier. Education and support are essential for proper use of a vaginal dilator.[14,33,134,135] See Appendix 24D for a self-care guide on the use of dilators.

The *EROS Therapy Device* is a small handheld device that creates gentle suction on the clitoris, increasing blood flow and sensation to the surrounding tissues. Patients with stage I and II cervical cancer treated with RT noted significant improvement in sexual desire, arousal, and lubrication with use of this device; dyspareunia was also decreased and sexual satisfaction was increased. Improved vaginal elasticity and moisture and decreased vaginal bleeding have been reported with continued use of the device.[33,136]

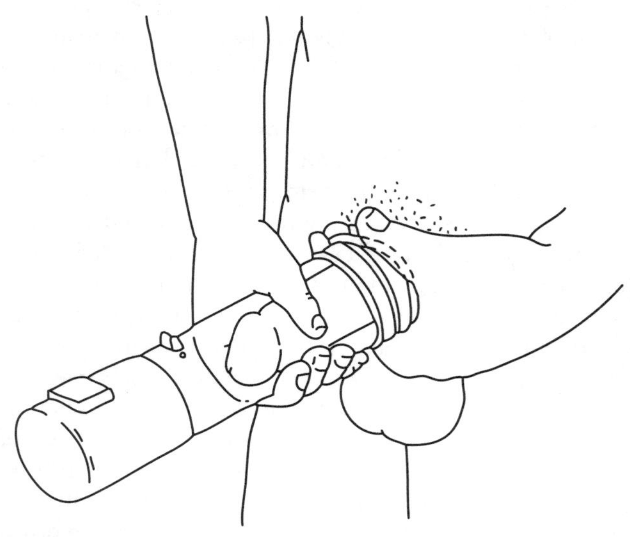

FIGURE 24-4

Placement of external vacuum device.

Physical interventions

Physical interventions to decrease sexual dysfunctions or defects caused by cancer treatment include surgery to repair tissues or restore function and the use of external products to improve body image and self-esteem.

Surgical interventions. The surgical interventions most commonly undertaken to affect sexual health include development of continent urinary reservoirs and neobladders, breast reconstruction, vaginal reconstruction, and the placement of penile implants to manage erectile dysfunction. Additionally, the use of testicular implants to enhance body image following orchiectomy, methods to repair nerve damage following radical prostatectomy, and techniques to create a penis have the potential to improve sexual health by both improving function and enhancing body image.

Urinary function. The impact of sexual health alterations due to cystectomy is decreased through the use of a continent reservoir (Koch or Indiana pouch made from a piece of bowel and placed behind the umbilicus), which improves sexual adjustment by decreasing concerns about leakage and odor,[137] or through construction of a neobladder that maintains normal bladder function and voiding patterns.[137,138] Even though the Koch or Indiana pouch requires catheterization, body image alterations are decreased due to absence of an external device for urinary drainage.[2] When compared to patients with an ileal conduit, those persons with a neobladder had increased quality of life and decreased sexual dysfunctions.[137–139] If the prostate is spared during cystectomy and a neobladder is created, potency is maintained in 75% to 100% of men and daytime continence is 95% to 100%.[139,140]

Breast reconstruction. Undergoing breast reconstruction may include not only creation of a new breast but also breast reduction or remodeling.[141,142] The presurgical size and shape of the breasts and overall body shape and anatomy influence the type and method of reconstruction to be used. Breast reconstruction may be immediate, may occur at the time of mastectomy, or may be done at a later date.

Breast reconstruction generally is done in two stages. In the first stage, a tissue expander is placed under the chest muscle, creating a space for the implant. Over weeks to months, the expander is gradually inflated with saline until the space is the right size for the implant to be placed. In the second stage, the expander is removed and the implant is placed. Widely used implants have a silicone shell and are filled with either saline or silicone.

Many women prefer to use their own tissue for reconstruction. The most common methods for "natural" reconstruction use a flap of skin, muscle, and fat from the transverse rectus abdominous muscle (TRAM) or the latissimus muscle to create the new breast. In both techniques, the skin, fat, and muscle are loosened and then tunneled under the skin up to the breast to make the new breast mound. The blood vessels remain intact, preserving blood supply. The TRAM flap technique has a double cosmetic effect in that it both reconstructs the breast and provides a tummy tuck.

The final step of all procedures is creation of a nipple, which usually occurs 3 or more months following breast reconstruction. A variety of procedures are available: (1) a partial graft from the remaining nipple may be used to create a new nipple or (2) a small area in the new breast may be raised to create a nipple. An areola can be created by tattooing the skin or grafting skin from the groin area that normally has a similar color to the areola. In some instances, nipple-sparing surgery may be used. In this procedure, the skin and nipple remain intact while the tumor, fat, and muscle are removed, leaving clean margins. The area may be radiated to minimize the risk of recurrence.[143,144]

Vaginal reconstruction. Multiple techniques for vaginal reconstruction are available. The large or small bowel, musculocutaneous flaps from the gracilis or rectus muscles, or a pedicle graft from the greater omentum can be used to construct a new vagina.[145–147] Following surgery, intercourse is possible and orgasmic sensations return in 30% to 70% of those women experiencing them prior to surgery.[145–147] Vaginal reconstruction following total pelvic exenteration allows for intercourse, but the physiological and psychological sequelae of exenteration surgery may preclude sexual activity due to lack of desire, fatigue, and other surgical side effects.[148] Vaginal reconstruction is not a panacea for sexual dysfunction, as vaginal dryness or persistent discharge, depending on the tissues used, is common and the new vagina may be seen as too big or too small, and rarely just right.[146,147] Additionally, lubrication may be needed for easier penile penetration and vaginal dilation is required for the rest of the woman's life to ensure the vagina remains patent.[149]

Penile implants. Insertion of a non-inflatable or inflatable prosthesis in the penis restores men's ability to have intercourse and increases desire and arousal, erectile ability, and frequency of intercourse. Three types of implants are available: non-inflatable, two-part inflatable, and three-part inflatable.[150–152] Selection of which implant will best meet the patient's needs is based on age of the patient and partner, size and shape of the penis, prior surgeries and implants, and a number of other factors to assure the best fit and functionality for the patient.[153]

The non-inflatable implant is the least expensive, involves the simplest surgical procedure, and is the easiest to use: It is bent up for sexual intercourse and bent down when not in use. Two silicone rods are placed in the corpora cavernosa, and an erection is always present, which may be embarrassing or bothersome. The use of elastic briefs may help to conceal the erection. Over time, thinning of penile tissue may occur and the implant may need to be removed or replaced.

The two-part inflatable implant consists of two cylinders with a pump and a reservoir. The cylinders are placed within the corpora cavernosa, and the pump and reservoir are in the scrotum. The pump is squeezed to move fluid from the reservoir into the cylinders. When an erection is no longer desired, the penis is held down to allow fluid to return to the reservoir. A partial erection is always present, which may be concealed by wearing elastic briefs. Those using this implant complain of the unnatural shape of the penis, as the implants are irregular in shape. As with the non-inflatable implant, over time the penile tissue may thin, requiring removal or replacement of the implant.[150–153]

The three-part inflatable implant consists of three parts: two cylinders placed in the corpora cavernosa, a reservoir implanted in the lower abdomen/groin, and the pump implanted in the scrotum. The pump is squeezed to move the fluid from the reservoir into the cylinders to obtain an erection; a release button on the pump allows the fluid to return to the reservoir and the penis to become flaccid. The penis has a normal look both when flaccid and when erect, and erections appear more normal. Because the penis is not constantly erect, there is less likelihood of thinning of the penile flesh requiring implant removal or replacement.[150–154]

The self-care guide in Appendix 24E provides information about the different penile implants and how to use them.[131]

COMPLEMENTARY AND ALTERNATIVE MEDICINE

Complementary and alternative medicine (CAM) remains a field filled with possibilities for management of sexual dysfunction. Cancer care programs across the United States are beginning or expanding integrative medicine programs to meet the needs of patients who want more than medicines to treat their cancers and manage side effects. Mind–body techniques such as hypnosis, relaxation, meditation, and guided imagery have shown value in decreasing stress and anxiety, minimizing treatment side effects such as nausea and vomiting, and promoting general relaxation. For those individuals with sexual dysfunctions, the end results of using these techniques may be increased intimacy and communication, and resolution of underlying factors that may affect sexual health.[155]

Many cancer patients use herbs, vitamins, minerals, and other supplements to relieve symptoms of cancer treatment and to promote general well-being. In the area of sexual health, some evidence supports the use of herbs for erectile dysfunction and the use of psychotherapy for overall sexual dysfunction. In particular, good to moderate scientific evidence is available for the use of DHEA, Panax ginseng, L-argenine, and L-carnitine for ED and for Yohimbe for both ED and general sexual dysfunction.[155] Further study is needed to define doses, length of treatment, and long-term side effects and safety profiles before these products can be recommended to cancer survivors. Ongoing and future research will provide answers for how best to use CAM therapies for all aspects of cancer care, including sexual health.

NURSING OUTCOMES

Nursing outcomes have been minimally identified for sexual health, body image, and sexual dysfunction. Neither the International Classification for Nursing Practice nor the Nursing Quality Forum has nursing-sensitive outcomes identified for sexual health. Outcomes are available from the Nursing Outcomes Classification (NOC),[156] which identifies patient outcomes that are sensitive to nursing interventions and evaluates the effects of nursing care as part of the nursing process. Each outcome includes a label, definition, and set of indicators and measures to achieve the nursing outcome. Three outcomes are identified for sexual health: body image (1200), sexual identity (1207), and sexual functioning (0119). Each has a series of indicators rated from "never demonstrated" to "consistently demonstrated."

To respond to the increasing number of patient-reported outcome (PRO) measures used in clinical practice, Hughes et al.[157] conducted a "multiphase, multidisciplinary, consensus process" to identify expert recommendations for addressing concerns seen in those patients with cancer that are commonly addressed in PRO questionnaires. Twenty domains were identified. The recommendations for the sexual function domain include (1) discussing the safety of sexual activity with the patient, (2) identifying contraceptive practices, and (3) assessing the patient and partner's levels of concern about sexual issues. Additional recommendations include (4) assessing prior and current sexual health, (5) treating underlying causes of sexual dysfunction when possible, and (6) considering referral to a person skilled in managing sexual health concerns.

The Oncology Nursing Society (ONS) has published a series of PEP (Putting Evidence into Practice) resources "designed to provide evidence-based care and teaching."[158] Six categories ranging from "recommended for practice" to "not recommended for practice" identify the level of evidence behind common interventions. Currently, 20 PEP resources are available. None specifically addresses sexual function, although one does address hot flashes and PEP resources are available for other symptoms likely to affect sexual health, intimacy, and body image such as pain and fatigue resources.[158]

PATIENT SELF-CARE

Information is available on sexual health from numerous organizations, the Internet, and a variety of print sources. The National Cancer Institute (NCI) and the American Cancer Society (ACS) both offer publications, available online or in booklet format, that address sexuality, body image, intimacy, and reproductive health. The NCI PDQ's *Sexuality and Reproductive Issues*[33] website contains a section specifically for patients and another specifically for healthcare providers, while the *Facing Forward: Life After Cancer Treatment*[159] publication has a section on sexuality, intimacy, and body image. The ACS has two publications, *Sexuality for the Man with Cancer*[160] and *Sexuality for the Woman with Cancer*,[161] that discuss sexual health issues in an easy-to-read and -understand format, providing answers to common patient concerns. Numerous organizations and foundations, such as Livestrong, ChemoCare, Us Too, and Susan G. Komen for the Cure, have information on their websites about sexual health issues. Patients also can find information through disease-specific organizations' online chat rooms, where sexuality is a common thread in discussion forums. Additionally, five self-care guides that may be given to patients with sexual health concerns are included in this chapter.

Management of body image and sexual health concerns has been discussed for decades but remains an area in need for major improvement in the delivery of comprehensive cancer care. Discussions of sexual concerns frequently are difficult for patients and healthcare providers alike, resulting in missed opportunities for interventions to promote better quality of life for patients and their caregivers. Incorporating sexual assessment, however brief, into the overall assessment legitimizes patient concerns and may make initiating more in-depth discussions easier for the nurse and the patient. Sexual health concerns impact quality of life. To ensure that the most comprehensive, best-quality care is provided, nurses should incorporate sexual assessment into their routine patient care practices and become familiar with potential interventions to meet any identified needs.

REFERENCES

1. Flynn KE, Jeffery DD, Keefe FJ, et al. Sexual functioning along the cancer continuum: focus group results from the Patient-Reported Outcomes Measurement Information System (PROMISTM) *Psychooncology.* 2011;20(4):378–386.
2. Krebs LU. Sexual and reproductive dysfunction. In: Yarbro CH, Wujcik D, Gobel BH, eds. *Cancer Nursing: Principles and Practice.* 7th ed. Sudbury, MA: Jones and Bartlett; 2011:879–911.
3. Krebs L. What should I say? Talking with patients about sexuality issues. *Clin J Oncol Nurs.* 2006;10:313–315.
4. Krebs LU. Sexual assessment: research and clinical. *Nurs Clin North Am.* 2007;42:515–529.
5. Krebs LU. Sexual assessment in cancer care: concepts, methods and strategies for success. *Semin Oncol Nurs.* 2008;24:80–90.
6. Tierney DK. Sexuality: a quality-of-life issue for cancer survivors. *Semin Oncol Nurs.* 2008;24:71–79.
7. Nishimoto PW. Sexuality. In: Gates RA, Fink RM, eds. *Oncology Nursing Secrets.* 3rd ed. St. Louis, MO: Mosby; 2008:488–501.
8. Katz A. *Breaking the Silence on Cancer and Sexuality: A Handbook for Survivors.* Pittsburgh, PA: Oncology Nursing Society; 2007.
9. Incrocci L. Cancer and sexual function: talking about sex to oncologists and about cancer to sexologists. *Sexologies.* 2007;16:265–266.
10. White ID. Oncosexology and the role of the nurse: integration, specialisation or isolation? *Sexologies.* 2007;16(4):304–308.
11. World Health Organization (WHO). *Health Topics: Sexual Health.* Geneva, Switzerland: WHO. http://www.who.int/topics/sexual_health/en/. Accessed August 19, 2012.
12. World Health Organization (WHO). *Sexual and Reproductive Health: Core Competencies in Primary Care.* Geneva, Switzerland: WHO; 2011. http://whqlibdoc.who.int/publications/2011/9789241501002_eng.pdf. Accessed August 19, 2012.
13. Hatzichristou D, Rosen RC, Derogotis LR, et al. Recommendations for the clinical evaluation of men and women with sexual dysfunction. *J Sex Med.* 2010;7:337–348.
14. Roth AJ, Carter J, Nelson CJ. Sexuality after cancer. In: Holland JC, Breitbart WS, Jacobsen PB, Lederberg MS, Loscalzo MJ, McCorkle, R. *Psycho-Oncology.* 2nd ed. New York: Oxford University Press; 2010:245–250.
15. Matulonis UA, Kornblith A, Lee H, et al. Long-term adjustment of early-stage ovarian cancer survivors. *Int J Gynecol Cancer.* 2008;18(6):1183–1193.
16. Lara LAS, DeAndrade JM, Consolo FD, Rom o APMS. Women's poorer satisfaction with their sex lives following gynecologic cancer treatment. *Clin J Oncol Nurs.* 2012;16(3):272–277.
17. Aerts L, Enzlin P, Verhaeghe J, Vergote I, Amant F. Sexual and psychological functioning in women after pelvic surgery for gynaecological cancer. *Eur J Gynaecol Oncol.* 2009:30(6):652–656.
18. Cleary V, Hegarty J, McCarthy G. Sexuality in Irish women with gynecologic cancer. *Oncol Nurs Forum.* 2011;38(2):E87–E96.
19. Diaz VA, Close JD. Male sexual dysfunction. *Prim Care Clin Office Pract.* 2010;37:473–489.
20. Ginsberg TB. Male sexuality. *Clin Geriatr Med.* 2010;26:185–195.
21. Thompson IM, Tangen CM, Goodman PJ, add back names. Erectile dysfunction and subsequent cardiovascular disease. *JAMA.* 2005;294:2996–3002.
22. DeRogatis LR, Burnett AL. The epidemiology of sexual dysfunctions. *J Sex Med.* 2008;5:289–300.
23. Mercadante S, Vitrao V. Sexual issues in early and late stage cancer: a review. *Support Care Cancer.* 2010;18:659–665.
24. Viatori M. Testicular cancer. *Semin Oncol Nurs.* 2012;28(3):180–189.
25. Albaugh A, Kellogg-Spadt S, Krebs LU, Lewis JH, Kramer-Levien D. Sexual function and sexual rehabilitation with GU cancer: what patients want to know. In: Held-Warmkessel J, ed. *Site-Specific Cancer Series: Urologic Cancers.* Pittsburgh, PA: Oncology Nursing Society; 2009:121–148.
26. Galbraith ME, Crighton F. Alterations of sexual function in men with cancer. *Semin Oncol Nurs.* 2008;24:102–114.
27. Cotrim H, Pereira G. Impact of colorectal cancer on patient and family: implications for care. *Eur J Oncol Nurs.* 2008;12:217–226.
28. Bruner GW, Calvano T. The sexual impact of cancer and cancer treatments in men. *Nurs Clin North Am.* 2007;42:555–580.
29. Li C-C. Sexuality among patients with a colostomy: an exploration of the influences of gender, sexual orientation, and Asian heritage. *J Wound Ostomy Continence Nurs.* 2009;36(3):288–296.
30. da Silva GM, Hull T, Roberts PL, et al. The effect of colorectal surgery in female sexual function, body image, self-esteem and general health: a prospective study. *Ann Surg.* 2008;248:266–272.
31. Liang JT, Lai HS, Lee PH, Chang KJ. Laparoscopic pelvic autonomic nerve-preserving surgery for sigmoid colon cancer. *Ann Surg Oncol.* 2008;15:1609–1616.
32. Tyler A. Urothelial cancer: ureter, renal pelvis, and bladder. *Semin Oncol Nurs.* 2012;28(3):154–162.
33. National Cancer Institute. *PDQ® Sexuality and Reproductive Issues.* Bethesda, MD: NCI. http://www.cancer.gov/cancertopics/pdq/supportivecare/sexuality/HealthProfessional. Accessed August 19, 2012.
34. Stilos K, Doyle C, Daines P. Addressing the sexual health needs of patients with gynecologic cancers. *Clin J Oncol Nurs.* 2008;12:457–463.
35. Krychman ML, Pereira L, Carter J, Amsterdam A. Sexual oncology: sexual health issues in women with cancer. *Oncology.* 2006;71:18–25.
36. Barton-Burke M, Gustason CJ. Sexuality in women with cancer. *Nurs Clin North Am.* 2007;42:531–554.
37. Davila HH, Weber T, Burday D, et al. Total or partial prostate sparing cystectomy for invasive bladder cancer: long-term implications on erectile function. *BJU Int.* 2007;100:1026–1029.
38. Fialka-Moser V, Crevenna R, Korpan M, Quittan M. Cancer rehabilitation, particularly with aspects on physical impairments. *J Rehabil Med.* 2003;35:153–162.
39. Pelusi J. Sexuality and body image. *AJN.* 2006;106(3 suppl):32–38.
40. Shell JA. Sexuality. In: Langhorne ME, Fulton JS, Otto SE, eds. *Oncology Nursing.* 5th ed. St. Louis, MO: Mosby; 2007:546–564.
41. Brotto LA, Yule M, Breckon E. Psychological interventions for the sequelae of cancer: a review of the literature. *J Cancer Surv.* 2010;4:346–360.
42. Brydoy M, Fossa SD, Dahl O, Bjoro T. Gonadal dysfunction and fertility problems in cancer survivors. *Acta Oncologica.* 2007;46:480–489.
43. Beard CJ. The risk of bladder, bowel, and sexual dysfunction after radiation therapy: what data tell us and how we can use it to counsel our patients. *Cancer J.* 2005;11:106–109.
44. Katz A. Quality of life for men with prostate cancer. *Cancer Nurs.* 2007;30:302–308.
45. Akbal C, Tinay I, Simsek F, Turkeri LN. Erectile dysfunction following radiotherapy and brachytherapy for prostate cancer: pathophysiology, prevention and treatment. *Int Urol Nephrol.* 2008;40:355–363.
46. Stipetich R, Abel L, Anderson RL, Butler WM, Wallner KE, Merrick GS. Nursing considerations in brachytherapy-related erectile dysfunction. *Urol Nurs.* 2005;25:249–254.

47. Morillo V, Guinot JL, Tortajada I, et al. Secondary effects and biochemical control in patients with early prostate cancer treated with 125-I seeds. *Clin Transl Oncol.* 2008;10:359–366.
48. Sadovsky R, Basson R, Krychman M, et al. Cancer and sexual problems. *J Sex Med.* 2010;7:349–373.
49. Van der Wielen GJ, van Putten WLJ, Incrocci L. Sexual function after three-dimensional conformal radiotherapy for prostate cancer: results from a dose-escalation trial. *Int J Radiat Oncol Biol Phys.* 2007;68:479–484.
50. Sklar C. Maintenance of ovarian function and risk of premature menopause related to cancer treatment. *J Natl Cancer Inst Monog.* 2005;34:25–27.
51. Bakewell RT, Volker DL. Sexual dysfunction related to the treatment of young women with breast cancer. *Clin J Oncol Nurs.* 2005;9:697–702.
52. Maher EJ, Denton A. Survivorship, late effects and cancer of the cervix. *Clin Oncol.* 2008;20:479–487.
53. White ID. The assessment and management of sexual difficulties after treatment for cervical and endometrial malignancies. *Clin Oncol.* 2008;20:488–496.
54. Krebs LU. Sexual health during cancer treatment. In: Quinn GP, Vadaparampil ST. *Reproductive Health and Cancer in Adolescents and Young Adults.* New York: Springer; 2012:61–76.
55. Fossa S, Dahl AA. Fertility and sexuality in young cancer survivors who have adult-onset malignancies. *Hematol Oncol Clin North Am.* 2008;22:291–303.
56. Franklin DJ, Packel L. Cancer-related fatigue. *Arch Phys Med Rehabil.* 2006;87(suppl 1):S91–S93.
57. Vistad I, Fossa SD, Kristensen GB, Dahl AA. Chronic fatigue and its correlates in long-term survivors of cervical cancer treated with radiotherapy. *BJOG.* 2007;114:1150–1158.
58. Wilkes GM, Barton-Burke M. *2012 Oncology Nursing Drug Handbook.* Burlington, MA: Jones & Bartlett Learning; 2012.
59. Otto S. Chemotherapy. In: Langhorne ME, Fulton JS, Otto SE, eds. *Oncology Nursing.* 5th ed. St. Louis, MO: Mosby; 2007:262–276.
60. Braun-Inglis C. Chemotherapeutic agents. In: Newton S, Hickey M, Marrs J, eds. *Mosby's Oncology Nursing Advisor: A Comprehensive Guide to Clinical Practice.* St. Louis, MO: Mosby; 2009:197–198, 223–238.
61. Blecher CS. Chemotherapeutic agents. In: Newton S, Hickey M, Marrs J, eds. *Mosby's Oncology Nursing Advisor: A Comprehensive Guide to Clinical Practice.* St. Louis, MO: Mosby; 2009:198–223.
62. Gobel BH, Mast D. Chemotherapeutic agents. In: Newton S, Hickey M, Marrs J, eds. *Mosby's Oncology Nursing Advisor: A Comprehensive Guide to Clinical Practice.* St. Louis, MO: Mosby; 2009:238–263.
63. Krebs LU. Chemotherapeutic agents. In: Newton S, Hickey M, Marrs J, eds. *Mosby's Oncology Nursing Advisor: A Comprehensive Guide to Clinical Practice.* St. Louis, MO: Mosby; 2009:263–286.
64. Thaler-deMers D. Endocrine and fertility effects in male cancer survivors. *AJN.* 2006;106:66–71
65. DiBlasio CJ, Malcolm JB, Derweesh IT, et al. Patterns of sexual and erectile dysfunction and response to treatment in patients receiving androgen deprivation therapy for prostate cancer. *BJU Int.* 2008;102:39–43.
66. Orbaugh K. Hormonal therapy agents. In: Newton S, Hickey M, Marrs J, eds. *Mosby's Oncology Nursing Advisor: A Comprehensive Guide to Clinical Practice.* St. Louis, MO: Mosby; 2009:317–325.
67. Schover LR. Premature ovarian failure and its consequences: vasomotor symptoms, sexuality and fertility. *J Clin Oncol.* 2008;26:753–758.
68. Remer SE. Targeted therapy/targeted therapy agents. In: Newton S, Hickey M, Marrs J, eds. *Mosby's Oncology Nursing Advisor: A Comprehensive Guide to Clinical Practice.* St. Louis, MO: Mosby; 2009:287–313.
69. Manolis A, Doumas M. Antihypertensive treatment and sexual dysfunction. *Curr Hypertens Rep.* 2012;14:285–292.
70. Costantini A, Navarra CM, Ashing-Giwa KT, Yeung S. Sexuality and gender: psychosocial implications in cancer patients: a multicultural perspective. In: Riba M, Grassi L. *Clinical Psycho-Oncology: An International Perspective.* Hoboken, NJ: John Wiley and Sons; 2012:39–54.
71. Katz A. *Surviving After Cancer: Living the New Normal.* Lanham, MD: Rowman & Littlefield; 2011:196–197.
72. Deneris A, Huether SE. Structure and function of the reproductive system. In: Huether SE, McCance KL, eds. *Understanding Pathophysiology.* 5th ed. St. Louis, MO: Mosby; 2012:774–798.
73. Latendresse G, McCance KL. Alterations of the reproductive system, including sexually transmitted disease. In: Huether SE, McCance KL, eds. *Understanding Pathophysiology.* 5th ed. St. Louis, MO: Mosby, 2012:799–870.
74. Dirksen SR. Nursing assessment: reproductive system. In: Lewis SL, Dirksen SR, Heitkemper MM, Buscher L, Camera IM. *Medical–Surgical Nursing: Assessment and Management.* 8th ed. St. Louis, MO: Mosby; 2011:1287–1305.
75. Masters W, Johnson V. *Human Sexual Response.* Boston, MA: Little Brown; 1966.
76. Basson R. Women's sexual function and dysfunction: current uncertainties, future directions. *Int J Imp Res.* 2008;20:466–478.
77. Kaplan HS. *Disorders of Desire.* New York: Simon & Schuster; 1974.
78. Robinson P. *The Modernization of Sex.* London: Paul Elek; 1976.
79. Lief H. Inhibited sexual desire. *Med Aspects Human Sex.* 1977;11(1):3–9.
80. Zilbergeld B, Ellison CR. Desire discrepancies and arousal problems in sex therapy. In: Leiblum S, Pervin L, eds. *Principles and Practice of Sex Therapy.* New York: Guilford Press;1980, 65-101.
81. Basson R. Using a different model for female sexual response to address women's problematic low sexual drive. *J Sex Marital Ther.* 2001;27:395–403.
82. Levin RJ. Critically revisiting aspects of human response cycle of Masters and Johnson: correcting errors and suggesting modifications. *Sex Relationship Ther.* 2008;23(4):393–399.
83. Southard NZ, Keller J. The importance of assessing sexuality: a patient's perspective. *Clin J Oncol Nurs.* 2009;13(2):213–217.
84. Southern S, Cade R. Sexuality counseling: a professional specialization comes of age. *Fam J.* 2011;19:246–262.
85. Price B. Sexuality: raising the issue with patients. *Cancer Nurs Pract.* 2010;9(5):29–35.
86. Hautamaki K, Miettinen M, Kellakumpu-Lehtinen P-K, Aalto P, Lehto J. Opening communication with cancer patients about sexuality-related issues. *Cancer Nurs.* 2007;30:399–404.
87. Katz A. The sounds of silence: sexuality information for cancer patients. *J Clin Oncol.* 2008;23:238–241.
88. Park ER, Norris RL, Bober SL. Sexual health communication during cancer care: barriers and recommendations. *Cancer J.* 2009;15(1):74–77.
89. Wylie K. Assessment and management of sexual problems in women. *JRSM.* 2007;100:547–550.
90. Bonierbale M. From sexual difficulties to sexual dysfunctions (SD). *Sexologies.* 2009;18:10–13.
91. Hughes MK. Sexuality and cancer: the final frontier for nurses. *Oncol Nurs Forum.* 2009;36(5):E241–E246.
92. Clayton AH, Hamilton DV. Female sexual dysfunction. *Obstet Gynecol Clin North Am.* 2009;36:861–876.
93. Incrocci L. Male cancer and sexual function. *Sexologies.* 2007;16:273–278.
94. Schover LR. Sexuality and fertility after cancer. *Hematology Am Soc Hematol Educ Program.* 2005:523–527.
95. Schover LR. Reproductive complications and sexual dysfunction in cancer survivors. In: Ganz PA, ed. *Cancer Survivorship: Today and Tomorrow.* New York: Springer; 2007:251–271.
96. Seftel AD, Miner MM, Kloner RA, Althof SE. Office evaluation of male sexual dysfunction. *Urol Clin North Am.* 2007;34:463–482.
97. Tsertsvadze A, Yazdi F, Fink HA, et al. *Diagnosis and Treatment of Erectile Dysfunction. Evidence Report/Technology Assessment No.171.* AHRQ publication no. 08(09)-E016. Rockville, MD: Agency for Healthcare Research and Quality; 2009.

98. Ratner ES, Foran KA, Schwartz PE, Minkin MJ. Sexuality and intimacy after gynecologic cancer. *Maturitas.* 2010;66:23–26.
99. Reese JB, Shelby RA, Keefe FJ, Porter LS, Abernethy AP. Sexual concerns in cancer patients: a comparison of GI and breast cancer patients. *Support Care Cancer.* 2010;18:1179–1189.
100. Rheaume C, Mitty, E. Sexuality and intimacy in older adults. *Geriatr Nurs.* 2008;29(5):342–349.
101. Shell JA. Including sexuality in your nursing practice. *Nurs Clin North Am.* 2007;42:685–696.
102. Adler NE, Page AEK, eds. *Cancer Care for the Whole Patient: Meeting Psychosocial Health Needs.* Washington, DC: National Academies Press; 2008;171–173.
103. Giraldi A, Rellini A, Pfaus JG, et al. Questionnaires for assessment of female sexual dysfunction: a review and proposal for a standardized screener. *J Sex Med.* 2011;8:2681–2706.
104. Rizvia SJ, Yeunga NW, Kennedy SH. Instruments to measure sexual dysfunction in community and psychiatric populations. *J Psychosom Res.* 2010;70:99–109.
105. Rosen RC, Riley A, Wagner G, Osterloh IH, Kirkpatrick J, Mishra A. The International Index of Erectile Function (IIEF): a multidimensional scale for assessment of erectile dysfunction. *Urology.* 1997;49(6):822–830.
106. Rosen RC, Cappelleri JC, Smith MD, Lipsky J, PenÄa BM. Development and evaluation of an abridged, 5-item version of the International Index of Erectile Function (IIEF-5) as a diagnostic tool for erectile dysfunction. *Int J Impot Res.* 1999;11:319–326.
107. Rosen R, Brown C, Heiman J, et al. The Female Sexual Function Index (FSFI): a multidimensional self-report instrument for the assessment of female sexual function. *J Sex Marital Ther.* 2000;26:191–208.
108. Isidori AM, Pozza C, Esposito K, et al. Development and validation of a 6-item version of the Female Sexual Function Index (FSFI) as a diagnostic tool for female sexual dysfunction. *J Sex Med.* 2010;7(3):1139–1146.
109. Derogatis LR. The Derogatis Interview for Sexual Functioning (DISF/DISF-SR): an introductory report. *J Sex Marital Ther.* 1997;23(4):291–304.
110. Clayton AH, McGarvey EL, Clavet GJ. The Changes in Sexual Functioning Questionnaire (CSFQ): development, reliability, and validity. *Psychopharmacol Bull.* 1997;33(4):731–745.
111. *Patient Reported Outcomes Measurement Information System (PROMIS).* http://www.nihpromis.org/. Accessed August 19, 2012.
112. Waterhouse J, Metcalfe MC. Development of the Sexual Adjustment Questionnaire. *Oncol Nurs Forum.* 1986;13(3):53–59.
113. Andersen BL, Lamb M. Sexuality and cancer. In: Murphy GP, Lawrence W, Lenhard RE, eds. *American Cancer Society Textbook of Clinical Oncology.* 2nd ed. Atlanta, GA: American Cancer Society; 1995:699–713.
114. Annon JS. *The Behavioral Treatment of Sexual Problems.* Honolulu, HI: Mercantile Printing; 1974:43–47.
115. Mick J, Hughes M, Cohen MZ. Using the BETTER model to assess sexuality. *Clin J Oncol Nurs.* 2004;8:84–86.
116. de Vocht HM, Notter J, van de Weil HBM. *Sexuality and Intimacy: Impact of Cancer and Discussion with Health Care Professionals from a Client's Perspective.* Paper presented at The 2nd Rotterdam Symposium on Cancer and Sexuality; June 2010; Rotterdam, Netherlands. http://www.issc.nu/uploads/07-hildedevocht.pdf. Accessed August 31, 2012.
117. National Cancer Institute (NCI)/National Institutes of Health (NIH). *Common Terminology Criteria for Adverse Events (CTCAE)* Ver. 4.03. NIH Publication No. 09-5410. http://evs.nci.nih.gov/ftp1/CTCAE/CTCAE_4.03_2010-06-14_QuickReference_8.5x11.pdf. Accessed August 19, 2012.
118. Wilmoth MC. Life after cancer: what *does* sexuality have to do with it? *Oncol Nurs Forum.* 2006;33:905–910.
119. Mick JM. Sexuality assessment: 10 strategies for improvement. *Clin J Oncol Nurs.* 2007;11:671–675.
120. Kendirci M, Bejma J, Hellstom WJ. Update on erectile dysfunction in prostate cancer patients. *Curr Opin Urol.* 2006;16:186–195.
121. Basson R. Pharmacotherapy for women's sexual dysfunction. *Expert Opin Pharmacother.* 2009;10(10):1631–1648.
122. van Staa TP, Sprafka JM. Study of adverse outcomes in women using testosterone therapy. *Maturitas.* 2009;62(1):76–80.
123. Padma-Nathan H. PDE-5 inhibitor therapy for erectile dysfunction secondary to nerve-sparing radical retropubic prostatectomy. *Rev Urol.* 2005;7(suppl 2):S33–S38.
124. Incrocci L, Slob AK, Hop WC. Tadalafil (Cialis) and erectile dysfunction after radiotherapy for prostate cancer: an open-label extension of a blinded trial. *Urology.* 2007;70:1190–1193.
125. Carson CC. PDE5 inhibitors: are there differences? *Can J Urol.* 2006;13(suppl 1):34–39.
126. Wang R. Penile rehabilitation after radical prostatectomy: where do we stand and where are we going? International Society for Sexual Medicine. April 2007. http://rejoynmedical.com/articles/penile-rehabilitation.html. Accessed August 19, 2012.
127. Lau DH, Kommu S, Mumtaz FH, Morgan RJ, Thompson CS, Mikhailidis DP. The management of phosphodiesterase-5 (PDE5) inhibitor failure. *Curr Vasc Pharmacol.* 2006;4(2):89–93.
128. Tsao AK, Nehra A. Intracavernosal injection of vasoactive agents. In: Mulchay JJ, ed. *Male Sexual Function: A Guide to Clinical Management.* Totowa, NJ: Humana Press; 2006:287–302.
129. Kava BR. Advances in the management of post-radical prostatectomy erectile dysfunction: treatment strategies when PDE-5 inhibitors don't work. *Rev Urol.* 2005;7(suppl 2):S39–S50.
130. Andersson KE. Mechanisms of penile erection and basis for pharmacological treatment of erectile dysfunction. *Pharmacol Rev.* 2011;63(4):811–859.
131. Bruner DW, Berk L. Altered body image and sexual health. In: Yarbro CH, Frogge MH, Goodman M, eds. *Cancer Symptom Management.* 3rd ed. Sudbury, MA: Jones and Bartlett; 2004:596–634.
132. Pahlajani G, Raina R, Jones S, Ali M. Zippe C. Vacuum erection devices revisited: its emerging role in the treatment of erectile dysfunction and early penile rehabilitation following prostate cancer therapy. *J Sex Med.* 2012;9(4):1182–1189.
133. Mazzola C, Mulhall JP. Penile rehabilitation after prostate cancer treatment: outcomes and practical algorithm. *Urol Clin North Am.* 2011;38(2):105–118.
134. Wolf JK. Prevention and treatment of vaginal stenosis resulting from pelvic radiation therapy. *Commun Oncol.* 2006;3:665–671.
135. Cullen K, Fergus K, DasGupta T, Fitch M, Doyle C, Adams L. From "sex toy" to intrusive imposition: A qualitative examination of women's experiences with vaginal dilator use following treatment for gynecological cancer. *J Sex Med.* 2012;9:1162–1173.
136. Schroder M, Mell LK, Hurteau JA, et al. Clitoral therapy device for treatment of sexual dysfunction in irradiated cervical cancer patients. *Int J Radiat Oncol Biol Phys* 2005;61(4):1078–1086.
137. Davila HH, Weber T, Burday D, et al. Total or partial prostate sparing cystectomy for invasive bladder cancer: long-term implications on erectile function. *BJU Int.* 2007;100:1026–1029.
138. Nieuwenhuijzen JA, de Vries RR, Bex A, et al. Urinary diversions after cystectomy: the association of clinical factors, complications and functional results of four different diversions. *Eur Urol.* 2008;53:834–844.
139. Horenblas S, Meinhardt W, Ijzerman W, et al. Sexuality-preserving cystectomy and neobladder: initial results. *J Urol.* 2001;166:837–840.
140. Puppo P, Introni C, Bertolotto F, Naselli A. Potency-preserving cystectomy with intrafascial prostatectomy for high-risk superficial bladder cancer. *J Urol.* 2008;179:1727–1732.
141. Atisha D, Alderman AK, Lowery JC, Kuhn LE, Davis J, Wilkins EG. Prospective analysis of long-term psychosocial outcomes in breast reconstruction. *Ann Surg.* 2008;247:1019–1028.
142. Warren AG, Morris DJ, Houlihan MJ, Slavin SA. Breast reconstruction in a changing breast cancer treatment paradigm. *Plast Reconstr Surg.* 2008;121:1116–1126.

143. American Cancer Society. Breast reconstruction after mastectomy. http://www.cancer.org/Cancer/BreastCancer/MoreInformation/BreastReconstructionAfterMastectomy/breast-reconstruction-after-mastectomy-toc. Accessed August 19, 2012.
144. Garcia-Etienne CA, Forcellini D, Sagona A, et al. Breast reconstruction: a quality measure for breast cancer care? *Breast.* 2012;21:105–106.
145. Abd El-Aziz S. Vaginal reconstruction using the ileocecal segment after resection of pelvic malignancy. *J Egypt Natl Cancer Inst.* 2006;18:1–7.
146. Imparato E, Alfei A, Aspesi G, Meus AL, Spinillo A. Long-term results of sigmoid vaginoplasty in a consecutive series of 62 patients. *Int Urogynecol J.* 2007;18:1465–1469.
147. Soper JT, Secord AA, Havrilesky LJ, Berchuck A, Clarke-Pearson DL. Comparison of gracilis and rectus abdominis myocutaneous flap neovaginal reconstruction performed during radical pelvic surgery: flap-specific morbidity. *Int J Gynecol Cancer.* 2007;17:298–303.
148. American Cancer Society. Surgery for vaginal cancer. http://www.cancer.org/Cancer/VaginalCancer/DetailedGuide/vaginal-cancer-treating-surgery. Accessed August 19, 2012.
149. Bridoux V, Kianfard B, Michot F, ReschB, Silbert L, Tuech JJ. Transposed right colon segment for vaginal reconstruction after pelvic exenteration. *Eur J Surg Oncol.* 2010;36:1080–1084.
150. Mayo Clinic. Penile implants. http://www.mayoclinic.com/health/penile-implants/MY00358. Accessed August 19, 2012.
151. Bettocchi C, Palumbo F, Spilotros M. Penile prosthesis implant: when, what and how. *J Men's Health.* 2009;6(4);299–306.
152. Drogo K, Montague DK. Penile prosthesis implantation in the era of medical treatment for erectile dysfunction. *Urol Clin North Am.* 2011;38:217–225.
153. Bettocchi C, Palumbo F, Spilotros M, et al. Penile prostheses. *Ther Adv Urol.* 2010;2(1):35–40.
154. Chung E, Brock G. Emerging and novel therapeutic approaches in the treatment of male erectile dysfunction. *Curr Urol Rep.* 2011;12:432–443.
155. Krebs LU. Sexuality alterations. In: Decker GM, Lee CO, eds. *Handbook of Integrative Oncology Nursing: Evidence-Based Practice.* Pittsburgh, PA: Oncology Nursing Society; 2010:133–140.
156. Moorhead S, Johnson M, Maas ML, Swanson E, eds. *Nursing Outcomes Classification (NOC).* St. Louis, MO: Mosby; 2008.
157. Hughs EF, Wu AW, Carducci MA, Snyder CF. What can I do? Recommendations for responding to issues identified by patient-reported outcomes assessments used in clinical practice. *Support Oncol.* 2012;10(4):143–148.
158. Oncology Nursing Society. Putting evidence into practice resources. http://www.ons.org/research/pep. Accessed August 19, 2012.
159. National Cancer Institute. *Facing Forward: life After Cancer Treatment.* Bethesda, MD: NCI. http://www.cancer.gov/cancertopics/coping/life-after-treatment/page5. Accessed September 2, 2012.
160. American Cancer Society. *Sexuality for the Man with Cancer.* Atlanta, GA: ACS. http://www.cancer.org/Treatment/TreatmentsandSideEffects/PhysicalSideEffects/SexualSideEffectsinMen/SexualityfortheMan/index. Accessed September 2, 2012.
161. American Cancer Society. *Sexuality for the Woman with Cancer.* Atlanta, GA: ACS. http://www.cancer.org/Treatment/TreatmentsandSideEffects/PhysicalSideEffects/SexualSideEffectsinWomen/SexualityfortheWoman/index. Accessed September 2, 2012.

Suggestions to Enhance Intimacy, Comfort, and Pleasure After Cancer Treatment

Name: ______________________________

Symptom and Description

Certain cancer treatments may leave you unable to maintain sexual contact or have intercourse in the same way you did before treatment. It may help to try out new ways of being intimate that you may not have thought of or tried before.

You will need to keep an open mind and look at your own thoughts on intimacy. Open communication with your partner will help you be successful. If you find the idea of new sexual positions interesting but feel that your upbringing, religion, or culture may prevent you from trying them, you may want to talk to your healthcare provider or a psychologist or sexual counselor. You also may wish to see a psychologist or counselor if you are having problems with your relationship or have a history of sexual abuse. Your healthcare provider should be able to give you a referral.

Management

Setting the Mood

Talking to your partner and creating a sensual environment or "setting the mood" with candlelight, wine, massage, bathing together, sensual or erotic clothing, or erotic pictures or movies (whatever appeals to you and your partner) are important parts of being intimate for most people. Foreplay and exploring each other's body with touching and caressing can increase sensations and pleasure.

Procedure

- Try sexual activities you may not have tried before, such as oral–genital sex or mutual masturbation. These may be pleasurable if you are unable to have intercourse.
- Anal intercourse is an alternative technique requiring the use of lubricants and gentle dilation. Talk with your healthcare provider to see if anal intercourse is safe for you.
- Try mechanical devices such as a vibrator to maintain sexual fulfillment or for vaginal or anal penetration when intercourse is not possible.
- Use touching, caressing, massage, or other forms of physical contact to maintain intimacy.
- Communicate with your partner what you like and do not like.

(continued)

Follow-Up

If you have tried some of these suggestions and not found them helpful, contact your healthcare provider. Continued problems with sex may require the help of a psychologist or sexual counselor.

Phone Numbers

Call your healthcare provider for any concerns.

Doctor: ______________________ Phone: ______________________

Nurse: ______________________ Phone: ______________________

Other: ______________________ Phone: ______________________

Comments

Source: Krebs LU. Altered Body Image and Sexual Health. In: Yarbro CH, Wujcik D, Gobel BH, eds. *Cancer Symptom Management.* 4th ed. Burlington, MA: Jones & Bartlett Learning; 2014.

Managing Vaginal Dryness

Name: ____

Symptom and Description

A woman's ovaries stop making estrogen at the time of normal menopause or because of some cancer treatments. These treatments may include surgical removal of the ovaries, radiation therapy to the pelvis, or some chemotherapy drugs. Without estrogen, the vagina becomes drier and less elastic and sexual intercourse or masturbation may become uncomfortable or even painful. The vagina may feel irritated or become infected. Using moisturizers may prevent vaginal dryness and restore vaginal moisture, while vaginal lubricants will make intercourse easier.

Management

- Use moisturizers to add moisture to the vagina. These products are *not* for use during intercourse, as they do not provide lubrication. Commonly used moisturizers are Replens and KY-Liquibeads.
- Vitamin E oil may be used to relieve vaginal dryness and is less expensive than products sold as moisturizers. Vitamin E products are available at grocery stores and pharmacies.
- Use only water-based lubricants such as K-Y Jelly, Astroglide, or similar products to help with intercourse or masturbation.
- Do *not* use Vaseline, baby oil, or other oil-based products, as they can irritate the vagina.
- Use lubricated condoms on the penis or vibrator.
- Encourage foreplay to increase normal vaginal lubrication.

Procedure

To add moisture:

- Insert the moisturizer into the vagina using the applicator that is supplied with the product.
- For vitamin E oil, pierce the capsule with a pin. Squeeze the oil onto your finger and gently rub the oil inside the vagina and on the vulva.
- Depending on the product, you will use it 3 to 4 times per week.
- After use, wash the applicator in warm soapy water, allow it to dry, and store it for reuse.

For intercourse or masturbation:

- Using the applicator, squeeze the lubricant into the vagina just before intercourse.
- If there is no applicator, you can use the plastic applicator that comes with medications for yeast infections or for contraceptive jellies or creams, if you have one.
- If you use an applicator, wash the applicator in warm soapy water, allow it to dry, and store it for reuse.

(continued)

- If one application of lubricant does not seem to last during intercourse, use more as needed.
- Cold lubricant can be uncomfortable. Keep the lubricant warm by wrapping the tube in a heating pad or setting it in a warm cup of water.
- Either partner can sensually apply warm lubricant to the labia, vagina, or penis using the fingers.

Follow-Up

- If vaginal dryness is still a problem, ask your healthcare provider if you can use estrogen vaginal cream or estrogen replacement therapy.
- Contact your healthcare provider if you have any vaginal irritation, itching, discharge, or bleeding.

Phone Numbers

Call your healthcare provider for any concerns.

Doctor: ______________________ Phone: ______________________

Nurse: ______________________ Phone: ______________________

Other: ______________________ Phone: ______________________

Comments

Source: Krebs LU. Altered Body Image and Sexual Health. In: Yarbro CH, Wujcik D, Gobel BH, eds. *Cancer Symptom Management.* 4th ed. Burlington, MA: Jones & Bartlett Learning; 2014.

Self-Injecting Medications to Have an Erection

Name: ____________________

Symptom and Description

Sometimes following cancer treatment, men are no longer able to have or maintain an erection. Because you are unable to have an erection, your healthcare provider has prescribed a medication for you. You inject this medication into the side of the penis at the base (the area farthest from the tip of the penis) to obtain an erection. An erection usually happens in 8 to 10 minutes and can last for 30 to 90 minutes. This medication will not cause any problems with having an orgasm or ejaculation.

You will learn how to give yourself the injection in your healthcare provider's office or clinic. Once you learn how to inject the medication, you will be able to do it yourself. Plan to inject the medication 5 to 10 minutes before sexual activity. *Use this medication not more than every 3 days and no more often than 10 times per month.*

Procedure

1. Store the medication as directed (some medications need to be refrigerated; others do not).
2. Gather equipment needed to inject the medication:
   - Medication bottle
   - Syringe and needle
   - Alcohol swabs
   - Cotton ball or gauze pad
3. Wash your hands with soap and water; dry them thoroughly .
4. Prepare the medication:
   - Using an alcohol swab, clean the rubber stopper on the top of the medication bottle.
   - Using the syringe and attached needle (30 gauge, ½ inch [13 mm]), withdraw the prescribed amount of medication into the syringe.
5. Select the site of injection along the left or right side of the penis where there are no veins, as shown in Figure 24-C1. It is important to alternate the areas where you inject the medication.
6. Grasp the penis firmly and stretch the skin taut by pulling the penis away from the body. You may lay the penis against the thigh. Avoid any area where a vein is clearly visible.
7. Wipe the injection site with an alcohol swab for about 1 minute.
8. Insert the entire length of the needle at a 90-degree angle, as shown in Figure 24-C2; the needle should not be leaning forward or back toward you.
9. Slowly inject the entire amount of medication into the penis.

(continued)

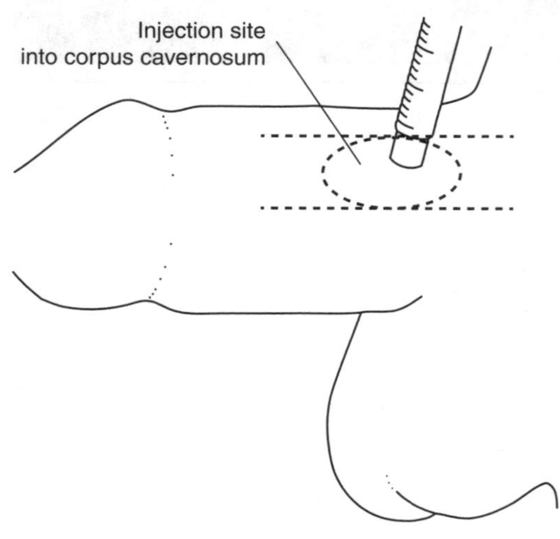

FIGURE 24-C1

Injection site.

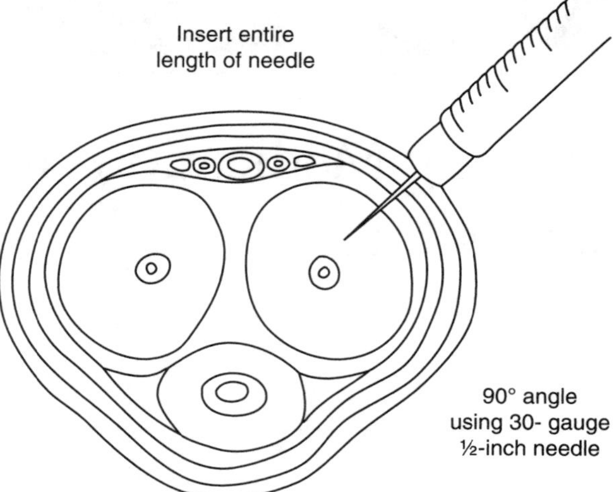

FIGURE 24-C2

Insert the needle at a 90-degree angle (cross section view).

10. Withdraw the needle and apply pressure to the injection site with a cotton ball or clean gauze for about 30 seconds or until any bleeding stops.
11. Dispose of the syringe and needle in a designated disposal box, and put the alcohol swab and cotton ball into the trash.

Management

- An erection usually occurs within 5 to 15 minutes after injection. Foreplay often helps achieve an erection.
- The medication may have some side effects. You need to watch for the following conditions:
  - Bleeding at the site of the injection: Apply pressure to the injection site until the bleeding stops, usually about 3 minutes (6 minutes if you take a blood thinner).
  - Pain or numbness at the tip of the penis: This temporary effect usually goes away in 2 to 3 minutes.
  - Penile pain: This side effect is rare, but is more common in men who have had a radical prostatectomy or have diabetes.
  - Swelling at the injection site: This problem usually happens only if the medication is injected into the skin instead of the base of the penis.
  - Flushing or dizziness: Lie down for 5 to 10 minutes or until the symptoms go away. Call your healthcare provider if the flushing or dizziness lasts longer than 20 minutes.
  - No erection: This generally is a result of poor self-injection technique or too low a dose of medication. Talk with your healthcare provider if this happens more than once.
  - Scars or areas of tenderness on the penis: These effects may happen as a result of poor technique, use of the medication over long periods of time, or possibly an infection or other medical problem. Call your healthcare provider for an examination.
  - Extreme bruising or swelling: Firmly compress the entire penis with your hand for 10 minutes, and do not perform self-injection again until instructed by your healthcare provider.
  - A prolonged erection (lasting longer than 4 hours): This condition can cause permanent damage to the penis. Contact your healthcare provider or go to the emergency room of your local hospital.

Follow-Up

Be sure you understand what to expect and what to do should problems occur. Notify your nurse and/or doctor if any of the following occurs

- Prolonged erection, lasting longer than 4 hours (contact your healthcare provider immediately or go to the emergency room)
- Flushing or dizziness lasting more than 20 minutes
- Prolonged bleeding (longer than 3 minutes or 6 minutes if you are on a blood thinner)
- Extreme bruising or swelling of the penis
- Scars or areas of tenderness on the penis

If you are unsure of any of these instructions, be sure to clarify them with your healthcare provider.

Phone Numbers

Call your healthcare provider for any concerns.

Doctor: ______________________________ Phone: __________________________

Nurse: ______________________________ Phone: __________________________

Other: ______________________________ Phone: __________________________

Comments

Source: Krebs LU. Altered Body Image and Sexual Health. In: Yarbro CH, Wujcik D, Gobel BH, eds. *Cancer Symptom Management.* 4th ed. Burlington, MA: Jones & Bartlett Learning; 2014.

Preventing Vaginal Shortening and Decreased Elasticity

Name: ______________________________

Symptom and Description

A possible effect of having radiation treatments to your vagina is decreased blood flow in the vagina. This condition may cause dry, tender, and less elastic feelings in the vagina. Radiation therapy to the vagina also may cause scar tissue to form, leading to a shortened or narrowed vagina. Pelvic surgery or menopause also may make the vagina feel shorter or less elastic. These conditions are called *vaginal stenosis* (sten-oh'-sis). Keeping the vagina open and elastic is important for comfort during sexual activity and during pelvic exams. It also allows your healthcare provider to see the treated area better.

Prevention

Regular sexual intercourse (three or more times per week) or use of a vaginal dilator will help prevent vaginal stenosis. Both will keep the vagina open (dilated) and the tissue more elastic. A vaginal dilator is a smooth plastic or rubber cylinder measuring approximately 6 inches in length. Vaginal dilators come in four different sizes (1–4) or widths (extra small, small, medium, and large). Your healthcare provider can help you get a dilator or suggest alternatives.

Ask your provider when you can resume intercourse or begin using a dilator. Usually you can begin about 1 to 2 weeks after your last radiation treatment (once the irritation is gone) or 4 to 6 weeks after your surgery. Some women may continue intercourse throughout their radiation treatments.

Procedure for Using a Dilator

1. Make sure you have privacy.
2. Stand with one leg up on a stool or toilet seat as if you were inserting a tampon, or lie back in bed or in a warm tub with your knees bent and apart (whichever is most comfortable for you).
3. If your doctor has ordered estrogen cream, spread it on the rounded end of the dilator. If you are not using estrogen cream, use a water-based lubricant such as K-Y Jelly or Astroglide. *Oil-based lubricants such as Vaseline or baby oil should not be used, as they can cause irritation that may lead to discomfort or infection.* Before applying the cream or jelly, warm the tube by running it under hot water so that the lubricant will be more comfortable.
4. Use your fingers to separate the skin at the opening to the vagina.
5. Insert the rounded end of the dilator into your vagina as far as possible using firm but gentle pressure.

6. There are two ways to use the dilator. Both are fine, but one may be more comfortable for you than the other:
   - Insert the dilator into the vagina and hold it in place for 20 to 30 minutes. You can try squeezing the dilator gently while in place and then relax your muscles.
   - Insert the dilator and hold it in place for 5 to 20 seconds. Remove and reinsert. Repeat this "in, hold, and out" motion for 10 to 15 minutes.
7. After use, wash the dilator with mild soap, dry it well, and store it until the next use.
8. Use the dilator 1 time a day for about 4 weeks, then 3 times a week for about 6 months. You may need to continue using a dilator 2 or 3 times per week for the rest of your life.

Follow-Up

Notify your healthcare provider if you have any of the following:

- Vaginal itching
- Vaginal discharge of any color with a strong odor
- Fever
- Heavy bleeding (spotting with beginning use is not uncommon)
- Painful intercourse
- Abdominal pain
- Difficulty inserting the dilator

Keep your regular follow-up appointments.

- Do not use your dilator for 3 days prior to a pelvic exam.
- Do not have intercourse 1 day prior to your exam.

Phone Numbers

Call your healthcare provider for any concerns.

Doctor: ________________________________ Phone: ____________________________

Nurse: ________________________________ Phone: ____________________________

Other: ________________________________ Phone: ____________________________

Comments

Source: Krebs LU. Altered Body Image and Sexual Health. In: Yarbro CH, Wujcik D, Gobel BH, eds. *Cancer Symptom Management.* 4th ed. Burlington, MA: Jones & Bartlett Learning; 2014.

Managing Your Penile Implant

Name: ______________________________

Symptom and Description

You have a penile implant because you are unable to have an erection due to your cancer treatment. You can use your penile implant whenever you want to have an erection. Three types of penile implants are available: non-inflatable, semi-inflatable (two-piece inflatable), and fully inflatable (three-piece inflatable). Infections and irritation of the penis can occur with a penile implant. You may need to have your implant replaced about every 10 or so years.

Procedure and Management

Use the following procedure and management suggestions based on the type of prosthesis you have implanted.

Procedure

Non-inflatable

1. When you wish to have sexual intercourse, gently position the penis forward and upward.
2. When sexual intercourse is completed, position the penis downward or up against the abdomen.
3. With this type of implant, you will have a continual erection. This can feel uncomfortable or be embarrassing. Wearing elastic briefs can help make the penis less obvious.

Semi-inflatable

1. To create an erection, firmly squeeze and release the combination pump several times. This moves the fluid from the reservoir to two cylinders located in the shaft of the penis. The combined pump and reservoir is located in the scrotum.
2. To deflate the erection, hold the penis in a downward position for 10 seconds and release. This will cause the fluid to return to the reservoir.
3. While not as obvious as the non-inflatable implant, the penis will look abnormal and be slightly rigid. Wearing elastic briefs can help make the penis less obvious.

Fully inflatable

1. To create an erection, squeeze the pump several times to move the fluid from the reservoir to the cylinders located in the shaft of the penis (see Figure 24-E). The pump is rectangular and located in the scrotum. The reservoir is located in the groin.
2. To deflate the implant, squeeze the sides of the pump to release the fluid from the cylinders back into the reservoir (see Figure 24-E).
3. The penis has a normal look when flaccid or erect; you will not need elastic briefs.

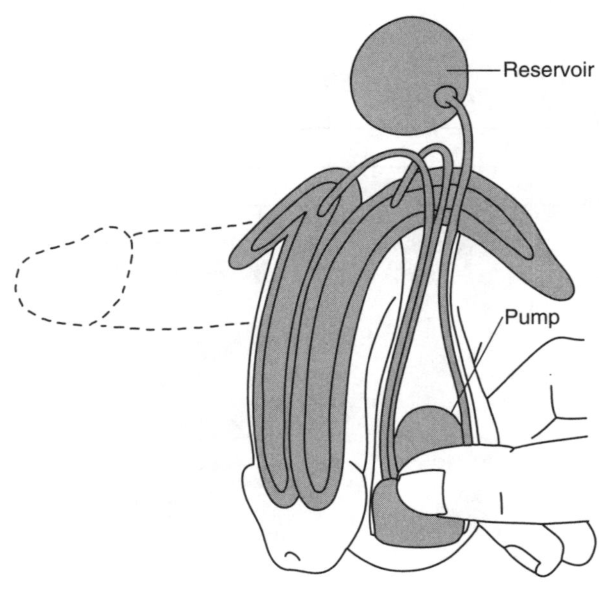

FIGURE 24-E

Fully inflatable prothesis. The fully inflatable prosthesis consists of three components: a reservoir placed under the rectus muscle, two cylinders placed in the corpora cavernosa, and a pump placed in the scrotal sac.

Management

- You may have pain for 1 to 2 weeks following surgery. Take pain medications as ordered to relieve the pain. You may have scrotal swelling for the first two weeks as well.
- You usually can begin sexual intercourse about 6 to 8 weeks after your surgery (check with your surgeon for specific instructions).
- Infections or problems with the implant working correctly happen in about 2% to 10% of patients. Your healthcare provider/surgeon will keep an eye on you for any infection. Implants that do not work correctly may need to be replaced.

Follow-Up

Careful observation can prevent serious problems with your implant. Report any of the following problems to your healthcare provider:

1. Tenderness or pain in the penis
2. Temperature greater than 100°F (38°C)
3. Discharge of pus from the urethra (the opening at the end of the penis)
4. Unusual swelling along the penis
5. Signs of penile irritation:
    - The skin of the penis appears as if you can almost see through it.
    - The implant is partly visible beneath the penile skin.

(continued)

Phone Numbers

Call your healthcare provider for any concerns.

Doctor: ______________________________ Phone: ___________________________

Nurse: ______________________________ Phone: ___________________________

Other: ______________________________ Phone: ___________________________

Comments

Source: Krebs LU. Altered Body Image and Sexual Health. In: Yarbro CH, Wujcik D, Gobel BH, eds. *Cancer Symptom Management.* 4th ed. Burlington, MA: Jones & Bartlett Learning; 2014.

Chapter 25

Extravasation

Colleen O'Leary, MSN, RN, AOCNS®
Kimberly Catania, MSN, RN, AOCN®

THE PROBLEM

Extravasation is defined by the Infusion Nursing Society (INS) as "the inadvertent leakage of a vesicant solution into surrounding tissue."[1] The Oncology Nursing Society (ONS) expands this definition of extravasation by including "the passage or escape of antineoplastic drugs into the tissue that may lead to necrosis in severe situations."[2] Extravasation can be a result of mechanical factors such as manipulation that can occur during the insertion of a catheter, while the catheter is in place, or as a result of preexisting or emerging vein problems.

Extravasation of vesicant chemotherapy has been referred to as both a "preventable catastrophe" and "a dreaded complication of chemotherapy."[3,4] It can result in significant distress and suffering to patients, and is thought to be the most severe acute complication that occurs with peripheral intravenous administration of vesicant drugs.[5] Tissue damage from extravasation can result in full-thickness skin loss as well as muscle and tendon necrosis, often requiring surgical intervention. This tissue damage can, in turn, lead to outcomes ranging from large scars to functional limitations to amputation.

A long-term effect of extravasation is a neurologic syndrome referred to as complex regional pain syndrome (CRPS), which requires chronic pain management.[6] CRPS typically develops after some sort of trauma to the tissue. Manifestations associated with CRPS include typical neuropathic pain characteristics such as intense burning pain, increased sensitivity to pain, and pain from stimuli that typically do not cause pain.[7]

Extravasation is also experienced with the use of central venous catheters when the catheter is damaged, ruptures, or migrates outside of the vein. This can result not only in tissue damage, but also in injury to the mediastinum, lung, and other regions.[8]

INCIDENCE

Incidence rates of extravasations have been difficult to capture due to the fact that there is not a formalized central reporting system for this complication. One small study conducted in 1979, which is often mentioned in the literature, estimates incidence rates for extravasation at approximately 6.5%.[9] Another commonly cited rate of chemotherapy extravasation is based on 2002 data from the M. D. Anderson Cancer Center, which provide a rate of 0.01%.[10] More accurate data should be available soon due to the 2009 creation of the Centers for Medicare and Medicaid Services International Classification of Diseases (ICD-9) code 999.81, extravasation of chemotherapy.[11]

Chemotherapy extravasation incidence in infants and children is estimated to be as high as 11%.[12] Small children's fragile veins, combined with their diminished ability to verbally communicate their pain, may leave pediatric patients particularly prone to infiltration and extravasation injuries.

ETIOLOGY

Possible etiologies of extravasation are different for peripheral and central venous catheters. Manipulation of the cannula during vein insertion can result in vein wall puncture, piercing, or trauma, which in turn leads to extravasation.[13] Administration of vesicants into a vein below a venipuncture site that is less than 24 hours old or into a vein below a recent or nonhealed vesicant extravasation site could allow the vesicant being administered to leak into surrounding tissue, resulting in extravasation.[13] Even when the cannula is properly placed in an appropriate site, displacement of the cannula from the vein itself can result in extravasation.[13]

Extravasation from a central venous access device (CVAD) can also occur. A difficult insertion of the CVAD that required additional probing and difficulty advancing the guidewire can increase the risk of extravasation. Inadvertent and undetected piercing, slicing, or nicking of the catheter during its insertion increases the risk for extravasation.[8] In addition, CVAD extravasation can result from displacement of the needle from an implanted venous access port (IVAP) when the needle is not properly inserted.[13] Incorrect needle placement is more common with the use of newly placed IVAPs, as increased edema and tenderness may prevent proper palpation of the site prior to the needle's insertion.

Although uncommon, extravasation can also occur due to damage to the catheter from mechanical difficulties such as thrombus formation, drug precipitate within the catheter, or internal pinch-off of the catheter.[13] Fibrin sheath and thrombosis formation in the CVAD may cause retrograde displacement of the CVAD, leading to extravasation.[13] Use of a syringe that contains less than 10 mL of fluid to flush a CVAD can generate high internal pressure that potentially could result in separation of the catheter from the portal body of an IVAP, leading to extravasation.[13]

TABLE 25-1

Classification of Agents

Non-Irritant Agents	Irritant Agents	Vesicant Agents
Aldesleukin (Interleukin-2)	Bleomycin	Cisplatin[a]
Asparaginase	Carboplatin	Dactinomycin
Busulfan	Carmustine	Daunorubicin
Cladribine	Cisplatin[a]	Docetaxel
Cyclophosphamide	Dacarbazine	Doxorubicin
Cytarabine	Daunorubicin	Epirubicin
Fludarabine	Daunorubicin liposomal	Idarubicin
Gemcitabine	Docetaxel	Mechlorethamine
Gemtuzumab ozogamicin	Doxorubicin liposomal	Melphalan
Ifosfamide	Etoposide	Mitomycin
Methotrexate	Floxuridine	Paclitaxel
Pentostatin	Irinotecan	Vinblastine
Rituximab	Mitoxantrone[b]	Vincristine
Thiotepa	Oxaliplatin[c]	Vindesine
Trastuzumab	Topotecan	Vinorelbine

[a]Cisplatin is reported as a vesicant if greater than 20 ml of 0.5 mg/ml concentration extravasates.
[b]Mitoxantrone may act as a vesicant depending on concentration; it is classified as a vesicant in the Oncology Nursing Society chemotherapy guidelines.
[c]Oxaliplatin has been reported to have vesicant properties.

Source: "Vesicant Extravasation Part I: Mechanisms, Pathogenesis, and Nursing Care to Reduce Risk" Sauerland C, Engelking C, Wickham R, Corbi D, 2006, *Oncology Nursing Forum, 33*, p. 1135. Copyright 2006 by the Oncology Nursing Society. Reprinted with permission[13].

PATHOPHYSIOLOGY

Regardless of whether the cause of extravasation is mechanical or physiologic, the pharmacologic characteristics and resulting tissue reaction of the extravasating agent determine the management of this condition. Drugs are categorized as being nonirritants, irritants, or vesicants (Table 25-1).[13,14]

Nonirritant drugs are those drugs that if they leak outside of a vessel wall cause no tissue damage. Venous flare is a localized hypersensitivity reaction, most often seen with doxorubicin, that is characterized by erythema, vein streaking, and itching along the vein through which the agent is infusing. The difference between venous flare and extravasation is that blood return is maintained with venous flare, and there is an absence of pain and swelling with the former condition.

Irritant drugs can cause local tissue reactions including phlebitis, pain, and venous irritation. Although these drugs do not generally cause tissue damage, they can cause ulceration in concentrated amounts.[13] The most common symptom associated with irritant drugs is an achy pain that subsides when the infusion stops.

Vesicants are the drugs that cause the most severe tissue damage. Both antineoplastic and non-antineoplastic agents may be classified as vesicants. Antineoplastic vesicants can cause cellular toxicity when in contact with tissue and are divided into two categories based on the mechanism of damage: non-deoxyribonucleic acid (DNA)–binding agents and DNA-binding agents (Table 25-2).[13–15]

Non-DNA-binding drugs

Vinca alkaloids including vinblastine, vincristine, vindesine, and vinorelbine; alkylating drugs including amasacrine, cisplatin, mechlorethamine, melphelan, and oxaliplatin;

TABLE 25-2

Non-DNA-Binding Vesicant Drugs and DNA-Binding Vesicant Drugs

Non-DNA-binding Drugs	DNA-binding Drugs
Vinca Alkaloids:	**Anthracyclines:**
• Vinblastine	• Daunorubicin
• Vincristine	• Doxorubicin
• Vindesine	• Epirubicin
• Vinorelbine	• Idarubicin
Alkyklating Drugs:	**Antitumor Antibiotics:**
• Amsacrine	• Bleomycin
• Cisplatin*	• Dactinomycin
• Mechlorethamine	• Mitomycin C
• Melphalan	• Mitoxantrone
• Oxaliplatin	
Taxanes:	**Alkylating Drugs:**
• Docetaxel*	• Mechlorethamine
• Paclitaxel*	

*Irritants with vesicant potential

Source: Data from Sauerland et al[13]; Polovich et al[14]; Schulmeister[15].

and taxanes including docetaxel and paclitaxel cause cell death by interrupting cells' ability to divide. Vinca alkaloids and taxanes are toxic to intracellular microtubules, which is the means by which they cause cell death. Microtubules are important for maintaining cell structure and forming the mitotic spindle, which is necessary for mitotic cell division. Vinca alkaloids inhibit microtubule formation in the mitotic spindle, which in turn inhibits cell division.[16] Microtubules must remain dynamic to change and duplicate; taxanes, however, enhance microtubule stabilization, thereby preventing cell division.[17]

Alkylating drugs may bind to nucleic acids, proteins, amino acids, or nucleotides. Depending on where the drug binds, it can stop DNA from forming or interfere with DNA function, such as by inactivating DNA repair enzymes or initiating cell membrane damage.[18] Non-DNA-binding drugs are metabolized in the tissue and are cleared more rapidly from sites of extravasation, so they cause less tissue damage than DNA-binding drugs.[19] Tissue injury from non-DNA-binding drugs usually remains localized, is mildly to moderately painful, and improves over time.

DNA-binding drugs

Anthracyclines, antitumor antibiotics, and some alkylating drugs are DNA-binding drugs. Anthracyclines including daunorubicin, doxorubicin, epirubicin, and idarubicin not only bind to the nucleic acids in DNA, but are also toxic to topoisomerase II. Topoisomerase II enzymes help to regulate the winding of the DNA helix. When the anthracyclines destroy topoisomerase II enzymes, it leads to breaks in the DNA strand. Additionally, anthracyclines generate a variety of free radicals that inhibit ribonucleic acid (RNA) and protein synthesis, which eventually causes cell death.[13]

The primary anthracycline for which extravasation has been studied is doxorubicin. The generally accepted theory regarding doxorubicin extravasation is that as affected cells die, the normal tissues surrounding the extravasated area take up the drug by engulfing the protein molecules. Engulfment creates larger molecules that do not easily exit from the tissue, which leads to a continuous cycle of tissue damage as the drug stays in the tissue for a long period of time. Tissue necrosis can progress over weeks to months, resulting in damage that is larger in size, deeper in depth, and more painful than damage from other DNA-binding drugs.[20,21]

Antitumor antibiotics including mitomycin, mitoxantrone, dactinomycin, and bleomycin bind to DNA, causing cross-linkage of DNA and inhibiting DNA synthesis.[22–24] DNA intra- and inter-strand cross-linking occurs, leading to apoptosis.[22–24] RNA and protein synthesis are also inhibited, albeit to a lesser extent.

Non-antineoplastic vesicant drugs

Drugs other than antineoplastic drugs may also demonstrate vesicant properties (Table 25-3). The extravasation of these drugs can result in extensive skin and soft-tissue damage that could require debridement, flap reconstruction, or skin grafting.[6,13,25] Pharmacologic characteristics that contribute to the vesicant properties of a drug include its potential hydrogen (pH), osmolarity and vasoconstriction.[25] Drugs that have vesicant properties related to their pH or osmolarity include 10% dextrose, 15% mannitol, parenteral nutrition, and phenytoin.[6,13,25]

Veins become irritated when the pH of the infused solution differs from the normal physiologic pH. When extreme pH differences occur, whether alkaline or acidic, cell proteins are damaged and cell death results.[25] Once cell death occurs, the endothelium of the vein is compromised and becomes more susceptible to rupture.

Osmolarity can also affect how tissue reacts to extravasation. When hypertonic solutions escape outside a vein, fluid shifts from inside the cell to the interstitial spaces, interrupting cell function.[25] The ensuing swelling and pressure can lead to skin necrosis and serious tissue damage. Conversely, solutions that are hypo-osmolar can cause cells to swell and eventually rupture.

Dobutamine, dopamine, epinephrine, and vasopressin are vasoconstrictive drugs that have vesicant properties.[6,13,25] The vasoconstrictive properties of these drugs come into play when they are in contact with tissue. The very nature of these drugs is to reduce blood flow and produce constriction of smooth muscle. Extravasation of these drugs, therefore, can result in ischemic necrosis.[13,22]

Agents with high electrolyte concentrations, such as calcium chloride 5.5%, calcium gluconate 10%, potassium chloride 7.45%, sodium bicarbonate 4.2% or 8.4%, and sodium chloride 10%, cause smooth muscle to contract.[25] This effect leads to prolonged exposure of tissue to the drug, which can result in ischemia and tissue necrosis.[25] Other drugs that can have vesicant properties include diazepam, fluoroquinolones, gentamycin, nafcillin, penicillin, promethazine, radiographic contrast media, and vancomycin.[6,13,25]

TABLE 25-3

Non-Antineoplastic Vesicant Drugs

pH/Osmolarity	Vasoconstriction
• 10% Dextrose • 15% Mannitol • Phenytoin • Parenteral nutrition	• Dobutamine • Epinephrine • Vasopressin • Dopamine
Concentrated Electrolyte Solutions	**Other**
• Calcium Chloride 5.5% • Calcium Gluconate 10% • Potassium Chloride 7.45% • Sodium Bicarbonate 4.2% or 8.4% • Sodium Chloride 10%	• Diazepam • Fluoroquinolones • Gentamycin • Nafcillin • Penicillin • Promethazine • Radiographic contrast media • Vancomycin

Source: Data from Hadaway[6]; Sauerland et al[13]; Doellman et al[25].

SYMPTOM ASSESSMENT

RISK FACTORS

Patients with cancer often have multiple factors that put them at high risk for extravasation. These factors can be procedure-related, materials or equipment-related, or patient-related. Procedure-related factors that can increase the risk of extravasation include factors associated with venipuncture as well as infusion procedures. Use of staff who are untrained or inexperienced in venipuncture puts a patient at increased risk for extravasation. Both the American Society of Clinical Oncology (ASCO) and the ONS recommend that chemotherapy should be administered by professional staff who are specifically trained in chemotherapy procedures.[26,27] Multiple attempts at venipuncture or the use of unfavorable venipuncture sites can also increase risk for extravasation.[28] Unfavorable venipuncture sites include areas with little subcutaneous fat, such as the back of the hand; veins over vital nerves and tendons, such as the antecubital fossa and wrist; areas close to bones; and areas of joint flexion.[12,28]

Use of appropriate equipment and materials for venipuncture and infusion is imperative in reducing the risk of extravasation. The choice of a needle that is less likely to become dislodged, yet allows blood to flow easily is recommended. This can be accomplished by using the smallest-gauge cannula in the largest vein possible.[3,6,28] Rigid intravenous (IV) catheters can easily puncture the vein if the patient moves. Therefore use of a small-bore plastic cannula is preferred.[8,28] Properly securing the IV cannula will reduce the risk of extravasation. The ability to visualize the IV insertion site to allow continual inspection is important to verify that the catheter is placed correctly in

TABLE 25-4

Risk Factors for Extravasation

Procedure Factors	Equipment/Materials Factors	Patient Factors
• Untrained or inexperienced staff • Multiple attempts at cannulation • Use of unfavorable cannulation sites (e.g., back of hand, antecubital fossa, wrist)	• Rigid intravenous catheters • Unsecured cannula • Wet, loose dressings • Dressing that obscures insertion site	• Small blood vessels (e.g., infants and children) • Fragile blood vessels (e.g., elderly and some patients with cancer) • Hard, sclerosed veins • Veins that easily move or roll • Reduced choice of veins (e.g., lymphedema, limb amputation) • Obstructed vena cava • Multiple previous intravenous cannulations or venipunctures • Obesity • Cormorbid conditions (e.g., diabetes, peripheral circulatory conditions like Raynaud's syndrome, eczema, psoriasis, and radiation damage) • Excessive patient movement in affected limb • Patients with sensory deficits (e.g., peripheral vascular disease, neuropathy, diabetes, paralysis, sedation, somnolence, cognitive deficits, and altered mental status)

Source: Data from Schulmeister[8]; American Society of Clinical Oncology[26]; Jacobson et al[27]; Wengstron et al[28]; Dougherty[29]; Dougherty[30].

the vein. Use of a clear dressing to secure the cannula without the use of additional gauze or other dressing to cover the actual insertion site, as well as keeping the dressing dry and tightly secured, decreases the risk of extravasation.[8,28]

Patient-related risk factors for extravasation include small blood vessels like those seen in infants and children, fragile blood vessels sometimes seen in the elderly or patients with cancer, veins that have become hard or thick as a result of frequent venipuncture, and veins that are mobile or "roll" when venipuncture is attempted.[8,28–30] Lymph node removal or dissection can result in fluid retention seen with lymphedema, which impairs lymph circulation and increases the risk of extravasation.[8,28–30] Limb amputation reduces the choice of available veins, thereby increasing the risk for extravasation.[8,28–30] An obstructed vena cava can result in elevated venous pressure and increased venous return. When systemic venous return is increased, right ventricular preload increases leading to a sudden increase in stroke volume and pulmonary blood flow, potentially causing leakage around smaller veins that can increase the risk of extravasation.

Once veins are punctured, they require adequate time for self-repair to ensure there is no leakage from the site of venipuncture. Multiple previous venipunctures immediately prior to obtaining adequate IV access increases the risk of extravasation when the IV is started below the sites of venipuncture.

Obesity may obscure veins from view and palpation. Comorbid conditions that increase the risk for extravasation include diabetes and peripheral circulatory conditions such as Raynaud's syndrome that impair circulation.[8,28–30] Conditions such as eczema, psoriasis, and radiation damage increase the risk for extravasation because of the difficulty experienced in accessing veins through damaged skin.[8,28–30]

Excessive patient movement can increase the risk for extravasation through inadvertent dislodgement of the IV cannula. Assuring that the IV is secured adequately and instructing the patient to use caution when moving the limb that is accessed is important in maintaining the IV site. Patients with sensory deficits due to conditions such as peripheral vascular disease, neuropathy, diabetes, and paralysis, as well as those with sedation, somnolence, cognitive deficits, and altered mental status, may have impaired ability to detect and report a change in sensation at the chemotherapy site, which in turn increases their risk for extravasation injury.[8,28–30] (See Table 25-4 for a review of risk factors related to extravasation.)

SELF-ASSESSMENT

It is vital to educate patients regarding the possible side effects of treatment, including the risk of extravasation. Patients should be taught to be aware of any pain or sensation at the site of the infusion and asked to report these symptoms as soon as they are aware of them. The most typical symptoms for assessing extravasation include pain, swelling, redness, discomfort, burning, stinging, tingling, or other acute changes at the site of extravasation.[28–30] Although these symptoms should be taken seriously, none of them is considered confirmation of extravasation on its own. All reports of such symptoms should be followed up with additional examination.

OBJECTIVE ASSESSMENT

In addition to patient reports, objective assessment is necessary to confirm an extravasation. Visual assessment is useful in validating the presence of extravasation. Although there may be no initial signs of extravasation, most often immediate indications of extravasation from a peripheral IV include mild erythema, pruritus and edema, IV flow that slows or stops, loss of blood return, and leaking around the IV catheter.[19,28,31] There is often accompanying discomfort or pain, sometimes described as burning or tingling, which ranges from mild to intense depending on the agent and the patient.[19,28,31]

Early physical symptoms usually appear immediately, but their onset can also be delayed for days to weeks.[27] Within 2 to 3 days, increased erythema, pain, discoloration, induration, dry desquamation, and/or blistering may appear.[19,31] Within 2 to 3 weeks, blistering, peeling, and sloughing of skin and tissue necrosis may be seen.[19,28]

Extravasation from a central venous catheter (CVC) can manifest differently due to the potentially larger areas of extravasation and tissue damage. Pain and stinging are common with both IVAPs and tunneled CVCs, occurring around the port, in the area of the dependent chest, or at the insertion site.[31] Additional objective manifestations of CVC extravasation include sudden swelling around the port pocket or dependent chest; palpable crepitus; fluid leaking around the needle or insertion site; erythema around the port, dependent chest, clavicular area, or neck area; and loss of blood return.[31] CVC tip displacement from the superior vena cava can also manifest as intractable cough with the infusion, pleural effusions, and abnormal chest radiography, resulting in substernal chest pain, dyspnea, and fatigue.[31] Because these cues can occur either early or late, careful monitoring of the site should be performed throughout the infusion and continue for 3 weeks or longer after completion of vesicant administration.[19,30]

Verification of line patency should be assured throughout the course of vesicant infusions and with any suspected extravasation. Lack of line patency should be suspected with increased resistance while administering medications, slow or sluggish infusions, change in the infusion flow, and lack or loss of blood return from the cannula.[14,28] Distinguishing between extravasation and other reactions, such as a flare reaction, vessel irritation, and venous shock, is important to determining continued management (Table 25-5). The major differences between these conditions and extravasation generally are determined by such issues as timing of symptoms and presence of pain, swelling, blood return, and

TABLE 25-5

Distinguishing Extravasation from Other Conditions

Characteristic	Flare Reaction	Vessel Irritation	Venous Shock	Extravasation
Pain	Uncommon	Aching and tightness, above administration site, as agent is infused	Vessel spasm	Common at and around administration site, burning, stinging, cool sensation during infusion. Pain increases in intensity over time.
Color	Red streaks or blotches, wheal formation along vessel, diffuse or irregular pattern, usually subsides within minutes	Reddened or darkened	No discoloration	Redness in area of needle or venipuncture site. Sometimes difficult to see if occurs deep in tissue (e.g., as result of needle dislodgement from implanted port). Redness intensifies over time.
Timing	Appears suddenly and dissipates within 30–90 minutes	Appears within minutes of vesicant administration. Color may only appear later.	Appears immediately after vesicant adminstration	Appears immediately after vesicant administration and intensifies over time.
Swelling	Unlikely	Unlikely	Unlikely	Occurs often; is easier to detect from superficial extravasation (e.g., from peripheral vein), increases over time.
Blood Return	Present	Present	Often absent	Not present
Ulceration	Does not occur	Does not occur	Does not occur	Immediately after vesicant administration, skin is intact. If untreated, blistering and sloughing begins within 1–2 weeks, followed by tissue necrosis that may require surgical debridement and skin grafting or flap placement.

Source: Data from Polovich et al[14].

ulceration.[8,12,13,28] With venous flare, there is generally no pain, swelling, or ulceration. Immediate blotches or streaks along with wheal formation appear along the vein where the agent is being infused; these signs dissipate within 30 to 90 minutes.[8,12,13,28] Aching, tightness, erythema, or dark discoloration that intensifies over time is typical of vessel irritation.[8,12,13,28] Blood return is maintained, and swelling and ulceration do not occur.[8,12,13,28] Venous shock is manifested as spasms of the muscular wall of the blood vessel that usually occur immediately after the infusion is started.[8,12,13,28] Blood return is often absent, but there is no discoloration or swelling.[8,12,13,28]

DEGREES OF TOXICITY

The National Cancer Institute (NCI) Common Terminology Criteria for Adverse Events (CTCAE) describes infusion site extravasation as well as several other conditions that are results of extravasation injury. The CTCAE describes a grading or severity scale for adverse events (AEs). Each AE is graded on a scale of 1–5, with 1 indicating mild symptoms and 5 indicating death resulting from the AE. In addition to infusion site extravasation, AEs that can occur with extravasation include venous injury, soft-tissue necrosis, and skin ulcerations (Table 25-6).[32] In addition, many institutions develop their own scales based on such items as severity of extravasation, degree of tissue damage, or level of care required for treatment of extravasation.

SYMPTOM MANAGEMENT STRATEGIES

THERAPEUTIC APPROACHES

The best approach to extravasation injury is prevention. Guidelines for the prevention of chemotherapy extravasation are available from professional organizations such as

TABLE 25-6

National Cancer Institute Common Terminology Criteria for Adverse Events (CTCAE)

Adverse Event	Grade				
	1	2	3	4	5
Infusion site extravasation		Erythema with associated symptoms (e.g., edema, pain, induration, phlebitis)	Ulceration or necrosis; severe tissue damage; operative intervention indicated	Life-threatening consequences; urgent intervention indicated	Death
Venous injury	Asymptomatic diagnostic finding; intervention not indicated	Symptomatic (e.g., claudication); repair or revision not indicated	Severe symptoms; limiting self-care activities of daily living (ADL); repair or revision indicated; disabling	Life-threatening consequences; evidence of end organ damage; urgent operative intervention indicated	Death
Soft tissue necrosis		Local wound care; medical intervention indicated (e.g., dressings or topical medications)	Operative debridement or other invasive intervention indicated (e.g., tissue reconstruction, flap or grafting)	Life-threatening consequences; urgent intervention indicated	Death
Skin ulceration	Combined area of ulcers <1 cm; nonblanchable erythema of intact skin with associated warmth or edema	Combined area of ulcers 1–2 cm; partial thickness skin loss involving skin or subcutaneous fat	Combined area of ulcers >2 cm; full-thickness skin loss involving damage to or necrosis of subcutaneous tissue that may extend down to fascia	Any size ulcer with extensive destruction; tissue necrosis, or damage to muscle, bone, or supporting structures with or without full thickness skin loss	Death

Source: Data from National Cancer Institute Common Terminology Criteria for Adverse Events (CTCAE)[32].

the ONS, the INS, and the European Oncology Nursing Society (EONS).[14,25,28] Included in these guidelines are recommendations regarding the choice of site for peripheral IV therapy, especially when administering vesicants; according to these protocols, the IV should be recently started (within 24 hours) and should be selected in order of preference from the forearm (basilic, cephalic, and median antebrachial), avoiding the dorsum of the hand, wrist, and antecubital.[8,12,14,33] The guidelines also recommend avoiding sites with sclerosis, thrombosis, or scar formation; limbs with impaired circulation; and sites below a previous venipuncture attempt.[8,12,14,33] Selecting an appropriately sized catheter for the vein is also important.[6] The IV should be stabilized by securing it to the skin using a clear dressing; this type of dressing covers the skin entry site while allowing visualization of the insertion site.

Patency of the IV line and brisk blood return should be verified just prior to drug infusion by flushing with 5 to 10 mL of normal saline or a 5% dextrose solution.[15] It is recommended that chemotherapy drugs be properly diluted and infused through the sidearm of a free-flowing IV with either normal saline or 5% dextrose.[14]

When administering vesicants using the direct push method, blood return should be checked every 2 to 5 mL by gently aspirating with the syringe. Vesicants may also be administered as a continuous infusion but only through a CVAD. Blood return should be checked by aspirating with a syringe at the port closest to the patient according to institutional policy and procedure.[14,33] The patient should be instructed to notify a clinician immediately if he or she experiences any pain, burning, leaking, or other changes in sensation at the infusion site.

Central venous access devices

To safeguard against vesicant extravasation with CVADs, proper placement should be verified radiologically following initial placement of the catheter and prior to drug administration. If there are any complaints of chest pain or dyspnea, inability to aspirate blood, or inability to infuse a solution, then positioning of the catheter should be reconfirmed before continuing with the infusion.[15]

Initial management

It is widely accepted that early identification and intervention upon the first signs and symptoms of extravasation are crucial in preventing potentially serious adverse outcomes. However, with the exception of dexrazoxane, which is approved to treat anthracycline extravasation, management recommendations are based primarily on anecdotal experience; definitive treatment has not been established.[19,25,31] Standard guidelines recommend the following steps at the first sign of drug infiltration or extravasation (Figure 25-1):[14,25,28,30,33]

1. Stop the infusion immediately. Do not flush the line, and avoid applying pressure to the extravasation site.
2. Disconnect the IV tubing from the IV device, but do not remove the IV device or noncoring port needle.
3. Attempt to aspirate residual fluid from the IV device using a small (1–3 mL) syringe.
4. Remove the peripheral IV device or port needle.
5. Assess the site of the suspected extravasation and note any symptoms experienced by the patient.
   a. Assessment and documentation should include drug extravasated, dose, volume, position and size of any apparent wound, presence of swelling, and extent and spread of erythema and pain.
   b. If possible, digital photographs should be obtained to help further document the injury and assess changes over time.
6. Notify the physician or advanced practice nurse.
7. Initiate appropriate management measures in accordance with professional practice guidelines and institutional policies.

Having an extravasation kit available may help expedite intervention for extravasations (Figure 25-2). An extravasation kit may include cold packs, warm packs, 3-mL syringes, 25-gauge needles, institution/practice setting extravasation policy, management algorithm or standing orders, documentation form, indelible pen for marking the area, and a digital camera to photograph the extravasation. Some institutions include antidotes that should be supplied, along with syringes and needles, diluents, and reconstitution instructions. If the antidotes are not included because of the drugs' cost or short shelf-life, the kit should provide information about how to quickly obtain antidotes.[14,15,25,31]

Cold application. Application of an ice pack to cool the site of extravasation is recommended for extravasation of anthracyclines (doxorubicin, daunorubicin, epirubicin, and idarubicin), alkylating agents (mechlorethamine), antitumor antibiotics (dactinomycin and mitomycin-C), and taxanes (docetaxel and paclitaxel).[14] Cooling causes vasoconstriction, which helps decrease the spread of the drug to other tissue while also reducing local inflammation and pain.

Heat application. Application of heat is indicated for extravasation of the plant alkaloids, such as vincristine, vinblastine, vindestine, and vinorelbine, to increase blood flow to the area. This step helps disperse the extravasated vesicant and promotes its absorption.[28] Heat should be applied to the affected area for 15 to 20 minutes 4 times per day for the first 24 to 48 hours.[14]

Limb elevation. Limb elevation has not been shown to decrease pain or resolve the extravasation. However, elevating the affected area may help with reabsorption of the extravasated drug and is recommended for the first 24 to 28 hours whenever possible.[25]

ANTIDOTES AND TREATMENTS

An antidote is an agent that is either applied or injected to the extravasated area to counteract the effects of the infiltrated agent. Antidotes can help prevent progression of the extravasation to ulceration, blistering, and necrosis. Most of the recommendations regarding extravasation management come from anecdotal reports, animal studies, or a small number of uncontrolled studies in humans. This type of evidence is the best available because chemotherapy extravasation rates are relatively low, and considerable ethical issues are involved with conducting controlled research on extravasation.[9,31] Although the evidence supporting the use of different antidotes is often inconclusive, several agents have been recommended to prevent tissue necrosis and ulceration following extravasation.

Sodium thiosulfate

While the exact mechanism of sodium thiosulfate is not known, it is thought to prevent alkylation and reduce subcutaneous tissue destruction.[34] Subcutaneous injection of sodium thiosulfate using a 25-gauge needle around the affected area is recommended for extravasation of mechlorethamine.[14,33] Sodium thiosulfate is supplied as a 10% or 25% solution and should be diluted to a 1/6 molar solution, by mixing 4 mL of the 10% solution with 6 mL of sterile water or 1.6 mL of the 25% solution with 8.4 mL of sterile water.[33,35] Using 2 mL for each milligram extravasated, multiple local subcutaneous injections of sodium thiosulfate should be administered as soon as possible after the extravasation, changing the needle for each injection, followed by ice application for 6 to 12 hours.[14,15]

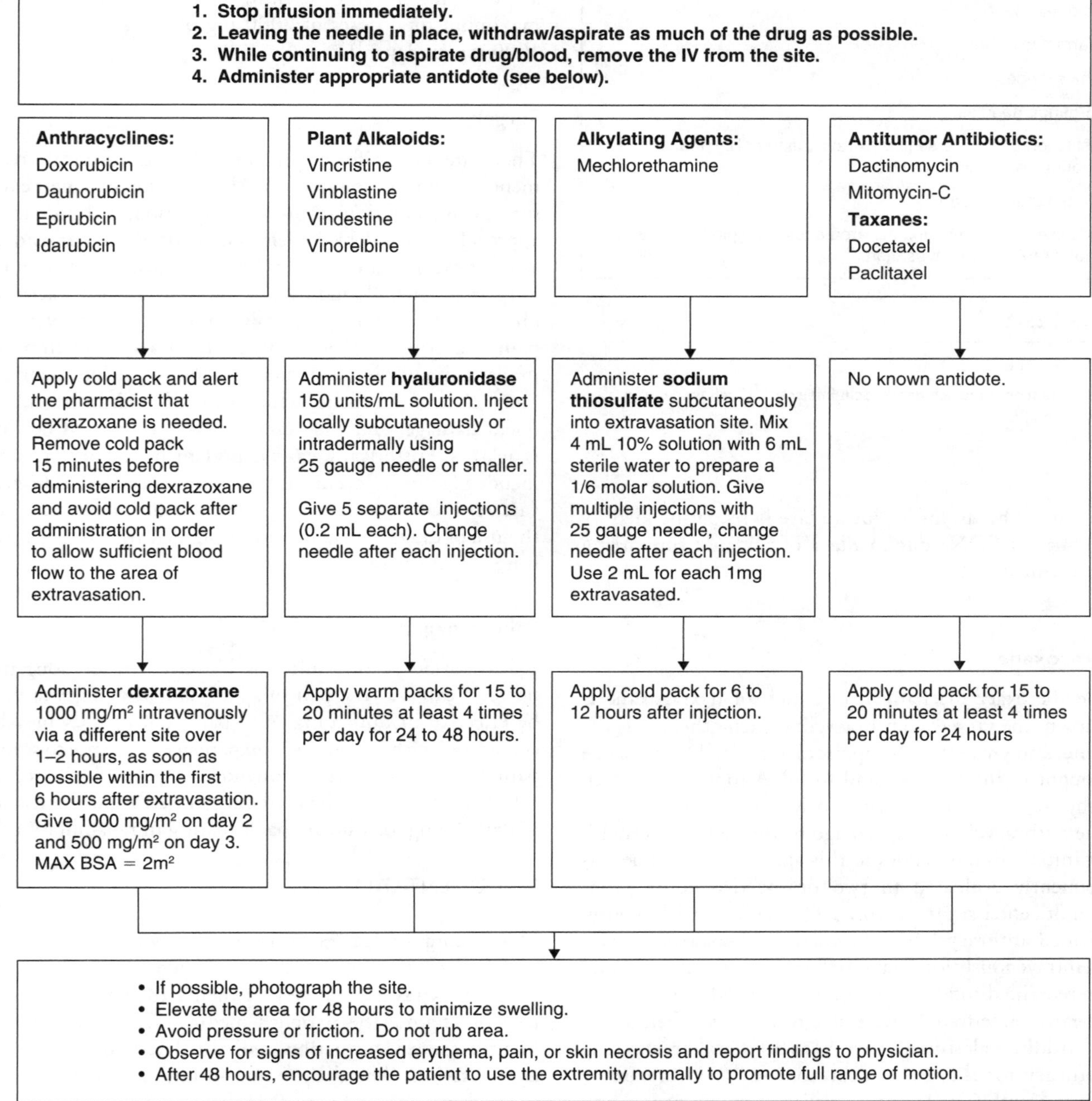

FIGURE 25-1

Extravasation management algorithm.

Source: Data from Polovich et al[14]; Doellman et al[25]; Wengstrom and Margulies[28]; Dougherty[30]; Wilkes[33].

Hyaluronidase

Hyaluronidase is an enzyme that breaks down hyaluronic acid in connective and soft tissue. This destruction of hyaluronic acid allows for the dispersion of the offending agent, thereby reducing local concentration of the damaging agent and increasing its rate of absorption.[25,36] Local subcutaneous injection of hyaluronidase has been recommended for extravasation of vinca alkaloids and can be used in combination with heat application. It is recommended to administer pain medication prior to this

- Cold packs
- Warm packs
- 3 ml syringes
- 25-gauge needles
- Institutional/practice setting extravasation policy, management algorithm or standing orders
- Documentation form
- Indelible pen for marking the area and/or a digital camera to photograph the extravasation.

FIGURE 25-2

Extravasation kit.

Source: Data from Polovich et al[14]; Schulmeister[15]; Doellman et al[25]; Wickham et al[31].

procedure. The use of hyaluronidase is recommended by ONS but not EONS due to a lack of evidence supporting this treatment.[14,28]

Dexrazoxane

While the exact mechanism of action of dexrazoxane is unknown, the target of anthracycline chemotherapy is the enzyme known as DNA topoisomerase II. Dexrazoxane is thought to inhibit and bind to DNA topoisomerase II, thereby disabling the enzyme so it is no longer affected by the anthracycline and damage to the cells is averted.[37] After initial animal studies of this agent, dexrazoxane was subsequently evaluated in two prospective nonrandomized multicenter studies involving 54 patients with biopsy-confirmed anthracycline extravasations. Dexrazoxane was given intravenously for 3 days. In 53 of the patients, skin and tissue remained intact; one required surgical intervention; and nearly three-fourths were able to continue chemotherapy.[38] Additional studies have been undertaken showing the efficacy for the use of dexrazoxane.[39,40] Dexrazoxane is effective with CVAD anthracycline extravasation as well as peripheral extravasation of these agents.[21] This antidote must be reconstituted with the supplied diluent to provide a concentration of 10 mg/mL. The patient's dose, based on body surface area, is injected into a 1000-mL infusion bag of 0.9% sodium chloride.[37] Topical cooling, such as ice packs, should be removed for at least 15 minutes prior to and during administration.[37]

Dexrazoxane is administered intravenously as three 1- to 2-hour infusions through a different venous access location.[38] The first dose should be given within 6 hours of the actual extravasation, and subsequent doses administered 24 and 48 hours after extravasation. The first and second doses are 1000 mg/m^2 and the third dose is 500 mg/m^2, up to maximum total doses of 2000 mg on days 1 and 2, and 1000 mg on day 3.[14,38]

Surgery

There are no uniform guidelines for the surgical treatment of extravasation injuries. Although some suggest early surgical intervention to prevent ulceration, a conservative approach such as debridement is more often recommended, as most extravasations heal without surgical intervention.[10] Surgery is generally indicated if there are areas of excessive blistering, ulceration, progressive induration, and persistent pain and erythema, or with major extravasation from an implanted port. Surgical interventions can include debridement of necrotic tissue, which can help minimize subsequent damage, and wide excision or skin grafts if healing is delayed. Historically, early debridement had been recommended for anthracycline extravasations as delayed surgical care resulted in poor functional outcomes; however, with the use of dexrazoxane in anthracycline extravasation, this is no longer the case.

Pain management

Extravasation accompanied by blistering, ulceration, and necrosis can be very painful. Non-opioid analgesics may be effective in mitigating mild pain, but opioids may be considered with patients who experience moderate to severe pain. Use of opioids is recommended for patients who report difficulty in moving the extremity or performing activities of daily living, or who are participating in rehabilitation.[31]

DOCUMENTATION

Documentation of extravasation is key in assessment and follow-up (Figure 25-3). When documenting a vesicant extravasation, key elements to include are the patient's name, the patient's medical record number or identification information, and the date and time of the extravasation. The drug name, dilution, and estimated volume extravasated as well as the method of administration and blood return should be included. The type and placement of vascular access, patient-reported symptoms including time in relation to drug administration, and a description of the affected area, including the size, swelling, erythema, blisters, and a photograph if possible, are other items that are important to include. Any immediate interventions that were employed should be documented, including the physician or advanced practice nurse who was notified and the instructions given. The follow-up plan should include patient teaching and reevaluation and any referrals such as to plastic surgery or physical therapy.[8,13,14,33]

- Patient name, medical record number, date and time of extravasation
- Drug name, dilution, and estimated volume extravasated
- Method of administration and blood return
- Type and placement of vascular access
- Pretreatment assessment of site and blood return
- Patient reported symptoms including time in relation to drug administration and description of affected area including size, swelling, erythema, blisters
- Include a photograph if possible
- Any immediate interventions (based on institutional policies, ONS, INS standards) that were employed including the physician or advanced practice nurse that was notified and instructions given
- The follow-up plan including patient teaching and re-evaluation and any referrals such as plastic surgery or physical therapy

FIGURE 25-3

Documentation of extravasation.

Source: Data from Sauerland et al[13]; Polovich et al[14]; Schulmeister[15]; Wilkes[33].

PATIENT FOLLOW-UP

When vesicant extravasations are untreated or undertreated, patients may develop complications requiring surgery or skin grafting. After the immediate management steps are followed, patients should continue to be monitored carefully. Arrangements should be made for the patient to return for periodic assessment of the extravasation site, including photographs based on institutional policies and the patient's needs.[14] Patients should be informed that the extravasation has occurred, the possible reasons for it should be explained, and the management of the complication should be identified.[30] Home instructions should include resources for care of the extravasation site, including instructions to observe the site closely, keep the area clean and dry, avoid sun exposure, and promptly report any changes.[14,30] Analgesics should be prescribed and administered as required. If blistering or tissue breakdown occurs, consider sterile dressings to prevent superimposed infection from occurring. If needed, assist with initiating a referral to plastic surgery, physical therapy, or pain service providers.[14]

While the prevention and initial management strategies are similar to those outlined earlier, treatment for children—like that for adults—is based on the anecdotal literature. The value of hot or cold compresses is debatable, and there is little evidence of efficacy and some risk of skin breakdown with heat.[22]

NURSING IMPLICATIONS

The primary responsibility for the prevention, early recognition, management, and patient education related to extravasation rests with nurses who are directly administering chemotherapy. Knowledge of risks and careful observation of patients throughout their course of treatment is critical to the prevention and effective treatment of this complication. Nurses need to be knowledgeable about the most current evidence-based treatment options as well as their institutional/practice setting protocols. They should be prepared to act promptly to prevent serious complications.[22] Careful adherence to proper procedures and timely identification of signs and symptoms are critical to avoid potentially life-altering complications. Because of the lack of evidence-based guidelines for extravasation, future nursing research should focus on first establishing benchmarks for quantifying chemotherapy extravasation.

PATIENT SELF-CARE

With increasing initiatives to improve quality of care, it is important to consider the role that patients play in their own care and outcomes. With effective self-care tools, patients are better able to actively participate in the management of their condition.[41] Self-care includes education and interventions to assist patients in managing their health. The evidence suggests that self-care not only increases patient self-efficacy, but also reduces patient costs related to both inpatient and outpatient contact.[42] Successful interventions include communicating the patient's and caregiver's roles, providing ongoing support, and ensuring appropriate follow-up. With extravasation, it is important to educate the patient about the type of chemotherapy that is being administered, the potential risks associated with extravasation, signs and symptoms to report to the nurse, and follow-up care that may be needed (see Appendix 25A).

REFERENCES

1. Dychter S, Gold DA, Carson D, Haller M. Intravenous therapy. *J Infus Nurs.* 2012;35(2)84–91.
2. Polovich M, White JM, Kelleher LO, eds. *Chemotherapy and Biotherapy Guidelines and Recommendations for Practice.* Pittsburgh, PA: Oncology Nursing Society; 2005.
3. Schrijers DL. Extravasation: a dreaded complication of chemotherapy. *Ann Oncol.* 2004;14(suppl 3):26–30.
4. Thakur JS, Chauhan GS, Diwana VK, et al. Extravasational side effects of cytotoxic drugs: a preventable catastrophe. *Indian J Plast Surg.* 2008;41(2):145–150.
5. Chanes DC, da Luz Goncalves Pedreira M, de Gutierrez MGR. Antineoplastic agents extravasation from peripheral intravenous line in children: a simple strategy for a safer nursing care. *Eur J Oncol Nurs.* 2012;16(1):17–25.

6. Hadaway L. Infiltrations and extravasation. *Am J Nurs.* 2008;107(8):64–72.
7. Bruehl S. An update on the pathophysiology of complex regional pain syndrome. *Anesthesiology.* 2010;113(3):713–725.
8. Schulmeister L. Extravasation management: clinical update. *Semin Oncol Nurs.* 2011;27(1):82–90.
9. Barlock AL, Howser DM, Hubbard SM. Nursing management of adriamycin extravasation. *Am J Nurs.* 1979;79(8):94–96.
10. Langstein HN, Duman H, Seeling D, et al. Retrospective study of the management of chemotherapeutic extravasation injury. *Ann Plast Surg.* 2002;49(4):369–374.
11. ICD-9-CM Index to diseases addenda (FY10). http://www.cdc.gov/nchs/data/icd9/icdidx10add(2).pdf. Accessed July 6, 2012.
12. Goolsby TV, Lombardo FA. Extravasation of chemotherapeutic agents: prevention and treatment. *Semin Oncol.* 2006;33(1):139–143.
13. Sauerland C, Engelking C, Wickham R, et al. Vesicant extravasation. Part I: mechanisms, pathogenesis, and nursing care to reduce risk. *Oncol Nurs Forum.* 2006;33(6):1134–1141.
14. Polovich M, Whitford W, Olsen M, eds. *Chemotherapy and Biotherapy Guidelines and Recommendations for Practice.* Pittsburgh, PA: Oncology Nursing Society; 2009.
15. Schulmeister L. Vesicant chemotherapy: the management of extravasation. *Cancer Nurs Pract.* 2009;8(3):34–37.
16. Vincristine [Package insert]. Hospira; Lake Forest, IL; December 2007. http://www.hospira.com/_docs/VinCRIStine-482805-PROMOWEB.pdf. Accessed September 8, 2012.
17. Hernandex-Vargas H, Palacios J, Moreno-Bueno G. Telling cells how to die: docetaxel therapy in cancer cell lines. *Cell Cycle.* 2007;6(7):780–783.
18. Oronsky BT, Reed T, Knox SJ, Scicinski JJ. The scarlet letter of alkylation: a mini review of selective alkylating agents. *Transl Oncol.* 2012;5(4):226–229.
19. Ener RA, Meglathery SB, Styler M. Extravasation of systemic hemato-oncological therapies. *Ann Oncol.* 2004;15(6):858–862.
20. Dorr RT. Antidotes to vesicant chemotherapy extravasations. *Blood Rev.* 1990;4:401–404.
21. Langer SW, Sehisted M, Jensen PB. Treatment of anthracycline extravasation with dexrazoxane. *Clin Cancer Res.* 2000;6(9):3680–3686.
22. Mitomycin [Package insert]. Bedford Laboratories; Bedford, Ohio; June 2000. http://www.fda.gov/ohrms/DOCKETS/ac/08/briefing/2008-4367b1-10_MEL%20Proposed%20Package%20Insert.pdf. Accessed September 8, 2012.
23. Novantrone [Package insert]. EMD Serono, Inc.; Rockland, MA; August 2008. http://www.accessdata.fda.gov/drugsatfda_docs/label/2009/019297s030s031lbl.pdf. Accessed October 1, 2012.
24. Bleomycin [Package insert]. Teva Parenteral Medicine, Inc.; Irvine, CA; July 2007. http://www.bdipharma.com/Package%20Insert/Teva/Bleomycin_7-2007.pdf. Accessed October 1, 2012.
25. Dollman D, Hadaway L, Bowe-Geddes LA, et al. Infiltration and extravasation: update on prevention and management. *J Infus Nurs.* 2009;32(4):203–211.
26. American Society of Clinical Oncology. American Society of Clinical Oncology statement regarding the use of outside services to prepare or administer chemotherapy drugs. *J Clin Oncol.* 2003;21(9):1882–1883.
27. Jacobsen JO, Polovich M, Gilmore TR, et al. Revisions to the 2009 American Society of Clinical Oncology/Oncology Nursing Society chemotherapy administration safety standards: expanding the scope to include inpatient settings. *J Oncol Pract.* 2011;8(1):2–6.
28. Wengstrom Y, Margulies A, European Oncology Nursing Society Task Force. European Oncology Nursing Society extravasation guidelines. *Eur J Oncol Nurs.* 2008;12(4):357–361.
29. Dougherty L. IV therapy: recognizing the differences between infiltration and extravasation. *Br J Nurs.* 2008;17(14):898–901.
30. Dougherty L. Extravasation: prevention, recognition, and management. *Nurs Stand.* 2010;24(52): 48–55.
31. Wickham R, Engelking C, Sauerland C, et al. Vesicant extravasation. Part II: evidence-based management and continuing controversies. *Oncol Nurs Forum.* 2006;33(6):1143–1149.
32. U.S. Department of Health and Human Services, National Institutes of Health, National Cancer Institute. Common terminology criteria for adverse events v.4.03; 2010. http://evs.nci.nih.gov/ftp1/CTCAE/CTCAE_4.03_2010-06-14_QuickReference_5x7.pdf. Accessed October 29, 2012.
33. Wilkes GM. Chemotherapy: principles of administration. In: Yarbro CH, Wujcik D, Gobel BH, eds. *Oncology Nursing Principles and Practice.* 7th ed. Burlington, MA: Jones & Bartlett Learning; 2011:390–457.
34. Dorr RT, Soble M, Alberts DS. Efficacy of sodium thiosulfate as a local antidote to mechorethamine skin toxicity in the mouse. *Cancer Chemother Pharmacol.* 1988;22(4):299–302.
35. Mustargen [Package insert]. Baxter Oncology for Lundbeck, Inc.; Deerfield, IL; November 2010. https://dailymed.nlm.nih.gov/dailymed/drugInfo.cfm?id=41157. Accessed October 8, 2012.
36. Kassmer E. Evaluation and treatment of chemotherapy extravasation injuries. *J Pediatr Oncol Nurs.* 2000;17(3):135–148.
37. Totect [Package insert]. TopoTarget A/S; Copenhagen, Denmark; December 2007.http://dailymed.nlm.nih.gov/dailymed/archives/fdaDrugInfo.cfm?archiveid=6565. Accessed October 8, 2012.
38. Mouridsen HT, Langer SW, Buter J, et al. Treatment of anthracycline extravasation with Savene (dexrazoxane): results from two prospective clinical multicentre studies. *Ann Oncol.* 2007;18(3):546–550.
39. Fontaine C, Noens L, Pierre P, et al. Savene® (dexrazoxane) use in clinical practice. *Support Care Cancer.* 2012;20(5):1109–1112.
40. Kane RC, McGuinn WD Jr, Dagher R, et al. Dexrazoxane (Totect): FDA review and approval for the treatment of accidental extravasation following intravenous anthracycline chemotherapy. *Oncologist.* 2008;13(4):445–450.
41. Institutes of Medicine. *Priority Areas for National Action: Transforming Health Care Quality.* Washington, DC: National Academies Press; 2003:52.
42. Kennedy AP, Nelson E, Reeves D, et al. A randomized controlled trial to assess the effectiveness and cost of a patient oriented self management approach to chronic inflammatory bowel disease. *Gut.* 2004;53(11):1639–1645.

Extravasation

Patient Name: ______________________________

This guide will help you learn about ways to prevent and manage chemotherapy that leaks into the tissues. It has helpful hints about what to report to your nurse and about follow-up care.

Symptom and Description

Chemotherapy drugs are given into a vein (intravenous or IV). Some of these drugs can cause problems if they leak from the vein or IV into the tissues. Some chemotherapy drugs are called *vesicants*. A vesicant drug may cause tissue damage if it leaks from the vein into tissues-this is called *extravasation*. This leak can happen due to many reasons:

- Past IV treatments
- Thin and fragile veins
- History of peripheral vascular disease
- The needle or catheter that is in your arm or chest can slip out of the vein
- A small number of veins where the IV can be placed due to skin changes from radiation treatments, or a condition called lymphedema (swelling of the arm)

The damage caused by extravasation can be mild or severe, based on the drug that has leaked into the tissue. It can cause a painful ulcer or sore. If the damage is not treated, the sore may not heal and it may get worse.

Prevention

You must tell your doctor or nurse if you see or feel any damage to the skin where the IV needle was placed to give your chemotherapy. Signs and symptoms can occur at the time you are getting your chemotherapy or days later. You should tell your nurse right away if you have any of these signs at or near the IV site:

- Redness
- Swelling
- Changes to your skin
- Pain, burning, or stinging
- Any other abnormal feelings

If this problem is found early, there is a lower risk of problems or damage caused by the drug leaking into the tissue.

Management

Treatment depends on which drug leaked out of your veins and into your tissues. Your nurse knows which drugs cause damage and how to treat the damage when it happens. Drugs, warm packs, cold packs, or putting your arm up on pillows may be used to treat the extravasation.

(continued)

Your nurse or doctor will explain the treatment to you—please do what the nurse or doctor tells you to do. Talk to your doctor or others on your healthcare team if you have questions.

Follow-up

Someone from the care team will call in 1 to 2 days to ask you how you are doing. If the area becomes worse, you will be asked to return to the clinic to see if you need more treatment.

Phone Numbers

Physician: ____

Nurse: ____

Office or inpatient unit number: _________________________

Source: O'Leary C, Catania K. Extravasation. In: Yarbro CH, Wujcik D, Gobel BH, eds. *Cancer Symptom Management*. 4th ed. Burlington, MA: Jones & Bartlett Learning; 2014.

CHAPTER 26

Lymphedema

Sheila H. Ridner, PhD, RN, FAAN

THE PROBLEM

Lymphedema has traditionally been viewed as a progressive, chronic condition that occurs when protein-rich fluid accumulates in the interstitial spaces because the lymphatic system either cannot accept or transport lymph fluid into the circulatory system.[1] Two types of lymphedema are distinguished: primary (idiopathic) lymphedema, which is related to genetic and familial abnormalities in the lymphatic structure or function, and secondary (acquired) lymphedema, which is caused by trauma, such as infection, surgery, radiation, or crush injuries. Classifications of primary lymphedema are based on the age when swelling first appears:

- Congenital lymphedema: present at birth
- Lymphedema praecox: after birth but before age 35
- Lymphedema tarda: after age 35

Secondary lymphedema does not have a similar classification system, but it can appear immediately or many years after the traumatic event. Secondary lymphedema is a well-known problem for patients who have cancer or who have undergone cancer treatment; however, this population may independently experience primary or secondary lymphedema, and some persons may experience both at the same time.

Therapeutic management of lymphedema has focused primarily on reduction of swelling. However, recent research suggests that swelling is only one of many symptoms experienced by individuals with this condition that may require nursing interventions; research also indicates that the failure of healthcare professionals to address the complex nature of the lymphedema experience is very frustrating to patients.[2] Depending on the location of a tumor and type of resultant treatment modalities, secondary lymphedema in patients who have experienced cancer may occur in the head and neck, trunk (shoulder, breast, back, chest, abdomen, genitals, groin), or limbs (upper and lower). This chapter addresses secondary lymphedema that occurs in any area of the human body.

INCIDENCE

Primary lymphedema affects approximately 1 in 10,000 people younger than the age of 20.[3] Although its prevalence in persons who are aged 20 and older is unknown, cancer patients who undergo cancer treatment and are at risk for secondary lymphedema may also have or develop primary lymphedema.

Secondary lymphedema, though most commonly associated with breast cancer treatment, remains a risk for many cancer patients despite refinements in surgical procedures and more tightly controlled radiation field exposure. Incidence of secondary lymphedema varies across cancer populations. Rates of lymphedema related to treatment of head and neck cancer may be as high as 75%, with these patients experiencing both internal and external swelling.[4] Incidence of truncal lymphedema in breast cancer survivors is not well documented, but a growing number of these survivors are reporting swelling in their breast, axilla, and back. A recent study found that 48.2% of 287 breast cancer survivors followed for six years after treatment had experienced arm swelling at least once, and 34% had clinical evidence of lymphedema.[5] Rates of lymphedema after gynecological cancer treatment range between 6% and 37%.[6]

ETIOLOGY

Lymphedema is a potential problem for anyone who has experienced a malignancy, surgery, or radiation-based treatment for cancer that has disrupted the lymphatic system.

PATHOPHYSIOLOGY

The lymphatic system is an essential part of both the circulatory and immune systems.[7] The role of growth factors in the embryonic development of the lymphatics is becoming more understood, as is the role that genetics plays in the development of primary lymphedema.[7,8] The lymphatic system has many functions, including maintenance of interstitial fluid homeostasis, fat absorption and transport from the intestines, and lymphedema prevention. A normally functioning lymphatic system works in tandem with the cardiovascular system to support fluid exchange at the blood capillary–interstitial–lymphatic interface. The lymphatic system is responsible for removing fluid that is not reabsorbed by the venous capillaries, cellular debris, large molecules, macrophages, lymphocytes, and erythrocytes out of the interstitial space.[7,8] The fluid and debris enter the lymphatic system through lymphatic vessels that begin as tubes that interface with the interstitium. Fluid and proteins move through the lymphatic collector vessels and nodes by three mechanisms: (1) contraction of segments between each valve; (2) compression of the vessel through external forces such as contraction of surrounding muscle tissue, extremity movement, respiratory effort, and arterial pulsation; and (3) auto-contraction of the lymphatic vessel endothelial cells. The small vessels in the interstitium empty into deeper vessels, which in turn empty into larger lymphatic trunks that drain into the left thoracic or right lymphatic ducts located in the head and neck region of the body.

Compromise of any of these mechanisms can impede lymph flow. In the case of patients who have received treatment for cancer, several factors a can impact these mechanisms. For example, a tumor can block lymph flow. Surgery causes actual physical/anatomic disruption of the lymphatic system and surrounding soft tissues. Radiation causes tissue damage that unleashes an acute inflammatory response. Damaged tissue may be replaced by normal cells, leading to good outcomes. This repair process can become pathogenic, however, when overproduction of extracellular matrix leaves a permanent fibrotic scar. The resulting loss of function can reduce the efficacy of muscle movement that assists lymph transport and causes lymph nodes to become fibrotic, also impeding movement. Radiation-induced scarring and fibrosis may directly impair lymphatic function as (1) lymph channels may become contracted or nonfunctional, (2) damaged muscles may not contract and extend with sufficient force to move fluid through vessels, and (3) fibrosed lymph nodes may obstruct lymph flow.

It remains unclear why some individuals who sustain damage to their lymphatic systems as a result of cancer or cancer treatment develop lymphedema, whereas others do not. Nevertheless, once lymphedema develops, hydrostatic forces interact with the excess fluid, an inflammatory response is triggered, venous reuptake may be compromised, and multiple pathological changes take place.[7,9,10] Cellular architecture is altered; proteins accumulate; the number of cells, fibroblasts, histocytes, and neutrophils increases; collagen predominates; and fibrosis again occurs. Thus untreated lymphedema actually triggers processes very similar to those that initially caused the condition, offering some explanation for the progressive nature of this problem. These underlying pathobiological processes—many of which have been identified only in the last decade—clarify why early treatment of lymphedema is so critical. Treatment that minimizes the progression of these pathological processes should improve patient outcomes. Although current treatment modalities focus primarily on movement of the stagnant fluid from the interstitium, as more becomes known about the underlying biological mechanisms concerning lymphedema, doorways will be opened to pursue biology-based therapies in the future.

SYMPTOM ASSESSMENT

RISK FACTORS

Possible risk factors for secondary lymphedema have been postulated. In general, increased risk is associated with the extent of surgery or nodal dissection. The greater the surgical field and the larger the number of nodes dissected, the higher the risk of developing lymphedema. This is true not only for surgery done in the axillary regions, but also with procedures in the groin and any other area of the body. Similarly, the larger size of the radiation field and the larger the radiation dose, the higher the risk. Obesity is also a known risk factor for lymphedema; this includes both having a body mass index (BMI) greater than 30 at time of initial treatment[11] and experiencing weight gain after treatment.[12] Development of seromas after breast cancer surgery is now also believed to be a risk factor for lymphedema,[13,14] as is infection and early swelling.[14]

SELF-ASSESSMENT

Individuals tend to be very aware of subtle changes in their bodies, so it is not surprising that self-report continues to be the most common method of identifying secondary lymphedema following cancer treatment. Breast cancer survivors may experience tingling, heaviness, or tightness of jewelry in their arms before noticeable swelling becomes evident. These self-reported symptoms should not be ignored in breast cancer survivors or any other cancer survivor.

Patients who report these problems should be referred to a lymphedema therapist for evaluation. Patients with lymphedema may experience odd sensations in the swollen areas, poor range of motion, weakness, fatigue, psychological distress, and functional impairments.[2,15,16] A recent qualitative study that addressed the thoughts and feelings that breast cancer survivors with lymphedema experienced related to their condition and its treatment identified both physical and psychological issues.[2] There was perceived lack of support from poorly informed healthcare providers and from a healthcare system that did not recognize the chronic nature of the disease or the need for insurance coverage for lymphedema treatment and supplies. Multiple losses were identified, including loss of a positive body image, function, time, and normalcy. Self-care was often discontinued because there was no perceived benefit from such actions and patients desired to return to a more normal life—that is, one without bandaging and compression garments.

Symptom-related difficulties are not confined to the breast cancer survivor population. Survivors of head and neck cancer who develop lymphedema also have similar odd sensations in the swollen area, tightness, and fatigue.[17] Additionally, these patients experience problems sleeping, swallowing difficulties, changes in their voice, and firmness in skin. Nurses need to directly ask patients about a variety of symptoms to solicit this information, as patients may not associate these symptoms with their swelling.

Few tools have been developed specifically to evaluate symptoms related to lymphedema. The Lymphedema Breast Cancer Questionnaire (LBCQ) is frequently used in research studies.[18] The Gynecologic Cancer Lymphedema Questionnaire is a modified version of the LBCQ for the lower limbs.[19] Symptom checklists for lymphedema occurring in the head and neck, arms, and trunk that include evaluation of the intensity and distress of each reported symptom are under development, and preliminary findings have been published using these instruments.[17,20,21] Nurses interested in using any of these tools should contact the first authors of these referenced publications to obtain permission to use these checklists as well as copies of the instruments.

OBJECTIVE ASSESSMENT

A complete medical history, coupled with a thorough physical examination, often generates enough information to correctly diagnose lymphedema.[22]

History

When eliciting a history from individuals with swelling, it is important to reassure them that you are asking questions to help determine the best course of care for them, not to form a judgment about the causation of the swelling. As many patients blame themselves for doing something that caused the swelling, emphasis should be placed on our lack of understanding as to why some people get lymphedema and others do not, and the message reinforced that it is not their fault they have swelling. As you assess the patient, remember you are trying to rule out differential diagnoses such as myxedema, lipedema, deep vein thrombosis, cancer recurrence, chronic venous insufficiency, cellulitis, or other infections.[22] When taking a history, do the following:

- Determine the trajectory and presentation of the current illness: new onset versus exacerbation of previous swelling; location of swelling; episodes of worsening or remission of symptoms; swollen area hot to touch.
- Review prior and current medical diagnoses.
- Determine whether the patient had seromas or infections immediately after cancer surgery.
- Review current medications.
- Evaluate possible causes, such as recent surgery, tumor, previous auto accident, heavy lifting, insect or dog bite, burns (including sunburn), cuts, puncture wounds, or no known event.
- Determine whether there is a family history of known primary lymphedema, "big legs" or "one leg bigger than the other," and limb or other body swelling.
- Inquire about other symptoms, including pain, heaviness, or other sensations in the swollen area; impaired mobility in joints or limbs; and tighter-fitting clothing or jewelry.
- Inquire about travel to foreign countries.
- Inquire about recent air travel.

For patients with head and neck cancers, ask about the following symptoms:

- New onset of difficulty swallowing
- Respiratory distress
- Change in hearing

Physical assessment

A thorough, high-touch, hands-on physical examination is critical to identifying lymphedema. Evaluate the following:

- Location and spread of swelling, paying close attention to asymmetry of the back, chest, limbs, face, and other areas
- Skin—redness, heat, cold, cracking, oozing fluid (with or without foul odor), turgor, necrosis, masses, thickness, scaling
- Nail beds
- Pulses in all extremities
- Range of motion
- Stemmer's sign test—difficulty lifting the skin from the dorsum of the fingers or toes
- Signs of infection
- Pain
- Determination of the grade of lymphedema
- Volume of the swollen area, if possible

Diagnostic evaluation

There is no "gold standard" for objective volumetric measurement of swelling associated with lymphedema. Measurement methods for lymphedema in the trunk or head and neck areas are currently very limited. Attempts to use tape measures to measure swelling in the anatomically difficult areas of the body have been undertaken, but measurement errors are common. Serial photographs offer a method to document visible change over time in these areas and should be considered. Despite these drawbacks, a number of existing methods are used to measure affected limbs: (1) water displacement, (2) limb girth via tape measurements in centimeters, (3) infrared laser perometry, and (4) bioelectrical impedance (BIA).

Water displacement. Water displacement is typically used to determine volume differences between limbs; it does not provide data about the location of the edema or the contours of the limb.[23] This method requires removal of any clothing covering the limb, followed by placement of the limb in a cylinder of water. The amount of water moved out of the cylinder by the limb is measured by weight or volume and used to estimate limb volume.

Circumferential measurement of limbs. Limb circumference measurements can be used to compare differences in girth between limbs or to calculate volume. Patients must remove all limb coverings and extend limbs while measurement increments are marked on the skin or on a strip of adhesive tape attached to the skin.[23] A nonstretch, flexible tape measure is recommended in assessing circumferences to ensure consistent tension over soft tissue, muscle, and bony prominences. The tape measure, which is calibrated in units of 0.1 cm, is placed around the limb at intervals of 4 to 10 cm from wrist to axilla, depending on the selected protocol. Many times both limbs are measured for comparison of circumferences at similar anatomic locations to compare differences in girth. At other times, limb volume is calculated using either a formula or a cylinder or a cone.

Perometry. Perometry employs an optoelectronic volumetry device that works similarly to computer-assisted tomography, but uses infrared light instead of x-rays.[24] Clothing covering a limb must be removed prior to measurement. This device allows for depiction of the shape of the limb, and calculations of changes in volume can be made in seconds, using computer software.

Bioelectrical impedance. Bioelectrical impedance devices can be used to estimate extracellular volume and assess presence of lymphedema.[25] These devices are most commonly used to evaluate arms, but more recently have been modified to measure legs. The devices can be either single or multiple frequency. Clothing does not have to be removed from the limb(s) with this technique. Instead, lightly adhesive electrodes are placed on each hand, each wrist, and one foot. The procedure takes less than one minute and is painless. The devices are portable, allowing measurements to be done in clinics and community settings.

If a through medical history coupled with a thorough physical examination does not generate enough information to correctly diagnose lymphedema or a differential diagnosis is not obvious, other diagnostic modalities may be indicated. In these cases, lymphoscintigraphy is the preferred method to evaluate lymphatic involvement.[26] However, the value of this technology in terms of determining the patient's prognosis and its impact on treatment decisions is somewhat controversial—a point that should be considered before ordering this diagnostic test.

Venous ultrasound is indicated for any lower limb swelling. Magnetic resonance imaging (MRI) or computed tomography (CT) scans are indicated if there is reason to suspect tumor recurrence or the presence of tumor invasion that has compressed the lymphatics.

DEGREES OF TOXICITY

Multiple staging/grading criteria for lymphedema have been introduced, with subtle differences noted among the published methods. For the purposes of this text, degrees of severity are presented based on the Common Terminology Criteria for Adverse Events version 4.03 (CTCAE v4.03),[27] a grading system with which many oncology nurses are highly familiar. The criteria for lymphedema in CTCAE v4.03 are described in the vascular section of this system. These criteria are not highly applicable to secondary lymphedema as seen in cancer patients. Instead, the following criteria categories best represent typical lymphedema presentations in cancer populations and should serve as the guidelines for evaluating degree of lymphedema toxicity when nurses are examining patients:

- Edema—face
- Neck edema
- Edema—trunk
- Genital edema
- Edema—limbs

Although the CTCAE v4.03 uses the term "edema," the criteria for severity (Table 26-1) and the treatment guide for this condition (Figure 26-1) also apply to lymphedema. These five criteria are classified as Grades 1, 2, and 3.

SYMPTOM MANAGEMENT STRATEGIES

THERAPEUTIC APPROACHES

There are currently no known medications that can successfully treat lymphedema, nor are there any data to support the effectiveness of any herbal remedies or other complementary or alternative therapies. Patients should be cautioned to consult with their physician before embarking on a course of treatment using any oral agent. Regardless of the length of time a patient has experienced lymphedema, if he or she has pain related to the condition, pain management interventions should be initiated.

TABLE 26-1

National Cancer Insitute Common Terminology Criteria for Adverse Events (CTCAE): Edema

Grade	Criteria
1	Mild, visible swelling that does not impact instrumental ADL, self-care ADL, or function
2	Moderate, visible swelling that obliterates some anatomical landmarks, and limits instrumental ADL and function
3	Severe and medically significant swelling that may be disabling, limiting instrumental ADL, self-care ADL, and function

Source: Data from National Cancer Institute Common Terminology Criteria for Adverse Events (CTCAE)[27].

Early or mild lymphedema

A recent study in breast cancer survivors strongly supported the fact that early identification and treatment of mild degrees of swelling—specifically, a 3% difference between affected and unaffected arms—in these survivors can potentially reverse or prevent subsequent chronic lymphedema.[24] This level is lower than the 5% to 10% inter-limb discrepancy set by the CTCAE v4.03 standard for labeling someone as experiencing Grade 1 edema of the extremity and represents a degree of volume change that is not likely to be discernible by circumferential measurement alone. Additional research has suggested that subtle changes in the 20- to 30-cm segment of affected arms above the wrist in breast cancer survivors post-treatment predict early-onset lymphedema.[28] Perometry was used in these sentinel studies to identify the volume change, but this technology is not available in most cancer clinics. Nevertheless, patients may complain of tightness or heaviness in a limb before visible swelling is noted; based on the previously mentioned research, a referral to a lymphedema therapist for breast cancer survivors reporting this symptom is highly desirable. While the Stout Gergich et al. study[24] has not been replicated in other types of cancer survivors at risk for lymphedema, given the underlying pathology for all cancer treatment related lymphedema there is reason to believe that early treatment could have similar benefits for other groups of cancer survivors.

Beyond the findings in the previously cited studies,[24,28] there is little evidence to support any specific risk-reduction strategies for cancer patients at risk for developing lymphedema.[29,30] A recent comprehensive review of data to support lymphedema risk-reduction strategies commonly taught to patients concluded that only maintaining a normal body weight and participating in supervised exercise programs had substantial evidence to support them as risk-reduction practices. Some have called for caution when educating at-risk individuals about risk-reduction practices, given the potential impact that such precautions may have on quality of life and the lack of evidence to support many of the precautions patients are being urged to take.[30]

Complete decongestive therapy. When there is identified swelling, even though there is little supporting evidence, the current gold standard of care for all grades of lymphedema is complete decongestive therapy (CDT), a two-phase treatment protocol for both primary and secondary lymphedema.[31,32] Phase I consists of intensive manual lymphatic drainage (MLD), two-way short-stretch compression bandaging, exercises, and meticulous skin care. Phase II, the maintenance phase, includes lifelong wearing of daytime elastic sleeves (routinely replaced based on updated measurements), nighttime compression wrapping, and exercises and skin care.

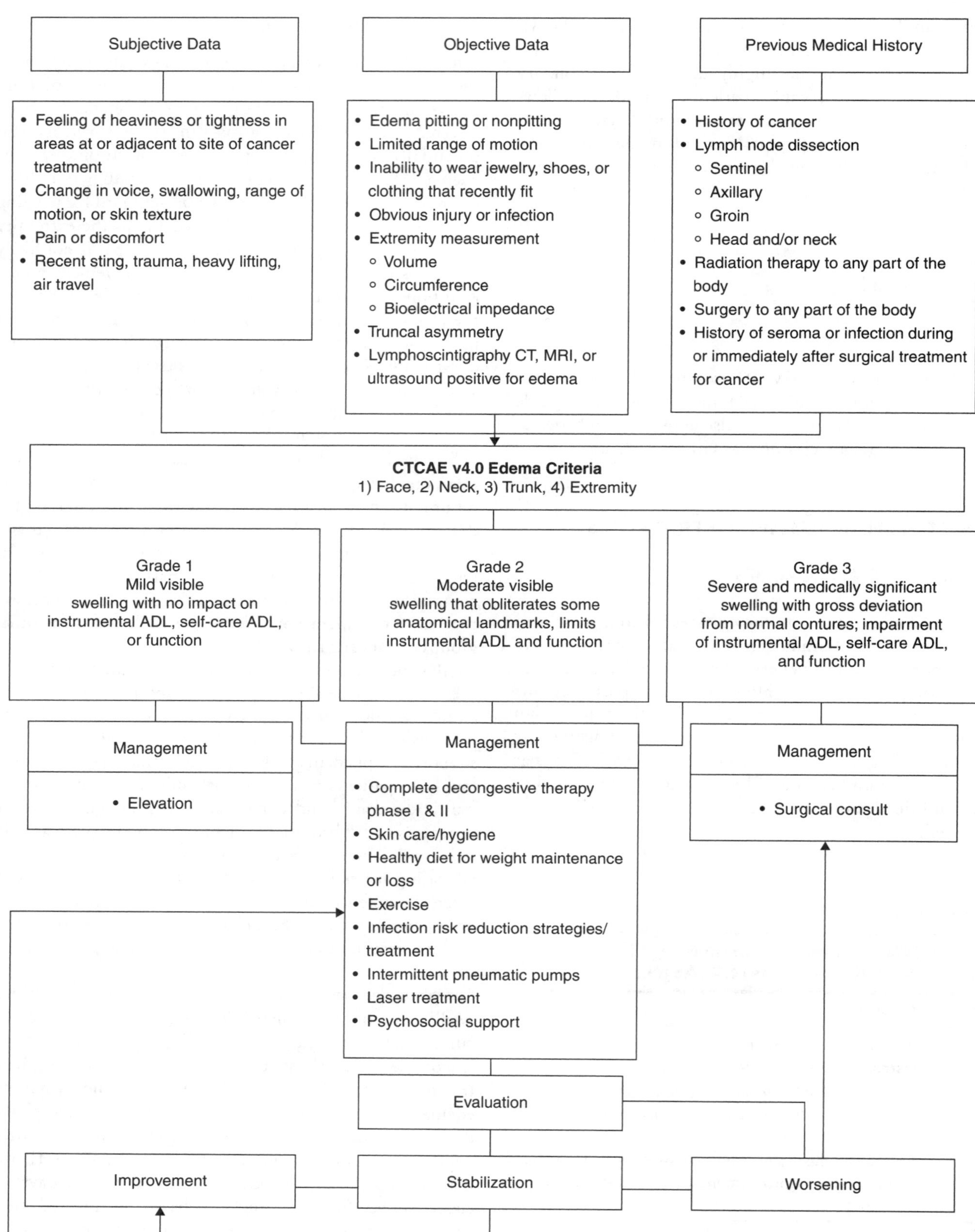

Abbreviations: ADL: activities of daily living; CT: computed tomography; MRI: magnetic resonance imaging.

FIGURE 26-1

Lymphedema assessment.

Ideally, Phase I treatment should be conducted by a certified lymphedema therapist or by a health professional who has attended a lymphedema treatment training school and is working on obtaining enough hands-on clinical hours to sit for certification. Certified therapists do not necessarily have to be physical therapists, and the certification status and lymphedema training status—not the type of degree—should be the primary factors in deciding who should treat the patient. Phase I therapy usually requires several sessions, and it is very important that the patient understand that the effectiveness of the therapy is highly dependent upon active patient participation in the plan of care. In general, the four components of Phase I care are administered as follows:

- Manual lymphatic drainage: includes lymph movement from the swollen areas into the lymphatic system for transport. Pressures and techniques may vary slightly from therapist to therapist, as different training schools teach slightly different techniques.
- Compression bandaging: application of bandages after MLD is completed to maintain the gains achieved from the massage itself. Patients may have to wear very bulky bandages at home while undergoing Phase I treatment and should remove them only as instructed by the therapist.
- Exercises: therapist-taught exercises to help move the lymphatic fluid. These will vary based on the area of body in which the swelling is occurring, but may include movement of limbs and breathing exercises.
- Meticulous skin care: keeping the skin clean and supple, using moisturizing creams to prevent cracking. Patients with lymphedema are at high risk for infection in the swollen areas. Constant observation for any signs of infection and prompt treatment of infection should any signs become evident are recommended.

Phase II therapy consists of patient self-care that incorporates, with some modification, the four components of Phase I therapy. Again, it is very important for patients to complete self-care as instructed; however, many do not do so. For example, data show that only half of all breast cancer survivors with lymphedema complete the prescribed self-care.[33]

In Phase II, patients are taught how to complete self-MLD. This may be very difficult for some patients to do, as reaching swollen areas is at times problematic because of the location of the swelling or range-of-motion difficulties. Many patients find that intermittent, pneumatic compression devices are helpful assistive devices for conducting MLD at home.[20,21] These devices require a prescription and are costly. They should be used only under the guidance of a healthcare professional knowledgeable about lymphedema.

The bulky bandages used in Phase I therapy may be replaced by compression garments for day wear, but some patients may require bandaging or other types of compression garments at night to maintain a reasonable level of arm volume. Good skin hygiene, moisturizing, and skin observation should continue. Exercises to enhance fluid movement should be performed as taught by a certified lymphedema therapist and should account for the patient's overall physical condition and location of swelling. Attention should be given to exercising the entire body to maintain health.[34]

Low-level laser therapy. Noninvasive, low-level (cold) laser treatment has been used for wound healing for decades. In the mid-1990s, investigators began to study its use as a method for treating lymphedema, primarily in the breast cancer population. This technology has been evaluated as both a stand-alone method and in conjunction with other methods such as pneumatic compression devices or MLD.[35–37] In one study that compared low-level laser treatment to treatment with pneumatic compression devices, those patients who received laser therapy had better long-term results.[36] A second study concluded that laser therapy combined with standard treatment produced additional benefits such as symptom relief and improved range of motion.[35] Although the laser is not curative, a growing body of evidence supports the hypothesis that it may both improve patient outcomes as a single modality and enhance the response to standard therapy. An increasing number of lymphedema therapists are incorporating this modality into their practice.

Late or severe lymphedema

Lymphedema is a chronic condition that requires lifelong self-care to maintain reasonable control over the volume of fluid and to reduce infection rates and functional impairment. In stages of severe lymphedema of limbs, where large skin folds and severe bulky fibrotic mass are present, liposuction can be used as a debulking procedure.[38] Although this therapy does not cure the lymphedema and compression garments must be worn continuously to maintain the reduction in limb girth, the procedure can assist some patients in regaining functional abilities, such as walking, that has become difficult simply due to body mass of the swollen areas. Other surgical approaches are being explored to improve lymphatic function.

Lymph node transplant. Transplantation of lymph nodes from nonsurgical areas of the body to affected areas, such as the wrist or axilla, of breast cancer survivors with lymphedema who had less than desirable outcomes with noninvasive therapeutic modalities is being explored.[39] The results to date appear promising for a subgroup of patients; however, concerns about the long-term morbidity of the donor site exist. Patients should be referred to surgeons who have experience in performing these procedures if they wish to be evaluated as candidates for such transplants.

Microsurgery. Lymphatic venous anastomosis techniques are being undertaken in some patients with secondary lymphedema who have not responded to traditional therapy.[38,40,41] Some positive results have been noted in patients who proved resistant to noninvasive therapeutic techniques. Should patients inquire about this surgical approach to treatment, they should be referred only to surgeons who have experience in performing the procedures.

In addition to the surgical approaches described previously, autologous stem cell therapy is being explored as a therapy for lymphedema. At least one randomized trial, conducted in a small group of breast cancer survivors with lymphedema, has compared the use of autologous stem cell injections to multiple sites in the swollen arm to traditional compression sleeve therapy.[42] Members of the stem cell group did not wear compression garments after the procedure. Those in the compression sleeve group wore their garments daily for 4 weeks, then removed the garments for 4 weeks, and reapplied them for 4 additional weeks. The compression group showed improvement only when the garment was being worn; the stem cell group showed improvement throughout the entire follow-up period (12 weeks). Symptomatic improvement in pain and arm sensitivity was noted in the stem cell group. Though highly experimental, this strategy represents a new approach to treatment that warrants further study.

Studies conducted in animal models that combined growth factor therapy with lymph node transplants have met with some success.[43] Although human studies using this approach to treat lymphedema are lacking, the results from animal studies underscore the importance of translating findings from bench science, where these growth factors were identified, to the bedside, as possible new lymphedema treatment modalities.

End-of-life care

Lymphedema is often present at the end of life, when tumor burden may be high and cause anatomic blockage to both lymphatic vessels and nodes, thereby initiating new swelling. Preexisting lymphedema may become more severe due to immobility or infection.[44,45]

Assessment of the patient's physical and mental status should guide the plan of treatment in such scenarios. Collaboration among patients and both lay and professional caregivers is needed to ensure the most appropriate plan of care is developed. Use of traditional lymphedema treatment techniques require the patient to be physically able to tolerate MLD, bandaging, compression sleeves, and exercise. While some patients may be able to tolerate this treatment, many will not be able to do so. Therefore, these approaches may need to be modified substantially in end-of-life settings, or the decision may be made to not treat the lymphedema at all.

In patients who desire treatment, use of MLD, bandaging, or compression sleeves alone—not in combination—may palliate symptoms. Repositioning the affected areas on pillows to support the additional weight may be required. Skin care should be undertaken to reduce infection risk. To enhance comfort, pain medication may need to be administered prior to initiating any type of treatment, and antibiotics should be prescribed if infection is present in the swollen areas. Reassessment of the patient's physical and mental status should be done on a regular basis, and lymphedema treatment should be discontinued upon request of the patient or when it becomes clear that the risks of treatment (e.g., pain or severe fatigue) outweigh the benefits.

NURSING IMPLICATIONS

Nurses are in a unique position to support patients with lymphedema to live as active, functioning members of society, and to experience a high quality of life despite having a chronic medical condition. Nurses can serve as patient advocates, educators, hands-on therapists, and symptom managers.

Reimbursement for lymphedema therapy and supplies is often problematic. Nurse advocates may influence patient outcomes, such as the cost of care, by helping patients draft letters to insurance carriers that describe the difficulties they are experiencing due to the lymphedema. These letters may assist patients in obtaining some reimbursement for supplies or lymphedema therapy.

The role of the nurse as a patient educator is critical to improving patient symptom outcomes. A holistic approach to patient education is indicated, given the implications for a healthy weight and exercise and the multiple symptoms associated with the swelling. It may be helpful to begin the education session by initially discussing with patients the need to focus on total physical and psychological health, not just the swelling. Some key topics to address are healthy diet, exercise/fitness, infection prevention, self-care, and symptoms related to lymphedema, including the psychological distress. Determine patients' level of knowledge in these areas and tailor the education to meet individual needs.

Healthy eating is the cornerstone of a physically fit person. This consideration is critical to ensure the patient has the necessary nutrients to maintain a healthy immune system and body weight and to maintain nutritional soundness. Weight management for patients with lymphedema is also important, as being overweight increases the risk of getting lymphedema and may worsen the swelling in those persons who already have lymphedema.

Likewise, physical fitness is important, as data now demonstrate that under supervision, breast cancer patients with lymphedema can engage not only in exercise such as walking or swimming, but, with appropriate supervision, in progressive resistance exercise as well.[34] The muscle movement associated with these activities can cause shifts in lymph fluid. Research involving breast cancer survivors with lymphedema found that some individuals cut back on physical activity when they develop lymphedema.[46] Patients who are active should be encouraged to stay physically active. If they are not physically active, suggest that they start with small, easy activities such as walking, and work their way up to a higher level of fitness. Exercise may be critical to improving the patient's overall health, diminishing the fatigue reported in conjunction with the patient's lymphedema, and (possibly) maintaining a lower volume of fluid.

Preventive care is needed to reduce the risk of infection in the lymphedema-affected areas and to promote overall good health. Many patients with lymphedema find it helpful to keep a topical antibiotic and bandages with them at all times. Keeping the skin clean and supple will reduce the risk of cracking skin. Although no study has examined the relationship between dental caries, poor dentition, oral infection, and lymphedema, many therapists and physicians have reported anecdotally that in patients with arm lymphedema, treatment of underlying dental problems has appeared to reduce the recurrence of infections in the swollen limb. Thus, as for any other person, brushing and flossing of teeth and regular visits to a dentist for teeth cleanings and examination should be encouraged.

Self-care related to lymphedema itself should not consume the patient's life; nevertheless, self-care is as important to this patient population as it is to those persons with other chronic illnesses such as high blood pressure and diabetes. Patients should be educated about the need to conduct Phase II CDT.

Many patients with lymphedema are unaware that odd sensations in the swollen areas, poor range of motion, weakness, fatigue, psychological distress, functional impairments, problems sleeping, swallowing difficulties, changes in their voice, and firmness in skin are symptoms of lymphedema. This lack of knowledge may be related to inadequacy or lack of education regarding the lymphedema experience; in other words, they may not have been informed that lymphedema is "more than swelling" and that management of all symptoms is necessary to maintain quality of life. Nurses are uniquely positioned to educate patients about the broad symptom issues faced by persons with lymphedema.

Finally, nurses can also directly affect the volume of swelling. Treatment of lymphedema does not have to be delegated to physical therapists. Advanced practice nurses, if trained as lymphedema therapists can, and do, provide hands-on CDT and bill for their services. Thus nurses can directly impact a very important patient outcome, reduction of volume of swelling, and slow the progression of lymphedema to Grade 3.

PATIENT SELF-CARE

There is no known cure for cancer-related lymphedema. Consequently, self-care is for three purposes: (1) to facilitate continued fluid movement from the affected areas; (2) to maintain skin integrity and physical function; and (3) to manage symptoms associated with lymphedema such as altered sensations, fatigue, psychological distress, loss of confidence in body image, and reduction of activity.[46] Each patient's self-care needs may vary, so a tailored approach to planning self-care is indicated, particularly as a recent systematic review found there is little evidence to inform specific self-care tasks.[47] Although each self-care plan may differ, in every case the importance of self-care should be emphasized and lymphedema self-care activities should be assessed at every patient visit. (See Appendix 26A.) Clearly, nurses play a vital role in the ongoing reinforcement and assessment of adherence to self-care activities.

REFERENCES

1. Bergan J, Bunke N. General considerations. In: Lee B-B, Bergan J, Rockson SG, eds. *Lymphedema: A Concise Compendium of Theory and Practice*. London: Springer; 2011:3–10.
2. Ridner SH, Bonner CM, Deng J, Sinclair VG. Voices from the shadows: living with lymphedema. *Cancer Nurs.* 2012;35(1):E18–E26.
3. Orphanet. Primary lymphedema. 2007. http://www.orpha.net/consor/cgi-bin/OC_Exp.php?lng+EN&Expert=77240. Accessed December 29, 2012.
4. Deng J, Ridner SH, Dietrich MS, et al. Prevalence of secondary lymphedema in patients with head and neck cancer. *J Pain Symptom Manage.* 2012;43(2):244–252.
5. Hayes S, Di Sipio T, Rye S, et al. Prevalence and prognostic significance of secondary lymphedema following breast cancer. *Lymphat Res Biol.* 2011;9(3):135–141.
6. Hareyama H, Ito K, Hada K, et al. Reduction/prevention of lower extremity lymphedema after pelvic and para-aortic lymphadenectomy for patients with gynecologic malignancies. *Ann Surg Oncol.* 2012;19(1):268–273.
7. Rockson S. Update on the biology and treatment of lymphedema. *Curr Treat Opt Cardiovasc Med.* 2012;14(2):184–192.
8. Olszewski WL. Anatomy of the lymphatic system and its disorders. In: Lee B-B, Bergan J, Rockson SG, eds. *Lymphedema: A Concise Compendium of Theory and Practice*. London: Springer; 2011:49–56.
9. Avraham T, Daluvoy S, Zampell J, et al. Blockade of transforming growth factor-β1 accelerates lymphatic regeneration during wound repair. *Am J Pathol.* 2010;177(6):3202–3214.

10. Montgomery LD, Dietrich MS, Armer JM, Stewart BR, Ridner SH. Segmental blood flow and hemodynamic state of lymphedematous and nonlymphedematous arms. *Lymphat Res Biol.* 2011;9(1):31–42.
11. Ridner S, Dietrich M, Stewart B, Armer J. Body mass index and breast cancer treatment-related lymphedema. *Support Care Cancer.* 2011;19(6):853–857.
12. Helyer LK, Varnic M, Le LW, Leong W, McCready D. Obesity is a risk factor for developing postoperative lymphedema in breast cancer patients. *Breast J.* 2010;16(1):48–54.
13. Fu MR, Guth AA, Cleeland CM, et al. The effects of symptomatic seroma on lymphedema symptoms following breast cancer treatment. *Lymphology.* 2011;44(3):134–143.
14. Bevilacqua J, Kattan M, Changhong Y, et al. Nomograms for predicting the risk of arm lymphedema after axillary dissection in breast cancer. *Ann Surg Oncol.* 2012;19(8):2580–2589.
15. Hayes SC, Rye S, Battistutta D, Newman B. Prevalence of upper-body symptoms following breast cancer and its relationship with upper-body function and lymphedema. *Lymphology.* 2010;43(4):178–187.
16. Rosedale M, Fu M. Confronting the unexpected: temporal, situational, and attributive dimensions of distressing symptom experience for breast cancer survivors. *Oncol Nurs Forum.* 2010;37(1):E28–E33.
17. Deng J, Ridner S, Murphy B Dietrich M. Preliminary development of a lymphedema symptom assessment scale for patients with head and neck cancer. *Support Care Cancer.* 2012;20(8):1911–1918.
18. Armer JM, Stewart BR, Shook RP. 30-month post-breast cancer treatment lymphoedema. *J Lymphoedema.* 2009;4(1):14–18.
19. Carter J, Raviv L, Appollo K, Baser RE, Iasonos A, Barakat RR. A pilot study using the Gynecologic Cancer Lymphedema Questionnaire (GCLQ) as a clinical care tool to identify lower extremity lymphedema in gynecologic cancer survivors. *Gynecol Oncol.* 2010;117(2):317–323.
20. Ridner SH, Murphy B, Deng J, Kidd N, Galford E, Dietrich MS. Advanced pneumatic therapy in self-care of chronic lymphedema of the trunk. *Lymphat Res Biol.* 2010;8(4):209–215.
21. Ridner S, Murphy B, Deng J, et al. A randomized clinical trial comparing advanced pneumatic truncal, chest, and arm treatment to arm treatment only in self-care of arm lymphedema. *Breast Cancer Res Treat.* 2012;131(1):147–158.
22. Piller NB. Differential diagnosis general considerations. In: Lee B-B, Bergan J, Rockson SG, eds. *Lymphedema: A Concise Compendium of Theory and Practice.* London: Springer; 2011:119–124.
23. Gjorup C, Zerahn B, Hendel HW. Assessment of volume measurement of breast cancer-related lymphedema by three methods: circumference measurement, water displacement, and dual energy x-ray absorptiometry. *Lymphat Res Biol.* 2010;8(2):111–119.
24. Stout Gergich NL, Pfalzer LA, McGarvey C, Springer B, Gerber LH, Soballe P. Preoperative assessment enables the early diagnosis and successful treatment of lymphedema. *Cancer.* 2008;112(12):2809–2819.
25. Ward LC, Dylke E, Czerniec S, Isenring E, Kilbreath SL. Confirmation of the reference impedance ratios used for assessment of breast cancer-related lymphedema by bioelectrical impedance spectroscopy. *Lymphat Res Biol.* 2011;9(1):47–51.
26. Andrade M. Laboratory/imaging diagnosis: general guidelines. In: Lee B-B, Bergan J, Rockson SG, eds. *Lymphedema: A Concise Compendium of Theory and Practice.* London: Springer; 2011:139–143.
27. U.S. Department of Health and Human Services, National Institutes of Health, National Cancer Institute. Common terminology criteria for adverse events (CTCAE) version 4.0. June 14, 2010. http://evs.nci.nih.gov/ftp1/CTCAE/CTCAE_4.03_2010-06-14_QuickReference_8.5x11.pdf. Accessed January 3, 2012.
28. Stout NL, Pfalzer LA, Levy E, et al. Segmental limb volume change as a predictor of the onset of lymphedema in women with early breast cancer. *PM R.* 2011;3(12):1098–1105.
29. Cemal Y, Pusic A, Mehrara BJ. Preventative measures for lymphedema: separating fact from fiction. *J Am Coll Surg.* 2011;213(4):543–551.
30. Nielsen I, Gordon S, Selby A. Breast cancer-related lymphoedema risk reduction advice: a challenge for health professionals. *Cancer Treat Rev.* 2008;34(7):621–628.
31. Földi E, Földi M. Complete decongestive therapy. In: Lee B-B, Bergan J, Rockson SG, eds. *Lymphedema: A Concise Compendium of Theory and Practice.* London: Springer; 2011:229–236.
32. Koul R, Dufan T, Russell C, et al. Efficacy of complete decongestive therapy and manual lymphatic drainage on treatment-related lymphedema in breast cancer. *Int J Radiat Oncol Biol Phys.* 2007;67(3):841–846.
33. Ridner S, Dietrich M, Kidd N. Breast cancer treatment-related lymphedema self-care: education, practices, symptoms, and quality of life. *Support Care Cancer.* 2011;19(5):631–637.
34. Schmitz KH, Ahmed RL, Troxel AB, et al. Weight lifting for women at risk for breast cancer–related lymphedema. *JAMA.* 2010;304(24):2699–2705.
35. Dirican A, Andacoglu O, Johnson R, McGuire K, Mager L, Soran A. The short-term effects of low-level laser therapy in the management of breast-cancer-related lymphedema. *Support Care Cancer.* 2011;19(5):685–690.
36. Kozanoglu E, Basaran S, Paydas S, Sarpel T. Efficacy of pneumatic compression and low-level laser therapy in the treatment of postmastectomy lymphoedema: a randomized controlled trial. *Clin Rehabil.* 2009;23(2):117–124.
37. Lau RW, Cheing GL. Managing postmastectomy lymphedema with low-level laser therapy. *Photomed Laser Surg.* 2009;27(5):763–769.
38. Campisi C, Eretta C, Pertile D, et al. Microsurgery for treatment of peripheral lymphedema: long-term outcome and future perspectives. *Microsurgery.* 2007;27(4):333–338.
39. Lin C-H, Ali R, Chen S-C, et al. Vascularized groin lymph node transfer using the wrist as a recipient site for management of postmastectomy upper extremity lymphedema. *Plast Reconstr Surg.* 2009;123(4):1265–1275.
40. Lee BB, Laredo J, Neville R. Reconstructive surgery for chronic lymphedema: a viable option, but. *Vascular.* 2011;19(4):195–205.
41. Damstra R, Voesten H, van Schelven W, van der Lei B. Lymphatic venous anastomosis (LVA) for treatment of secondary arm lymphedema: a prospective study of 11 LVA procedures in 10 patients with breast cancer related lymphedema and a critical review of the literature. *Breast Cancer Res Treat.* 2009;113(2):199–206.
42. Maldonado GEM, Pérez CAA, Covarrubias EEA, et al. Autologous stem cells for the treatment of post-mastectomy lymphedema: a pilot study. *Cytotherapy.* 2011;13(10):1249–1255.
43. Lähteenvuo M, Honkonen K, Tervala T, et al. Growth factor therapy and autologous lymph node transfer in lymphedema: clinical perspective. *Circulation.* 2011;123(6):613–620.
44. Murphy BA, Cmelak A, Bayles S, et al. Palliative issues in the care of patients with cancer of the head and neck. In: Hanks G, Cherny NI, Christakis NA, Fallon M, Kaasa S, Portenoy RK., eds. *Oxford Textbook of Palliative Medicine.* New York: Oxford University Press; 2010;1145–1172.
45. Ridner SH. Lymphedema. In: Esper P, Kuebler KK, eds. *Palliative Practices from A–Z for the Bedside Clinician.* Pittsburgh, PA: Oncology Nursing Society; 2008;179–186.
46. Ridner S. Quality of life and a symptom cluster associated with breast cancer treatment-related lymphedema. *Support Care Cancer.* 2005;13(11):904–911.
47. Ridner SH, Fu MR, Wanchai A, et al. Self-management of lymphedema: a systematic review of the literature from 2004 to 2011. *Nurs Research.* 2012;61(4):291–299.

Swelling (Lymphedema)

Patient Name: ____

This guide will help you learn about your swelling, its treatment, and the importance of becoming and staying actively involved in managing the swelling.

Symptom and Description

You might have had some swelling right after surgery or during your radiation. That was normal, and it got better as you healed. Now you are noticing swelling that is different from that initial swelling. You have swelling of your (circle all that apply) face, neck, breast, chest, back, underarm, arm, hand, leg, or foot—a condition that is sometimes called *lymphedema*. This swelling can happen any time after surgery or radiation treatment for cancer. In some people, if it is treated very early, the swelling may disappear. In others, it may come and go, or it may stay. It is hard to predict what will happen with your swelling as time goes on. Very little is understood about why some people never get swelling (lymphedema) while others do, or why the swelling is not exactly the same in every person who has it. The swelling happens because the surgery or radiation that you had reduced the ability of your lymphatic system to move fluid out of the space between the cells in your body.

You may feel tight or heavy in the area that is swollen. Depending on where the swelling occurs, it may be hard to turn your head or to raise or lower your arms or legs. You may not like how the swelling makes you look. You may feel tired. You may not want to stay active and engage in social or recreational activities because you are afraid of making your swelling worse. These things happen to some, but not all, people with this kind of swelling.

It is important to take care not only of the swelling, but also of the rest of your body. If you see a therapist for your swelling, it is very important to do what you are told to do to take care of yourself, such as to wear compression garments and take care of your skin. You may not want to do this because it takes time or you do not think it helps. In fact, these measures reduce your risk of getting infection in the swollen area and help to keep the swelling from getting worse—so it is very important to perform the self-care. Try hard to complete the self-care activities that you are taught to do. It is also very important to maintain a normal body weight, because people who are overweight tend to have more trouble with the swelling.

Remember—the swelling can be managed. Try not to let it keep you from living an active, social life.

Management

1. If you have swelling, your doctor or nurse practitioner should refer you to a trained lymphedema therapist as soon as any amount of swelling, no matter how small, is noticed. This referral is very important because some research now shows that very early treatment may reverse the swelling. It is very important that the person be trained in lymphedema management—contact the National Lymphedema Network if you or your

(continued)

healthcare team have problems finding a trained therapist. You may need to check with your insurance provider about how to document a referral for the insurance company.

2. You should plan to have an evaluation and examination by the therapist and several appointments to reduce your swelling. You should have a fully developed plan for self-care at home by the end of your treatment. The treatments may include the following steps:
   a. Massage
   b. Bandaging
   c. Exercise
   d. Skin care
   e. Compression garments
   f. Pumps
   g. Education about how to take care of your swelling, whether you need to follow any restrictions, and how to know when to come back for additional treatments
3. Report *any* sign of infection in your swollen area immediately to your healthcare team. If you are traveling or unable to reach your team, go to the nearest emergency room and tell them you have lymphedema and are concerned you may be getting an infection. Signs are:
   a. Red streaks going up or down an arm or leg
   b. General redness in your swollen area
   c. Heat or skin that is hot to touch in the swollen area
   d. Increase in swelling
   e. Sudden pain or soreness in the swollen area
   f. Nausea, aching, and vomiting with a fever (this can occur before other signs develop)
4. Contact your doctor or nurse if you notice any changes in your swelling:
   a. Clothes, shoes, or jewelry becoming tighter
   b. Compression garments starting to feel "too tight"
   c. New numbness, pain, or tingling in the swollen area
5. Eat a healthy diet. If you are overweight, try to lose weight by following a healthy diet plan.
6. If you have pain or odd, bothersome sensations in your swollen areas, talk to your healthcare team about ways to reduce the discomfort. These ways could include options such as positioning changes or medications for pain.
7. Follow the individualized self-care plan you were taught by your therapist. Maintain good hygiene, wear sunscreen, keep moving (walking is an excellent exercise), and if you find yourself angry or depressed about your swelling, ask for a referral to a mental health counselor or locate a lymphedema support group (live or on the web).
8. Special instructions for you:

   ____

   ____

   ____

   ____

Follow-up

Phone Numbers

Nurse: ____

Physician: ____

Lymphedema Therapist: ____

Website

National Lymphedema Network: www.lymphnet.org

Source: Ridner SH. Lymphedema. In: Yarbro CH, Wujcik D, Gobel BH, eds. *Cancer Symptom Management.* 4th ed. Burlington, MA: Jones & Bartlett Learning; 2014.

Chapter 27

Ocular and Otic Complications

Colleen O'Leary, MSN, RN, AOCNS®

THE PROBLEM

Cancer therapies, including systemic chemotherapy and biotherapy as well as radiation therapy, can produce acute and chronic organ damage. The eye has generally been considered protected from such damage.[1] Although ocular side effects are relatively uncommon, the oculo-visual system has a potentially high degree of sensitivity to toxic substances. The development of more aggressive treatment regimens and the introduction of newer agents and combination therapies have collectively contributed to an increase in reported cases of ocular side effects. A number of drugs in clinical use are also considered ototoxic, having the potential to cause inner ear damage as a side effect. In addition, radiotherapy is a common modality in the management of brain and head and neck neoplasms. Due to the complex anatomy of this area, radiation exposure to nontarget structures during irradiation of the brain, head, and neck is often unavoidable. As a result, ototoxicity is often seen as a complication after radiotherapy to these areas.

Advancements in treatment have resulted in longer survival for patients with cancer. Consequently, healthcare professionals are seeing more patients with adverse ocular and otic side effects secondary to their treatment. Understanding these side effects will help to recognize them early and intervene before permanent damage occurs. Anticipation of treatment-related toxicities may provide the opportunity to develop or provide interventions that could minimize an expected side effect.

INCIDENCE AND ETIOLOGY

Ocular toxicities

Although relatively uncommon, ocular toxicities occur with a variety of anticancer agents (Table 27-1).[1–33] Toxicities can occur in the adnexia, which is composed of the accessory visual structures including the eyebrows, eyelids, and lacrimal structures; in the anterior segment, including the crystalline lens, iris, and cornea; in the posterior segment, including the retina, choroid, optic disc, and vitreous humor; and in neuro-ophthalmic areas of the eye.[1–3] General neurotoxic side effects of chemotherapy occur frequently and often result in limiting the patient's dose of chemotherapy. Although most neurotoxicities are peripheral neuropathies, central neurotoxicities can occur as well. Central neuropathies affecting vision include disc edema, retinal edema, optic neuritis, optic atrophy with vision loss, and neuro-ophthalmic lesions.[1,4] Most of the optic toxicities are relatively specific to certain drugs and are often dose or administration related.

An estimated 25% to 50% of patients receiving 5-fluorouracil experience ocular toxicities, with blepharitis (inflammation of the eyelid) being one of the most common side effects.[1,4,6,8] Cetuximab is associated with ocular cutaneous toxicities, including blepharitis, in 80% of patients, with 15% of these cases being severe.[9,10] Other antineoplastic agents that have been associated with blepharitis include high-dose methotrexate, fludarabine, and cladrabine. This side effect has occurred in only a small number of cases, however.[4,8]

TABLE 27-1

Agents Causing Ocular Toxicities

Toxicity	Agent
Blepharitis	5-Fluorouracil Cetuximab High-Dose Methotrexate Fludarabine Cladrabine
Epiphora	5-Fluorouracil High-Dose Cytarabine Doxorubicin Bevacizumab Imitanib
Dry Eye Syndrome	5-Fluorouracil Tretinoin
Conjunctivitis	Doxorubicin 5-Fluorouracil Capecitabine Carmustine Methotrexate Erlotinib Epirubicin
Trichomegaly	Cetuximab Erlotinib Gefitinib
Cataract	Prednisone Dexamethasone Tamoxifen Total Body Irradiation
Photophobia	Procarbazine Vincristine Vinblastine 5-Fluorouracil

Source: Data from Ernest and Edijana[1]; Ananth[2]; Ananth[3]; Foroozan[4]; Schmid et al[5]; Singh and Singh[6]; Hardten[7]; Blomquist[8]; Criado[9]; Ramirez-Soria et al[10]; Butovich[11]; Kaercher and Bron[12]; Hazin et al[13]; Smith et al[14]; Lemp[15]; Eisman et al[16]; Alexandrescu et al[17]; Foerster et al[18]; Kerob et al[19]; Bouche et al[20]; Carser and Summers[21]; Lane and Goldsein[22]; Symonds et al[23]; Perry[24]; Howell et al[25]; Schneider et al[26]; Li et al[27]; Chandler et al[28]; Gupta et al[29]; Gianni et al[30]; Conill et al[31]; Fard-Esfahani et al[32]; Gunduz et al[33].

Epiphora (excessive tearing) is associated with a variety of antineoplastic agents. It occurs in as many as 50% of patients receiving 5-fluorouracil, then gradually subsides after treatment is discontinued.[1,4,11,12] Although no ocular toxicities have been reported with low-dose cytarabine, at high doses 40% to 100% of patients experience ocular toxicities, including epiphora and conjunctivitis.[4,6,8,12] In patients who are treated with doxorubicin, 25% experience epiphora.[5,12,13] Other agents that are known to contribute to epiphora include bevacizumab and imitinab.[12,13]

Dry eye syndrome, also known as keratoconjunctiva sicca, is the most common condition treated by ophthalmologists.[7,13,14] It is most often seen with the use of 5-fluorouracil and retinoids. The retinoid tretinoin, used in the treatment of acute promyelocytic leukemia, has been associated with dry eye syndrome.[13,14] In addition, in a small study of 52 patients receiving 5-fluorouracil for a variety of cancers, 6% of the patients complained of dry eyes.[16]

Noninfective conjunctivitis is reported in 2% to 25% of patients receiving a variety of chemotherapeutic agents.[12] As many as 25% of patients receiving doxorubicin, 12.5% receiving 5-fluorouracil, and 10% receiving capecitabine have reported experiencing conjunctivitis at some time during their treatment.[13] Other agents that have been associated with conjunctivitis include carmustine, methotrexate, erlotinib, and epirubicin. The percentages of patients experiencing conjunctivitis with these agents have been shown to be 3%, 8%, 12%, and 15%, respectively.[13]

Trichomegaly (excessive growth of eyelashes) has been described as a toxicity associated with epidermal growth factor receptor inhibitors (EGFRIs). However, the incidence of trichomegaly related to other cancer therapies has not been widely evaluated, and it is thought that only a small minority of patients experience this complication.[17] Trichomegaly has been reported most often with the use of cetuximab, erlotinib, and gefitinib.[18–22] Trichomegaly has also been shown to occur along with trichiasis and conjunctivitis in 12% of patients with cancer.[17] The development of corneal ulcerations resulting from trichomegaly is infrequent and seems to be associated with contact lens use.[17]

Cataracts can also develop secondary to cancer therapy, as a side effect of chemotherapeutic agents as well as supportive medications used in treatment. Cataracts have been reported in 1% to 9% of lymphoma and leukemia patients receiving long-term prednisone and dexamethasone as part of their treatment.[23,24] Tamoxifen has also been associated with cataract development. In a clinical trial of 60 postmenopausal women receiving tamoxifen for breast cancer, 6.8% of the participants developed cataracts during treatment.[25] A connection between radiation and the development of cataracts was also observed in 6.6% of 257 patients receiving total-body irradiation with bone marrow transplantation.[26]

Although they are uncommon, a variety of other ocular conditions may arise as a result of anticancer therapy. Paclitaxel and docetaxel, for example, have been linked to the onset of glaucoma.[27] A rare side effect of treatment with procarbazine, vincristine, vinblastine, and 5-fluorouracil is photophobia.[23–25,27–30] Less common ocular side effects related to a variety of chemotherapeutic agents include periorbital edema, pain, nystagmus, foreign body sensation, vision field loss, ptosis, Stevens-Johnson syndrome, and retinal detachment.[5,8]

Radiation therapy can also produce adverse ocular symptoms. Because structures of the eye are sensitive to irradiation, long-term exposure to high doses of radiation can result in ocular complications. These complications range from mild reversible symptoms to more severe irreversible complications including trichiasis, epiphora, ectropian, nasolacrimal duct obstruction, dry eye, iritis, cataract optic neuropathy, and retinopathy.[15,31,32] Patients receiving whole-brain radiation (WBRT) have been shown to be at risk for radiation-induced ocular toxicities.[31–33] In one study, 5.4% of patients receiving WBRT experienced ocular complications.[31]

A connection between iodine-131 therapy and ocular complications has also been reported. In one study, 51% of patients receiving at least 3 months of therapy with this isotope exhibited signs of dry eye, burning, and redness.[32]

Otic toxicities

The ototoxicity of drugs reflects the effects that the drug has either on the cochlea and vestibular cells of the inner ear or on the acoustic nerve (Table 27-2).[1,34–39] The otic damage is manifested in a variety of disorders, ranging from tinnitus and vertigo to hearing loss. Antitumor drugs categorized as ototoxic, meaning they were associated with hearing loss as well as potential tinnitus and vertigo, include vinblastine (incidence of less than 0.1%), oxaliplatin (less than 0.1%), carboplatin (4.5%), and cisplatin (more than 10%, with a number of studies showing an average of 62% of patients receiving cisplatin experience hearing loss).[35–37]

TABLE 27-2

Agents Causing Otic Toxicities

Toxicity	Agent
Hearing Loss	Cisplatin
Tinnitus	Dasatinib
	Imatinib
	Sorafinib
	Vinblastine
	Oxaliplatin
	Carboplatin
	Cisplatin
Vertigo	Dasatinib
	Imitanib
	Sunitinib
	Trastuzumab
	Cetuximab
	Vinblastine
	Oxaliplatin
	Carboplatin
	Cisplatin

Source: Data from Ernest and Edijana[1]; Mick et al[34]; Cianfrone et al[35]; Knoll et al[36]; Reavis et al[37]; Riga et al[38]; Jehanne et al[39].

A few reports indicate that vincristine given at high doses (2–2.5 mg/m^2) may cause bilateral sensorineural hearing loss.[38] However, other studies report no statistically significant difference in the incidence of ototoxicity with low- or high-dose vincristine, although there was a slight decline in audiometry results when higher doses were administered.[39] Etoposide has also been identified as ototoxic, but there are no published incidence rates.[35] Some antineoplastic agents cause less severe otic disturbances, such as tinnitus alone. These drugs include dasatinib and imatinib (incidence of less than 0.1%), as well as sorafanib (1%–10%).[35] Drugs that cause vertigo include desatinib and imatinib (incidence of less than 0.1%), sunitinib and trastuzumab (1%–10%), and cetuximab (more than 10%).[35]

The use of radiation therapy to treat cancer of the head and neck may also cause hearing loss. The frequency of radiation-induced damage to ear function has been found to be as high as 54% in treatment of nasopharyngeal cancer, with this side effect being the most common complication associated with this therapy.[40] Exposure of the middle ear to radiation can lead to otitis media with effusion (OME), a complication that occurs 26% of the time.[41] OME is characterized by deafness, tinnitus, and pain in the ear that can be lifelong.[41]

PATHOPHYSIOLOGY

OCULAR COMPLICATIONS

Blepharitis

Blepharitis is an ocular condition characterized by inflammation of the eyelids. The most frequent patient complaint is of ongoing eye irritation, often accompanied by eye redness.[42] Blepharitis is categorized according to where the condition arises. The less common anterior blepharitis is found mainly around the eyelashes and follicles. Posterior blepharitis involves inflammation of the inner portion of the eye around the meibomian glands. The meibomian glands are similar to sebaceous glands, in that they secrete an oily layer of the tear film.[43] This layer helps to prevent evaporation of tears and allows them to spread over the ocular surface. Given that this secretion is critical to ocular surface lubrication, posterior blepharitis often occurs with other conditions such as dry eye syndrome, conjunctivitis, and keratitis.[42]

Epiphora

When there is an increased production of tears or tears cannot drain properly from the eyes, individuals experience what is known as epiphora or watery eyes. Epiphora may result from a variety of conditions, but generally can be attributed to one of four categories: lid-globe growth abnormalities, obstructive lacrimal drainage disorders, ocular surface disorders, and (rarely) neurogenic lacrimal hypersecretory disorders.[11,14] Epiphora as a result of cancer treatment most likely is due to ocular surface disorders. Many other conditions can contribute to epiphora, including blepharitis, foreign bodies, droopy lower eyelids, and allergies.[11,14]

Dry eye

When the eye fails to produce a sufficient amount of tears to function properly, dry eye or keratoconjunctiva sicca is seen. Tears are an important source of moisture, oxygen, and nutrients for the eye. Any decrease in tear production can result in irritation. Such a decrease in tear formation is often the result of lacrimal aqueous insufficiency.[11,13,16]

Conjunctivitis

When the membrane lining the sclera and inside of the eye becomes inflamed, the condition is called conjunctivitis. Cellular infiltration, vascular engorgement, and diffuse exudation accompany this condition. Viral infections are the most common cause of conjunctivitis, but noninfectious causes are also seen with the administration of chemotherapeutic agents. In these cases, conjunctivitis is often accompanied by itching and irritation. Rarely is it a source of pain or photophobia.[13]

Trichomegaly

Trichomegaly is characterized by increased maturation of the hair of the eyelashes and eyebrows. Cetuximab, gefitinib, and erlotinib are monoclonal antibodies that signal block transduction pathways, including epidermal growth factor receptors. These receptors are important in the normal development of the epidermis and hair follicles.[20] Alteration in the negative growth regulator p27 has been indicated as the mechanism that affects follicular and epidermal growth. The up-regulation of p27 seen with the monoclonal antibodies could explain the increase in maturation of hair follicles leading to trichomegaly.[20]

Cataracts

Cataracts are a clouding of the lens of the eye. The normally clear lens allows light to pass through to the retina, where it is changed into nerve signals that are sent to the brain. As cataracts develop, part of the lens becomes more opaque, so that light does not pass through as easily and the patient's vision becomes blurry. The lens is made mostly of water and protein. This protein is arranged in a particular pattern that allows light to pass through it and the lens to remain clear. As the protein changes, it may begin to clump together, thereby causing the opacities that are seen with cataracts.[44] Most cataracts develop symmetrically in bilateral eyes.

Glaucoma

Glaucoma is actually a group of diseases that affect the optic nerve. Two types of glaucoma are distinguished: primary open-angle glaucoma (POAG) and angle-closure glaucoma. The aqueous humor, which is produced in the ciliary body of the eye, flows through the posterior and anterior chambers of the eye and eventually drains out of the eye via outflow mechanisms, thereby preserving the integrity and functioning of vital ocular structures. When a problem with the eye's drainage mechanisms arises, fluid can build up in the eye, producing increased intraocular pressure (IOP). This increased pressure can damage the optic nerve, resulting in irreversible loss of vision. When there is an anatomical open angle, which increases the IOP and damages the optic nerve, the condition is referred to as POAG.[13] The less common angle-closure glaucoma is an ocular emergency where the IOP suddenly increases, resulting in optic nerve damage.[12] Glaucoma associated with chemotherapy administration is related to capillary protein leakage that develops into glaucoma.[13]

Photophobia

When the rapidly dividing cells of the corneal epithelium are exposed to chemotherapeutic agents, destruction of pinpoint areas of the outer layer of the epithelium can occur. This condition, which is referred to as superficial punctuate keratitis, is the cause of chemotherapy-induced photophobia, which results in the eyes becoming overly sensitive to light.[13,45]

OTIC COMPLICATIONS

The human ear is divided into outer, middle, and inner ear areas. The outer ear is made up of the pinna and external auditory canal. The tympanic membrane and the boney ossicles are found in the middle ear, and the inner ear consists of the oval window, the cochlea, the semicircular canals, and the vestibule.[46] The cochlea houses the organ responsible for hearing, the organ of Corti, and the semicircular canals and vestibule are responsible for balance and equilibrium.[46]

In a normal healthy ear, hearing is accomplished through a series of vibrations and impulses. A sound wave travels through the external auditory canal to the middle ear, where the tympanic membrane begins to vibrate.

This vibration causes the ossicles to vibrate and press upon the oval window of the inner ear. Vibration of the oval window forces fluid in the cochlea to oscillate along the organ of Corti, which is lined with hair cells. These hair cells, which serve as hearing receptors, are stimulated by the fluid movement, which causes a nerve impulse to travel through the cochlear nerve to the vestibulocochlear nerve (cranial nerve VIII). The impulse then travels to the temporal lobe auditory processing centers of the brain, which allows us to hear.[46]

Hearing loss is classified into one of two categories: conductive or sensorineural. When there is a malfunction (usually a blockage) of the outer or middle ear, conductive hearing loss occurs. When there is malfunction of the inner ear, sensorineural hearing loss occurs.[47]

Most of the research regarding chemotherapy-induced ototoxicity is based on the use of cisplatin, as this agent has the highest incidence of associated hearing loss. It has been suggested that cisplatin causes damage to the hair cells lining the organ of Corti, resulting in sensorineural hearing loss.[46–51] Some researchers believe that this injury occurs due to the effects of cisplatin on the capase-3/7 enzyme. Cisplatin appears to increase the activity of capase-3/7, which initiates events that lead to apoptosis.[51] Other researchers are studying the role of reactive oxygen species (ROS), also called oxygen free radicals, that are produced by cisplatin. Using animal studies, it is hypothesized that the ROS decrease antioxidant enzymes found in the cochlea, rendering it more susceptible to damage from cisplatin.[48,49]

SYMPTOM ASSESSMENT

RISK FACTORS

The most common risk cited for ocular or ototoxicities is the dose or intensity of the treatment. As with many toxicities, the higher the dose or intensity of treatment, the more likely a patient is to experience toxicities. There are a few specific risk factors reported for ototoxicities. The major risk factors include preexisting hearing loss, younger age, higher cumulative dose of cisplatin, dose schedule, coexisting renal dysfunction, central nervous system (CNS) tumors, and concomitant or previous CNS radiation.[52–54] Studies have shown that young age may be most detrimental, with children younger than the age of 5 years having a relative risk of hearing loss that is 20-fold greater than those older than the age of 20 years who receive the same cisplatin dose.[54]

There also appears to be a genetic relationship to cisplatin-induced ototoxicity. The polymorphic glutathione-S-transferase (GST) enzymes are encoded on certain human genes. The risk of having hearing loss associated with cisplatin was four times greater in patients with certain GST patterns.[55] Another study showed that pediatric patients with null genotype for GST-M1 or GST-T1 had a fourfold increased risk of higher-grade ototoxicity.[56]

SELF-ASSESSMENT

Ocular complications

Although often disturbing, optic toxicities are generally well tolerated and do not interfere excessively with a patient's activities of daily living. When a patient has blepharitis, the eyelids become reddened, itchy, and swollen, with a scaly appearance at the base of the eyelashes. As scales become coarser, the surface of the eye becomes irritated and forms crusts, which may cause the lids to stick together when waking up in the morning. If this crust falls into the eye, the patient may experience a foreign body or gritty sensation. Blepharitis is usually transient and relatively well tolerated.[42,43]

The patient with epiphora will have increased tearing when not crying. The epiphora itself is usually painless but may occur in conjunction with irritations that cause the eye to itch or have a foreign body sensation. Patients with dry eyes typically complain of blurred vision that improves with blinking, irritation, chronic tearing, burning, and difficulty watching television or reading.[12,13]

The patient with conjunctivitis will notice redness and swelling of the eyelids, along with scratchy, watery, or itchy eyes. The conjunctivitis will usually resolve several days after the source of irritation is removed.[7]

Trichomegaly manifests itself as an overgrowth of eyelashes. As long as the lashes remain smooth, they may cause only minor irritation, along with some interference when wearing glasses. However, often the lashes become wiry and corkscrew-like. In this case, the lashes may become ingrown and cause more pain and irritation to the eye.[7,20]

Patients with photophobia will avoid light due to the pain experienced with pupil constriction. They will notice pain when changing from dark to light environments, often experiencing this problem when going outside during the day.[45]

More serious and often irreversible toxicities include cataracts and glaucoma. Common symptoms of cataracts are gradual blurring of vision, fading color vision, decreased night vision, decreased sensitivity to contrast, and photophobia.[7] Nighttime driving may be difficult, colors may appear to be faded or dull, and lights may appear to be too bright or with halos around them. Patients with cataracts may have to change eyeglass prescriptions frequently and double vision may occur. which can worsen over time.[7] Glaucoma often has no apparent symptoms other than a loss of side vision over time.[7]

Otic complications

Tinnitus is described as a roaring, hissing, or humming sound in the ears. It may interfere with a patient's ability to rest or concentrate, and the patient may be unable to sleep at night.[34,35] Nausea and vomiting may be associated with tinnitus as well. Severe nausea over an extended period of time may also cause the patient to feel dizzy.

With vertigo, patients may feel dizzy when they change positions or move their head. They may describe feeling as if the room is spinning or that they themselves may be spinning.[35,36] In severe cases, people may fear that they may fall down when they stand up. Nausea, vomiting, and tinnitus may accompany vertigo.

Patients who experience hearing loss will notice that sounds are muffled or not as loud. Most hearing loss is progressive and painless; it can be either unilateral or bilateral.[46–48]

OBJECTIVE ASSESSMENT

Ocular complications

There are no laboratory or diagnostic tests that confirm the majority of ocular toxicities. However, with epiphora, tear cultures and Schirmir's test may help to rule out mechanical causes.[11,12] A Schirmir's test uses filter paper placed inside the lower lid to test for moisture content.

Obtaining a thorough assessment is important to help diagnose the etiology of the toxicity as well as to make the differential diagnosis. The history should include questions about symptom initiation, duration, and exacerbation. In addition, smoking history, questions regarding allergens that induce or exacerbate the symptoms, and history of light sensitivity and eye pain are warranted.[7,11–13,15,42,43] The physical exam should include a thorough eye exam including visual acuity and visual field testing. Eye structures should be examined for erythema, edema, and crusting of eyelashes or lid margin.[11–13,15,42,43] Eyelashes should be carefully evaluated for misdirected eyelashes, loss of lashes, loss of pigmentation of lashes, and abnormal growth of eyelashes from meibomian gland orifices.[42,43] Because chronic inflammation of the eye can lead to structural changes, malposition of the eyelids should be evaluated.[42,43] Given that visual fields are the first to be affected by glaucoma, examination for glaucoma should also include optic nerve examination and evaluation of IOP.[13,57] If glaucoma is suspected, a complete ophthalmoscopic exam, including examination of the optic disc, can assist with determining progression of the disease.[57]

Otic complications

When ototoxic treatments are necessary, it is important to complete audiologic examinations throughout treatment. The exam should include a thorough history and physical. The patient history should include determining the onset, location, and pattern of the toxicity as well as exacerbating and alleviating factors.[58–60] Associated symptoms, including nausea, vomiting, pain, or neurologic symptoms, should be identified. Medical history to be addressed includes previous ear disease, noise exposure, and head injury. All medications should be reviewed to determine any additional ototoxic medications.[58–60] A complete head and neck examination, including cranial nerve examination and evaluation of the external canal and tympanic membrane, should be performed on all patients. If a vascular component of hearing loss is suspected, auscultation over the neck, periauricular area, temple, orbit, and mastoid is warranted.[58–60]

Hearing evaluation can be conducted using a whispered voice test, Weber test, and Rinne test.[60] To perform the whispered voice test, stand an arm's length behind the patient and occlude the ear canal. Whisper a short sentence or sequence of numbers, and ask the patient to repeat them. Repeat the test in the other ear. A systematic review of four studies on the whisper test showed that hearing impairment could be detected 90% to 100% of the time with this approach.[60] The Weber and Rinne tests both use tuning forks to evaluate hearing. The Weber tuning fork test is performed by pressing the handle of the tuning fork into the forehead or bridge of nose and asking the patient if the sound is louder in one ear or the other; the sound is heard equally in a patient with normal hearing. The Rinne test compares bone conduction and air conduction of sound. To perform the test, the handle of the tuning fork is placed on the mastoid bone. When the patient can no longer hear the sound emitted, the vibrating end of the tuning fork is placed near the external auditory canal. If the patient can again hear the tuning fork, the test is positive or normal.

Additional audiologic assessments completed by an audiologist may be warranted to provide accurate and detailed information regarding the patient's hearing ability. These assessments include audiography, speech determination testing, and tympanometry. The baseline audiogram can help to determine hearing loss over time.

Laboratory tests including blood sugar, complete blood count, and thyroid studies can help to determine whether other medical abnormalities are contributing to the hearing loss.[60] Imaging studies, including magnetic resonance imaging and computed tomography, can be helpful in cases of CNS involvement when neurologic symptoms accompany hearing loss.[58–60]

DEGREES OF TOXICITY

Grading of ocular and otic toxicities is essential for the ongoing monitoring of anticancer therapies. In clinical trials as well as routine oncologic therapy, the National Cancer

Institute's (NCI) Common Terminology Criteria for Adverse Events (CTCAE) is the most widely accepted and used tool for assessing toxicities of cancer treatment. The CTCAE rates toxicity on a scale of 1–5. In general, Grade 1 is defined as mild, such that the patient experiences no or mild symptoms that do not require interventions.[61] Grade 2 adverse events are considered moderate, with minimal, local, or noninvasive interventions indicated and where the symptoms limit age-appropriate instrumental activities of daily living (ADL). Grade 3 adverse events are severe or medically significant but not immediately life threatening; hospitalization is indicated and these symptoms limit self-care ADLs. Grade 4 adverse events have life-threatening consequences, so urgent intervention is indicated. Grade 5 adverse events lead to death. Some symptoms do not have a Grade 5, as death would not occur due to the symptom.

Clinicians can use the CTCAE to grade ocular toxicities including blurred vision, cataracts, conjunctivitis, photophobia, keratitis, glaucoma, dry eyes, and watery eyes (Table 27-3).[61] The otic toxicities described previously, including tinnitus, vertigo, and hearing loss, are included in CTCAE grading (Table 27-4).[61] The otic toxicity grading also delineates differences between adult and pediatric findings.

The previous version of CTCAE for ototoxicity had been criticized for not including lower-frequency hearing loss, which occurs most often in children. To address this issue, other grading tools were developed specifically for children. These include the Brock criteria, the American Speech-Language Hearing Association (ASHA) ototoxic criteria, and the Davis-Silverman criteria.[62–64] The Brock criteria were developed specifically to address platinum-induced hearing loss in children and are used widely in Europe and internationally.[65] Using a scale of 0–4, this instrument measures hearing loss in children based on pure tone audiologic frequencies. As a 0 on the Brock criteria indicates hearing loss, a limitation of these criteria is that

TABLE 27-3

National Cancer Institute Common Terminology Criteria for Adverse Events (CTCAE): Eye Disorders

	Grade				
Adverse Event	**1**	**2**	**3**	**4**	**5**
Blurred vision	Intervention not indicated	Symptomatic: limiting instrumental activities of daily living (ADL)	Limiting self-care ADL		
Cataract	Asymptomatic; clinical or diagnostic observations only; intervention not indicated	Symptomatic: moderate decrease in visual acuity (20/40 or better)	Symptomatic with marked decrease in visual acuity (worse than 20/40 but better than 20/200); operative intervention indicated (e.g., cataract surgery)	Blindness (20/200 or worse) in the affected eye	
Conjunctivitis	Asymptomatic or mild symptoms; intervention not indicated	Symptomatic; topical intervention indicated (e.g., antibiotics); limiting instrumental ADL	Limiting self-care ADL		
Dry eye	Asymptomatic; clinical or diagnostic observations only; mild symptoms relieved by lubricants	Symptomatic; multiple agents indicated; limiting instrumental ADL	Decrease in visual acuity (<20/40); limiting self-care ADL		
Glaucoma	Elevated intraocular pressure (EIOP) with single topical agent for intervention; no visual field deficit	EIOP causing early visual filed deficits; multiple topical or oral agents indicated; limiting instrumental ADL	EIOP causing marked visual field deficits (e.g., involving both superior and inferior visual field); operative intervention indicated; limiting self-care ADL	Blindness (20/200 or worse) in the affected eye	
Photophobia	Symptomatic but not limiting ADL	Limiting instrumental ADL	Limiting self-care ADL		
Watering eyes	Intervention not indicated	Intervention indicated	Operative intervention indicated		

Source: Data from National Cancer Institute Common Terminology Criteria for Adverse Events (CTCAE)[61].

TABLE 27-4

National Cancer Institute Common Terminology Criteria for Adverse Events (CTCAE): Ear and Labyrinth Disorders

	Grade				
Adverse Event	**1**	**2**	**3**	**4**	**5**
Hearing impaired	Adults enrolled in a monitoring program: Threshold shift of 15–25 dB averaged at 2 contiguous test frequencies in at least one ear. Adults not enrolled in monitoring program: subjective change in hearing in the absence of documented hearing loss. Pediatric: Threshold shift >20 dB at 8 kHz in at least one ear.	Adults enrolled in monitoring program: Threshold shift of >25 dB averaged at 2 contiguous test frequencies in at least one ear. Adults not enrolled in monitoring program: hearing loss but hearing aid or intervention not indicated; limiting instrumental activities of daily living (ADL). Pediatric: Threshold shift >20 dB at 4 kHz and above in at least one ear.	Adults enrolled in monitoring program: Threshold shift of >25 dB averaged at 3 contiguous test frequencies in at least one ear. Adults not enrolled in monitoring program: hearing loss with hearing aid or intervention indicated; limiting self-care ADL. Pediatric: Hearing loss sufficient to indicate therapeutic intervention, including hearing aids; threshold shift >20 dB at 3 kHz and above in at least one ear; additional speech-language related services indicated	Adults: Decrease in hearing to profound bilateral loss; non-servicable hearing. Pediatric: Audiologic indication for cochlear implant and additional speech-language related services indicated.	
Vertigo	Mild symptoms	Moderate symptoms; limited instrumental ADL	Severe symptoms; limiting self-care ADL		
Tinnitus	Mild symptoms	Moderate symptoms; limited instrumental ADL	Severe symptoms; limiting self-care ADL		

Source: Data from National Cancer Institute Common Terminology Criteria for Adverse Events (CTCAE)[61].

the system does not distinguish between normal hearing and mild hearing loss.[62–64] The ASHA criteria define ototoxicity as a 20 dB threshold elevation at specific frequencies, a 10 dB elevation at two consecutive frequencies, or absent responses at three consecutive frequencies in post-therapy testing.[62–64] These criteria require a baseline audiogram to compare post-therapy results, which can sometimes be difficult to obtain in very young or acutely ill children.[63] The Davis and Silverman criteria grade hearing loss at a specific threshold. Normal hearing is defined as 0–20 dB, mild hearing loss as 21–40 dB, moderate hearing loss as 41–70 dB, severe hearing loss as 71–90 dB, and profound loss as more than 95 dB.[63,64]

SYMPTOM MANAGEMENT STRATEGIES

THERAPEUTIC APPROACHES

Ocular complications

Therapeutic approaches for ocular complications are focused on symptom management and interventions to minimize further discomfort or damage. Some of the complications resolve when the offending agent is discontinued while others require additional interventions.

Blepharitis. The goal of treating blepharitis is to alleviate the acute symptoms and provide some interventions to help alleviate future exacerbations. As the foundation of treatment, good lid hygiene should be emphasized. No randomized trials have been conducted on specific interventions for blepharitis, so much of the information is based on clinical experiences.[66] Applying heat to the lids and meibomian gland can help to liquefy the abnormal secretions. Warm compresses held in place for 5 to 10 minutes four times a day can accomplish this.[66–68] Following the application of warm compresses, massaging the lids can assist with emptying the meibomian gland and improving secretion.[66] Cleansing the lids following the compresses can be helpful with patients who have a large accumulation of debris. Commercially available eyelid scrubs can be used for this purpose, but equally as effective is the use of very dilute baby shampoo applied with a clean wash cloth, gauze pad, or cotton swab.

Antibiotics can be used to help reduce the population of bacteria in the lashes and conjunctiva. Topical azithromycin ophthalmic solution and erythromycin or bacitracin ointments have been shown to be effective for this purpose.[66,69] With severe long-term cases of blepharitis, oral antibiotics have been shown to be effective in reducing the bacterial colonization in the lid and conjunctiva.[66] Doxycycline 100 mg or tetracycline 1000 mg daily in divided doses for 2 to 4 weeks is frequently used.[66] It is important to educate the patient regarding potential side effects of tetracycline, including photosensitivity, gastrointestinal upset, interference with warfarin, and decreased effectiveness of oral contraceptives. Tetracycline can also cause permanent tooth discoloration and affect bone development. Therefore, in women who are pregnant or nursing or with children younger than the age of 12 with developing bones, erythromycin should be used instead of tetracyline.[66]

Tacrolimus ointment 0.03% twice daily is effective for chronic blepharitis.[67,68] If the patient has only a minimal response, 0.1% tacrolimus cream can be used. With either formulation, tacrolimus should not be used for longer than 6 months.[67,68]

Epiphora. If there is no identifiable mechanical cause of epiphora, the use of artificial tears or antihistamine drops can be effective.[13,15,67,68] Antibiotic eye drops are indicated when there is a bacterial infection involved with the epiphora.[13,15] If the epiphora is a result of nasolacrimal duct obstruction, a new tear duct can be created by connecting the lacrimal sac directly to the nasal cavity; this procedure is known as dacryocystorhinostomy.[13]

Dry eye. In most cases of dry eye, the use of artificial tears is very effective.[70] When dry eyes are not relieved with artificial tears, punctual occlusion, topical cyclosporine, and topical steroids can be therapeutic.[67,68,71] With severe dry eye, such as that seen with autoimmune conditions, systemic immunomodulatory agents such as methotrexate or rituximab can result in significant improvement in tear production and symptom relief.[72]

Conjunctivitis. Patients with viral conjunctivitis require supportive treatment through duration of their symptoms. Antihistamine drops are effective in reducing symptoms throughout the course of the disease.[73,74] Antibiotic eye drops are the mainstay of treatment for bacterial conjunctivitis, and can be used along with antihistamine drops to reduce symptoms and irritation.[74] Because the majority of drug-induced conjunctivitis is manifested with redness, irritation, and serous discharge, treatment with artificial tears, withdrawal of the offending agent, and a short course of topical steroids usually resolve the issue.[74]

Trichomegaly. Although there is no specific treatment for trichomegaly at this time, trimming of the eyelashes with scissors is the most frequent intervention utilized by patients experiencing trichomegaly.[20,67,68,75–83] Some patients elect to have their eyelashes removed using electrolysis, laser, photodynamic therapy, or waxing.[76,79,82,84–87]

Cataracts. The preferred method to remove cataracts is phacoemulsification, which involves inserting an ultrasonic needle into the crystalline lens, breaking apart the cataract, and aspirating it out.[13] An artificial lens is then placed into the lens capsular bag. As with any ophthalmic surgery, there is a risk of persistent inflammation, macular edema, or retinal detachment.[13]

Glaucoma. Glaucoma can be treated with medication, laser procedures, and surgical interventions.[88] Most of the medications used to treat glaucoma work by decreasing the production of aqueous humor in the eye.[88] The exception to this are the prostaglandin medications that work to increase the outflow of aqueous humor from the eye.[88,89] Trabeculoplasty is the most common procedure used to treat glaucoma.[13] This relatively simple and painless procedure, which is performed in an outpatient facility, involves aiming a laser beam at the eye's main outflow structure called the trabecular meshwork.[13]

Photophobia. When treating photophobia, it is important to correct the underlying condition. With chemotherapy-induced photophobia, studies have shown that abrupt withdrawal of the offending agent is effective in reversing photophobia.[13,45,90]

Otic complications

Much of the research involving ototoxicity management focuses on the prevention of symptoms. Given that ROS formation is thought to be a key factor in ototoxicity, prevention strategies include the administration of free-radical scavengers. These scavengers, including amifostine, acetylcysteine, salicylates, and vitamin E, prevent the damaging effects of ROS on proteins, lipids, and DNA.[50,91,92] Amifostine is the only one of these agents that has been used in clinical practice thus far. However, in several studies using amifostine as an otoprotectant, the ototoxicity of cisplatin was not reduced significantly.[50,52,93]

Studies of the treatment of tinnitus have found that the administration of melatonin is associated with a perceptible reduction in tinnitus.[94–96] At a dose of 3 mg daily for 30 days, the improvement was most significant in patients with bilateral tinnitus and those whose sleep was disturbed due to the tinnitus.[95,96] Melatonin is also sleep inducing, which may have added to the effectiveness in some of the patients, as they may just have been able to sleep better and thus not perceive the tinnitus.[95,96]

Management of hearing loss depends on the severity of loss. Moderate to severe hearing loss may require the use of hearing aid devices, whereas mild hearing loss does not.[47] In children with hearing loss, classroom and educational accommodations should be made. Cochlear implants have been effective in children with severe sensorineural hearing loss.[97] Cochlear implants have two parts that are implanted into the child's cochlea. The external part acts as a processor and transmitter of acoustic signals that are received by the internal part, which then translates the information into electrical signals that are read by the cranial nerve.[98] Not all children are candidates for cochlear implants; they have to undergo extensive testing to determine their eligibility for these devices. Other management interventions specifically for children with hearing loss include the use of assistive devices to amplify sounds in group situations such as classrooms as well as school support for children and parents.

NURSING IMPLICATIONS

The majority of optic and otic toxicities, although not life threatening, can cause drastic changes in a patient's lifestyle and quality of life. Ocular toxicities can range from minor irritation to severe problems causing loss of independence. Otic toxicities affect communication, with the ensuring disruption sometimes leading to isolation and depression. It is imperative that the nurse educate the patient and family about the short- and long-term optic and otic toxicities that may potentially arise with anticancer therapies.

PATIENT SELF-CARE

Providing education to patients about their condition is an important role of the nurse. The use of self-care tools allow patients to actively participate in managing their conditions.[99] The evidence indicates that self-care not only increases patient self-efficacy, but also decreases the number of inpatient and outpatient visits, thereby reducing patient costs.[100] With ocular toxicities, including blepharitis, epiphora, dry eye, conjunctivitis, trichomegaly, cataracts, glaucoma, and photophobia, providing patient education regarding self-care interventions, the necessity of continued follow-up, and available resources is imperative (Appendix 27A). Likewise, educating patients about common ear or hearing problems, including ototoxicity, dizziness, and vertigo, is crucial. Self-care tools that assist patients with sensory loss can be invaluable to obtaining more positive outcomes (Appendix 27B).

REFERENCES

1. Ernest A, Edijana C. Ocular toxicity of systemic anticancer chemotherapy. *Pharm Pract.* 2006;4:55–59.
2. Ananth L. Eye anatomy and eye structure: an overview of ocular anatomy. Suite101.com. http://lakshmiananth.suite101.com/eye-anatomy-and-eye-structure-an-overview-of-ocular-anatomy-9261403. Accessed December 29, 2012.
3. Ananth L. Lacrimal gland anatomy: how the lacrimal apparatus works. Suite101.com. http://lakshmiananth.suite101.com/lacrimal-gland-anatomy-how-the-lacrimal-apparatus-works-9267924. Accessed December 29, 2012.
4. Foroozan R. North American Neuro-ophthalmology (NANO) annual meeting: neuro-ophthalmic complications of chemotherapy. 2010. http://content.lib.utah.edu/utils/getfile/collection/ehsl-nam/id/283/filename/image. Accessed December 29, 2012.
5. Schmid KE, Kornek GV, Scheithauer W, Binder S. Update on ocular complications of systemic cancer chemotherapy. *Surv Ophthalm.* 2006;51(1):19–40.
6. Singh P, Singh A. Ocular adverse effects of anti-cancer chemotherapy and targeted therapy. *J Cancer Res Ther.* 2012;1(1):5–12.
7. Hardten DR. Dry eye disease in patients after cataract surgery. *Cornea.* 2008;27(7):855.
8. Blomquist PH. Ocular complications of systemic medications. *Am J Med Sci.* 2011;342(1):62–69.
9. Criado PR. Blepharitis and trichomegaly induced by cetuximab. *An Bras Dermatol.* 2010;85(6):919–920.
10. Ramirez-Soria MP, Espana-Gregori E, Avino-Martinez J, Pastor-Pascual F. Blepharitis related to cetuximab treatment in an advanced colorectal cancer patient. *Arch Soc Esp Oftalmol.* 2008;83(11):665–668.
11. Butovich IS. On the lipid composition of human meibum and tears: comparative analysis of nonpolar lipids. *Invest Ophthalmol Vis Sci.* 2008;49(9):3779–3789.
12. Kaercher T, Bron AJ. Classification and diagnosis of dry eye. *Dev Ophthalmol.* 2008;41:36–53.
13. Hazin R, Abuzetun JY, Daoud YJ, Abu-Khalaf MM. Ocular complications of cancer therapy: a primer for the ophthalmologist treating cancer patients. *Curr Opin Ophthalmol.* 2009;20(4):308–317.
14. Smith J, Nichols KK, Baldwin EK. Current patterns in the use of diagnostic tests in dry eye evaluation. *Cornea.* 2008;27(6):656–662.
15. Lemp MA. Management of dry eye disease. *Am J Manag Care.* 2008;14(3):S88–S101.
16. Eiseman AS, Flanagan JC, Brooks AB, et al. Ocular surface, ocular adnexal, and lacrimal complications associated with the use of systemic 5-fluorouracil. *Ophthal Plast Reconstr Surg.* 2003;19(3):216–224.
17. Alexandrescu DT, Kauffman CL, Dasanu CA. Persistent hair growth during treatment with the EGFR inhibitor erlotinib. *Dermatol Online J.* 2009;15(3):4–8.
18. Foerster CG, Cursiefen C, Knuse FE. Persisting corneal erosion under cetuximab (Erbitux) treatment (epidermal growth factor receptor antibody). *Cornea.* 2008;27(5):612–614.
19. Kerob D, Dupuy A, Reygagne P, et al. Facial hypertrichosis induced by cetuximab, an anti-EGFR inhibitor. *Arch Dermatol.* 2006;142(12):1656–1657.
20. Bouche O, Brixi-Benmansour H, Bertin A, et al. Trichomegaly of the eyelashes following treatment with cetuximab. *Ann Oncol.* 2005;16(10):1711–1712.
21. Carser JE, Summers YJ. Trichomegaly of the eyelashes after treatment with erlotinib in non-small cell lung cancer. *J Thorac Oncol.* 2006;1(9):1040–1041.
22. Lane K, Goldstein SM. Erlotinib-associated trichomegaly. *Ophthal Plast Reconstr Surg.* 2007;23(1):65–66.

23. Symonds JG, Lovicu FJ, Chamberlain CG. Differing effects of dexamethasone and diclofenac on posterior capsule opacification-like changes in a rat lens explants model. *Exp Eye Res.* 2006;83(4):771–782.
24. Perry MC, ed. *The Chemotherapy Source Book,* 4th ed. Philadelphia, PA: Lippincott Williams & Wilkins; 2007.
25. Howell A, Cuzick J, Baum M, et al. Results of the ATAC (Arimidex, Tamoxifen, Alone or in Combination) trial after completion of 5 years' adjuvant treatment for breast cancer. *Lancet.* 2005;365(9453):60–62.
26. Schneider RA, Schultze J, Jensen JM, Hebbinghaus D, Galalae RM. Long-term outcome after static intensity-modulated total body radiotherapy using compensators stratified by pediatric and adult cohort. *Int J Radiat Oncol Biol Phys.* 2008; 70(1):194–202.
27. Li J, Tripathi RC, Tripathi BJ. Drug-induced ocular disorders. *Drug Saf.* 2008;31(2):127–141.
28. Chandler HL, Barden CA, Lu P, Kusewitt DF. Colitz CM. Prevention of posterior capsular opacification through cyclooxygenase-2 inhibition. *Mol Vis.* 2007; 13:677–691.
29. Gupta A, Kaliaperumal S, Sengupta S, Babi RL. Bilateral cataract following lightning injury. *Eur J Ophthalmol.* 2008;16(4):624–626.
30. Gianni L, Panzini I, Li S, et al. Ocular toxicity during adjuvant chemoendocrine therapy for early breast cancer: results from International Breast Cancer Study Group trials. *Cancer.* 2006;106(3):505–513.
31. Conill C, Berenguer J, Vargas M, et al. Incidence of radiation-induced leukoencephalopathy after whole brain radiotherapy in patients with brain metastases. *Clin Transl Oncol.* 2007;9(9):590–595.
32. Fard-Esfahani A, Mirshekarpour H, Fallahi B, et al. The effect of high-dose radioiodine treatment on lacrimal gland functions in patients with differentiated thyroid carcinoma. *Clin Nucl Med.* 2007;32(9): 696–699.
33. Gunduz K, Pulido JS, McCannel CA, et al. Ocular manifestations and treatment of central nervous system lymphomas. *Neurosurg Focus.* 2006;21(5):1–7.
34. Mick P, Weswterberg BD. Sensorineural hearing loss as a probable serious adverse drug reaction associated with low-dose oral azithromycin. *J Otolaryngol.* 2007;36(5):257–263.
35. Cianfrone G, Pentangelo D, Cianfrone E, et al. Pharmacological drugs inducing ototoxicity, vestibular symptoms and tinnitus: a reasoned and updated guide. *Eur Rev Med Pharmacol Sci.* 2011;15(6):601–636.
36. Knoll C, Smith RJ, Shores, Blatt J. Hearing genes and cisplatin deafness: a pilot study. *Laryngoscope.* 2006;116(1):72–74.
37. Reavis KM, McMillan G, Austin D, et al. Distortion-product otoacoustic emission test performance for ototoxicity monitoring. *Ear Hear.* 2010;32(1):61–74.
38. Riga M, Psarommatis I, Korres S, et al. The effect of treatment with vincristine on transient evoked and distortion product otoacoustic emissions. *Int J Pediatr Otorhinolaryngol.* 2006;70(6):1003–1008.
39. Jehanne M, Lumbroso-Le Rouic L, Savignoni A, et al. Analysis of ototoxicity in young children receiving carboplatin in the context of conservative management of unilateral or bilateral retinoblastoma. *Pediatr Blood Cancer.* 2009;52(5):637–643.
40. Yeh SA, Tang Y, Lui CC, Huang YJ, Huang EY. Treatment outcomes and late complications of 849 patients with nasopharyngeal carcinoma treated with radiotherapy alone. *Int J Radiat Oncol Biol Phys.* 2005;62(3):672–679.
41. Wang SZ, Yan XJ, Guo M, Jiang J. Clinical analysis of otitis media with effusion after 3D planning system based radiotherapy of nasopharyngeal carcinoma. *China Oncol.* 2006;16:503–507.
42. Lowery RS. Adult blepharitis. Medscape.com. June 17, 2011. http://emedicine.medscape.com/article/1211763-overview. Accessed December 29, 2012.
43. American Academy of Ophthalmology. Blepharitis: preferred practice pattern. October 2011. http://one.aao.org/CE/PracticeGuidelines/Snippet.aspx?cid=7802696a-baaa-4b10-afda-f95992f81784. Accessed December 29, 2012.
44. National Eye Institute. Facts about cataracts. September 2009. http://www.nei.nih.gov/health/cataract/cataract_facts.asp. Accessed December 29, 2012.
45. Das S, Seitz B. Recurrent corneal erosion syndrome. *Surv Ophthalmol.* 2008;53:3–15.
46. Fontana S, Porth C. Disorders of hearing and vestibular function. In: Porth C, ed. *Pathophysiology: Concepts of Altered Health States.* Philadelphia, PA: Lippincott Williams & Wilkins; 2005:1329–1353.
47. Helt-Cameron J, Allen PJ. Cisplatin ototoxicity in children: implications for primary care providers. *Pediatr Nurs.* 2009;35(2):121–128.
48. Rybak LP, Mukherjea D, Jajoo S, Ramkumar V. Cisplatin ototoxicity and protection: clinical and experimental studies. *Tohoku J Exp Med.* 2009;219(3):177–186.
49. Rybak LP, Whitworth CA, Mukherjea D, Ramkumar V. Mechanisms of cisplatin-induced ototoxicity and prevention. *Hear Res.* 2007;226(1):157–167.
50. van den Berg JH, Beijnen JH, Balm AJ, Schellens JH. Future opportunities in preventing cisplatin induced ototoxicity. *Cancer Treat Rev.* 2006;32(5):390–397.
51. Garcia-Berrocal J, Nevado J, Ramirez-Camacho R, et al. The anticancer drug cisplatin induces an intrinsic apoptotic pathway inside the inner ear. *Br J Pharmacol.* 2007;152(7):1012–1020.
52. Grewal S, Merchant T, Reymond R, McInerney M, Hodge C, Shearer P. Auditory late effects of childhood cancer therapy: a report from the children's oncology group. *Pediatrics.* 2010;125(4):e938–e951.
53. Knight KRC, Kraemer DF, Neuwelt EA. Ototoxicity in children receiving platinum chemotherapy: underestimating a commonly occurring toxicity that may influence academic and social development. *J Clin Oncol.* 2005;23(34):8588–8596.
54. Sullivan MJ. Hepatoblastoma cisplatin and ototoxicity. *Cancer.* 2009;115(24):5623–5626.
55. Oldenburg J, Kraggerud SM, Cvancarova M, Lothe RA, Fossa SD. Cisplatin-induced long-term hearing impairment is associated with specific glutathione-s-transferase genotype in testicular cancer survivors. *J Clin Oncol.* 2007; 25(6):708—714.
56. Barahmani N, Carpentieri S, Li XN, et al. Glutathione S-transferase M1 and T1 polymorphisms may predict adverse effects after therapy in children with medulloblastoma. *Neuro Oncol.* 2009;11(3):292–300.
57. Vorwerk C, Thelen U, Buchholz P, Kimmich F. Treatment of glaucoma patients with insufficient intraocular pressure control: a survey of German ophthalmologists in private practice. *Curr Med Res Opin.* 2008;24(5):1295–1301.
58. Labuguen RH. Initial evaluation of vertigo. *Am Fam Physician.* 2006;3(2):244–251.
59. Shargorodsky J, Curhan GC, Farwell WR. Prevalence and characteristics of tinnitus among US adults. *Am J Med.* 2010;123(8): 711–718.
60. Bagai A, Thavendiranathan P, Detsky AS. Does this patient have hearing impairment? *JAMA.* 2006;295(4):416–428.
61. National Institutes of Health, National Cancer Institute. Common terminology criteria for adverse events (CTCAE). Cancer.gov. June 14, 2010. http://evs.nci.nih.gov/ftp1/CTCAE/CTCAE_4.03_2010-06-14_QuickReference_5x7.pdf. Accessed December 29, 2012.
62. Neuwelt EA, Brock P. Critical need for international consensus on ototoxicity assessment criteria. *J Clin Oncol.* 2010;28(10):1630—1632.
63. Chang KW. Clinically accurate assessment and grading of ototoxicity. *Laryngoscope.* 2011;121(12):2649–2657.
64. Schultz C, Goffi-Gomez MVS, Liberman PHP, Carvalbo AL. Report on hearing loss in oncology. *Braz J Otorhinolaryngol.* 2009;75(5):634–641.
65. Brock PR, Bellman SC, Yeomans EC. Cisplatin ototoxicity in children: a practical grading system. *Med Pediatr Oncol.* 1991;19(4): 295–300.
66. Lindsey K, Sueko M, Elham H, et al. Interventions for chronic blepharitis. *Cochrane Database System Rev.* 2012;16(5):1–128 (CD005556).

67. Basti S. Ocular toxicities of epidermal growth factor receptor inhibitors and their management. *Cancer Nurs.* 2007;30(1 suppl 1):10–16.
68. Burtness B, Anadkat M, Basti S, et al. NCCN task force report: management of dermatologic and other toxicities associated with EGFR inhibition in patients with cancer. *J Natl Compr Canc Netw.* 2009;7(suppl 1): S5–S21.
69. Luchs J. Efficacy of topical azithromycin ophthalmic solution 1% in the treatment of posterior blepharitis. *Adv Ther.* 2008;25(9):858–870.
70. Paugh JR, Nguyen AL, Ketelson HA, et al. Precorneal residence time of artificial tears measured in dry eye subjects. *Optom Vis Sci.* 2008;85(8):725–731.
71. Perry HD, Solomon R, Donnenfeld ED, et al. Evaluation of topical cyclosporine for the treatment of dry eye disease. *Arch Ophthalmol.* 2008;126(8):1046–1050.
72. Dias AC, Modulo CM, Jorge AG, et al. Influence of thyroid hormone on thyroid hormone receptor beta-1 expression and lacrimal gland and ocular surface morphology. *Invest Ophthalmom Vis Sci.* 2007;48(7):3038–3042.
73. Attas-Fox L, Barkana Y, Iskhakov V, et al. Topical tacrolimus 0.03% ointment for intractable allergic conjunctivitis: an open-label pilot study. *Curr Eye Res* 2008;33(7):545–549.
74. Choi H, Lee SB. Nonseasonal allergic conjunctivitis in the tropics: experience in a tertiary care institution. *Ocul Immunol Inflamm.* 2008;16(4):141–145.
75. Osio A, Mateus C, Soria JC, et al. Cutaneous side-effects in patients on long-term treatment with epidermal growth factor receptor inhibitors. *Br J Dermatol.* 2009;161(3):515–521.
76. Marquez G, Herrara-Acosta E, Vidal I, et al. A case of trichomegaly of the eyelashes and facial hypertrichosis induced by erlotinib (Tarceva) [Letter]. *Int J Dermatol.* 2009;48(1):97–98.
77. Robert C, Soria J-C, Spatz A, et al. Cutaneous side-effects of kinase inhibitors and blocking antibodies. *Lancet Oncol.* 2005;6(7):491–500.
78. Lacouture ME, Melosky BL. Cutaneous reactions to anticancer agents targeting the epidermal growth factor receptor: a dermatology–oncology perspective. *Skin Ther Lett.* 2007;12(6):1–5.
79. Shah NT, Kris MG, Pao W, et al. Practical management of patients with non-small-cell lung cancer treated with gefitinib. *J Clin Oncol.* 2005;23(1):165–174.
80. Carser JE, Summers YJ. Trichomegaly of the eyelashes after treatment with erlotinib in non-small-cell lung cancer. *J Thorac Oncol.* 2006;1(9):1040–1041.
81. Braiteh F, Kurzrock R, Johnson FM. Trichomegaly of the eyelashes after lung cancer treatment with the epidermal growth factor receptor inhibitor erlotinib. *J Clin Oncol.* 2008;26:3460–3462.
82. Lane K, Goldstein, SM. Erlotinib-associated trichomegaly. *Ophthal Plast Reconstr Surg.* 2007;23(1):65–66.
83. Bagazgoitia L, Aboin S, Bea A, et al. Trichomegaly due to cetuximab. *Med Clin (Barc).* 2009;133(8):323.
84. Bovenschen HJ, Alkemade JA. Erlotinib-induced dermatologic side-effects [Letter]. *Int J Dermatol.* 2009;48(3):326–328.
85. Papadoupoulos R, Chasapi V, Bachariou A. Trichomegaly induced by erlotinib. *Orbit.* 2008;27(4):329–330.
86. Monti M, Motta S. Clinical management of cutaneous toxicity of anti-EGFR agents. *Int J Biol Markers.* 2007;22(suppl 4):S53–S61.
87. Morse L, Calarese P. EGFR-targeted therapy and related skin toxicity. *Semin Oncol Nurs.* 2006;22(3):152–162.
88. Hazin R, Hendrick AM, Kahook MY. Primary open angle glaucoma: diagnostic approach and management. *J Natl Med Assoc.* 2009;101(1):46–50.
89. Moore W, Nischal KK. Pharmacologic management of glaucoma in childhood. *Paediatr Drugs.* 2007;9(2):71–79.
90. De Marinis M, Rinalduzzi S, Accornero N. Impairment in color perceptions in migraine with and without aura. *Headache.* 2007;47(6):895–904.
91. Paksoy M, Ayduran E, Sanli A, Eken M, Aydin S, Oktay ZA. The protective effects of intratympanic dexamethasone and vitamin E on cisplatin-induce otoxicity are demonstrated in rats. *Med Oncol.* 2011; 28(2):615–621.
92. Bird PA, Begg EJ, Zhang M, Keast AT, Murray DP, Balkany TJ. Intratympanic versus intravenous delivery of methylprednisolone to cochlear perilymph. *Otol Neurotol.* 2007; 28(8):1124–1130.
93. Fouladi M, Chintagumpala M, Ashley D, et al. Amifostine protects against cisplatin-induced ototoxicity in children with average-risk medulloblastoma. *J Clin Oncol.* 2008;26(22):3749–3755.
94. Neri G, De Stefano A, Baffa A, et al. Treatment of central sensorineural stimulus with orally administered melatonin and sulodexide: personal experience from a randomized controlled study. *Acta Otorhinolaryngol Ital.* 2009;29(2):86–91.
95. Reiter RJ, Tan D-X, Korkmaz L, Fuentes-Broto L. Drug-mediated ototoxicity and tinnitus: alleviation with melatonin. *J Physiol Pharmacol.* 2011;62(2):151–157.
96. Lopez-Gonzalez MA, Santiago AM, Estaban-Ortego F. Sulpiride and melatonin decrease tinnitus perception modulating the autolimbic dopaminergic pathway. *J Otolaryngol.* 2007;36(4):213–219.
97. Children's Hearing Institute. Treatments. Childrenshearing.org. 2012. http://www.hearinglosseducation.com/treatments/cochlear-implants. Accessed December 29, 2012 .
98. American Speech-Language Hearing Association (ASHA). Assistive technology: what are assistive listening devices? ASHA.org. 2009. http://www.asha.org/public/hearing/treatment/assist_tech.htm. Accessed December 29, 2012, 2009.
99. Institutes of Medicine. *Priority Areas for National Action: Transforming Health Care Quality.* Washington, DC: National Academies Press; 2003:52.
100. Kennedy AP, Nelson E, Reeves D, et al. A randomized controlled trial to assess the effectiveness and cost of a patient oriented self management approach to chronic inflammatory bowel disease. *Gut.* 2004;53(11):1639–1645.

APPENDIX 27A SELF-CARE GUIDE

Common Eye Problems

Patient Name: ____

Symptom and Description: Blepharitis

Blepharitis is an inflammation of the eyelid that may include reddened eyelids with drainage and crusting around the eyelashes. Common symptoms of blepharitis include the following:

- Red eyes
- Gritty sensation
- Burning sensation
- Excessive tearing
- Itchy eyelids
- Red, swollen eyelids
- Crusting or matting of eyelashes
- Flaking or scaling of the eyelid
- Light sensitivity
- Blurred vision

Management

- Warm compresses
  - o Soak a wash cloth in warm (not scalding) water and place it over your eyes.
  - o As the wash cloth cools, rewarm it and replace it for a total of 5–10 minutes of soaking.
  - o Repeat 2–4 times a day.
- Lid massage
  - o Perform lid massage immediately after applying warm compresses.
  - o Use the cloth you used for your compress or your fingertips.
  - o Gently massage the edge of your eyelid toward the eye with a gentle circular motion.
- Lid washing
  - o Use warm water or warm water with small amount of baby shampoo.
  - o Moisten a clean wash cloth, gauze pad, or cotton swab.
  - o Gently clean along the lashes and lid to remove any accumulated crusts.
  - o Be careful not to touch the eye itself.
  - o Avoid vigorous washing.
- Antibiotic ointment
  - o Your doctor may prescribe an ointment to be used in your eye.
  - o Place the ointment directly onto the eyelid in a thin line.
  - o Use at bedtime since the ointment can cause blurring.

(continued)

Symptom and Description: Watery Eyes

Watering of the eyes, or excessive tearing (called epiphora), occurs when tears spill out of your eyes, even when you are not crying. You may produce tears as a reflex, such as if an object is in your eye, or to lubricate your eye. A patient with watery eyes may experience excessive tearing when not crying that is most often painless.

Management

- Use warm compresses to help your eye to drain if you have any type of eye infection.
- Try to eliminate any additional irritants to your eye such as dust. An air cleaner may be necessary.
- Protect your eyes from light by wearing dark or colored glasses.

Symptom and Description: Dry Eye Syndrome

Dry eye syndrome occurs when your eyes do not produce enough tears. Your eyes may produce excessive tearing, but dry eye syndrome may be causing a lack of important chemicals to lubricate your eyes, which may make them feel dry.

Common symptoms of dry eye syndrome include:

- Dry or gritty feeling in your eye
- Sensation of foreign object in eye
- Excessive watering of eyes

Management

- Use artificial tears or ointments during the day.

Symptom and Description: Conjunctivitis

Many people know conjunctivitis as "pink eye." The name "conjunctivitis" refers to the redness and inflammation that occurs around the conjunctiva—a clear, thin membrane that covers the white of the eye. Conjunctivitis can be caused by allergies, bacteria, or viruses. It is easy to get from dirty hands, washcloths, cosmetics, or towels that have bacteria or viruses attached to them. Most types of conjunctivitis go away on their own in 5–7 days. However, conjunctivitis caused by bacteria may require antibiotic eye drops.

Common symptoms of conjunctivitis include:

- Redness or swelling of eyelids
- Scratchy, watery, itchy eyes
- Pus or discharge from the eye
- Sensitivity to light

Management

- Wash your hands often and avoid contact with family members or others with an impaired immune system.
- Avoid rubbing or touching your eyes.
- Do not share eye makeup or eye cosmetics with anyone.
- If you wear contact lenses, they should be cleaned regularly.
- Avoid wearing contact lenses while you have conjunctivitis.
- Do not share towels or sheets with anyone while your eye problems continue.

- If you have only one eye that is affected, use a separate washcloth and towel for that eye.
- Gently wash your eyelids with a warm, clean moist towel to remove pus and drainage.
- You may receive antihistamine pills or eye drops to relieve your symptoms.
- Do not go swimming in a public pool while you have conjunctivitis.

Symptom and Description: Trichomegaly

Trichomegaly is an excessive growth of eyelashes as a result of your cancer treatment.

Management

- Carefully trim eyelashes with small scissors.
- Pay careful attention to avoid the eye itself.
- You may want to have your eyelashes removed with electrolysis, laser or photo treatments, or waxing.

Symptom and Description: Cataracts

Cataracts are painless and lead to progressive loss of vision occurring over time. A cataract is a cloudy area in the lens of your eye that prevents light from passing through. Cataracts do not spread from one eye to the other.

Common symptoms of cataracts include:

- Cloudy or blurry vision
- Trouble seeing in the dark or at night
- Difficulty with nighttime driving
- Lights appear to be bright or to have a halo around them
- Need to change your eye glass prescription often
- Double vision, which worsens over time

Management

- Notify your healthcare provider about any change in your vision.
- Use a bright light when trying to read.
- Wear corrective lenses to improve your vision.
- Surgery may be recommended by your doctor if your vision gets extremely cloudy.

Symptom and Description: Glaucoma

There are several types of glaucoma. The most common type, open angle, occurs over time, while closed-angle glaucoma occurs suddenly. With glaucoma, the optic nerve is damaged from increased eye pressures. The fluid in your eye, which normally drains out, may build up with glaucoma. Without treatment, pressure on the optic nerve may cause irreversible blindness. Glaucoma cannot be cured but it can be managed. The only symptom of glaucoma is the loss of side vision over time.

Management

- Get regular eye exams yearly.
- Medicines, eye drops, or surgery may be used to reduce eye pressure.
- Surgery, including laser procedures, may need to be repeated every few years.

(continued)

Symptom and Description: Photophobia

Photophobia is the avoidance of light due to pain. It is a common result of injury to the cornea. The pupils are the dark circles in the center of your eye that constrict or get smaller when exposed to light. As a result of injury, swelling of any eye structure may cause pain when your pupils are constricting.

You may notice pain in your eye when you move from a dark to light area. Most people experience photophobia when going outside into the bright light.

Management

- Wearing dark or colored glasses will decrease the amount of light that enters your eye and make you less sensitive to light.
- The most common treatment is to remove the underlying cause of photophobia.

Follow-up

Be sure to call your doctor or nurse:

- If you have eyelashes that are growing in toward your eye
- If you develop any sudden severe eye pain
- If you have sudden loss of vision
- If your eyes become sensitive to light or if you see halos around your eyes
- If your symptoms worsen or do not improve with treatment

Phone Numbers

Nurse: ____________________ Phone: ____________

Doctor: ____________________ Phone: ____________

Other: ____________________ Phone: ____________

Source: O'Leary C. Ocular and Otic Complications. In: Yarbro CH, Wujcik D, Gobel BH, eds. *Cancer Symptom Management.* 4th ed. Burlington, MA: Jones & Bartlett Learning; 2014.

Common Ear/Hearing Problems

Patient Name: ____

Symptom and Description: Ototoxicity

Ototoxicity occurs after you take medications that cause damage to the inner ear; it results in temporary or permanent loss of hearing. Ototoxicity may cause your loss of hearing, if you have one, to become worse. Your risk of ototoxicity increases as the drug accumulates in your body. This side effect may also occur after you receive high doses of drugs that may damage certain cells in your inner ear. The hearing loss you experience as a result of medications may be reversible.

The first sign of ototoxicity may be dizziness. Other symptoms of ototoxicity include:

- Ringing, roaring, hissing, or humming sounds in your head known as tinnitus
  - o Tinnitus may interfere with your ability to rest or concentrate.
  - o You may be unable to sleep at night.
  - o As ototoxicity becomes worse, the sounds become louder.
- Pressure or fullness in your head or ears, like you have a cold
- Loss of hearing
- Existing hearing loss that becomes worsen
- Feeling as if the room is spinning around you or as if you are spinning (vertigo)
- Nausea and vomiting

Management

- Notify your healthcare provider if you notice any dizziness, any change in pattern of dizziness, or any ringing in your ears.
- Drink 2–3 liters of fluid per day to prevent dehydration.
- Carry a sipper cup of your favorite drinks with you.
- Change position slowly.
- Stress or anxiety may increase your tinnitus.
- If your tinnitus increases with stress, relaxation techniques may help.
- Using a quiet radio, television, or low-level sounds when you are trying to rest may help you to ignore tinnitus and make it easier to sleep or relax.

Symptom and Description: Dizziness and Vertigo

Dizziness is a term that describes when you feel "woozy" or "faint." *Vertigo* is a term that describes the feeling that the room is spinning around you. Dizziness may be a sign that the balance mechanism in your inner ear is not working properly. Some causes of dizziness include:

- Medications, including chemotherapy
- If you are dehydrated and change positions
- Stress, tiredness, fever, fatigue, anemia, heart problems, or stroke

(continued)

- Depression
- Breathing hard (hyperventilation)
- Inflammation in your inner ear caused by infection
- Infections in your brain or central nervous system
- Tumors found in your brain or canal of the ear

Common symptoms of dizziness include:

- Most people notice dizziness when they change position or move their heads.
- You might feel like the room is spinning around you.
- Severe dizziness is when you fear that you will fall down if you stand up.
- Some people may lose hearing or vision with dizziness.
- Nausea, ringing in the ear, and vomiting may occur with dizziness.

Management

- Drink 2–3 liters of fluid per day to prevent dehydration.
- Change position slowly.
- With moderate dizziness, walk slowly and often.
- Walk with assistance for severe dizziness.
- If you have vertigo, your healthcare provider may teach you "vestibular exercises" to try to get rid of your dizziness.
- Vestibular exercises involve you sitting down and changing into different positions.

Follow-up

Contact your doctor or nurse about your ototoxicity, dizziness, or vertigo in any of the following circumstances:

- If you develop any sudden severe ear pain
- If you have a temperature greater than 100.5°F
- If you experience vomiting more than 4–5 times in 24 hours
- If you have sudden loss of vision or if you lose your hearing

Phone Numbers

Nurse: ______________________________ Phone: ______________

Doctor: _____________________________ Phone: ______________

Other: ______________________________ Phone: ______________

Source: O'Leary C. Ocular and Otic Complications. In: Yarbro CH, Wujcik D, Gobel BH, eds. *Cancer Symptom Management.* 4th ed. Burlington, MA: Jones & Bartlett Learning; 2014.

CHAPTER 28

Skin and Nail Bed Changes

Linda Morse, RN, MSN

THE PROBLEM

Cancer therapies have a myriad of side effects. Because treatment is traditionally aimed at rapidly replicating cells, side-effect management and research have focused on gastrointestinal and hematopoietic toxicities, targeting events such as bone marrow suppression, nausea, vomiting, and diarrhea. With the exception of alopecia, adverse effects involving the skin, hair, and nails have received less attention until recently. The increased development of molecularly targeted therapies has resulted in unique toxicities involving sensitive areas. Minimization of adverse events of the integumentary system is critical to maintenance of quality of life (QOL) and patient comfort. More than 50 dermatologic toxicities associated with 30 different treatment agents have been described in the literature, making this a significant issue.[1] Some skin changes are merely cosmetic; others interfere with the ability to comfortably walk, work, and even dress.

Cutaneous toxicities can lead to patient discomfort, reluctance to adhere to the treatment schedule, interrupted and delayed drug or radiation schedules, and dose reductions. Furthermore, the financial cost of treating dermatological toxicities is significant. In one study, the mean cost of treating rash associated with cetuximab (including drugs, clinic visits, and other services) came to $2842 per patient with colon cancer; the mean cost for patients with lung cancer receiving erlotinib was $2715 per patient.[2,3] Fortunately, patient education and empowerment, practical prevention strategies, and early evidence-based intervention may make a significant difference in the outcomes associated with these side effects.

Few prospective, randomized trials exploring side effects related to the skin and nails have been published to date, although studies in this area are currently under way. In the meantime, clinicians and scientists have convened to review results of clinical trials and develop consensus statements to provide guidance and recommendations.

In this chapter, a variety of changes in the skin and nails related to cancer treatment are discussed, along with therapeutic approaches for the prevention and management of these changes. Some of the recommendations are evidence based; others are based on anecdotal reports because there are many unanswered and under-researched questions remaining. The terms in Table 28-1 may be helpful, as some of the skin and nail changes may be unfamiliar.

PATHOPHYSIOLOGY OF THE SKIN

The skin is the largest organ of the body. Together with the hair, nails, sebaceous glands, and sweat glands, it constitutes the integument system. The function of the skin is to provide the first line of defense against invasion of foreign substances and loss of fluid, to moderate temperature, and to eliminate waste.[4,5] Skin thickness varies from 0.05 mm (eyelids) to 4 mm on the soles and palms.[4]

The anatomy of the skin is detailed in Figure 28-1. Skin is composed of three layers: the epidermis (most superficial), the dermis (provides support and strength), and the hypodermis (fat tissue).[6] Four types of cells are distributed throughout the epidermis. Melanocytes contain skin pigment called melanin. Langerhans cells help activate the immune system; Merkel cells perform sensory functions.[4]

TABLE 28-1

Definition of Terms
Papule: Palpable, discrete lesion of less than 5 mm. May occur in groups or be isolated. Contains no visible fluid.
Pustule: Small, solid skin elevation containing purulent material.
Desquamation: Shedding of the epidermis. Superficial shedding will lead to flaking or peeling skin. Loss of the entire epidermal layer will result in moisture and weeping of serous fluid.
Paronychia: Inflammation involving the folds of skin surrounding the lateral and proximal finger or toe nail.
Hyperkeratosis: Thickening of the stratum corneum.
Trichomegaly: Abnormally long eyelashes and/or eyebrows.
Hypertrichosis: Kinking of the eyelashes, causing them to turn toward the eye and causing irritation.
Fissure: A narrow, deep skin split extending to the dermis.
Folliculitis: Superficial bacterial infection of the hair follicle. Multiple small, raised, itchy, red lesions less than 5 mm in diameter. Pustules may also be present.

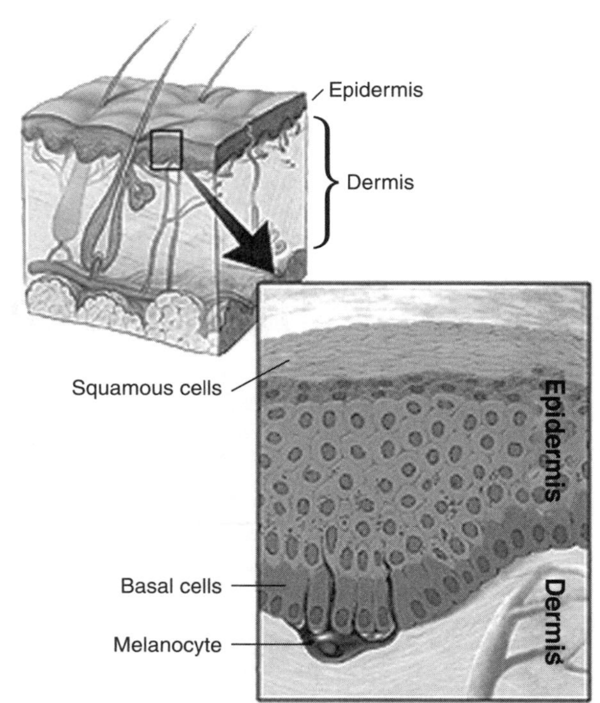

FIGURE 28-1

Skin anatomy.

Source: Data from National Cancer Institute. Don Bliss, Illustrator.

Keratinocytes proliferate and migrate toward the cell surface, ultimately forming the outermost layer.[4,5]

The epidermis is made up of stratified squamous epithelium in three layers: the stratum corneum, the keratinocyte layer, and the basal layer. The stratum corneum, also known as the horny layer, is made up of mature keratinocytes that contain fibrous proteins (keratins). This outer protective barrier is continuously shed, requiring its ongoing replacement. The horny layer is relatively thin, but thicker on the palms of the hands and soles of the feet.[7]

The inner layer is made up of basal cells. These germinal or stem cells continuously divide and form new keratinocytes that mature over time and join the stratum corneum. The life cycle from basal cell layer to stratum corneum is thought to be approximately 3 weeks.[7] Approximately 10% of basal cells divide each day. The basal layer is contiguous with the sheath lining the hair follicle, sharing high epidermal growth factor receptor (EGFR) expression. EGFR expression is lost as keratinocytes migrate from the basal layer to the stratum corneum. High expression is also found in sebaceous glands.[6]

PAPULOPUSTULAR SKIN RASH

Papulopustular rash (PPR) is the most common toxicity associated with both tyrosine kinase inhibitors (TKIs) and monoclonal antibodies (MAbs) that target and inhibit the epidermal growth factor receptor. As development of a rash may be a surrogate marker for response to treatment, it is especially important to take steps to minimize the impact of the rash on the patient and develop successful treatment strategies.[8] The rash can affect the patient's QOL and ability to adhere to the treatment plan.[9] Approximately 32% of healthcare providers report discontinuing treatment, and as many as 76% withholding treatment, which may influence the patient's response to therapy,[10] making it imperative that PPR be optimally managed.

INCIDENCE

The rash resulting from MAbs is slightly more severe and the incidence higher than rash associated with EGFR-TKI agents.[11–13] As many as 80% to 90% of colorectal patients treated with MAbs develop rash, including 9% to 14% with grade 3 or 4.[14–16] In a meta-analysis, the rate of rash with the single-agent EGFR-TKI, erlotinib, was 67.2% to 73.4% for all grades, with 8.0% to 11.0% experiencing high-grade rash.[15] Rash may also occur with multikinase inhibitors (MKIs) such as lapatinib, sorafenib, and sunitinib, although it usually takes a milder form. Some evidence indicates that individuals with a more severe rash are more likely to respond to EGFR inhibitor therapy.[8,17]

Late changes related to PPR include post-inflammatory changes such as hyperpigmentation and telangiectasia.

This outcome is not particular to PPR, but rather may occur in response to cutaneous injury due to many causes. The incidence of this problem is not known at this time.[18]

PATHOPHYSIOLOGY

Papulopustular rash is commonly called "acne-like" or "acneiform," creating confusion because EGFR-related rash is histologically unlike acne and its treatment is different.[14,19–21] EGFR is strongly expressed in normal epidermal and follicular keratinocytes (i.e., the basal layer of the epidermis), with lower expression in the sebaceous epithelium, the outer root sheath of the hair follicle, and eccrine epithelium.[12,21] EGFR stimulates the normal differentiation and development of epidermal keratinocytes, enhances epidermal growth, protects the skin against ultraviolet (UV)-induced damage, inhibits inflammation, and promotes wound healing. It is not well understood why this rash develops. The inhibition of EGFR by TKIs and MAbs seems to lead to abnormal keratinization of the epidermis, rupture of follicles, an increase in inflammation, cytokine release, and the characteristic inflammatory rash.[12,20,22,23] Rash pustules are initially microscopically sterile with no signs of infection.[11,20] However, disruption of the skin barrier may lead to secondary infection with bacteria,[14] often *Staphylococcus aureus*.[20] Microscopic examination also reveals a superficial inflammation surrounding hyperkeratotic or dilated follicular shafts, or neutrophilic folliculitis with rupture of epithelial lining.[24]

SYMPTOM ASSESSMENT

Risk factors

There does not seem to be any association between the risk of developing rash and history of other skin abnormalities such as acne or rosacea.[14] Host characteristics that have been implicated as risk factors for developing erlotinib-related rash include nonsmoking history, fair skin,[25] and age greater than 70 years. Risk factors associated with a cetuximab rash include male gender and age less than 70 years.[24] Exposure to UV radiation may contribute to the development of PPR.[5,13] The incidence and severity of PPR are dose dependent, with higher doses producing more severe rashes.[8]

Self-assessment

Skin changes may occur soon after beginning treatment, making it important to reinforce patient education about reporting any changes to the physician or nurse. Patients may note changes in sensation (burning, tenderness), erythema, and edema preceding the appearance of PPR.[13,14] Rash usually appears within 2 to 4 weeks[24], with MAb-associated rash appearing 1 to 3 weeks after treatment begins.[14] The PPR can wax and wane from day to day or even throughout the day, with exacerbation or spontaneous resolution occurring for no apparent reason.[11,26,27] Ultimately, PPR lesions dry and form crusts.[13]

The PPR develops in cosmetically sensitive areas such as the face, upper chest, scalp, and back.[21] Inhibition of the EGFR-derived UV protection may explain why the rash tends to occur in areas exposed to sun.[28] Less frequently, it may appear on the arms and legs, abdomen, or buttocks.[21] Lapatinib tends to cause rash localized to the trunk and less often on the face.[23] Itchy, tender erythematous papules and pustules emerge.

A late-onset PPR eruption is probably a different entity. This rash has a similar appearance, but occurs approximately 200 days after targeted therapy is started and appears mainly on the trunk (chest, back, buttocks, or thighs). In one study, all patients with this late-onset rash had positive cultures for *S. aureus*. Lesions were larger and more pruritic than those associated with earlier-onset PPR.[19]

The PPR has a significant impact on patient-reported QOL, especially in younger patients. In one trial, patients were asked to complete a dermatology-specific QOL questionnaire.[29] Younger patients (younger than 50 years) were found to have lower QOL than older patients with similar toxicities. The study revealed that higher rates of rash result in lower QOL (grade 1, median score 41.7; grade 2, median score 52.6; grade 3, median score 69.8). There was a more marked effect on emotions as compared to symptoms and functioning.[29] The most bothersome symptoms seem to be pain, burning, stinging, and irritation as well as feelings of depression.[30]

Objective assessment

Physical exam. A baseline assessment of preexisting skin conditions should be documented. It is important to ask each patient to return to the clinic for another examination 1 to 2 weeks after the first treatment when the rash tends to appear or peak. It may be necessary to reinforce preemptive treatment or institute additional remedies as described later in this section.

At the baseline visit, a thorough exam of the skin should be performed, with special attention paid to high-risk areas and any signs of rash, infection such as the presence of purulent material, and small abscesses. PPR is also often accompanied by xerosis (dry skin), pruritus, and discomfort.

The nurse should ask patients if the rash is affecting their body image and QOL. Often people are able to work, shop, exercise, and be socially active while receiving treatment. Other patients may be uncomfortable with their appearance and the questions and comments from other individuals. Every visit is a chance to reinforce teaching, review what is working and what is not, and provide emotional support.

Degrees of toxicity

A limitation in conducting clinical trials is the inadequacy of grading systems. Most authors have used some form of the Common Terminology Criteria for Adverse Events (CTCAE)[31] to assess this side effect (Table 28-2). Some common EGFR-related toxicities are included in Table 28-2, including rash acneiform and dry skin. Although this system is widely used in research, it may not be practical for clinical care. A major problem is that it is not descriptive of this particular rash and does not describe variations in subjective symptoms or the effect of the rash on patient QOL. The only measures included are pain, the need for intervention (or not), and the amount of body surface area involved. This lack of specificity for toxicities related to this class of drugs is true not only for the rash but for other cutaneous effects as well.[13,18]

A new grading system for EGFR-induced toxicities (Table 28-3) has been suggested by the Multinational Association of Supportive Care in Cancer (MASCC).[18] The goal of the MASCC grading system is to classify a particular toxicity according to severity, which should then trigger recommendations for intervention. It should also standardize descriptions of toxicities so clinical trials can be compared. The MASCC system is specific to EGFR-induced dermatologic events.[18,32] It is hoped that adoption of such a scale will facilitate research and that the scale will be more meaningful to clinicians when recommending interventions.

Typical EGFR-related rashes are shown in Color Plate 28-1 (EGFR grade 1 papulopustular rash) and Color Plate 28-2 (grade 3 EGFR papulopustular rash).

TABLE 28-2

National Cancer Institute Common Terminology Criteria for Adverse Events (CTCAE): Selected Skin-Related Toxicities

Rash Acneiform

Grade 1: Papules and/or pustules covering < 10% BSA, which may or may not be associated with symptoms of pruritus or tenderness

Grade 2: Papules and/or pustules covering 10%–30% BSA, which may or may not be associated with symptoms of pruritus or tenderness; associated with psychosocial impact; limiting instrumental ADL

Grade 3: Papules and/or pustules covering >30% BSA, which may or may not be associated with symptoms of pruritus or tenderness; limiting self-care ADLs; associated with local superinfection with oral antibiotics indicated

Grade 4: Papules and/or pustules covering any percent BSA, which may or may not be associated with symptoms of pruritus or tenderness, and which are associated with extensive superinfection with IV antibiotics indicated; life-threatening consequences

Dry Skin

Grade 1: Covering < 10% BSA and no associated erythema or pruritus

Grade 2: Covering 10%–30% BSA and associated with erythema or pruritus; limiting instrumental ADLs

Grade 3: Covering >30% BSA and associated with pruritus; limiting self-care ADLs

Nail Discoloration

Grade 1: Asymptomatic; clinical or diagnostic observations only; intervention not indicated

Nail Loss

Grade 1: Asymptomatic separation of the nail bed from the nail plate or nail loss

Grade 2: Symptomatic separation of the nail bed from the nail plate or nail loss; limiting instrumental ADLs

Nail Ridging

Grade 1: Asymptomatic; clinical or diagnostic observations only; intervention not indicated

Palmar–Plantar Erythrodysesthesia Syndrome

Grade 1: Minimal skin changes or dermatitis (erythema, edema, or hyperkeratosis) without pain

Grade 2: Skin changes (peeling, blisters, bleeding, edema, or hyperkeratosis) with pain; limiting instrumental ADLs

Grade 3: Severe skin changes (peeling, blisters, bleeding, edema, or hyperkeratosis) with pain; limiting self-care ADLs

Abbreviations: ADLs: activities of daily living; BSA: body surface area.

Source: Data from National Cancer Institute Common Terminology Criteria for Adverse Events (CTCAE)[31].

TABLE 28-3

Proposed MASCC EGFR Inhibitor Dermatologic Grading System (Selected Toxicities)

Papulopustular Eruption (Grade individually: scalp, face, chest, back)

Grade 1A: Papules or pustules <5 or 1 area of erythema or edema <1cm in size

Grade 1B: Papules or pustules <5 or 1 area of erythema or edema <1cm in size AND pain or pruritus

Grade 2A: Papules or pustules 6–20; OR 2–5 areas of erythema or edema <1cm in size

Grade 2B: Papules or pustules 6–20; OR 2–5 areas of erythema or edema <1cm in size AND pain, pruritus, or effect on emotions or functioning

Grade 3A: Papules or pustules >20; OR more than 5 areas of erythema or edema <1cm in size

Grade 3B: Papules or pustules >20; OR more than 5 areas of erythema or edema <1cm in size; AND pain, pruritus, or effect on emotions or functioning

Nail Changes: Nail Plate

Grade 1: Onycholysis or ridging without pain

Grade 2: Onycholysis with mild/moderate pain; any nail plate lesion interfering with instrumental activities of daily living (ADLs)

Grade 3: Nail plate changes interfering with self-care ADLs

Nail Changes: Nail Fold

Grade 1: Disruption or absence of cuticle; OR erythema

Grade 2: Erythematous/tender/painful; OR pyogenic granuloma; OR crusted lesions OR any fold lesion interfering with instrumental ADLs

Grade 3: Periungual abscess; OR fold changes interfering with self-care ADLs

Nail Changes: Digit Tip

Grade 1: Xerosis AND/OR erythema without pain

Grade 2: Xerosis AND/OR erythema with mild/moderate pain or stinging; OR finger tip fissures; OR any digit tip lesion interfering with instrumental ADLs

Grade 3: Digit tip lesions interfering with self-care ADLs

Erythema

Grade 1: Painless erythema, blanching; erythema covering <10% body surface area (BSA)

Grade 2: Painful erythema, blanching; erythema covering 10%–30% BSA

Grade 3: Painful erythema, nonblanching; erythema covering >30% BSA

Xerosis (Dry Skin)

Grade 1: Scaling/flaking covering < 10% BSA; NO erythema/pruritus/effect on emotions or functioning

Grade 2A: Scaling/flaking covering 10%–30% BSA + pruritus OR effect on emotions/functioning

Grade 2B: Scaling/flaking + pruritus covering 10%–30% BSA AND effect on emotions/functioning

Grade 3A: Scaling/flaking covering >30% BSA AND pruritus AND erythema AND effect on emotions/functioning AND fissuring/cracking

Grade 3B: Scaling/flaking covering >30% BSA AND pruritus AND erythema AND effect on emotions/functioning AND fissuring/cracking + signs of superinfection

Hair Changes: Scalp Hair Loss or Alopecia

Grade 1: Terminal hair loss < 50% of normal

Grade 2A: Hair loss associated with marked increase in shedding and 50%–74% of normal

Grade 2B: Marked loss of at least 75% of hair compared to normal; may affect functioning in social, personal, or professional situations

(continued)

TABLE 28-3

Proposed MASCC EGFR Inhibitor Dermatologic Grading System (Selected Toxicities) (*continued*)
Hair Changes: Disruption of Normal Hair Growth (Specify): Facial Hair (Diffuse, Not Just Male Beard/Mustache), Eyelashes; Eyebrows, Body Hair, Beard, and Moustache Hair
Grade 1: Distortion of hair growth; does not cause symptoms or require intervention
Grade 2A: Distortion of hair growth in many hairs in given area that cause discomfort or symptoms that may require individual hairs to be removed
Grade 2B: Distortion of hair growth of most hairs in a given area; symptoms or resultant problems requiring removal of multiple hairs
Hair Changes: Increased Hair Changes (Specify): As Above
Grade 1: Increase in length, thickness, and/or density of hair; able to camouflage by periodic shaving, bleaching, or removal of individual hairs
Grade 2A: Increase in length, thickness, and/or density of hairs that is very noticeable and requires regular shaving or removal of hairs to camouflage; may cause symptoms related to hair overgrowth
Grade 2B: Marked increase in density, thickness, and/or length of hair that requires either frequent shaving or destruction of the hair to camouflage; may cause symptoms related to hair overgrowth; without hair removal, inability to function normally in social, personal, or professional situations

Abbreviations: ADLs: activities of daily living; BSA: body surface area; EGFR: epidermal growth factor receptor; MASCC: Multinational Association of Supportive Care in Cancer.

Source: Data adapted from Lacouture ME, Maitland ML, Segaert S, et al. A proposed EGFR inhibitor dermatologic adverse event-specific grading scale from the MASCC skin toxicity study group. *Support Care Cancer.* 2010;18:509–522.[18] Reprinted with kind permission from Springer Science and Business Media.

THERAPEUTIC APPROACHES

Much of what is available to guide clinical practice is a result of the work of experts who have developed practice guidelines.[26,33,34] However, some research findings exist to guide practice, especially in the area of prophylactic or preemptive treatment.[28,35,36]

Prevention

The Skin Toxicity Evaluation Protocol with Panitumumab (STEPP) was a randomized trial comparing the impact of preemptive skin care on toxicity and QOL in patients with colorectal cancer being treated with panitumumab, a MAb directed at EGFR.[28] Of the 95 patients enrolled in this trial, 48 received preemptive treatment, consisting of a skin moisturizer applied to high-risk areas each morning, sunscreen to all sun-exposed areas, topical steroid cream to high-risk areas each night, and doxycycline 100 mg twice a day. The 47 other patients received reactive treatment as the provider deemed necessary. The treatment regimen was chosen for the anti-inflammatory properties of hydrocortisone cream; the anti-inflammatory action (through lymphocyte inhibition) of the tetracycline analogue, doxycycline, as well as its antibacterial properties; a moisturizer to maintain skin integrity; and sunscreen to prevent UV-induced skin damage. Patients on the preemptive regimen experienced a significant reduction of approximately 50% in the development of moderate (grade 2 or higher) skin toxicity (29% versus 62% in the reactive group). Grade 2 or higher skin toxicity was delayed in the preemptive group.[28]

The benefit of prophylactic minocycline has also been demonstrated.[35] In one study, patients receiving cetuximab were randomized to receive either oral minocycline (n = 24) or placebo (n = 24). Patients also used topical tazarotene on one side of the face. Tazarotene was not found to be helpful, leading to significant skin irritation in some patients. Patients receiving minocycline had a lower incidence of severe rash (20% versus 42% with placebo).[35]

Tetracycline has also been tested as a prevention strategy for PPR.[36] In the study investigating this prophylactic regimen, eligible patients were randomly assigned to receive either tetracycline 500 mg twice a day for 28 days (n = 16) or placebo (n = 22). Although tetracycline did not prevent the rash, the antibiotic seemed to reduce rash severity. Patients on tetracycline reported a better QOL as measured by a dermatology-specific questionnaire, especially in such parameters as skin burning or stinging, skin irritation, and being troubled by the persistence or recurrence of skin changes.[36]

The remaining evidence for preemptive or reactive treatment is derived from algorithms developed by expert consensus panels.[26,33,34,37] A summary of recommendations is presented in Table 28-4.[6,11,14,24,27,33,34]

TABLE 28-4

Recommendations for Prevention and Treatment of EGFR Inhibitor Papulopustular Rash
Prevention
• Apply moisturizers, preferably emollients, at least 2 times each day. Suggested products include Eucerin, Aveeno (fragrance-free), Aquaphor, Neutrogena Norwegian formula, SARNA Ultra, Vaseline Intensive Care Advanced Healing Lotion, and Vanicream. • Avoid lotions that contain alcohol. • Apply hydrocortisone 1% to the face, upper chest, and back. • Apply sunscreen of at least SPF 30 to sun-exposed areas. Avoid prolonged sun exposure. • Consider doxycycline 100 mg BID for the first 6 weeks of treatment or minocycline 100 mg daily for 8 weeks. Doxycycline is preferred if renal impairment is present; minocycline is less photosensitizing. • Provide patient education regarding appropriate skin care products, gentle care of skin, and need to notify the doctor or nurse at the first signs of skin rash.
Management of Grade 1 PPR
• Continue treatment at full dose. • Provide psychological support. • Continue preemptive treatment. • Consider topical antibiotic treatment to the affected area (clindamycin 1% gel, erythromycin 3% gel/cream, metronidazole 0.75% to 1% cream/gel). • Consider treatment to the affected area with topical hydrocortisone 1% or 2.5% cream if not used preemptively.
Management of Grade 2 PPR
• Continue treatment at full dose. Provide more intensive follow-up. • Provide psychological support. • Provide topical antibiotic treatment to affected area if not already initiated. • Apply erythromycin 2% lotion for scalp lesions if present. Consider adding triamcinolone acetonide 0.1%. Mix erythromycin and triamcinolone in equal parts of propylene glycol and water. • If pustules are present, consider oral semisynthetic tetracycline (minocycline 100 mg/day or doxycycline 100 mg/day for up to 4 weeks). • Initiate hydrocortisone 2.5% cream or pimecrolimus 1% cream to affected area if not already initiated.
Management of Grade 3 PPR
• Interrupt treatment for up to 21 days or until PPR is improved to grade 2. Restart treatment at full dose or consider whether dose reduction is required, especially if there is recurrent rash. Provide intensive follow-up. • Provide psychological support. • Consider referral to a dermatologist. • Give analgesics. • Give topical and oral antibiotics as above; give steroid or pinecrolimus cream as above. • Consider oral corticosteroids (methylprednisolone 0.4 mg/kg, prednisone 0.5 mg/kg) for up to 10 days and wean patient from the dose. • Consider clindamycin powder 2% in amcinonide lotion. Apply BID.
Management of Grade 4 PPR
• Interrupt treatment immediately. Consider discontinuation of therapy. • Provide psychological support. • Provide referral to a dermatologist. • Give analgesics. • Give intensive topical wound treatment. • Consider systemic treatment with oral retinoids (isotretinoin 0.3–0.5 mg/kg), IV corticosteroids (methylprednisolone, dexamethasone), IV/IM antihistamines, IV broad-spectrum antibiotics (amoxicillin/clavulanic acid, gentamycin), and IV hydration.

Abbreviations: BID: twice daily; EGFR: epidermal growth factor receptor; IV: intravenous; IM: intramuscular; SPF: sun protective factor.

Source: Data from Li and Perez-Soler[6]; Robert et al[11]; Melosky et al[14]; Lacouture et al[24]; Lynch et al[27]; Pinto et al[33]; Thatcher et al[34].

Management

Currently, it is thought that topical corticosteroids are ineffective for treating severe PPR. However, it is possible that they may be useful in minimizing PPR in the early stages due to the anti-inflammatory effect.[17,26,37] This therapy may also be useful after a more severe rash has been treated with antibiotics.[26,37] There have been no clinical trials to test this approach, however. High-potency steroid agents such as clobetasol propionate are also untested. Some believe that topical corticosteroids can be used on the face without significant skin thinning, especially if used for limited time periods. There are no data to support the use of systemic steroids or to confirm that their use does not interfere with the efficacy of EGFR inhibitors.[26] However, administration of systemic steroids in the absence of pustules has been recommended.[17,38]

Topical immunomodulatory agents such as pimecrolimus are interesting due to their anti-inflammatory activity. These agents have anecdotally been found to reduce the severity of rash.[26] To date, no data from clinical trials have been published that support their use.[6,38] Topical retinoids and acne medications should not be used for this indication, as these agents may cause further irritation and exacerbation of the rash.[26]

Practitioners have reported success using shampoos such as Tegrin and Selsun Blue for scalp dryness and irritation. If irritation progresses, clobetasol foam or fluocinolone acetonide shampoo may be helpful.[5] Patients should allow the shampoos to remain on the scalp for 5 minutes, and then rinse thoroughly with water. If pustules or folliculitis appears on the scalp, systemic antibiotics may be necessary.[39]

Antibiotics should be considered for prevention of PPR or treatment of any secondary infection. As noted earlier, some evidence indicates that the use of minocycline for PPR prophylaxis may be useful, both for its antibiotic effect and as an anti-inflammatory agent.[35] Tetracyclines such as minocycline have reasonable activity against *S. aureus*, although other antibiotics, such as topical mupirocin may be used.[11,26,33] Anecdotal evidence suggests that topical antibiotic creams or gels, such as clindamycin, may be useful,[17,38] although no clinical trials have confirmed this benefit.

Xerosis (dry skin) can be minimized with the use of moisturizers. However, as treatment progresses, patients may experience cracking of skin or fissures on the fingertips, similar to "paper cuts." Several remedies have been tried, including continued moisturizing, soaking finger tips in 50% white vinegar with 50% water, and applying Zim's Crack Cream, heavy emollients, or heavy-zinc oxide hand cream to the finger tips.[5,39] Sealing fissures with cyanoacrylate (liquid bandage) or adhesive, high-potency steroid flurandrenolide tape may be helpful.[5]

Crusting or dryness in the nose can be managed with saline nasal spray, moisturized air, and petroleum jelly gently applied to mucous membranes with a cotton-tip applicator.[38,39] To help prevent secondary infection, intranasal mupirocin 2% may be useful.[5]

HAIR CHANGES

Many chemotherapy and targeted agents cause changes in the growth or character of hair. Although alopecia is the change that immediately comes to mind, newer agents, such as EGFR inhibitors, can cause other unique toxicities.

Hair is produced by a group of epidermal cells located at the base of the hair follicle. This follicle extends from the skin surface to the dermis or even deeper. As the epidermal cells divide, the oldest cells progress to the cell surface, become keratinized, and die. Thus hair is actually made up of dead epidermal cells.[4]

PATHOPHYSIOLOGY

Treatment with EGFR inhibitors can lead to several changes in the quality and distribution of the patient's hair. EGF receptors are found in the highest concentration in the basal layer of the skin and the outer root sheath of the hair follicle, where keratinocytes are dividing and undifferentiated.[40] EGFR acts like a switch that turns the growth phase of the hair follicle on and off. These signals vary depending on the normal rate of growth of any particular area of hair, resulting in changes in normal patterns of growth.[11] Hair changes occur in 9% of patients receiving EGFR targeted therapies, typically appearing after 2 to 3 months of treatment.[5]

Trichomegaly—that is, abnormally long hair growth—presents after several months of treatment and can affect both lashes and (less commonly) eyebrows (Color Plate 28-3). Lashes grow and may curl, turning back toward the cornea and irritating the eye (hypertrichosis).[5,38] Due to the sometimes extreme length, lashes may brush against eyeglasses.

Scalp hair may become thin, brittle, curly, or unruly, and diffuse alopecia may occur.[41] Hair loss may also be androgen-like (frontal) and may indicate modification of androgen signaling.[40] Generally, patients will notice minimal hair loss on the scalp, arms, and legs, although women may note an increase in hair growth on the face and upper lip.[42] Hair loss is more common 7 to 10 weeks into treatment and occurs in 5% to 6% of patients.[27]

Alopecia is found in 27% of patients treated with sorafenib and in 6% of patients receiving sunitinib, generally after 3 to 15 weeks of treatment.[43] Hair may regrow during treatment, although it may be brittle, thin, and curly during this period. Sunitinib causes hair depigmentation in 10% of patients after 5 to 6 weeks of treatment. Due to cyclic dosing of sunitinib, bands of depigmented hair may develop.[43] Hair appears grayish in color, but this effect is reversed after sunitinib is discontinued.[44]

THERAPEUTIC APPROACHES

Patient preparation and education are important. Treatments may include depilation of unwanted facial hair. The only known treatment for trichomegaly is to have the lashes cut periodically by a friend, cosmetologist, or ophthalmologist. Lashes may need to be removed by an ophthalmologist to avoid corneal abrasion, ulceration, and erosion.[5,18,21,41]

HAND–FOOT SYNDROME AND HAND–FOOT SKIN REACTION

Hand–foot syndrome (HFS), also known as palmar–plantar erythrodysesthesia (PPE) or acral erythema, is a painful, erythematous inflammation of the skin. Although the palms of the hands and the soles of the feet are most commonly affected, other areas of the body may be involved, such as skin areas exposed to pressure (e.g., the belt line, under the breasts, the groin). Inflammation can progress to blistering and superficial desquamation. After withdrawal of the agent causing the reaction, tissue regenerates.[45,46] Color Plate 28-4 (erythema and desquamation of the palms) and Color Plate 28-5 (erythema and edema of the plantar surface of the foot) show typical HFS.

Hand–foot skin reaction (HFSR) is a distinct syndrome.[47–49] Even so, HFSR and HFS share some qualities, such as distribution pattern, dose dependency, and discomfort. Compared to HFS, HFSR is associated with different anticancer drugs, is generally less diffuse, and is complicated by the development of areas of hyperkeratosis that resemble thick calluses. Hyperkeratosis may occur without other associated signs and symptoms.[49] Typical hyperkeratosis on the foot of someone with HFSR is seen in Color Plate 28-6.

INCIDENCE AND ETIOLOGY

Hand–foot syndrome is seen with anthracyclines and antimetabolites and drugs with prolonged serum levels either due to a long half-life or due to schedules that involve prolonged dosing. HFS is also dose dependent. Chemotherapy regimens associated with HFS include liposome-encapsulated doxorubicin (PLD), 5-fluorouracil (5-FU) given as a prolonged infusion, capecitabine, bleomycin, docetaxel, methotrexate, thiotepa, cytarabine, lomustine, hydroxyurea, 6-mercaptopurine, and interleukin-2.[46,50,51] As many as 50% of patients receiving PLD are affected by HFS, although the numbers reported are quite variable.[52] HFS incidence is correlated with higher PLD doses and increased number of cycles.[53]

Hand–foot skin reaction is a similar entity to HFS, but is associated with a different class of anticancer agents—the multikinase inhibitors, such as sunitinib and sorafenib. MKIs target multiple molecular pathways, blocking uncontrolled cell division. Sunitinib causes HFSR in 18.9% of patients treated, with 5.5% developing more severe reactions. Sorafenib is associated with HFSR in 33.8% of patients treated with this agent, with 8.9% developing more severe reactions.[48,54–56] Both drugs are administered orally, providing continuous, prolonged exposure to drug. It is possible that inhibition of one or more of the pathways targeted by the MKIs is involved in HFSR development.[57] The incidence and severity of HFSR have been found to be higher when sorafenib is combined with vascular endothelial growth factor (VEGF) antibody, bevacizumab, with this regimen resulting in HFSR in 79% of recipients.[58] In an interesting twist, drugs that inhibit single pathways are not associated with HFSR.[55] More recently, a new BRAF inhibitor, vemurafenib, has been used in clinical trials for patients with lung cancer and has been FDA approved for the treatment of malignant melanoma. This agent has been found to be associated with the development of squamous cell skin carcinoma and MKI-like cutaneous skin changes such as HFSR.[59]

HFS and HFSR are compared and contrasted in Table 28-5.[40,45,48,49,52,55,56,60]

PATHOPHYSIOLOGY

It is not well understood why HFS and HFSR occur, but some researchers hypothesize that pressure on the palmar and plantar surfaces leads to capillary rupture and extravasation of the drug, causing an inflammatory reaction. Others have noted that the drug is found in higher concentrations in the eccrine sweat glands in affected areas, leading to the hypothesis that the reactions may be a direct toxicity from chemotherapy.[46,50,52,60] Histologically, the hyperkeratotic lesions characteristic of HFSR contain band-like areas of necrotic keratinocytes, telangiectasias, and inflammatory infiltrate. The depth of keratinocyte changes varies, with patients initiating MKI therapy fewer than 30 days earlier having changes in lower levels of the epidermis and patients treated for 30 or more days demonstrating changes in the stratum corneum.[61]

SYMPTOM ASSESSMENT

Risk factors

Body areas experiencing repetitive pressure, such as the palms and soles, are at higher risk for HFS. Other high-risk areas include the belt line, under the breasts, and the groin.[45,46] Body areas with excess sweating may be at increased risk, and individual sweat patterns may make some patients more susceptible to this syndrome. In one study, patients who produced more sweat in the palms and soles were more likely

TABLE 28-5

Comparison of HFS and HFSR

	Hand–Foot Syndrome (HFS)	Hand–Foot Skin Reaction (HFSR)
Associated agents	Liposomal doxorubicin 5-Fluorouracil infusion Capecitabine Bleomycin Docetaxel Paclitaxel Methotrexate Thiotepa Cytarabine Lomustine Hydroxyurea 6-Mercaptopurine Interleukin-2 Etoposide Cyclophosphamide Melphalan Daunorubicin Idarubicin Cisplatin Vincristine Mitomycin	Sunitinib Sorafenib Vemurafenib
Signs and symptoms	Pain Swelling Numbness/tingling Dysesthesia Symmetrical erythema and edema Blistering, fissuring Desquamation that can progress to ulceration and crusting Any high-pressure area (e.g., groin, buttocks) More diffuse and symmetric	Pain Edema Numbness/tingling Dysesthesia Flat blisters with erythematous halo Desquamation Painful, hyperkeratotic lesions Scaly skin calluses More localized lesions, usually on heels and forefoot but can be on any high-pressure area such as joints and fingertips
Incidence	2%–56% Dose and schedule dependent	19%–60% Dose dependent
Time to onset	2–12 days after infusion May require repeated exposure	14–28 days after initiating therapy Rare after 6 weeks

Source: Data from Lacouture et al[40]; Sanborn and Sauer[45]; Anderson et al[48]; Balagula et al[49]; Payne et al[52]; Gomez and Lacouture[55]; Kollmannsberger et al[56]; Lorusso et al[60].

to develop HFS.[60] The incidence of HFS also increases as the dose of drug and number of cycles given increase.[53] HFSR is most commonly found on the palms and soles, although it may involve lateral sides of the fingers and toes.[55,62]

Self-assessment

As HFS develops, patients may describe numbness and tingling of the hands and feet, and discomfort when handling hot objects. Symptoms usually appear from 2 to 12 days after administration of the chemotherapy. HFS may have an impact on the ability to perform usual activities and on QOL. If chemotherapy is not delayed or the dose reduced, patients may experience further deterioration.[45,46,60] Patient education is of prime importance so changes are detected and treated early. Patients should be encouraged to not minimize the severity of symptoms.[63]

A similar presentation occurs with HFSR: erythema, paresthesias, and dysesthesias of the palms and soles. During the first month of treatment with an MKI, patients should examine their feet daily for callus formation or buildup of existing calluses. After the first month, the patient should examine these areas at least weekly. Patients should report any changes, as blistering and the emergence of thick, painful, hyperkeratotic lesions may follow.[47,62,64] These lesions may be especially difficult for elderly persons, who often have problems with balance, ambulation, and accomplishing daily tasks.

Objective assessment

Physical exam. The physical exam of a person with HFS may reveal a dry, furrowed skin appearance of the hands and feet, sometimes with fissuring. This condition can progress to edema and diffuse erythema of the palms and plantar surfaces, sometimes including the dorsal areas of the hands and feet. Other areas of high pressure should also be examined, such as the belt line, sacral area, and elbows. Recovery from HFS usually occurs within 1 to 2 weeks. If chemotherapy is not delayed or the dose reduced, earlier symptoms of HFS may be followed by blistering desquamation, crusting, ulceration, and necrosis of the skin, with associated discomfort and significant changes in the ability to perform activities of daily living.[12,45,46,55,60] Figures 28-5 and 28-6 show the characteristic appearance of HFS.

MKIs are often used in the elderly, who may have preexisting calluses. Calluses protect skin from the effects of constant friction and are most often found on the heels and balls of the foot. Calluses are more common in women, black individuals, and people older than age 65. It may be useful to construct a baseline "foot map" of preexisting calluses. Baseline evaluation should also include assessment for diabetes, peripheral neuropathy, peripheral vascular disease (PVD), and immunosuppression. These comorbidities place patients at risk for altered skin integrity and infection, and patients should be cautioned against self-treatment of such conditions.[62]

Patients with signs and symptoms of HFSR will have a more localized presentation. Blisters may be found over high-pressure areas of the feet or hands. These can progress to hyperkeratosis, typically evidenced as an area of yellowish, painful plaque found especially on the heel and metatarsals. The area may be surrounded by an erythematous, edematous halo.[48,55,56,63] Plaques can be quite painful and can severely interfere with functional status.[65] Desquamation may also be present, especially with sunitinib treatment.[57] The reaction can appear as early as 1 to 2 weeks after beginning drug treatment.[47,48,54,57,65]

Degrees of toxicity

The most recent version of the National Cancer Institute's Cancer Therapy Evaluation Program (CTEP) Common Terminology Criteria for Adverse Events, Version 4.0 (CTCAE v4.0),[31] does not differentiate between HFS and HFSR. Version 4.0 includes one adverse event, palmar–plantar erythrodysesthesia (PPE) syndrome, although hyperkeratosis is not characteristic of PPE. (See Table 28-2.) While the CTCAE does capture the subjective experience of pain, the symptoms associated with HFS and HFSR are omitted. Likewise, the impact on functional status is present, but QOL is omitted. Future editions may capture differences between the syndromes and describe the experience more accurately; precise categorization is imperative in clinical trials investigating symptom management.

THERAPEUTIC APPROACHES

At present, there are no evidence-based guidelines for the prevention and management of HFS or HFSR. In clinical practice, management strategies for HFS and HFSR include patient education, prevention, early detection, and maintenance of optimal comfort and skin integrity. Education is critical in the management of this skin reaction. Although many of the recommendations for prevention and treatment of HFSR and HFS are the same, care of calluses is particular to HFSR.

Prevention

A consensus panel reviewed 56 abstracts related to MKI-associated HFSR. None of the prevention or management strategies were from randomized, controlled trials. The authors combined this review with their personal experiences or recommendations. The result was a "3C" approach for prevention and management of HFSR associated with MKIs: control calluses, comfort feet with cushions, and cover with creams.[48,57,62] Although its recommendations were specifically for HFSR, with the exception of issues relating to callus control, the panel's findings are likely useful for patients at risk for HFS.

Preventive strategies include a pretreatment manicure and pedicure, or treatment by a podiatrist prior to beginning therapy for removal of preexisting hyperkeratotic areas. Use of emollients to moisturize callused areas and use of keratolytic agents to exfoliate them are recommended, using products such as salicylic acid and urea.[48,57,62]

Prevention of both HFSR and HFS should include wearing well-fitting shoes and slippers, using a cushioning gel or silicone shoe insert, and avoiding pressure on the palms and soles. Shoes should be fitted late in the day when feet are most swollen, allowing ample room. Laced shoes will facilitate adjustments in refitting as the feet change size. Shoes should not rub on the heels, as this may lead to irritation and callus formation. Care should be made that socks fit well and are seamless, absorbent, cushioned, and moisture wicking.[62]

Hot water baths and showers should be avoided, as well as long walks and running. Hands can be protected with gloves and avoidance of repetitive activities. Patients should be encouraged to wear loose-fitting underclothing and natural fibers. Foot soaks with warm water Epsom salts (magnesium sulfate) may be soothing. Overheating and sun exposure cause sweating, which can increase reactions. In such a case, wash gently and pat skin dry.[48,56,57,62,66]

Persons at risk for HFSR should also be taught debridement techniques for managing calluses. If not in the special group of people at increased risk for complications (e.g., persons with diabetes, peripheral neuropathy, peripheral vascular disease, or immunosuppression), patients should soak their feet for 20 to 30 minutes followed by gentle debridement with a tool such as a fine- to medium-grade pumice stone or an emery board. Any vigorous debridement should be performed by a professional. Any person at increased risk for alterations in skin integrity, ulceration, and infection should avoid pumice stones, emery boards, razor blades, and over-the-counter remedies containing salicylic acid. Individuals with diabetes should maintain good blood sugar control and perform prophylactic foot care.[62]

Although vitamin B_6 (pyridoxine) in doses of 50–150 mg daily may be helpful in preventing HFSR, this therapy has not been found to be helpful in the management of the syndrome once it occurs.[55] Other researchers have found pyridoxine ineffective in preventing HFS. A randomized, double-blind, placebo-controlled study of 360 patients receiving capecitabine therapy revealed no difference in incidence of HFS between participants receiving placebo and those receiving pyridoxine 100 mg BID. The incidence of HFS of all grades was 81.7% in the placebo arm and 77.8% in the treatment arm. HFS grades 2 and 3 occurred in 30.6% of patients in the placebo arm and 31.7% of treated patients.[67] Pyridoxine was also found to be ineffective in a double-blind, randomized, placebo trial in patients receiving PLD. Patients ($n = 18$) receiving pyridoxine demonstrated HFS (52%) at a rate similar to patients ($n = 16$) receiving placebo (50%). No differences were found in the toxicity grades.[68] Until further data about the role of pyridoxine in the prevention of HFSR and HFS become available, many healthcare providers are prescribing it due to its low probability of causing harm and its low cost.[60] However, there are no data supporting this treatment approach.

Also among the consensus panel's recommendations for prevention of HFSR were glucocorticoids and cyclooxygenase-2 (COX-2) inhibitors. Glucocorticoids are recommended based on expert opinion; there is no evidence from clinical trials to support their use. COX-2 inhibitors are recommended based on successful prophylaxis of HFS when used with capecitabine.[48]

One randomized trial of 137 patients receiving capecitabine failed to show efficacy from the use of a keratolytic agent. No difference was found at the end of one cycle in the incidence of moderate or severe HFS between use of a urea/lactic acid-based keratolytic agent versus a placebo cream.[69] Other sources suggest that patients who are at risk for HFSR begin using over-the-counter–strength salicylic acid and/or urea-containing lotions twice daily at the first sign of changes in sensation in the hands or feet to provide natural exfoliation.[66] Maintaining soft, pliable skin may help preserve skin integrity.

Researchers have investigated the effect of cooling the hands and feet while infusing PLD on the incidence of HFS. Results have been mixed. A prospective, nonrandomized trial studied 53 patients who received either single-agent PLD or PLD combined with carboplatin and paclitaxel; all participants received dexamethasone and pyridoxine premedication. In addition, 28 patients used ice packs on their hands and feet during infusion. PLD doses ranged from 30 mg/m^2 to 50 mg/m^2 every 21 to 28 days. Cold was found to significantly delay the onset of HFS only if the PLD dosage was in the range of 30–35 mg/m^2. Overall, the treatment was well tolerated.[71]

A second trial looked retrospectively at 330 patients who received single-agent PLD, some of whom used hand and foot cooling. HFS occurred in 102 patients. Predictors for HFS included higher PLD dose and more PLD cycles. One interesting finding was that patients who used cooling developed HFS more often (39%; 48 of 123) than those who did not (26%; 54 of 207).[54]

Patients need to be aware of the signs and symptoms of HFS and HFSR, and know to contact the nurse or doctor when symptoms or skin changes. As noted earlier, patients with comorbidities such as diabetes, peripheral vascular disease, peripheral neuropathy, or compromised immunity should be cautioned against self-treatment without professional supervision. Recommendations for the prevention of HFSR are listed in Table 28-6.[39,49,55,62,66]

Management

The HFSR consensus panel also made recommendations for the management of HFSR treatment according to grade. The following discussion is based on its results.

Grade 1 toxicity is characterized by minimal skin changes without pain. Usual activities are not disrupted. Recommendations include no interruption in anticancer treatment, control of callused areas, moisturizing skin with creams, continued patient education, and cushioning affected areas. To control hyperkeratosis, a keratolytic agent such as 20% to 40% urea or 6% salicylic acid may be used for exfoliation. Alpha hydroxyl acid (5% to 8%) twice a day may also provide chemical exfoliation.[48]

TABLE 28-6

Preemptive Recommendations for Hand–Foot Skin Reaction

- Patient education is of prime importance to minimize this complication and initiate early treatment.
- Perform a baseline skin examination for hyperkeratotic areas (especially palms and soles). Examine the feet and hands, making note of existing skin lesions. Teach the patient to examine the hands and feet.
- Ensure removal of calluses by a qualified individual (minor calluses can be removed by manicure/pedicure; more extensive calluses should be treated by a podiatrist).
- Encourage a manicure and pedicure prior to initiation of treatment. Educate patients about exfoliation of skin, to be done weekly.
- Instruct patients to avoid hot water in the shower and bath and to use tepid water with dish washing. Patients should not use hot tubs.
- Instruct patients to use mild soaps such as Aveeno, Cetaphil, or Dove products.
- Vigorous rubbing of the skin should be avoided. Instruct patients to pat skin dry after a shower or bath and to avoid constrictive clothing.
- Excessive pressure on the feet should be avoided. Instruct patients to avoid long walks, running, or other activities that can cause excessive pressure on the feet. Advise patients to wear well-fitting shoes with padded insoles; soft, thick socks; and slippers and to avoid walking in bare feet.
- Excessive pressure on the hands should be avoided. Protect hands with gloves during gardening. Avoid repetitive motions such as raking, shoveling, and cutting with scissors. Avoid carrying heavy bags.
- Instruct patients to use moisturizing creams twice a day. Creams containing ammonium lactate (Amlactine) or urea are recommended. Alternatively, use a heavy moisturizer such as Vaseline. Maintain skin integrity by keeping skin soft and pliable.
- Skin should be protected from sun exposure with shading and/or sunscreen. Sunscreen should have a SPF of at least 30. If wearing sandals, patients should be taught to apply sunscreen to the feet or to cover them to protect the feet from sunlight.
- Encourage frequent communication, especially during the first month of treatment. Reinforce teaching in each discussion. Patients should be aware of contact information and the need to inform the doctor or nurse at the first symptoms of HFSR.

Source: Data from Balagula and Lacouture[49]; Gomez and Lacouture[55]; Wood et al[62]; Pyle et al[66].

Reactions may progress to the more serious grade 2, which is characterized by skin changes such as peeling, blisters, bleeding, edema, or pain, but does not interfere with function. Patients will notice painful redness and swelling of the hands and feet, and possible discomfort. Skin may be thickened and edematous. Recommendations are the same as for grade 1 reactions, with the possible addition of anticancer drug dose modification.[48,62]

Grade 3 reactions involve skin changes and pain that affect the ability to function. Skin may scale or shed, resulting in open sores, blisters, and skin thickening. Callused areas may be quite thick and painful. In addition to the recommendations for grade 2 reactions, the HFSR consensus panel recommended using topical therapies including cortisone creams, topical antibiotics, wet disinfectants, emollients, and urea-based cream. Systemic pyridoxine 50–150 mg each day may be implemented; systemic steroids are not recommended at this time. Treatment with the anticancer agent should be held, and the dose reduced when treatment is ultimately resumed.[48,62]

There is little evidence to guide practice related to HFSR. An uncontrolled study of 12 patients suggested improvement of painful hyperkeratotic lesions with 40% urea cream, a keratolytic agent (produces loosening of the horny or outer skin layer and skin shedding), 0.1% tazarotine cream (reduces epidermal growth and reduces inflammation), and 5% fluorouracil cream (when applied topically, has been used successfully to treat inherited tender hyperkeratotic skin lesions). All patients treated with one or more of these agents had improvement in their lesions and dermatologic QOL.[61] Anecdotal evidence suggests that this cream with fluocinonide 0.05% (a high-potency steroid) may help.[62]

Once the hyperkeratotic area is treated, it is important to keep the area moisturized to prevent recurrence. Non-urea-based creams such as Eucerin, Vaseline, and CeraVe may be helpful and should be applied liberally to hands and feet.[54,62] Table 28-7 lists several skin care products from a variety of sources that may be useful in the care of patients with HRS and HFSR.[44,48,57]

Although not life-threatening, HFS and HFSR can lead to significant patient discomfort and disability. In a study of 91 women receiving chemotherapy for breast or gynecological cancer, skin changes were the most frequently reported unpleasant side effect (34.1%). Of the women who developed HFS, 47% reported it to be the most unpleasant side effect.[71] Its occurrence can lead to treatment interruption or dose reduction, potentially leading to lower treatment response rates.[49] Unlike some other skin changes due to cancer treatment, there are many recommendations for prevention and treatment of HFS and HFSR that make it possible for the patient to participate in self-care.

TABLE 28-7

Selected Skin Care Products for Hand–Foot Reactions

Over-the-Counter Product	Product Information
Cetaphil skin cleansers, Aveeno shower gel, Dove products	Nondeodorant, perfume-free products
Udderly Smooth Extra Care Cream	Thicker for more intense moisturization than lotions; anti-itch formulations available; contains allantoin, dimethicone, and 10% urea
Gold Bond Triple Action Relief Cream	Thicker for more intense moisturization than lotions; anti-itch formulations available; contains 5% dimethicone, 0.15% menthol, aloe, and vitamin E
Norwegian Formula Smoothing Relief Anti-itch Moisturizer by Neutrogena	Contains 5% dimethicone, camphor 0.1%, and lidocaine
Norwegian Formula Foot Cream by Neutrogena	Contains cetearyl alcohol, dimethicone, methol, and urea
Bag Balm	Cooling effect; contains 8-hydroxyquinoline sulfate 0.3% in petroleum lanolin; eucalyptus
Eucerin cream	Use at night due to greasy formulation; contains mineral oil and lanolin
Eucerin Dry Skin Therapy	Contains urea and alpha hydroxyl acid
Aquaphor Healing Ointment	41% petrolatum
Kerasal	5% salicylic acid softens skin; 10% urea exfoliates and moisturizes
Blue Lizard	UVA and UVB sunblock, water resistant

Source: Data from Schwandt et al[44]; Anderson et al[48]; Manchen et al[57].

NAIL TOXICITY

Nails protect the ends of the fingers and toes. The nail plate consists of a hard keratin cover protecting an epithelial layer made of rapidly proliferating cells. These cells differentiate and keratinize to form the nail plate. The rapidly dividing cells are sensitive to chemotherapy damage, which can result in abnormal nail growth.[51] The cuticle protects the surrounding area from infection and trauma.

INCIDENCE AND ETIOLOGY

Nail changes are a relatively uncommon consequence of chemotherapy. Some changes are more characteristic of molecularly targeted agents. Presentation depends on the nail structure affected and the severity of the insult. The taxanes and anthracyclines are the cytotoxic drugs most commonly implicated.[73] Docetaxel leads to nail changes in 88% of patients, with 43% experiencing challenges in carrying out normal activities.[73] Nail toxicity, usually paronychia, has been observed in 10% to 15% of patients receiving EGFR inhibitors, generally no earlier than 4 to 8 weeks after treatment begins.[74]

Changes can be divided into three categories: changes caused by damage to the nail bed, damage to the nail plate, and damage to the fold surrounding the nail.[47] Changes may be simply cosmetic, or may have significant impact on functioning and QOL.

Damage to the nail bed

Onycholysis is separation of the nail plate from the nail bed. This toxicity is thought to be caused by damage to the nail bed epithelium by either direct cytotoxic effects or antiangiogenic effects of chemotherapy.[46,47] The separation may be painful or may cause no discomfort. Onycholysis occurs more commonly in the great toes and resolves when chemotherapy stops.[45] It may also occur only in the fingernails when combined with exposure to ultraviolet light.[46] Drugs associated with onycholysis include the taxanes, bleomycin, capecitabine, doxorubicin, fluorouracil, methotrexate, etoposide, mitoxantrone, and hydroxyurea.[45,52,72]

Interventions include keeping nails short to avoid traumatic removal of the nail, protecting the nail with a bandage, applying topical antimicrobial agents, and avoiding irritating substances. Use of local cooling of the hands or feet may significantly decrease the incidence and severity of this problem.[72,75]

Subungual hemorrhages or splinter hemorrhage are tiny areas of bleeding under the nails. They appear as painless black or red lines under the nails, and are more common on the hands than the feet. The hemorrhages actually occur in the epidermis of the nail bed and adhere to the underside

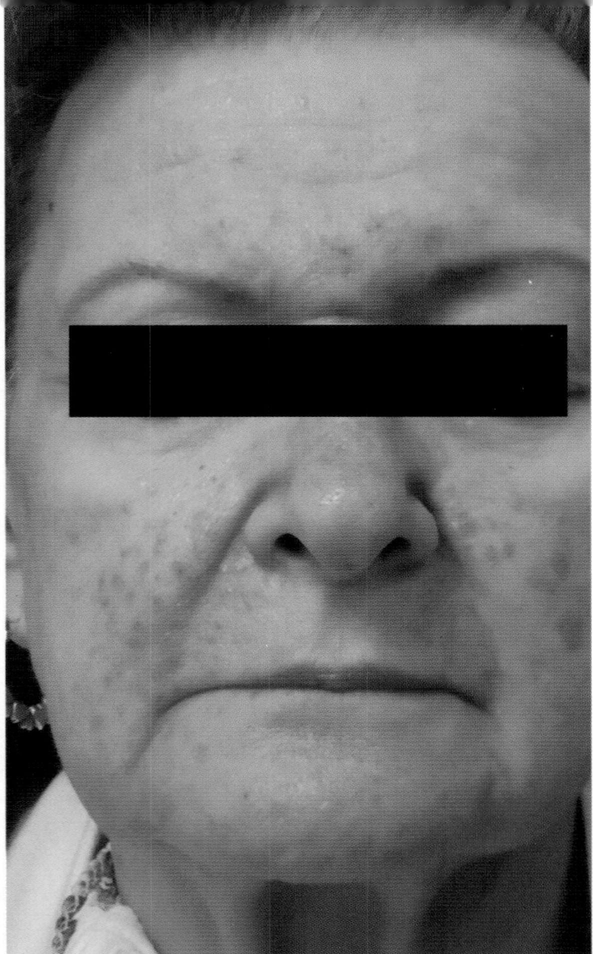

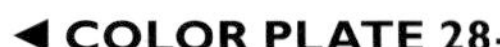

◄ COLOR PLATE 28-1

Grade 1 EGFR papulopustular rash.

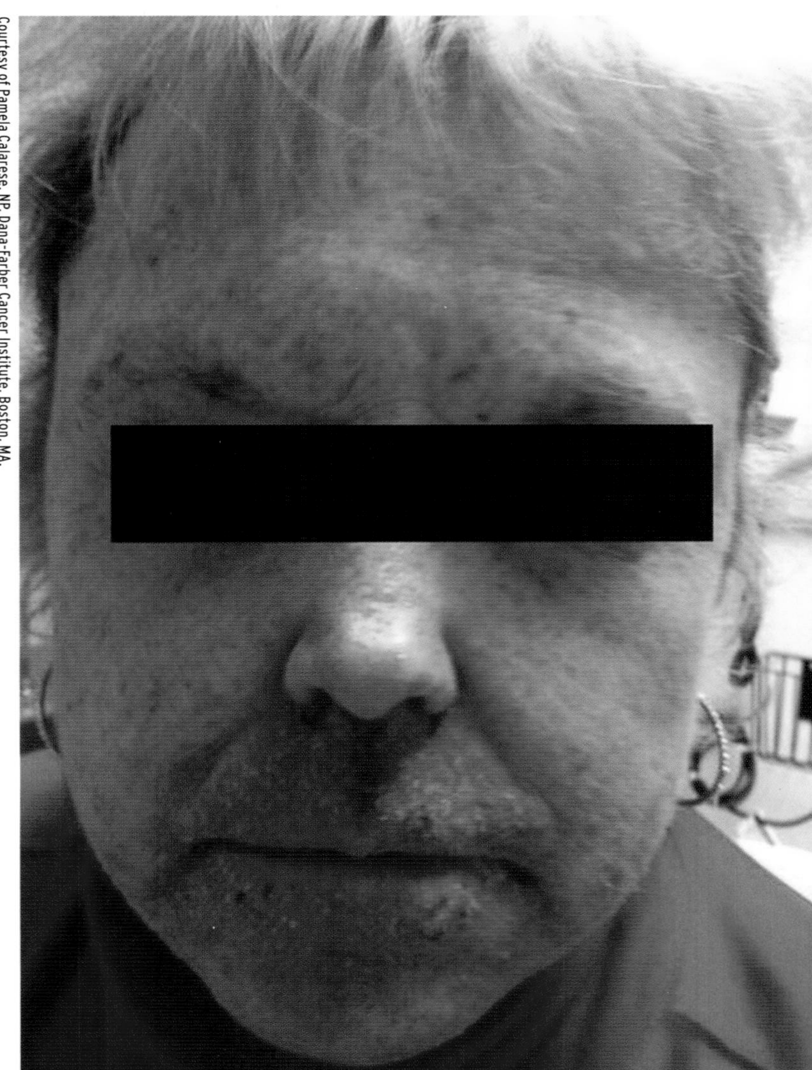

Courtesy of Pamela Calarese, NP, Dana-Farber Cancer Institute, Boston, MA.

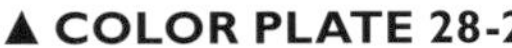

▲ COLOR PLATE 28-2

Grade 3 EGFR papulopustular rash.

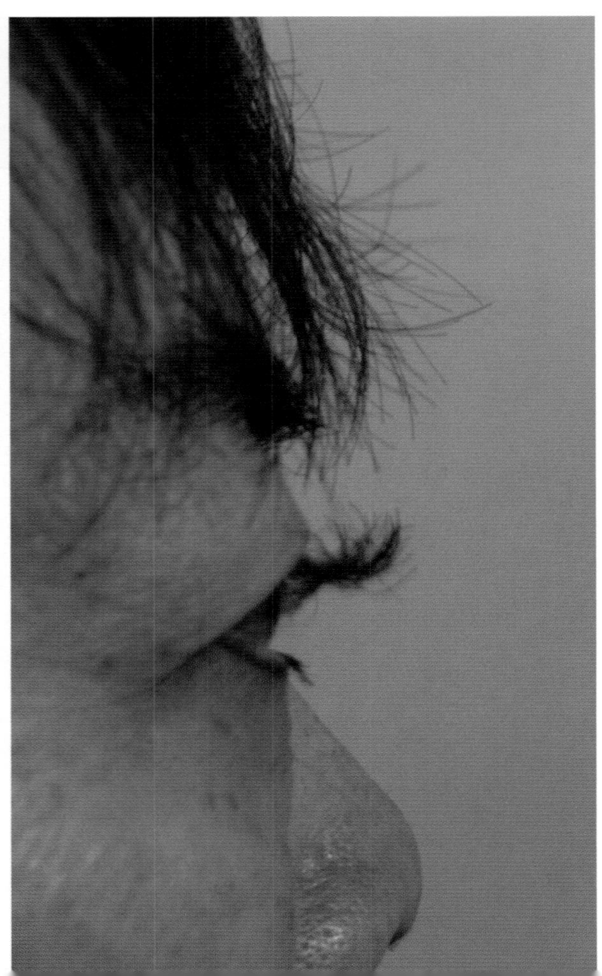

◄ COLOR PLATE 28-3

EGFR-related trichomegaly.

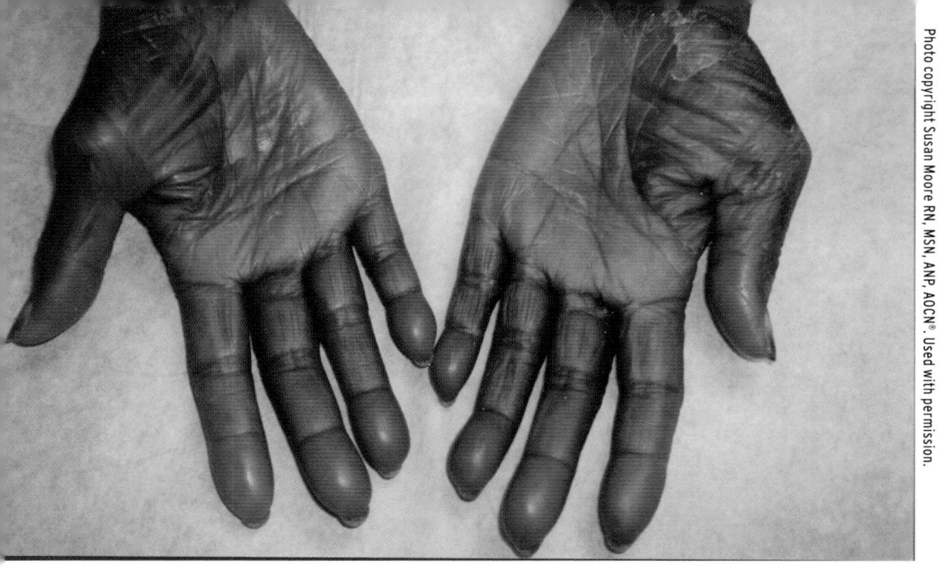

◀ COLOR PLATE 28-4

Hand-Foot Syndrome (HFS). Erythema and desquamation of the palms.

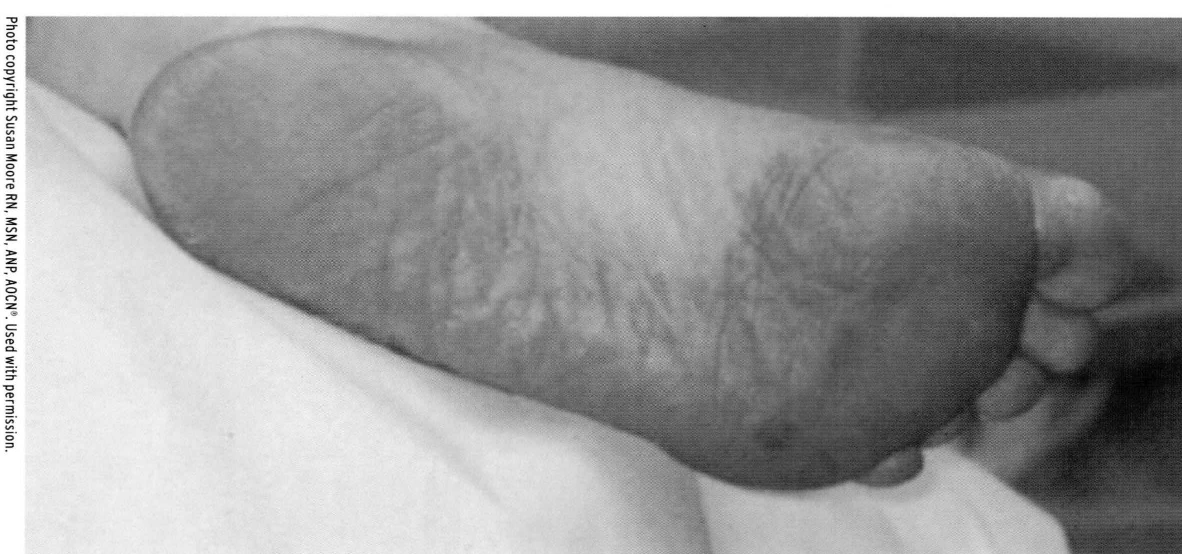

▲ COLOR PLATE 28-5

Hand-Foot Syndrome (HFS). Erythema and edema of the plantar surface of the foot.

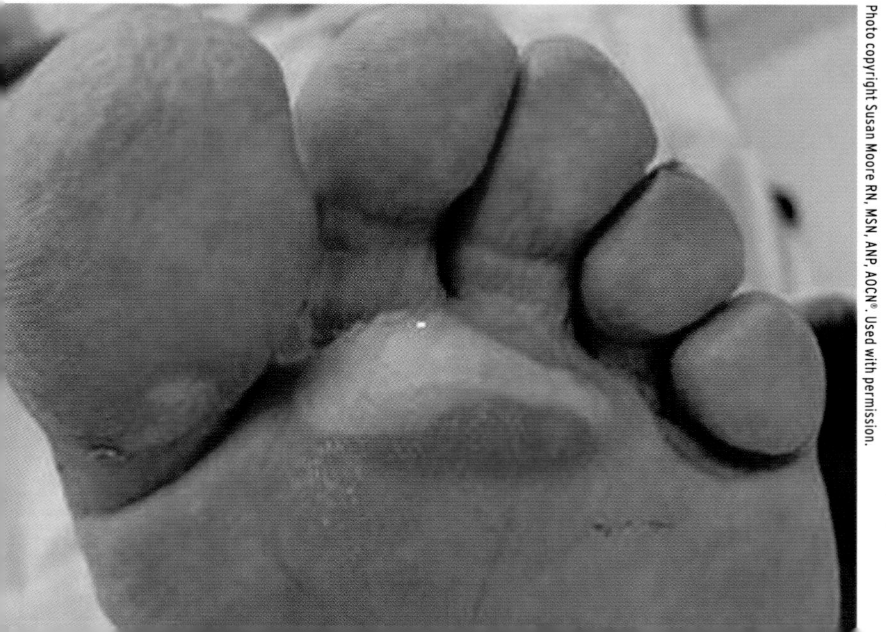

◀ COLOR PLATE 28-6

Hand-Foot Skin Reaction (HFSR). Keratosis of the foot.

of the nail. They may vary in pattern, color, location (distal or proximal), and frequency, and may or may not be associated with pain. The hemorrhages move forward as the nail grows and can be scraped away with a nail file when they reach the free end of the nail.[11,40]

These hemorrhages are associated with drugs that target the VEGF receptor and platelet-derived growth factor receptor, including sunitinib and sorafenib. VEGF may be involved in the constant repair of microscopic trauma to the nails, and blockage of the VEGF receptor may interfere with capillary repair and lead to the appearance of the tiny hemorrhages.[11] The hemorrhages do not require treatment. Nail polish will cover the discoloration.

Damage to the nail plate

Changes in nail pigment exhibit a variety of patterns depending on the offending agent. Cyclophosphamide, fluorouracil, and cisplatin have been shown to cause diffuse nail hyperpigmentation.[45,47] Longitudinal bands of hyperpigmentation are more common and associated with cyclophosphamide, hydroxyurea, melphalan, busulfan, and doxorubicin. Also possible are transverse bands of darkening. These changes are cosmetic;[47] appearance of the nails can be improved with polish.

Nail grooves and lines come in several varieties. Beau's lines appear when growth of the nail slows or terminates. Interruption of growth results in transverse depressions. The depressions move forward as the nail grows and is trimmed.[47] The grooves provide a record of treatment cycles. Ridges may be solitary or multiple, typically spaced 2 to 3 mm apart.[45]

Mees' lines (true leukonychia) are transverse opaque lines that indicate damage to the nail matrix; these lines move as the nail grows. Little is known about their etiology, although they may be due to cessation of nail growth related to chemotherapy.[45] They are associated with administration of docetaxel, cisplatin, anthracyclines, vincristine, cyclophosphamide, and sorafenib.[45,47] No treatment is required.

Muehrcke's lines are apparent leukonychia and are caused by damage to the nail bed. They appear as horizontally white lines with a normal-colored nail bed. They resolve without intervention when treatment is stopped.[47]

Brittle nails are commonly associated with cytotoxic agents and EGFR inhibitors. Nail growth may also be slowed. Biotin 2.5 mg each day may strengthen nails.[13,47]

Damage to the nail fold (paronychia)

Paronychia, or periungual inflammation, is an erythematous inflammation of the nail fold. All of the EGFR inhibitors (cetuximab, erlotinib, gefitinib, panitumumab, and lapatinib) have been shown to cause this toxicity.[13] It is seen in 12% to 25% of patients receiving these agents and can occur in any toenail or fingernail, usually occurring 1 to 4 months after therapy begins.[38,41,47] It may take several months for paronychial lesions to resolve.[42]

PATHOPHYSIOLOGY

The exact mechanism by which EGFR inhibitors lead to paronychia is unknown,[11,41] but may be due to the effect of EGFR inhibition on nail keratinocytes.[41] It may also be due to skin fragility. Epidermal changes noted with cetuximab include thinning of the stratum corneum and slowed rates of keratinocyte proliferation. The resulting fragility may make it easier for nail fragments to penetrate and desquamate the periungual tissues, leading to inflammation.[13] This inflammation is not always associated with infection and, therefore, is not always responsive to topical antibiotics.[42]

SYMPTOM ASSESSMENT

Patients may first describe tenderness of the skin surrounding the nails on the fingers or toes. Although paronychia does not significantly disrupt function if the toxicity is grade 1, this condition can become quite painful to the point of interfering with activities of daily living with significant impact on QOL. It can become difficult to work, care for the house or children, walk comfortably, or even wear usual shoes. Patients need to be taught preventive care, and to report early signs of inflammation and infection.

If preventive measures are not successful, paronychia may progress to a painful, red inflammation of the lateral and proximal nail folds. This can result in very painful pyogenic granuloma-like lesions. Secondary infection with *S. aureus* or gram-negative bacteria may occur.[47] Wearing shoes may become impossible, such that patients are forced to wear sandals. The CTCAE grading[31] (Table 28-2) does not capture this toxicity. The MASCC system[18] details paronychia as well as other nail changes (Table 28-3).

THERAPEUTIC APPROACHES

There have been no randomized controlled trials to guide recommendations. Preventive measures may include avoiding rubbing and pressure on nail folds, avoidance of harsh chemicals and prolonged water immersion, and moisturization with creams. Patients should avoid nail biting, pushing back the nail cuticle overzealously, tearing skin around the nail, and cutting nails too short.[11,12,37,47] Artificial or acrylic nails are discouraged. Nails can be polished, but polish remover should be used sparingly because it can dry nails.[12]

Treatment may include soaking in aluminum acetate (Burow's solution) or vinegar solution (1 part white vinegar to 3 parts water), washing with antiseptics (diluted hydrochloric acid solution or boric acid solution 3%), and protecting and cushioning the area. Creams containing corticosteroids and antiseptics have been suggested (betamethasone 0.05% plus cliochinol 3% ointment; betamethasone 0.1% plus gentamicin 0.05% or 0.1% cream; bethamethasone valerate 0.1% plus fusidic 2% acid cream; triamcinolone acetonide 3% plus chlortetracycline 0.1% ointment; or triamcinolone benetonide 2% plus fusidic acid 0.03% cream). Topical or systemic antibiotics may been useful (e.g., minocycline; doxycycline).[33,37,41] If secondary infection is suspected, the areas should be cultured and systemic antibiotics initiated. Severe paronychia may require temporary interruption of treatment.[37]

The National Comprehensive Cancer Network (NCCN) Task Force recommends that the area be cultured for bacteria and fungi and that oral antibiotics be used as appropriate.[76] For fissuring, the NCCN recommends Monsel's solution (ferric subsulfate liquid), silver nitrate, or zinc oxide cream.[76] Nonsteroidal anti-inflammatory drugs (NSAIDs) have been suggested to relieve discomfort.[33] Most patients improve with topical antibiotics and gentle care.[77] Painful granulation tissue may be treated with silver nitrate sticks or aqueous potassium permanganate;[37,47,77] the affected nail may require removal. Severe lesions may also be treated with tissue excision under anesthesia followed by electrocautery and intralesional triamcinolone.[41] Patients with severe paronychia should be seen by a dermatologist.[37]

ACUTE RADIATION DERMATITIS

INCIDENCE

More than 60% of all patients treated for cancer in North America will receive radiation therapy (RT) at some point. Although skin toxicity has been improved by modern technology, some degree of skin reaction is expected in the majority of patients, varying from skin redness to painful skin breakdown.[7] In fact, an estimated 90% to 95% of patients will experience some degree of skin reaction.[78,79] This reaction can lead to significant discomfort, difficulty sleeping, and impaired limb movement; diminish the ability to perform usual activities; and negatively impact QOL.[79,80]

After tissue destruction ceases, tissue repair begins, as a result of homeostatic feedback where cells are stimulated to proliferate and differentiate from the basal layer. Epithelial cells migrate from outside the treatment field, filling in damaged areas.[80]

PATHOPHYSIOLOGY

The epithelial cells of the skin divide rapidly and are sensitive to the effects of radiation. Irradiation of the skin leads to direct tissue injury and inflammatory cell recruitment. A fixed percentage of epidermal basal cells, endothelial cells, and vascular structures experience damage. Keratinocyte damage leads to DNA damage and inflammatory cytokine release due to the generation of free radicals. Each dose of radiation prevents normal cells from repopulating the epidermis, thereby compounding the skin reaction. As basal cells replicate in an attempt to replace injured cells, the skin becomes dry and flaky (dry desquamation). If cells are not replaced rapidly enough, desquamation will become moist as the epidermis is shed, and the basal cell layer, sweat, and sebaceous glands sustain further damage.[78,79,81–83]

SYMPTOM ASSESSMENT

Risk factors

Skin response to radiation therapy varies. A variety of treatment-related factors influence this response, including the size of the daily dose (fraction), the type of energy used (e.g., photon, electron, proton), the volume treated, the length of the treatment course, and the use of bolus doses (an additional dose of radiation to a particular area). Patient characteristics may influence response, including genetic predisposition for less robust healing, personal factors (e.g., areas of skin friction, overlapping skin folds), areas of thin skin (e.g., axilla, face, perineum), existing skin integrity, comorbidities (e.g., diabetes, renal failure), nutritional status, race and ethnicity, concomitant medications, sun exposure, smoking, obesity, older age, and functional status.[7,78–81] The use of radiation sensitizers as a factor in increasing skin reactions is well known, and the timing of their administration is critical.[81]

Newer radiation techniques also influence skin toxicity. Studies support a decrease in skin toxicity with the use of intensity-modulated radiation therapy (IMRT) over conventional techniques.[84,85]

Self-assessment

During the first few day of receiving radiation, patients may notice transient flushing of the skin in the treated area, a result of histamine and serotonin release, extracapillary cell injury, and dilation of vessels.[79] Sustained erythema becomes apparent after approximately two weeks of therapy. Lighter skin becomes blanchable with a more intense pink color; darker skin may become more pigmented. The surface of the skin is otherwise normal in appearance. Although patients do not experience any discomfort in the early stages, as the skin reddens and becomes more inflamed, tenderness may occur.[78] Patients may describe sensations such as sensitivity or tightness.[79,80]

As cellular destruction continues, melanin cells migrate toward the cell surface, causing hyperpigmentation. Hair falls as follicles shed hair and move into the resting phase of the cell cycle. Skin becomes dry and itchy as sweat and sebaceous glands are affected.[79] Later, skin may become more intensely pink with itching and discomfort. As skin dries, the outer surface will flake and peel. This may be the extent of the skin reaction. However, areas where skin folds or friction occurs between skin surfaces or between skin and clothing are at risk for further loss of the epidermis, resulting in moist desquamation. This degree of reaction is more uncomfortable and usually requires a rest from treatment.[81]

Re-epithelialization of skin begins 10 to 14 days after treatment ends. In this process, epithelial cells migrate from the basal layer. The migration of cells across the irradiated skin is encouraged by a moist wound-healing environment; wounds have been found to heal 50% faster in a moist versus a nonmoist environment.[79,80]

Patients are typically seen daily with the exception of weekends. They should be educated to report changes in skin sensation and skin integrity. Personnel in the department must also be alert to changes. Certainly, moist desquamation is reason for concern as the protective barrier has been broken, putting the patient at risk for infection and further discomfort. Dealing with skin care in areas where skin folds can create a challenge for both the patient and the staff.

Objective assessment

Physical exam. Assessment of skin in the treatment-affected area should be performed prior to beginning treatment to establish a baseline, and such examination should be repeated at least weekly by a doctor or nurse. Evaluation should include changes in physical symptoms as well as changes in the patient's experience. The assessment should identify any color changes, erythema, dry desquamation, moist desquamation, drainage, odor, suspected infection, and patient descriptions of itching, dryness, or pain. This exam is also an opportunity to reinforce teaching, and to adjust strategies for preventing or minimizing skin reaction. The impact of radiation dermatitis on discomfort, quality of life, functional status, and ability to perform activities of daily living, to apply prescribed topical treatment and dressings, and to pay for expensive dressing supplies should be assessed.[78]

Skin typically exhibits sustained erythema and edema with radiation doses in the range of approximately 2000 to 4000 cGy. The outline of the treatment field may be visible and the skin in the area hot to the touch. With doses beyond 3000 cGy, skin may become dry and flaky with itching. Inflammatory reactions occur after 4 to 5 weeks of treatment and doses exceeding 4000 cGy. Areas of moist desquamation, especially skin folds, should be observed for signs of infection and treatment instituted as appropriate.[78]

Degrees of toxicity

Information from CTCAE version 4.0[31] pertaining to radiation dermatitis is found in Table 28-8. Although this grading tool is useful for classifying the degree of skin reaction, it does not capture symptoms or the impact of the reaction on the patient's life.

THERAPEUTIC APPROACHES

Although radiation has been used for many years in the treatment of cancer, there is little evidence-based information to guide the management of skin reactions. Many of the measures used in the prevention and treatment of skin reactions are based on anecdotal evidence, and care standards vary widely from institution to institution.[86] Clinical trials are plagued by methodological problems, small sample sizes, conflicting results, a variety of measurement tools and outcomes measured, and a focus on prevention rather than treatment.[78,79,81] Nevertheless, simply paying attention to developing a standard approach can lead to positive results. One study showed that adoption of a skin care protocol based on literature review and evidence, use of moist wound-healing principles, and stopping outdated practices resulted in practice improvements.[87]

Some sources have raised concerns that using products on irradiated skin will create a bolus effect, increasing skin dose and irritation. Although many radiation centers restrict the use of products on skin in the treatment field, research evidence does not support this practice.[88]

The Oncology Nursing Society's Radiodermatitis Putting Evidence into Practice (PEP) team did an extensive review of the literature, including clinical practice guidelines, systematic reviews, and clinical research studies, looking for evidence to guide interventions for dermatitis.[78]

TABLE 28-8

National Cancer Institute Common Terminology Criteria for Adverse Events (CTCAE): Radiation Therapy Toxicities: Dermatitis Radiation
Grade 1: faint erythema or dry desquamation
Grade 2: moderate to brisk erythema; patchy moist desquamation, mostly confined to skin folds and creases; moderate edema
Grade 3: moist desquamation in areas other than skin folds and creases; bleeding induced by minor trauma or abrasion
Grade 4: life-threatening consequences; skin necrosis or ulceration of full-thickness dermis; spontaneous bleeding from involved site; skin graft indicated
Grade 5: Death

Source: Data from National Cancer Institute Common Terminology Criteria for Adverse Events (CTCAE)[31].

They found evidence supporting washing with mild soap and water, along with the use of deodorant. In the studies reviewed, not only did washing increase patient comfort, but irradiated skin either suffered no harm or sustained significantly less damage.[78,79,87] It is generally recommended that patients avoid irritating or perfumed products, although there is little evidence to support application of any particular product. It is recommended that the soap be pH neutral or nonalkaline. In a study investigating the irritant properties of 18 soap products, only Dove soap was found to be mild.[79,80]

The use of deodorant on intact, treated skin remains controversial. In a study of 84 women receiving radiation to the breast, patients were randomized to no deodorant versus non-aluminum-containing deodorant. Results demonstrated a reduction in grade 2 axillary desquamation, axillary moist desquamation, axillary pain and discomfort, axillary pruritus, grade 2 breast dermatitis, and pain for women using deodorant when compared to those using no deodorant.[89] In another study, 15 products including deodorants, powders, and creams were found to have little effect on the radiation surface at any application of product depth. No differences were found between metallic and nonmetallic products.[78] Aistar[90] reviewed studies evaluating skin care protocols for women with breast cancer and found no evidence that deodorant should be avoided during treatment. The PEP recommendation is to allow the use of deodorant without aluminum in the treated field.[78]

Creams are often recommended for the prevention of skin reactions. A large ($n = 208$) study compared commonly used products (e.g., Aquaphor, Biafine RK, and RadiaCare) to water-mist placebo for dermatitis prevention in women receiving whole-breast radiation. The researchers found no differences in the development of dermatitis among the groups. Patients preferred the cream-based Biafine.[83]

The PEP team reported on agents with some evidence supporting their use as dermatitis interventions. In a randomized study, *Calendula officinalis* was found to be superior to Biafine in the reduction of grade 2 dermatitis, pain, and dose interruption. *Calendula* is a medicinal herb with antimicrobial properties. Although the thick cream was difficult to apply, the product is now available in a petroleum base.[78–80] In another large randomized trial,[82] hyaluronic acid cream was found to be superior to placebo in preventing radiodermatitis. PEP has classified *Calendula* cream and hyaluronic acid/sodium hyaluronate cream in the "likely to be effective" category.[78]

The PEP team failed to find sufficient evidence warranting the recommendation of other topical agents. Studies were reviewed looking at aloe vera, trolamine, MAS065D, topical steroids, dexpanthenol, glutathione and anthocyanin, sucralfate, moisturizing creams, urea lotion, anionic polar phospholipid, vitamin C, chamomile cream, almond ointment, and sodium sucrose octasulfate. In all of these studies, either the results were mixed or the trials very small.[78,80,86,91]

Results of studies using hydrocolloid dressings have been mixed, although some patients expressed comfort from dressings. Dressings also have the potential to decrease eschar formation, improve conditions for epidermal growth, and improve overall wound healing.[79,80]

Studies of silver leaf dressings have been of limited value due to their very small sample sizes. This product is a nonadherent rayon and polyester dressing that offers several benefits, including moisture retention, management of exudate, greater comfort, and less frequent dressing changes, which results in reduced wound bed disruption. One study examined the use of silver leaf dressings for radiation-induced wounds. Patients were found to have a significant reduction in grades 3 and 4 desquamation.[79,80] Studies of no-sting barrier film (Cavilon), granulocyte/macrophage colony-stimulating factor (GM-CSF)–impregnated gauze, and honey-impregnated gauze also were hampered by small samples.[78,91] Application of Cavilon did statistically reduce the frequency and duration of moist desquamation and pruritus.[79] It is difficult to study dressings during treatment because they need to be removed daily prior to therapy to avoid a bolus effect. Therefore, if a dressing is designed to remain in place for more than a day, its benefit is lost.[79]

Studies of oral zinc, red wine, sucralfate, and proteolytic agents have also failed to produce sufficient evidence to recommend these interventions' use. Five studies investigating trolamine failed to demonstrate any advantage from using this agent over *Calendula*, best supportive care, or Lipiderm. Gentian violet is not recommended.[78,91]

An international consensus panel developed guidelines for management of radiation dermatitis combined with EGFR inhibitor rash. Recommendations included maintaining clean, dry skin as prophylaxis. For grade 1 dermatitis, the panel members suggested use of perfume-free moisturizers, as well as use of antibacterial agents if anti-infective measures if appropriate. However, they warned that overuse of antiseptic cream can be irritating.[82]

For grades 2 and 3 dermatitis, the consensus panel suggested continued cleaning and gentle drying and consideration of a number of topical remedies. The latter agents included drying gels, possibly antiseptics, hydrophilic dressings, anti-inflammatory emulsions (e.g., trolamine, hyaluronic acid cream), and zinc oxide paste. If infection is suspected, clinical judgment may lead to culture, with topical antibiotics being given for superinfection (not prophylactically). In such cases, management by a team consisting of a radiation oncologist, medical oncologist (if appropriate), nurse, and dermatologist is necessary. Grade 4 dermatitis is rarely seen and requires specialized wound care.[82] Specific recommendations are listed in Table 28-9.[78–80,82,89]

TABLE 28-9

Recommendations for Prevention and Management of Radiation-Induced Dermatitis

Prevention

- Gentle skin washing with soap and lukewarm water, and drying of skin in radiation portal. Use mild soap (Dove) and pat skin dry.
- Instruct patients to avoid the following in the irradiated field: scratching, vigorous rubbing, irritating fabrics or binding clothing, exfoliation, strong detergents/
- Use of moisturizers is optional: non-alcohol, lanolin-free, fragrance-free, water-based cream has been recommended. However, the choice of product can be based on cost and ease of application.
- The use of non-aluminum-containing deodorant on intact skin is acceptable.
- Do not use heating pads or ice packs in treated areas.
- If shaving, use only an electric razor on treated areas.
- Avoid sun exposure. Use sunscreen with sun protection factor of at least 30.
- Examine irradiated skin at least weekly for signs of toxicity.
- Consider the use of calendula cream or hyaluronic acid/ sodium hyaluronate cream.

Management

Grade 1

- Gentle skin washing and drying, even if irritated or ulcerated.
- Use of moisturizers is optional (see "Prevention").
- Consider antibacterial moisturizers (triclosan or chlorhexidine-based cream).
- Continue to follow directions for prevention.

Grades 2 and 3

- Determine that the skin reaction is not due to a concomitant medication.
- Validate the accuracy of the radiation dose and its distribution.
- If there is no evidence of infection, use topical treatments.
- If there are signs of infection, consider culture and topical or systemic antibiotics.
- The following may be considered:
  - Topical steroids: mometasone, methylprednisolone, beclomethasone, betamethasone creams
  - Anti-inflammatory emulsion (trolamine)
  - Zinc oxide paste
  - Drying gels
  - Antiseptics (such as chlorhexidine)
  - Hydrophilic dressings, Cavilin No-Sting Barrier Film, or Silver Leaf Nylon Dressing for moist desquamation
  - Blood cultures if fever or other signs of sepsis

Source: Data from Feight et al[78]; McQuestion[79,80]; Bernier et al[82]; Theberge et al[89].

The international panel also discussed the difficulty of using current grading systems, which are subjective and make it difficult to compare studies. They recommended that photography become a standard part of care to document toxicity in clinical trials.

Without evidence to guide clinical practice, practices may continue to vary widely even within single departments. Further research should be built on previous studies. Some interventions have shown promise, but without replication of the results supporting their use, they cannot be recommended. The question being asked must be clearly defined. Is the intervention supposed to prevent the symptom, delay its appearance, or improve the rate of healing?[78,82] To date, there has been little study of how people of different ages and from diverse groups respond to skin treatments. Skin can vary tremendously across racial and ethnic lines. Nurses are present in nearly all radiation therapy departments, involved in patient teaching and symptom management, so nursing research in this area is encouraged.

NURSING IMPLICATIONS

Molecularly targeted agents are becoming increasingly common in the treatment of cancer. Changes to the skin, hair, and nails are among the major toxicities associated with these drugs. In addition, radiation therapy has long been known to result in skin changes. The vast majority of patients are treated in the outpatient setting, and the nurses caring for them must be knowledgeable about our current understanding of preemptive treatment and evidence-based remedies according to toxicity grade, and must possess expert patient teaching skills. Patients need to be well-informed to participate in self-care, and nurses can provide guidance along the way.

Although progress has been made, much remains to be done to develop evidence-based interventions for the care of the skin and nails. Many patients are living with cancer as a chronic illness, working and raising children. Effective management of toxicities that affect appearance, quality of life, and the ability to carry on with day-to-day activities is critical, as patients may continue taking chemotherapeutic drugs for many years. We are just beginning to understand the impact on psychological coping and social functioning of such side effects. The little research that has been done notes there may be significant embarrassment with physical appearance, inhibited displays of affection, and the fear that the appearance of the rash will lead to a need to reveal the diagnosis. This research is in its infancy, relying on tools that have not been validated. Research results are conflicting, and there are many gaps in knowledge about what patients need to know and need for support.[30,92]

It is important to explore what skin, hair, and nail changes mean to each individual patient, as patients' perceptions may vary widely. Some people are severely embarrassed by a mild skin rash; others seem hardly to notice a much more severe rash. Nurses are symptom management experts and, in collaboration with their medical colleagues, need to lead the way in exploring new remedies for skin toxicity, and in developing and following standard protocols related to these side effects.

PATIENT SELF-CARE

Prevention and early detection of toxicity by exam or patient self-report are of critical importance in managing the skin effects of chemotherapy and the effects of molecularly targeted therapy on the skin and nails. These toxicities have a significant impact on the treatment experience, and their management is of critical importance. Informing patients of techniques they can employ to minimize or manage toxicities is critical for patient empowerment and comfort. Patients may self-administer molecularly targeted agents for years and, in partnership with the healthcare team, become adept at managing the side effects of such therapy. Successful side effect management has the potential to avoid unnecessary interruptions in therapy and dose reductions. Without management strategies and open lines of communication, however, patients may avoid informing their healthcare providers of toxicities, fearing that treatment will be stopped. The self-care tools in the appendices that follow may be helpful in patient education about papulopustular rash (Appendix 28A), hand–foot syndrome and hand–foot skin reaction (Appendix 28B), and radiation dermatitis (Appendix 28C).

REFERENCES

1. Balagula Y, Rosen ST, Lacouture ME. The emergency of supportive onco-dermatology: the study of dermatologic adverse events to cancer therapies. *J Am Acad Dermatol.* 2011;65(3):624–635.
2. Abraham A, Rademaker A, Ortiz S, et al. Economic impact associated with the management of dermatologic adverse drug reactions (dARDs) induced by EGFR inhibitors (EGFRIs) in lung cancer [abstract]. *J Clin Oncol.* 2008;26(15S):19094.
3. Borovicka JH, Mulcahy MF, Calahan C, West DP, Lacouture ME. Economic impact in the management of dermatologic toxicities (dTs) induced by the epidermal growth factor receptor inhibitor (EGFRI) cetuximab in colorectal cancer [abstract]. *J Clin Oncol.* 2008:26(15):3569.
4. Hogle WP. Overview of skin issues related to the oncology patient. In: Haas ML, Moore-Higgs GJ, eds. *Principles of Skin Care and the Oncology Patient.* Pittsburgh, PA: ONS Publishing Division; 2010:1–32.
5. Lacouture, ME. Insights into the pathophysiology and management of dermatologic toxicities to EGFR-targeted therapies in colorectal cancer. *Cancer Nurs.* 2007;30(4S):S17–S26.
6. Li T, Perez-Soler R. Skin toxicities associated with epidermal growth factor receptor inhibitors. *Target Oncol.* 2009;4:107–119.
7. FitzGerald TJ, Jodoin MB, Tillman G, et al. Radiation therapy toxicity to the skin. *Dermatol Clin.* 2008;26:161–172.
8. Saif MW, Merikas I, Tsimboukis S, Syrigos K. Erlotinib-induced skin rash, pathogenesis, clinical significance and management in pancreatic cancer patients. *J Pancreas.* 2008;9(3):267–274.
9. Haley AC, Calahan C, Gandhi M, West DP, Rademaker A, Lacouture ME. Skin care management in cancer patients: an evaluation of quality of life and tolerability. *Support Care Cancer.* 2011;19:545–554.
10. Boone SL, Rademaker A, Liu D, Pfeiffer C, Mauro DJ, Lacouture ME. Impact and management of skin toxicity associated with anti-epidermal growth factor receptor therapy: survey results. *Oncology.* 2007;72:152–159.
11. Robert C, Soria JC, Spatz A, et al. Cutaneous side-effects of kinase inhibitors and blocking antibodies. *Lancet Oncol.* 2005;6(7):491–500.
12. Dest VM. Systemic therapy-induced skin reactions. In: Haas ML, Moore-Higgs GJ, eds. *Principles of Skin Care and the Oncology Patient.* Pittsburgh, PA: ONS Publishing Division; 2010:141–166.
13. Balagula Y, Garbe C, Myskowski PL, et al. Clinical presentation and management of dermatological toxicities of epidermal growth factor receptor inhibitors. *Int J Dermatol.* 2011;50:129–146.
14. Melosky B, Burkes R, Rayson D, Alcindor T, Shear N, Lacouture M. Management of skin rash during EGFR-targeted monoclonal antibody treatment for gastrointestinal malignancies: Canadian recommendations. *Curr Oncol.* 2009;16(1):16–26.
15. Jia Y, Lacouture ME, Su X, Wu S. Risk of skin rash associated with erlotinib in cancer patients: a meta-analysis. *J Support Oncol.* 2009;7(6):211–217.
16. Mittmann N, Seung SJ. Rash rates with EGFR inhibitors: meta-analysis. *Curr Oncol.* 2011;18(2):e54–e63.
17. Oishi K. Clinical approaches to minimize rash associated with EGFR inhibitors. *Oncol Nurs Forum.* 2008;35:103–111.
18. Lacouture ME, Maitland ML, Segaert S, et al. A proposed EGFR inhibitor dermatologic adverse event-specific grading scale from the MASCC skin toxicity study group. *Support Care Cancer.* 2010;18:509–522.
19. Amitay-Laish I, David M, Stemmer SM. *Staphylococcus* coagulase-positive skin inflammation associated with epidermal growth factor receptor-targeted therapy: an early and a late phase of papulopustular eruptions. *Oncologist.* 2010;15:1002–1008.
20. Tan EH, Chan A. Evidence-based treatment options for the management of skin toxicities associated with epidermal growth factor receptor inhibitors. *Ann Pharmacol.* 2009;43:1658–1666.
21. Agero ALC, Dusza SW, Benvenuto-Andrade C, Busam KJ, Myskowski P, Halpern AC. Dermatologic side effects associated with the epidermal growth factor receptor inhibitors. *J Am Acad Dermatol.* 2006;55(4):657–670.
22. Lacouture ME, Lai SE. The PRIDE (papulopustules and/or paronychia, regulatory abnormalities of hair growth, itching and dryness due to epidermal growth factor receptor inhibitors) syndrome. *Br J Dermatol.* 2006;155(4):852–854.
23. Frankel C, Palmieri FM. Lapatinib side-effect management. *Clin J Oncol Nurs.* 2010;14(2):223–233.
24. Lacouture ME, Anadkat MJ, Bensadoun R-J, et al. Clinical practice guidelines for the prevention and treatment of EGFR inhibitor-associated dermatologic toxicities. *Support Care Cancer.* 2011;19:1079–1095.
25. Lai SE, Minnelly P, O'Keeffe A, et al. Influence of skin color in the development of erlotinib-induced rash: a report from the SERIES clinic [abstract]. *J Clin Oncol.* 2007;25(suppl 18S):9127.
26. Perez-Soler R, Delord JP, Halpern A, et al. HER1/EGFR inhibitor-associated rash: future directions for management and investigation outcomes from the HER1/EGFR inhibitor rash management forum. *Oncologist.* 2005;10(5):345–356.
27. Lynch TJ, Kim ES, Eaby B, Garey J, West DP, Lacouture ME. Epidermal growth factor receptor inhibitor-associated cutaneous toxicities: an evolving paradigm in clinical management. *Oncologist.* 2007;12(5):610–621.

28. Lacouture ME, Mitchell EP, Piperdi B, et al. Skin toxicity evaluation protocol with panitumumab (STEPP): a Phase II, open-label, randomized trial evaluating the impact of a pre-emptive skin treatment regimen on skin toxicities and quality of life in patient with metastatic colorectal cancer. *J Clin Oncol.* 2010;28(8):1351–1357.
29. Joshi SS, Ortiz S, Witherspoon JN, et al. Effects of epidermal growth factor receptor inhibitor-induced dermatologic toxicities on quality of life. *Cancer.* 2010;116(16):3916–3923.
30. Wagner LI, Lacouture ME. Dermatologic toxicities associated with EGFR inhibitors: the clinical psychologist's perspective. Impact on health-related quality of life and implications for clinical management of psychological sequelae. *Oncology.* 2007;21(11 suppl 5):34–36.
31. U.S. Department of Health and Human Services. *Common Terminology Criteria for Adverse Events (CTCAE) Version 4.0.* NIH Publication No. 09-5410. 2009.
32. Boucher J, Olson L, Piperdi B. Preemptive management of dermatologic toxicities associated with epidermal growth factor receptor inhibitors. *Clin J Oncol Nurs.* 2011;15(5):501–508.
33. Pinto C, Barone CA, Girolomoni G, et al. Management of skin toxicity associated with cetuximab treatment in combination with chemotherapy and radiotherapy. *Oncologist.* 2011;16(2):228–238.
34. Thatcher N, Nicolson M, Groves RW, et al. Expert consensus on the management of erlotinib-associated cutaneous toxicity in the U.K. *Oncologist.* 2009;14(8):840–847.
35. Scope A, Agero ALC, Dusza SW, et al. Randomized double-blind trial of prophylactic oral minocycline and topical tazarotine for cetuximab-associated acne-like eruption. *J Clin Oncol.* 2007;25(34):5390–5396.
36. Jatoi A, Rowland K, Sloan JA, et al. Tetracycline to prevent epidermal growth factor receptor inhibitor-induced skin rashes: results of a placebo-controlled trial from the North Central Cancer Treatment Group. *Cancer.* 2008;113(4):847–853.
37. Regulai Z, Bachet JB, Bachmeyer C, et al. Management of cutaneous adverse events induced by anti-EGFR (epidermal growth factor receptor): a French interdisciplinary therapeutic algorithm. *Support Care Cancer.* 2012;20:1395–1404.
38. Eaby B, Culkin A, Lacouture ME. An interdisciplinary consensus on managing skin reactions associated with human epidermal growth factor receptor inhibitors. *Clin J Oncol Nurs.* 2008;12:283–290.
39. Eilers RE, Gandhi JD, Patel MF, et al. Dermatologic infections in cancer patients treated with epidermal growth factor receptor inhibitor therapy. *J Natl Cancer Inst.* 2010;102(1):47–53.
40. Lacouture ME, Boerner SA, LoRusso PM. Non-rash skin toxicities associated with novel targeted therapies. *Clin Lung Cancer.* 2006;8 (suppl 1):S36–S42.
41. Choi JN. Chemotherapy-induced iatrogenic injury of skin: new drugs and new concepts. *Clin Dermatol.* 2011;29:587–601.
42. Hammond-Thelin LA. Cutaneous reactions related to systemic immunomodulators and targeted therapeutics. *Dermatol Clin.* 2008;26:121–159.
43. McLellan B, Kerr H. Cutaneous toxicities of the multikinase inhibitors sorafenib and sunitinib. *Dermatol Ther.* 2011;24:396–400.
44. Schwandt A, Wood LS, Rini B, Dreicer R. Management of side effects associated with sunitinib therapy for patients with renal cell carcinoma. *Onco Targets Ther.* 2009;2:51–61.
45. Sanborn RE, Sauer DA. Cutaneous reactions to chemotherapy: commonly seen, less described, little understood. *Dermatol Clin.* 2008;26:103–119.
46. Huang V, Anadkat M. Dermatologic manifestations of cytoxic therapy. *Dermatol Ther.* 2011;24:401–410.
47. Balagula E, Lacouture ME. Dermatologic toxicities. In: Olver IN, ed. *The MASCC Textbook of Supportive Care and Survivorship.* New York: Springer; 2011:361–380.
48. Anderson R, Jatoi A, Robert C, Wood L, Keating KN, Lacouture ME. Search for evidence-based approaches for the prevention and palliation of hand–foot skin reaction (HFSR) caused by the multikinase inhibitors (MKIs). *Oncologist.* 2009;14(4):291–302.
49. Balagula Y, Lacouture ME, Cotliar JA. Dermatologic toxicities of targeted anticancer therapies. *J Support Oncol.* 2010;8(4):149–161.
50. Wilkes GM, Doyle D. Palmar–plantar erythrodysesthesia. *Clin J Oncol Nurs.* 2005;9(1):103–106.
51. Viale PH. Chemotherapy and cutaneous toxicities: implications for oncology nurses. *Semin Oncol Nurs.* 2006;22(3):144–151.
52. Payne AS, James WD, Weiss RB. Dermatologic toxicities of chemotherapeutic agents. *Semin Oncol.* 2006;33:86–97.
53. Tanyi JL, Smith JA, Ramos L, Parker CL, Munsell MF, Wolf JK. Predisposing risk factors for palmar–plantar erythrodysesthesia when using liposomal doxorubicin to treat recurrent ovarian cancer. *Gynecol Oncol.* 2009;114:219–224.
54. Lacouture ME, Wu S, Robert C, et al. Evolving strategies for the management of hand–foot skin reaction associated with the multitargeted kinase inhibitors sorafenib and sunitinib. *Oncologist.* 2008;13(9):1001–1011.
55. Gomez P, Lacouture ME. Clinical presentation and management of hand–foot skin reaction associated with sorafenib in combination with cytotoxic chemotherapy: experience in breast cancer. *Oncologist.* 2011;16(11):1508–1519.
56. Kollmannsberger C, Bjarnason G, Burnett P, et al. Sunitinib in metastatic renal cell carcinoma: recommendations for management of noncardiovascular toxicities. *Oncologist.* 2011;16(5):543–553.
57. Manchen E, Robert C, Porta C. Management of tyrosine kinase inhibitor-induced hand–foot skin reaction: viewpoints from the medical oncologist, dermatologist, and oncology nurse. *J Support Oncol.* 2011:9(1):13–23.
58. Asad NS, Aragon-Ching JB, Dahut WL, et al. Hand–foot skin reaction increases with cumulative sorafenib dose and with combination anti-vascular endothelial growth factor therapy. *Clin Cancer Res.* 2009;15(4):1411–1416.
59. Huang V, Anadkat M, Cornelius L. Cutaneous toxic effects associated with vemurafenib and inhibition of the BRAF pathway. *Arch Dermatol.* 2012;148(5):628–633.
60. Lorusso D, Di Stefano A, Carone V, Fagotti A, Pisconti S, Scambia G. Pegylated liposomal doxorubicin-related palmar–plantar erythrodysesthesia ("hand–foot" syndrome). *Ann Oncol.* 2007;18(7):1159–1164.
61. Lacouture ME, Reilly LM, Gerami P, et al. Hand foot skin reaction in cancer patients treated with the multikinase inhibitors sorafenib and sunitinib. *Ann Oncol.* 2008;19:1955–1961.
62. Wood LS, Lemont H, Jatoi A, et al. Practical considerations in the management of hand–foot skin reaction caused by multikinase inhibitors. *Comm Oncol.* 2010;7(1):23–29.
63. Berg DT. Capecitabine: a new adjuvant option for colorectal cancer. *Clin J Oncol Nurs.* 2006;10(4):479–486.
64. Autier J, Escudier B, Wechsler J, Spatz A, Robert C. Prospective study of the cutaneous adverse effects of sorafenib, a novel multikinase inhibitor. *Arch Dermatol.* 2008;144(7):886–892.
65. Wood L, Manchen B. Sorafenib: a promising new targeted therapy for renal cell carcinoma. *Clin J Oncol Nurs.* 2007;11(5):649–656.
66. Pyle L, Beirne D, Bird J, Hoggarth L, Jamieson C, Lane L. Managing the side effects of sunitinib: a guide to empowering the patient. *Cancer Nurs Pract.* 2008;7(4):42–47.
67. Kang Y-K, Lee SS, Yoon DH, et al. Pyridoxine is not effective to prevent hand–foot syndrome associated with capecitabine therapy: results of a randomized, double-blind, placebo-controlled study. *J Clin Oncol.* 2010;28(24):3824–3829.
68. Von Gruenigen V, Frasure H, Fusco N, et al. A double-blind, randomized trial of pyridoxine versus placebo for the prevention of pegylated liposomal doxorubicin-related hand–foot syndrome in gynecologic oncology patients. *Cancer.* 2010;116(20):4735–4743.
69. Wolf SL, Qin R, Menon SP, et al. Placebo-controlled trial to determine the effectiveness of a urea/lactic acid-based topical keratolytic agent for prevention of capecitabine-induced hand–foot syndrome: North

Central Cancer Treatment Group Study (N05C5). *J Clin Oncol.* 2010; 28(35):5182–5187.

70. Mangili G, Petrone M, Gentile C, De Marzi P, Vigano R, Rabaiotti E. Prevention strategies in palmar–plantar erythrodysesthesia onset: the role of regional cooling. *Gynecol Oncol.* 2008;108:332–335.
71. Hackbarth M, Haas N, Fotopoulou C, Lichtenegger W, Sehouli J. Chemotherapy-induced dermatological toxicity: frequencies and impact on quality of life in women's cancer. Results of a prospective study. *Support Care Cancer.* 2008;16(3):267–273.
72. Gilbar P, Hain A, Peereboom VM. Nail toxicity induced by cancer chemotherapy. *J Oncol Pharm Pract.* 2009;15(3):143–155.
73. Winther D, Saunte DM, Knap M, Haahr V, Jensen AB. Nail changes due to docetaxel: a neglected side effect and nuisance for the patient. *Support Care Cancer.* 2007;15:1191–1197.
74. Heidary N, Naik H, Burgin S. Chemotherapeutic agents and the skin: an update. *J Am Acad Dermatol.* 2008;58:545–570.
75. Scotte F, Tourani J-M, Banu E, et al. Multicenter study of frozen glove to prevent docetaxel-induced onycholysis and cutaneous toxicity of the hand. *J Clin Oncol.* 2005;23(19):4424–4429.
76. Burtness B, Anadkat M, Basti S, et al. NCCN task force report: management of dermatologic and other toxicities associated with EGFR inhibition in patients with cancer. *J Natl Compr Canc Netw.* 2009;7(suppl 1):S5–S21.
77. Roe E, Muret MPG, Marcuello E, Capdevila J, Pallares C, Alomar A. Description and management of cutaneous side effects during cetuximab or erlotinib treatments: a prospective study of 30 patients. *J Am Acad Dermatol.* 2006;55(3):429–437.
78. Feight D, Baney T, Bruce S, McQuestion M. Putting evidence into practice: evidence-based interventions for radiation dermatitis. *Clin J Oncol Nurs.* 2011;15(5):481–492.
79. McQuestion M. Radiation-induced skin reactions. In: Haas ML, Moore-Higgs GJ, eds. *Principles of Skin Care and the Oncology Patient.* Pittsburgh, PA: ONS Publishing Division; 2010:115–135.
80. McQuestion M. Evidence-based skin care management in radiation therapy: clinical update. *Semin Oncol Nurs.* 2011;27(2):1–17.
81. Hymes SR, Strom EA, Fife C. Radiation dermatitis: clinical presentation, pathophysiology, and treatment 2006. *J Am Acad Dermatol.* 2006;54(1):28–46.
82. Bernier J, Bonner J, Vermorken JB, et al. Consensus guidelines for the management of radiation dermatitis and coexisting acne-like rash in patients receiving radiotherapy plus EGFR inhibitors for the treatment of squamous cell carcinoma of the head and neck. *Ann Oncol.* 2008;19(1):142–149.
83. Gosselin TK, Schneider SM, Plambeck MA, Rowe K. A prospective randomized, placebo-controlled skin care study in women diagnosed with breast cancer undergoing radiation therapy. *Oncol Nurs Forum.* 2010;37(5):619–626.
84. Pignol JP, Olivotto I, Rakovitch E, et al. A multicenter randomized trial of breast intensity-modulated radiation therapy to reduce acute radiation dermatitis. *J Clin Oncol.* 2008;28(13):2085–2092.
85. Freedman GM, Li T, Nicolaou N, Chen Y, Ma, C, Anderson PR. Breast intensity-modulated radiation therapy reduces time spent with acute dermatitis for women of all breast sizes during radiation. *Int J Radiat Oncol Biol Phys.* 2009;74(3):689–694.
86. Elliott EA, Wright JR, Swann S, et al. Phase III trial of an emulsion containing trolamine for the prevention of radiation dermatitis in patients with advanced squamous cell carcinoma of the head and neck: results of radiation therapy oncology group trial 99-13. *J Clin Oncol.* 2006;24:2092–2097.
87. Nystedt KE, Hill JE, Mitchell AM, et al. The standardization of radiation skin care in British Columbia: a collaborative approach. *Oncol Nurs Forum.* 2005;32(6):1199–1205.
88. Bieck T, Phillips S. Appraising the evidence for avoiding lotions or topical agents prior to radiation therapy. *Clin J Oncol Nurs.* 2010;14(1):103–105.
89. Theberge V, Harel F, Dagnault A. Use of axillary deodorant and effect on acute skin toxicity during radiotherapy for breast cancer: a prospective randomized non-inferiority trial. *Int J Rad Oncol Biol Physics.* 2009;75(4):1048–1052.
90. Aistars J. The validity of skin care protocols followed by women with breast cancer receiving external radiation. *Clin J Oncol Nurs.* 2006;10(4):487–492.
91. Kedge EM. A systemic review to investigate the effectiveness and acceptability of interventions for moist desquamation in radiotherapy patients. *Radiology.* 2009;15:247–257.
92. White KJ, Roydhouse BA, Scott K. Psychosocial impact of cutaneous toxicities associated with epidermal growth factor receptor-inhibitor treatment. *Clin J Oncol Nurs.* 2011;15(1):88–96.

Papulopustular Rash

Patient Name: ______________________________

This self-care guide is intended to help you prevent and manage this side effect of cancer treatment. The guide also will help you decide when to notify a member of your healthcare team of your symptoms.

Papulopustular rash is a skin condition that can occur when people receive molecularly targeted drugs such as cetuximab, erlotinib, and panitumumab. A milder version can occur with sorafenib and sunitinib. The rash is caused by an inflammatory reaction of the skin to the action of the drug. Although the rash can sometimes look like acne, it is a different kind of rash and is treated very differently. Do not use medicines you would usually use for acne, which will make the rash worse.

The rash is not life threatening and can get better with proper care and time, even while still taking your anticancer medicine. The sooner your healthcare team is aware of skin changes, the more likely they are to help you successfully manage the changes.

One of the medications you are taking, ______________________________, can cause this skin reaction. This guide may help prevent or decrease the side effect. It is important that you let your healthcare team know what you are feeling so they can make suggestions and follow this side effect.

The schedule for taking your medication is

____

____

Symptom and Description

Papulopustular rash may be very mild with just a few red spots, or it can become quite severe with many large, red pustules and even bleeding. The rash can be itchy or painful. It usually appears within 2 to 3 weeks of beginning treatment and can get either better or worse with time. The rash is most common on the face, the upper chest, upper back, and scalp, but it can occur on any part of the body. It may begin with tenderness and redness of the skin.

Prevention

There are some things that can be done to help prevent or minimize the rash. It is important to follow the instructions of your doctor and nurse. They will be aware of how to prevent and manage this rash. Some things that may help include these steps:

- Protect your skin from the sun. Wear protective clothing, sunglasses, and sunscreen when outdoors. Use sunscreen with a sun protective factor (SPF) of at least 15. Look for products that contain titanium dioxide or zinc oxide. Reapply frequently. Sun can make the rash worse.
- Bathe with bath oil or very mild soap and shampoo. Use only products on your skin that contain no perfume, alcohol, or dye. Pat skin dry.

(continued)

- Wear loose-fitting clothing that allows your skin to breathe.
- Avoid using hot water for the bath or shower.
- Apply moisturizers at least two times each day to your whole body, especially right after you dry your skin. Apply the moisturizer all over the body. Suggested products include Eucerin, Aveeno (fragrance-free), Aquaphor, Neutrogena Norwegian formula, SARNA Ultra, Vaseline Intensive Care Advanced Healing Lotion, and Vanicream. Avoid lotions that contain alcohol, which can dry the skin.
- Avoid laundry detergent with strong perfumes.
- Makeup is fine to use but use only hypoallergenic products.
- Drink at least eight 8-ounce glasses of fluid each day to keep skin well hydrated.
- Do not use acne medicine. It is not recommended for this rash and will dry your skin.
- Use creams and preventive antibiotics as instructed by your doctor and nurse.
- Avoid heavy beard growth. Use a sharp multiblade razor, pre-shaving emollients, and moisturizing aftershave. Do not use alcohol-containing products or an electric shaver.
- If you are taking a pill medicine, avoid grapefruit products while being treated. Also, carefully follow the instructions given to you by the doctor and nurse. Whether you take the pill with or without food can change the amount of drug you absorb and its side effects.
- Do not take any over-the-counter medicine or use products on your skin without first discussing them with your doctor or nurse.
- Call your nurse or doctor if you develop a rash. Your care will be reviewed, and informing them will allow them to follow your condition.

Management

Most people eventually develop a rash. It is important for you to contact your doctor or nurse when a rash appears so they can monitor the rash and change or add medicine as needed to keep the rash from getting too bad. It is also important to follow their directions so the anticancer medicine can be continued and you can remain comfortable.

- Continue all of the care you have used to prevent the rash. Continue your use of moisturizer creams, but not in an area of pustular rash.
- It is very likely that your doctor or nurse will prescribe creams and even antibiotics to help minimize the rash. Carefully follow directions for their use.
- The rash can be covered with makeup or a cover-up such as Dermablend. Remove make-up with a hypoallergenic liquid cleanser such as Neutrogena, Dove, or Ivory Skin Cleansing Liquid-Gel.
- If your rash is uncomfortable, speak with your doctor or nurse about appropriate medicine to help with the pain.
- Remember to keep in frequent contact with your doctor or nurse if you have any questions or concerns. There may be something that can be changed about your care that would help make you more comfortable.
- Having a rash can affect you socially or psychologically. If you feel you would benefit from talking more about this issue, contact your doctor or nurse.

Follow-up

If you are having difficulty with a rash, it is important to remain in close contact with members of your healthcare team. Follow their instructions as closely as possible. If you have questions about these instructions, or are concerned that you may not be able to follow the instructions, let your healthcare team know so they can help.

Phone Numbers

Nurse: ________________________________ Phone: ______________

Office: ________________________________ Phone: ______________

Return appointment: ____

Source: Morse L. Skin and Nail Bed Changes. In: Yarbro CH, Wujcik D, Gobel BH, eds. *Cancer Symptom Management.* 4th ed. Burlington, MA: Jones & Bartlett Learning; 2014.

Hand–Foot Syndrome and Hand–Foot Skin Reaction

Patient Name: ______________________________

This self-care guide is to help you prevent and manage this side effect of cancer treatment. The guide also will help you decide when to notify a member of your healthcare team about your symptoms.

Hand–foot syndrome is a condition caused by some drugs used to treat cancer. The palms of the hands and soles of the feet may burn and tingle. This sensation may progress to swelling and redness of these areas. The problem may resolve or may become more painful, making it difficult to handle objects, wear your shoes, or even walk comfortably. In severe cases, the skin will blister, may peel, and may cause sores. This skin reaction may occur on other parts of your body, especially where there is pressure and warmth, such as the groin, under the breasts, and in the armpits.

Hand–foot skin reaction is similar to hand–foot syndrome but is associated with different medicines. Unlike patients with hand–foot syndrome, patients with hand–foot skin reaction develop painful, yellowish-colored patches on the heels and the balls of the feet and sometimes the palms of the hands. These patches may appear without other skin changes, usually beginning after 2 to 3 weeks of treatment.

These side effects are not life threatening and will reverse with proper care and time away from treatment. The sooner your healthcare team is aware of the changes, the more likely they are to help you successfully manage the changes.

One of the medications you are taking, ______________________, can cause this skin reaction. Following the recommendations in this guide may help prevent or decrease the side effect. It is important that you let your healthcare team know what you are feeling so they can make suggestions and monitor this side effect.

The schedule for taking your medication is

____

____

Symptom and Description

Hand–foot syndrome and hand–foot skin reaction usually start with numbness and tingling of the palms of the hands and soles of the feet. The skin looks red and slightly swollen. The hands or feet may feel uncomfortable and you may find that touching warm objects causes more discomfort than usual. It is fine to continue to take your medicine, but you should notify a member of your healthcare team about what you are feeling and seeing so the side effect can be monitored.

If this condition progresses, the skin will become more red, swollen, and painful. Your skin may become dry and crack. It may become difficult to perform your usual activities. Wearing shoes and walking may be difficult. It is very important to notify your doctor or nurse if you are having any of these problems. Do not take any more medicine until you have talked to them. If the condition continues to worsen, the skin may blister and peel, leaving ulcers and sores that will severely limit your activities.

Prevention

We do not know exactly how or why these syndromes occur. However, we think that gentle care of the hands and feet will prevent or decrease the severity of the side effect. If you are receiving intermittent treatments, avoid the activities (discussed below) for the day before and 3 days after the treatment. If you are receiving more daily treatment, avoid the activities for the entire time you are taking the medicine.

- It is recommended that you obtain a manicure and pedicure before beginning treatment to make sure your skin is in excellent baseline condition. Examine your feet each day. If instructed to do so, use a pumice stone once a week after a shower or bath to remove rough spots.
- Avoid hot water. This will make the sensations worse. Take tepid baths and showers. Use tepid water to wash dishes.
- Soak feet in Epsom salts (magnesium sulfate) for 20 to 30 minutes each day.
- Avoid activities that increase pressure on the hands, feet, and other skin surfaces that may be affected. Wear loose-fitting, cotton undergarments. Do not run or take long walks.
- Avoid vigorous skin rubbing or long periods of pressure on any skin surface. Pat skin to dry it.
- Wear well-fitting shoes with no pressure points, and soft, absorbent socks. Avoid walking in bare feet. Wear shoes or padded slippers.
- Avoid sun exposure.
- Drink at least 8 glasses of fluid daily (8-ounce glasses; about 2 liters).
- Protect hands by wearing gloves when gardening. Avoid repetitive activities such as shoveling, raking, and use of scissors. Avoid carrying heavy bags for long periods of time.
- Keep skin soft and moisturized with creams and emollients. Make certain these products do not contain alcohol. Apply moisturizers immediately after bathing and periodically throughout the day. It may help to apply lanolin under cotton gloves and socks at bedtime, especially during winter months. Discuss recommended products with your healthcare team.

Management

If you develop more discomfort of the hands or feet, notify your doctor or nurse. They will give you suggestions and may ask you to come to the clinic to be checked. Follow their instructions. In addition, you may find the following suggestions to be helpful:

- Follow directions for prevention.
- Continue to treat your hands and feet gently. Applying cold cloths may help relieve any discomfort.
- Soak hands and feet in cool water or Epsom salts (magnesium sulfate), 3 to 4 times each day. Pat skin dry and use a moisturizer. Udderly Smooth, Bag Balm, or Aquaphor may be helpful.
- Wear cotton socks and well-padded shoes. Pressure-relieving, cooled-gel shoe inserts may be soothing. Protect hands with gloves.
- Report any signs of infection immediately. Signs of infection may include fever or sores on the hands or feet.

(continued)

Follow-up

If you are having symptoms of hand–foot syndrome or hand–foot skin reaction, it is important to remain in close contact with members of your healthcare team. Follow their instructions as closely as possible. If you have questions about these instructions, or are concerned that you may not be able to follow the instructions, let your healthcare team know so they can help.

Phone Numbers

Nurse: ______________________________ Phone: ______________

Office: ______________________________ Phone: ______________

Return appointment: ______________________________________

Source: Morse L. Skin and Nail Bed Changes. In: Yarbro CH, Wujcik D, Gobel BH, eds. *Cancer Symptom Management.* 4th ed. Burlington, MA: Jones & Bartlett Learning; 2014.

Skin Care During Radiation Therapy

Patient Name: ____

This self-care guide is to help you prevent and manage skin changes that can occur as a result of radiation treatment. The guide also will help you decide when to notify a member of your healthcare team about your symptoms.

To reach the area being treated, radiation must pass through your skin. The skin protects our bodies from invasion by foreign matter such as bacteria. Skin can be damaged by radiation. Although some degree of skin reaction is likely, there are several things you can do to help keep skin soft and comfortable. Following the recommendations in this guide may be helpful. It is important that you let your healthcare team know what you are feeling so they can make suggestions and monitor side effects.

The schedule for your radiation treatment is

____

____

Symptom and Description

Radiation treatments affect only the skin in the area being treated. You may not notice a difference in the sensation or appearance of your skin until you have received several treatments. However, eventually the skin may look inflamed and red, and feel uncomfortable. Some people compare it to having a sunburn. This condition may progress to dry flaking of the skin in the treatment area, and if the skin reaction progresses, loss of the outermost layer of skin.

Certain areas of the body are at more risk for severe skin reaction. These include areas of skin fold such as the armpit, under the breast, and in the groin. Skin surfaces rub against each other in these skin folds, and the area may be moist. This rubbing can lead to skin breakdown.

It is important to remember that the skin reaction may continue to get worse after the radiation stops. Eventually, with time away from treatment, the skin will improve.

Prevention

You can take some steps to help prevent or minimize the skin reaction. It is important to follow the instructions of your doctor and nurse about how to prevent and manage this skin reaction. Some measures that may help include in the following:

- Wash the treatment area gently with warm water and a mild soap such as Ivory, unscented Neutrogena, or unscented Dove. Soap should be fragrance free and contain no deodorant. Soap should not contain lanolin. Pat the skin dry.
- Moisturizing with skin cream is acceptable. Apply the cream after daily radiation treatment and on the weekend. Avoid areas with skin folds. Use plain, unscented, lanolin-free creams There is no particular cream or lotion that has been found to be especially helpful.
- Use calendula cream if your breast is being irradiated. If you are having another part of the body treated, discuss the use of this cream with your doctor or nurse. Another type of cream that may be helpful for skin reaction is cream containing hyaluronic acid. Both calendula and hyaluronic acid-containing creams are widely available as over-the-counter products.

(continued)

- If your scalp is in the treatment area, use gentle shampoo and pat your hair dry. Air-dry your hair or use a hairdryer on the cool setting. Avoid gels, mousses, and hairspray.
- If you need to shave in the radiation area, use an electric razor.
- It is fine to use deodorant in the treatment area. There is no evidence that this practice increases the skin reaction. It may be better to use a deodorant that does not contain aluminum. Kiss My Face and Tom's of Maine are among the companies that make deodorant without metal. Do not use deodorant if you have any breaks in your skin. You may wish to use cream with no metal or perfume in the treatment area.
- Avoid excessive heat or cold in the treated area. Do not use a hot tub, heating pad, or ice on the treated skin.
- Avoid friction on the treated skin. Wear soft, loose-fitting clothing. Women should avoid wearing tight, constricting, or underwire bras if they will be in the treatment area. A loose-fitting sports bra may be more comfortable.
- It is especially important to keep areas with treated skin folds clean and dry.
- If there is a dressing in the treatment area, use netting to hold the dressing in place rather than tape.
- If you are a swimmer and the pool has chlorinated water, rinse with fresh water after leaving the pool.
- Avoid sun exposure in the treated area. Cover skin with soft clothing. Use sun blocks with at least 30 SPF.
- Avoid scratching or rubbing the skin in the treated area.

Management

In spite of your best skin care, a skin reaction may develop. In this case, let your doctor or nurse know at your next radiation visit. You should continue careful skin care, but other creams and cleaners may be added or substituted for those you are now using.

- If you develop red, sore skin, and especially if the skin is flaking or moist and painful, notify a member of your healthcare team and keep in close contact with the team.
- Maintain skin care with gentle cleansing and patting the skin dry.
- Apply skin creams, remedies, and dressings as instructed.
- Discuss the use of a low-dose corticosteroid cream for itching or irritation with your doctor or nurse.

Follow-up

If your skin becomes irritated, it is important to remain in close contact with members of your healthcare team. Follow their instructions as closely as possible. If you have questions about these instructions, or are concerned that you may not be able to follow the instructions, let your healthcare team know so they can help.

Phone Numbers

Nurse: ________________________________ Phone: ____________

Office: ________________________________ Phone: ____________

Return appointment: ________________________________

Source: Morse L. Skin and Nail Bed Changes. In: Yarbro CH, Wujcik D, Gobel BH, eds. *Cancer Symptom Management.* 4th ed. Burlington, MA: Jones & Bartlett Learning; 2014.

PART X

ALTERATIONS IN PSYCHOSOCIAL FUNCTION

CHAPTER 29

Anxiety

Yvonne Rucker, RN, MSN, OCN®
Barbara Holmes Gobel, RN, MS, AOCN®

THE PROBLEM

The diagnosis and management of cancer can cause a number of stresses. One of the most commonly identified responses to the cancer experience, in addition to depression, is that of anxiety.[1] Anxiety can be described as vague, uneasy, and unpleasant feelings of potential harm or distress; these feelings are accompanied by an arousal that is due to real or perceived threats to one's physical or mental well-being.

Cancer-related anxiety is considered to be a normal reaction to the diagnosis and management of a potentially life-threatening illness. Anxiety is experienced along a continuum from mild anxiety to severe anxiety.[2] Mild anxiety can be beneficial, as it serves as a motivator. For example, a woman's anxiety regarding the potential for recurrence of breast cancer following breast surgery may motivate her to initiate the adjuvant chemotherapy and radiation therapy that were recommended. Increased or unrelieved anxiety, in contrast, can be harmful both psychologically and physiologically. This type of anxiety may interfere with a patient's ability to understand necessary information about the diagnosis and treatment of the cancer. At times, levels of anxiety and distress related to cancer may be severe and exceed what is considered normal. Psychiatric assistance may be required in these circumstances.

Patients with cancer commonly experience toxicities related to treatment that increase in intensity over time. The dose escalation associated with many chemotherapy regimens and the multimodal treatment received by patients puts these individuals in the position of accepting higher risks and potential deficits in exchange for the possibility of living longer. Patients may experience psychological distress such as anxiety at the time of diagnosis, before and during treatment, and over an extended period of time as they adjust to the changes and long-term effects of treatment.

Nurses are challenged to help patients cope with the experience of cancer. Positive coping involves the patient's ability to adapt functionally in the face of distress. Patients need to learn to cope with not only their natural response of anxiety, but also with many of the symptoms that accompany it, including insomnia, fatigue, and depression.[3] Anxiety may intensify when combined with somatic symptoms.[4] The effective management of anxiety may help to improve the patient's quality of life throughout the cancer continuum, from reducing toxicities during treatment (e.g., by teaching relaxation and guided imagery to help reduce nausea, vomiting, and anxiety) to improving adherence to treatment regimens, and finally, to helping patients accept death with grace and dignity.

Much of the recent research regarding anxiety in patients with cancer identifies anxiety as one part of a cluster of symptoms, with each symptom potentially impacting the existence and severity of other symptoms. This cluster of symptoms includes various psychological symptoms (e.g., anxiety and depression) and quality of life symptoms (e.g., fatigue and insomnia).[5] For example, sleep disturbance is associated with a negative impact on quality of life, poorer functional performance, and mental health and emotional dimensions, as well as physical functioning, bodily pain, and vitality dimensions of quality of life.[6–9] Insomnia, fatigue, depression, and anxiety are positively correlated with one another and negatively correlated with quality of life.[10]

INCIDENCE

The incidence of anxiety in patients with cancer varies greatly, ranging from 2% to 48%.[2,4,11,12] Explanations as to why this variation in incidence exists include the somatic characteristics of anxiety (e.g., fatigue and insomnia), which may be a result of the diagnosis and treatment of cancer and not an outgrowth of the anxiety response itself.[4] The psychological distress varies with the type of cancer and cancer treatment.[13,14] Mao et al. found that, when adjusted for cancer type and sociodemographic variables, most patients' psychological distress decreases over time, and that after two years, there is no appreciable difference in psychological distress in cancer survivors.[13]

ETIOLOGY

Anxiety is often a response to a threat, and it is found in all clinical populations. Anxiety can be experienced at diagnosis, during treatment, or over a long period of time following diagnosis and treatment. Although the symptoms of anxiety are a highly personal experience that can be affected by past feelings and situations, anxiety does produce a number of typical signs and symptoms—namely, sweating, trembling, worry, tachypnea, shortness of breath, tachycardia, palpitations, muscle tension, restlessness, apprehension, poor concentration, insomnia, loss of appetite, and dizziness or lightheadedness.[12,15]

Anxiety can be acute or chronic in nature. Acute anxiety is usually related to the stress of cancer and its treatment. For example, a patient may experience acute episodes of anxiety related to upcoming chemotherapy treatments or to periods of uncontrolled pain. Chronic anxiety generally predates the cancer diagnosis, but may be exacerbated during treatment.[16]

In addition to occurring on its own, anxiety can be accompanied by almost any other psychiatric illness. Depression frequently accompanies anxiety, and there is a great deal of symptom overlap between depression and anxiety.[1] Difficulty sleeping, poor appetite, and difficulty concentrating can be key symptoms for either anxiety or depression, or both. Effective treatment of anxiety that is accompanied by depression requires management of the depression as well.

PATHOPHYSIOLOGY

The four types of anxiety typically seen in patients with cancer are (1) reactive anxiety related to the disease, (2) anxiety related to treatment, (3) preexisting anxiety disorders that predate the diagnosis of cancer, and (4) anxiety related to medical factors.

ANXIETY RELATED TO THE DISEASE

Most individuals who receive a diagnosis of cancer demonstrate what are considered normal responses to stress. These responses can include an initial period of shock and disbelief, followed by a time of turmoil accompanied by symptoms of anxiety and depression. Disruption of sleep and appetite commonly occur during this time. The mood of the individual is often sad or anxious, with a sense of despair and hopelessness. In the absence of a crisis such as a cancer diagnosis, these responses would likely be considered pathologic.[17] In the context of adjustment to the diagnosis of cancer, however, the behaviors are signs of normal and adaptive coping. This exaggerated response generally diminishes over a period of a week.[17] Encouragement and support by family and friends during this period of time can help to promote the individual's emotional well-being. The treating physician or advanced practice nurse is also in a position to help the individual by offering support, compassion, and reassurance, while detailing the facts of the medical situation. Cancer recurrence or progression of the disease is associated with a higher prevalence of anxiety.[18]

Some individuals may find the anxiety caused by cancer-related stress to be intolerable. If the individual considers the levels of anxiety to be intolerable or if the stress level persists for several weeks or months, psychiatric treatment may be required.

ANXIETY RELATED TO TREATMENT

Cancer treatment can cause anxiety in some patients.[15] For some patients, cancer treatment is seen as a positive event that may hold promise for providing a cure of the cancer or control of symptoms. Others may view cancer treatment as a threat and an event wrought with significant toxicities, such as nausea and vomiting, alopecia, and painful diagnostic procedures (e.g., bone marrow biopsy, lumbar puncture). This negative view may cause anxiety. In addition, a lack of treatment, such as occurs with inoperable forms of cancer or cancer that is refractory to treatment, may cause significant anxiety.[17]

PREEXISTING ANXIETY DISORDERS

Many patients face the diagnosis and treatment of cancer with a history of a preexisting anxiety disorder. Knowledge of this preexisting disorder is important in the care and management of a patient with cancer because the disorder can be reactivated during the cancer experience.[17] The chronic disorders seen most often in cancer include generalized anxiety disorder (GAD), specific phobias, panic disorder with or without agoraphobia, adjustment disorder with anxious mood, and post-traumatic stress disorder.[1] Anxiety related to phobias and panic disorders complicates the care of patients with cancer. Phobias are usually related to specific situations or fears, including fear of blood, needles, doctors, and hospitals. A diagnosis of a generalized anxiety disorder requires the existence of chronic (over a period of greater than 6 months) tension, worry, and feelings of apprehension.[15]

ANXIETY RELATED TO MEDICAL FACTORS

The most common medical factors causing anxiety in patients with cancer include medication side effects, substance abuse and withdrawal, uncontrolled pain, and delirium.[2] Some of the abnormal metabolic states that cause anxiety in patients with cancer include bleeding, infection, hypoxia, hypocalcemia, hypoglycemia, and pulmonary embolism.[2] A number of medications taken by patients with cancer have anxiety as a side effect. These include central nervous system (CNS) stimulants, withdrawal from CNS depressants, psychotropic and cardiovascular medications, as well as a variety of other medications. Table 29-1 lists some of the medications that may cause anxiety.[17,19,20]

Substance abuse and associated withdrawal can occur with tobacco, alcohol, narcotics, or other addictive substances. Eliciting information on the use of tobacco and other addictive substances is vital for completing a thorough history of a patient. The existence of severe pain can increase the chance of the development of anxiety.[17]

Delirium may be misdiagnosed as anxiety, depression, or psychosis.[16] Due to the distressing nature of delirium to the patient and family, it should be diagnosed early and treated aggressively. Notably, delirium may occur as a terminal event in patients with advanced disease.[21] Benzodiazepines and tricyclic antidepressants have the potential to cause delirium in patients with advanced cancer.[22] The cardinal symptoms of delirium include disorientation; altered levels of consciousness and attention; disorders of perception, emotion, psychomotor capabilities, and behavior; and disturbances of sleep patterns.[22,23] Cautious use of benzodiazepines and tricyclic antidepressants may help to prevent the symptom of delirium when treating patients with cancer for anxiety.

TABLE 29-1

Medications That May Cause Anxiety

Central nervous system (CNS) stimulants	Caffeine, amphetamines, cocaine
CNS depressant withdrawal	Barbiturates, benzodiazepines
Psychotropics	Antipsychotics, buspirone
Other	Steroids, theophylline

Source: Data from NCI[17]; Clark[19]; Satterfield[20].

SYMPTOM ASSESSMENT

Unfortunately, there appears to be a discrepancy between healthcare professionals' ratings of anxiety and patients' own ratings of their anxiety.[24] This discrepancy may reflect a lack of training or education of nurses and other healthcare professionals regarding signs and symptoms of anxiety. There is a need for a "user-friendly" (e.g., not cumbersome or time-consuming) assessment scale that can help to detect the presence of cancer-related anxiety. Once anxiety is detected, interventions can then be provided to those patients who are experiencing psychological distress and anxiety, especially those with moderate to high levels of anxiety at the time of diagnosis. Ongoing assessment of the patient's psychological distress is important, as patients may continue to experience elevated levels of distress, including anxiety years after diagnosis.[13]

RISK FACTORS

The level of distress that a patient experiences depends on three types of factors: medical, psychological, and social. Medical factors include the site of the cancer, stage of the disease, clinical course of the disease, type of treatment, and other medical problems, including the presence of pain.[14,25]

Psychological factors include coping ability, emotional maturity, disruption of life goals, and the ability to modify life plans. Higher levels of anxiety are generally experienced at the time of diagnosis and in conjunction with a change in the treatment plan or prognosis.[15] Cancer and its treatment can lead to situations that may increase the potential for psychological distress. These conditions include changes in appearance, role transition dilemma, functional impairment, and sexual dysfunction.[26–28]

Social factors include support from friends, family, and significant others. Younger survivors, persons without a living partner, and less educated patients have a higher prevalence of anxiety.[29,30] The presence of side effects related to either the disease process or its treatment may increase the risk for anxiety in patients with cancer. The side effects most observed to coexist with anxiety are fatigue, dyspnea, nausea, and pain.[4]

SELF-ASSESSMENT

Almost immediately after diagnosis, the patient is inundated with new information and is expected to make difficult decisions regarding treatment.[31] These demands can be overwhelming due to the many life changes that a person with cancer faces. A patient experiencing anxiety may have physical symptoms such as a racing heart, sweating, headaches, a feeling of restlessness, stomach upset, or loss of appetite. Hypervigilance, trouble concentrating, fear of death, and fear for the future are all psychological responses to anxiety.[15] Changes in body image related to surgery (e.g., mastectomy or prostatectomy), alopecia, financial concerns, and existential concerns are also commonly experienced along the cancer trajectory.[32–34] Research has shown that older individuals with cancer have decreased levels of anxiety compared to younger patients with cancer.[30] Mild anxiety will often increase patients' alertness to their environment, but moderate to severe anxiety can impair their ability to comprehend education.[2] A patient's anxiety can, however, impede the processing of information that healthcare professionals share with the patient or even affect a patient's willingness to start or continue treatment.

OBJECTIVE ASSESSMENT

A number of tools are available to detect and measure anxiety. Some of the more commonly used tools include the State-Trait Anxiety Inventory (STAI), the Hospital Anxiety and Depression (HAD) scale, the Beck Anxiety Inventory (BAI), the Distress Thermometer, and the Impact of Event (IES) scale.[35–39]

The STAI is a 40-item scale, with 20 items assessing state anxiety and 20 items assessing trait anxiety.[40,41] State anxiety is situational, whereas trait anxiety is a tendency to be anxious in stressful situations.[42]

The HAD scale consists of two subscales, one assessing depression (7 items) and one assessing anxiety (7 items).[43,44]

The Distress Thermometer is a one-item tool that rates distress on a continuum ranging from no distress (0) to severe distress (10) in the past week.[38] Although this instrument is not specific in detecting anxiety, it is helpful in identifying and monitoring for emotional distress, which includes depression, anxiety, and a combination of anxiety and depression.[45]

The Beck Anxiety Inventory is a 21-item tool that helps to differentiate physical and emotional symptoms of anxiety from those of depression.[46]

The IES assesses current subjective distress due to a specific life event. The IES was developed to assess concepts central to the diagnosis of post-traumatic stress disorder (PTSD), as described in the *Diagnostic and Statistical Manual of Mental Disorders*, fourth edition, text revision (DSM-IV-TR).[47] The DSM-IV-TR is the primary resource used for identifying mental health disorders, including anxiety.[48,49]

None of the tools described here is specific for anxiety in patients with cancer. As a consequence, the identification of anxiety must be generalized to the cancer experience. Table 29-2 provides more information on these tools.[35–49]

In most situations, patients with cancer are not assessed with these tools unless they are a part of a research program

TABLE 29-2

Review of Commonly Used Tools to Assess and Measure Anxiety

Name of Tool	Scale Used	Specific Features	Measurement
State-Trait Anxiety Inventory (STAI)	20-item scale measuring A-state scale	Measure of state (transitory) anxiety	Self-report tool measures transitory anxiety characterized by feelings of apprehension, tension, and autonomic-induced symptoms
	20-item scale measuring A-trait scale	Measure of trait anxiety	Measures general arousal and tendency to anxiety
Diagnostic and Statistical Manual of Mental Disorders, Fourth Edition (DSM-IV)	Classification system	Classifies anxiety into primary and secondary disorders Used most frequently in psychiatric setting	Tool administered by psychiatrist or trained mental health professional
Hospital Anxiety and Depression Scale (HAD)	14-item scale, 7 concerning anxiety	Excludes somatic symptoms of disease Widespread use in cancer and other physical illnesses	Self-report tool
Impact of Event Scale (IES)		Developed to assess concepts central to the diagnosis of posttraumatic stress disorder (PTSD)	Tool administered by psychiatrist or trained mental health professional
Beck Anxiety Inventory (BAI)	21-item scale concerning anxiety	Helps in the differentiation between anxiety and depression	Used to distinguish between somatic and cognitive symptoms of anxiety
Distress Thermometer	1-item scale	Not specific to anxiety but to all areas of distress	Self-report tool

Source: Data from Spielberger et al[35]; Zigmund et al[36]; Beck et al[37]; Jacobsen et al[38]; Horowitz et al[39]; Kase et al[40]; Seki-Nakamura et al[41]; Lin et al[42]; Arving et al[43]; Meraner et al[44]; Zwahlen et al[45]; Hopko et al[46]; Haagsma et al[47]; American Psychiatric Association[48]; Kawa et al[49].

or have sought psychological or psychiatric assistance. Assessment of anxiety in daily clinical practice differs from the assessments and measurements done for the purposes of research. The clinician at the bedside does not have easy access to or the time to use sophisticated measurement tools. Because of the lack of clinically useful and objective tools and their high workloads, many clinicians use their own judgment to assess the presence or absence of anxiety.[27]

A review of the medical record includes a thorough review of medications that the patient is currently taking and the dates when any medications were started. Many medications can induce symptoms of anxiety (see Table 29-1). The medical record or discussion with the patient may reveal certain medications that have been discontinued, perhaps inadvertently. Sudden withdrawal of sedatives or alcohol in a patient who is physically dependent on those substances may precipitate withdrawal symptoms, which may incorrectly appear to be severe anxiety. Individuals who smoke more than 2 packs of cigarettes per day and who must stop smoking while in the hospital may also experience withdrawal symptoms including anxiety, irritability, and restlessness.[2]

DEGREES OF TOXICITY

Anxiety toxicity can be graded using the National Cancer Institute's Common Terminology Criteria for Adverse Events (CTCAE). The CTCAE grading scale is used to standardize the evaluation of adverse events that occur with cancer treatments and therapies. The grading scale ranges from 0 (no adverse events) to 5 (death) (Table 29-3).[50] Although there may be times when patients experience no anxiety, it is anticipated that patients will experience anxiety during certain periods, such as at diagnosis or when beginning a new therapy. At these times, individuals with progressively severe anxiety may experience increases in symptoms such as tachycardia, sensations of dyspnea, and restlessness. Suicide rates for individuals with cancer are elevated relative to those for the general population, but are especially high in the first 5 years after diagnosis.[51]

SYMPTOM MANAGEMENT STRATEGIES

THERAPEUTIC APPROACHES

It is essential that every treatment plan be individualized and based on an accurate assessment. If a person's anxiety does not interfere with decision making or initiating or maintaining treatment and is not intolerable to the patient, then no specific interventions may be required other than reassurance and continual efforts to build a therapeutic relationship.[52] Once it is identified that an individual has problems with anxiety, it is appropriate for the clinician either to intervene with resources from within the cancer care arena or to refer the patient to a mental health professional. Figure 29-1 provides an algorithm for the management of anxiety in the patient with cancer.

Talking with the patient and reviewing the medical record may provide valuable information regarding the presence of anxiety. Opening communication by simply asking, "How are you feeling?" can provide a great deal of information. For example, if the patient responds by stating that eating or sleeping is a problem, the clinician can provide input into managing the problem, thereby potentially reducing anxiety. Attentive listening is the best communication style that can be used, including showing interest and maintaining a nonjudgmental focus on what the person is expressing.[12] Asking the patient directly whether he or she has ever been treated for anxiety, "nerves," or depression can help to determine whether the symptoms of anxiety preceded the diagnosis of cancer. Using a calm, reassuring approach when communicating with a patient may lessen the sense of anxiety. This approach is demonstrated through both verbal and nonverbal behavior.

TABLE 29-3

National Cancer Institute Common Terminology Criteria for Adverse Events (CTCAE): Anxiety

Adverse Event	1	2	3	4	5
Anxiety	Mild symptoms; intervention not indicated	Moderate symptoms; limiting instrumental activities of daily living (ADL)	Severe symptoms; limiting self-care ADL; hospitalization not indicated	Life-threatening; hospitalization indicated	Death

Anxiety: a disorder characterized by apprehension of danger and dread accompanied by restlessness, tension, tachycardia, and dyspnea unattached to a clearly identifiable stimulus.
Source: Data from National Cancer Institute Common Terminology Criteria for Adverse Events (CTCAE)[50].

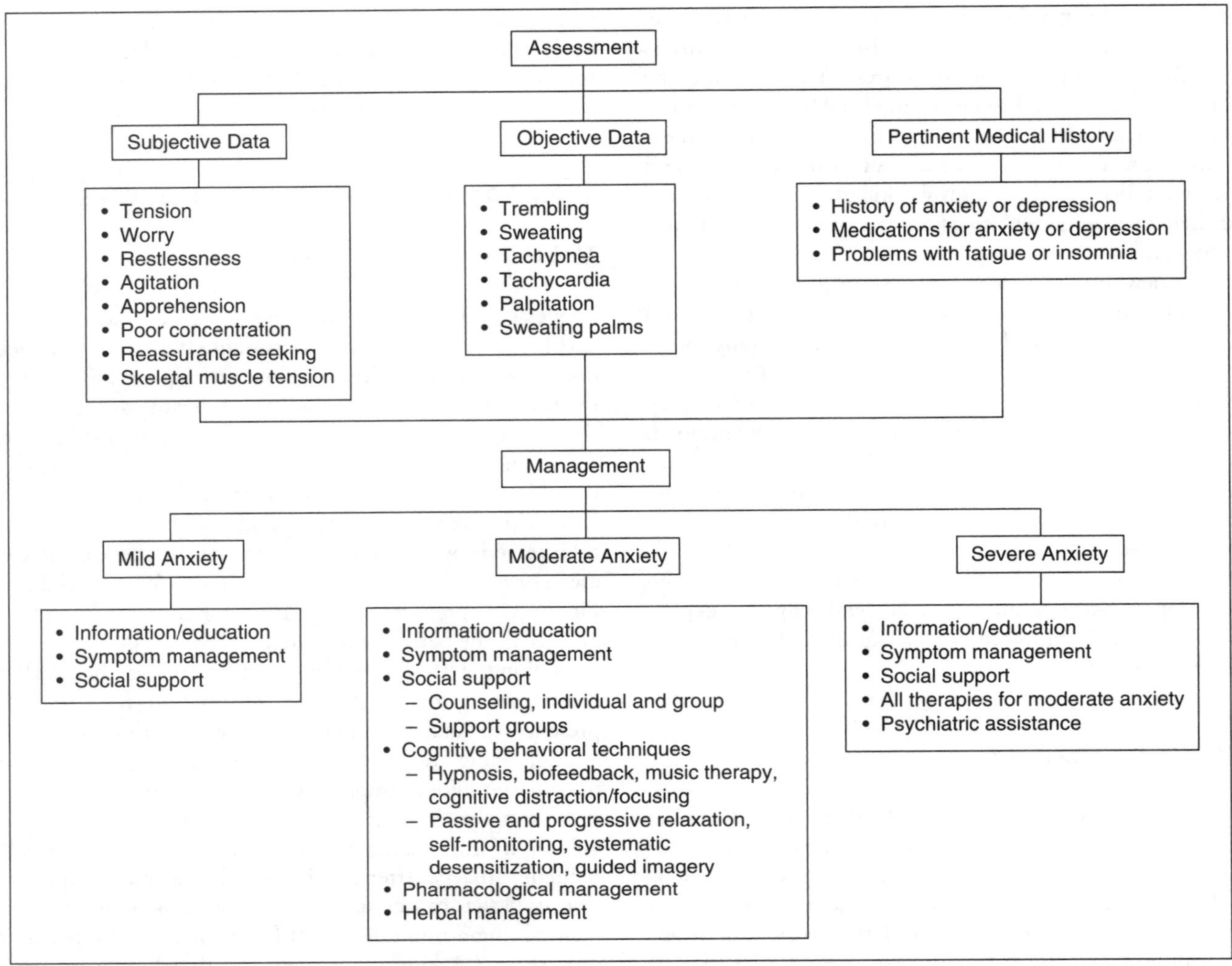

FIGURE 29-1

Algorithm for the management of anxiety in the patient with cancer.

The family also needs this same empathic approach to the management of their anxiety.[12] Journaling and participating in support groups are interventions that individuals can easily use and that are beneficial in decreasing anxiety.[2]

Patient education

Information-seeking behavior is a strategy that many people use as a means of coping with and relieving stress and anxiety. Studies show that "structured" (verbal, written, audiovisual, or computer-based) patient information and education can positively affect the patient's coping abilities.[53–56] Information serves many purposes; it helps patients understand the meaning of the diagnosis of cancer, different treatments and outcomes, side effects of treatments, and alternatives and consequences to treatment.[53,54] The National Comprehensive Cancer Network (NCCN) standards of care state that education is an important strategy for any level of cancer-related anxiety, particularly after psychotherapy has been initiated.[57] Providing information in a caring and compassionate manner can promote a sense of control in a person's life.[58]

A systematic review of the research on information needs and sources of information among patients with cancer found that the most frequently encountered information need of patients was treatment-related (38.1%) and the most frequently accessed source of health information was health professionals (27.3%), followed closely by printed materials (26.6%).[59] Within the treatment-related information category, the most frequently requested subcategories of information dealt with available treatments and treatment options (17.2%) and side effects of treatment/risks and benefits of treatment (20.5%).[59] According to this systematic review, information needs change over time for patients with cancer. During the diagnosis and treatment phase, patients are most interested in finding out about their specific diagnosis, exploring their treatment options, and understanding side effects associated with treatment. During the post-treatment phase, in addition to finding out about treatment and side effects, patients have a significant need for information related to rehabilitation. Physicians and printed materials were found to be the most relied-upon sources of information during the diagnosis and treatment phase. In addition to physicians, nurses and other healthcare professionals represented equally important sources of information in the post-treatment phase.[59]

Treatment selection for many cancers is complex. This complexity can be confusing and anxiety provoking, yet patients are expected to be active participants in their treatment decisions and rehabilitation options. When a woman is considering treatment for breast cancer, a multitude of choices must be understood. Some of these treatment decisions include whether she should have a modified radical mastectomy versus lumpectomy plus irradiation, immediate versus delayed reconstruction, or preoperative versus postoperative adjuvant chemotherapy. During this period of information seeking, a woman may receive information from a variety of sources. Traditional sources of information include discussions with physicians and nurses and written and audiovisual materials. Patients may also obtain information from the American Cancer Society (ACS), the National Cancer Institute (NCI), and the Internet.

The ACS provides an array of services, support programs, and informational resources. The NCI provides up-to-date information to both healthcare professionals and the general public. The NCI has an open-access website (www.cancer.gov) that makes available a variety of cancer information resources. One of the major resource programs established by the NCI to allow easy access to updated information is the Physician Data Query (PDQ) program. Although the PDQ was initially intended for physician use, a patient component has been added, called the Patient version of PDQ. Through this website, patients are able to conduct cancer and cancer treatment research/literature searches, seek information about cancer clinical trials, and learn about their disease.[60]

Patient education at any point along the cancer continuum should be individualized based on a number of factors: the amount and type of information desired by the patient, the patient's preferred style of learning (oral or written, group or individual), and the presence of factors that may impede learning (e.g., pain, fatigue, anxiety). The support that patients receive in an information-giving encounter may also contribute positively to patients' coping abilities.[58]

Social support

Cancer affects not only the individual with the disease, but all members of the individual's social support system. The individual's coping abilities and the availability to receive support from significant others (e.g., family, friends), in turn, influences the capacity to adjust and adapt to a cancer diagnosis and its treatment.[17] This social support system is unique to each individual. For many individuals, their primary support system is the family. Regardless of the composition of the family, members of this group are impacted by the patient's cancer diagnosis and treatment, and support is needed to help them cope with this situation.[61] Open and honest communication with both the patient and the family and structured time designed to enhance their communication with one another are critical to the success of any treatment plan. If appropriate, the family may be encouraged to participate in counseling or psychotherapy with the patient.

Some patients may seek their social support outside of the family. They may look for a new social network composed of patients facing similar problems, such as in group psychotherapy or support groups.[62] This psychotherapeutic support provides a necessary social connection. Studies have found evidence that in illness social support can actually accelerate recovery and protect against the health consequences of life stress.[17] Conversely, lack of social support can be detrimental to psychological health.[63]

Counseling and support groups

At times during the cancer experience, individuals and families may need support via counseling and support groups. The support needs can be unique to the situation and the person. The available support could include individual or interpersonal counseling, support groups, sex counseling, grief counseling, and cognitive-behavioral therapies.[64] Pharmacologic management may be used in addition to counseling.[16] The use of a mental health professional for individual counseling is not always a viable option. Some drawbacks to the use of a counselor include insurance considerations and lack of available mental health professionals in all settings.[65,66] In the absence of a counselor, support groups may provide the needed support.

Different types of support groups are available, and there is no clear definition of what constitutes a support group. Some groups are self-led or facilitated by a patient, whereas other groups are facilitated by healthcare professionals. A number of studies suggest that the problems that patients with cancer experience, such as anxiety and depression, can be reduced through participation in support groups.[67] When a patient with cancer participates in a support group composed of understanding people who have experienced or are experiencing similar problems, the patient may receive emotional and social support, as well as assistance in coping with the day-to-day stresses of living with cancer. Talking with another experienced patient may facilitate coping by providing a credible source of information.

Self-help groups are often independent of medical care but can act to link the healthcare system and the public. Support groups run by healthcare professionals are common in cancer care. Discussion of problems that arise in the course of daily living and adapting to illness are amenable to the group setting. Goals of support groups include sharing, providing education, socializing, and receiving affirmation. Daniels and Kissane report that studies have shown the effectiveness of both individual and group therapy for the psychological treatment of patients with anxiety or depression.[64]

A vast array of professionally led support groups can be found in many settings. In many communities, support groups have been set up for specific diseases (e.g., breast cancer support groups) or for specific points along the disease trajectory (e.g., grief support groups). If a support group is not available where a patient is being treated, the local ACS office usually offers a list of local support groups.

The ACS has designed several programs for the education and support of patients with cancer and their families. Two examples of these widely used programs include "I Can Cope" and "Man to Man." "I Can Cope" is a structured education program that offers support to patients and families through group discussions and socialization.[68] "Man to Man" is an educational/support program designed for men who have prostate cancer. It incorporates three initiatives: information programs, group programs for the partners of men with prostate cancer and their families, and a one-to-one visitation program.

Consideration must also be given to those patients who may be geographically isolated or unable to travel, yet are able to verbalize concerns and may benefit from interaction with a support group. Advances in telecommunications and computer technologies may help to remedy this problem.[66] Benefits of this type of telecommunication-based support group includes connecting persons with cancer who would not otherwise be able to participate in a support group, allowing participants to remain in familiar and informal surroundings while supporting one another, and maintaining privacy and enhanced continuity because participants may be able to continue in the group regardless of their setting of care.[64]

Electronic networks and computer-based support systems are other examples of useful communications technology in the cancer setting. Not only do various organizations and institutions place information on electronic networks, but some networks are set up specifically for cancer patient support.

Group support has limitations that may impede reliance on group intervention. Limitations include the difficulty of forming a group at exactly the time that a particular patient is in need of assistance, the large number of counselors prepared with an individual rather than a group orientation, and the preference of many patients for privacy. Problems of attendance at group meetings may occur as well. The number of participants in a group may fluctuate for various reasons, including inability to attend due to feeling ill, other commitments on the day of the therapy, inclement weather, and potentially a lack of interest. Group dynamics may change as the size and composition of the group changes.

Cognitive and behavioral interventions

Cognitive and behavioral techniques are well suited to the treatment of anxiety because these techniques are often effective not only in managing symptoms, but also in restoring or enhancing a sense of self-control. The perception of having increased control over a situation may lead to decreased feelings of helplessness and hopelessness, thereby promoting an improved psychological affective state (mood).[12] Examples of cognitive techniques include hypnosis, biofeedback, music therapy, mindfulness-based stress reduction, and cognitive distraction or focusing. Passive relaxation, progressive muscle relaxation, self-monitoring, and systematic desensitization are examples of behavioral techniques used for the management of anxiety.[17,64] Techniques such as hypnosis, biofeedback, and music therapy use elements from both cognitive and behavioral interventions. Often these techniques are used in combination.[17,64] For example, the use of progressive muscle relaxation is frequently combined with guided or controlled imagery.

Cognitive techniques. Cognitive interventions are based on how an individual interprets life events and bodily sensations. The goal of cognitive interventions is to identify dysfunctional automatic thoughts and underlying beliefs so as to allow for a more rational response.[12] When individuals are facing difficult problems, such as the diagnosis and treatment of cancer, cognitive therapy may help them to see the situation from a new point of view. Life-threatening problems may continue to seem real but not overwhelming. Challenging self-defeating thoughts, demonstrating the fallacies in the belief structure, stressing realistic goals, and establishing a plan that ensures incremental successes are basic cognitive strategies relevant to the treatment of anxiety in the individual with cancer.[12] Enabling hope is another way of reinterpreting negative thought processes. The act of planning, encouraging humor, and finding a reason for living are among the underused techniques to develop and maintain hope.

Behavioral techniques. Behavioral techniques are aimed at modulating patterns of behavior that help individuals cope. One of the most fundamental behavioral techniques to manage anxiety is self-monitoring. When an individual is able to monitor his or her own behavior, the individual can identify dysfunctional reactions and then learn to control them.[12] For example, a patient may experience an extreme anxiety reaction every time the needle to a vascular access device needs to be changed. The patient can be taught to monitor his or her reaction and the outcome of that reaction. With assistance from a nurse, the patient may identify that the reaction is causing a delay in care. The patient may then learn new approaches or techniques to control the reaction. It may be necessary to combine self-monitoring with other behavioral techniques.

Music therapy

Music has been used to promote health and well-being for many years in different cultures. The healing power of music has been used to address an array of social, physical, emotional, and spiritual concerns for people all over the world. More recently, patients with cancer have been introduced to music as a healing modality. Music in cancer care has been used to aid in symptom relief (e.g., cancer-related pain and discomfort) and reduce the adverse effects of cancer treatment. Music has also been used to aid in the relief of anxiety in patients with cancer.[69] Even if a music therapist is not available, the act of listening to music is a simple, low-cost intervention that may help to lessen anxiety.

Relaxation and imagery techniques

Relaxation and imagery techniques are behavioral techniques commonly used in the management of anxiety to achieve an anti-stress response, with resulting mental and physical relaxation. Specific relaxation techniques include meditation, progressive muscle relaxation, guided imagery, rhythmic breathing, and passive progressive muscle relaxation.[3]

Consider the patient who perceives a bone marrow aspirate and biopsy procedure to be highly threatening. When thinking about this procedure, the patient may experience feelings of anxiety as well as physiologic responses of tachypnea, tachycardia, profuse sweating, and skeletal muscle tension. This stress response could potentially be altered by teaching the patient progressive muscle relaxation or guided imagery. It is important to teach these techniques well in advance of the next bone marrow procedure, as both progressive muscle relaxation and guided imagery are skills that must be practiced to develop proficiency in their use.[3] Some people find it helpful to make audiotapes of a relaxation teaching session. Others find it helpful to listen to soothing music or nature sounds while practicing these skills. Table 29-4 reviews the techniques and patient characteristics related to relaxation techniques.[69–72]

Relaxation techniques used primarily for symptom control are most helpful when combined with distracting or focusing imagery. The focus of attention on a negative factor, such as pain, can be diverted using distracting or focusing imagery. A patient may begin to relax using progressive muscle relaxation and then add a pleasant image to focus attention. Perhaps this image is a beautiful, warm, white sandy beach. The patient may use this image to "escape" and imagine warm sand being gently poured over areas of discomfort.

Complementary and alternative therapies

Complementary therapies have become more popular in cancer symptom management. Acupuncture, for example, is a complementary therapy based on traditional Chinese medicine. Several types of acupuncture are practiced, including patient-administered acupuncture,

TABLE 29-4

Relaxation Techniques

Type	Techniques	Patient Characteristics
Progressive muscle relaxation	Focus on contraction and relaxation of various muscle groups Progression moves up or down the body Focus on breathing	Good muscle control to isolate muscle groups Patient is able to comfortably focus on breathing
Verbal relaxation	Relaxation from head to toe Focus on deep breathing	Patient is able to comfortably focus on breathing Good for patients in pain
Guided imagery	Focus on pleasant activity Uses all 5 senses to "live" the pleasant experience	Requires concentration Good for patients who are not comfortable focusing on breathing

Source: Data from Lin et al[69]; Leon-Pizarro et al[70]; Demiralp et al[71]; Chapman[72].

electro-acupuncture, auricular acupuncture, and acupressure.[73] Acupuncture has been shown to provide relief for anxiety and other symptoms that have been associated with increased anxiety (e.g., pain, nausea and vomiting, fatigue).[73]

Reiki is an energy therapy. Although research is required to support its use on a broader scale, some patients do express anecdotal relief of anxiety symptoms by releasing the blocked energy flows.[74] In a systematic review completed by Wilkinson et al., massage therapy was shown to give short-term relief to patients with cancer experiencing symptoms of anxiety.[75]

More research needs to be done on the effectiveness of complementary and alternative therapies in the treatment of cancer symptoms, but it is important to be aware that many cancer survivors will use complementary and alternative therapies along their cancer course.[76]

Pharmacologic treatment

Pharmacologic agents are often used in conjunction with psychotherapy in treating moderate to severe anxiety. Antianxiety and antidepressant medications are frequently prescribed to treat anxiety, but other medications are also commonly used in the treatment of other conditions that may be beneficial in decreasing levels of anxiety.

Benzodiazepines are the most commonly used anxiolytics (Table 29-5).[17,77] The agents in this class that are most frequently prescribed for cancer-related anxiety include alprazolam, chlordiazepoxide, clonazepam, clorazepate, diazepam, lorazepam, and oxazepam.[78] Benzodiazepines are beneficial in treating acute cases of anxiety because they are able relieve symptoms quickly, whereas many of the other medications must be taken for weeks before symptoms are lessened. The disadvantages of using benzodiazepines are that they can be heavily sedative in nature and that they have an addictive potential.[79,80] For this reason, these agents are often used for short-term relief of anxiety, or in cases where other medications have been ineffective.[17] The sedation associated with benzodiazepines is most severe in patients with impaired liver function. Other side effects of benzodiazepines include confusion, decreased motor coordination, sedation, headache, and problems with visual accommodations.[79,81] These side effects are dose dependent and reversible. Tolerance to benzodiazepine-related sedation often occurs during long-term therapy, while the anxiolytic effects continue.[81] Benzodiazepines have additive effects if combined with other medications that have CNS depressant properties, such as opioids. Abrupt withdrawal of benzodiazepines can lead to a withdrawal syndrome similar to alcohol withdrawal.[81]

Although antidepressants are used primarily to decrease depression, some are also effective in treating anxiety as well as depression with an anxiety component. Selective serotonin reuptake inhibitors (SSRIs) and serotonin-norepinephrine reuptake inhibitors (SNRIs) are considered the first-line antidepressants because of their efficacy in treating anxiety.[78] SSRIs include fluoxetine, sertraline, escitalopram, paroxetine, and citalopram; commonly used SNRIs include venlafaxine and duloxetin.[78,79,82] Both SSRIs and SNRIs have fewer side effects than are typically seen with benzodiazepines, although there is commonly a

TABLE 29-5

Commonly Used Benzodiazepines to Treat Anxiety in Patients with Cancer

Drug (trade name)	Half-life (hours)	Usual Daily Dose	Usual Maximum Recommended Daily Dose	Comments
Chlordiazepoxide (Librium)	24–48	10–20 mg/day	100 mg/day	Long half-life leads to accumulation of active metabolites
Diazepam (Valium, Valrelease)	35	5–15 mg/day	30 mg/day	Same as chlordiazepoxide; rapid oral absorption
Oxazepam (Serax)	4–15	10–30 mg/day	60 mg/day	Short half-life reduces risk of excessive plasma accumulation
Clorazepate (Tranxene, Tranxene-SD)	48	15–30 mg/day	60 mg/day	Same as chlordiazepoxide
Lorazepam (Ativan)	10–20	2–4 mg/day	4 mg/day	Short half-life reduces risk of excessive plasma accumulation
Alprazolam (Xanax)	9–20	0.5 mg/day	4 mg/day	Short half-life reduces risk of excessive plasma accumulation

Source: Data from NCI[17]; Martel et al[77].

delay of 4 to 6 weeks before they become effective due to their slow onset of action.[17] Side effects noted with these agents include headache, nausea, drowsiness, insomnia, and decreased sexual drive or performance.[79]

Beta blockers, such as propranolol and nadolol, are helpful in decreasing social phobia (also known as performance anxiety or stage fright).[78] The effects of beta blockers help ameliorate physical symptoms, such as trembling associated with elevated catecholamine levels.[83] Beta blockers may be beneficial to diminish symptoms of anxiety that can be anticipated before administration of chemotherapy or prior to invasive procedures such as bone marrow biopsies.[78] One limiting factor in using beta blockers is hypotension.[78] Other side effects of beta blockers include dizziness and fatigue.

Buspirone is also useful in treating anxiety and has fewer side effects than other medications; for example, it avoids the addictive potential seen with benzodiazepines, though it takes at least 2 weeks for the drug to begin to work.[79] Several of the older antidepressant medications, such as tricyclic antidepressants (e.g., imipramine) and monoamine oxidase inhibitors (MAOIs; e.g., phenelzine, tranylcypromine, and isocarboxazid), are still used to treat anxiety, but they tend to have more side effects than the newer antidepressants.[79] Tricyclics may cause dry mouth, constipation, and decreased sexual drive or performance. Drinking or eating foods or taking medications that contain tyramine should be avoided when using MAOIs because of the potential for dangerous elevations in blood pressure.[64,79] Antihistamines (e.g., diphenhydramine, hydroxyzine, and promethazine) are also occasionally used to treat anxiety, but are not as effective as the benzodiazepines. They may be used when it is preferred to avoid benzodiazepines due to the patient's alcohol or substance abuse.[78]

The treatment of elderly patients with benzodiazepines requires special care. With advancing age comes changes in hepatic enzyme function that affect the metabolism of benzodiazepines. The pathways of hepatic detoxification of benzodiazepines involve microsomal oxidation, glucuronide conjugation, and nitroreduction. Although conjugation and nitroreduction do not change appreciably as age increases, oxidation becomes less efficient with age.[84] Diazepam, alprazolam, and triazolam are examples of benzodiazepines that are oxidized. Lorazepam, oxazepam, and temazepam are benzodiazepines that are metabolized by conjugation and may be better choices in the treatment of elderly patients because they provide for improved clearance.[84] These medications can be used to treat anxiety, but special attention should be paid to their dose, schedule, and signs of accumulation. With increasing age, many aspects of brain function are more vulnerable to benzodiazepines. As a consequence, side effects that may be more pronounced in the elderly include disorientation, memory disturbance, excessive drowsiness, and changes in gait and balance.[78,80]

Herbal management of anxiety

Herbs and nutritional supplements are not regulated as pharmaceuticals, but rather are considered dietary supplements. A dietary supplement is a product (e.g., vitamin, mineral, herb) taken in effort to augment or act as a substitute dietary intake for that product.[85] Although herb therapy is most often self- or patient-regulated, it is important to recognize that herbs used in the medicinal sense are, in reality, drugs. Many people equate the word "herb" with "safe," which implies that herbs represent a better kind of medicine. Nutritional supplements, because they are not regulated as pharmaceuticals, may cause adverse events due to the action of the herb or supplement due to a contaminant in the compound, or due to interactions with other medications that are being taken concomitantly.[86] Table 29-6 lists herbs used for the management of anxiety.[87–89]

NURSING IMPLICATIONS

The two most important nursing actions with respect to anxiety are communication and assessment. Communication that is therapeutic involves developing a trusting relationship that will be facilitated through nonjudgmental communication.[12] Building trust helps patients feel comfortable enough to have difficult conversations about their concerns related to such topics as fertility, sexuality, and role transition. Assessment across the cancer illness trajectory will allow for early detection of anxiety and can be beneficial in identifying distress before it evolves into severe anxiety. The nurse's assessment is integral in recognizing anxiety at the time of the cancer diagnosis, intermittently throughout treatment and post treatment, at the time of reccurrence, and/or when transitioning to palliative care; such assessment provides an opportunity for the nurse to identify anxiety during transitional phases in the cancer journey when anxiety levels are likely to escalate.[12] Patient-centered interventions are built on the nurse's ability to identify the needs that are unique to the patient and create a plan of care that prevents the development of severe anxiety or manages anxiety with a focus on the individual's needs.[3]

PATIENT SELF-CARE

Anxiety, like most responses to cancer, is highly personal and is affected by past feelings and experiences. The anxiety response may be mild and time limited, or it may be prolonged and require psychiatric assistance. Regardless of the level of the response, the presence of anxiety can affect the patient's quality of life. As such, healthcare professionals

TABLE 29-6

Herbs Used to Manage Anxiety

Name	Plant	Commonly Known Uses	Administration Considerations	Side Effects/Contraindications
Ginseng (Asian or American)	Dried root of several species of the genus *Panex*	Improve learning and memory Anti-cancer Anti-diabetes Immunomodality	Daily dosage: 50–300 mg Available as tea, capsules, extracts, other edible products	Contraindicated in pregnancy, Use with caution with cardiovascular disease or diabetes (potential hypoglycemia) "Ginseng Abuse Syndrome" (elevated blood pressure, sleeplessness, restlessness) Significant interactions with drugs, including antidiabetic agents, warfarin, digoxin
Kava (aka Kava Kava)	Dried root of *Piper methysticum*	Anxiety Stress Insomnia	Daily dosage: Capsules: 50–400 mg of root extract Available as capsule, tincture and tea	May cause sedation effect, gastrointestinal upset, dizziness, decreased reaction time and impaired motor skills, hepatotoxicity, and rash, temporary yellowing of the skin, hair and nails
St. John's wort	Leaves and flowering tops of *Hypericum perforatum*	Depression Anxiety Sleep disorders Wound healing	Daily dosage: 300–1800 mg Available as a tea, tincture, and capsule	Significant interactions with drugs- antihypertensive medications, immunosuppressants (e.g., decreased serum concentrations of cyclosporine and tacrolimus), certain selective serotonin reuptake inhibitors (risk for potentiation), digoxin, and benzodiazepines. May cause dizziness, restlessness, photosensitivity, dry mouth, gastrointestinal upset, allergic reaction, and confusion
Valerian	Dried rhizome and roots of a tall perennial herb, *Valerian officinalis*	Anxiety Insomnia	Daily dosage: Extract: 60–900 mg Root powder: 15 g Available as a liquid, extract, and capsule	Central nervous system depressants can potentiate effects Sedative effect May cause gastrointestinal upset, headache, restlessness, decreased motor activity, and dizziness

Source: Data from Benzie et al[87]; Dasgupta[88]; Tracy et al[89].

need to be aware of the potential for the presence of anxiety and have support interventions in place to assist patients in their coping process. This range of interventions is necessary to help meet the needs of each patient.

See Appendix 29A for a self-care guide that teaches a combination of progressive muscle relaxation, passive progressive muscle relaxation, and guided imagery.

REFERENCES

1. Brown LF, Kroenke K, Theobald DE, Wu J, Tu W. The association of depression and anxiety with health-related quality of life in cancer patients with depression and/or pain. *Psychooncology.* 2010;19(7):734–741.
2. Stephenson PL. Before the teaching begins: managing patient anxiety prior to providing education. *Clin J Oncol Nurs.* 2006;10(2):241–245.
3. Kwekkeboom KL, Cherwin CH, Lee JW, Wanta B. Mind–body treatments for the pain–fatigue–sleep disturbance symptom cluster in persons with cancer. *J Pain Symptom Manage.* 2011;39(1):126–138.
4. Greer JA, Park ER, Prigerson HG, Safren SA. Tailoring cognitive-behavioral therapy to treat anxiety comorbid with advanced cancer. *J Cogn Psychother.* 2010;24(4):294–313.
5. So WKW, Marsh G, Ling WM, et al. The symptom cluster of fatigue, pain, anxiety, and depression and the effect on the quality of life of women receiving treatment for breast cancer: a multicenter study. *Oncol Nurs Forum.* 2009;36(4):E205–E214.
6. Otte JL, Carpenter JS. Theories, models, and frameworks related to sleep–wake disturbances in the context of cancer. *Cancer Nurs.* 2009;32(2):90–104.
7. Roscoe JA, Kaufman ME, Matteson-Rusby SE, et al. Cancer-related fatigue and sleep disorders. *Oncologist.* 2007;12(suppl 1):35–42.
8. Barsevick A, Beck SL, Dudley WN, et al. Efficacy of an intervention for fatigue and sleep disturbance during cancer chemotherapy. *J Pain Symptom Manage.* 2010;40(2):200–216.

9. Coleman EA, Goodwin JA, Coon SK, et al. Fatigue, sleep, pain, mood, and performance status in patients with multiple myeloma. *Cancer Nurs.* 2011;34(3):219–227.
10. Byar KL, Berger AM, Bakken SL, Cetak MA. Impact of adjuvant breast cancer chemotherapy on fatigue, other symptoms, and quality of life. *Oncol Nurs Forum.* 2006;33(1):E18–E26.
11. Smith AB, Wright EP, Rush R, Stark DP, Velikova G, Selby PJ. Rasch analysis of the dimensional structure of the Hospital Anxiety and Depression Scale. *Psychooncology.* 2006;15(9):817–827.
12. Miovic M, Block S. Psychiatric disorders in advanced cancer. *Cancer.* 2007;110(8):1665–1676.
13. Mao JJ, Armstrong K, Bowman MA, Xie SX, Kadakia R, Farrar JT. Symptom burden among cancer survivors: impact of age and comorbidity. *J Am Board Fam Med.* 2007;20(5):434–443.
14. Andrykowski MA, Lykins E, Floyd A. Psychological health in cancer survivors. *Semin Oncol Nurs.* 2008;A24(3):193–201.
15. Sheldon LK, Swanson S, Dolce A, Marsh K, Summers J. Putting evidence into practice®: evidence-based interventions for anxiety. *Clin J Oncol Nurs.* 2008;12(5):113–120.
16. National Comprehensive Cancer Network. NCCN clinical practice guidelines in oncology: management (version 1.2013). 2012. http://www.nccn.org. Accessed September 19, 2012.
17. National Cancer Institute: *PDQ® Adjustment to Cancer*. Bethesda, MD: National Cancer Institute. June 14, 2012. http://cancer.gov/cancertopics/pdq/supportivecare/adjustment/HealthProfessional. Accessed September 19, 2012.
18. Kenne Sarenmalm E, Ohlén J, Odén A, Gaston-Johansson F. Experience and predictors of symptoms, distress and health-related quality of life over time in postmenopausal women with recurrent breast cancer. *Psychooncology.* 2008;17(5):497–505.
19. Clark CP, Moore PJ, Gillin JC. Sleep disorders. In: Ebert MH, Loosen PT, Nurcombe B, Leckman JF, eds. *Current Diagnosis and Treatment: Psychiatry*. 2nd ed. New York: McGraw-Hill; 2008. 470–495.
20. Satterfield JM, Rollman BL. Anxiety. In: Feldman MD, Christensen JF, eds. *Behavioral Medicine: A Guide for Clinical Practice*. 3rd ed. New York: McGraw-Hill; 2008, 227–239.
21. Bush S, Bruera E. The assessment and management of delirium in cancer patients. *Oncologist.* 2009;14(10):1039–1049.
22. Okamura M, Akizuki N, Nakano T, et al. Clinical experience of the use of a pharmacological treatment algorithm for major depressive disorder in patients with advanced cancer. *Psychooncology.* 2008;17(2):154–160.
23. Bruera E, Bush SH, Willey J, et al. The impact of delirium and recall on the level of distress in patients with advanced cancer and their family caregivers. *Cancer.* 2009;115(9),2004–2011.
24. Merckaert L, Libert Y, Messin S, Miani M, Slachmuylder JL, Razovi D. Cancer patients' desire for psychological support: prevalence and implications for screening patients' psychological needs. *Psychooncology.* 2010;19(2):141–149.
25. Hinz A, Krauss O, Hauss JP, et al. Anxiety and depression in cancer patients compared with the general population. *Eur J Cancer Care.* 2010;19(4):522–229.
26. Borsellino M, Young MM. Anticipatory coping. *Clin J Oncol Nurs.* 2011;15(3):311–315.
27. Meraner V, Giesinger J, Kemmler G, et al. Development of a screening tool for the identification of psychooncological treatment need in breast cancer patients. *Psychooncology.* 2009;18(9):974–983.
28. Roulston A, Bickerstaff D, Haynes T, Rutherford L, Jones, L. A pilot study to evaluate an outpatient service for people with advanced lung cancer. *Int J Palliat Nurs.* 2012;18(5):225–233.
29. Hoffman KE, McCarthy EP, Recklitis CJ, Ng AK. Psychological distress in long-term survivors of adult-onset cancer: results from a national survey. *Arch Intern Med.* 2009;169(14):1274–1281.
30. Nelson CJ, Weinberger MI, Balk E, Holland J, Breitbart W, Roth AJ. The chronology of distress, anxiety, and depression in older prostate cancer patients. *Oncologist.* 2009;14(9):891–899.
31. DuBenske LL, Gustafson DH, Shaw BR, Cleary JF. Web-based cancer communication and decision making systems: connecting patients, caregivers, and clinicians for improved health outcomes. *Med Decis Making.* 2010;30(6):732–744.
32. Den Oudsten BL, Van Heck GL, Van der Steeg AF, Roukema JA, De Vries J. Clinical factors are not the best predictors of quality of sexual life and sexual functioning in women with early stage breast cancer. *Psychooncology.* 2010;19(6):646–656.
33. Lund-Nielsen B, Müller K, Adamsen L. Malignant wounds in women with breast cancer: feminine and sexual perspectives. *J Clin Nurs.* 2005;14(1):56–64.
34. van den Hurk CJ, Mols F, Vingerhoets AJ, Breed WP. Impact of alopecia and scalp cooling on the well-being of breast cancer patients. *Psychooncology.* 2010;19(7):701–709.
35. Spielberger CD, Gorsuch RL, Lushene R, Vagg PR, Jacobs GA. *Manual for the State-Trait Anxiety Inventory*. Palo Alto, CA: Consulting Psychologists Press; 1970.
36. Zigmund AS, Snaith RP. The hospital anxiety and depression scale. *Acta Psychiatr Scand.* 1983;67(6):361–370.
37. Beck AT, Epstein N, Brown G, Steer RA. An inventory for measuring clinical anxiety: psychometric properties. *J Consult Clin Psychol.* 1988;56(6):893–897.
38. Jacobsen PB, Donovan KA, Trask PC, et al. Screening for psychologic distress in ambulatory cancer patients: *a* multicenter evaluation of the Distress Thermometer. *Cancer.* 2005;103(7):1494–1502.
39. Horowitz M, Wilner N, Alvarez W. Impact of Event Scale: a measure of subjective stress. *Psychosom Med.* 1979;41(3):209–218.
40. Kase L, Ledley DR. *Wiley Concise Guide to Mental Health: Anxiety Disorders*. Weiner IB, ed. Hoboken, NJ: John Wiley and Sons; 2007.
41. Seki-Nakamura K, Maebayashi K, Nasu-Izumi S, Akimoto T, Mitsuhashi N. Evaluation of anxiety and salivary chromogranin a secretion in women receiving breast conserving surgery followed by radiation therapy. *J Radiat Res.* 2011;52(3):351–359.
42. Lin JM, Brimmer DJ, Maloney EM, Nyarko E, Belue R, Reeves WC. Further validation of the Multidimensional Fatigue Inventory in a US adult population sample. *Popular Health Metrics.* 2009;7(18):1–12.
43. Arving C, Glimelius B, Brandberg Y. Four weeks of daily assessments of anxiety, depression and activity compared to a point assessment with the Hospital Anxiety and Depression Scale. *Qual Life Res.* 2008;17(1):95–104.
44. Meraner V, Gamper EM, Grahmann A, et al. Monitoring physical and psychosocial symptom trajectories in ovarian cancer patients receiving chemotherapy. *BMC Cancer.* 2012;12(77):1–10.
45. Zwahlen D, Hagenbuch N, Carley MI, Recklitis CJ, Buchi S. Screening cancer patients' families with the Distress Thermometer (DT): a validation study. *Psychooncology.* 2008;17(10):959–966.
46. Hopko DR, Armento MEA, Robertson SMC, et al. Brief behavioral activation and problem-solving therapy for depressed breast cancer patients: randomized trial. *J Consult Clin Psychol.* 2011;79(6):834–849.
47. Haagsma JA, Polinder S, Olff M, Toet H, Bonsel GJ, vanBeeck EF. Posttraumatic stress symptoms and health-related quality of life: a two year follow up study of injury treated at the emergency department. *BMC Psychiatry.* 2012;12(1):1–8.
48. American Psychiatric Association. *Diagnostic Criteria from DSM-IV-TR*. 4th ed. Washington, DC: American Psychiatric Association; 2000.
49. Kawa S, Giordano J. A brief historicity of the *Diagnostic and Statistical Manual of Mental Disorders*: issues and implications for the future of psychiatric canon and practice. *Philos Ethics Humanit Med.* 2012;7(2):1–9.
50. National Cancer Institute. *Common Terminology Criteria for Adverse Events, v4.0*, Bethesda, MD: National Cancer Institute. May 29, 2009. http://evs.nci.nih.gov/ftp1/CTCAE/CTCAE_4.03_2010-06-14_QuickReference_5x7.pdf. Accessed September 19, 2012.
51. Misono S, Weiss NS, Fann JR, Redman M, Yueh B. Incidence of suicide in persons with cancer. *J Clin Oncol.* 2008;26(29):4731–4738.

52. Ching LC, Devi MK, Emily ANK. Anxiety in patients with breast cancer undergoing treatment: a systematic review. *JBI Lib System Rev.* 2010;8(25):1016–1057.
53. Deshler AM, Fee-Schroeder KC, Dowdy JL, et al. A patient orientation program at a comprehensive cancer center. *Oncol Nurs Forum.* 2006;33(3):569–578.
54. Hoff AC, Haaga DA. Effects of an education program on radiation oncology patients and families. *J Psych Oncol.* 2005;23(4):61–75.
55. Jones RB, Pearson J, Cawset AJ, et al. Effect of different forms of information produced for cancer patients on their use of the information, social support, and anxiety: randomised trial. *BMJ.* 2005;332(7547):942–948.
56. Katz MR, Irish JC, Devins GM. Development and pilot testing of a psychoeducational intervention for oral cancer patients. *Psychooncology.* 2004;13(9):642–653.
57. National Comprehensive Cancer Network. NCCN clinical practice guidelines in oncology: distress management (version 1.2013). 2012. http://www.nccn.org. Accessed September 23, 2012.
58. Cohen MZ, Bankston S. Cancer-related distress. In: Yarbro CH, Wujcik D, Gobel BH, eds. *Cancer Nursing Principles and Practice.* 7th ed. Burlington, MA: Jones & Bartlett Learning; 2011:667–684.
59. Rutten LJF, Arora HK, Bakos AD, Aziz N, Rowland J. Information needs and sources of information among cancer patients: a systematic review of research (1980–2003). *Patient Ed Counsel,* 2005; 57:250–261.
60. National Cancer Institute. National Institutes of Health. Comprehensive cancer information: National Cancer Institute. http://www.cancer.gov. Accessed September 23, 2012.
61. Shaw J, Harrison J, Young J, et al. Coping with newly diagnosed upper gastrointestinal cancer: a longitudinal qualitative study of family caregivers' role perception and supportive care needs. *Support Care Cancer.* August 30, 2012. (Epub ahead of print).
62. Öster I, Oliver Hedestig O, Johansson M, Nina Klingstedt N, Lindh J. Sharing experiences in a support group: men's talk during the radiotherapy period for prostate cancer. *Palliat Support Care.* 2012; 27:1–9.
63. Mehnert A, Lehmann C, Graefen M, Huland H, Koch U. Depression, anxiety, post-traumatic stress disorder and health-related quality of life and its association with social support in ambulatory prostate cancer patients. *Eur J Cancer Care.* 2010;19(6):736–745.
64. Daniels J, Kissane DW. Psychosocial interventions for cancer patients. *Curr Opin Oncol.* 2008;20:367–371.
65. Klimmek R, Snow D, Wenzel J. Insurance-related and financial challenges reported by managed care enrollees with breast cancer. *Clin J Oncol Nurs.* 2010;14(5):598–606.
66. O'Brien M, Harris J, King R, O'Brien T. Supportive-expressive group therapy for women with metastatic breast cancer: improving access for Australian women through use of teleconference. *Counsel Psychother Res.* 2008;8(1):28–35.
67. Breitbart WS, Alici Y. Psychooncology. *Harv Rev Psychiatry.* 2009;17(6):361–375.
68. Martin MY, Pollack LA, Evans MB, et al. Tailoring cancer education and support program for low-income, primarily African American cancer survivors. *Oncol Nurs Forum.* 2011;38(1):E55–E59.
69. Lin M, Hsieh Y, Hsu Y, Fetzer S, Hsu MC. A randomised controlled trial of the effect of music therapy and verbal relaxation on chemotherapy-induced anxiety. *J Clin Nurs.* 2011;20(7/8):988–999.
70. Leon-Pizarro C, Gich I, Barthe E, et al. A randomized trial of the effect of training in relaxation and guided imagery techniques in improving psychological and quality-of-life indices for gynecologic and breast brachytherapy patients. *Psychooncology.* 2007;20(11):971–979.
71. Demiralp M, Oflaz F, Komurcu S. Effects of relaxation training on sleep quality and fatigue in patients with breast cancer undergoing adjuvant chemotherapy. *J Clin Nurs.* 2010;19(7–8):1073–1083.
72. Chapman S. Cancer pain part 2: assessment and management. *Nurs Stand.* 2012;26(48):44–49.
73. O'Regan D, Filshie J. Autonomic neuroscience: basic and clinical. *Auton Neurosci.* 2010;157(1–2):96–100.
74. Burden B, Herron-Marx S, Clifford C. The increasing use of Reiki as a complementary therapy in specialist palliative care. *Int J Palliat Nurs.* 2005;11(5):248–253.
75. Wilkinson S, Barnes K, Storey L. Massage for symptom relief in patients with cancer: systematic review. *J Adv Nurs.* 2008;63(5):430–439.
76. Gansler T, Kaw C, Crammer C, Smith T. A population-based study of prevalence of complementary methods use by cancer survivors: a report from the American Cancer Society's studies of cancer survivors. *Cancer.* 2008;113(5):1048–1057.
77. Cloos J, Ferreira V. Current use of benzodiazipines in anxiety disorders. *Curr Opin Psychiatry.* 2009; 22(1): 90–95.
78. O'Donnell JM, Shelton RC. Drug therapy of depression and anxiety disorders. In: Brunton LL, Chabner BA, Knollmann BC, eds. *Goodman & Gilman's The Pharmacological Basis of Therapeutics.* 12th ed. New York: McGraw-Hill; 2011:397–416.
79. National Institute of Mental Health. *Mental Health Medications.* Bethesda, MD: National Institute of Mental Health; 2010. http://www.nimh.nih.gov/health/publications/mental-health-medications/nimh-mental-health-medications.pdf. Accessed April 3, 2012.
80. Smith AJ, Tett SE. Improving the use of benzodiazepines: is it possible? A non-systematic review of interventions tried in the last 20 years. *BMC Health Serv Res.* 2010;10(321):1–12.
81. Vinkers CH, Olivier B. Mechanisms underlying tolerance after long-term benzodiazepine use: a future for subtype-selective GABA receptor modulators? *Adv Pharmacol Sci.* 2012;2012:1–19.
82. Marrs JA. Stress, fears, and phobias: the impact of anxiety. *Clin J Oncol Nurs.* 2006;10(3):319–322.
83. Baker JG, Hill SJ, Summers RJ. Evolution of -blockers: from anti-anginal drugs to ligand-directed signaling. *Trends Pharmacol Sci.* 2011;32(4):227–234.
84. Bulat T, Castle SC, Rutledge M, Quigley P. Clinical practice algorithms: medication management to reduce fall risk in the elderly. Part 3: benzodiazepines, cardiovascular agents, and antidepressants. *J Am Acad Nurse Pract.* 2008;20(2):55–62.
85. U.S.FoodandDrugAdministration. *Regulatoryinformation:DietarySupplement Health and Education Act of 1994.* Silver Spring, MD: U.S. Food and Drug Administration; May 20, 2009. http://www.fda.gov/RegulatoryInformation/Legislation/FederalFoodDrugandCosmeticActFDCAct/SignificantAmendmentstotheFDCAct/ucm148003.htm. Accessed April 1, 2012.
86. Bent S. Herbal medicine in the United States: review of efficacy, safety, and regulation. *J Gen Intern Med.* 2008;23(6):854–859.
87. Benzie IFF, Wachtel-Galor S, eds. *Herbal Medicine: Biomolecular and Clinical Aspects.* 2nd ed. Boca Raton, FL: CRC Press; 2011.
88. Dasgupta A. *Effects of Herbal Supplements in Medicine.* Berlin: Walter de Gruyton;2011.
89. Tracy TS, Kingston, RL, eds. *Herbal Products: Toxicology and Clinical Pharmacology.* 2nd ed. Totowa, NJ: Humana Press; 2007.

Relaxation and Guided Imagery

Patient Name: ____________________

This guide will help you learn the many things that you can do to help your stress. Two things that are easy to learn are called *progressive muscle relaxation* and *guided imagery.* They may also help with pain, and nausea and vomiting.

These skills take practice. The more you practice these skills, the more helpful they are. Some people find it helpful to make a tape to listen to as they practice. A soothing tape of music may help. Many libraries have "relaxation tapes" or quiet, soothing music.

Symptom and Description

It is common to feel stress or anxiety when you have cancer. Anxiety can be a vague or uneasy feeling of distress. There are many things that can bring on these feelings, such as trips to your doctor's office, treatments for your cancer, or fears about your cancer.

Management

Preparation

1. Find a quiet, comfortable spot to practice.
2. Sit up or lie down while you practice.
3. Have a blanket or sheet handy. Often when people are relaxed, they find they are cooler and need a light blanket.
4. Take a few minutes to think about your breathing. (You can keep your eyes open or closed.) Try to do stomach breathing. Fill your stomach as you breathe in and then breathe out. Begin to slow down, and slow your breathing down. Try to focus on your breathing.

Progressive Muscle Relaxation

1. Take in a deep breath. Hold that breath for a count of four, let it out, and begin to relax. Do this about four times. As you breathe in, think about good, soothing energy flowing in. As you breathe out, breathe out your stress and bad thoughts.
2. Allow your mind to focus on one body part at a time. Move from the top of your head all the way down to your toes.
3. Relax your head and your scalp. Repeat this two or three times.
4. Move down to your eyes. Relax your eyes and the muscles around your eyes. Squeeze your eyes tight for four counts, then relax. Notice the difference in your eyes and face when your eyes are squeezed and tense, and when they are relaxed.
5. Focus on your mouth. Relax your mouth. Allow it to go limp. . . . Move down your neck, relax your neck. . . . Relax your shoulders. . . .
6. When you get to your arms, you may relax them one at a time or both at the same time. You may even choose to relax each finger, one at a time.
7. Move all the way down to your toes using this skill.

(continued)

Extra Tips (tips that may help body areas that are tense or painful)

1. As you move down your body, you may want to tighten and then relax certain body parts. This helps to show how different your body feels when it is tense and when it is relaxed. You can tense and then relax your eyes, hands, toes, mouth, and shoulders. You should get more relaxed as you move down your body. If you feel relaxed, you may not feel like doing this part past your mouth or shoulders.
2. Warm often feels good. Think about any part of your body being warmed by the sun. For example, if your right arm has pain, you can focus on this arm. Think about warm rays of sun on your arm as you relax.
3. Tense or sore muscles may feel better with the "knot" method. Think about your sore spot, such as your shoulder, as a big, tight knot. In your mind, slowly untie the knot. As you untie the knot, the sore spot becomes less and less sore. When you untie the knot all the way, you can focus on how your body is more relaxed.
4. Try the "sandbag" method for a body part that hurts. Think about the area that hurts as an empty sandbag. Slowly fill up the sandbag with warm sand. As you fill the bag, push out the hurt. Fill the bag until you can't put any more sand in it. Slowly pour out the sand. Any hurt that is left flows out with the sand. Enjoy the soothing feeling of the bag when it is again empty.

Guided Imagery

1. It is best to do this skill after you have done the progressive muscle relaxation. Once your body is relaxed, you can allow your mind to rest.
2. Before you begin, think about a special image or place. This can be a place where you have been or it can be a made-up place. Choose a relaxing place. Think about the whole scene. What does it look like? What do you hear? What do you taste or smell? Be as detailed as you like.
3. Some examples of pleasant places might include a warm, sunny beach, a sparkling lake, a walk in the woods, or a lovely snow-capped mountain.
4. Your image should be a place where you can be very relaxed. It is a place with no stress or worry. You can go to this place when you need a break.

Example of a Guided Imagery Scene

I am lying alone on a beach in the late afternoon sun. It is nice and warm, but not too hot. The water is aqua blue, with small white caps close to the shore. The sky is light blue, with a few white puffy clouds. I am lying with my feet to the water, with the sun moving to the right of me. I can feel my warm beach towel under me and warm sand on my hands and feet. I feel the soothing sun on my body. I hear seagulls flying over me. I hear sea grass swaying in the breeze behind me. I hear some children playing in the sand, but I can't hear what they are saying. The water is gently lapping on the shore, over and over and over . . .

Follow-up

1. These skills are not to be used instead of pain medicine or any other type of medicine that you need. They should be used *with* your current treatment.
2. It is okay to fall asleep during either progressive muscle relaxation or guided imagery. It does not mean that it is not working. It may mean that you need the sleep. Give yourself the rest that comes with a relaxed body and mind.
3. Progressive muscle relaxation and guided imagery take practice to help you relax. When you feel good with these skills, they may also help with pain or nausea and vomiting.
4. Talk with your doctor, nurse, or someone you trust about your stress. They may be able to give you other ideas.

Phone Numbers

Nurse: ________________________________ Phone: ________________

Physician: ______________________________ Phone: ________________

Other: ________________________________ Phone: ________________

Comments

Source: Rucker Y, Gobel BH. Anxiety. In: Yarbro CH, Wujcik D, Gobel BH, eds. *Cancer Symptom Management.* 4th ed. Burlington, MA: Jones & Bartlett Learning; 2014.

Chapter 30

Cognitive Dysfunction

Marlene Z. Cohen, RN, PhD, FAAN
Nicole A. Shonka, MD
Terri S. Armstrong, PhD, ANP-BC, FAANP
Jeffrey S. Wefel, PhD, ABPP

THE PROBLEM

It is becoming increasingly well recognized that alterations in cognitive function frequently occur in patients as a consequence of cancer or its therapy. These signs and symptoms are important because of the impact they have on functional independence, their effect on both quality of life (QOL) and adherence to follow-up care, the distress they create for patients and their families, and their relationship with survival. Cognitive dysfunction is alarming to both patients and their families, and it may impair judgment and endanger safety. In the past, cognitive changes were primarily identified in patients with known central nervous system (CNS) disease, those receiving treatments administered directly to the CNS, or those acutely ill from disease or intensive chemotherapy. Recently, more widespread and subtle problems with cognitive function have been recognized in patients who have completed therapy and are in remission, as well as in those individuals currently receiving treatment. A growing body of published literature is clarifying the neurobiological mechanisms underlying cognitive changes in cancer patients, although effective therapies are still being investigated.

Cognitive functioning refers to a set of mental processes under the control of the brain that are involved in processing, interpreting, and acting on internal and external stimuli. The word "cognition" comes from the Latin *cognoscere*, meaning "get to know."[1] Common examples of cognitive functions include attention, memory, language reasoning, and perception; collectively, they allow people to make sense of their experiences and to interact with others and the environment.

The Diagnostic and Statistical Manual of Mental Disorders 5[2] is in the process of being updated, and is expected to be finalized in May of 2013. This fifth revision is the most recent version of psychiatric nomenclature. In DSM-5 development, the diagnostic category that was formerly known as "delirium, dementia, amnestic, and other cognitive disorders" is now labeled "neurocognitive disorders" and is divided into three broad syndromes: (1) delirium, (2) mild neurocognitive disorder, and (3) major neurocognitive disorder. The work group revising the DSM categories recommended using "major neurocognitive disorder" as the name for one of these syndromes because the term "dementia" had a pejorative or stigmatizing connotation and was not commonly used to describe younger adults with cognitive disturbance.

"Delirium," from the Latin *delirare*, meaning "deviate or be deranged,"[3] is the diagnostic term to describe an organic mental disorder that usually has an acute onset and is characterized by a disturbance in awareness or attention that follows a fluctuating course. Delirium is often reversible, except when it occurs during the last 24 to 48 hours of life. However, delirium may be prolonged. A recent systematic review of 21 observational studies[4] found prolonged delirium was associated with dementia, increasing numbers of medical conditions, increasing severity of delirium, hypoactive symptoms, and hypoxic illnesses. In a study of 99 persons with cancer, the main identified causes of delirium were opioids, infection, brain metastases, hypercalcemia, and dehydration.[5]

In delirium, both alertness and cognition are disturbed. The four DSM-5 criteria for the diagnosis of delirium are as follows:

1. Disturbance in level of awareness and reduced ability to direct, focus, sustain, and shift attention.
2. A change in cognition, such as deficits in orientation, executive ability, language, perception, learning, and memory. However, when level of awareness is greatly reduced, this change may be difficult to assess. Also, a preexisting neurocognitive disorder should not account for disturbances.
3. History, physical examination, or laboratory findings that provide evidence indicating that the disturbance is caused by direct physiologic consequences of a general medical condition.
4. Development of the disturbance over a short period of time (usually hours to a few days), and its tendency to fluctuate in severity during the course of a day.

In addition, the following supportive features are commonly present in delirium but are not key diagnostic features: sleep–wake cycle disturbance, psychomotor disturbance, perceptual disturbances (e.g., hallucinations, illusions), emotional disturbances, delusions, labile affect, dysarthria, and electroencephalography (EEG) abnormalities (i.e., generalized slowing of background activity).

Delirium can take either a hyperactive or a hypoactive form. The hyperactive form is characterized by loud, aggressive behavior, often including hallucinations, agitation, and disorientation. The hypoactive form is associated with quiet, passive behavior, including sedation and confusion. In some individuals, delirium may involve a combination of both forms (mixed features).

Mild neurocognitive disorders may be associated with several diseases, including Alzheimer's disease, vascular disease, traumatic brain injury, HIV infection, and substance use. Major neurocognitive disorders also include disorders associated with these diseases, as well as a category of "other specified major neurocognitive disorders," which were formerly labeled dementia. Although the DSM-5 development team suggests that the term "dementia" should not be used, it is commonly found in the literature. "Dementia," from the Latin *dementare*, meaning "insane,"[6] is the diagnosis for chronic and irreversible cognitive disorders with a more gradual onset. A simple definition of dementia is an acquired deterioration of cognitive abilities that hinders people from performing activities of daily living.[7] Dementia is usually irreversible and may not have identified precipitating factors.

The DSM-5 development version includes four criteria for major neurocognitive disorder:

A. Evidence of significant cognitive decline from a previous level of performance in one or more of the following domains: complex attention, executive ability, learning and memory, language, visuoconstructional–perceptual ability (construction and visual perception) and social cognition (recognition of emotions). Decline in these domains is determined by concerns of the patient, a knowledgeable informant, or the clinician that cognitive function has significantly declined AND neurocognitive performance has clearly declined, typically 2 or more standard deviations below appropriate norms (i.e., below the 3rd percentile) on formal testing, or equivalent clinical evaluation.
B. The cognitive deficits are sufficient to interfere with independence (i.e., requiring assistance at a minimum with instrumental Activities of Daily Living [more complex tasks such as paying bills or managing medications]).
C. The cognitive deficits do not occur exclusively in the context of delirium.
D. The cognitive deficits are not wholly or primarily attributable to another Axis I disorder (e.g., Major Depressive Disorder, Schizophrenia).

Criteria for mild neurocognitive disorders are similar to those for major disorders except that the evidence of decline is modest for mild disorder as opposed to significant in the major disorder category.

INCIDENCE

Conflicting reports have arisen regarding the frequency of cognitive dysfunction related to cancer and therapy, likely due to the heterogeneity of cancer treatments and inadequate study design and analysis. Nevertheless, cognitive dysfunction—including disruptions in information processing, attention, memory retrieval, and executive function—is commonly noted in cancer patients. These symptoms often accompany fatigue, anemia, and depression, but can also occur independently. Cancer survivorship is associated with disability and poor health, particularly in older adults.[8] As many as 75% of cancer patients experience problems with memory, executive functioning, and attention during cancer therapy, and as many as 35% of survivors report symptoms in these areas persisting for months or years.[9]

ETIOLOGY

Manifestations of cognitive deficits vary greatly from subtle, acute, and temporary to dramatic, chronic, and progressive. Cognitive impairments can originate from the tumor itself, chemotherapy and supportive medications, or radiation therapy—the last of which can be broken down into early and delayed effects on cognition.

Effect of tumor

First, the tumor itself may affect functioning. In patients with primary or metastatic brain tumors, cognitive deficits are affected by factors such as lesion type, lesion momentum (i.e., speed of tumor growth), tumor location, and tumor-related epilepsy.[10] At baseline, patients with low-grade glioma have been noted to have significant impairment of selective and divided attention when compared to age-matched healthy cohorts.[11] In another study, 23% of women had cognitive deficits prior to treatment with chemotherapy for breast cancer.[12] Evaluation of patients with brain metastases who underwent whole-brain radiotherapy (WBRT) actually showed improvement in delayed recall over time, supporting the contention that baseline function was adversely affected by the metastases themselves.[13] The stress of a cancer diagnosis may confound the baseline cognitive assessment in some individuals, but cognitive abilities have been shown to be largely independent of affective distress when tools to measure depression and anxiety are employed.[14–16]

Chemotherapy

Chemotherapy and supportive drugs can also affect cognition. Hess and colleagues found that among patients treated with chemotherapy for ovarian cancer, 92% developed cognitive impairments in areas including attention, processing speed, and reaction time by their third cycle of chemotherapy.[17] Shilling and colleagues longitudinal study of breast cancer patients revealed declines in working memory and verbal learning 6 months after chemotherapy,[18] and Hurria et al.[19] found a similar decline in domains of psychomotor speed, visual–spatial abilities, and visual memory in women aged 65 and older 6 months after chemotherapy. Men with prostate cancer who receive androgen therapy have been reported to experience declines in executive function.[20] Another study of breast cancer patients found that patients who were treated for hypertension and diabetes and those who reported fewer hours spent in "cognitive activities" had worse cognitive performance at baseline.[21]

Chemoendocrine therapy such as tamoxifen adds to cognitive difficulties.[22,23] Deprez and colleagues[24] recently published a longitudinal study of 34 breast cancer patients and compared neuropsychologic testing and magnetic resonance diffusion tensor imaging (MR-DTI) with two control groups—one consisting of 16 breast cancer patients not given chemotherapy and one including 19 age-matched healthy controls. Those individuals who were treated with chemotherapy had significant decline in measures of attention, psychomotor speed, and memory from baseline to 3 to 4 months after treatment compared to both control groups.

A recent publication evaluated breast cancer survivors who had received cyclophosfamide, methotrexate, and fluorouracil (CMF) 20 years previously and compared them to age-matched controls without history of malignancy.[25] The CMF group had significantly worse immediate and delayed verbal memory as well as processing speed, executive functioning, and psychomotor speed. Their memory complaints on two of the three measures, however, were not supported by their test performance. Interestingly, both exercise and simultaneous fluoxetine have been shown in rodent models to ameliorate the detrimental cognitive effects of fluorouracil,[26,27] although these modalities have yet to be tested in humans.

A study of allogeneic stem cell transplant recipients followed patients longitudinally with neuropsychological testing done at baseline, 80 days, 1 year, and 5 years post-transplant. Between 80 days and 5 years post-transplant, most functions were recovered except verbal recall. Even so, survivors had poorer motor dexterity and 41.5% had mild or greater global deficit scores, compared to 19.7% of case-matched controls, at 5 years.[28]

Although significant, these losses may not always be permanent; indeed, many patients appear to regain the lost function. Cross-sectional studies of cognition in breast cancer patients revealed post-chemotherapy cognitive impairment ranging from 17% to 75%, but with relatively stable or improved performance evident by 12 to 18 months after the end of therapy.[29] A recent longitudinal study of 61 postmenopausal breast cancer patients evaluated before and then 6 and 12 months after chemotherapy revealed that only motor functioning declined over the long term.[30] However, in a study of twins, only one of whom was a cancer survivor, survivors were more likely to experience cognitive dysfunction and dementia than their twin.[31] These studies emphasize the need for extended follow-up testing.

Immunochemotherapy with interleukin-2 (IL-2) and interferon (IFN) alpha has been correlated with neuropsychological changes for which the mechanism, timing, and persistence of deficits remain unclear. IFN-alpha, which is used to treat several types of malignancies, is often associated with cognitive dysfunction as well as mood disorders, with rates of depression approaching 50%.[32] Patients have experienced acute dysphoria, depression, and delirium with features of Parkinsonism. Pretreatment depression not surprisingly predicts mood disorders during interferon therapy. Cognitive dysfunction frequently presents concurrently with mood disorders, and can manifest as impaired executive function and slowed processing speed. Intravenous administration seems to correlate more often with neuropsychiatric effects compared to subcutaneous administration, as do higher doses and longer time of therapy.[32] Pegylated interferon may result in fewer adverse neuropsychiatric effects, but this outcome has not been thoroughly investigated.[33] A study comparing 47 patients receiving IFN-alpha alone versus IL-2 alone or with IFN-alpha tested patients' spatial working memory, reaction time, and planning. Tests were administered before treatment, after 5 days of treatment, and again after 1 month. Those individuals who received IFN-alpha alone had longer reaction times but no impairments in accuracy.

By day 5, those treated with IL-2 had impaired spatial working memory and planning—deficits that persisted 1 month later.[34]

Supportive medications

Supportive medications such as corticosteroids, antiepileptic drugs, narcotics, and benzodiazepines can add to cognitive dysfunction in cancer patients. There is great variability in the incidence (range: 1.8% to 57%) of cognitive impairment due to corticosteroids cited in the literature.[35] Deficits in episodic memory have been widely noted with corticosteroid therapy, and have been attributed to reversible atrophy of neurons in the hippocampus, which can occur after only 4 to 5 days of therapy. Distractibility has been seen in as many as 79% of patients and intermittent memory impairment in 71%. Occasionally patients may have persistent memory impairment consistent with steroid-induced dementia, although this effect is rare.[35]

Antiepileptic drugs (AEDs) can also have deleterious effects on cognition. These effects are usually acute, and patients most often habituate over time. AEDs have been shown to impair memory by as much as 15% to 20%.[36] A recent double-blind study comparing continuation of monotherapy versus withdrawal of an AED resulted in a 17% improvement in neuropsychological testing, particularly in the domains of concentration, memory, and complex motor coordination, in the group that stopped their use of AEDs. Patients in the withdrawal group had primarily been taking carbemazepine (57%), valproate (21%), and phenytoin (11%).[37] Patients with low-grade glioma are the cancer population most likely to require AEDs.

Patients continuously taking moderate doses of opioids for chronic pain have shown delays in information processing and impairments in attention, memory, problem solving, psychomotor performance, and reaction time.[38,39] In a blinded study comparing cognitive effects of the benzodiazepine lorazepam with placebo, patients taking 2 mg twice daily had significant cognitive impairment on task performance measures as well as on cerebral electrophysiologic indices.[36]

Radiation therapy

As with chemotherapy, while radiation therapy (RT) is largely accepted as causing cognitive decline, studies have shown varied results regarding the severity and longevity of the ensuing cognitive deficits. Effects on cognition, characterized by progressive dementia, motor slowing, and gait impairment, have been reported. The likelihood of CNS damage depends on the total dose (measured in grays [Gy]), the dose delivered with each treatment (Gy per fraction), and the volume irradiated.[40] The maximum "safe" dose is generally accepted to be 60 Gy given in 1.8–2.0 Gy daily fractions.

Neurological side effects of radiation are divided into three chronological categories: acute (occurring during RT), early-delayed (up to 6 months after RT), and late-delayed (from 6 months to several years after RT). High fractions—greater than 3 Gy—can lead to headache, drowsiness, vomiting, fever, and focal neurologic deficits in as many as 50% of patients; [41] however, these doses are not often used. Somnolence syndrome, manifested by drowsiness, nausea, and anorexia, is most commonly seen in children but can also occur in adults within the first 2 months after beginning RT.[41]

In one study, repeat neurocognitive evaluations were done in patients with small-cell lung cancer given prophylactic cranial irradiation (PCI). Compared to baseline, a significant decline in language was observed 250 to 449 days after PCI. However, from 450 to 1400 days after PCI, this function normalized and then improved over baseline.[42] Conversely, a recent study comparing patients who received PCI to a control arm of patients who were not radiated revealed that while global functioning was intact at 1 year, greater decline in learning and memory was apparent in the PCI arm.[43] Another large, multigroup study involving more than 700 patients compared those receiving standard 25 Gy versus 36 Gy PCI; the researchers found a mild, yet significant deterioration over 3 years of follow-up in patient-reported communication and memory in both groups.[44] However, in the subset of patients ($N = 265$) enrolled and assessed in Radiation Therapy Oncology Group (RTOG) 0212,[45] the higher-dose PCI arms were associated with a greater incidence of cognitive decline on objective cognitive tests. This discrepancy in findings between objective and subjective measures of cognitive function underscores the importance of objectively testing cognitive function in clinical trials and clinical practice to draw valid inferences from the data with regard to this neurotoxicity. Of course, it is also important to recognize that patients' experiences may differ from the results of measures and these experiences need to be taken seriously by clinicians.

Recent studies have supported an early (1 to 4 months) component of cognitive function decline, including diminished verbal and short-term memory recall, which may have some regenerative capacity.[46–49] A detailed evaluation of more than 200 patients receiving whole-brain radiation therapy in an international randomized trial revealed that while tumor response (i.e., local control) was correlated with time to neurocognitive deterioration, the same was not true for the domain of memory. Those persons surviving to 4 months had a significant decline in memory regardless of tumor reduction.[47]

Gondi et al. reviewed studies published throughout the 1990s and early 2000s and reported that hippocampal irradiation led to learning and memory impairments among those individuals receiving radiation for skull base, maxillary, nasopharyngeal, and pituitary tumors.[50] Patients radiated for primary brain tumors experienced a dose-response correlation between learning and memory impairment and the maximum radiation dose to the left hippocampus.[51] In light of these findings, the RTOG is accruing patients to a study that will spare the hippocampus from radiation therapy.

A study conducted in the Netherlands on patients with low-grade glioma 6 years after radiation therapy initially concluded that cognitive deficits were primarily attributable to the underlying tumor and that fractions of less than 2 Gy were "safe."[52] After a mean of 12 years post-therapy, however, those persons with stable disease within the original study were reassessed; patients who had undergone RT had significantly greater deficits in attention, executive functioning, and information processing speed regardless of fraction dose compared to patients who did not have RT. Fifty-three percent of those patients who had received RT, compared with 27% of those who did not, developed cognitive decline in 5 or more of 18 neuropsychological test parameters. Decreased cognitive function also correlated with white matter hyperintensity and cortical atrophy seen on MRI.[52]

A large retrospective study of 184 patients with primary central nervous system lymphoma (PCNSL) treated from 1985 to 2000 at a single institution showed that 24% of patients developed neurotoxicity after chemotherapy and radiation 5 years after treatment. Neurotoxicity manifested as rapidly progressive subcortical dementia, with the median time to death after diagnosis being 1.8 years. A multivariate analysis revealed only RT as a significant contributor to this outcome, supporting the use of current therapies, which focus on avoidance of RT in this population when possible.[53] The majority of these patients likely had leukoencephalopathy.

The most severe late-delayed complication of RT is leukoencephalopathy—a constellation of periventricular white matter abnormalities, ventricular dilation, and cortical atrophy with associated frontal cognitive deficits such as those involving executive function, attention, and judgment. Risks for leukoencephalopathy include large RT doses, large radiated brain volume, advanced age, diabetes, hypertension, and concurrent chemotherapy, especially intrathecal or high-dose intravenous methotrexate.[41] The risk of developing this condition is lower when methotrexate is given before starting radiation therapy and greatest when the two treatments are given concurrently. These patients may improve, stabilize, or develop debilitating and fatal dementia.[54]

IMPACT ON QUALITY OF LIFE

Even mild disruption in cognitive function from either tumor or the effects of therapy can impair daily social and work functioning as well as overall quality of life.[55] Interestingly, recent studies have demonstrated cognitive dysfunction in as many as 23% of breast cancer patients[12] and 44% of patients with acute myelogenous leukemia (AML) or myelodysplastic syndromes.[56] Several recent studies have also reported treatment-associated cognitive deficits (chemobrain) in patients receiving active treatment for a variety of solid tumors, including ovarian, testicular, and breast cancers,[12,57–59] in both long-term survivors[29] and those in hospice care,[60] as well as in those with tumors directly involving the CNS.[61–64]

In the most widely studied group—women with breast cancer—it has been well established that a subset of patients experience cognitive changes after therapy. The extent of the problem has been debated, with small cross-sectional studies reporting wide variations in occurrence, and suggestions being made that some patients may have exhibited deficits prior to the initiation of treatment.[65] Recently, a longitudinal comparison of breast cancer survivors who were treated with chemotherapy found that these patients exhibited significantly more cognitive symptoms than both those breast cancer survivors who received radiation and noncancer controls.[66] The majority of patients reported that these declines had negatively impacted their relationships at home and work, as well as their physical functioning. These studies also reported that neurocognitive dysfunction precedes QOL declines, but showed a relationship between the degree of alteration in neurocognition and overall QOL.

PATHOPHYSIOLOGY

Cognitive dysfunction in the broad oncology population varies in association with the primary disease, with a much higher incidence of cognitive dysfunction being linked to brain tumors and less cognitive dysfunction being associated with cancers occurring outside the CNS. A number of other issues create challenges in determining the scope of neurotoxicity, including the following: (1) different treatment regimens have different neurotoxicities; (2) the time since treatment affects the development, resolution. and progression of cognitive side effects for different therapies; and (3) methodological differences between studies, such as the variety of cognitive tests and classification criteria that have been used, may lead to different estimates.[67]

As noted earlier, manifestations of cognitive deficits vary greatly from subtle, acute, and temporary to dramatic, chronic, and progressive. Genetic variations in apolipoprotein E (ApoE) and catechol-*o*-methyltransferase (COMT) have been shown to increase an individual's likelihood of developing cognitive changes due to cancer therapy, as these substances influence neural plasticity and neurotransmission.[68,69] Such differences may explain, in part, why cognitive changes are not universally seen among patients receiving the same cancer therapy. Also as noted earlier, cognitive impairments can originate from the tumor itself, surgery, chemotherapy and supportive medications, or radiation therapy—the last of which can be broken down into early and delayed effects on cognition.

The risk of developing neurotoxicity associated with chemotherapy increases when patients experience the following aspects of treatment: (1) exposure to higher doses due to planned use of high-dose regimens or high concentrations of the parent drug and/or its metabolite due to impaired systemic clearance and/or pharmacogenetic modulation of drug pharmacokinetics; (2) additive or synergistic effects of multiagent chemotherapy; (3) additive or synergistic effects of multimodality therapy that includes administration of chemotherapy either concurrent or subsequent to cerebral radiation; (4) intra-arterial administration with blood–brain barrier disruption; and (5) intrathecal administration.[54]

Animal[70] and imaging[54] studies are beginning to elucidate the mechanisms underlying changes in cognition and behavior that have been reported in numerous observational studies in a variety of cancer patient populations treated with chemotherapy (including 5-fluorouracil, methotrexate, doxorubicin, paclitaxel, cisplatin, BCNU and cyclophosphamide). Experimental animal studies have observed increased cell death and decreased cell division among neural stem cells, with associated decrements on behavioral tasks dependent on hippocampal and frontal systems. The cognitive effects of fluorouracil have been extensively studied, as this agent has been used for several decades for breast and colorectal cancer. Fluorouracil passively diffuses across the blood–brain barrier. In mice models, this agent has been demonstrated to decrease cell proliferation in the hippocampal subgranular zone and to decrease oligodendrocytes in white matter tracts.[71] However, not all chemotherapies have demonstrated adverse effects on brain structure or function. For example, several targeted agents, such as an epidermal growth factor tyrosine kinase inhibitor (erlotinib) and a proteasome inhibitor (bortezomib), decrease glioma stem-like cell viability, yet have minimal impact on neural stem cells.

Several recent studies that included imaging studies of the brain have demonstrated (1) decreased white matter integrity in the frontal, parietal, and occipital regions after treatment, which were associated with changes in attention and verbal memory;[24] (2) gray matter volume decrease within a month after completion of chemotherapy, which did not recover in all regions at 1 year post treatment;[72] and (3) decreased total brain volume and gray matter volume, as well as deficits in immediate and delayed verbal memory, processing speed, executive functioning, and psychomotor speed in breast cancer survivors who had received cyclophosfamide, methotrexate, and fluorouracil 20 years previously.[25,73] Furthermore, studies using magnetoencephalography have demonstrated abnormal organization in brain networks that is widespread and associated with cognitive dysfunction in brain tumor patients.[74] However, persistent and late emerging cognitive dysfunction has not always been found—an inconsistency that emphasizes the need for extended follow-up in the survivorship period.

Many women with breast cancer also receive endocrine therapy as part of their adjuvant treatment. These therapies may also influence cognitive functioning,[23] but these effects are difficult to separate out from the effects of chemotherapy alone in the current literature due to the small sample sizes and methodological designs of studies carried out to date.[22,23]

Biological response modifiers (BRMs; also known as immunotherapies) have been demonstrated to (1) directly or indirectly augment the patient's immunological defenses, (2) modify tumor cells such that the patient's immunologic response is increased, or (3) bolster the patient's ability to manage toxicities secondary to other cancer treatments.[55] Immunochemotherapy with IL-2 and IFN-alpha have been correlated with neuropsychological changes for which the mechanism, timing, and persistence of deficits remain unclear.

While the etiology of cognitive impairment after chemotherapy remains unknown, a number of mechanisms have been postulated to be involved.[65] These include direct neurotoxic effects (e.g., injury to neurons or surrounding cells, altered neurotransmitter levels), oxidative stress and DNA damage, induced hormonal changes, immune dysregulation and/or release of cytokines, and blood clotting in small CNS vessels. In addition, some patients may have a genetic predisposition to developing cognitive impairment.

RADIATION THERAPY

Neuropathological studies of the irradiated brain have demonstrated adverse effects of radiation on white matter tracts and cerebral vasculature secondary to damaged oligodendrocytes, resulting in axonal demyelination and disruption of vascular endothelial cells, and contributing to coagulative necrosis, vessel-wall thickening, and focal mineralization. Chronic radiation toxicity has also been associated with alterations in neurogenesis as well as metabolic abnormalities and inflammatory responses.[75]

Risk factors for CNS damage from radiation therapy include age greater than 60 years, greater total dose, greater total dose delivered with each treatment, greater volume of brain irradiated, hyperfractionated schedules, shorter overall treatment time, concomitant or subsequent use of chemotherapy, and presence of comorbid vascular risk factors (e.g., diabetes).[40,41] Effects on cognition, characterized by progressive dementia, motor slowing, and gait impairment, have been reported.

Recent studies have documented acute and subacute cognitive decline, including diminished episodic memory in patients with brain metastases.[46–49] Detailed evaluation of more than 200 patients receiving whole-brain radiation therapy in an international randomized trial revealed that while tumor response (i.e., local control) was associated with time to neurocognitive deterioration, this was not true for the domain of memory. Those participants surviving to 4 months had a significant decline in memory regardless of tumor reduction.[47]

SYMPTOM ASSESSMENT

Management of cognitive dysfunction, which is described in more detail later, relates to treating the underlying cause of the symptoms. Potential barriers to management include problems making an accurate assessment and diagnosis, including differentiating from other symptoms. It is especially important and challenging to distinguish among delirium, dementia, and depression. Assessing changes, especially subtle changes, requires relying on patient and family reports, and formal neuropsychological testing when it is available. As we have learned with other symptoms, clinicians may not trust these "subjective reports" as they need to. Data from the Nurses' Health Study found subjective memory complaints were associated with objective cognitive status.[76] However, there is often discordance between subjective reports of cognitive dysfunction and objective evidence of cognitive dysfunction, with numerous studies demonstrating stronger relationships between subjective patient-reported cognitive difficulties, mood disturbance, and fatigue than between subjective patient-reported cognitive difficulties and objective cognitive dysfunction.[54] Additionally, data are limited on the clinical course of cognitive dysfunction associated with cancer and cancer therapy, although it is recognized that the impact of this side effect can continue for years after treatment is completed.

The importance of early identification and assessment of cognitive dysfunction in patients undergoing chemotherapy has been emphasized in recent review articles.[9,41] Assessment can be difficult, however, when comorbid conditions such as fatigue, mood disorders, and delirium are present. The propensity for misdiagnosis and the failure to diagnose behavioral abnormalities can have serious consequences and actually lead to worsening of conditions if inappropriate treatment is initiated.

Perhaps the most important clinical tool is a baseline, or prior to cancer therapy, measurement of cognition with which to compare future test results. Longitudinal testing is critical for identifying baseline or preexisting deficits and monitoring progress or decline over time. The International Cognition and Cancer Task Force (ICCTF) currently recommends the use of objective tools that can measure frontal subcortical functions of learning and memory, processing speed, and executive function, as these represent commonly impaired cognitive domains in patients with non-CNS cancer.[67] We recommend referral to a clinical neuropsychologist whenever possible. Ideally, patients should be assessed for difficulty at each clinical evaluation because the time until cognitive difficulties occur after therapy varies.[9,41]

OBJECTIVE ASSESSMENT

Assessing for potential confounding factors, described earlier, is important. It is important to know if symptoms can be attributed to delirium, dementia, depression, anxiety, or level of functioning before the diagnosis and treatment of cancer. In addition, cognitive symptoms may result from the cancer itself, from its treatment, and from other physical factors and symptoms such as fatigue and anemia. Clinicians can use several simple questions to screen for cognitive dysfunction (Figure 30-1). A physical assessment should be conducted and a medical history taken. Cognitive assessment questions should be included, and appropriate diagnostic evaluation and lab tests should be conducted.

A variety of screening tools exist; however, they were not designed to detect mild cognitive disturbance of the type typically encountered in cancer patients. The most commonly used screening test is the Mini-Mental State Exam (MMSE), developed by Folstein, Folstein, and McHugh.[77] The MMSE evaluates five categories of cognition (orientation, registration, attention and calculation, recall, and language) and takes less than 5 minutes to administer. It is important to remember that sociodemographic factors such as age, education, and culture influence normative performances on the MMSE. Patients who demonstrate difficulties on this screening test can be referred for formal neuropsychological evaluation. One drawback of this tool is that it detects profound dysfunction and is not a sensitive measure of subtle alterations in learning, memory, executive functioning, and other areas.[42] PAR, Inc., owns the copyrights to this screening test and charges for its use.

If there is concern for cognitive dysfunction based on clinical interview or screening measures, referral to a clinical neuropsychologist for a formal evaluation is warranted. Clinical neuropsychologists have an armamentarium of objective, standardized tests with known reliability- and validity-related evidence that assess all domains of cognitive function.[78] Additionally, a neuropsychological evaluation will include assessment of mood, personality, and other relevant symptoms, as well as the psychosocial background and current setting in which the individual is reporting or manifesting cognitive deficits. Differential diagnostic conclusions and treatment recommendations can then be tailored to the specific needs and circumstances of the individual.

There is no set of proscribed tests that should be used in the clinical evaluation of cancer patients. Instead,

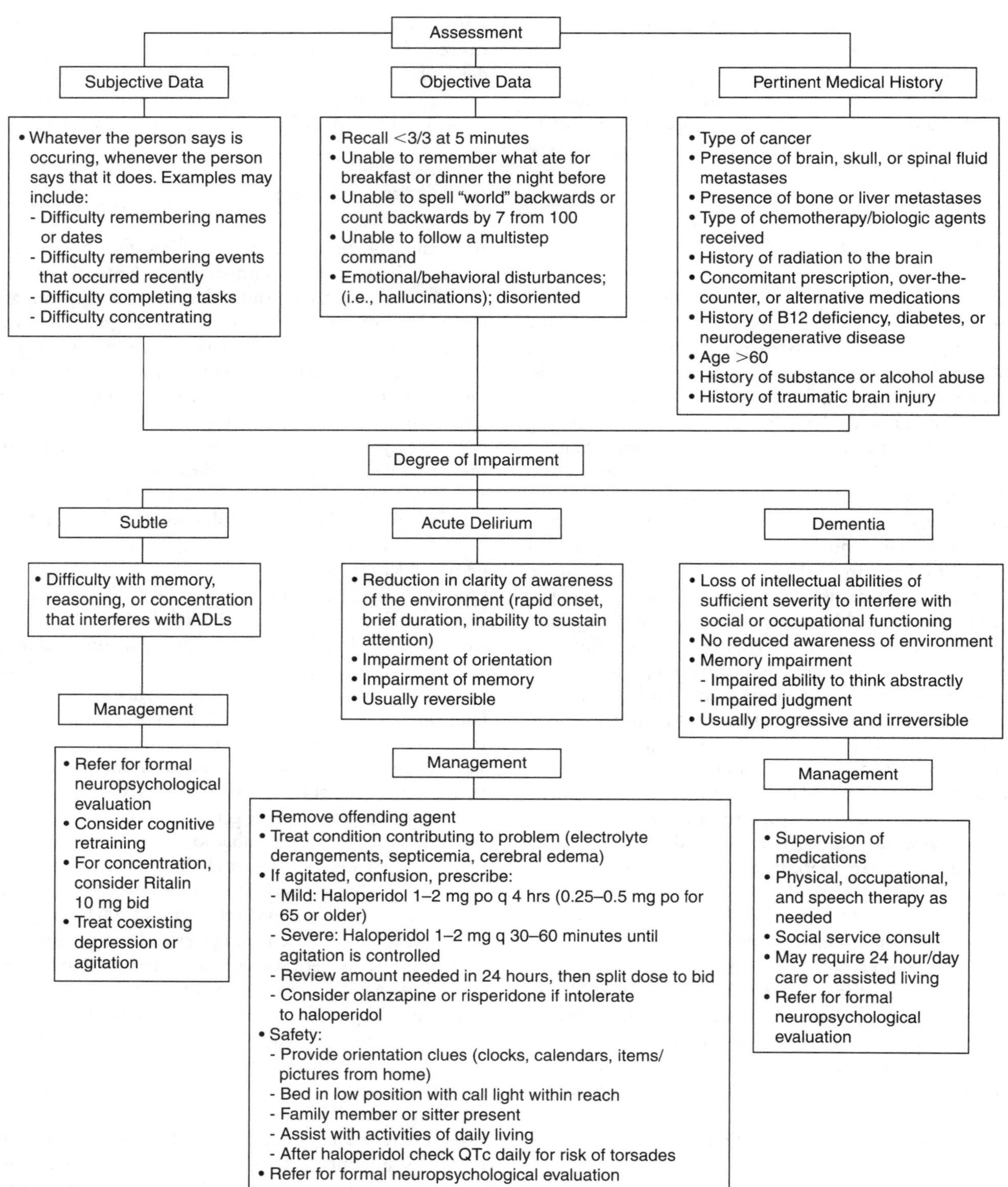

FIGURE 30-1

Assessment and management of cognitive dysfunction.

the neuropsychologist should consider the purpose of the evaluation (e.g., rule out dementia, return to work), the frequency of reevaluation (the need for consideration of tests with alternative forms and tests robust to practice effects), the domains of cognition most frequently impacted by the cancer or cancer therapy the patient has received, and the general stamina of the patient, as cancer patients frequently have multiple symptom comorbidities including fatigue and may require more brief and tailored evaluations or evaluations broken up across multiple assessment days. As noted earlier, the ICCTF has published recommendations underscoring the importance of using objective tools to measure learning and memory, processing speed, and executive function in research studies assessing the impact of chemotherapy on cognition—these areas represent commonly impaired cognitive domains in patients with non-CNS cancer.[67] The same set of cognitive tests and domains has also been recommended by the Response Assessment in Neuro-Oncology group for use in brain tumor clinical trials.[79,80]

DIAGNOSTIC EVALUATION

Several recent developments in imaging hold promise for future application in evaluating the cognitive effects of cancer and cancer therapy. Applying volumetric measurement to standard MRI displayed reversible reductions of the cingulate, parahippocampal, and prefrontal gyri that correlated with attention and visual memory in a study of breast cancer patients before and after chemotherapy.[81] Another study that evaluated the volume of the hippocampus in patients after chemotherapy compared with chemotherapy-naïve controls did not find a significant difference in this measure, although imaging was not performed at baseline.[82]

Deprez and colleagues[24] published the first longitudinal study investigating chemotherapy-induced changes in cerebral white matter. Intact axonal membranes and myelin in normal white matter guide diffusion of water molecules in specific direction. Damage to this tissue will cause increased random motion, leading to decreased fractional anisotropy (FA). In the Deprez et al. study, 34 women with breast cancer underwent neurocognitive testing with magnetic resonance diffusion tensor imaging (MR-DTI) at baseline and again after chemotherapy. Significant decreases in attention and verbal memory correlated with decreases in FA on MR-DTI.

Positron emission tomography (PET) scanning has also been shown to detect changes that correlate with neurocognition. In one study, patients who were treated for breast cancer with chemotherapy 5 to 10 years previously were evaluated with neurocognitive testing and PET scans and were compared with chemotherapy-naïve controls. Short-term memory deficits in the chemotherapy group correlated with changes in metabolism within the inferior frontal gyrus, and metabolism in the basal ganglia was decreased in the subgroup of those who also had received tamoxifen.[83]

Although these radiographic tools are not yet ready for widespread clinical application, the ability to correlate structural and functional changes in the brain with cognition is on the horizon.

DEGREES OF TOXICITY

As stated previously in this chapter, cognitive dysfunction can occur as a result of the cancer or can be associated with its treatment. The National Cancer Institute's (NCI) Cancer Therapy Evaluation Program (CTEP) developed Common Terminology Criteria for Adverse Events (CTCAE) to provide a standard language for reporting toxicity occurring in cancer trials sponsored by the NCI. For each event, grades are assigned using a scale from 0 to 5, with the following descriptors:

0 = No adverse event or within normal limits
1 = Mild adverse event
2 = Moderate adverse event
3 = Severe and undesirable adverse event
4 = Life-threatening or disabling adverse event
5 = Death related to adverse event

Several categories of adverse events with the CTCAE may apply to patients experiencing cognitive dysfunction. Specific criteria for each grade associated with an adverse event are provided in Table 30-1.[84] The NCI notes that this grading scale should be used in individual protocols to determine and assign a dose-limiting toxicity associated with the particular therapy. These criteria should be used to grade toxicity related to cancer treatments, but they are not designed to determine care or other treatment decisions.

SYMPTOM MANAGEMENT STRATEGIES

Primary prevention of impaired memory and concentration begins with recognition of conditions associated with impaired memory and concentration and avoidance of their causes if possible. Patients who receive agents that affect cognitive function should be aware of the possible effects on cognitive function, and the healthcare team should monitor patients for these effects.

A variety of measures to prevent delirium in the hospitalized older patient population,[85] in the intensive care unit,[86]

TABLE 30-1

National Cancer Institute Common Terminology Criteria for Adverse Events (CTCAE)

Toxicity	Grade 0	Grade 1	Grade 2	Grade 3	Grade 4
NEUROLOGY					
Ataxia (incoordination)	Normal	Asymptomatic but abnormal on physical exam	Moderate symptoms limiting instrumental activities of daily living	Severe symptoms limiting self-care activities of daily living; mechanical assistance indicated	—
Cognitive disturbance/ learning problems	None	Mild disability; not interfering with work/school performance; preservation of intelligence	Moderate disability; interfering with work/ school/life performance; but capable of independent living	Severe disability; resulting in significant impairment of work/ school/life performance	—
Confusion	Normal	Mild confusion	Moderate disorientation; limiting instrumental activities of daily living	Severe disorientation; limiting self-care activities of daily living	Harmful to others or self; requiring hospitalization
Delusions	Normal	—	Moderate	Severe but hospitalization not indicated	Harmful to others or self; requiring hospitalization
Depressed level of consciousness	Normal	Decreased level of alertness	Sedation; slow response to stimuli limiting instrumental activities of daily living	Obtundation or stupor; difficult to arouse	Life-threatening consequences
Hallucinations	Normal	Mild hallucinations (distorted perception)	Moderate hallucinations	Severe hallucinations but hospitalization not indicated	Harmful to others or self; requiring hospitalization
Leukoencephalopathy associated radiological findings	None	Asymptomatic; mild increase in SAS (subarachnoid space) and/or mild ventriculomegaly; and/or small (± multiple) focal T2 hyperintensities, involving periventricular white matter or <1/3 of susceptible areas of cerebrum	Moderate increase in SAS; and/ or moderate ventriculomegaly; and/or focal T2 hyperintensities extending into centrum ovale; or involving 1/3 to 2/3 of susceptible areas of cerebrum	Severe increase in SAS; severe ventriculomegaly; near total white matter T2 hyperintensities or diffuse low attenuation CT; focal white matter necrosis (cystic)	Life-threatening; severe increase in SAS; severe ventriculomegaly; diffuse low attenuation with calcification CT; diffuse white matter necrosis MRI
Memory impairment	Normal	Mild; not interfering with function	Moderate; limiting instrumental activities of daily living	Severe; limiting self-care activities of daily living	—
Anxiety	Normal	Mild apprehension not associated with a defined stimulus	Moderate mood alteration limiting instrumental activities of daily living	Severe mood alteration interfering with self-care activities of daily living	Suicidal ideation or danger to self, hospitalization indicated
Depression	Normal	Mild mood alteration not interfering with function	Moderate mood alteration limiting instrumental activities of daily living	Severe mood alteration interfering with self-care activities of daily living	Suicidal ideation or danger to self, hospitalization indicated
Euphoria	Normal	Mild mood elevation	Moderate mood elevation	Severe mood elevation/hypomania	—
Personality	Normal	Mild change, but not disruptive to patient or family	Moderate change	Severe; requiring mental health intervention	Harmful to others or self; requiring hospitalization
Seizure(s)	None	Brief partial seizure; no loss of consciousness	Brief generalized seizure	Multiple seizures despite medical intervention	Life-threatening; prolonged and/or repetitive seizures
Speech impairment (e.g., dysphasia or aphasia)	Normal	Awareness of receptive or expressive dysphasia, not impairing ability to communicate	Moderate receptive or expressive dysphasia; impaired ability to communicate spontaneously	Severe receptive or expressive dysphasia; impairing ability to read, write or communicate intelligibly	Inability to communicate

Abbreviations: CT: computed tomography; MRI: magnetic resonance imaging.

and in the postoperative setting[87] have been reported. General measures to reduce the occurrence of delirium include reducing medications to a minimum, frequently reorienting patients, and scheduling their activities. Encouraging mobility, self-care, and independence as much as possible and avoiding restraints and disruptions also may reduce the severity of delirium. Increasing sleep and reducing agitation with relaxation methods, such as music, relaxation tapes, and massage, are also helpful tools. Breitbart and Alici[88] and Valentine and Duffy[89] provide recent reviews of the diagnosis and management of delirium in cancer patients.

Limited data are available on the prevention of subtle alterations in neurocognition in the cancer patient. Preoperative neuropsychological evaluations, functional MRI, and intraoperative testing are routinely used to minimize postoperative morbidity.[90] Several preclinical studies have shown that *N*-acetyl cysteine (an antioxidant) and fluoxetine (an antidepressant) can prevent chemotherapy-related cognitive dysfunction in animals.[91] Risk factors have also been identified that increase the risk of altered cognition during chemotherapy—including use of high-dose regimens, additive or synergistic multiagent chemotherapy regimens, and direct intrathecal administration of chemotherapeutic agents, as well as concomitant medications known to have neurocognitive effects.[55]

Recently, attention has focused on the use of complementary or alternative therapy to either prevent or treat memory problems both in the general population and in patients with cancer. Ginkgo biloba is derived from ginkgo fruits and seeds and has been used in traditional Chinese medicine for millennia.[92] Earlier studies reported improved cognition and memory with its use, but a recent *Cochrane Database Systematic Review*[93] reported inconsistent results for reduction in cognitive impairment or dementia.

THERAPEUTIC APPROACHES

In patients with cancer, treating the underlying disease or complications of cancer and cancer therapy often results in improved cognition. Such treatment measures can include surgery for brain tumors or metastases, correction of electrolyte abnormalities, treatment of infection, transfusions for anemia, corticosteroids for cerebral edema, and dose reduction or change of chemotherapy or other medications that may be causing the cognitive problems. Discontinuing use of alcohol and illicit drugs should be addressed if necessary. Nonessential medications known to reduce cognitive function should be avoided. Testing for comorbid psychological or mood disorders should also be considered. Dementia is often underdiagnosed in persons aged 65 and older; its estimated prevalence is 6% to 10% and approaches 50% in those older than age 80 years living independently. As many as 20% of geriatric cancer patients have tested positive for cognitive disorders.[94–96]

While cobalamin (vitamin B_{12}) deficiency has been shown to correlate with cognitive decline and dementia, randomized trials have failed to demonstrate an improvement in cognitive or mood symptoms after replacement.[97,98] However, one study did show improvement in delirium with cobalamin replacement, so this possibility should be kept in mind when treating delirium.[98]

Specific treatment

Although most therapeutic approaches are broad spectrum in nature, some specific treatments are available for adverse cognitive effects from the tumor itself, chemotherapy, supportive medications, and radiation therapy.

Methylphenidate has been shown to increase attention in childhood cancer survivors[99,100] and to improve cognition in cancer patients with hypoactive delirium.[101] The largest nonrandomized study of 30 patients with glioblastoma who received this medication showed improvement in stamina, cognitive function, and motivation independent of disease progression with doses of 10 mg twice daily.[102,103] A recent review described several studies that have tested methylphenidate for depression in cancer patients with positive results; improvement in depressive symptoms ranged from 46% to 73% of patients, including one study of patients receiving hospice care and one study of hospitalized patients.[103] Methylphenidate, which has been shown to increase cognition and decrease depression, can also be used to alleviate some of the adverse effects of opioids—namely, somnolence—and may also allow higher doses to be tolerated. Three randomized, double-blind trials using methylphenidate showed increased activity and decreased drowsiness in patients using doses of 15–20 mg/day.[103]

Cognitive changes from chemotherapy can be acute and reversible, and when symptoms present during therapy, the side-effect profile of each drug should be thoroughly investigated. Some chemotherapeutic agents can cause reversible posterior leukoencephalopathy syndrome (RPLS). Patients can also present with cortical blindness, headache, and altered mental status, which is often associated with hypertension. Magnetic resonance imaging (MRI) reveals bilateral hyperintense T2 signal in the occipital and parietal lobes. Removal of the offending agent and treatment of concurrent hypertension usually leads to symptom resolution.[41] In a 2009 literature review, Marinella and colleagues[104] found that the most frequent offenders were (in order of decreasing frequency) gemcitabine, doxorubicin, cyclophosphamide, vincristine, cisplatin, bevacizumab, methotrexate, and cytarabine.

Animal studies have demonstrated that dextromethorphan (a glutamate receptor antagonist) and exercise can ameliorate chemotherapy-related cognitive dysfunction in animals.[105,106] A recent review has summarized much of the literature to date examining interventions for chemotherapy-associated cognitive decline.[106]

As mentioned earlier, steroids are frequently used as supportive medications in cancer therapy; they can cause a myriad of neurocognitive complaints, ranging from insomnia to depression and even psychosis. If cessation or taper is medically contraindicated and symptoms are severe, an atypical antipsychotic, such as olanzapine or risperidone, is recommended.[35,107] Preventive administration of corticosteroids have been suggested to decrease the acute cognitive effects of RT but this practice has not been validated. In a study of 34 patients with primary or secondary brain tumor who were 6 months or longer post RT, donepezil was given for 24 weeks and produced significant improvement of cognitive functioning, mood, and health-related quality of life.[108]

Cerebral radionecrosis can occur 6 months to years after therapy and cause symptoms similar to those associated with tumor. Treatment for radionecrosis includes steroids, surgical resection, and, in two recent studies, a limited course of bevacizumab.[109,110] One trial has shown some efficacy for heparin or warfarin in this indication.[111] Leukoencephalopathy—a serious delayed complication of cerebral RT—can include periventricular white matter abnormalities, cortical atrophy, and ventricular dilation. No specific therapy exists for this side effect, but in cases of significant ventricular dilation suggestive of normal-pressure hydrocephalus (NPH), ventriculoperitoneal shunting may result in a mild and transient improvement in cognition and motor function.[53] Unfortunately, options to treat neurotoxicity remain of limited value.

Cancer treatments can impair cognition and have been modified because of cognitive and late effects in children. CNS-directed chemotherapy has largely replaced cranial irradiation in the treatment of acute lymphoblastic leukemia (ALL), as the detrimental effects of cranial irradiation on intellectual function and learning ability have become evident. Subtle long-term neurocognitive deficits have been found in survivors of childhood ALL after treatment with chemotherapy.[112]

Few studies have been conducted with children who have recently completed cancer treatment, and limitations exist in the current research such as use of unvalidated questionnaires, lack of appropriate statistical analysis, and small sample sizes.[113] A variety of psychosocial effects were found in those studies that have been carried out, including learning difficulties. Qualitative studies have identified cognitive impacts and issues for children related to school.[114–116] In a fascinating review of the history of pediatric neuropsycho-oncology, Ris noted that the bias has been toward prevention of CNS damage, so that interventions have been slow to be developed and tested. Some exceptions to this rule are interventions that include cognitive rehabilitation/retraining, use of methylphenidate for cognitive deficits, and optimizing educational interventions.[117]

Nonspecific treatment

Nonspecific treatments are designed to improve comfort or preserve remaining cognitive function. These treatments include medication to relieve agitation or depression and behavioral techniques to provide safety or improve overall function.[118]

Medications can be used in the nonspecific treatment of concentration and memory disturbances to treat coexisting depression, anxiety, or agitation. Haloperidol is a neuroleptic commonly used to treat the agitation that may occur with acute delirium. Haloperidol in low doses, typically 0.5 mg to 1.0 mg, may be given PO, IV, or IM for mild confusion. The dose is titrated every 45 to 60 minutes against the target symptoms and generally does not exceed 20 mg in 24 hours. Other drugs used for this indication include olanzapine, risperidone, lorazepam, propofol, and midazolam. For confusion and agitation at the end of life, low-dose haloperidol given on an around-the-clock basis is recommended.[118] A recent study at Memorial Sloan-Kettering Cancer Center found that aripiprazole may be as effective as haloperidol in the management of delirium and its subtypes, although treatment with haloperidol resulted in more side effects.[119] However, a *Cochrane Database* review found only three studies that met its criteria and examined the use of antipsychotics to treat delirium. These studies compared haloperidol with risperidone, olanzapine, and placebo in the management of delirium. Delirium scores were not significantly different among these drugs, and low-dose haloperidol did not have a higher incidence of adverse effects compared with other antipsychotics.[120]

Safety is an issue for patients with any cognitive impairment. Notably, it is important to improve the safety and orientation of hospitalized patients with acute delirium. One way to do so is to provide orientation clues such as clocks, calendars, nightlights, family pictures, and other items from home. Reintroducing staff and place at each interaction, not confronting patients with cognitive tasks beyond their capabilities, and reducing sensory input are all useful steps. Additional mechanical safety measures include keeping the bed in a low position, placing the call bell within reach, offering assistance with ADLs, making sure hearing aids and glasses are used if needed, and encouraging relatives to be present or provide a sitter if family is unavailable.[118] Safety can be a problem for patients with even subtle cognitive deficits. Inability to remember or difficulty concentrating can prevent persons from driving or completing tasks at work. A formal neuropsychological evaluation can identify such deficits and help determine patients' ability to work and care for themselves safely. Many rehabilitation facilities offer formal driving evaluations in a simulated driving environment to ascertain difficulties that patients may have.

There are currently no proven treatments for cognitive impairment. Although potential therapies have been identified, research about them is limited. Fardell et al.'s[106] recent review of this literature noted several potential interventions. These measures include use of erythropoietin (EPO), which increases hemoglobin levels. The relationship between cognition and hemoglobin is not clear, but several studies have reported that reduced hemoglobin predicted decline in cognitive function. A variety of methodological issues with this research have been identified, however. It is unclear if EPO treatment is important during chemotherapy to predict cognitive function after therapy, and studies have not been adequately powered or have lacked appropriate control groups to establish a clear effect of EPO on cognition. The stimulant methylphenidate may also reduce cancer-related fatigue, and has been found to enhance memory in healthy persons and cognitive function in patients with primary brain tumors. Again, these studies lack sufficient power to detect differences, and it is unclear how methylphenidate might affect late cognitive outcomes.

Modafinil, a CNS stimulant, has been found to enhance cognition in healthy adults, and to reduce fatigue in cancer patients. Preliminary research is promising, and needs to be confirmed with larger, longitudinal, randomized controlled studies.

Donepeil, a cholinesterase inhibitor, is used to treat cognitive impairment in persons without cancer. It slows dementia progression. Animal research points to its potential usefulness in cancer patients. Only one study, carried out by Jatoi et al.,[121] has studied the effects of donepezil on cognitive function in persons with cancer, but this study closed early because of poor accrual; thus its results remain inconclusive.

Fluoxetine, a selective serotonin reuptake inhibitor (SSRI) used to treat depression, increases serotonin levels in the brain. Animal research has found it to be beneficial in mitigating chemotherapy-induced cognitive impairment. However, these findings need to be replicated in persons with cancer.

Antioxidants and specific diets appear to reduce the rate of cognitive decline in both humans and rodents. However, little clinical work has been done on the usefulness of antioxidants and supplements in treatment of chemotherapy-induced oxidative stress and cognitive deficit. The Chinese herb, Ginkgo biloba, is used to treat dementia, memory loss, and difficulties in concentration. Kaschel's review of 29 placebo-controlled randomized trials with Ginkgo biloba found benefits in cognitive function.[122] Current research is underway to examine this herb.

Behavioral techniques

In addition to the use of medication and safety measures, therapeutic interactions may have a role in improving memory and concentration or assisting in adaptation to existing deficits. In patients with mild or circumscribed impairments, cognitive retraining may be effective, and other patients may benefit from using behavioral compensation techniques.[118] Formal evaluation by trained professionals, such as neuropsychologists or therapists, allows deficits to be explored and appropriate therapies prescribed.

Cognitive rehabilitation consists of behavior-oriented interventions in which persons receive noninvasive training designed to improve cognitive and functional performance. Cognitive rehabilitation may include any of the following: (1) retraining to retrieve cognitive abilities that may be lost, (2) teaching compensatory techniques that encourage the use of residual abilities to develop alternative ways to perform cognitive tasks, and (3) holistic methods that address social, emotional, and functional issues related to cognitive impartment. These approaches have been used in many clinical populations, but experience with them is limited in cancer populations. Two examples produced different results. Ferguson et al.[123] found improvements in self-reported cognitive function and other factors 6 months after Memory and Attention Adaption Training, which focused on compensatory strategies. These participants had completed chemotherapy 18 months to 3 years previously. A second study did not find improved cognitive functioning after cognitive training in persons immediately after chemotherapy.[124]

Finally, physical activity has been shown to mitigate fatigue in cancer survivors. These programs based on this precept have also been shown to improve cognitive function in both healthy and otherwise ill persons (those with depression and Alzheimer's disease). Animal research has also found physical activity to be associated with improved cognition. The impact of physical activity on chemotherapy-induced cognitive impairments has yet to be studied.

PATIENT SELF-CARE

Patients, their families, and healthcare providers may attribute different meanings to the symptoms of cognitive dysfunction, seeing them as medical problems, spiritual events, or a normal part of the dying process. Cognitive symptoms are particularly important and distressing to patients and their families, so careful assessment, education of the patient and family, and interventions to keep patients comfortable, safe, and functioning are as important with cognitive symptoms as with all cancer-related symptoms. Resources, such as the self-care guide (Appendix 30A) that follows, may be useful for educating and counseling patients and their families.

REFERENCES

1. Oxford Dictionaries Online. Origin of cognition. n.d. Available at: http://oxforddictionaries.com/definition/cognition?region=us&q=cognition. Accessed February 28, 2012.
2. American Psychiatric Association. DSM-5 development: neurocognitive disorders. 2012. Available at: http://www.dsm5.org/proposedrevision/pages/neurocognitivedisorders.aspx. Accessed February 28, 2012.
3. Oxford Dictionaries Online. Origin of delirium. n.d. Available at: http://oxforddictionaries.com/definition/delirium?region=us&q=delirium. Accessed February 28, 2012.
4. Dasgupta M, Hillier LM. Factors associated with prolonged delirium: a systematic review. *Int Psychogeriatr.* 2010;22(3):373–394.
5. Bruera E, Bush SH, Willey J, et al. Impact of delirium and recall on the level of distress in patients with advanced cancer and their family caregivers. *Cancer.* 2009;115(9):2004–2012.
6. Oxford Dictionaries Online. Origin of dementia. n.d. Available at: http://oxforddictionaries.com/definition/dementia?region=us&q=dementia. Accessed February 28, 2012.
7. Seeley WW, Miller BL. Dementia. In: Longo DL, Fauci AS, Kasper DL, Hauser SL, Jameson JL, Loscalzo J, eds. *Harrison's Principles of Internal Medicine.* 18th ed. New York: McGraw-Hill; 2012: 3300–3316.
8. Ness KK, Wall MM, Oakes JM, Robison LL, Gurney JG. Physical performance limitations and participation restrictions among cancer survivors: a population-based study. *Ann Epidemiol.* 2006;16(3): 197–205.
9. Janelsins MC, Kohli S, Mohile SG, Usuki K, Ahles TA, Morrow GR. An update on cancer- and chemotherapy-related cognitive dysfunction: current status. *Semin Oncol.* 2011;38(3):431–438.
10. Wefel JS, Armstrong TA, Kohli S. Neuropsychological function and quality of life. In: Norden AD, Reardon DA, Wen PYC, eds. *Primary Central Nervous System Tumors: Current Clinical Oncology.* New York: Springer Science Media; 2011:143–170.
11. Ruge MI, Ilmberger J, Tonn JC, Kreth FW. Health-related quality of life and cognitive functioning in adult patients with supratentorial WHO grade II glioma: status prior to therapy. *J Neurooncol.* 2011;103(1):129–136.
12. Jansen CE, Cooper BA, Dodd MJ, Miaskowski CA. A prospective longitudinal study of chemotherapy-induced cognitive changes in breast cancer patients. *Support Care Cancer.* 2011;19(10):1647–1656.
13. Khuntia D, Brown P, Li J, Mehta MP. Whole-brain radiotherapy in the management of brain metastasis. *J Clin Oncol.* 2006;24(8):1295–304.
14. Bender CM, Sereika SM, Berga SL, et al. Cognitive impairment associated with adjuvant therapy in breast cancer. *Psychooncology.* 2006;15(5):422–430.
15. Vardy J, Rourke S, Galica J, et al. Cytokine levels in patients (pts) with localized colorectal cancer (CRC) after surgery and their relationship to fatigue and cognitive function. 2006 ASCO Annual Meeting proceedings. *J Clin Oncol.* 2006;24(18S Pt I):3623.
16. Jenkins V, Shilling V, Deutsch G, et al. A 3-year prospective study of the effects of adjuvant treatments on cognition in women with early stage breast cancer. *Br J Cancer.* 2006;94(6):828–834.
17. Hess LM, Chambers SK, Hatch K, et al. Pilot study of the prospective identification of changes in cognitive function during chemotherapy treatment for advanced ovarian cancer. *J Support Oncol.* 2010;8(6): 252–258.
18. Shilling V, Jenkins V, Morris R, Deutsch G, Bloomfield D. The effects of adjuvant chemotherapy on cognition in women with breast cancer: preliminary results of an observational longitudinal study. *Breast.* 2005;14(2):142–150.
19. Hurria A, Rosen C, Hudis C, et al. Cognitive function of older patients receiving adjuvant chemotherapy for breast cancer: a pilot prospective longitudinal study. *J Am Geriatr Soc.* 2006;54(6):925–931.
20. Mohile SG, Lacy M, Rodin M, et al. Cognitive effects of androgen deprivation therapy in an older cohort of men with prostate cancer. *Crit Rev Oncol Hematol.* 2010;75(2):152–159.
21. Schilder CM, Seynaeve C, Linn SC, et al. Cognitive functioning of postmenopausal breast cancer patients before adjuvant systemic therapy, and its association with medical and psychological factors. *Crit Rev Oncol Hematol.* 2010;76(2):133–141.
22. Palmer JL, Trotter T, Joy AA, Carlson LE. Cognitive effects of tamoxifen in pre-menopausal women with breast cancer compared to healthy controls. *J Cancer Surviv.* 2008;2(4):275–282.
23. Schilder CM, Seynaeve C, Beex LV, et al. Effects of tamoxifen and exemestane on cognitive functioning of postmenopausal patients with breast cancer: results from the neuropsychological side study of the tamoxifen and exemestane adjuvant multinational trial. *J Clin Oncol.* 2010;28(8):1294–1300.
24. Deprez S, Amant F, Smeets A, et al. Longitudinal assessment of chemotherapy-induced structural changes in cerebral white matter and its correlation with impaired cognitive functioning. *J Clin Oncol.* 2012;30(3):274–281.
25. Koppelmans V, Breteler MM, Boogerd W, Seynaeve C, Gundy C, Schagen SB. Neuropsychological performance in survivors of breast cancer more than 20 years after adjuvant chemotherapy. *J Clin Oncol.* 2012;30(10):1080–1086.
26. Fardell JE, Vardy J, Shah JD, Johnston IN. Cognitive impairments caused by oxaliplatin and 5-fluorouracil chemotherapy are ameliorated by physical activity. *Psychopharmacology (Berl).* 2012;220(1):183–193.
27. El Beltagy M, Mustafa S, Umka J, et al. Fluoxetine improves the memory deficits caused by the chemotherapy agent 5-fluorouracil. *Behav Brain Res.* 2010;208(1):112–117.
28. Syrjala KL, Artherholt SB, Kurland BF, et al. Prospective neurocognitive function over 5 years after allogeneic hematopoietic cell transplantation for cancer survivors compared with matched controls at 5 years. *J Clin Oncol.* 2010;29(17):2397–2404.
29. Correa DD, Ahles TA. Neurocognitive changes in cancer survivors. *Cancer J.* 2008;14(6):396–400.
30. Tager FA, McKinley PS, Schnabel FR, et al. The cognitive effects of chemotherapy in post-menopausal breast cancer patients: a controlled longitudinal study. *Breast Cancer Res Treat.* 2010;123(1):25–34.
31. Heflin LH, Meyerowitz BE, Hall P, etal. Cancer as a risk factor for long-term cognitive deficits and dementia. *J Natl Cancer Inst.* 2005;97(11):854–856.
32. Valentine AD, Meyers CA. Neurobehavioral effects of interferon therapy. *Curr Psychiatry Rep.* 2005;7(5):391–395.
33. Dickinson MD, Barr CD, Hiscock M, Meyers CA. Cognitive effects of pegylated interferon in individuals with primary brain tumors. *J Neurooncol.* 2009;95(2):231–237.
34. Capuron L, Fornwalt FB, Knight BT, Harvey PD, Ninan PT, Miller AH. Does cytokine-induced depression differ from idiopathic major depression in medically healthy individuals? *J Affect Disord.* 2009;119(1–3): 181–185.
35. Warrington TP, Bostwick JM. Psychiatric adverse effects of corticosteroids. *Mayo Clin Proc.* 2006;81(10):1361–1367.
36. Meador KJ, Gevins A, Leese PT, Otoul C, Loring DW. Neurocognitive effects of brivaracetam, levetiracetam, and lorazepam. *Epilepsia.* 2011;52(2):264–272.
37. Lossius MI, Hessen E, Mowinckel P, et al. Consequences of antiepileptic drug withdrawal: a randomized, double-blind study (Akershus study). *Epilepsia.* 2008;49(3):455–463.
38. Verdejo A, Toribio I, Orozco C, Puente KL, Perez-Garcia M. Neuropsychological functioning in methadone maintenance patients versus abstinent heroin abusers. *Drug Alcohol Depend.* 2005;78(3):283–288.
39. Perez-Alvarez S, Cuenca-Lopez MD, de Mera RM, et al. Methadone induces necrotic-like cell death in SH-SY5Y cells by an impairment of mitochondrial ATP synthesis. *Biochim Biophys Acta.* 2010;1802(11):1036–1047.
40. Lawrence YR, Li XA, el Naqa I, et al. Radiation dose-volume effects in the brain. *Int J Radiat Oncol Biol Phys.* 2010;76(3 suppl):S20–S27.

41. Soussain C, Ricard D, Fike JR, Mazeron JJ, Psimaras D, Delattre JY. CNS complications of radiotherapy and chemotherapy. *Lancet.* 2009;374(9701):1639–1651.
42. Grosshans DR, Meyers CA, Allen PK, Davenport SD, Komaki R. Neurocognitive function in patients with small cell lung cancer: effect of prophylactic cranial irradiation. *Cancer.* 2008;112(3):589–595.
43. Sun A, Bae K, Gore EM, et al. Phase III trial of prophylactic cranial irradiation compared with observation in patients with locally advanced non-small-cell lung cancer: neurocognitive and quality-of-life analysis. *J Clin Oncol.* 2011;29(3):279–286.
44. Le Pechoux C, Laplanche A, Faivre-Finn C, et al. Clinical neurological outcome and quality of life among patients with limited small-cell cancer treated with two different doses of prophylactic cranial irradiation in the intergroup phase III trial (PCI99-01, EORTC 22003-08004, RTOG 0212 and IFCT 99-01). *Ann Oncol.* 2010;22(5):1154–1163.
45. Wolfson AH, Bae K, Komaki R, et al. Primary analysis of a phase II randomized trial radiation therapy oncology group (RTOG) 0212: impact of different total doses and schedules of prophylactic cranial irradiation on chronic neurotoxicity and quality of life for patients with limited-disease small-cell lung cancer. *Int J Radiat Oncol Biol Phys.* 2011;81(1):77–84.
46. Chang EL, Wefel JS, Hess KR, et al. Neurocognition in patients with brain metastases treated with radiosurgery or radiosurgery plus whole-brain irradiation: a randomised controlled trial. *Lancet Oncol.* 2009;10(11):1037–1044.
47. Li J, Bentzen SM, Renschler M, Mehta MP. Regression after whole-brain radiation therapy for brain metastases correlates with survival and improved neurocognitive function. *J Clin Oncol.* 2007;25(10):1260–1266.
48. Welzel G, Fleckenstein K, Schaefer J, et al. Memory function before and after whole brain radiotherapy in patients with and without brain metastases. *Int J Radiat Oncol Biol Phys.* 2008;72(5):1311–138.
49. Meyers CA, Brown PD. Role and relevance of neurocognitive assessment in clinical trials of patients with CNS tumors. *J Clin Oncol.* 2006;24(8):1305–1309.
50. Gondi V, Tome WA, Mehta MP. Why avoid the hippocampus? A comprehensive review. *Radiother Oncol.* 2010;97(3):370–376.
51. Mahajan A, Dong L, Prabhu S. Application of deformable image registration to hippocampal doses and neurocognitive outcomes [abstract]. *Neuro Oncol.* 2007;9:538.
52. Douw L, Klein M, Fagel SS, et al. Cognitive and radiological effects of radiotherapy in patients with low-grade glioma: long-term follow-up. *Lancet Neurol.* 2009;8(9):810–818.
53. Omuro AM, Ben-Porat LS, Panageas KS, et al. Delayed neurotoxicity in primary central nervous system lymphoma. *Arch Neurol.* 2005;62(10):1595–1600.
54. Wefel JS, Schagen SB. Chemotherapy-related cognitive dysfunction. *Curr Neurol Neurosci Rep.* 2012;12(3):267–275.
55. Wefel JS, Witgert ME, Meyers CA. Neuropsychological sequelae of non-central nervous system cancer and cancer therapy. *Neuropsychol Rev.* 2008;18(2):121–131.
56. Meyers CA, Albitar M, Estey E. Cognitive impairment, fatigue, and cytokine levels in patients with acute myelogenous leukemia or myelodysplastic syndrome. *Cancer.* 2005;104(4):788–793.
57. Batalo M, Nagaiah G, Abraham J. Cognitive dysfunction in postmenopausal breast cancer patients on aromatase inhibitors. *Exp Rev Anticancer Ther.* 2011;11(8):1277–1282.
58. Correa DD, Hess LM. Cognitive function and quality of life in ovarian cancer. *Gynecol Oncol.* 2012;124(3):404–409.
59. Skaali T, Fossa SD, Dahl AA. A prospective study of cognitive complaints in patients with testicular cancer. *Clin Genitourin Cancer.* 2011;9(1):6–13.
60. Black B, Herr K, Fine P, et al. The relationships among pain, nonpain symptoms, and quality of life measures in older adults with cancer receiving hospice care. *Pain Med.* 2011;12(6):880–889.
61. Corn BW, Moughan J, Knisely JP, et al. Prospective evaluation of quality of life and neurocognitive effects in patients with multiple brain metastases receiving whole-brain radiotherapy with or without thalidomide on Radiation Therapy Oncology Group (RTOG) trial 0118. *Int J Radiat Oncol Biol Phys.* 2008;71(1):71–78.
62. Correa DD, Shi W, Thaler HT, Cheung AM, DeAngelis LM, Abrey LE. Longitudinal cognitive follow-up in low grade gliomas. *J Neurooncol.* 2008;86(3):321–327.
63. Li J, Bentzen SM, Li J, Renschler M, Mehta MP. Relationship between neurocognitive function and quality of life after whole-brain radiotherapy in patients with brain metastasis. *Int J Radiat Oncol Biol Phys.* 2008;71(1):64–70.
64. Correa DD, Rocco-Donovan M, DeAngelis LM, et al. Prospective cognitive follow-up in primary CNS lymphoma patients treated with chemotherapy and reduced-dose radiotherapy. *J Neurooncol.* 2009;91(3):315–321.
65. Vardy J, Wefel JS, Ahles T, Tannock IF, Schagen SB. Cancer and cancer-therapy related cognitive dysfunction: an international perspective from the Venice cognitive workshop. *Ann Oncol.* 2008;19(4):623–629.
66. Phillips KM, Jim HS, Small BJ, Laronga C, Andrykowski MA, Jacobsen PB. Cognitive functioning after cancer treatment: a 3-year longitudinal comparison of breast cancer survivors treated with chemotherapy or radiation and noncancer controls. *Cancer.* 2012;118(7):1925–1932.
67. Wefel JS, Vardy J, Ahles T, Schagen SB. International Cognition and Cancer Task Force recommendations to harmonise studies of cognitive function in patients with cancer. *Lancet Oncol.* 2011;12(7):703–708.
68. Small BJ, Rawson KS, Walsh E, et al. Catechol-*O*-methyltransferase genotype modulates cancer treatment-related cognitive deficits in breast cancer survivors. *Cancer.* 2011;117(7):1369–1376.
69. Ahles TA, Saykin AJ, Noll WW, et al. The relationship of APOE genotype to neuropsychological performance in long-term cancer survivors treated with standard dose chemotherapy. *Psychooncology.* 2003;12(6):612–619.
70. Seigers R, Fardell JE. Neurobiological basis of chemotherapy-induced cognitive impairment: a review of rodent research. *Neurosci Biobehav Rev.* 2011;35(3):729–741.
71. Han R, Yang YM, Dietrich J, Luebke A, Mayer-Proschel M, Noble M. Systemic 5-fluorouracil treatment causes a syndrome of delayed myelin destruction in the central nervous system. *J Biol.* 2008;7(4):12.
72. McDonald BC, Conroy SK, Ahles TA, West JD, Saykin AJ. Gray matter reduction associated with systemic chemotherapy for breast cancer: A prospective MRI study. *Breast Cancer Res Treat.* 2010;123(3):819–828.
73. Koppelmans V, de Ruiter MB, van der Lijn F, et al. Global and focal brain volume in long-term breast cancer survivors exposed to adjuvant chemotherapy. *Breast Cancer Res Treat.* 2011; 132(3):1099–1106.
74. Bosma I, Reijneveld JC, Klein M, et al. Disturbed functional brain networks and neurocognitive function in low-grade glioma patients: a graph theoretical analysis of resting-state MEG. *Nonlinear Biomed Phys.* 2009;3(1):9.
75. Fike JR, Rola R, Limoli CL. Radiation response of neural precursor cells. *Neurosurg Clin North Am.* 2007;18(1):115–127.
76. Amariglio R, Townsend M, Grodstein F, Sperling, R., Rentz, D. Specific subjective memory complaints in older persons may indicate poor cognitive function. *J Am Geriatrics Soc.* 2011;59:1612–1629.
77. Folstein MF, Folstein SE, McHugh PR. "Mini-Mental State": a practical method for grading the cognitive state of patients for the clinician. *J Psychiatr Res.* 1975;12(3):189–198.
78. Lezak MD, ed. *Neuropsychological Assessment.* 4th ed. New York: Oxford University Press; 2004.
79. Reardon DA, Galanis E, DeGroot JF, et al. Clinical trial end points for high-grade glioma: the evolving landscape. *Neuro Oncol.* 2011;13(3):353–361.
80. van den Bent MJ, Wefel JS, Schiff D, et al. Response assessment in neuro-oncology (a report of the RANO group): assessment of outcome in trials of diffuse low-grade gliomas. *Lancet Oncol.* 2011;12(6):583–593.
81. Inagaki M, Yoshikawa E, Matsuoka Y, et al. Smaller regional volumes of brain gray and white matter demonstrated in breast cancer survivors exposed to adjuvant chemotherapy. *Cancer.* 2007;109(1):146–156.

82. Yoshikawa E, Matsuoka Y, Inagaki M, et al. No adverse effects of adjuvant chemotherapy on hippocampal volume in Japanese breast cancer survivors. *Breast Cancer Res Treat.* 2005;92(1):81–84.
83. Silverman DH, Dy CJ, Castellon SA, et al. Altered frontocortical, cerebellar, and basal ganglia activity in adjuvant-treated breast cancer survivors 5–10 years after chemotherapy. *Breast Cancer Res Treat.* 2007;103(3):303–311.
84. National Cancer Institute. Common terminology criteria for adverse events, v. 4.03. 2010. Available at: http://evs.nci.nih.gov/ftp1/CTCAE/CTCAE_4.03_2010-06-14_QuickReference_5x7.pdf.
85. Rathier MO, Baker WL. A review of recent clinical trials and guidelines on the prevention and management of delirium in hospitalized older patients. *Hosp Pract (Minneap).* 2011;39(4):96–106.
86. Morandi A, Jackson JC. Delirium in the intensive care unit: a review. *Neurol Clin.* 2011;29(4):749–763.
87. Steiner LA. Postoperative delirium. Part 2: detection, prevention and treatment. *Eur J Anaesthesiol.* 2011;28(10):723–732.
88. Breitbart W, Alici Y. Evidence-based treatment of delirium in patients with cancer. *J Clin Oncol.* 2012;30(11):1206–1214.
89. Valentine AD, Duff JD. Assessment and management of psychological symptoms. In: Duffy JD, Valentine AD, eds. *MD Anderson Manual of Psychosocial Oncology.* New York: McGraw-Hill Professional; 2011:87–98.
90. Blonski M, Taillandier L, Herbet G, et al. Combination of neoadjuvant chemotherapy followed by surgical resection as a new strategy for WHO grade II gliomas: a study of cognitive status and quality of life. *J Neurooncol.* 2012;106(2):353–366.
91. Konat GW, Kraszpulski M, James I, Zhang HT, Abraham J. Cognitive dysfunction induced by chronic administration of common cancer chemotherapeutics in rats. *Metab Brain Dis.* 2008;23(3):325–333.
92. Ernst E. The risk–benefit profile of commonly used herbal therapies: ginkgo, St. John's wort, ginseng, echinacea, saw palmetto, and kava. *Ann Intern Med.* 2002;136(1):42–53.
93. Birks J, Grimley Evans J. Ginkgo biloba for cognitive impairment and dementia. *Cochrane Database Syst Rev.* 2009;1(1):CD003120.
94. Rodin MB, Mohile SG. A practical approach to geriatric assessment in oncology. *J Clin Oncol.* 2007;25(14):1936–1944.
95. Plassman BL, Langa KM, Fisher GG, et al. Prevalence of cognitive impairment without dementia in the United States. *Ann Intern Med.* 2008;148(6):427–434.
96. Kelley BJ, Petersen RC. Alzheimer's disease and mild cognitive impairment. *Neurol Clin.* 2007;25(3):577–609, v.
97. van Dyck CH, Lyness JM, Rohrbaugh RM, Siegal AP. Cognitive and psychiatric effects of vitamin B_{12} replacement in dementia with low serum B_{12} levels: a nursing home study. *Int Psychogeriatr.* 2009;21(1):138–147.
98. Kwok T, Lee J, Lam L, Woo J. Vitamin B_{12} supplementation did not improve cognition but reduced delirium in demented patients with vitamin B_{12} deficiency. *Arch Gerontol Geriatr.* 2008;46(3):273–282.
99. Conklin HM, Khan RB, Reddick WE, et al. Acute neurocognitive response to methylphenidate among survivors of childhood cancer: a randomized, double-blind, cross-over trial. *J Pediatr Psychol.* 2007; 32(9):1127–1139.
100. Conklin HM, Reddick WE, Ashford J, et al. Long-term efficacy of methylphenidate in enhancing attention regulation, social skills, and academic abilities of childhood cancer survivors. *J Clin Oncol.* 2010;28(29):4465–4472.
101. Gagnon B, Low G, Schreier G. Methylphenidate hydrochloride improves cognitive function in patients with advanced cancer and hypoactive delirium: a prospective clinical study. *J Psychiatry Neurosci.* 2005;30(2):100–107.
102. Meyers CA, Weitzner MA, Valentine AD, Levin VA. Methylphenidate therapy improves cognition, mood, and function of brain tumor patients. *J Clin Oncol.* 1998;16(7):2522–2527.
103. Sood A, Barton DL, Loprinzi CL. Use of methylphenidate in patients with cancer. *Am J Hosp Palliat Care.* 2006;23(1):35–40.
104. Marinella M, Markert R. Reversible posterior leucoencephalopathy syndrome associated with anticancer drugs. *Intern Med J.* 2009;39(12):826–834.
105. Vijayanathan V, Gulinello M, Ali N, Cole PD. Persistent cognitive deficits, induced by intrathecal methotrexate, are associated with elevated CSF concentrations of excitotoxic glutamate analogs and can be reversed by an NMDA antagonist. *Behav Brain Res.* 2011;225(2):491–497.
106. Fardell JE, Vardy J, Johnston IN, Winocur G. Chemotherapy and cognitive impairment: Treatment options. *Clin Pharmacol Ther.* 2011;90(3):366–376.
107. Ularntinon S, Tzuang D, Dahl G, Shaw RJ. Concurrent treatment of steroid-related mood and psychotic symptoms with risperidone. *Pediatrics.* 2010;125(5):e1241–e1245.
108. Shaw EG, Rosdhal R, D'Agostino RB.Jr, et al. Phase II study of donepezil in irradiated brain tumor patients: effect on cognitive function, mood, and quality of life. *J Clin Oncol.* 2006;24(9):1415–1420.
109. Torcuator R, Zuniga R, Mohan YS, et al. Initial experience with bevacizumab treatment for biopsy confirmed cerebral radiation necrosis. *J Neurooncol.* 2009;94(1):63–68.
110. Levin VA, Bidaut L, Hou P, et al. Randomized double-blind placebo-controlled trial of bevacizumab therapy for radiation necrosis of the central nervous system. *Int J Radiat Oncol Biol Phys.* 2011;79(5): 1487–1495.
111. Glantz MJ, Burger PC, Friedman AH, Radtke RA, Massey EW, Schold SC JR. Treatment of radiation-induced nervous system injury with heparin and warfarin. *Neurology.* 1994;44(11):2020–2027.
112. Buizer AI, de Sonneville LM, Veerman AJ. Effects of chemotherapy on neurocognitive function in children with acute lymphoblastic leukemia: a critical review of the literature. *Pediatr Blood Cancer.* 2009;52(4):447–454.
113. Wakefield CE, McLoone J, Goodenough B, Lenthen K, Cairns DR, Cohn RJ. The psychosocial impact of completing childhood cancer treatment: a systematic review of the literature. *J Pediatr Psychol.* 2010;35(3):262–274.
114. McGrath P, Suppiah R, Patton MA. Re-entering life: paediatric acute myeloid leukaemia at one year post treatment. *Aust J Holist Nurs.* 2005;12(2):23–34.
115. Duffey-Lind EC, O'Holleran E, Healey M, Vettese M, Diller L, Park ER. Transitioning to survivorship: a pilot study. *J Pediatr Oncol Nurs.* 2006;23(6):335–343.
116. Ortiz MC, de Lima RA. Experiences of families with children and adolescents after completing a cancer treatment: support for the nursing care. *Rev Lat Am Enfermagem.* 2007;15(3):411–417.
117. Ris MD. Lessons in pediatric neuropsycho-oncology: What we have learned since Johnny Gunther. *J Pediatr Psychol.* 2007;32(9):1029–1037.
118. Maldonado JR. Delirium in the acute care setting: characteristics, diagnosis and treatment. *Crit Care Clin.* 2008;24(4):657–722, vii.
119. Boettger S, Friedlander M, Breitbart W, Passik S. Aripiprazole and haloperidol in the treatment of delirium. *Aust N Z J Psychiatry.* 2011;45(6):477–482.
120. Lonergan E, Britton A, Luxenberg J, Wyller T. Antipsychotics for delirium. *Cochrane Database Syst Rev.* 2007;18(2):CD005594.
121. Jatoi A, Kahanic SP, Frytak S, et al. Donepezil and vitamin E for preventing cognitive dysfunction in small cell lung cancer patients: preliminary results and suggestions for future study designs. *Support Care Cancer.* 2005;13(1):66–69.
122. Kaschel R. Ginkgo biloba: specificity of neuropsychological improvement: a selective review in search of differential effects. *Hum Psychopharmacol.* 2009;24(5):345–370.
123. Ferguson RJ, Ahles TA, Saykin AJ, et al. Cognitive-behavioral management of chemotherapy-related cognitive change. *Psychooncology.* 2007;16(8):772–777.
124. Poppelreuter M, Weis J, Bartsch HH. Effects of specific neuropsychological training programs for breast cancer patients after adjuvant chemotherapy. *J Psychosoc Oncol.* 2009;27(2):274–296.

Cognitive Dysfunction, Delirium, and Dementia

Patient Name: ____

This self-care guide will help you learn about changes in thinking skills and what you can do to manage these problems.

Symptom and Description

Problems with "thinking," including problems with concentration and memory, delirium, and dementia, can occur as a result of cancer, cancer treatment, or other medications or conditions both related and unrelated to your cancer.

Many people think problems with concentration or memory are related to the stress of having cancer or a normal part of aging. Although this may be true, other conditions or medications may also contribute to the problem. Identifying such problems can help find their cause. If you are finding it difficult to concentrate or remember things, you should tell your doctor or nurse. Although the doctor or nurse may examine you, a routine examination may not reveal subtle problems unless you bring them up. Identifying such problems early may allow your healthcare team to begin treatment and provide techniques that may improve your quality of life.

Prevention

Sometimes it is necessary to give patients cancer treatments known to affect thinking skills. To help prevent cognitive dysfunction:

- Alert your healthcare team to any difficulties with your thinking skills you notice. Keep a log of specific examples to share with them during each clinic visit.
- Tell your healthcare team about all over-the-counter and prescription medications and any complementary therapies (such as vitamins and herbs) you are taking.
- Get plenty of sleep. Sleep deprivation may reduce your cognitive function. Adequate rest may not alleviate the problem but might lessen its severity.

Management

Experiencing difficulties with thinking skills can be both frightening and frustrating. Communication with your healthcare team is important for appropriate evaluation and treatment. Assessment by a clinical neuropsychologist can help determine the nature and severity of cognitive changes, and this healthcare provider may make recommendations for interventions to minimize the adverse effects of these cognitive changes on your daily life.

- Alert your healthcare team to any difficulties with your thinking skills. Keep a log of specific examples to share with them during your next clinic visit.
- Review all medications that you take, including over-the-counter and complementary therapies, with your doctor or nurse, as these medications may be contributing to your problem.

(continued)

- If your doctor prescribed medications to improve your thinking skills or to treat depression or anxiety, take them as ordered. Do not change the dose or stop the medication without speaking to your doctor or nurse.
- If your short-term memory is affected, use tools to help organize your life. Examples include daily pill dispensers, calendars showing specific activities that need to be done, electronic organizing devices or date planners, and watches with alarms that can be set to remind you of when to take medication.
- Avoid activities that may be dangerous if you are alone. For example, avoid cooking, using tools with which you can injure yourself, or traveling to unfamiliar places.
- If problems are acute, ask your family to watch for safety issues.

Follow-up

- Continue to track any difficulties you have, and alert your doctor or nurse when you have problems.
- When you start taking any new medication, ask your doctor how long it may be until you see a response and when the drug should be evaluated.

Phone Numbers

Nurse: ______________________________ Phone: __________

Physician: ______________________________ Phone: __________

Other: ______________________________ Phone: __________

Comments

Source: Cohen MZ, Shonka NA, Armstrong TS, Wefel JS. Cognitive Dysfunction. In: Yarbro CH, Wujcik D, Gobel BH, eds. *Cancer Symptom Management.* 4th ed. Burlington, MA: Jones & Bartlett Learning; 2014.

CHAPTER 31

Depression

Caryl D. Fulcher, MSN, RN, CNS-BC

THE PROBLEM

Receiving a diagnosis of cancer is a catastrophic event for the individual patient and for the family, confronting them with fears of pain, suffering, and uncertainty about the future. Shock, disbelief, anger, and sadness are common reactions. For most patients, these feelings give way within a couple of weeks to the process of adjusting to the news and proceeding with treatment decisions. For some patients, however, the "normal and expected" emotions become more disruptive or even debilitating, and they develop depressive symptoms. The range of emotion experienced by patients can be viewed on a continuum with "normal sadness" at one end and "psychiatric disorder, major depression" at the other end (Figure 31-1).[1,2]

Depressed feelings are not restricted to the time of diagnosis, but can occur at any period of time during the cancer trajectory. Some periods are considered more vulnerable than others; in addition to the period during which the initial diagnosis is made, other vulnerable times include the discovery of a suspicious symptom, a change to a different treatment modality, and recurrence or progression of disease (Table 31-1).[2]

DEFINITIONS OF DEPRESSION

Definitions of psychiatric disorders can be found in the *Diagnostic and Statistical Manual of Mental Disorders*, fourth edition, text revision (DSM-IV-TR).[3] In DSM-IV-TR, depressive disorders are categorized as adjustment disorders, major depressive disorders, or dysthymia. An adjustment disorder is defined as a reaction to an identifiable psychosocial stressor (e.g., cancer diagnosis) with a degree of psychopathology that is less severe than a major depressive disorder but that exceeds what would usually be expected, or that results in significant impairment in social/occupational functioning; this is the most common type of depression in people with

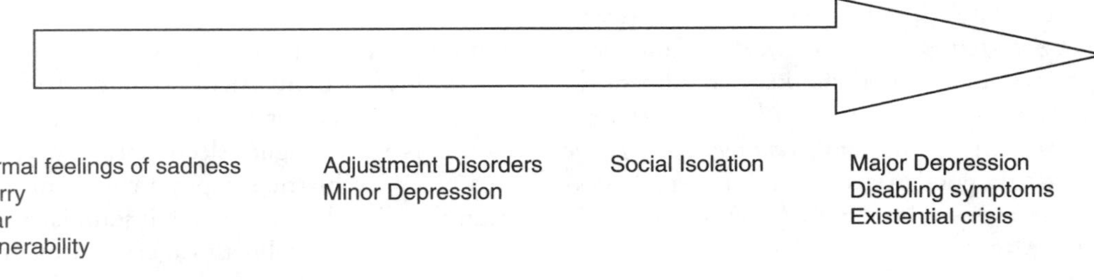

FIGURE 31-1

Continuum of depression and distress.

TABLE 31-1

Periods of Increased Vulnerability for Depression or Distress
• Finding a suspicious symptom
• During disease work-up
• Hearing the diagnosis
• Awaiting treatment
• Changing treatment modality
• Ending treatment
• Discharge from hospital
• Post-treatment survivorship
• Medical follow-up and surveillance
• Treatment failure
• Disease recurrence/progression
• Advanced cancer
• End of life

Source: Adapted with permission from the NCCN Clinical Practice Guidelines in Oncology (NCCN Guidelines®) for Distress Management (V.3.2012). © 2012 National Comprehensive Cancer Network, Inc[2].

TABLE 31-2

Symptoms of Adjustment Disorder
• Emotional or behavioral symptoms in response to an identifiable stressor (e.g., cancer diagnosis, treatment)
• Occurring within 3 months of onset of the stressor
• Symptoms are clinically significant, evidenced by:
Marked distress, in excess of what would be expected
Or
Significant impairment in social or occupational functioning
• Subtype of predominant symptom may be depressed mood

Source: Data from American Psychiatric Association[3].

TABLE 31-3

Symptoms of Major Depression
Present for most of the day, every day, for ≥ 2 weeks
1. Depressed mood
Or
2. Loss of interest or pleasure in most activities
And ≥4 of the following:
• Significant weight or appetite change (loss or increase)
• Insomnia or hypersomnia
• Fatigue or loss of energy
• Worthlessness or excessive guilt
• Diminished concentration, ability to think, or indecisiveness
• Recurrent thoughts of death or suicide

Source: Data from American Psychiatric Association[3].

cancer (Table 31-2).[3] A major depressive disorder includes symptoms lasting most of the day, every day, for 2 weeks or more and includes a depressed mood and additional symptoms that are described in Table 31-3.[3] Dysthymia refers to a chronic condition of depressive symptoms lasting much of the time for 2 years or longer. In addition to being a label for psychiatric disorders, the term "depression" is also used to describe a mood and a feeling.

It should be apparent that many of the symptoms described as being related to depression, such as fatigue, insomnia, and appetite change, are also common in cancer patients and associated with their disease or treatment, even when no evidence of clinical depression is apparent. For this reason, attention must be paid to the psychological symptoms that do not overlap with those resulting from treatment or disease. These symptoms include feelings of hopelessness and worthlessness, loss of self-esteem, guilt, and the inability to experience pleasure.[4] Alternative criteria have been explored in an attempt to identify the severity of major depression among cancer patients. Akechi et al.[5] found that *not participating in medical care* and *social withdrawal* appeared to be good markers of moderately severe major depression and that *fearfulness* or *depressed facial expression or body posture* and *brooding, self-pity, or pessimism* appeared to be good markers for mild major depressive disorder. These authors also reported that *inability to be cheered up, to smile, and to respond to good news or humor* may be a marker for severe major depression in patients with cancer;[5] these terms are descriptors of anhedonia.

Distress is a term often used to describe patients experiencing depression and anxiety; the National Comprehensive Cancer Network (NCCN) elected to use this word as part of its terminology because it was viewed as less psychiatric and, therefore, less stigmatizing or embarrassing. NCCN defines distress as "a multifactorial unpleasant emotional experience of a psychological, social, and/or spiritual nature that may interfere with the ability to cope effectively with cancer."[2] Thus "distress" is a broader term than "depression," although in many cases the two are used synonymously.

SYMPTOMS CLUSTER

Some symptoms are known to occur together or in clusters of three or more. Anxiety and depression, for example, often occur together in cancer patients.[6] Depression also co-occurs with fatigue, sleep disturbance, and pain,[7] and in a neuropsychiatric symptom cluster of depressed mood, cognitive disturbance, fatigue, insomnia, and pain as found in women receiving breast cancer treatment.[8] Perhaps even more important is the finding that higher levels of depression and poorer mental quality of life are significantly related to higher "symptom bother" from seven symptom clusters affecting older adult breast cancer survivors.[9] This result supports the saying, "Depression makes everything worse."

PREVALENCE OF DEPRESSION

The prevalence of depression in people with cancer is reported to range from 20% to 50% for solid tumors[10] and as low as 8% in other cancers.[11] The range is wide because of the many definitions of depression and the varying times when depression is assessed in cancer patients. Most prevalence studies include all the depressive disorders and cite occurrence at any time in the cancer trajectory. Some patients are assessed at the time of their diagnosis, others during active treatment, and some at intervals such as one year post-treatment or at disease recurrence. Burgess et al. found that among breast cancer patients, prevalence of depression was 33% at diagnosis, 15% after one year, and 45% after recurrence was diagnosed.[12] Miovic and Block report that approximately 50% of patients who have advanced cancer meet the criteria for either an adjustment disorder (11% to 35%) or major depression (5% to 26%).[13]

Cancer patients who are depressed report a poorer quality of life, are less likely to adhere to medical interventions, and often have longer hospital stays and higher use of healthcare services.[14,15] Many have poorer functional status, and some studies attribute increased mortality to patients with cancer and coexisting depression. In a meta-analysis examining the effect of depression on recurrence and mortality in cancer patients, Satin and colleagues found reasonable evidence that depression predicts mortality but not disease progression.[16] This relationship is thought to arise because patients with depression are more likely to be noncompliant with treatment. A study of 293 patients with early-stage breast cancer who were treated for depressive symptoms showed they were more likely to complete adjuvant therapy than those in the placebo (untreated) arm.[17]

Depression affects treatment adherence in several significant ways:

- Depressed patients are unable to integrate their cancer diagnosis and treatment information.
- They demonstrate reduced motivation toward self-care.
- They have difficulty making plans.
- Depressed individuals hold negative health beliefs and are pessimistic about treatment.
- They avoid health-promoting behaviors.
- They demonstrate social withdrawal and isolation.
- They use community resources to a lesser extent.
- They have greater difficulty tolerating the side effects of treatment.[18]

PATHOPHYSIOLOGY AND ETIOLOGY

Several theories about the etiology of depression have been proposed. According to the biopsychosocial model, a preexisting vulnerability exists that is activated with the occurrence of a stressful event such as cancer or its treatment.[19] At a physiologic level, this perspective translates to the monoamine hypothesis of depression, which suggests that insufficient neurotransmitter activity—namely, dopamine, norepinephrine, and serotonin—contribute to the development of depression.

Recent research on pathophysiology of depression in cancer has focused on psychoneuroimmunologic pathways. An association has been found between low natural killer cell (NK) activity and depression; factors contributing to even greater decline in NK activity, such as anxiety, smoking, psychomotor retardation, insomnia, and alcohol dependency, are common in depressed cancer populations.[14]

Activation of pro-inflammatory cytokines can result in a "sickness syndrome" characterized by symptoms that overlap with those of major depression: anhedonia, fatigue, anorexia, weight loss, insomnia, cognitive impairment, psychomotor retardation, and hyperalgesia.[14] Cytokines may cause this "sickness behavior" by altering the metabolism of monoamines, tryptophan, or thyroid hormones, as well as by activating corticotrophin-releasing factor and thereby stimulating the hypothalamic–pituitary–adrenal axis.[14] Tissue destruction in malignant disease may also play a role in prompting the activation of pro-inflammatory cytokines. Some neoplastic cells produce cytokines and some cancer treatments provoke extensive tissue damage and lead to significant immune activation and release of pro-inflammatory cytokines.[19]

SYMPTOM ASSESSMENT

Despite the high prevalence of depression in people with cancer, fewer than one-third of affected patients are identified by medical providers.[14] The following barriers may all impede the diagnosis of depression:

- Busy oncology practitioners often do not ask about emotional concerns. They may instead expect the patient to initiate a discussion of any concerns, and they may feel uncomfortable pursuing emotional topics and lack time and privacy in the office.
- Many patients have inadequate insurance to cover mental health needs, and oncology providers may lack awareness about free or low-cost community resources.
- Many patients do not want to bother their provider with emotional symptoms; they may feel embarrassed or think the oncology specialists are not interested. Stigma is often associated with mental health issues.
- Poor coordination often exists between different treatment settings, so psychosocial symptoms observed in one setting may not be followed up in another setting.
- Many believe depression is "normal" with cancer and that displaying a "fighting spirit" is expected and "negative feelings" should be hidden.
- Cultural difference may influence the reporting of psychological symptoms; older adults and some ethnic groups are more likely to report and focus on physical symptoms rather than psychological concerns.[14]

RISK FACTORS

Depression risk factors for the general public include a prior history of depression, suicide attempts, substance abuse, concurrent life stressors, a family history of depression, younger age, and single marital status. Cancer-related risk factors include the aforementioned as well as advanced disease, poorly controlled pain, increased physical impairment/disability, and perceived lack of support. Certain cancers, including those affecting the pancreas, head and neck, lung, and brain, as well as lymphomas, are associated with higher prevalence of depression or distress,[14] and certain chemotherapeutic agents are known to contribute to depression (Table 31-4).[1,14]

SELF-ASSESSMENT: THE PATIENT'S EXPERIENCE

Patients rarely come to their oncology provider saying, "I'm depressed." Some recognize their low mood, but others may be more aware of coexisting symptoms such as frequent tearfulness, loss of interest in doing anything, irritability, frustration, or preoccupation with details and loss of "big picture" vision. In a study of patients with cancer and major depressive disorder, Kleiboer and colleagues found that 94% of the patients reported psychological symptoms, which included loss of interest, low mood, a sense of guilt, lack of control, anxiety, loss of confidence, and irritability.[20] Family members may notice the symptoms even if the patient is not aware of the changes. Nurses may observe that hospitalized patients have become more withdrawn and stopped using their laptop or phone to communicate with friends and family. A change in affect or demeanor to one that is "flat" may be apparent, and the amount of verbal interaction may lessen. Increased focus on physical symptoms is common, particularly in older patients. Figure 31-2 illustrates assessment and management of depression.

TABLE 31-4

Anticancer Medications Associated with Depression
Amphotericin-B
Asparaginase
Corticosteroids
Cyproterone
Docetaxel
Interferon-alpha
Interleukin-2
Leuprolide
Paclitaxel
Procarbazine
Tamoxifen
Vinblastine
Vincristine
Vinorelbine

Source: Data from National Cancer Insitute[1]; Miller and Massie[14].

SUICIDE IN CANCER

A chapter on depression must include discussion of suicide, and several recent reviews provide insight into the risks and rate of suicide in cancer. A review of 39 articles concluded that despite the prevalence of suicidal ideation in a cancer population being comparable to that of the general population, the prevalence of *completed* suicide is higher in cancer patients.[21] In fact, another review concluded that the incidence of suicide among persons with cancer is approximately double the incidence in the general population.[22] Suicide rates are difficult to estimate in cancer patients, as occurrences such as medication overdoses and cessation of necessary treatments and nourishment by patients and families are not always reported. In seeking to understand suicide, clinicians must also appreciate the broader concept often underlying suicide: a desire for hastened death. In such a case, instead of wishing to harm oneself, the person wishes to die sooner than might occur by natural disease progression.[23] Desire for hastened death may take the form of a passive wish for death with no active plan, a request for assistance in hastening death, or an active desire and plan to commit suicide. Feeling like a burden to others is a common risk factor.[24]

In patients with cancer, clinicians may find that a fleeting wish to die is relatively common and not necessarily a cause for alarm.[23] Persistent thoughts of suicide, an actual plan or attempt, and self-injurious behaviors warrant intervention.

Suicide risk assessment

Suicide risk factors have been identified that are relevant to the general population as well as factors that are specific to people with cancer. (Table 31-5).[1,21,22,25] Many studies have reported that the highest risk for completed suicide occurs during the first year after diagnosis.[26–28] A recent large cohort found that of the 5875 patients who committed suicide, 2111 (36%) did so within the first year of diagnosis, and 1 in 3 of those did so within one month of diagnosis.[29] However, suicide risk also remains high among some survivors long after seemingly successful treatment. In one study, 12% of a sample of adult survivors of childhood cancer reported thoughts of or suicide attempts 20 years after treatment.[25] Factors associated with suicidal symptoms in these survivors included younger age at diagnosis, a longer time since diagnosis, and radiation treatments to the head.[25] Cranial radiation has been associated with impaired memory and cognitive function, retarded growth, and physical disfigurement; these effects may also contribute to development of suicidal symptoms.[25] Late life effects are also more common in this group of patients.

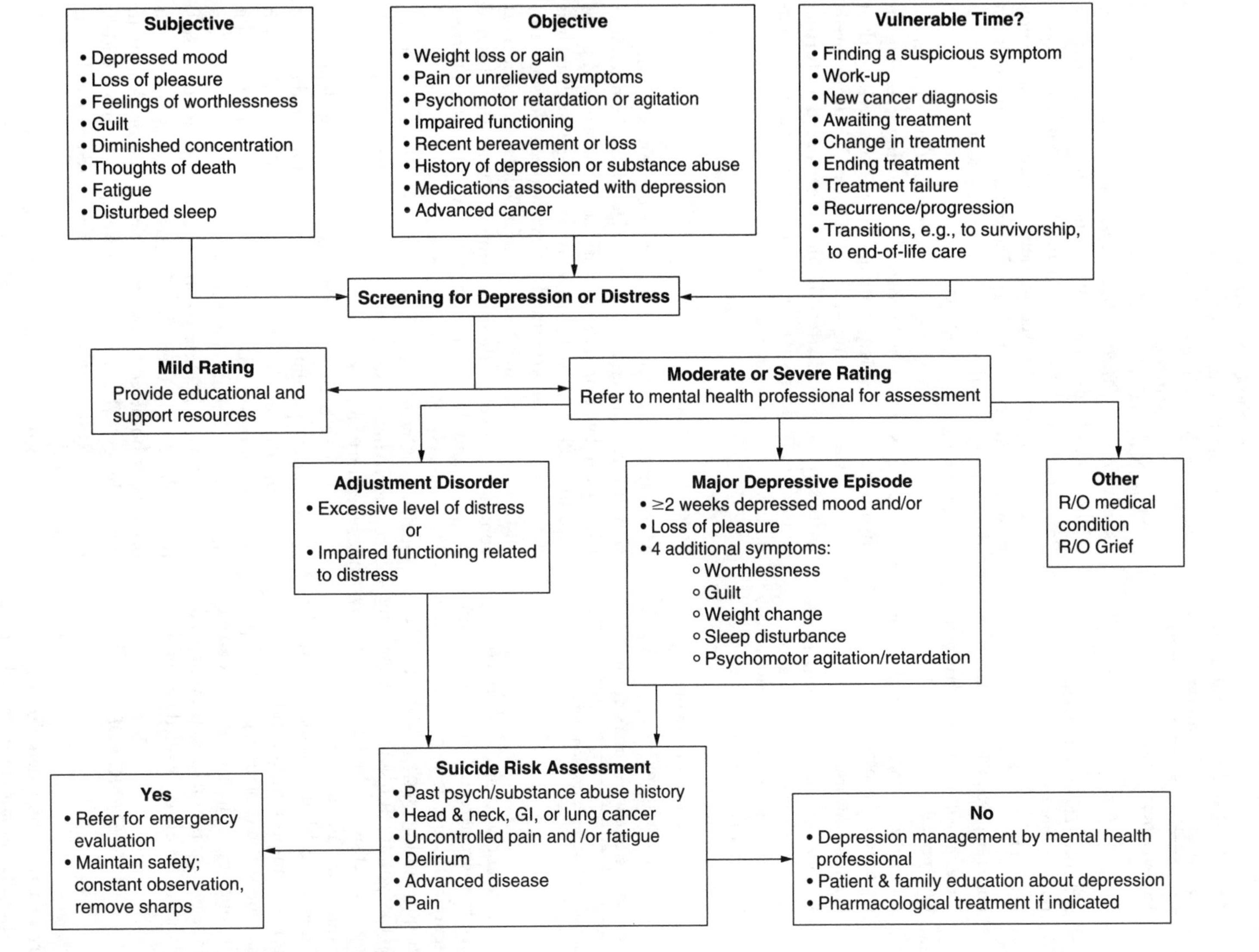

FIGURE 31-2

Assessment and management of depression.

Abbreviations: GI: gastrointestinal; R/O: rule out.

TABLE 31-5

Risk Factors for Suicide

General Population and Patients with Cancer	Specific Risk Factors Related to Patients with Cancer
History of psychiatric disorder or substance abuse	Hopelessness
Family history of suicide	Advanced stage of disease, poor prognosis
Few social supports	Fear of the future
Chronic disease	Impaired physical functioning
Pain	Time since diagnosis; risk greatest in first months
Older age or youth	Cancer type: lung, oral, pharyngeal, prostate and pancreatic
Living alone	Confusion/delirium
Unemployment	Presence of deficit symptoms, (e.g., loss of mobility, loss of bowel and bladder control, amputation, sensory loss, paraplegia, inability to eat and to swallow)
Male gender	Feeling like a burden to others
	Loss of autonomy
	Desire to control one's death

Source: Data from National Cancer Institute[1]; Robson et al[21]; Amgioano et al[22]; Recklitis et al[25].

Suicidal thoughts represent a crisis, and emergency action is indicated when they are detected. It is not uncommon for patients contemplating suicide to give clues about their thoughts. Direct questioning, such as asking, "Have you been feeling so bad that you are thinking about harming yourself?" is an appropriate action. If the patient responds affirmatively, further questions about plans are necessary to determine risk and mental health involvement should be pursued. Family input is also important in making plans to assure safety. Whereas true suicidal plans represent a psychiatric emergency, the oncology clinician also has a role. Effective symptom management is crucial to prevent a suicide driven by despair due to poorly controlled symptoms.

OBJECTIVE ASSESSMENT: SCREENING FOR DEPRESSION

Cancer patients report that their providers do not understand their psychosocial needs, do not consider such needs integral to cancer care, and fail to recognize, adequately treat, or offer referral for depression or other sequelae of stress due to illness.[30] This under-recognition of depression is widely documented in clinical oncology settings.[31,32]

Widespread screening is recommended to improve recognition of depressive symptoms. Screening differs from assessment in that it is a rapid method to identify individuals with psychosocial distress. It is typically done using a self-report tool as a means to determine which patients would benefit from referral to a mental health professional for further assessment.

The National Comprehensive Cancer Network published *Clinical Practice Guidelines in Oncology: Distress Management* beginning in 1999, and screening for distress has consistently been recommended as a standard of care.[2] In these consensus-based guidelines, screening is recommended at an early oncology visit and at appropriate intervals thereafter. Vulnerable times are listed as prompts for repeated screening (Table 31-1).

The American College of Surgeons Commission on Cancer[33] has established a standard requiring screening for distress for all oncology patients in facilities seeking their accreditation beginning in 2015. "Distress" is an umbrella term; screening for distress should trigger a need for further assessment of depression in affected individuals with referral offered to those in need.

Screening tools

Many screening tools are available for distress or depression. It is recommended that the selected tool be brief, user friendly, and validated for use with cancer patients. Mitchell identified 45 short tools that were tested against distress as defined by a semi-structured interview (the gold standard) and found only six methods had been validated.[34] The most commonly used of those instruments were the Hospital Anxiety and Depression Scale (HADS),[35] the Distress Thermometer (DT),[2] and a screen consisting of two verbal questions. Given that all tools had approximately the same accuracy, Mitchell suggests tool selection be based on client acceptability and cost-effectiveness.

Tools have been used to assess and monitor depression in noncancer patients for many years. One widely used tool is the Patient Health Questionnaire (PHQ-9),[36] which asks nine questions utilizing the DSM-IV criteria for major depression. It has also been used in a shorter, two-question form (PHQ-2):[37] "Have you been feeling down, depressed, or hopeless?" and then, "In the past two weeks, have you often been bothered by having little interest or pleasure in doing things?" Table 31-6 lists several of the more widely known screening tools that have been used in psychiatric and medical settings.[2,35–44]

Each oncology facility or practice needs to establish a process for screening and triage of those patients with moderate to severe distress or depressive symptoms. A list of mental health professionals to whom referrals can be made is necessary as well; ideally, these providers will be professionals who understand the unique needs of people with cancer.

TABLE 31-6

Common Self-Report Screening Tools for Depression and Distress in Cancer Patients

Name of Tool (Reference)	# of Items	Focus of Measurement
Distress Thermometer & Problem List (DT)(2)	0–10 rating plus 38 problems	Distress and problems related to distress
Brief Symptom Inventory (BSI-18) (38)	18	Somatization, anxiety, depression, general distress
Hospital Anxiety & Depression Scale (HADS) (35)	14	Clinical depression and anxiety
Functional Assessment of Chronic Illness Therapy (FACIT) (39)	27	4 domains of quality of life
Profile of Mood States (POMS) (40)	65	6 mood states
Beck Depression Inventory (BDI) Also BDI-short form (41)	21 13	Behavioral, cognitive, and somatic components of depression
Geriatric Depression Scale(GDS) Also GDS-short form (42)	30 15	Depression
Patient Health Questionnaire (PHQ-9) (36) Also PHQ 2 (37)	9 2	Depression
Center for Epidemiological studies-Depression Scale (CES-D) (43)	20	Depression
Zung Self-Rating Depression Scale (44)	20	Depression

The mental health professional assessing depression in the cancer patient must consider the pathology of the cancer, the sequelae of chemotherapy and other biological treatments, and the psychological impact that the patient is experiencing. The relationship between physical symptoms and mood must be considered, as pain can exacerbate depressive symptoms and fatigue can mimic depression through its impact on activity level, sleep, and concentration.[14] Grief must also be distinguished from depression, although the two may occur together. Grief is a distressing but normal emotional response to loss, and people with cancer face many losses along their cancer journey. Grieving individuals are usually able to enjoy people and activities at times; in contrast, in depressed individuals, their anhedonia is persistent.

SYMPTOM MANAGEMENT STRATEGIES

Once depression is identified, treatment options must be considered. First, the benefits of treating depression must be reviewed with the patient and family:

- Improved self-concept and sense of control
- Reduced distress, and often reduced pain, anxiety, and fatigue
- Improved ability to participate in medical treatment
- Reduced distress for family members who are concerned about changes in the patient's mood and functioning

Next, medications that may be contributing to the patient's depression must be reviewed and, when possible, discontinued or changed to an alternative that does not affect mood. Medications that can contribute to depressive symptoms include steroids, methyldopa, reserpine, barbiturates, propranolol, and some antibiotics such as amphotericin B.[1] Attention to pain control is also important, as depression often accompanies pain, and each symptom exacerbates the other. Attention to sleep and nutrition is another important factor in depression management, as fatigue is another often comorbid symptom with depression.

THERAPEUTIC APPROACHES

Psychosocial interventions

Oncology nurses have long recognized that their patients display evidence of their psychosocial and emotional needs, but in the past decade more science has endorsed the importance of identifying and integrating psychosocial needs into oncology care. The 2008 publication by the Institute of Medicine, *Cancer Care for the Whole Person, Meeting Psychosocial Needs*, reported strong evidence supporting the value of psychosocial interventions and recommended a standard for integrating such interventions to achieve quality cancer care.[30] Research efforts in this area continue to expand; however, to date, research on the effectiveness of specific interventions for patients with cancer and depression is scarce, is often of poor quality, and has produced ambiguous results.[45–47] Lack of evidence should not be interpreted as implying lack of efficacy, but rather indicates the need for more quality research. Interventions with the most evidence of effectiveness are listed in Table 31-7[45] and Table 31-8[48].

Cognitive-behavioral therapy

Cognitive-behavioral therapy (CBT) is based on the premise that cancer poses a severe threat to the patient's life; core positive beliefs are challenged and core negative beliefs are activated in this therapeutic approach. The individual's adjustment to the disease involves the interaction between the interpretation of the stresses and the coping strategies available. Identifying and correcting inaccurate thoughts, feelings, and behaviors, which are often associated with depressed and anxious feelings, allows for symptom improvement. In patients with cancer, the goal is to foster an optimistic but realistic attitude toward their situation, with a focus on modifying dysfunctional or irrational thoughts about cancer and its effect on their life. Techniques for relaxation and problem solving are also taught in CBT sessions, and homework is assigned to provide practice and ultimately aid symptom relief. CBT is effective in both group and individual modalities, and strong evidence supports its effectiveness.[46,47] Advanced training in CBT is needed to treat patients.

TABLE 31-7

Common Psychosocial Interventions to Manage Depression

Intervention	Description
Cognitive-behavioral therapy	Psychotherapy focusing on identifying and changing maladaptive thoughts and behaviors to reduce negative emotions and facilitate psychological adjustment. Stress management and problem-solving are usually included.
Counseling	Psychosocial care provided by a qualified professional. Can be delivered individually, in groups or in family groups; good communication and trust-building are essential for successful outcomes.
Psychoeducation	Information provided to increase knowledge of a particular subject and likely decrease uncertainty and increase well-being. Print, audiovisual, and interpersonal methods can be used.
Psychotherapy	Interpersonal treatment of emotional, relationship, or life situation disturbances provided by a qualified mental health professional in the context of a contracted relationship.
Stress management	Instruction in techniques to manage stress, including relaxation training, breathing exercises, meditation, imagery, writing, and others; goal is effective coping.

Source: Data from Li et al[45].

Supportive psychotherapy

Supportive counseling is the most widely used intervention for cancer-related depression. The focus is on helping patients in their immediate situation by reinforcing current support and coping options and teaching new ones as necessary. The goal is to help the patient manage mood and symptoms rather than to explore and uncover past issues. Worries and fears related to cancer are normalized, and strengths are positively reinforced. Supportive counseling can be delivered to patients individually, in groups, or with a partner/family.

Advanced training is required to provide psychotherapy, but nurses are instrumental in helping to identify and address concerns of both patients and caregivers. Quality nursing practice includes asking "What are your concerns today?" and listening attentively to the patient's response. Providing emotional support can be as simple as asking regularly about the patient's emotional state, addressing disturbing or embarrassing topics directly and with sensitivity, acknowledging the family's role and need for support, and providing resources for psychotherapy, home care, financial aid, and other support services.[49] Peer volunteers—often survivors of a similar cancer—can provide patients with hope in seeing that others have faced similar challenges with success. Nurses can help patients to problem solve, support adaptive coping strategies, and promote provider–patient communication by rehearsing difficult topics or scenarios. For many oncology nurses, this is the heart and reward of their practice.

Psychoeducational interventions

Seeking information is one important way that individuals cope with their cancer. Providing patients and families with information about the disease, its treatment, the diagnostic tests, and the usual side effects help them to anticipate, prepare, and feel less overwhelmed. Orienting new patients to the clinic or hospital, providing tours, describing procedures, and offering resources and contact information are helpful strategies for reducing anxiety and depression, especially when patients are also given an opportunity to ask questions and express concerns.[46]

Antidepressant medications

The efficacy of antidepressant medication has been proven both in patients with depression and in patients

TABLE 31-8

Antidepressants Commonly Used in the Cancer Setting

Drug	Dose (mg/day PO)	Possible Unique Benefits	Possible Side Effects
Buproprion/ Buproprion ER (Norepinephrinergic)	75–450	May be helpful for concentration and low energy; fewer sexual side effects	Seizures, headache, nausea, likely impedes tamoxifen's efficacy
Citalopram (SSRI)	10–40	Few P450 interactions	Headache, diarrhea, constipation, restlessness, sexual dysfunction
Duloxetine (SNRI)	20–60	Management of neuropathic pain	Worsening of narrow-angle glaucoma and hepatic insufficiency, nausea, dizziness, fatigue, sexual dysfunction
Ecitalopram (SSRI)	10–20	Few P450 interactions	Headache, diarrhea, constipation, restlessness, sexual dysfunction
Fluoxetine (SSRI)	10–80	Long-action so (1) may be dosed once weekly at 90 mg and (2) least likely to trigger discontinuation syndrome	Nausea, nervousness, weight gain, headache, insomnia, strong inhibition of tamoxifen and other CYP2D6 substrates
Mirtazapine (SSRI)	15–45	Sleep aid at low doses; appetite stimulant; antiemetic; less gastrointestinal side effects;	Dry mouth, sedating at low doses, weight gain
Paroxetine/Paroxetine CR (SSRI)	5–60 (62.5 if CR)	Management of hot flashes	Headache, somnolence, dizziness, sexual dysfunction, gastrointestinal upset, dry mouth, prominent discontinuation syndrome, strong inhibition of tamoxifen and other 2D6 substrates
Sertraline (SSRI)	25–200		Headache, diarrhea, constipation, restlessness, sexual dysfunction
Trazodone (Atypical)	25–250	Sleep aid	Sedation, orthostasis, riapism, sexual dysfunction
Venlafaxine/Venlafaxine SR (SNRI)	37.5–300	Possibly helpful for hot flashes and neuropathic pain; least interaction with tamoxifen; few P450 interactions	Blood pressure increases, sexual dysfunction, prominent discontinuation syndrome

Abbreviations: CR: controlled release; SR: sustained release.

Source: Data from Braun and Pirl[48].

with depression and medical illness.[50] However, the data on using antidepressants in patients with cancer remain scarce.[46,51,52] Evidence related to depression in other populations may be applicable to cancer patients, but the diagnostic overlap of some depression symptoms with those of cancer, as well as the higher rates of side effects related to medication and treatment withdrawal in the cancer populations, must be considered.[52] Comorbid cancer pain can exacerbate depression and hopelessness, so pain treatment is essential when pain and mood disturbance coexist.[52]

Selective serotonin reuptake inhibitors and serotonin norepinephrine reuptake inhibitors. The agents most studied and most commonly used in the cancer setting are selective serotonin reuptake inhibitors (SSRIs) and serotonin-norepinephrine reuptake inhibitors (SNRIs). They are first-line choices due to their tolerability and safety profiles; all are equally efficacious.

In selecting an antidepressant, it is useful to question whether a blood relative of the patient has been successfully treated with a particular agent; if so, that may be a good choice. Consider the side-effect profile, drug interactions, and cost as well (Table 31-8). SSRIs share a similar side-effect profile, with gastrointestinal disturbance, headache, fatigue or insomnia, sexual dysfunction, and increased anxiety being the most common risks. An important difference is the long half-life of fluoxetine, which makes its potential for drug interactions a greater risk. The other SSRIs and SNRIs have shorter half-lives; the challenge in using these medications is that abrupt cessation may result in a *discontinuation syndrome* with symptoms that may include malaise, light-headedness, dizziness, and lightning-like pains in the extremities.[48] Such abrupt cessation may occur, for example, when patients experience severe mucositis or a bowel obstruction and they are unable to consume oral preparations. This syndrome is most often seen with paroxetine, venlafaxine, and duloxetine, although extended-release venlafaxine may be less likely to cause withdrawal effects. Gradual discontinuation over several weeks to months reduces this withdrawal syndrome. Most antidepressants act by increasing the levels of one or more monoamine neurotransmitters in the synaptic cleft between neurons.[19]

In prescribing antidepressant medications for cancer patients, there are several key principles to follow:

1. Start at a low dose and increase the dose slowly to avoid unwanted side effects.
2. Educate and reassure the patient while waiting for the medication's therapeutic benefit to occur; this can take up to 3 weeks for mood improvement, although sleep and appetite benefits may be seen sooner with some antidepressants.
3. Symptom improvement may be achieved with lower doses in cancer patients than are required for other depressed patients.
4. Monitor side effects and target symptoms carefully, as cancer symptoms and effects of other drugs may compound the picture.
5. Continue treatment for 4 to 6 months after symptom improvement to avoid relapse of depression.
6. When ready to discontinue, gradually decrease the dose by 50% over several weeks to minimize withdrawal effects.[53]

Tricyclic antidepressants. Tricyclic antidepressants (TCAs) are seldom used to treat depression in people with cancer. They have more side effects than SSRIs and SNRIs, such as orthostatic hypotension, weight gain, sedation, cardiac arrhythmias, and anticholinergic delirium, but in low doses they are sometimes used as a sleep aid. This is particularly true for amitriptyline and trazodone.

Atypical antidepressants. Atypical antidepressants such as bupropion and mirtazapine are valuable to the cancer patient. Bupropion does not induce sexual dysfunction and is useful in helping fatigue. Mirtazapine helps stimulate appetite, a desirable effect for patients with anorexia. Its sedative effect benefits those individuals with sleep difficulty, and the medication is available in a rapidly dissolving tablet for those with difficulty swallowing oral preparations.

Psychostimulants. Psychostimulants (methylphenidate and dextroamphetamine) are used for their energizing effect in depressed cancer patients. It should be noted that psychostimulants are approved by the Food and Drug Administration primarily for use in attention-deficit/hyperactivity disorder, so other uses are considered off-label. Most often these medications are used in patients with advanced or terminal disease because their onset of action is rapid—hours or days, rather than weeks. Some evidence indicates that, along with their impact on mood, psychostimulants reduce anorexia and fatigue, improve attention and concentration, and counteract opiate-induced sedation.[14] The most common side effects with these agents are insomnia and agitation, and rarely psychosis.

Nontraditional uses of antidepressants. Oncology clinicians have discovered that some antidepressant medications are useful beyond the treatment of depression and anxiety. In recent years they have shown benefit in treating neuropathic pain, chronic pain, and hot flashes. Trials with venlafaxine, fluoxetine, and paroxetine have shown significant hot flash reduction compared to placebo.[54] Tricyclic antidepressants have been studied most in providing effective treatment for neuropathic pain in patients with cancer and at doses lower than those required for depression management.[55]

Significant drug interactions. Several important drug interactions between antidepressant medications and cancer treatments have emerged that require attention. In particular, a growing number of studies have raised questions about the interaction of antidepressants and tamoxifen. Tamoxifen is converted to its active metabolites—4-hydroxytamoxifen and endoxifen (4-hydroxy-*N*-desmethyltamoxifen)—by cytochrome P450 enzymes, the most clinically relevant of which is CYP2D6. Strong CYP2D6 inhibitors reduce the serum levels of endoxifen and may significantly interfere with the clinical efficacy of tamoxifen.[56] Strong CYP2D6 inhibitor antidepressants include paroxetine and fluoxetine, and other indirect evidence suggests bupropion also has considerable effects on the metabolism of tamoxifen.[57] The emerging consensus is that clinicians should use antidepressants with lower CYP2D6 inhibition properties (citalopram, escitalopram, duloxetine) or CYP2D6 noninhibitor antidepressants (venlafaxine, mirtazapine) in patients concurrently taking tamoxifen.[56]

St. John's wort, an herb used to treat mild depression, is known to interact with the drug-metabolizing enzyme CYP 3A4 and lowers the efficacy of irinotecan and tamoxifen[58] as well as imatinib.[59]

Serotonin syndrome is a potentially life-threatening condition that can occur when serotonin reaches toxic levels in the body. At risk are cancer patients taking an SSRI or SNRI and narcotics and/or antiemetics, (e.g., 5-HT_3 antagonists, such as ondansetron and granisetron). Excessive serotonergic agonism results from either therapeutic drug use, overdose, or drug interactions.[54] Likewise, linezolid, an antibacterial agent and monoamine oxidase inhibitor, should not be administered to patients taking SSRIs, TCAs, or SNRIs due to the risk of serotonin syndrome.[60] Linezolid inhibits the action of monoamine oxidase A, an enzyme that breaks down serotonin, thus allowing serotonin buildup. Symptoms of serotonin syndrome include hyperreflexia, myoclonus, tremor, tachycardia, hypertension, hyperthermia, sweating, shivering, nausea, diarrhea, agitation, confusion, and delirium, and can progress to coma.[53]

Many oncology providers feel comfortable beginning or continuing their patients on antidepressant medication, but it is important to seek a psychiatric consult in the following circumstances:

- Severe or worsening depression when suicidal risk may be present
- Adequate dose and time on antidepressant has produced no clinical benefit
- Psychotic or manic symptoms are present
- Lithium or neuroleptic treatment is contemplated
- Severe anxiety symptoms are present.

Complementary approaches

Complementary therapies are believed to be widely used by cancer patients, but as noted earlier, herbs and dietary supplements may produce dangerous interactions when used in conjunction with prescription medications. Studies report benefits of complementary therapies, but unfortunately many studies are of poor quality and use heterogeneous samples, so further research is required to truly understand the role of such therapies in managing symptoms such as depression.[61–66] The Oncology Nursing Society has created a resource called *Putting Evidence into Practice: Improving Oncology Patient Outcomes*.[67] In this resource, intervention studies for depression are reviewed and categorized in terms of their weight of evidence, including the following complementary therapies as shown in Table 31-9.

The paucity of evidence makes selecting an intervention for the depressed cancer patient difficult. Combining interventions—particularly psychotherapy with antidepressant treatment—is most likely to be effective; indeed, that is the standard for treating depression in noncancer populations. Many clinicians select psychosocial and psychoeducational interventions for mild to moderate depression, and add pharmacological agents for those with more severe symptoms.

TABLE 31-9

Complementary Therapies and Weight of Evidence

Intervention	Weight of Evidence
Relaxation therapy	Likely to be effective
Massage	Effectiveness not established
Exercise	Effectiveness not established
Hypnosis	Effectiveness not established
Reflexology	Effectiveness unlikely
Reiki	Effectiveness not established

SPECIAL POPULATIONS

Elderly

Cancer is predominantly a disease of the elderly, and the U.S. population is aging in greater numbers than ever before. Some evidence reports the risk of depression plateaus from ages 65 to 75 years, but then increases again.[68] Risk factors for depression in the elderly include the same risks as for all adults, but also include loss of spouse, functional disability, inadequate emotional support, and medications known to contribute to depression.[68] Elderly patients are more likely to complain of somatic signs of depression (sleep disturbance, general aches) than emotional signs (sad mood, loss of interest or pleasure).[69] Antidepressant medication risks such as the cardiac arrhythmias, hypotension and anticholinergic effects of the TCAs and the long half-life and P450 effects of some SSRIs make them less desirable for elderly patients.

Compliance with antidepressant medication may also be an issue. Givens et al.[70] found four themes related to poor antidepressant adherence among older adults: the fear of dependence, resistance to viewing depressive symptoms as a medical illness, concern that antidepressant medication would prevent natural sadness, and prior negative experience with medication for depression.

Mental health providers integrated into medical care clinics are often well accepted by older adults. Such integration provides accessibility and allows collaboration between primary providers and mental health experts.

Nurses must be aware that elderly patients are likely to have more comorbid health conditions, lower functional status, and caregiver partners who also have health concerns. At the same time, more treatment is being delivered in outpatient settings with prominent emphasis on participation in one's care.

Post-treatment survivors

Cancer symptoms or treatment effects, which persist and lead to chronic conditions, are becoming more common as the population of cancer survivors grows. Coping on a long-term basis with the stresses of chronic illness presents another opportunity for emotional deterioration and depression. Although most research is done with cancer patients in early treatment, evidence indicates that long-term survivors experience serious psychological distress,[71,72] and randomized trials reveal that cognitive-behavioral, psychoeducational and stress management interventions benefit depression in survivors in the post-treatment period.[71,72] Supportive care interventions may need to be focused differently for such individuals than for those patients who have been recently diagnosed. One breast cancer patient relayed her discouragement when members of her support group asked when her treatment would end; in her case, the treatment would always be ongoing.

Family caregivers are also at risk for developing depression as they attempt to cope with a never-ending role of providing care to their loved ones. Cancer surveillance visits after treatment completion are an opportunity for assessment and referral for psychosocial care, and nurses have a prominent role in survivorship clinics, which should include psychosocial care as a standard offering.

NURSING IMPLICATIONS

Patients' reluctance to report emotional reactions and the barriers to recognizing distress have been described. Oncology nurses are well positioned to integrate psychosocial aspects of care into oncology practice. Often nurses are the ones observing the patient in relation to the family, and can assess changes in family dynamics. Patients may perceive the physician as too busy or not interested in their psychosocial issues, yet see the nurse as an understanding listener and helpful problem-solver. Nurses may be the ones assigned to review the screening tools after administration, but screening alone is insufficient. Assuring resources are provided is essential, and nurses often act as the liaison in making referrals to other disciplines. Developing a relationship in which the patient feels comfortable sharing concerns is a fundamental objective for nurses, and this relationship is the gateway to achieving integration of psychosocial care and meeting the needs of the "whole patient."

Nurses can evaluate their therapeutic approach to managing depression by assuring that the following goals are met:

- Screening for distress or depression is occurring and is documented; referrals are made when appropriate; and supportive resources, including online information, are provided.
- Opportunity for patients to express emotional concerns is provided. The nurse also pays attention to any changes in the patient's appearance, activity level, and family dynamics.
- The patient and family understand depression as an illness and can list the patient's target symptoms and an intervention for management.
- The patient and family have sufficient knowledge of any antidepressant medication prescribed, including dose, side effects, time necessary for therapeutic response, and effects of abrupt cessation.
- Coexisting symptoms that affect depression are managed, such as pain and fatigue.
- Self-care strategies are emphasized to assure safety, optimal functional status, and regular inclusion of pleasant activities to enhance quality of life.

PATIENT SELF-CARE

Providing written resources, including facility-specific and local contacts for support groups and educational information and opportunities, is important so that patients can refer to these materials later. Several national organizations represent valuable resources for patients and families who are dealing with cancer and depression:

- CANCER CARE: www.cancercare.org.
- American Psychosocial Oncology Society Helpline: 866-276-7443. Helpline is a toll-free hotline for cancer patients to obtain referrals for local counseling and support services throughout the United States.
- National Cancer Institute—Depression: http://www.cancer.gov/cancertopics/pdq/supportivecare/depression/Patient.
- People Living with Cancer: www.plwc.org.
- The Wellness Community: www.thewellness-community.org.
- Disease-specific organizations usually have resources on coping; see their websites.

Symptom management is the focus and pride of oncology nurses. Including interventions to identify and manage depression as part of their care will help patients experience improved quality of life, enhance treatment adherence, and demonstrate responsiveness to patient emotional needs. Along with these resources, nurses can provide patients with the self-care guides in Appendix 31A and Appendix 31B to augment teaching and monitor symptoms.[73,74]

REFERENCES

1. National Cancer Institute. Depression (PDQ®) health professional version. 2011. Available at: http://www.cancer.gov/cancertopics/pdq/supportivecare/depression/HealthProfessional/. Accessed February 6, 2012.
2. National Comprehensive Cancer Network (NCCN). *Clinical Practice Guidelines in Oncology (NCCN Guidelines®) for Distress Management* (V.3.2012). 2012. Available at: NCCN.org. Accessed May 31, 2012.
3. American Psychiatric Association. *Diagnostic and Statistical Manual of Mental Disorders.* 4th ed., text revision. Washington, DC: American Psychiatric Association; 2000.
4. Miller K, Massie MJ. Depression and anxiety. *Cancer J.* 2006;12(5): 388–397.

5. Akechi T, Ietsugu T, Sukigara M, et al. Symptom indicator of severity of depression in cancer patients: a comparison of the DMS-IV criteria with alternative diagnostic criteria. *Gen Hosp Psychiatry.* 2009;31:225–232.
6. Massie, MJ, Lloyd-Williams M, Irving G, Miller, K. The prevalence of depression in people with cancer. In: Kissane DW, Maj M, and Sartorius N, eds. *Depression and Cancer.* Oxford, UK: John Wiley & Sons, Ltd; 2011: 1–36.
7. Miaskowski C, Cooper BA, Paul SM, et al. Subgroups of patients with cancer with different symptom experiences and quality-of-life outcomes: a cluster analysis. *Oncol Nurs Forum.* 2006;33:E79–E89.
8. Kim HJ, Barsesvick A, Beck, SL, Dudley W. Clinical subgroups of a psychoneurologic symptom cluster in women receiving treatment for breast cancer: a secondary analysis. *Oncol Nurs Forum.* 2012;39:E20–E29.
9. Roiland RA, Heidrich SM. Symptom clusters and quality of life in older adult breast cancer survivors. *Oncol Nurs Forum.* 2011;38:672–680.
10. Pasquini M, Biondi M. Depression in cancer patients: a critical review. *Clin Pract Epidemiol Ment Health.* 2007;3. Available at: http://www.cpementalhealth.com/content/3/1/2.
11. Sharpe M, Strong V, Allen K, et al. Major depression in outpatients attending a regional cancer centre: screening and unmet treatment needs. *Br J Cancer.* 2004;90(2):314–320.
12. Burgess C, Cornelius B, Love S, Graham J, Richards M, Ramirez A. Depression and anxiety in women with early breast cancer: five year observational cohort study. *Br Medl J.* 2005; 330: 702–707.
13. Miovic M, Block S. Psychiatric disorders in advanced cancer. *Cancer.* 2007;110:1665–1676.
14. Miller K, Massie MJ. Depressive disorders. In: Holland JC, Breitbart WS, Jacobsen PB, Lederberg MS, Loscalzo MJ and McCorkle R, eds. *Psychooncology.* 2nd ed. New York: Oxford University Press; 2010:311–318.
15. Muskin PR. Major depressive disorder and other medical illness: a two-way street. *Ann Clin Psychiatry.* 2010;22 (4 suppl):S15–S20.
16. Satin JR, Linden W, Phillips MJ. Depression as a predictor of disease progression and mortality in cancer patients: a meta-analysis. *Cancer.* 2009;115:5349–5361.
17. Tuma RS. Untreated depressive symptoms interfere with patient compliance. *Oncol Times.* June 10, 2005: 5–6.
18. DiMatteo MR, Haskard-Zolnierek KB. Impact of depression on treatment adherence and survival from cancer. In: Kissane DW, Maj M, Sartorius N, eds. *Depression and Cancer.* Oxford, UK: John Wiley & Sons; 2011:101–124.
19. Musselman DL, Miller AH, Royster EB, McNutt MD. Biology of depression and cytokines in cancer. In: Kissane DW, Maj M, Sartorius N, eds. *Depression and Cancer.* Oxford, UK: John Wiley & Sons; 2011:51–79.
20. Kleiboer A, Bennett F, Hodges L, Walker J, Thekkumpurath P, Sharpe M. The problems reported by cancer patients with major depression. *Psychooncology.* 2011; 20: 62–68.
21. Robson A, Scrutton F, Wilkinson L, MacLeod F. The risk of suicide in cancer patients: a review of the literature. *Psychooncology.* 2010;19:1250–1258.
22. Anguiano L, Mayer DK, Piven ML, Rosenstein D. A literature review of suicide in cancer patients. *Cancer Nurs.* 2012;35(4)1314–1316.
23. Breitbart W, Pessin H, Kolva E. Suicide and desire for hastened death in people with cancer. In: Kissane DW, Maj M, Sartorius N, eds. *Depression and Cancer.* Oxford, UK: John Wiley & Sons; 2011:125–150.
24. Hudson PL, Kristjanson LJ, Ashby M, et al. Desire for hastened death in patients with advanced disease and the evidence base of clinical guidelines: a systematic review. *Palliat Med.* 2006;20:693–701.
25. Recklitis CJ, Lockwood RA, Rothwell MA, Diller LR. Suicidal ideation and attempts in adult survivors of childhood cancer. *J Clin Oncol.* 2006;24(24):3852–3857.
26. Hem E, Loge JG, Haldorsen T, Dedberg O. Suicide risk in cancer patients from 1960–1999. *J Clin Oncol.* 2004; 22(20): 4209–4216.
27. Robinson D, Renshaw C, Okello C, Moller H, Davies A. Suicide in cancer patients in southeast England from 1996–2005: a population-based study. *Br J Cancer.* 2009; 101(1): 198–201.
28. Yousaf U, Christensen ML, Engholm G, Storm HH. Suicides among Danish cancer patients 1971–1999. *Br J Cancer.* 2005;92(6):995–1000.
29. Johnson TV, Garlow SJ, Brawley OW, Master VA. Peak window of suicides occurs within the first month of diagnosis: implications for clinical oncology. *Psychooncology.* 2012;21;351–356.
30. Adler NE, Page AEK, eds. *Cancer Care for the Whole Patient: Meeting Psychosocial Health Needs.* Washington, DC: National Academies Press; 2008.
31. President's Cancer Panel. *Living Beyond Cancer: Finding a New Balance. President's Cancer Panel 2003–2004 Annual Report.* Bethesda, MD: National Cancer Institute, National Institutes of Health, Department of Health and Human Services; 2004.
32. Maly RC, Umezawa Y, Leake B, Silliman RA. Mental health outcomes in older women with breast cancer: impact of perceived family support and adjustment. *Psychooncology.* 2005;14(7):535–545.
33. American College of Surgeons Commission on Cancer. Cancer program standards 2012: ensuring patient centered care, V1.0. 2012. Available at: http://www.facs.org/cancer/coc/cocprogramstandards2012.pdf. Accessed May 10, 2012.
34. Mitchell A. Short screening tools for cancer-related distress: a review and diagnostic validity meta-analysis. *J Natl Compre Canc Netw.* 2010;8(4):487–494.
35. Zigmond AS, Snaith RP. The hospital anxiety and depression scale. *Acta Psychiatr Scand.* 1983;67(6):361–371.
36. Kroenke K, Spitzer RL, Williams JBW. The PHQ-9: validity of a brief depression severity measure. *J Gen Intern Med.* 2001;16(9):606–613.
37. Kroenke K, Spitzer RL, Williams JBW. The patient health questionnaire-2: validity of a two-item depression screener. *J Gen Intern Med.* 2003;14(11):1284–1292.
38. Derogatis LR, Melisaratos N. The brief symptom inventory: an introductory report. *Psychol Med.* 1983;13(3):596–605.
39. Cella DF, Tulsky DS, Gray G, et al. The functional assessment of cancer therapy scale: development and validation of the general measure. *J Clin Oncol.* 1993;11(3):570–579.
40. McNair DM, Lorr M, Droppleman LF. *Profile of Mood States Manual.* San Diego, CA: Educational and Industrial Testing Service; 1992.
41. Beck AT, Ward CH, Mendelson M, Mock J, Erbaugh J. An inventory for measuring depression. *Arch Gen Psych.* 1961;4;561–571.
42. Yesavage JA, Brink TS, Rose TL, et al. Development and validation of a geriatric depression screening scale: a preliminary report. *J Psych Res.* 1983;17(1):37–49.
43. Radloff LS. The CES-D scale: a self-report depression scale for research in the general population. *App Psychol Meas.* 1977;1:385–401.
44. Zung WW. A self-rating depression scale. *Arch Gen Psych.* 1965;12:63–70.
45. Li M, Fitzgerald P, Rodin G. Evidence-based treatment of depression in patients with cancer. *J Clin Oncol.* 2012;30(11):1187–1196.
46. Jacobsen P, Jim HS. Psychosocial interventions for anxiety and depression in adult cancer patients: achievements and challenges. *CA Cancer J Clin.* 2008;58(4):214–230.
47. Fulcher CD, Badger TA. Depression. In: Eaton LH, Tipton JM, eds. *Putting Evidence into Practice: Improving Oncology Patient Outcomes.* Pittsburgh, PA: Oncology Nursing Society; 2009:105–118.
48. Braun IM, Pirl WF. Psychotropic medications in cancer care. In: Holland JC, Breitbart WS, Jacobsen PB, Lederberg MS, Loscalzo MJ, McCorkle R, eds. *Psychooncology.* 2nd ed. New York: Oxford University Press; 2010:378–385.
49. Kaplan M. Cancer survivorship: meeting psychosocial needs. *Clin J Oncol Nurs.* 2008;121(6):989–992.
50. Rayner L, Price A, Evans A, Valsraj K, Higginson IJ, Hotopf M. Antidepressants for depression in physically ill people [Review]. *The Cochrane Collaboration.* John Wiley & Sons, Ltd.; 2010: 1–23.

51. Williams S, Dale J. The effectiveness of treatment for depression/depressive symptoms in adults with cancer: a systematic review. *Br J Cancer.* 2006;94:372–390.
52. Rodin G, Lloyd N, Katz M, Green E, Mackay JA, Wong RKS. The treatment of depression in cancer patients: a systematic review. *Support Care Cancer.* 2007;15:123–136.
53. Grassi L, Nanni MG, Uchistomi Y, Riba M. Pharmacotherapy of depression in people with cancer. In: Kissane DW, Maj M, Sartorius N, eds. *Depression and Cancer.* Oxford, UK: John Wiley & Sons; 2011:151–176.
54. Kim HF, Fisch MJ. Antidepressant use in ambulatory cancer patients. *Curr Oncol Rep.* 2006;8:275–281.
55. Saarto T, Wiffen PT. Antidepressants for neuropathic pain. *Cochrane Database Syst Rev.* 2007;4:CD0054554.
56. Breitbart W. Do antidepressants reduce the effectiveness of tamoxifen? *Psychooncology.* 2011;20:1–4.
57. Desmarais JE, Looper KJ. Interactions between tamoxifen and antidepressants via cytochrome P450 2D6. *J Clin Psychiatry.* 2009;70:1688–1699.
58. Deng G, Cassileth BR. Integrative oncology: complementary therapies for pain, anxiety and mood disturbance. *CA Cancer J Clin.* 2005;55(2):109–116.
59. Novartis Pharmaceuticals Corporation. Package insert: Gleevec®: drug interactions. Available at: http://www.pharma.us.novartis.com/product/pi/pdf/gleevec_tabs.pdf.
60. U.S. Department of Health and Human Services. FDA drug safety communication: serious CNS reactions possible when linezolid is given to patients taking certain psychiatric medications. Available at: http://www.fda.gov/Drugs/DrugSafety/ucm265305.htm. Accessed April 12, 2012.
61. Rajasekaran M, Edmonds PM, Higginson IL. Systematic review of hypnotherapy for treating symptoms in terminally ill adult cancer patients. *Palliat Med.* 2005;19:418–426.
62. Hofmann SG, Sawyer AT, Will AA, Oh D. The effect of mindfulness-based therapy on anxiety and depression: a meta-analytic review. *J Consult Clin Psychol.* 2010;78(2):169–183.
63. Listing M, Reiβhauer A, Krohn M, et al. Massage therapy reduces physical discomfort and improves mood disturbances in women with breast cancer. *Psychooncology.* 2009;18:1290–1299.
64. Danhauer, SC, Mihalko SL, Russell GB, et al. Restorative yoga for women with breast cancer: findings from a randomized pilot study. *Psychooncology.* 2009; 18: 360–368.
65. Smith KB, Pukall CF. An evidence-based review of yoga as a complementary intervention for patients with cancer. *Psychooncology.* 2009;18:465–475.
66. Ledesma D, Kumano H. Mindfulness-based stress reduction and cancer: a meta-analysis. *Psychooncology.* 2009;18:571–579.
67. Fulcher CD, Badger T, Gunter AK, Marrs J, Reese JM. Putting Evidence into Practice: Interventions for Depression. *Clin J Oncol.* 2008;12(1):131–140.
68. Winell J, Roth AJ. Psychiatric assessment and symptom management in elderly cancer patients. *Oncology.* 2005;19(11): 1479–1490.
69. Weinberger MI, Roth AJ, Nelson CJ. Untangling the complexities of depression diagnosis in older cancer patients. *Oncologist.* 2009;14: 60–66.
70. Givens JL, Datto CJ, Ruckdeschel K, et al. Older patients' aversion to antidepressants: a qualitative study. *J Gen Intern Med.* 2006;21:146–151.
71. Stanton AL. Psychosocial concerns and interventions for cancer survivors. *J Clin Oncol.* 2006;24(32):5132–5137.
72. Hoffman KE, McCarthy EP, Recklitis CJ, Ng AK. Psychological distress in long-term survivors of adult-onset cancer. *Arch Intern Med.* 2009;169(14):1274–1281.
73. Barsevick AM, Much JK. Depression self-care guide. In: Yarbro CH, Frogge MH, Goodman M, eds. *Cancer Symptom Management.* 3rd ed. Sudbury, MA: Jones and Bartlett Publishers; 2004:685–686.
74. Pleasurable activities. University of Michigan Depression Center. Available at: http://www.depressioncenter.org/MDOCC/self-management/pleasurable-activities.asp. Accessed May 7, 2012.

Recognizing Depression

Patient Name: ______________________________

This guide will help you and your loved ones recognize depression and learn things you can do to help yourself.

Description

Everyone feels depressed at some time in their life. Depression can be fleeting, lasting minutes or hours before resolving. It is normal to feel sad and depressed after a loss, such as the loss of one's health. An individual usually feels the worst immediately after this type of loss. The depressed feelings gradually lift and resolve over a period of weeks.

When the depression does not improve over time, is not related to a specific problem, lingers for weeks or months after the problem has resolved, or is out of proportion to the problem, it could indicate the presence of depression. Depression usually does not resolve without help. The most effective way to deal with depression is to see a professional.

The following self-test can help you to recognize the signs of depression. A self-test such as this does not diagnose depression, but indicates that you may need further assessment. If you take this test, bring it to your nurse and discuss the results with him or her. If you are depressed, treatment is available to help you.

Self-Test

Check off any symptoms you have had for 2 weeks or longer. Check symptoms that affect you almost every day for most of the day. Check all the statements about your mood that apply to you:

☐ I feel sad or depressed most of the time nearly every day.

☐ I have lost interest in most or all of the activities I used to enjoy.

☐ I feel worthless most of the time.

☐ I feel guilty; I blame or criticize myself.

☐ I have repeated thoughts of death or suicide.

☐ I have trouble concentrating or making decisions.

☐ I am eating more and have gained weight; or, I am eating less and have lost weight.

☐ I am sleeping more than usual; or, I am sleeping less than usual.

☐ I have no energy or feel tired most of the time.

☐ I feel agitated and nervous; or, I feel sluggish and slow.

☐ I have a plan to commit suicide.

☐ I have tried to kill myself in the past.

Scoring the Test

The first five statements describe feelings related to depressed mood. The next statements describe physical signs that are often present when a person in good health is depressed. However, if you have cancer, these symptoms could be related to either depression or your cancer

(continued)

therapy. If you checked two or more statements about your mood or a total of five statements from the complete list, you could be suffering from depression. Discuss this checklist with your nurse. If you checked the statements about suicide, you should discuss this test with your doctor or nurse immediately.

Management

You can do the following to deal with depression:

- Make a list of all the medications you take. Show it to your doctor or nurse. Some medicines may have to be stopped.
- Ask your doctor or nurse which side effects can be caused by the cancer and its treatment. Learn as much as you can to help to manage those side effects.
- Ask your doctor or nurse for help managing the side effects.
- Get plenty of rest, and exercise when you feel you have the energy.
- Eat a balanced diet. Do not try to lose weight at this time. Foods should be good for you and have lots of nutrition. Ask your nurse or dietitian for help if you are having problems with eating.
- Recognize that you are not alone. Depression in cancer is common; it does not mean you are weak. Talk about how you are feeling with your doctor or nurse. A support group may be helpful.
- Avoid alcohol. It can make you depressed.
- If medications have been ordered for you for depression, take them as directed. Let your doctor or nurse know of any side effects you may be experiencing.

Follow-up

As your depression goes away, you should experience the following:

- Better sleep patterns
- A decrease in grouchiness
- Better focus on tasks
- Ability to withstand stresses without overreacting
- Ability to think positively
- An improvement in mood
- Enjoyment in living

Treatment of depression is not quick. It may take weeks to months to notice improvement. Continue to take your medication.

Depression may come back. But knowing what it feels like, you will be able to recognize it.

Phone Numbers

Nurse: ____________________ Phone: __________

Physician: ____________________ Phone: __________

Other: ____________________ Phone: __________

Source: Fulcher CD. Depression. In: Yarbro CH, Wujcik D, Gobel BH, eds. *Cancer Symptom Management.* 4th ed. Burlington, MA: Jones & Bartlett Learning; 2014.

Pleasurable Activities

Patient Name: ______________________________

People who are depressed often lose interest in activities they have previously enjoyed. These activities are the ones that bring enjoyment; they may use your talents and abilities, or they may provide comfort and memories. Such activities have a positive effect on mood and feelings about oneself.

For people with depression and cancer, it can be a challenge to find pleasurable activities due to the cancer and treatment effects.

Scheduling time for fun and enjoyment is an important way to lift one's spirits. Depression operates in a circle: the less you do, the more depressed you feel, and the more depressed you feel, the less you do. Therefore, even when you are not in the mood, you may benefit from scheduling some pleasurable moments into your day. Without an effort to include pleasurable time, it's easy to forget or ignore it and the circle continues.

Pleasurable activities are those that can also be considered:

- Rewarding
- Meaningful
- Inspiring
- Relaxing

Such activities don't have to be a "big deal." Small, simple things that bring joy, humor, or comfort may help. If you are limited in your physical ability or attention span, choose activities that are within your capability. Be creative. If you are not able to tend your garden, spend some time designing a flower bed. A round of golf may be too taxing, but time on the putting green or even a ride in the golf cart may be fun. If you are having trouble thinking of things, ask a close friend or family member to help identify things you have enjoyed in the past. There are also lists available online by searching "pleasurable activities." Then, proceed to incorporate several into each day's plan.

Some Ideas

Listen to music	Wear a favorite outfit	Do artwork, color a picture
Read a story	Solve a puzzle	Soak in a tub or shower
Listen to comedy	Sit outside, "smell the roses"	Go for a ride
Be with friends/family	Look through a photo album	Call a friend
Write in a journal	Hold/stroke a pet	Read to a child

Follow-up

Keep track of the activities you are enjoying each day. After one week, and on the same day each week after that, take the depression self-test (Appendix 31A). Note whether your depressive symptoms are improving, and report this information to your doctor, nurse, or counselor.

(continued)

Phone Numbers

Nurse: ______________________________ Phone: ______________

Doctor: ______________________________ Phone: ______________

Counselor: ______________________________ Phone: ______________

Source: Fulcher CD. Depression. In: Yarbro CH, Wujcik D, Gobel BH, eds. *Cancer Symptom Management.* 4th ed. Burlington, MA: Jones & Bartlett Learning; 2014.

CHAPTER 32

Grief

Cheryl Brohard, PhD, RN, AOCN®

THE PROBLEM

The word *grief* originated in the early thirteenth century from the Anglo-French word *gref,* meaning "hardship or sorrow." Grief is defined as a normal response to loss and a unique, complex individualized human experience. There is no universal way of grieving. To prevent grief would be a contradiction to the nature of humanity. It is an internal response that occurs over time, and gives a person the time to deal with the loss and begin the process of healing. This chapter focuses on the patient's grief from the experience of being diagnosed with cancer. The etiology and incidence of grief, pathology, models and theories, symptoms of grief, and management strategies are discussed, and a self-care guide to grief is provided for the patient.

ETIOLOGY

The loss or losses for a person with cancer can occur at any point during the cancer trajectory. The etiologies of grief follow the cancer trajectory of an initial diagnosis, treatment, and either end-of-life or survivorship. The causes of grief during the diagnosis and treatment periods are temporary change in functionality or permanent disability due to the cancer or the cancer treatment, change or loss of job, loss of independence, change of self-image or self-identity, and shifting of roles within the work setting, family, or community.[1] These same causes of grief can extend to the patient's end-of-life, along with the additional losses of physical functioning, cognitive abilities, and hope for a future. The patient's abilities decline gradually, with the ultimate loss being life itself.[2] Cancer survivors may experience extended periods of grief after completion of treatment, as they may be dealing with permanent disabilities from cancer or the cancer treatment, such as lymphedema in women with breast cancer, a tracheostomy, pulmonary fibrosis from chemotherapy and radiation, chronic pain, and psychosocial issues.[3]

INCIDENCE

If we consider that every person with cancer is at risk for grief, then the reported 12 million people living with cancer in the United States are at risk.[4] Included in this number are the most vulnerable people for developing a grief response—namely, patients initially diagnosed with cancer (1.6 million) and those at the end-of-life (577,000).[4] It is important to consider all patients at risk for grief and to determine the patient's specific losses to recommend suited and targeted adaptive strategies.[5]

TERMINOLOGY COMMON TO GRIEF

Words and phrases associated with grief are confusing. Table 32-1 lists the most common terms associated with grief and their definitions.[6] It bears repeating that grief is a process and a normal response to loss. Mourning is the outward expression of grief. Bereavement is the period of time during which a person grieves his or her loss.

TABLE 32-1

Terminology Common to Grief

Definitions
- Grief is a process of experiencing the psychological, behavioral, social, and physical reactions to the perception of loss.
- Loss is having something valuable taken away or reduced.
- Mourning is the outward social expression of loss and is a process of adapting to the loss governed in part by the social, cultural, and spiritual beliefs and rituals.
- Bereavement is the time period given to grief and mourning.

Types of Grief
- Anticipatory Grief is loss that has not occurred, loss that has happened, loss currently being experienced.
- Preparatory Grief is the grief associated with a person who is facing impending death.
- Complicated Grief is an intensified grief experience or a prolonged grief period when the patient fails to return to pre-loss state.[13]
- Prolonged Grief Distress is a severe reaction to loss and may manifest itself as psychopathologies such as phobias, anxieties, somatic symptoms; intense longing for the loss; bitterness toward the loss; or ruminations of the loss.

TYPES OF GRIEF

The types of grief need to be identified as early as possible for assessment, treatment, and interventions. Four types of grief are distinguished: (1) anticipatory grief, (2) preparatory grief, (3) complicated grief, and (4) prolonged grief disorder. This chapter focuses on anticipatory grief, preparatory grief, and complicated grief as they pertain to the patient with cancer.

ANTICIPATORY GRIEF

Anticipatory grief is a reaction that occurs in advance of death when patients mourn the loss of their life or the life they expected to live. Anticipatory grief deals with the perceived or real losses associated with diagnosis, acute and chronic illnesses, and terminal illness. Not every patient with cancer experiences anticipatory grief, and there is no way of determining who will go through this process.

Anticipatory grief has three distinct foci of time.[7] The temporalities of anticipatory grief are oriented to the past, to the present, and to the future. The patient may experience grief over past experiences and events that were shared with others, knowing that these past experiences can never be regained. Enjoyable camping trips with the family or a 50th birthday party are in the past. The loss of the present or diminution of an experience can be heard in the patient's speech with "I cannot" or "I wish I could" phrases or "I cannot participate in life as I know it." This fear of loss of the patient's current life or the continued erosion of the present situation brings forward this type of grief. Anticipated grief related to the loss of future events can be observed in patients who state, "I have lost so much" or "A small part of me died when I was diagnosed with cancer" or "I fear that I will not get to see my daughter graduate from high school." Death or the loss of self falls into this foci.

Experiencing sadness, having concern for others and self, preparing for death, and adjusting to changes caused by the dying process are all symptoms of anticipatory grief. According to one theory, anticipatory grief makes the grief experience less difficult, but empirical evidence cannot confirm this theory.[8] However, experiencing anticipatory grief may provide time for the patient to accept the loss, complete unfinished business, perform a life review, resolve conflicts, or reshuffle priorities. Anticipating that one's life goals cannot be completed is a step toward recognition that life will be ending. Anticipatory grief finds the person anticipating future losses, processing the past and present losses.

PREPARATORY GRIEF

Slightly different is preparatory grief, which finds the terminally ill patient still living while facing impending death.[9] Mystakidou and colleagues evaluated 94 patients with a terminal diagnosis of cancer living in Greece, assessing them for factors influencing preparatory grief.[10] Multiple regression analysis found that young age (19 to 25 years), poor performance functioning as measured by Eastern Cooperative Oncology Group (ECOG) performance status, and the impact of the diagnosis event, as indicated by the intrusion variable and hyperarousal symptoms of grief, were significantly correlated ($p < .01$) with advanced cancer.[10] Depression, hopelessness, and anxiety were found to be predictors of preparatory grief, with anxiety being the strongest predictor.[11] Using multiple regression, the researchers found that more females than males diagnosed with terminal cancer, who were recruited from the palliative care service, reported increased preparatory grief.[12,13]

Mystakidou and others used three tools in their research study to identify advanced cancer patients with preparatory grief responses, including their own Preparatory Grief in Advanced Cancer Patients (PGAC) scale—a 31-item instrument aimed at assessing the concept of preparatory grief.[10] Anxiety and depression were measured by the Greek version of the Hospital Anxiety and Depression Scale (HADS).[14] Impact of Event Scale—Revised (IES-R) was used to measure the psychological impact of intrusion and avoidance on a traumatic event.[15] These researchers found that the IES-R score was significantly associated with anxiety and preparatory grief.[10] Thus it is important for the oncology nurse to screen patients for anxiety and depression.

COMPLICATED GRIEF

Some situations intensify or prolong the grieving period. Complicated grief is a failure to return to a new-normal, pre-loss state.[5] How to identify these people has not been part of the standard of practice. Especially vulnerable to complicated grief are people who suffered early separations as a child, were diagnosed with psychiatric disorders, came from dysfunctional families, or experienced sudden death situations. Ongoing monitoring of the grief response is needed to determine whether the patient has a normal grief response or progresses into complicated grief. Complicated grief of a patient manifests itself as early as 6 months after the loss. This reaction increases the risk of a prolonged grief disorder, depression, and anxiety.[16]

Multiple risk factors are known to be associated with complicated grief, but little evidence-based research has been undertaken to confirm the associations of the factors or the interventions to lower the risk. The incidence of complicated grief in patients with cancer is virtually unknown. Losses described in the cancer survivorship literature originate immediately after diagnosis and continue as unresolved losses well into the survivorship phase of the cancer trajectory.[3,17,18] Losses put aside during the diagnosis and treatment phases, such as losses of physical or body function—for example, infertility related to cancer treatment or urinary and sexual dysfunction related to prostate cancer treatment—or the loss of oneself—such as self-identity as a healthy sexual partner—will resurface during the long-term survival phase of the cancer survivor's life.[3,17,18]

Five types of complicated grief have been identified: chronic, delayed, exaggerated, masked, and disenfranchised.[7] Chronic grief indicates that the person is taking an extensive or excessive amount of time to process through the grief. Delayed grief indicates that the person is avoiding the normal feelings of grief and chooses to express the grief and feelings at a point later on. Exaggerated grief indicates a person's sense of being overwhelmed by grief may lead to a major psychiatric disorder. Masked grief indicates a person's physical manifestation (i.e., headaches, stomach pains, ulcers) may appear unrelated to the death. Disenfranchised grief is a loss that is not socially accepted and is not acknowledged.

MODELS AND THEORIES OF GRIEF

Several models and theories of grief provide the means to understand grief pathology. The most widely recognized model for nurses is the Five Stages of Grief developed by Kübler-Ross.[19] These stages—denial, anger, bargaining, depression, and acceptance—are not static, nor do they occur in a linear manner.[20,21] These symptoms fall within the emotional dimension of grief. It is theorized that the stages of grief overlap with one another and can accumulate for more than one loss during a given time frame.

A second major theory of grief comes from Worden. He suggested that humans have four basic tasks of mourning to be accomplished: (1) accept the reality of the loss, (2) experience the pain of grief, (3) adjust to the new environment where the loss is no longer present, and (4) emotionally relocate the loss and reinvest energy in other opportunities.[6] As part of this model, which he reported as a process theory, Worden proposed counseling and therapy for the four basic tasks. It has been theorized that people express their grief in one of two patterns: intuitive or affective (i.e., through emotions) or instrumental (i.e., through physical and cognitive ways). Although more males than females exhibit instrumental grief, these patterns are influenced by gender but not determined by it.[22]

Berger theorized that five distinct personalities of grievers exist.[23] The Nomads have not yet resolved their grief and do not seem to understand the loss that has affected their lives. The Memorialists are committed to preserving the memory of the loved one whom they have lost. The Normalizers are committed to recreating a sense of family and community. The Activists focus on helping other people who are dealing with the same disease or issues that caused their loved one's death. The Seekers adopt religious, philosophical, or spiritual beliefs to create meaning in their lives.

The social dimension of grief consists of cultural, language, practices, and norms of grief. Three theories of grief are based on the strength of the social relationship between people, and their ability to move forward after experiencing a loss. The attachment theory, formalized by Bowlby, is based on the relationships made during childhood.[24] Psychodynamic theory is based on the mother–child relationship, whereas interpersonal relationship theory is based on the quality of the relationship. The person who formed and secured a consistent relationship during early childhood demonstrates the ability to cope with loss and move forward, as compared to the person without these strong bonds and attachments, whose position becomes stagnant. The four overlapping phases of Bowlby's theory of attachment are shock, yearning and protest, despair, and recovery.[25]

Some theories of grief are gender free, such as the theory of completing the tasks of living by asking for forgiveness, saying "Thank you," and saying "I love you."[26] The Dual-Process Model of Coping with Bereavement is a process in which patients oscillate between loss-oriented processes of grief intrusions and breaking ties, and restoration-oriented processes of attending to life changes and establishing new roles and relationships.[27]

Spiritual distress has been part of the dimensions of grief recognized by hospice care for 40 years.[28] In one recent study, 44% of oncology patients on an acute palliative care unit (n = 113) were found to be in spiritual distress, which resulted in physical and emotional symptoms such as pain and depression.[29] Lee notes that people search for the existential meaning of life, formerly known as existential plight, which is one of the first tasks encountered by the patient with a new diagnosis of cancer.[30]

PATHOLOGY

Most researchers agree that grief has many aspects, factors, domains, or dimensions.[31–33] Domains of grief vary by professional perspective and may include either psychological, social, and spiritual factors[31] or psychological, biological, and sociocultural factors.[32] For patients with cancer, five human dimensions may be cited to represent a comprehensive perspective of grief (Figure 32-1). This model depicts the physical, cognitive, social, spiritual, and emotional dimensions of grief as overlapping and interacting.[33]

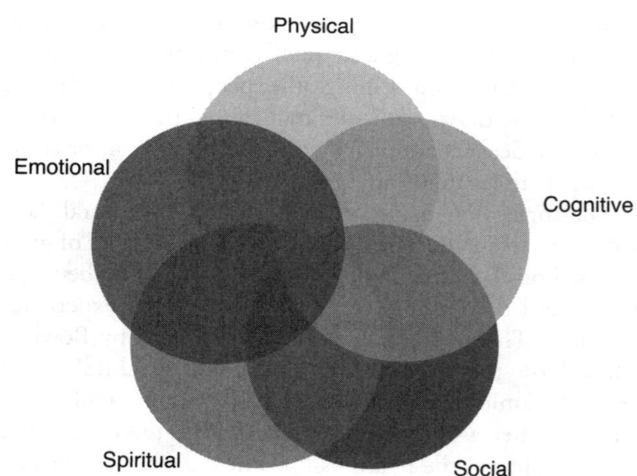

FIGURE 32-1

Dimensions of grief.

Cheng and colleagues conducted a series of focus groups with seven women living in Hong Kong about their grief experiences at the time of initial diagnosis. One woman described her inability to cope with a diagnosis of incurable cancer; she developed pain and became immobile.[34] This is an example of the physical dimension of grief. Another woman described her shock in terms of apathy and indecision, which are examples of the cognitive dimension. The experience of reuniting an estranged family, shifting roles from wife to husband, and having a daughter distance herself from her mother are examples of the social dimension of grief. Yet another woman showed the emotional expression of grief with her description of overwhelming fear and heightened anxiety upon hearing the diagnosis of cancer. Symptoms within the spiritual dimension were exhibited by several women in the focus group; that state was described as "no hope, no cure" by one woman.[34]

Accepted North American Nursing Diagnosis Association (NANDA) diagnoses within the coping and stress tolerance domain for grief are death anxiety, complicated grieving (and risk of), and chronic sorrow.[35] The definitions and defining characteristics of these three nursing diagnoses correspond with the terminology and descriptions of anticipatory grief, complicated grief, and prolonged grief.[35] Unlike for other cancer symptoms, there is no toxicity scale for grief. Numerous scales for grief, loss, and bereavement have been developed for the family members of patients with advanced cancer, but no instrument can be found in the literature that incorporates all five dimensions of grief for the patient with cancer.

SYMPTOM ASSESSMENT

An initial assessment of grief is needed at the time of diagnosis to identify the issues of grief. The nursing history should include questions about the patient's previous history of losses and experiences, dates and timing of the events with respect to the cancer diagnosis, and the patient's previous effective coping mechanisms. Losses and intensity of feelings associated with the cancer diagnosis are best described by the patient, even though the clinician may be aware of losses that the patient is not identifying. It is the person who defines the loss, experiences the loss, and draws meaning from the loss, whether the loss is perceived or actual.[36]

ASSESSMENT BY THE DIMENSIONS OF GRIEF

Oncology professionals are in the best position to assess patients for the symptoms of grief. The grief assessment should cover all five dimensions of grief; these dimensions have corresponding symptoms that require careful assessment by the oncology nurse (Table 32-2). It is common for patients to have symptoms from one or more dimensions of grief. Asking detailed questions about the existence and intensity of these symptoms listed in Table 32-2 will aid the oncology nurse in the assessment process.

The past history and source of physical symptoms are important to establish at the onset of the cancer trajectory. Physical symptoms not associated with the diagnosis of cancer, treatment, or other illnesses may be factors in determining the intensity of the grief response. Cognitive and emotional dimensions can be assessed by asking questions about the patient's perception of cancer, factors that influence the cancer, the losses that have accompanied the diagnosis, and what this experience means for the patient. It is important to include in the social history changes in the patient's role within the family, the meaning of cancer to the patient and family, cultural implications, changes in employment, and effects on self-identity. It is also important to assess the impact of the cancer diagnosis on the individual's spiritual beliefs.

DURATION AND ONGOING ASSESSMENT

A grief risk assessment can identify patients at risk for complicated grief. The duration of grief is unpredictable, as the "work of grief" is never completely finished. Ongoing monitoring of the grief response is needed to determine whether the patient has a normal grief response or progresses into complicated grief. The work of grief is a series of tasks that a person must endure to live with the loss. This work is neither orderly nor predictable.[16]

Unfortunately, no evidence-based research has identified or established the "normal grieving period" for a patient experiencing grief and loss. Instead, what the literature shows is that a normal grieving period for bereaved family members ranges from 6 to 13 months.[37] Feelings of depression are common in the first year. A sign that grief is healing is when the pain lessens. Integration of the losses into one's self is a cognitive process. People who are able to incorporate the loss into their reality are better able to cope with the change and move forward.

From the initial diagnosis until surveillance or end-of-life, the cancer trajectory provides the oncology nurse with a longitudinal perspective of the patient's ability to cope with loss. Ongoing assessments of the patient's grief are important. Observing for the patient's adjustment to the losses, anticipating new losses if the cancer progresses, and anticipating new losses if the cancer is cured provide the oncology nurse with opportunities to get to know the patient and understand the individual's adaptation and coping mechanism of loss. Simply speaking, the typical feelings, behaviors, and reaction to a loss needs to be

TABLE 32-2

Dimensions of Grief

Dimensions	Symptoms
Physical	Unable to relax
	Sleep disturbances
	Changes in bodily functions including bowels
	Changes in appetite, anorexia
	Changes in weight
	Tightness in the chest and throat
	Palpitations
	Dyspnea
	Headaches
	Fatigue
	Xerostomia
	Muscle aches
	Over-activity
	Crying
	Weeping
	Changes in body image
	Hair loss
	Not feeling within your body
Cognitive	Disbelief
	Preoccupation
	Difficulty concentrating
	Difficulty with simple tasks
	Absent-mindedness
	Confusion
	Disorientation
	Hallucinations
	Disorganization
	Preoccupation with the deceased
	Disturbed thinking
	Short-term memory loss
	Apathy
	Low self-esteem
	Accept the cancer diagnosis
Social	Loss of identity
	Vulnerability
	Feelings of being judged
	Withdraw from society
	Social isolation
	Over-activity
	Keeping busy
	Selective isolation
	Financial insecurity
	Role changes
	Discordant roles
	Clashing responsibilities
	Antagonistic roles
	Reintegration

(continued)

TABLE 32-2

Dimensions of Grief (continued)	
Dimensions	**Symptoms**
Emotional	Shock
	Disbelief
	Denial
	Anger
	Anxiety
	Sadness
	Helplessness
	Guilt
	Bargaining
	Numbness
	Ambivalence
	Yearning
	Shame
	Fear
	Bewilderment
	Loneliness
	Readjustment
	Acceptance
	Relief
	Emanicipation
Spiritual	Abandoned by God due to the disease
	Anger toward God
	Loss of faith
	Hope for a cure
	Spiritual restlessness
	Spiritual despair
	Brokenness
	Meaninglessness
	Dread
	Helplessness
	Alienation
	Guilt/shame

monitored by the oncology nurse, and observation of complicated grief must begin early for patient interventions to be effective.

SYMPTOM MANAGEMENT STRATEGIES

THERAPEUTIC APPROACHES

Just as symptoms overlap, so do management strategies for grief. Grief work begins with the care and compassion of being human and utilizing basic supportive-expressive techniques to facilitate communication between the nurse and the patient. It is vital that oncology nurses give the patient permission to feel all feelings of grief and loss. Just as important is the expression of those feelings to the healthcare team. The nurse should encourage the patient to be honest with others about his or her sorrow, as this communication will help shift the loss toward reconciliation and integration into one's self-identity. The patient with cancer may experience multiple losses at one time, and more than one strategy may need to be employed.[2]

Some fundamental interventions are for the oncology nurse to spend time and be present for the patient. Concise, directed, and meaningful interaction before chemotherapy or radiation therapy or at the clinic visit will give the nurse insight into the patient's ability to cope and process his or her grief. It is important for the oncology nurse to allocate time for listening to the patients, validating their expresses of grief, answering questions about the grief process, providing helpful, targeted interventions for the grief symptoms, and asking how well they are handling the physical, cognitive, social, spiritual, and emotional dimensions of their life.

Supportive nursing actions may include the following patient questions: How has cancer impacted your life? What would have been different about your life if you had never been diagnosed with cancer? The patient may respond with negative or positive answers. The oncology nurse should listen to the answers carefully to recognize the grief experience from the patient's perspective. Interventions to help people with cancer grieve their losses are very personal and unique.

Some of the basic approaches used by oncology nurses are to provide a supportive environment for open, honest conveyance of feelings, acknowledging that these feelings are important and commonly felt and actively listening to the person's concerns. The oncology nurse should help patients define what is important to them; assist them with communication methods such as a letter, video, or talks; and recognize that adaptation is a method of coping and integrating the grief into their self-portrait.[2] Recognizing that time is limited with patients, the oncology nurse needs to delegate aspects of psychosocial support that can be accomplished by other disciplines and coordinate the efforts of support with a coordinated effort.[38]

Referrals

Oncology nurses are instrumental in making referrals to other members of the patient's healthcare team. Physical dimensions are more problematic, because a variety of specialist and diagnostic tests could reveal no abnormalities. Previously mentioned were referrals to mental health counselors, bereavement counselors, and social workers for support with the cognitive, social, and emotional dimensions of grief. Chaplains and clergy are in the best position to counsel and advise patients on the spiritual dimension. Self-help groups are a gathering of people with like experiences, such as breast cancer survivor, who provide support on a common experience.

Formal grief interventions

Formal grief interventions may include one-on-one interaction with the individual, group therapy, or family therapy. Expertise in the field of psychotherapy is needed when the patient is experiencing complicated or prolonged grief disorder. Among the possible psychotherapies are cognitive-behavioral, psychodynamic, interpersonal, and group therapy; other interventions include music and art therapy, support groups, pharmacology, and guided mourning. The role of the nurse with patients in counseling is to facilitate communication whenever needed between disciplines, provide support and recognition for seeking help, and encourage the patient to continue the therapy.

Spiritual interventions aimed at discovering the meaning of life's purpose, reducing suffering, and improving self-esteem include supportive expressive group therapy, meaning-making intervention, and dignity therapy.[39] In a study conducted in four hospice centers in Australia, 12 terminally ill patients were asked how they expressed their spirituality and religion.[40] Qualitative analysis discovered four themes that were identified by these patients: supportive relationships; feeling uplifted by God, religion, nature, or music; spiritual practices such as prayer and forgiveness; and having hope.[40]

A limited number of studies have been conducted in patients with terminal cancer. A pilot study ($n = 15$) using a structured life review showed a significant increase in self-esteem and a decrease in depression in the reminiscence group.[41] A secondary analysis of these patients, who were recruited in a Japanese hospital, aimed to clarify the characteristics of a life review according to gender, age, and stage of disease with a group ($n = 16$) of patients with cancer.[42] This study revealed that males in the terminal stage of cancer were concerned about their physical condition, desire for death, and how to confront death, while females were concerned with resignation to life.

NURSING IMPLICATIONS

When the patient speaks freely about the losses from cancer or its treatment, then the nurse has evidence that reinvesting in new relationships, reengaging in prior roles and responsibilities, and moving forward with life plans or goals will be the next steps in the healing process of grief. Reorganizing, recovery, and personal growth are indicators that patients are working through their grief. The nurse can intervene with supportive words and encouragement as the patient engages in these steps. Recognizing the patient's progress forward into healing or the patient's risk for complicated grief and early intervention is important for the patient's well-being. Observing for manifestations of complicated grief or symptoms of prolonged grief disorder is important to oncology nurses as they manage the symptoms of the disease, treatment, and survivorship needs.

PATIENT SELF-CARE

It is important for patients to recognize that grief manifests itself in a uniquely personal way. Patients should understand that grief is a natural, normal part of accepting a cancer diagnosis, but it takes work to process and adapt to the experienced losses from this diagnosis. The self-care guide for grief (Appendix 32A) is a helpful handout that will aid the patient in recognizing the common symptoms of grief that can occur in the five dimensions of grief.

REFERENCES

1. Lichtenthal WG, Cruess DG, Prigerson HG. A case for establishing complicated grief as a distinct mental disorder in DSM-V. *Clin Psychol Rev.* 2004;24:637–662.
2. Hottensen D. Anticipatory grief in patients with cancer. *Clin J Oncol Nurs.* 2010;14(1):106–107.
3. Boyle D. Survivorship. *Clin J Oncol Nurs.* 2006;10(3):407–416.
4. American Cancer Society. *Cancer Facts and Figures 2012.* Atlanta, GA: American Cancer Society; 2012. Available at: http://www.cancer.org. Accessed June 30, 2012.
5. Fisch MJ. Grief during the course of illness. *J Support Oncol.* 2009;7 (1 suppl):20–21.
6. Worden JW. *Grief Counseling and Grief Therapy: A Handbook for the Mental Health Practitioner.* 2nd ed. London: Springer; 1991.
7. Rando T. *Treatment of Complicated Mourning.* Champaign, IL: Research Press; 2000.
8. Rando T. ed. *Loss and Anticipatory Grief.* Lexington, MA: Lexington Books; 1986.
9. Block SD. Assessing and managing depression in the terminally ill patient. ACP-ASIM End-of-Life Care Consensus Panel. American College of Physicians—American Society of Internal Medicine. *Ann Intern Med.* 2000;132:209–218.
10. Mystakidou K, Tsilika E, Parpa E, Panagiotou I, Galanos, Gouliamos A. The mediation effect of anxiety between post-traumatic stress symptoms and preparatory grief in advanced cancer patients. *J Pain Symptom Manage.* 2011;41(3):511–521.
11. Tsilika E, Mystakidou K, Parpa E, Galanos A, Sakkas P, Vlahos L. The influence of cancer impact on patients' preparatory grief. *Psychol Health.* 2009;24(2):135–148.
12. Mystakidou K, Athanasouli P, Pagoropoulou A, Vlahos L. Preparatory grief, psychological distress and hopelessness in advanced cancer patients. *Eur J Cancer.* 2008;17(2):145–151.
13. Mystakidou K, Tsilika E, Parpa E, et al. Demographic and clinical predicators of preparatory grief in a sample of advanced cancer patients. *Psychooncology.* 2006;15(9):823–833.
14. Zigmond A, Snaith RP. The hospital anxiety and depression scale. *Acta Psychiatr Scan.* 1983;67(6):361–370.
15. Weiss DS, Marmar CR. The impact of event scale—revised. In: Wilson J, Keane TM, eds. *Assessing Psychological Trauma and PTSD.* New York: Guilford; 1996:399–411.

16. Maddocks I. Grief and bereavement. *Med J Aust.* 2003;179(6 suppl): S6–S7.
17. Galbraith ME, Hays L, Tanner T. What men say about surviving prostate cancer: complexities represented in a decade of comments. *Clin J Oncol Nurs.* 2012;16(1):65–72.
18. Wittmann D, Foley S, Balon R. A biopsychosocial approach to sexual recovery after prostate cancer surgery: the role of grief and mourning. *J Sex Marital Ther.* 2011;37(2):130–144.
19. Kübler-Ross E. *On Death and Dying.* New York: Simon and Schuster; 1997.
20. Brown C, Wood A. Oncology nurses' grief: a literature review. *Clin J Oncol Nurs.* 2009;13(6):625–627.
21. Kübler-Ross E, Kessler D. *On Grief and Grieving: Finding the Meaning of Grief Through the Stages of Loss.* New York: Simon & Schuster; 2005.
22. Doka KJ, Martin TL. *Grieving Beyond Gender: Understanding the Ways Men and Women Mourn.* New York: Taylor and Francis Group; 2010.
23. Berger SA. *The Five Ways We Grieve: Finding Your Personal Path to Healing After the Loss of a Loved One.* Boston, MA: Shambhala Publications; 2009.
24. Bowlby J. *A Secure Base: Clinical Applications of Attachment Theory.* London: Routledge; 2005.
25. Buglass E. Grief and bereavement theories. *Nurs Stan.* 2010;24(41):44–47.
26. Byock I. *The Four Things That Matter Most.* New York: Simon & Schuster; 2004.
27. Stroebe MS, Schut H. The dual process model of coping with bereavement: overview and update. *Grief Matters: Austral J Grief Bereave.* 2008;11(1):4–10.
28. Saunders C. Spiritual pain. *J Palliat Care.* 1988;4(3):29–32.
29. Hui D, de la Cruz M, Thorney S, Parsons HA, Delgado-Guay M, Bruera E. The frequency and correlates of spiritual distress among patients with advanced cancer admitted to an acute palliative care unit. *Am J Hosp Palliat Care.* 2011;28(4):264–270.
30. Lee V. The existential plight of cancer: meaning making as a concrete approach to the intangible search for meaning. *Support Care Cancer.* 2008;16(7):779–785.
31. Jacobsen JG. Distinguishing symptoms of grief and depression in a cohort of advanced cancer patients. *Death Studies.* 2010;34(3):257–273.
32. Kacel E, Gao X, Prigerson HG. Understanding bereavement: what every oncology practitioner should know. *J Support Oncol.* 2011;9(5):172–180.
33. Ashton J. Bereavement care in home care and hospice. *Home Health Care Manage Pract.* 2008;20(5):394–399.
34. Cheng JO, Lo RS, Chan FM, Kwan BH, Woo J. An exploration of anticipatory grief in advanced cancer patients. *Psychooncology.* 2010;19(7),693–700.
35. NANDA International. *Nursing Diagnoses: Definitions and Classification 2012–2014.* 9th ed. Kaukauna, WI: Wiley-Blackwell; 2011:356–379.
36. Wenzel J, Shaha M, Klimmek R, Krumm S. Working through grief and loss: oncology nurses' perspectives on professional bereavement. *Oncol Nurs Forum.* 2011;38(4):E272–E282.
37. Zisook S, Shear K. Grief and bereavement: what psychiatrists need to know. *World Psychiatry.* 2009;8(2):67–74.
38. Gosselin T, Crane-Okada R, Irwin M, Tringali C, Wenzel J. Measuring oncology nurses' psychosocial care practices and needs: results of an Oncology Nursing Society psychosocial survey. *Oncol Nurs Forum.* 2011;38(6):729–738.
39. LeMay K, Wilson KG. Treatment of existential distress in life threatening illness: a review of manualized interventions. *Clin Psychol Rev.* 2008;28(3):472–493.
40. Tan HM, Grief M, Couns PC, Brauack-Mayer A, Beilby J. The impact of the hospice environment on patient spiritual expression. *Oncol Nurs Forum.* 2005;32(5):1049–1055.
41. Ando M, Tsuda A, Moorey S. Preliminary study of reminiscence therapy on depression and self-esteem in cancer patients. *Psychol Rep.* 2006;98(2):339–346.
42. Ando M, Morita T, O'Connor SJ. Primary concerns of advanced cancer patients identified through the structured life review process: a qualitative study using a text mining technique. *Palliat Support Care.* 2007;5(3):265–271.

Grief

Patient Name: ____

This self-care guide will help you know that grief is a normal process of dealing with loss. Having a diagnosis of cancer may put you at risk for experiencing loss.

Symptom and Description

Grief is defined as a normal response to loss and a unique, personal experience. You may experience none, one, or more symptoms of grief. Some of these symptoms may include the following:

- Inability to relax or trouble sleeping
- Loss of appetite
- Headaches, muscle aches, tightness in chest and throat
- Frequently crying
- Forgetfulness
- Difficulty concentrating
- No interest in social activities
- Anger, frustration
- Anxiety, sadness, depression
- Loneliness
- Anger toward God
- Loss of faith
- Spiritual restlessness

Prevention

There is nothing you can do to prevent grief. It is normal to grieve for a loss you experience.

Management

There is not one way of grieving. There is no procedure that shows you how to handle your grief. Grief is often a series of tasks that you must undertake to live with the loss and is orderly or predictable. The normal grieving period is usually 6 to 13 months, but it can last longer.

There are things that you can do to help with your grief:

- Give yourself permission to feel.
- Accept that all feelings of grief and loss are real.
- Be honest with others about your sorrow and disappointments.
- Think about how cancer has affected your life. What would be different if you had never been diagnosed with cancer?
- Express your feelings to your nurse.

(continued)

- Talk with someone who will listen and validate these feelings.
- Write your feelings in a journal or share them with a support group.
- Think about your past illnesses and how you were able to cope.
- Ask for help.
- Meet with a social worker or chaplain or bereavement counselor.
- In some situations, a psychologist or psychiatrist can help with your grief.

Follow-up

If you have strong feelings of loss for more than 6 months and the grief is not lessening, talk with your nurse and doctor, as they may be able to advise further counseling.

Phone Numbers

Nurse: ______________________________ Phone: ______________

Physician: ______________________________ Phone: ______________

Social Worker: ______________________________ Phone: ______________

Chaplain: ______________________________ Phone: ______________

Source: Brohard C. Grief. In: Yarbro CH, Wujcik D, Gobel BH, eds. *Cancer Symptom Management.* 4th ed. Burlington, MA: Jones & Bartlett Learning; 2014.

Chapter 33

Spiritual Distress

Elizabeth Johnston Taylor, PhD, RN

"I lost a lot of my spirituality watching her die." (Patient with stage II vaginal cancer, describing her experience of watching her mother suffer meaninglessly with cancer)

"Did I do something wrong? . . . Why me? . . . I think it is a disease from Satan. . . . What is it for . . . it's to kill people. And I feel like Satan put it inside of a person. . . . I want to know what did I do wrong in order to get this cancer. Is it a punishment or what?" (Incarcerated woman receiving chemotherapy for breast cancer)

"Cancer is a trial of my faith. . . . That's what I feel. He [God] is not going to put no more on us than we can bear. Maybe that was the trial of my faith, because I had got weak." (Religious African American woman with recurrent lung cancer)

"Worst of my whole illness is not being able to control my emotions. I was raised in Scotland where I had ground in to me 'men don't cry.' . . . I can keep my spirits up all I want; I can keep up a healthy attitude. I can appear normal, but then BANG!" (Retired Scottish gentleman hospitalized with lymphoma)

THE PROBLEM

Spiritual well-being appears to be associated with a fighting spirit, hope, life satisfaction, happiness, and other positive moods, as well as adjustment and overall quality of life among persons with and surviving cancer.[1–4] Conversely, spiritual distress among cancer patients has been found to be associated with depression and other negative mood states, as well as poor adjustment.[1,2,5,6] A review of research examining spiritual quality of life among persons with cancer noted that several studies have produced evidence indicating that spiritual quality of life is important to overall well-being.[1] Patients are not the only ones who experience spiritual distress while living with cancer; studies indicate that family carers' spiritual status frequently mirrors that of their loved one with cancer.[7–9] Given the integral nature of spiritual well-being to overall health, its significant relationship to psychological well-being, and its salience for many patients and family carers, it is important to support those experiencing spiritual distress.

SPIRITUAL DISTRESS DEFINED AND DESCRIBED

In common parlance, spiritual distress describes patients who report that their "spirits are down" or they feel "broken-hearted." Spiritual distress, an accepted nursing diagnosis, refers to "a disturbance in the belief or value system that provides strength, hope, and meaning to life."[10] The North American Nursing Diagnosis Association International's list of defining characteristics helps nurses understand this abstract definition and observe for spiritual distress. Manifestations of spiritual distress can include the following:[10]

- Expressions of lack of hope, meaning, and purpose in life, and forgiveness of self
- Expressions implying being abandoned by or having anger toward God
- Refusals of interaction with friends and family
- Sudden changes in spiritual practices
- Requests to see a religious leader
- No interest in nature
- Reading spiritual literature

No list could be complete, however, considering the complexity and variability of people and their spiritual dimensions. As the chapter-opening quotes from various persons living with cancer illustrate, spiritual distress can vary from a struggle to bear the burden of a "trial" of faith to bewilderment about meaningless suffering and mortal finiteness. It can also encompass the psychic trauma of believing that cancer is given by a demonic force as a punishment. Moreover, both loss of control and emotional lability can influence one's spirit titer.

INCIDENCE

Several substantial studies of persons with cancer have overtly quantified patients' perceptions of spiritual/religious need.[11–14] Researchers have observed from 42% to 73% of patients endorse the view that they experience at least one spiritual/religious need.[14] Alcorn and colleagues noted that 51% of 68 patients with advanced cancer identified four or more religious/spiritual concerns; they found there was no difference in the number or reported concerns based on whether the patient self-identified spirituality/religion as important.[12] Some reports note that the cancer experience often brings (or at least creates the perception of) greater awareness or intensification of spiritual experience for patients.[15,16] Many descriptions of the cancer experience note that existential suffering often accompanies those living with this threat to lifestyle, personal control, and even life itself.[17] Whether the terminology used is that of "spiritual need" (or "spiritual concerns," or some other term) or "existential suffering," it is logical to assume that these terms are at least overlapping with "spiritual distress."

It has often been assumed that spiritual distress may be particularly prevalent among persons experiencing cancer. Only recently, however, has "spiritual distress" been quantified among cancer patients. Spiritual distress, as determined by a chaplain, was observed in 44% of 113 cancer patients admitted to a Texan palliative care unit.[18] This spiritual distress presented as despair (32%), dread (29%), brokenness (27%), helplessness (25%), alienation (16%), meaninglessness (15%), and guilt or shame (8%). Contrasting these findings are those of a multisite study that asked patients whether they had "concerns about spiritual life"; these 441 participants reported no more than "a slight problem."[19] Similarly, communication experts found spiritual concerns mentioned in only 2% of 125 "pain talk utterances" among family carers of hospice patients who were having intervention discussions with social workers.[9] Clearly, incidence of spiritual distress will vary with the definition used, with the method for quantification employed, and with context.

Although these studies provide a small glimpse into the variation in how often spiritual distress occurs among those living with cancer, more credible evidence may be found from the considerable number of studies that have recently measured spiritual well-being using the Functional Assessment of Chronic Illness—Spiritual Well-Being Scale (FACIT-Sp).[20] Consistently across these studies, the average total score when combining the FACIT-Sp's meaning and faith subscales is approximately 30 ± 6, indicating a moderate amount of spiritual well-being—not what would be thought to be spiritual distress.[19,21–25]

This evidence that persons with cancer report fairly good levels of spiritual well-being may mean several things. First, spiritual well-being may not be the opposite of spiritual distress. Indeed, the two experiences may coexist. For example, one's spiritual "distress" may be the harbinger of or catalyst for continued spiritual growth—that is, an indicator of wellness. Second, self-reporting spiritual distress may be too painful for persons to undertake; perhaps there is a human defense mechanism that guards people from spiritual self-incrimination, as that incrimination would undermine one's very essence. Regardless of the mounting evidence suggesting that spiritual well-being may remain moderately high throughout the cancer and survivorship experiences, there remain ample circumstances for patients and family carers to experience spiritual distress given its etiology.

ETIOLOGY

Spiritual distress "arises from unmet needs and . . . the greater the degree to which a spiritual need remains unmet, the greater the disturbance in spiritual state and the greater the level of spiritual distress experienced by the patient." [26(p 89)] All humans have a spirit that deeply yearns for meaningfulness, inner peace, love, and connection with a transcendent Other—that Something More, the numinous holy, the sacred. So what would create distress for the human spirit? What might prevent one from satisfactorily experiencing meaningfulness, peace, love, and connection with an Ultimate Other? Presumably, multiple factors contribute to spiritual distress. Perhaps personality or even biological predispositions influence whether one's spirit is distressed by an event such as cancer. Previous life experiences, assumptions one holds about the world, and cultural and religious beliefs undoubtedly all contribute to spiritual distress.

What is it about the cancer experience that can distress the spirit? Based on a review of research, Taylor identified possible contributors to the increased spiritual awareness that many cancer patients report.[27] By considering what increases spiritual awareness for cancer patients, insights into what creates spiritual distress may be gained. The experiences inherent in living with cancer typically include the following:

- Loss and change (known to initiate a search for meaning)
- A realization of mortality (may lead one to seek immortality via afterlife beliefs and leaving legacies)
- Having existential questions (cause one to examine theological or philosophical answers)
- Feeling powerless and vulnerable (initiates a seeking for ultimate security and comfort, and a way to transcend self)
- Isolation and loneliness (prompt one to reconnect with others or a Greater Other, to search for love)
- Guilt or shame (leads to seeking forgiveness and acceptance)

Thus losses and changes to which a patient cannot assign meaning or reconcile with basic beliefs about the world will contribute to spiritual distress. Being unable to sense that one's existence will continue in some manner after death may also exacerbate spiritual distress. Unanswered existential questions, a continued sense of vulnerability, loneliness, and guilt may have the same effect.

PATHOLOGY

There is scanty evidence to describe the pathological pathways of spiritual distress. Nevertheless, a large number of studies have found that negative religious coping is related to poor adjustment to illness.[28] Examples of negative religious coping include believing that God is punishing the individual, feeling abandoned by God, viewing cancer as an act of the devil, and passive deferring of decisions to the divine. For instance, in the chapter-opening quotes, the daughter who infers God did not protect her mother from poor care and suffering portrays negative coping. Both this daughter and the incarcerated woman who felt punished display spiritual distress. Indeed, a positive image of God appears associated with less distress among women with breast cancer.[3,5]

A few studies have suggested that spiritual distress occurs when patients who have not had a healthy religious experience prior to diagnosis then encounter difficulty when trying to mobilize religious experience to cope with the illness.[3,5,29] Perhaps the situation is analogous to an adult digging out stored clothes from childhood, trying to wear them, and finding that they no longer fit. To illustrate, Hollywell and Walker observed that frequent prayer is usually associated with positive health outcomes (and often inversely related to anxiety and depression).[29] They noted that this association is particularly strong for those who already have a religious faith and regularly experienced prayer prior to their illness. Conversely, research documents that pleading, bargaining, and passive prayers (like wishful thinking) may be associated with negative health outcomes.

CAVEAT

Spiritual distress is not necessarily pathological. It may be a necessary and vital part of the spiritual journal, just as a harsh winter or fire can be essential to certain plants thriving in the biosphere. Although the experience will still be experienced as painful, it can produce new spiritual growth. To use a Christian example, it may be a "dark night of the soul"—a sense of God as noncommunicative, all the while cerebrally knowing that God is present and that this experience will mature the relationship. To use a Buddhist example, spiritual distress may arise from abandoning attachments, yet all the while knowing that this step is necessary to eliminate inner suffering.

Unlike other cancer symptoms, therefore, spiritual distress may not always be something to avoid. The wisdom of spiritual sages, clinical observations of mental health professionals, and empirical evidence suggest that spiritual distress may be a natural part of a process that can lead to spiritual transformation.[30] Although some persons may get "stuck," those who embrace and learn from the inwardly painful spiritual distress may experience transformation. This transformation explains why some cancer patients are heard to say, "Cancer made me a better person," or "I'm more in tune spiritually," or "I'm closer to God now because of my cancer."

SYMPTOM ASSESSMENT

RISK FACTORS

Although no studies have focused on identifying the risk factors for spiritual distress, clinical observations and findings from a few investigations suggest some possible risk factors. African American and Latino American cancer patients are often more likely to recognize themselves as having spiritual needs and to desire assistance with them.[14,31] These cultural groups are also more likely to use prayer and other spiritual practices to cope with cancer, and may be at more risk for spiritual distress if these practices are disturbed by illness. Even so, they may be at less risk overall because they utilize religious coping resources. Women are often found to be more religious than men or perceive themselves as spiritual[32,33] and may likewise be at risk for spiritual distress if their religiosity is challenged by cancer. It is also possible that younger adult cancer patients may be at higher risk for spiritual distress than older adults,[18] as are those persons who are receiving care for terminal illness or are hospitalized in an inpatient unit.[6,18,19,33]

Being religious (e.g., attending services regularly) is also associated with greater awareness of spiritual need and desire for nursing support with these needs.[33] The wisdom of spiritual sages would posit that the person who plants roots deeply in a spiritual community or religious tradition will have stronger spiritual health and be more spiritually disease resistant. As noted in a review by Taylor, a few studies of persons with cancer support the contention that, among whites at least, those for whom religion is an intrinsic (rather than extrinsic) phenomenon may also be at lower risk for spiritual disease.[14] That is, when religious beliefs provide life with meaning (rather than simply being social or self-serving), the patient may be at lower risk for spiritual distress.

In addition to certain groups of individuals characterized by demographic factors such as ethnicity, gender, and age, persons with certain spiritual beliefs or backgrounds may be at risk for spiritual distress. As described in the "Pathology" section, how patients attribute the cause of their cancer or how they believe that God views them may place them at risk. Cancer patients struggling with religious beliefs may be more likely to experience spiritual distress.

SELF-ASSESSMENT

The patient and family carer's experience of spiritual distress will likely have both cognitive and emotional dimensions. An intellectual struggle would be expected to contribute to emotional distress. For example, patients and their families may ask a form of "Why me/us?" Or they may wonder if there is an afterlife, if there is a deity who cares for them, and if this deity is powerful enough to affect their circumstances. Such questions, doubts, and struggles inherently bring, at least to some degree (depending on the strength of the denial mechanisms), emotional discomfort, anxiety, or depression. Conversely, because people typically expect that healthy spirituality should mean having good feelings, the lack of an affective spiritual experience can cause an intellectual questioning. For example, "I prayed, so why don't I feel happier now? Is God really there?"

These feelings and thoughts involved in spiritual distress reflect a relational nature as well. Some have pictured spirituality as involving both horizontal (or interpersonal) and vertical (or transpersonal) relationships. For those persons living with cancer, for example, spiritual distress may be manifested as the need to right wrongs in a relationship with others or with the divine. Given the broad definition of spiritual distress as "a disturbance in the belief or value system that provides strength, hope, and meaning to life,"[10] spiritual distress can manifest in a myriad of ways (see the definition and etiology discussions earlier in this chapter for other examples).

OBJECTIVE ASSESSMENT

Now that The Joint Commission mandates that all patients must be assessed for spiritual beliefs and practices (http://www.jointcommission.org/standards_information/jcfaqdetails.aspx?StandardsFaqId=290&ProgramId=1), it is essential for nurses to understand how to efficiently and effectively assess cancer patients for spiritual distress. Taylor[34] recommends a two-tiered approach to spiritual assessment:

- Tier 1 is a brief, superficial, initial assessment that will obtain data to determine whether any distress is present that requires further focused assessment. This assessment can be limited to asking the patient about general spiritual status (e.g., "How are you—inside?") and spiritual resources (e.g., "What do you think might help you with these concerns?" or "In what way can your healthcare team boost your spirits?").
- Tier 2 is a focused assessment that engages the patient to describe the specific type(s) of spiritual distress being experienced. For example, during the initial assessment the nurse may learn that the patient is wondering "why?" Tier 2 assessment questions would then reflect this specific problem of meaning. Follow-up questions could include "Tell me more about your 'why' questions" or "What answers are you finding for 'why'?"

Extensive lists of spiritual assessment questions are available,[34] and more can be found in Figure 33-1. In addition, the nurse can craft original questions to reflect the patient's immediate concerns and language.

Indeed, when talking with patients about their spiritual distress, it is important for nurses to be aware of the language utilized.[35] To introduce the topic of spiritual distress, nurses will be less likely to offend or disengage the patient if they avoid phrases such as "spiritual need." Although many understand the term "spiritual," it is often misunderstood as religiosity—which occasionally carries negative emotional meaning. The term "need or problem" conveys

Tier 1 Questions

Select a question from both section A and B.

A. Questions to elicit broad information:

- How are you—inside?
- How is being sick affecting your spirits?
- What spiritual concerns are bothering you the most now?
- How does your faith/spirituality affect the way you cope with being sick?

B. Follow-up questions to elicit information about how to provide care:

- In what way can your healthcare team boost your spirits?
- What or who do you think might help you with these spiritual concerns?
- What spiritual beliefs or practices are important to you when you are sick? How can I/we support these?

Tier 2 Questions

Select pertinent question(s) to elicit information about the specific spiritual concern assessed previously. Examples of more focused assessment questions are:

- How is religion important to you now?
- How does God work in your life now?
- How do you make sense of feeling angry at God/nature/the world?
- Tell me more about how prayer does or doesn't help you.
- How do you find yourself explaining suffering? Are these beliefs helpful?
- What do you see as the mission or purpose of your life?
- What motivates you to get well?
- Do you feel the need to "get right" with God or with someone else? What do you want to do to become forgiven or at peace?

FIGURE 33-1

Assessing for spiritual distress.

that a deficiency exists. For many individuals, therefore, acknowledging a spiritual need or problem or distress would be embarrassing or threatening. A nurse can employ more neutral phrases or use the language proffered by the patient. For example, if a patient remarks that it is "faith and family who are getting me through this," the nurse can create an assessment question using "faith." Neutral phrases such as "matters of the heart" or "spiritual interests" may also be helpful.

Other aspects of spiritual assessment are important to consider. First, the quality of the data collected during a spiritual assessment will be determined by the rapport and trust the nurse has established with the patient. Patients will more likely speak freely of their spiritual concerns to a nurse whom they perceive as warm, kind, respectful, and personally interested.[36] Rapport can be developed rapidly by a nurse who is genuinely caring. A nurse's presence, nonverbal messages, and behaviors can convey readily the qualities a patient needs to talk openly about spirituality.

Assessment data can also be collected from sources other than verbal interactions with patients. For example, the nurse must consider the nonverbal messages a patient sends. Objects such as religious jewelry or spiritually oriented books in the patient's environment can signal information about a patient's spirituality. Assessment data can be collected using paper-and-pencil surveys that ask about spiritual interests and assets. When retrieving a written assessment form from a patient, it is beneficial if the nurse debriefs the patient about his or her response to the survey. This debriefing, in fact, could become the springboard for spiritual care.

A spiritual assessment questionnaire that nurses can use, known as the Spiritual Health and Life-Orientation Measure (SHALOM), is offered by Fisher and Brumley.[37] This 20-item scale allows comparison between one's self-perceived and desired spiritual well-being. Other standardized tools used in research that may have potential for clinical assessment purposes include the FACIT-Sp,[20,38] the Daily Spiritual Experiences scale,[39] the DUREL,[40] and the Brief RCOPE (which measures positive and negative religious coping).[41] These instruments contain fewer than 20 items and can be easily administered. However, the scores that would constitute spiritual distress in a clinical population remain undetermined.

Cautions

Given the potential for psychospiritual damage if an untrained or inept nurse engages a patient in exploring spiritual distress, much caution should be observed by any nurse trying to ameliorate spiritual distress.[42,43] The following criteria offered by Hodge[44] can assist nurses to determine whether they should proceed from a tier 1 assessment to tier 2:

- Relevance. Is my assessment about spiritual distress important to this patient?
- Autonomy. Does the patient want to go deeper into this topic of spiritual distress with me? (Does the patient imply consent?)
- Clinician competence. Am I personally and professionally capable of entering this territory? (Am I culturally safe for this patient? Do I have countertransference issues?)
- Relevance to health or health care. Is my assessment of this patient's spiritual distress relevant to the patient's health and my delivery of health care?

It is vital that nurses recognize their role as spiritual care generalists, not specialists. With deep spiritual distress, especially that involving personal faith, the role of a nurse is to assess for its presence and then make a referral.[43]

Caution must also prevail when considering whether to assess spiritual distress using standardized measures. Although there are always benefits to standardized measurement of a symptom, and it has been recommended that spiritual health be measured using standardized tools among all patients receiving palliative care,[45] serious considerations arise that should balance such recommendations. Standardized measurement of spiritual distress assumes that it is a universal phenomenon that is, in fact, measurable. Furthermore, many of the measures assume a deistic worldview. Measurement assumes that there is a norm against which to compare findings and that nurses or other professionals can know which spiritual experiences are good and best for a patient. Each of these assumptions can be challenged.

SYMPTOM MANAGEMENT STRATEGIES

Spiritual distress cannot be fixed, cured, solved, or manipulated. Rather, the nurse's spiritually sensitive care for this symptom must be one that seeks to accompany, support, nurture, and be an "in-courage-ment."[35,46] The nurse can offer "interventions" such as those listed in the appendices to this chapter, but must do so while recognizing that spiritual work is done interiorly by the individual. Indeed, the nurse can care by promoting an environment that is safe for the patient to recognize and address spiritual distress. The outcome of this work is not controllable or predictable; rather, any spiritual healing or growth is a gift of grace.

THERAPEUTIC APPROACHES

A number of approaches to addressing spiritual distress have been identified by nurses. These include allowing patients to discuss their spiritual concerns and listening empathically; using full or transcendent presence; offering spiritually nurturing books, videos, or other visual materials; educating about and supporting spiritually healing nonreligious rituals; facilitating the expression of the spirit through art (e.g., body movement, painting, sculpting, music, quilting); supporting religious practices; introducing journal writing, prayer, meditation, or guided spiritual imagery; allowing reflection on dreams ("the avenue of the soul"); and making appropriate referrals.[47]

Although these approaches to addressing spiritual distress are helpful, they may not always be possible in the outpatient setting where nurse contact with patients is limited. In the outpatient setting, the oncology nurse's role may more often involve informing the patient about spiritual self-care and making an appropriate referral. Likewise, research findings indicate that therapeutics such as those listed previously are not always appreciated. A survey of 156 cancer patients and 68 family carers showed that nurse spiritual care therapeutics that were less intimate, commonly used, and not overtly religious were most welcomed by patients.[8] These study participants preferred interventions such as a nurse's private prayers and help with finding a quiet time and space, but gave low ratings to interventions such as teaching about writing or drawing their spirituality, discussing difficulties of praying when sick, and help with thinking about dreams.

Patients frequently report prayer is a significant source of comfort during illness.[14] Given that cancer often creates spiritual distress related to prayer and meditation (e.g., "Why aren't my prayers being answered?" "Am I praying the right way?"), and given that patients prefer a more oblique nurse approach to this challenge, the self-care guide in Appendix 33A can be beneficial to those who pray. This self-care guide may be especially helpful to those persons whose prayer or meditation practices lapsed prior to illness.[29]

Several healthcare teams have tested the efficacy of interventions that affect cancer patient spirituality. Most of these tested programs support patients to find meaningfulness amidst their illness (e.g., through life reviews, meaning-centered therapy, and "dignity therapy").[19,23,48] These therapies, reflected in the self-care guides developed in Appendices 33B and 33C, show much promise in supporting spiritual well-being among persons with cancer.

A patient may also benefit from a referral that should be selected based on the patient's spiritual need. Numerous spiritual care experts may be available to assist the patient:

- Chaplains (trained in clinical pastoral education, have pastoral counseling expertise—a fusion of theological and psychological knowledge)
- Clergy (depending on the religious denomination, have various levels of theological training; may have very limited counseling experience)
- Mental health professionals (have counseling expertise, and if spiritually sensitive, may be able to assist those who struggle with questions of meaning and purpose, guilt, or relational aspects of spiritual distress)
- Parish nurses (have some pastoral counseling training and understand the varieties of spiritual distress amidst illness)
- Spiritual directors (clergy or lay persons with some training in becoming "holy listeners" or "soul friends")
- Spiritual healers (shamans, medicine men, curanderos, and other folk healers may be considered spiritual care experts, particularly by many patients from non-Western cultures)

These spiritual care experts can be contacted by the patient or a chaplain at your healthcare institution. Nurses can assist clients to find information about how to contact such experts. Chaplains are generally employed or volunteer for healthcare institutions. Clergy and parish nurses are typically employed by a denomination's local parish, which may be found online or in the local telephone book. Spiritual directors are typically affiliated with a religious retreat center, which will also be listed in a telephone directory or on the internet. (Visit Spiritual Directors International online at www.sdiworld.org.) Spiritual healers are often learned about through "word of mouth," but may also list themselves in a directory. National centers for complementary therapies (found on the Internet) may be able to identify a spiritual healer for a patient.

NURSING IMPLICATIONS

The eradication of spiritual distress may be an inappropriate outcome, as it is an outcome over which a nurse has no control. However, a nurse will do well to monitor whether the patient's spiritual response to cancer is a holistically healthful one. In evaluating a patient's journey through spiritual distress, the nurse considers the following questions:

- Is the patient avoiding, minimizing, or denying the spiritual distress or the effect of this distress?
- Is the patient using healthful coping strategies to deal with the spiritual distress?
- If religious, are the patient's religious beliefs or practices rigid, toxic, or in any way harmful?
- Is the patient appreciative of the spiritual growth that can occur from struggling with matters that distress the spirit?

Such an evaluation is best done in person by asking sensitively worded questions and listening empathically.[35,43]

PATIENT SELF-CARE

In addition to spiritual care experts, other resources exist for those with spiritual distress. See Appendices 33A, 33B, and 33C for suggestions. Chapels in the hospital, retreat centers, and natural wildernesses can all provide a person with space for the introspection and meditation necessary for addressing spiritual distress. Numerous spiritual self-help books have been written and can be found in most bookstores and libraries. Biographies about how others have been transformed by suffering may also be helpful to a patient. Other spirit-nurturing tools can include movies about how persons triumphed over tragedy, inspirational music or recorded sounds of nature, physical objects that aid meditation (e.g., yantra, incense, floor pillow), and religious videos. The genre and content of the book, music, or other material need to match the personal needs and stylistic preferences of the patient, of course. This is one reason why it is usually best to have the patient select specific spiritual self-care materials if possible.

REFERENCES

1. Taylor EJ, Davenport F. Spiritual quality of life. In: King C Hinds P, eds. *Quality of Life: From Nursing and Patient Perspective.* 3rd ed. Burlington, MA: Jones & Bartlett Learning; 2012:83–104.
2. Krikorian A, Limonero JT, Maté J. Suffering and distress at the end-of-life. *Psychooncology.* October 11, 2011. [Epub ahead of print].
3. Schreiber JA, Brockoff DY. Twenty-five years later: what do we know about religion/spirituality and psychological well-being among breast cancer survivors? A systematic review. *J Cancer Surviv.* 2012;6(1):82–94.
4. Yanez B, Edmondson D, Stanton AL, et al. Facets of spirituality as predictors of adjustment to cancer: relative contributions of having faith and finding meaning. *J Consult Clin Psychol.* 2009;77(4):730–741.
5. Gall TL, Kristjansson E, Charbonneau C, et al. A longitudinal study on the role of spirituality in response to the diagnosis and treatment of breast cancer. *J Behav Med.* 2009;32(2):174–186.
6. Lo C, Zimmerman C, Rydall A, et al. Longitudinal study of depressive symptoms in patients with metastatic gastrointestinal and lung cancer. *J Clin Oncol.* 2010;28(18):3084–3089.
7. Murray SA, Kendall M, Boyd K, et al. Archetypal trajectories of social, psychological, and spiritual wellbeing and distress in family care givers of patients with lung cancer: secondary analysis of serial qualitative interviews. *BMJ.* 2010;340:c2581.
8. Taylor EJ, Mamier I. Spiritual care nursing: what cancer patients and family caregivers want. *J Adv Nurs.* 2005;49(3):260–267.
9. Wittenberg-Lyles E, Demiris G, Oliver DP, et al. Reciprocal suffering: caregiver concerns during hospice care. *J Pain Symptom Manage.* 2011;41(2):383–393.
10. NANDA International. *NANDA Nursing Diagnoses: Definitions and Classification 2007–2008.* Philadelphia: NANDA International; 2007.
11. Moadel A, Morgan C, Dutcher J. Psychosocial needs assessment among an underserved, ethnically diverse cancer patient population. *Cancer.* 2007;109(2 suppl):446–454.
12. Alcorn S, Balboni M, Prigerson H, et al. "If God wanted me yesterday, I wouldn't be here today": religious and spiritual themes in patients' experiences of advanced cancer. *J Palliat Med.* 2010;13(5):581–588.
13. Astrow A, Wexler A, Texeira K, et al. Is failure to meet spiritual needs associated with cancer patients' perceptions of quality of care and their satisfaction with care? *J Clin Oncol.* 2007;25(36):5753–5757.
14. Taylor EJ. Religion and patient care. In: Fowler M, Kirkham-Reimer S, Sawatzky R, et al., eds. *Religion, Religious Ethics, and Nursing.* New York: Springer; 2011:313–338.
15. Taylor EJ. Spiritual responses to cancer. In: Yarbro CH, Wujcik D, Gobel BH, eds. *Cancer Nursing: Principles and Practice.* 7th ed. Sudbury, MA: Jones and Bartlett; 2010.
16. Thuné-Boyle IC, Stygall J, Keshtgar MR, et al. The impact of a breast cancer diagnosis on religious/spiritual beliefs and practices in the UK. *J Religion Health.* 2010:50:203–218.
17. Boston P, Bruce A, Schreiber R. Existential suffering in the palliative care setting: an integrated literature review. *J Pain Symptom Manage.* 2011;41(3):604–618.
18. Hui D, de la Cruz M, Thorney S, et al. The frequency and correlates of spiritual distress among patients with advanced cancer admitted to an acute palliative care unit. *Am J Hosp Palliat Care.* 2011;28(4):264–270.
19. Chochinov B, Kristjanson LJ, Breitbart W, et al. Effect of dignity therapy on distress and end-of-life experience in terminally ill patients: a randomized controlled trial. *Lancet Oncol.* 2011;12(3):753–762.
20. Peterman AH, Fitchett G, Brady MJ, et al. Measuring spiritual well-being in people with cancer: the Functional Assessment of Chronic Illness

Therapy—Spiritual Well-Being Scale (FACIT-Sp). *Ann Behav Med.* 2002;24(1):49–58.
21. Frost MH, Johnson ME, Atherton PJ, et al. Spiritual well-being and quality of life of women with ovarian cancer and their spouses. *J Support Oncol.* 2012;10(2):72–80.
22. Rodin G, Yuen D, Mishitelle A, et al. Traumatic stress in acute leukemia. *Psychooncology.* 2013;22(2):299–307.
23. Breitbart W, Poppito S, Rosenfeld B, Jobin G, Martin E, Spencer B. Pilot randomized controlled trial of individual meaning-centered psychotherapy for patients with advanced cancer. *J Clin Oncol.* 2012;30(12):1304–1309.
24. Kandasamy A, Chaturvedi SK, Desai G. Spirituality, distress, depression, anxiety, and quality of life in patients with advanced cancer. *Indian J Cancer.* 2011;48(1):55–59.
25. Trinkaus M, Burman D, Barmala N, et al. Spirituality and use of complementary therapies for cure in advanced cancer. *Psychooncology.* 2011;20(7):746–754.
26. Monod SM, Rochat E, Büla CJ, Jobin G, Martin E, Spencer B. The spiritual distress assessment tool: an instrument to assess spiritual distress in hospitalized elderly persons. *BMC Geriatr.* 2010;10:88.
27. Taylor EJ. Caring for the spirit. In: Burke C, ed. *Psychosocial Dimensions of Oncology Nursing Care.* 2nd ed. Pittsburgh, PA: Oncology Nursing Press; 2009:59–77.
28. Ano G, Vasconcelles E. Religious coping and psychological adjustment to stress: a meta-analysis. *J Clin Psychol.* 2005;61(4):461–480.
29. Hollywell C, Walker J. Private prayer as a suitable intervention for hospitalized patients: a critical review of the literature. *J Clin Nurs.* 2008;18(5):637–651.
30. Park CL, Calhoun LG, Tedeshi RG. *Posttraumatic Growth: Positive Changes in the Aftermath of Crisis.* Mahwah, NJ: Lawrence Erlbaum Associates; 1998.
31. Buck H, Meghani S. Spiritual expressions of African Americans and whites in cancer pain. *J Holist Nurs.* 2012;30(2):107–116.
32. Shahibi L, Powell LH, Musick MA, et al. Correlates of self perceptions of spirituality in American adults. *Ann Behav Med.* 2002;24(1):59–68.
33. Taylor EJ. Prevalence of spiritual needs among cancer patients and family caregivers. *Oncol Nurs Forum.* 2006;33(4):729–735.
34. Taylor EJ. Spiritual assessment. In: Ferrell BR, Coyle N, eds. *Textbook of Palliative Nursing Care.* 3rd ed. New York: Oxford University Press; 2010:647–662.
35. Taylor EJ. *What Do I Say? Talking with Patients About Spirituality.* Philadelphia, PA: Templeton Press; 2007.
36. Taylor EJ. Client perspectives about nurse requisites for spiritual caregiving. *Appl Nurs Res.* 2007;20(1):44–46.
37. Fisher J, Brumley D. Nurses' and carers' spiritual wellbeing in the workplace. *Australian J Adv Nurs.* 2008;25(4):49–57.
38. Johnson ME, Piderman KM, Sloan JA, et al. Measuring spiritual quality of life in patients with cancer. *J Support Oncol.* 2007;5:437–442.
39. Underwood LG, Teresi JA. The Daily Spiritual Experience Scale: development, theoretical description, reliability, exploratory factor analysis, and preliminary construct validity using health-related data. *Ann Behav Med.* 2002;24(1):22–33.
40. Koenig H, Parkerson GR, Meador KG. Religion index for psychiatric research. *Am J Psychiatry.* 1997;154(6):885–886.
41. Pargament K, Feuille M, Burdzy D. The Brief RCOPE: current psychometric status of a short measure of religious coping. *Religions.* 2011;2:51–76.
42. Pesut B, Fowler M, Riemer-Kirkham S, et al. Particularizing spirituality in points of tension: enriching the discourse. *Nurs Inquiry.* 2009;16(4):337–346.
43. Taylor EJ. *Religion: A Clinical Guide for Nurses.* New York: Springer; 2012.
44. Hodge D. A template for spiritual assessment: a review of the JCAHO requirements and guidelines for implementation. *Social Work.* 2006;51:317–326.
45. Ferrell B, Virani R, Otis-Green S, et al. Improving the quality of spiritual care as a dimension of palliative care: the report of the Consensus Conference. *J Palliat Med.* 2009;12(10):885–904.
46. Pesut B, Thorne S. From private to public: negotiating professional and personal identities in spiritual care. *J Adv Nurs.* 2007;58(4): 396–403.
47. Taylor EJ. *Spiritual Care: Nursing Research, Theory, and Practice.* Upper Saddle River, NJ: Prentice Hall; 2002.
48. Ando M, Morita T, Akechi T, et al. Efficacy of short-term life-review interviews on the spiritual well-being of terminally ill cancer patients. *J Pain Symptom Management.* 2010;39(6):993–1002.

Prayer and Meditation

Patient Name: ____

This guide will help you to think about some ways you can nurture your spirit. It includes helpful hints about how you can pray or meditate while you are feeling sick or anxious.

Description

Many people who live with cancer (or with a loved one with cancer) have a hard time keeping their spirits up. Praying and meditating are sometimes hard to do when you have pain, worry, or other problems. You may be thinking something like this:

- "I don't have time to sit and be quiet, to think about what is happening."
- "I can't concentrate when I try to pray."
- "Why aren't my prayers being answered?"
- "I shouldn't pray for specific things or big things."
- "I'm trying to let God have control over my life, but sometimes I wish I could stay in control!"
- "Why me? I don't deserve it. It's not fair. Why would God allow this?"
- "Sometimes I wonder if God can hear me or if God really has the power to cure me."
- "I have asked God for one big thing, so I won't ask God for anything else."
- "I hope my prayers work, but sometimes I wonder."
- "Sometimes I wonder if I am good enough for God to give me what I'm asking."
- "Are my prayers said in the right way? Maybe I'm not very good at praying."

Suggestions for Self-Care

Prayer and meditation are ways of being with that which you believe is the Ultimate Other, the Divine. These practices also help you to listen to yourself. By listening to your authentic self, you can become more aware of the Divine's presence. Try some of these specific things that may help you to pray or meditate during tough times:

- Ask yourself why it is hard to pray or meditate now. You may find that writing about this issue in a journal or talking to a spiritual counselor will help (e.g., Is it because you can't concentrate? Is it because you feel angry? Is it because you are wondering if it does any good?). Knowing what your problems are with prayer and meditation will help you to choose more helpful approaches.
- Remember that there are different ways to pray or meditate. Choose the way that you like. For example, a social person may prefer prayers that are conversations. A shy, quiet person may like meditating on a passage from sacred writings.

(continued)

- Short, repeatable, or memorized prayers are useful when you are anxious and want to pray. Wording phrases in a positive way is helpful. For example, when you have lots of pain, you may want to try "God has mercy on me" or "The Lord is my Shepherd" over and over.
- When you want to be able to concentrate, you might find an object that helps you to focus. Feeling prayer beads or looking at a picture that makes you think of the Divine are examples.
- Remember there are various ways you can express yourself to the Divine. You may, for example:
  - Create art (e.g., a drawing that "says" how you see or relate to the Divine)
  - Sing, make noise or music somehow (e.g., scream into a pillow "Why, God?")
  - Body movement (e.g., dance about your anger at God)
  - Keep a journal (e.g., write your prayers, questions, and fears to the Divine with your strongest hand; responses that emerge from within can be written down with your other hand)
- Remember there are also many different ways the Divine communicates with you. You may, for example, experience the Divine in the following settings:
  - Nature (e.g., sitting on a log in the forest, listening to birds, planting flowers)
  - Your dreams
  - Daily life, when you have one of those spontaneous "aha" moments
  - Music or artwork others have created to portray the Divine
  - Everyday life that has evidence of the Divine (e.g., the laughter of a child, the kindness of others)
  - Reading sacred writings
- Breathing is an important part of some approaches to prayer and meditation. Slow, deep breaths can help one to feel better and more spiritually aware. You may combine your breathing in with an image of the Divine light or love coming into your body. As you breathe out, imagine your stress going out of you.
- While meditating, you may want to do the following:
  - Be in an upright or comfortable position, close your eyes, relax your muscles, and allow yourself time—even just 3 to 5 minutes
  - Select a short phrase on which to focus; repeat this phrase during your meditation or use it as a topic for reflection
  - Notice and put aside mental distractions (or decide that they are messages from which to learn)
  - Be aware of your breathing
- For more information, check the religion/spirituality section at your library or bookstore. Examples of books that might help include these:
  - *The Direct Path: Creating a Personal Journey to the Divine Using the World's Spiritual Traditions* by Andrew Harvey: Broadway Books; 2000)
  - *Praying Our Goodbyes* by Joyce Rupp, OSM: Ave Maria Press (Notre Dame, IN 46556); 1998
  - *Dreams and Spiritual Growth: A Judeo-Christian Way of Dreamwork* by Louis M. Savary, P. H. Berne, and S. K. Williams: Paulist Press (Ramsey, NJ 07446); 1984
  - *Beginning to Pray* by Anthony Bloom: Paulist Press (Ramsey, NJ 07446); 1970

Follow-up

Most nurses will be pleased to support your prayer and meditation practices. Let them know how they can help you. You may also find help from an expert in spiritual care, such as a chaplain, clergy person, counselor, or spiritual director. (Spiritual directors are trained holy listeners or soul friends. One can be found by looking on www.sdiworld.org.) A recommended spiritual care expert is:

Name/Title: ____

Contact Information (e.g., e-mail, phone): ______________________

Source: Taylor EJ. Spiritual Distress. In: Yarbro CH, Wujcik D, Gobel BH, eds. *Cancer Symptom Management.* 4th ed. Burlington, MA: Jones & Bartlett Learning; 2014.

Transforming Tragedy

Patient Name: ______________________________

This guide is only for those who often ask "why?" (perhaps secretly) or wonder how to make sense of cancer. It includes hints about how you can rethink the tragedy of cancer so that it can become a positive event in your life.

Description

Many people who live with cancer (or with a loved one with cancer) struggle with why such a bad thing has happened to them. You, too, may be thinking:

- "Why me? I don't deserve this."
- "It's unfair, unlucky."
- "Why did this happen?"
- "There's got to be a reason for it, but I haven't figured it out yet. Wish I could!"
- "Am I being punished?"
- "Why not me?"

Being able to think about the good aspects of having cancer will help you to feel better.

Suggestions for Self-Care

Many people who have cancer say that although they wish they had never gotten cancer, they found that it was "the best thing that ever happened." This is because having cancer can put energy into a spiritual journey. Things that may help you to change your tragedy into a triumph include the following pieces of advice:

- Recognize that this process is a struggle. It is also normal. Everyone who faces a serious loss or change will need to find a way to make sense of it, to find meaning.
- To find a satisfactory response to "why?" questions, you may have to engage in the painful process of asking these questions. To keep your emotions healthy, you will need to balance these painful questions with time-outs from the questioning.
- Don't accept that you should never ask these questions or that your God is not able to work with this struggle with you.
- Once you have thought of all of your "why?" questions, you may find some answers that satisfy you. It is more likely, however, that you will decide your questions can't be answered for now. You need to live with this mystery.
- Healing inside may begin when you arrive at a question like "No matter the why's, now how am I going to live?" or "How do I choose to respond to this tragic event in my life?"

Other questions that may be helpful to you in this process are the following:

- What have I learned about myself, thanks to cancer?
- How has cancer improved the way I relate to others?

- How has cancer strengthened me?
- How can I be more helpful to others now because of this experience?
- How am I growing spiritually because of cancer?
- What are the good things that have resulted from having cancer?
- Which lessons have I learned from this experience about living?

People who survive tragedy often use one of these ways of thinking to cope:

- Find a side benefit (e.g., "Having cancer has brought my family closer together")
- Compare yourself with someone who is worse off
- Be glad that your situation is not as bad as it could have been
- Realize that there are others who accompany you (i.e., your family, God, or a universal community of sufferers)
- Accept that your life is part of a bigger story that has a happy ending

You can do things that will help you to create meaning for your new life with cancer. For example:

- Do something that helps others (e.g., volunteer, participate in research, show kindness)
- Dedicate yourself to a cause—political, social, religious, or other
- Be creative (e.g., art)
- Leave a memory; create or give something so others can remember you later
- Enjoy what pleasures life can still bring to you (e.g., attend a concert, eat favorite foods, hold a baby)
- Pray or meditate to increase your sense of purpose and connection with the Divine (e.g., traditional forms of prayer, walking or centering prayers, journal writing)

In addition, you may wish to do the following:

- Discuss your spiritually painful questions with a spiritual care expert or trusted friend
- Consider reading or watching a movie about how people triumph over tragedy

Follow-up

Most nurses will be pleased to support your struggle to transform your tragedy. Let them know how they can help you. You may also find help from an expert in spiritual care, such as a chaplain, clergy person, spiritual director, or a counselor with spiritual sensitivity. A recommended spiritual care expert is:

Name/Title: ______________________________

Contact Information (e.g., e-mail, phone): ______________________________

Source: Taylor EJ. Spiritual Distress. In: Yarbro CH, Wujcik D, Gobel BH, eds. *Cancer Symptom Management.* 4th ed. Burlington, MA: Jones & Bartlett Learning; 2014.

Leaving a Legacy

Patient Name: ______________________________

This guide will help you to think about how you want leave a legacy. It offers ideas on how you can give something meaningful to others, or make the world a better place.

Description

Whether the cancer you have will shorten your life or not, having a serious illness often causes people to think about what makes life have meaning. One way people make their lives meaningful is to leave a legacy. Your legacy may involve giving something special to those you love; it could also mean doing something for your neighborhood or others you do not know. You may have found yourself thinking thoughts like these:

- "Is my life making a difference to others? To the world?"
- "I hope my family will remember [certain things about me]."
- "How can I give away things that I treasure?"

Suggestions for Self-Care

Giving something back to the world often returns to the giver a sense of purpose and joy. There are many ways to leave a legacy. Choose a way that is right for you.

- Create a work of art that leaves beauty in the world—for example, a poem, recipe, song, design, or knitted or sewn garment. It could be anything you make that will bring joy to others.
- Help a social or political or religious cause. Make a difference for others by lending your hand or voice or financial resources to a cause you think will make life better for others.
- Advance knowledge through science. Even if you are not a scientist, you can choose to be in a study or make a donation that will help people in the future. You can also share what you know from the "case study" of your life with others needing it. For example, you may be able to share how to have a healthy relationship, how to grow organic food, or what not to do when. . . .
- Tell your story or tell family stories so that the younger members of your family will understand you and their own family better. Stories share more than facts about you or your family background. Hidden in stories are values, morals, and beliefs that you cannot avoid sharing when telling them (e.g., "Grandma married Grandpa for love, even though her parents wanted her to marry a rich man"),

  There are several ways to tell your story so others will have it. Here are some ideas:

  - Record your stories to create an oral history.
  - Create a scrapbook (or a treasure box) with memorabilia from your life.
  - Write your story, or tell it to someone who can write up your story.
  - Draw your story; you may choose to use a timeline or as a graph with short written snippets to tell your story.

- o Depending on what you feel like doing, you may tell the facts of your life following a chronological order, or you may focus on themes throughout your life. Or you may want to just tell your favorite stories.

No matter how you tell your story, telling it will give you a bird's-eye view of your life. This perspective can bring a sense of thanks and meaning. It also will help those who have heard it.

Questions that may help you to think about telling your story include these:

- o What is most important for others to know about me?
- o What are the times in my life when I felt most alive?
- o What are the most important roles I have had? What did I accomplish in these roles?
- o Are there things I still need to tell (or retell to) my family or others?
- o What might be best to not include in my life story?
- o Which advice do I want to pass on? What are my hopes and dreams for my family?

- Remember that you have already left a legacy with the life you have lived thus far. You may want to reflect on the ways you have made a difference in the world. For example, you are likely to leave a legacy through your parenting, your friendships, your work, your gifts, your citizenship, your unseen good deeds, and so forth.
- Often we leave part of our legacy by giving away items that we treasure. For example, you may want to give special furniture, artwork, books, or jewelry to friends, family, or a museum. In addition to choosing who will get which items, you will want to think about when and how these gifts are given. Do you want to give them personally? Do you want to tell or write in a card why the item is special?

Follow-up

Most nurses will be pleased to support you as you think about how to leave your legacy. Let them know how they can help you. You may also find help from a counselor, chaplain, or a person trained to write biographies. A recommended expert is:

Name/Title: ______________________________

Contact Information (e.g., e-mail, phone): ______________________________

Source: Taylor EJ. Spiritual Distress. In: Yarbro CH, Wujcik D, Gobel BH, eds. *Cancer Symptom Management.* 4th ed. Burlington, MA: Jones & Bartlett Learning; 2014.

Chapter 34

Symptoms When Death Is Imminent

Marie Bakitas, DNSc, APRN, AOCN®, FAAN
Margaret Firer Bishop, MS, APRN
Margaret E. Hahn, MSN, FNP, APRN, ACHPN

"How people die remains in the memory of those who live on."

—*Dame Cicely Saunders (1918–2005)*

THE PROBLEM

"Imminent death" refers to the period of time when "death is expected to occur within hours to days based on the person's condition, disease progression, and symptom constellation."[1(p527)] As death approaches, there are usually a predictable series of observable changes that signal death is near. These include diminished cognition and mental clarity (usually due to increasing hypoxia of the brain and other vital organs, metabolic consequences of renal failure, or other aspects of physical changes), changes in breathing (due to respiratory acidosis, profound weakness, and inability to clear secretions), and changes in skin temperature, color, and turgor.

Two critical nursing concerns during this period are (1) expert management of symptoms at end-of-life and (2) family preparation for what to expect as death approaches (including assessing family needs and anticipatory grief responses) and in the post-death period. Nurses and other interdisciplinary team members should also determine an appropriate post-death bereavement plan to help with religious/spiritual practices and funeral arrangements.[2] Domain 7 of the National Consensus Guidelines for Palliative Care describes standards of care that apply to the patient who is imminently dying (Table 34-1).[2] Care of the imminently dying patient requires equal attention to the needs of the patient and the family.

Since Cicely Saunders made her prophetic quote (cited at the introduction to this chapter), a substantial body of literature has documented that lack of family preparation and witnessing a traumatic death event are linked to adverse family consequences during bereavement.[3] Therefore the quality of care, symptom relief, and circumstances of the imminently dying patient can have a profound positive or negative impact not only on the patient's final days, but also on the adjustment of the family for days and years to come.

Nursing involvement and care of the patient who is approaching death and the patient's family will vary in intensity based on the setting where end-of-life care is provided (e.g., home with hospice care, hospital, intensive care unit, assisted-living facility, nursing home, or residential hospice). It is important for the nurse to be committed to helping the patient and family achieve a comfortable and dignified environment for the dying patient, regardless of the setting. While this can be more difficult to achieve in a hospital or intensive care unit (ICU), assessing and respecting patient and family preferences can make this possible. The ability to provide expert symptom management may also determine whether patients are able to die in the setting of their choice.

TABLE 34-1

DOMAIN 7: Care of the Imminently Dying Patient, Clinical Practice Guidelines for Quality Palliative Care
Guideline 7.1 Signs and symptoms of impending death are recognized and communicated in developmentally appropriate language for children and patients with cognitive disabilities with respect to family preferences. Care appropriate for this phase of illness is provided to patient and family. Criteria: • The patient's and family's transition to the dying phase is recognized when possible and is documented and communicated appropriately, with attention to population-specific issues and age appropriateness, to patient, family, and staff. • End-of-life concerns, hopes, fears, and expectations are addressed openly and honestly in the context of social and cultural customs and within a developmentally appropriate manner. • Symptoms at the end of life are assessed and documented on a timely basis and are treated based on patient-family preferences. • The care plan is revised to meet the unique needs of the patient and family at this phase of the illness. The need for higher intensity and acuity of care during the active dying phase is met by the interdisciplinary team and documented. • Patient and family wishes regarding care setting for the death are documented. Any inability to meet these needs and preferences is reviewed and addressed by the palliative care team. • As patients decline, the hospice referral option will be introduced (or reintroduced) for those who have not accessed hospice services as appropriate. • The family is educated regarding the signs and symptoms of approaching death in a developmentally, culturally, and age-appropriate manner. • Ideally, sensitive communication is done around autopsy and organ donation decision making before the time of death as appropriate.
Guideline 7.2 Postdeath care is delivered in a respectful manner. Cultural and religious practices particular to the postdeath period are assessed and documented. Care of the body postdeath is delivered with respect to these practices, as well as in accordance to both organizational practice and local law.
Guideline 7.3 A postdeath bereavement plan is activated. An interdisciplinary team member is assigned to the family in the postdeath period to help with religious practices, funeral arrangements, and burial planning.

Source: Reprinted with Permission: National Consensus Project[2].

This chapter discusses the common progression of end-of-life cognitive, respiratory, and symptom management strategies (including palliative sedation for refractory symptoms), and other important care and education considerations for the family of the patient who is approaching death.

DELIRIUM

THE PROBLEM

Progressively decreasing awareness and delirium frequently occur in patients who are approaching death.[4–6] "Terminal delirium," "terminal restlessness," "terminal agitation," and "terminal psychosis" are all terms that have been used to describe diminished mental clarity and awareness in the waning days of life. Delirium may also manifest and be identified as a state of "near death awareness" (described later).[7,8] In a prospective series of 104 patients with advanced cancer consecutively admitted to a tertiary palliative care unit, terminal delirium was present in 88% of patients who died.[9]

Delirium, also termed "confusion," "agitation," or "forgetfulness," is defined by the American Psychiatric Association as an acute, altered level of consciousness with changes in cognition and attention caused by physiological disturbance.[10] It may present as reduced ability to focus, hold, or shift attention; a lack of environmental awareness; hypervigilance; memory deficits; perceptual disturbances (delusions and hallucinations); incoherent speech; and altered sleep–wake cycles. These changes in attention and cognition at the end of the individual's life may fluctuate over short periods of time. At end-of-life, delirium usually presents in one of three ways: (1) as a hyperactive state with agitated behavior, picking at clothes and bed covers, and rambling and loud incoherent speech; (2) as a hypoactive state with lethargy, little spontaneous movement, soft incoherent speech, anxiety, or fearfulness; or (3) as a mixed form, with features of both hyperactive and hypoactive states.[5,11] Most patients present with a mixed form of delirium.[12]

Delirium is distinct from dementia and psychoses.[12] Dementia is a chronic and progressive loss of intellectual (executive) function. Psychosis is a severe mental disorder in which thought and emotions are so impaired that contact is lost with external reality. It, too, can present as relapsing and remitting hallucinations and delusions. In both dementia and psychosis, patients maintain a normal state of arousal/level of consciousness, in contrast to the waxing and waning level of awareness common in delirium.[6]

"Near death awareness," which was originally described in a book of hospice nurses' anecdotes about end-of-life, entitled *Final Gifts*,[8] is a state in which the patient describes what dying is like, including visions of life after death and communication with relatives or others who have died. These utterances can be either comforting or frightening to the patient and family. Nonetheless, there is a lack of consensus about whether this state is another manifestation of delirium or is connected to another level of cognition. Suggestions for helping families and caregivers recognize and attend to a patient whom they believe may be experiencing near death awareness are described in Table 34-2.[7,8]

A key concept in defining "terminal delirium" is irreversibility.[13] Evaluation for potential reversible precipitating factors is key to delirium management.[11] Reversibility is more likely when psychoactive medications are used or dehydration is present, in contrast to when hypoxic encephalopathy, multi-organ system failure, or metabolic factors exist.[13] Therefore recognizing the features of terminal delirium is important to providing appropriate symptom management and family counseling. Appendix 34A, "Understanding, Managing, and Coping with Delirium as Death Approaches," is a useful handout that can be provided to family members to help explain this challenging end-of-life symptom.[14,15]

Etiology

The factors that are most likely to increase the risk of developing delirium in general include age older than 65 years, a history of dementia, a prior episode of delirium, depression, declining functional status, sensory impairments, decreased oral intake, drug or alcohol abuse, and a combination of multiple precipitating factors.[9] The Delirium Etiology Checklist[16] (Table 34-3) is a structured tool that identifies 12 potential contributing etiologies according to the likelihood of their being a cause for delirium (e.g., present, contributing, likely, or definite) based on clinical history and investigation. Hyperactive and mixed delirium is often attributable to medication reactions (e.g., benzodiazepines, opioids, anticholinergic agents), whereas dehydration and encephalopathies are more likely to induce hypoactive delirium.[17] As described earlier, the value in determining the etiology of a terminal delirium is to determine reversibility,[6] although there is some debate as to whether all causes of delirium ultimately result in a final common neurophysiological pathway.[18]

TABLE 34-2

Near Death Awareness: Tips for Listening and Attending to the Patient

Near death awareness (NDA) is a state in which the patient is describing what dying is like, including visions of life after death, communicating with relatives or others who have died and the like. Attentive listening may allow others to decipher messages that a patient may be trying to communicate as death approaches.

Two broad categories of messages have been described:

- Attempts to describe what dying is like:
  - Communicating with or experiencing the presence of someone who is not alive or visions of spiritual beings (e.g., seeing angels).
  - Preparing for travel or a change.
  - Describing a place they can see in another realm (e.g., describing a beautiful place or heaven, or a peaceful light).
  - Knowing when death will occur.
- Requests for something to ensure a peaceful death:
  - Achieve closure in a personal or spiritual relationship, or in an ethical matter.
  - Remove a barrier to achieving closure.
  - Prepare for death via specific items or rituals.

Pearls for Listening for NDA Phenomena:

Healthcare professionals should evaluate for causes of reversible delirium and treat when appropriate. In some cases it may be that agitation can be occurring from a NDA message that is not being understood or addressed. However, if it is determined that no reversible cause can be found and NDA is the source of the patients' utterances and behavior, some tips that can be helpful as you relate to your loved one are:

1. Gently ask patient about messages you do not understand.
2. Accept and validate what the patient is telling you; do not challenge or argue.
3. Be honest when you do not understand, but let patient know you will keep trying.
4. If you do not know what to say, say nothing – but be present.
5. Try to keep an open mind and listen carefully for messages they might try to convey through symbol or suggestion.
6. Consider if the message is trying to prepare loved ones for the future.

Source: Data from Marchand[7]; Callahan and Kelley[8].

TABLE 34-3

Delirium Etiology Checklist
Drug intoxication
Drug withdrawal
Metabolic-endocrine
Traumatic brain injury
Seizure-related
CNS infection
Systemic infection
CNS neoplasm
Systemic neoplasm
Cerebrovascular
Organ failure
Other CNS causes
Other systemic causes

Abbreviation: CNS: central nervous system.
Source: Data from Trzepacz and Meagher[16].

PATHOPHYSIOLOGY

Determining the cause and reversibility of delirium in the patient with advanced cancer can be challenging. Many different processes at end-of-life can affect the central nervous system and thereby impair thinking and occasionally cause seizures. Neurological function is impaired as end-of-life processes such as hypoxia, azotemia, hepatic encephalopathy, impaired cerebral blood flow or lesions, drug side effects, depression, and fever progress. Regardless of the etiology involved, some common pathophysiology pathways likely underlie this process, involving changes in brain neurotransmitters and inflammatory mechanisms.[5] For example, hypoxia from reduced lung capacity in end-stage lung cancer can lead to release of the excitatory neurotransmitter glutamate; the resultant increased oxygen requirements of nearby structures then lead to disorganized thought. Hypoxia is also known to cause increased dopamine levels, thereby compounding the problems created by high glutamate levels. Haloperidol may decrease the severity and duration of delirium by blocking the damage induced by dopamine and glutamate.[18,19]

SYMPTOM ASSESSMENT

Risk factors

Despite the prevalence of delirium in patients with serious, life-limiting illness, this symptom is often under-recognized and under-treated.[6] Assessment of the patient's history for risk factors for delirium includes medication use or changes, other medical problems, and results of recent diagnostic studies including hematology, chemistries, radiology, and microbiology. Physical examination may reveal fever, changes in blood pressure, oxygen saturation, lung congestion, or wounds. Clinical assessment includes recognizing the clinical features of delirium and evaluating precipitating factors. In some cases, psychiatric evaluation and consultation may be helpful in assessment, diagnosis, and management.

Objective assessment

Many assessment tools are available to assist in screening and monitoring, including the Confusion Assessment Method (CAM),[20] Delirium Rating Scale,[21] Memorial Delirium Assessment Scale,[20] and the Mini-Mental State Exam (MMSE).[20]

While it is important to understand assessment methods to accurately characterize delirium in the dying patient, goals of care will determine the amount and type of diagnostic testing used to identify potentially reversible etiologies and the interventions used to treat the cause(s). If the primary goal is symptom relief, diagnostic testing and cause-directed interventions might be minimal.

Degrees of toxicity

The Revised Delirium Rating Scale (DRS-R-98) is the most widely used diagnostic and assessment tool to measure delirium symptom severity.[21] This 16-item clinician-rated scale includes 13 severity items and 3 diagnostic items (temporal onset of symptoms, fluctuation of symptoms, and physical disorder). The 13-item severity section can be scored separately from the 3-item diagnostic section; their sum constitutes the total scale score. The severity of individual items is rated from 0 to 3 points so that scores range from 0 to 39, with higher scores indicating more severe delirium, and a cut-off score of 15 or greater being consistent with a diagnosis of delirium. The total scale can be scored initially to enhance the differential diagnosis by capturing characteristic features of delirium, such as acute onset and fluctuation of symptom severity. All items are anchored by text descriptions as guides for rating cognition along a continuum from normal to severely impaired. The DRS-R-98 has high interrater reliability, validity, sensitivity, and specificity for distinguishing delirium from mixed neuropsychiatric populations including dementia, depression, and schizophrenia.[21]

Assessment over time is critical to recognize delirium early in its course and to monitor for response to therapies. A continuous delirium assessment instrument, the Nursing Delirium Screening Scale (Nu-DESC), is an observational

DSM-IV criteria-designed, five-item scale that can be completed quickly and was created to assess patients for delirium over time[22] (Table 34-4). The advantages of the Nu-DESC are that it is easy to use, time-efficient, and accurate, and could lead to prompt delirium recognition and treatment.[22]

SYMPTOM MANAGEMENT STRATEGIES

When delirium is suspected, the first parameters of assessment are environmental safety and identifying a patient-appointed proxy decision maker. The latter point is key but often overlooked. Although patients with mild delirium may maintain capacity to make simple choices, a proxy decision maker should be consulted on more complex issues regarding overall treatment considerations.[5]

At end-of-life, the goals in managing delirium are to reverse or minimize the symptom if possible, to maintain safety for the patient and caregivers, to reduce caregiver burden, and to preserve quality of life for both the patient and home caregivers.[6] Delirium management is multifaceted. Treatment should be consistent with the patient's goals of care, which may include elimination and modification of previously used medications, hydration, and other therapies. Decisions such as whether to use antibiotics to treat infection when death is imminent can be controversial. Pharmacologic and nonpharmacologic approaches for symptom relief are often used in combination. In some cases, consultation with psychiatry may be indicated.

Therapeutic approaches

Pharmacologic. Although there are no Food and Drug Administration (FDA)–approved drugs for delirium, antipsychotics are the mainstay of delirium management, as they can relieve perceptual disturbances and agitation.[5,17,19] Both

TABLE 34-4

Nursing Delirium Screening Scale (Nu-DESC)

Features and descriptions	**Symptoms Rating (0–2)**		
Symptom / **Time Period**	**Midnight – 8 AM**	**8 AM – 4 PM**	**4 PM – Midnight**
I. Disorientation Verbal or behavioral manifestation of not being oriented to time or place or misperceiving persons in the environment.			
II. Inappropriate behavior Behavior inappropriate to place and/or for the person; e.g., pulling at tubes or dressings, attempting to get out of bed when that is contraindicated, and the like.			
III. Inappropriate communication Communication inappropriate to place and/or for the person; e.g., incoherence, uncommunicativeness, nonsensical or unintelligible speech.			
IV. Illusions/hallucinations Seeing or hearing things that are not there; distortions of visual objects.			
V. Psychomotor retardation Delayed responsiveness, few or no spontaneous actions/words; e.g., when the patient is prodded, reaction is deferred and/or the patient is unarousable.			
Total score			

The Nursing Delirium Screening Scale (Nu-DESC). Symptoms are rated from 0 to 2 based on the presence and intensity of each symptom and individual ratings are added to obtain a total score per shift. The first four items of the Nu-DESC are included in the Confusion Rating Scale (CRS).

Source: Data from Gaudreau et al[22].

conventional antipsychotics and newer atypical antipsychotics are effective. Drug selection is based on availability, dosing forms, side-effect profiles, and cost. Haloperidol is most commonly used in doses of 0.5–2 mg IV or PO every 1 to 6 hours, up to a total 24-hour dose of 20 mg.[12,17] The adverse effects of antipsychotics include sedation, extrapyramidal effects (e.g., akathesia, dystonia, tremor, anxiety), hypotension, anticholinergic effects, weight gain, and QTc prolongation (seen on electrocardiogram). However, the last issue is rarely a consideration in the patient imminently approaching death.

Benzodiazepines are not considered a first-line treatment unless delirium is related to alcohol withdrawal. These agents often cause paradoxical worsening of delirium.[6] Control of hyperactive delirium may require a combination of an antipsychotic and benzodiazepine, but benzodiazepines alone should be avoided.

The incidence of delirium is high in actively dying patients.[9] This symptom is distressing for family and patient, and the usual management strategies may prove ineffective. Delirium may be a contraindication to home management if it is not well-controlled, as comfort and safety may be difficult to establish.[6] In addition to nonpharmacologic therapies, palliative sedation may be considered in extreme cases. [23]

Nonpharmacologic. Nonpharmacologic interventions have demonstrated a reduced incidence of delirium, faster symptom relief, and improved cognition and quality of life without any effect on mortality.[6] A restful environment decreases extraneous stimuli. Such a setting may include soft lighting to avoid shadows and music if soothing to the patient, but not television or radio as background noise. The presence of a familiar person such as a family member or caregiver may be calming, as may verbal reassurance about the personal safety. Clocks and calendars can provide reorientation, as can verbal reminders about day of week and time of day and familiar objects from home (e.g., a favorite blanket or pillow, pictures). Use of eyeglasses and hearing aids increases accuracy of sensory inputs. Nonconfrontational redirection is a useful strategy to manage hallucinations and delusions. Acknowledge the patient's experience. Even routine care such as providing hygiene should be explained. Physical restraints at end-of-life are rarely indicated, and family presence is usually the primary strategy to ensure safety. Supporting the family provides reassurance and assists in maintaining the restful environment.[6]

Nursing implications

Delirium at end-of-life is one of the most distressing symptoms that a family may face. Patients' utterances when they are delirious can be upsetting to the family if the utterances are interpreted as patient expressions of distress. In some cases, as when utterances are interpreted as "near death awareness," families may feel comforted if patients are able to reminisce or express feelings of peace in "seeing" that they are going to a peaceful place. Expert pharmacologic and nonpharmacologic management is a critical component of end-of-life care so that family memories of the patients last days and hours are peaceful.

NOISY AIRWAY SECRETIONS/INEFFECTIVE AIRWAY CLEARANCE

THE PROBLEM

Noisy airway secretions (NAS) at the end of a patient's life are often referred to as "the death rattle." NAS are produced by oscillatory movements of secretions in the upper airways associated with the inspiratory and expiratory phases of expiration. These secretions occur in imminently dying patients who are obtunded or are too weak to expectorate.[24]

Incidence and etiology

Noisy airway secretions are reported to occur in 23% to 93% of patients in their last hours before death.[25] Patients who have an increased risk of respiratory congestion (e.g., patients with a diagnosis of lung cancer, cerebral metastases, pneumonia, and dysphagia) or any pulmonary pathology are more likely to have this symptom. The incidence of NAS increases the closer a patient is to death. The median time to death, once NAS are noted, is 8 to 23 hours.[25]

PATHOPHYSIOLOGY

The respiratory tract is lined with ciliated epithelial cells that continuously move mucus up the respiratory tract to be either subconsciously swallowed or coughed out. Mucus is produced by submucosal glands. Resting glands secrete mucus at a rate of approximately 9 mL/min.[25] When secretions are unable to be processed normally and begin to pool, audible breathing is heard as the turbulent air passes over the secretions. An increase in ventilatory rate and airway resistance increases the amount of turbulence.

SYMPTOM ASSESSMENT

Risk factors

Factors that contribute to the presence of NAS include excessive secretion of respiratory mucus, abnormal quality of mucus secretions inhibiting clearance, cilia dysfunction, inability to swallow, diminished cough reflex, and recumbent position. It is unclear whether hydration plays any role in the development or degree of NAS. Additionally, some speculation has focused on whether there are two subtypes of NAS.

Type I NAS is described as predominately an accumulation of salivary secretions related to a decline in consciousness and swallowing reflexes. Type II NAS is characterized by accumulation of bronchial secretions over several days as the patient becomes too weak to cough. Bronchial secretory glands are largely innervated by cholinergic nerve fibers, but other mechanisms (adrenergic nerves, cough receptor stimulation, and inflammatory changes) can also stimulate these glands. This theoretical distinction between Type I and Type II secretions has not been associated with clinicians' responses to NAS or choice of treatment.[24]

Objective assessment

A focused and thorough history and physical examination are key to evaluate for any treatable underlying causes. If physical findings associated with fluid overload are identified, a trial of diuretic should be considered. If pneumonia is thought to be the cause, a trial of antibiotics might be appropriate. Table 34-5 illustrates a recently validated assessment tool, the Victoria Respiratory Congestion Scale (VRCS),[26] which may be helpful in providing objective assessment regarding the intensity of the NAS and the effectiveness of interventions.

Objective signs of NAS include audible gurgling, rattling, or crackling sounds in the upper airway with each breath. Vibrations may be palpated across the chest, and percussion is likely to yield dullness. On auscultation, it is common to hear prominent rhonchi in the upper lung fields and trachea with wheezing in the lower bases.

In addition to physical assessment, it is important to assess how family members, friends, and loved ones interpret or respond to the NAS.

SYMPTOM MANAGEMENT STRATEGIES

Therapeutic approaches

Pharmacologic. If there is a suspected reversible cause of the NAS and it is in accordance with prognosis and family wishes, this condition should be the first focus of treatment. Therapy may include the use of diuretics for suspected fluid overload or antibiotics for infection. More often, if the patient is near death, these interventions are less useful and anticholinergic drugs become the primary mode of treatment. Some speculation suggests that anticholinergic agents are more effective with non-expectorated salivary or bronchial secretions, but less effective when NAS are caused by respiratory pathology including infection, tumor, fluid retention, and aspiration.[24] The most recent Cochrane Review reports no conclusive evidence for the effectiveness of anticholinergic therapy; nevertheless, because the practice of treating NAS with anticholinergics is so deeply ingrained in hospice care,

TABLE 34-5

The Victoria Respiratory Congestion Scale (VRCS)

VRCS Score	Observation
0	Congestion absent
1	Congestion audible at 12 inches(30 cm) from patient's chest but not further
2	Congestion audible at the end of the bed but not further
3	Congestion audible at the doorway of the room

Instructions:

- The staff member stands beside the patient's bed, bends slightly over the patient's chest, turns his or her head at 12 inches(30 cm) from the chest, and listens for several breaths. The staff then moves to the end of the bed and listens again for several breaths, and similarly at the door of the room
  - If no congestion is heard at the chest, the score is 0/3
  - If congestion is heard at the chest but not the foot of the bed, the score is 1/3
  - If congestion is heard at the chest and at the foot of the bed only, the score is 2/3
  - If congestion is heard at the doorway, the score is 3/3
- Distinction should be made between 'congested breathing' and 'snoring' or 'tachypnea,' which are not counted as congestion.
- Room noise should be reduced as possible (e.g., radio or television turned down) during assessment
- The room size is based on an approximate single room. If in a larger four-bed ward, the distance from the bed to where an average doorway would be is used.
- Whatever the room size or ambience, repeated measurements should replicate as best as possible the same conditions in order to compare changes in the VRCS.

Source: Data from Downing and Wainwright[26].

it is likely to continue.[27,28] The report underlines that there is no compelling evidence that one anticholinergic drug is superior to another, and it urges close monitoring for lack of therapeutic benefit and adverse effects so that futile treatments can be discontinued.[28] The anticholinergic medications typically used for this indication include hyoscine hydrobromide (scopolamine), atropine sulfate, and glycopyrrolate (Robinul). Atropine sulfate ophthalmic drops are often administered via an oral route in unconscious patients.

Nonpharmacologic. Reposition the patient onto his or her side with the head slightly elevated. Consider decreasing or stopping IV fluids. Suctioning is usually not recommended, as it is thought to cause more discomfort and agitation. If copious secretions are apparent in the oropharynx, gentle oral suctioning may be indicated. Patient and family teaching is an important mainstay of treatment. Appendix 34B offers some helpful suggestions for family members who are helping to care for a loved one with NAS.

Nursing implications

Though there is a dearth of evidence to suggest that NAS are distressing to patients at end-of-life, this symptom is often extremely upsetting for the family. Preventing or reducing NAS through pharmacologic use of antisecretory agents, reducing or eliminating parenteral hydration, and positioning can be a comfort to family. Nurses must be diligent in the care of patients with NAS by following evidence-based treatments and avoiding suctioning except for gentle oral suctioning.

INTRACTABLE SYMPTOMS AND PALLIATIVE SEDATION

THE PROBLEM

Intractable symptoms and suffering are concepts that can only be defined by the patient. Intractable symptoms or conditions of suffering are ones that the patient finds intolerable and that have not responded to treatment.[29–31] For a symptom to be defined as intractable, it must have been treated with all available remedies that have an acceptable risk to the patient.

As many as 35% of patients at end-of-life report "severe" pain and as many as 25% describe "intolerable" dyspnea.[32] As defined by Cecily Saunders, spiritual pain, psychosocial suffering, and physical pain are all components of "total pain."[33] For the purpose of management of intractable symptoms and intolerable suffering, there is generally a distinction made among symptoms that are physical, emotional, or existential. In the absence of intractable physical symptoms such as pain, delirium, or dyspnea, there is a lack of consensus regarding the use of strategies such as palliative sedation.[34,35]

Definition

Palliative sedation (PS) is the use of medications to provide decreased consciousness for the purpose of limiting suffering due to intractable symptoms in the imminently dying patient.[31,36] Palliative sedation is one therapeutic tool that may be used, with patient consent, for the treatment of refractory symptoms such as pain or dyspnea or, most commonly, for terminal delirium or agitation. Delirium, or terminal restlessness, that is not responsive to treatments such as haloperidol or other antipsychotics has been identified as the primary symptom for which PS is used.[30] With careful attention to patient values, palliative sedation can be used with appropriateness and dignity.

Palliative sedation to treat intractable symptoms or intolerable suffering has been described in the literature using a variety of terms, including "sedation," "terminal sedation," "sedation for intractable distress," "end-of-life sedation," "total sedation," "palliative sedation," and "palliative sedation therapy."[29–31,37] Currently, PS is the preferred term because it more accurately reflects the intent to provide relief or palliate intractable symptoms or suffering through sedation, rather than using sedation to hasten death in the terminally ill patient.[38] Conversely, "terminal sedation" might be interpreted to mean that the intent of the sedation is to terminate the patient's life.[30] De Graeff and Dean prefer the use of the term "palliative sedation therapy" because it provides the indication that it is a therapy to be used in palliative care, distinct from other forms of sedation.[30] Levy and Cohen use the term "palliative sedation" to indicate the deliberate use of sedative agents to provide either a temporary or permanent, light to deep level of sedation in consenting patients with terminal illness who are suffering with intractable symptoms.[29] Importantly, they note that the goal of this therapy is the relief of intractable symptoms, but not the hastening of death.

Incidence and etiology

Because so many different terms have been used in the literature to refer to PS in the terminally ill patient, it is difficult to determine the frequency of its use. Sources suggest an incidence ranging from 2% to 63%.[31,37,39] The wide variation in these numbers may be accounted for by the inclusion of U.S. and European studies and variations in practice due to differences in culture and practice laws. Generally, PS use is limited to the hospital or inpatient hospice setting, although some authors note its use in the home hospice setting.[29]

ETHICAL PRINCIPLES UNDERLYING THE USE OF PALLIATIVE SEDATION

Proportionality of sedation is a crucial concept in PS. Proportionality implies an ethical sense of degree that is applied to the action. In PS, this is the degree of sedation used for initial and ongoing medication titration to treat the symptom. Because the intention of PS is to relieve intractable symptoms and suffering, sedating medications are administered in proportional doses to induce a level of sedation required to relieve the patient-defined level of suffering. Proportionality also implies that the patient and family have been involved in the decision making about the depth of sedation desired. Mild sedation may allow for the relief of suffering caused by the intractable symptom while maintaining the patient's ability to be aroused and participate in ongoing assessments, decision-making, and interactions with loved ones. Some advocate for the minimum level of sedation to be used so that ongoing assessments of consent and symptom management can be accomplished. The National Hospice and Palliative Care Organization position statement refers to this as "controlled administration" of sedative agents so as to reduce a patient's consciousness minimally with the goal of rendering "intolerable and intractable suffering tolerable."[31] At times, proportionality would require deeper sedation without the opportunity to have ongoing intervals of arousal and consent due to the severity of the symptom being treated, such as with palliative sedation for intractable seizures, bleeding, delirium, or pain. With deep sedation, the patient is no longer able to participate in life closure activities that may have meaning to both patient and family. However, if suffering is severe, the peace of deep sedation may be a benefit that outweighs the burden.

Other foundational ethical principles to consider when discussing the appropriate use, risks, and benefits of PS with a patient or family include autonomy or self-determination, fidelity, beneficence and nonmaleficence, "double effect," and substituted judgment (in cases of patients who lack capacity for medical decision-making).[40] Autonomy or self-determination, defined as the informed patient's right to choose or refuse offered treatments, is the primary consideration underlying the appropriate use of PS in end-of-life care.[41] By obtaining informed consent prior to the start of PS, patient autonomy is respected. Appendix 34C provides a sample informed consent document for PS.[42] If a patient lacks capacity to participate in decision making, a family meeting is recommended to ensure that all members have an opportunity to participate in this critically important decision process. Table 34-6 provides a documentation template for capturing the essential components of such

TABLE 34-6

Family Meeting Agenda/Documentation When Using Palliative Sedation
Patient name: ________________ DOB: ________
DATE: ________ Time: ________ Location: ________
Attendees:
Facilitator:
Person documenting:
Durable Power of Attorney for Health Care: ________________
Patient's Attending Physician: ________________
Description of discussion of patient's condition and prognosis:
Description of discussion of patient's symptoms, interventions to date, possible additional interventions, and risk and benefits of these interventions:
Description of discussion about definition and initiation of palliative sedation:
• Document patient or surrogate decision about palliative sedation.
Description of discussion about the use of medically administered hydration or nutrition:
• Document patient or surrogate decision about medically administered hydration and nutrition.
Description of the plan for palliative sedation:
• Start date/time; location; clinicians involved; other individuals to be present
• Medications, tests, and interventions to be discontinued
• Medications, tests, and interventions to be continued.

Source: Data from Dartmouth Hitchcock Medical Center[42].

a family meeting.[42] Ongoing assessment of the patient or surrogate's agreement with the plan of care demonstrates continued respect for patient autonomy. Continued and meaningful communication between the patient, surrogate decision maker, and the clinical team forms the basis of providing informed consent prior to the use of PS.

Fidelity, or non-abandonment, concerns the need for healthcare providers to provide clear and truthful information and to be "present." Physical presence and emotional accessibility are aspects of "presence" and a component of fidelity. To truly be present—to "not abandon" the patient—requires emotional, intellectual, and physical presence. This consideration is especially salient for the patient with intractable symptoms who wishes to obtain the relief that PS could provide.

Beneficence and nonmaleficence imply an obligation to keep a patient's interests in the foreground while avoiding causing harm. Beneficence and nonmaleficence guide providers as they assess the patient and determine appropriate medication titration, patient comfort, and overall symptom control. Family involvement, education, and support also demonstrate the principle of beneficence.

The principle of double effect, which originated in Roman Catholic theology, considers the intent of an action to take primacy over the possible outcomes.[31] This principle applies in situations where an intended effect "runs the foreseeable danger of harm."[29,40] The intended benefit of PS is the relief of suffering, even though a foreseeable, unintended effect may be the possibility of hastening death. Several tenets or conditions must be met for an action to be considered acceptable under the principle of double effect. First, the act itself must be morally neutral or good. Second, the intent of the act must be good or beneficial. Third, a bad effect or negative outcome is possible and acknowledged. Fourth, the good effect follows from the action. Lastly, the intended benefit must be of significant value to the patient to have him or her put at risk.[40]

Participation in PS may evoke strong feelings for all involved, including nurses and other disciplines. Clinicians' religious or moral beliefs may not be consistent with participation in PS. As such, providing staff members with an opportunity to withdraw from participation in the administration of PS is appropriate. Institutions may choose to have a written policy and educate their staff about this issue at orientation as well as prior to the PS procedure itself.

SYMPTOM ASSESSMENT

Terminal delirium, terminal agitation, nausea, vomiting, pain, and confusion are the most common symptoms for which PS has been used. Prior to a symptom being labeled as "intractable," it must have been treated with all available pharmacologic and psychosocial treatments that are acceptable to the patient and the provider. Consultation with palliative care specialists or the bioethics committee is strongly suggested to assure that all acceptable and available treatments for the intractable symptom have been employed. Table 34-7 provides a comprehensive checklist to consider before proceeding with PS.[42]

SYMPTOM MANAGEMENT STRATEGIES

Institutional policy and procedure for patient consent (see Appendix 34-C for a sample informed consent form for patients undergoing palliative sedation),[42] care, and documentation of mandatory and advisable actions for PS should be accessible to all staff. The use of PS creates responsibilities both for families and for the healthcare team. Families value the provision of clear, understandable, and meaningful information about the procedure and their loved one.[43] Table 34-6 provides a guideline for a family meeting agenda that is an important and mandatory step prior to initiating PS. Staff will benefit from clear guidelines, the support of other staff members, and the option to conscientiously object to participation in the procedure. Knowledgeable and skilled staff are needed to carry out PS. The availability of knowledgeable staff may be one factor in initiating clinically indicated PS.

Prior to initiating PS, there may be a number of other important care decisions to be addressed with the patient and family—for example, decisions regarding the discontinuation of medical treatments such as medically administered nutrition and hydration, implantable cardiac defibrillators (ICDs) and pacemakers, use of vasopressors, continuation of close monitoring of vital signs, and lab assessments.[44] Few patients will remain capable of taking oral nutrition; however, if medically administered nutrition and hydration have been discontinued, and the patient is able, feeding of favored foods in small amounts may be acceptable. For all patients, careful oral hygiene is needed and can be taught to family, who may find this offering of care for their loved one to be a healing experience. The decision to continue or discontinue medically administered nutrition and hydration is independent of the PS decision.[45] As with other interventions, the risks and benefits of medically administered nutrition and hydration require monitoring and discussion with the patient and family as the situation evolves.[45]

Implanted cardiac defibrillators are a more common medical intervention than medically administered nutrition and hydration, as evidenced by a doubling of these devices' insertion rates from 46,000 in 2001 to 114,000 in 2006.[46]

TABLE 34-7

Palliative Sedation Checklist

- Allergy(s) and adverse drug reactions verified in medical record
- Weight: ____________________ kg
- CODE STATUS:
  - DNR/DNI order placed
- PALLIATIVE SEDATION CRITERIA (check all)
  - Terminal illness present as defined by prognosis of 6 months or less
  - Refractory symptoms present and
    - Concerted efforts short of sedation have failed to provide relief
    - AND
    - Additional interventions are unlikely to provide adequate relief within reasonable time from OR will likely cause unacceptable morbidity
  - Severe refractory symptoms are primarily physical
    - Although, psychological distress may be contributing to patient's suffering
  - Palliative Care Service assessment has been performed and documented by ____________________ MD/DO/APRN/PA
  - Palliative Care Service facilitated a family meeting that occurred and is documented by ____________________ MD/DP/APRN/PA on ____________________ date.
  - Patient or surrogate has signed an informed consent for palliative sedation
  - Involved staff have been informed of the plan and concerns regarding conscientious objection are accommodated.
- CONSULTS COMPLETED as needed
  - Psychiatry (should occur if severe psychological symptoms are refractory to treatments)
  - Palliative Care Service (mandatory)
- PATIENT CARE ORDERS
  - Bedrest with side rails in place
  - Hydration and nutrition as decided in family/patient meeting
- PATIENT MONITORING
  - Vital signs (temperature, heart rate, respiratory rate and blood pressure) every 8 hours
    - If comfort measures only (CMO), no vital signs monitoring need be done.
  - Level of sedation (Ramsay score) and comfort at least hourly
    - Document in appropriate areas of medical record

Source: Data from Dartmouth Hitchcock Medical Center[42].

Pacemaker insertions have increased as well. The majority of patients receiving these devices are older than 65 years, making it likely that discussion of the continued use of these devices as end-of-life approaches will be needed. Because ICDs can prolong life by preventing cardiac sudden death from abnormal tachyarrhythmias and treating bradyarrhythmias,[46] there is the risk that such a device may critically alter the dying experience. ICDs' continued activation during the active dying phase presents the potential for multiple cardiac shocks, which are both painful and inconsistent with a "do not resuscitate" (DNR) or "comfort measures only" (CMO) status. Criteria for the continued use or deactivation of these devices are lacking. Moreover, few patients or families understand their choices in having the device deactivated. Careful discussions of the associated risks and benefits are needed. The continued use of a pacemaker may improve quality of life during a terminal illness, but when a patient is actively dying or when PS is being considered, discussion of deactivation of both the ICD and the pacemaker should be considered.[46]

Providing and documenting all appropriate physical comfort care, such as mouth care, skin care, bowel and bladder management, and pain management, continues to be needed. Individual institutions may wish to have a protocol that identifies the frequency of these assessments and their documentation. Table 34-7[42] and Table 34-8[47] provide guidelines for documentation to accompany the palliative sedation procedure.

Therapeutic approaches

Medications used for palliative sedation. There are no clinical trials on which to base palliative sedation drug selection for end-of-life patients.[48] Categories of medications often used for PS include benzodiazepines, barbiturates, and anesthetics. Benzodiazepines are usually part of a PS regimen because they are commonly used to manage anxiety, are effective anticonvulsants, and work synergistically with opioids and antipsychotics. As a result, benzodiazepines have become the most frequently used drugs for PS in the United States.[34] Midazolam is the most frequently used benzodiazepine for the purpose of PS because of its short half-life and its ease of titration.[48]

TABLE 34-8

Nursing Documentation During Palliative Sedation

Prior to onset of Palliative Sedation

- Indication for implementation of palliative sedation
- Informed consent signed
- Goals of therapy
  - Depth of sedation
  - Refractory symptom being treated
- Medication ordered
- Family desire to be present
- Appropriate nursing documentation specific to patient situation and care.

During course of Palliative Sedation

- Medication use and administration
  - Initiation dose
  - Titrations – dose, patient assessments, time
- Depth of sedation achieved
  - Ramsay score (or similar assessment of sedation)
- Distress level/relief of distress
- Satisfaction of patient and/or family
- Patient care interventions for comfort

Frequency of assessment and documentation to be determined by the institution. A suggested minimal interval is every 8 hours and as indicated by patient condition. Mandatory documentation when a dose adjustment is made.

Source: Data from Dartmouth Hitchcock Medical Center[42].

Sedatives such as propofol and barbiturates such as pentobarbital have also been used for this indication, although many clinicians have less experience using these medications.[48] These medications have the advantages of a rapid onset of action and anticonvulsant properties. In general, barbiturates are reliable, cause a rapid onset of sedation, and have a different action from opioids and benzodiazepines; the last feature may be helpful for patients with tolerance or intolerance issues. However, sedatives do not provide analgesia, so ongoing analgesia with opioids is essential.[34] Paralytic agents are not used for PS because they lack efficacy for symptom relief.[48]

Consideration of side effects and institutional requirements are important in drug selection. State regulatory agencies may need to be contacted to determine the nurse's practice parameters regarding administration of agents for PS. Nurses will need to continue to assess the patient's comfort, degree of control of the intractable symptom, and proportional medication use. Checklists or guidelines that identify the frequency of assessments, symptoms to be assessed, and use of validated measures for assessment of sedation (such as the Ramsay Sedation Scale [Table 34-9][49]) can be used to create a palliative sedation policy to guide nursing care. Table 34-10 outlines common medications used for PS[32,34,49] and Table 34-11 illustrates a palliative sedation medication order sheet.[42]

Nursing implications

Palliative sedation for intractable symptom management is an uncommon treatment. However, when it is indicated, nurses are in a key position to provide ethical, diligent, and compassionate care for the patient and family. Transparency and communication among staff, patient, and family will ensure that all concerned are able to feel comfortable with this difficult care choice.

TABLE 34-9

Ramsay Sedation Scale

Score	Responsiveness
1	Patient is anxious and agitated or restless, or both.
2	Patient is cooperative, oriented, and tranquil.
3	Patient responds to commands only.
4	Patient exhibits brisk response to light glabellar tap or loud auditory stimulus.
5	Patient exhibits sluggish response to light glabellar tap or loud auditory stimulus.
6	Patient exhibits no response.

Source: Data from Cohen et al[49].

TABLE 34-10

Palliative Sedation Medications

	MIDAZOLAM Rapid, short-acting benzodiazepine	PENTOBARBITAL Long-acting barbiturate
ONSET OF ACTION	1 – 5 minutes	30 – 60 seconds (IV)
DURATION OF ACTION	60 – 120 minutes	60 – 180 minutes
HALF LIFE	1 – 4 hours	Average 22 hours
PEAK EFFECT	20 – 60 minutes	120 minutes
LOADING DOSE	1 – 5 mg	2 – 3 mg/kg slow IV push (no faster than 50 mg/min)
INITIAL DOSE	0.5 – 1 mg/hour	1 – 2 mg/kg/hour following initial bolus (loading dose)
TITRATION	1 – 2 mg/hour every 20 minutes to achieve minimal effective dose to maintain desired level of sedation	0.5 mg/kg/hour every 20 minutes to achieve minimal effective dose to maintain desired level of sedation
MAXIMUM DOSE	20 mg/hour	Not available
ROUTE	IV or SC	IV
INTERMITTENT DOSING SCHEDULE	Use 50% of hourly dose as an IV bolus every 30 minutes PRN signs of discomfort or awakening	Not available

Source: Data from Storey and Knight[32]; Cherney and Radbruch[34]; Cohen et al[49].

TABLE 34-11

Palliative Sedation Medication Orders

The ordering provider MUST be present at initiation of orders and remain readily accessible to nursing staff until a state of stable sedation of Ramsay Sedation Scale of 4–5 is achieved.

- Midazolam
  - Initial bolus
    - (2 – 5 mg) ________________ mg IV push
    - Followed by (1 – 2 mg) ____________ mg every 10 minutes until sedated.
  - Continuous infusion:
    - Begin hourly rate at half total initial dose required to sedate patient.
    - Titrate by (1 – 2 mg) ____________ mg/hr every 20 minutes to achieve minimal effective dose to maintain sedation.
    - Rate NOT to exceed 20 mg/hr.
  - Intermittent dose:
    - 50% of hourly dose as an IV bolus every 30 minutes PRN signs of discomfort or awakening.
- Pentobarbital
  - Initial bolus:
    - 2 mg/kg = ____________ mg slow (infuse over ____________ minutes IV infusion to induce sedation).
  - Continuous infusion (4 mg/mL)
    - 1 mg/kg/hour following initial bolus
    - Titrate by 0.5 mg/kg/hour every 20 minutes to achieve minimal effective dose to maintain sedation (per Ramsay Scale)
  - For signs of discomfort or awakening, call ordering provider for additional orders

Signature __________________________ MD/DO/APRN/PA Date ____________________ Time: ____________________

Print Name: __________________________ Pager # ___________________________

Source: Data from Dartmouth Hitchcock Medical Center[42].

CARE OF THE PATIENT AND FAMILY WHEN DEATH IS IMMINENT

THE PROBLEM

In the weeks and months prior to death, many indicators of the body's failure are apparent. Lab tests may reveal a decreased albumin and total protein level due to decreased food intake and declining hepatic function. The patient may exhibit outward signs of approaching death. Physically, the patient may become weaker and have longer and more frequent periods of sleep. The desire for food and fluids generally decreases, and the gastrointestinal tract function declines as end-of-life approaches. Feeding is often seen as an act of love and caring; when the patient has little or no desire for food, the family may need guidance to understand the physical basis for this symptom.

Closer to the time of death, breathing becomes less regular and increasingly shallow, resulting in respiratory acidosis. Cheyne-Stokes respirations (a pattern of shallow respirations alternating with deep respirations) may present. Informing the family of this pattern can help them as they observe their loved one. Airway congestion and noisy airway secretions may occur, resulting in increased sounds of respiration (described earlier in this chapter). Circulation changes occur as the heart beats less vigorously and more erratically. Blood pressure decreases, the pulse becomes erratic, and the skin may show signs of mottling. These changes may also be accompanied by decreased body temperature that may be detected starting at the extremities and moving toward the torso.

SYMPTOM ASSESSMENT

Objective assessment: patient

Dying patients continue to have physical, medical, psychosocial, emotional, and spiritual needs.[50] Approaching death is different for each person in each of these domains. The presence of caregivers, family, and friends can assist and support the patient during this journey. Physical symptoms associated with imminent death may include cool extremities, mottling of the skin, Cheyne-Stokes respirations, decreased urine output, and restlessness. As described earlier, patients may develop periods of delirium as death approaches. They may also experience near death awareness and talk of others who have already died, or about travel (i.e., "going home") or change. It may help family members to understand this process and be aware that their loved one may ask for permission to die (Table 34-2).[7,8]

Social needs may relate to unfinished business and the maintenance of important relationships. The need to love, give love, extend forgiveness, and accept forgiveness are part of the completion of life's tasks.[51] Hope and inner peace can be supported through rituals, religious practices, or cultural practices known to be of value to the patient.[50]

Prior careful discussion of personal values and decisions made regarding the use or deactivation of medical devices such as ICDs can prove helpful to maintaining the dignity of the patient as death approaches. These prior discussions are best made with the patient's loved ones so their grief and bereavement will be moderated by the knowledge that the patient's wishes were known and respected.

Objective assessment: family

As families adjust to the impending loss of a loved one, the roles of various members of the family may evolve and change. Death of a family member may cause individuals to face fears of their own mortality, which can result in a time of reflection that results in personal growth. Periods of loneliness and alienation may also become apparent as individuals process their own changing life circumstances.[50] Nurses can be aware of these aspects of coping and guide the family through this process with information and compassionate presence.

While most family members primarily want assurance that their loved one is comfortable and free from pain, other needs related to emotional, psychological, and spiritual domains may arise. Communication between clinicians and families during the dying process is essential at this time.[43] Essential communication includes coaching on patient care, allowing time to be with their loved one to process grief, and providing postdeath care with dignity. Another aspect of importance to families is interdisciplinary conversations. Bereaved families have reported that being prepared by clinicians about the dying process was an important part of their loved ones' end-of-life care.[43] However, providers should take care to discuss patient care matters privately where they cannot be overheard when speaking among themselves, as this can be very upsetting to the patient and family.[43]

Assessing the family's understanding of the physical signs of dying, the means of providing comfort, and their own ability to comfort and support one another becomes a priority for the nurse. Knowledge of and attention to the family's cultural and spiritual beliefs becomes an important aspect of the nursing assessment.

SYMPTOM MANAGEMENT STRATEGIES

Therapeutic approaches: patients

Physical symptoms can be managed with medications, physical care, massage, and positioning, as well as with energy therapies such as Reiki or Therapeutic Touch.[52]

Music may also be very helpful in active and passive participation in transitions and grief.[53] Music can assist the relaxation response and decrease anxiety, thereby decreasing physical pain. Coping can be supported through speech, singing, or playing of meaningful religious, spiritual, or culturally significant music.

In the last days or hours of life, vital signs are usually not taken; ICDs and pacemakers may be deactivated.[46] Gently assessing patients' needs for oral care and providing sips of fluid for hydration can be done with family assistance, while supporting the family's need to physically care for their loved one. Consistent with patient and family wishes, comfort measures and do not resuscitate orders should be in place.[54]

After death, supporting the family in their bereavement and maintaining the patient's dignity while providing care of the body become the goals of care. Table 34-12 provides helpful information for nurses and families in recognizing that death has occurred.[55]

Therapeutic approaches: family

Acknowledging the dynamic changes within family members and the family unit can help with family adjustment and grief. Normalizing grief, fear, and sometimes guilt and identifying family and individual strengths can be helpful in guiding families through this process. When a patient and family are cared for by hospice services, they have access to ongoing bereavement support after the patient's death; in contrast, families of patients dying without hospice care may not have been made aware of bereavement support. Families without this support may benefit from assessments by their own primary care provider or therapist, who can help to discern between normal grief and depression that may need treatment.

After the patient's death, family members can spend time with their loved one as desired. System issues particular to the location where death has occurred may have importance. Prior to death, the nurse can identify those issues and develop a plan of care to minimize the impact of those issues on the experience of the family. Identifying who can pronounce the death, having access to items for care of the body in the immediate postmortem period, and obtaining contact phone numbers for the funeral provider, for example, are all important considerations that should ideally be addressed in advance of the death. Prior understanding of the family's cultural and religious considerations, both during and immediately after death, will guide the nurses' care plan. Table 34-13 provides some basic steps in providing care of the body after death has occurred.[55]

TABLE 34-12

Identifying That Death Has Occurred

Physical transitions that may occur at the time of death:

- Respirations stop.
- Heart may beat for a short period after breathing stops.
- No response to verbal or physical stimuli
- Skin changes take place.
  - Pallor, cyanosis, greyness
- Body temperature drops.
- Muscle tone changes.
  - Seizure or muscle twitches may occur briefly.
  - Limbs become limp.
  - Jaw may drop open.
  - Eyes may remain open and pupils become fixed.
  - Bowels and bladder may relax causing defecation and voiding.

Death is determined when:

- Pupils do not respond to light
- No response to verbal or physical stimuli
- No respirations
- No pulse
- No heartbeat

Source: Data from EPEC Education for Physicians for End-of-Life Care[55].

Nursing implications

Caring for patients who are dying and their families can be an extremely meaningful, important, and rewarding experience.[56] Unfortunately, the concept of vicarious trauma—that is, the exposure to traumatic experiences of another—can affect the ability of the nurse to tolerate other stressful situations and can lead to interpersonal difficulties.[57] Nurses who care for dying patients and their families may also experience "compassion fatigue" or "burnout," leading to difficulty coping.[58] Symptoms of compassion fatigue are listed in Table 34-14.[58,59] Risk factors for compassion fatigue are listed in Table 34-15 and include high levels of empathy and exposure to traumatic experiences.[58,59] These traumatic experiences can trigger memories of or feelings about unresolved traumatic experiences or losses the nurse has previously endured, leading to increased stress and the possibility of compassion fatigue coping.[58] Elevated stress levels from vicarious trauma have been found in 38% of oncology nurses.[59] Hospice nurses have been found to be at moderate or high risk (52% and 26%, respectively) for compassion fatigue.[60]

Strategies to develop resilience can be employed through personal, professional, and institutional means. Personal strategies to enhance resilience may include spiritual practices such as meditation or prayer, having a sense of humor, and developing a "personal philosophy of nursing care."[58]

TABLE 34-13

Care of the Body After Death

Core principles:

- Maintain privacy and dignity while providing immediate postmortem care.
- Management of the body and the decedents' possessions are of utmost importance to the bereaved.
- Be aware of cultural, social, and religious requirements related to death and the care of the deceased.
- Prepare the family for viewing the body of their loved one.
  - Provide information about appearance of the body.
  - Remain with family until such time as the nurse is comfortable that the family is managing appropriately with their grief.

Basic guidelines for care of the body after death:

- Wear gloves.
- Elevate head of bed slightly or place head on pillow.
- Close eyes gently.
- Comb or arrange hair.
- Clean oral cavity and replace dentures.
- Wash body gently with mild soap and water and dry.
- Place a rolled towel under the chin to support jaw in closed position.
- Remove medical devices (prior to death, make note of devices that should not be removed according to local system regulations).
- Place clean colostomy bag.
- Cap IV lines or remove if appropriate.
- Remove catheters, tubes, and tape.
- Place absorbent pad at perineum.
- Place adhesive bandages on any puncture wounds.
- Jewelry
  - Consider leaving in place until family can view body.
  - Then, remove jewelry as possible, document to whom it was given.
  - If items not able to be removed, document as such.
- Document any items left with or removed from the body.
- Cover body with a clean sheet and blanket or dress in light clothing.

Considerations before family viewing:

- Determine individuals' comfort level and support decision to view or not view the body.
- Remain with family as needed.
- Allow privacy and encourage talking to and touching the decedent.

Source: Data from EPEC Education for Physicians for End-of-Life Care[55].

Within this text, there are many references for managing grief and loss that can be applied to the nurse's personal practice of self-reflection and that may be part of building resilience.

PATIENT AND FAMILY SELF-CARE

As patients approach death, nurses and family will often need to take over all responsibilities for their personal care, because fatigue and overall debility may prevent patients from performing the self-care activities that allowed them maintain independence during the cancer trajectory. At this phase of care, the nurse's role of encouraging self-care will shift to the family. There are many strategies that nurses can use to encourage family members to aid in the patient's care as well as their own self-care. The self-care guides at the end of this chapter deal with issues that may arise at end-of-life and are particularly challenging. Appendix 34A provides a care guide for families who are dealing with the difficult symptom of delirium. Noisy secretions at end-of-life are also common and distressing; Appendix 34B details helpful information for families to better understand and care for the patient when "death rattle" occurs. Finally, Appendix 34C provides a sample informed consent form for palliative sedation that should be provided to families

TABLE 34-14

Symptoms of Compassion Fatigue
• Increased negative arousal
• Difficulty separating from work and patient issues
• Lowered tolerance to frustration
• Decreased sense of self-competence
• Decreased ability to self-soothe
• Feelings of helplessness
• Decreased activity level
• Changes of sleep patterns

Source: Data from Beck[58]; Quinall et al[59].

TABLE 34-15

Risk Factors for Compassion Fatigue
• Younger age
• Unresolved personal trauma or loss
• Lack of professional or institutional supports
• High level of empathy
• Frequent exposure to trauma or loss

Sources: Data from Beck[58]; Quinall et al[59].

of patients in the rare situation when palliative sedation is needed. Transparency and detailed communication with the family and among healthcare providers will ensure that all patients, even those with intractable symptoms, have a means for peaceful, dignified dying that respects their autonomy.

ACKNOWLEDGMENT

The authors wish to thank Andrew C. Quinn, University of New Hampshire—Nursing/New Hampshire IDeA Network of Biomedical Research Excellence (NH-INBRE) Summer Undergraduate Research Fellow, Dartmouth-Hitchcock Medical Center, for his thoughtful review and suggestions.

REFERENCES

1. Knight P, Espinosa LA. Sedation for refractory symptoms and terminal weaning. In: Ferrell B, Coyle N, eds. *Oxford Textbook of Palliative Nursing.* 3rd ed. Oxford, UK: Oxford University Press; 2012:525–543.
2. National Consensus Project. *Clinical Practice Guidelines for Quality Palliative Care.* 2nd ed. Brooklyn, NY: National Consensus Project for Quality Palliative Care; 2009.
3. Wright AA, Keating NL, Balboni TA, Matulonis UA, Block SD, Prigerson HG. Place of death: correlations with quality of life of patients with cancer and predictors of bereaved caregivers' mental health. *J Clin Oncol.* 2010;28(29):4457–4464.
4. Chirco N, Dunn KS, Robinson SG. The trajectory of terminal delirium at the end of life. *J Hosp Palliat Nurs.* 2011;13(6):411–418.
5. Breitbart W, Alici Y. Delirium. In: Holland J, Breitbart W, Jacobsen P, et al., eds. *Psycho-oncology.* 2nd ed. New York: Oxford University Press; 2010:322–339.
6. Breitbart W, Alici Y. Agitation and delirium at the end of life: "we couldn't manage him." *JAMA.* 2008;300(24):2898–2910, E2891.
7. Marchand L. Near death awareness. *Fast Facts and Concepts* #118. 2009. Available at: http://www.eperc.mcw.edu/fastfact/ff_118.htm. Accessed June 27, 2012.
8. Callahan M, Kelley P. *Final Gifts: Understanding the Special Awareness, Needs, and Communications of the Dying.* New York: Bantam Books; 1992.
9. Lawlor PG, Gagnon B, Mancini IL, et al. Occurrence, causes, and outcome of delirium in patients with advanced cancer: a prospective study. *Arch Intern Med.* 2000;160(6):786–794.
10. American Psychiatric Association. *Diagnostic and Statistical Manual of Mental Disorders-IV-TR.* 4th ed. Arlington, VA: American Psychiatric Association; 2000.
11. de Rooij SE, Schuurmans MJ, van der Mast RC, Levi M. Clinical subtypes of delirium and their relevance for daily clinical practice: a systematic review. *Int J Geriatr Psychiatry.* 2005;20(7):609–615.
12. Heidrich DE, English N. Delirium, confusion, agitation. In: Ferrell B, Coyle N, eds. *Textbook of Palliative Nursing.* 3rd ed. New York: Oxford University Press; 2010:449–468.
13. Leonard M, Raju B, Conroy M, et al. Reversibility of delirium in terminally ill patients and predictors of mortality. *J Palliat Med.* 2008;22(7):848–854.
14. cancer.net Editorial Board. Care during the final days. 2011. Available at: http://www.cancer.net/coping/end-life-care/care-during-final-days. Accessed October 30, 2012.
15. American Cancer Society. *Caring for the Patient with Cancer at Home: A Guide for Patients and Families.* Atlanta, GA: American Cancer Society; 2009.
16. Trzepacz P, Meagher D. Neuropsychiatric aspects of delirium. In: Yodofsky S, Hales R, eds. *Textbook of Neuropsychiatry.* Washington, DC: American Psychiatric Publishing; 2007:445–517.
17. Bush SH, Bruera E. The assessment and management of delirium in cancer patients. *Oncologist.* 2009;14(10):1039–1049.
18. Schrader SLP, Wellik KE, Demaerschalk BM, Caselli RJ, Woodruff BK, Wingerchuk DM. Adjunctive haloperidol prophylaxis reduces postoperative delirium severity and duration in at-risk elderly patients. *Neurologist.* 2008;14(2):134–137.
19. Siddiqi N, Stockdale R, Britton AM, Holmes J. Interventions for preventing delirium in hospitalised patients. *Cochrane Database Syst Rev.* 2007;2:CD005563.
20. Wong CL, Holroyd-Leduc J, Simel DL, Straus SE. Does this patient have delirium? Value of bedside instruments. *JAMA.* 2010;304(7):779–786.
21. Trzepacz PT, Mittal D, Torres R, Kanary K, Norton J, Jimerson N. Validation of the delirium rating scale—revised—98: comparison with the delirium rating scale and the cognitive test for delirium. *J Neuropsychiatry Clin Neurosci.* 2001;13(2):229–242.
22. Gaudreau J-D, Gagnon P, Harel F, Tremblay A, Roy M-A. Fast, systematic, and continuous delirium assessment in hospitalized patients: The nursing delirium screening scale. *J Pain Symptom Manage.* 2005;29(4):368–375.
23. Rietjens JA, van Zuylen L, van Veluw H, van der Wikj L, van der Heide A, van der Rijt CC. Palliative sedation in a specialized unit for acute palliative care in a cancer hospital: comparing patients dying with and without palliative sedation. *J Pain Symptom Manage.* 2008;36(3):228–234.
24. Wildiers H, Menten J. Death rattle: prevalence, prevention and treatment. *J Pain Symptom Manage.* 2002;23(4):310–317.
25. Dudgeon D. Dyspnea, death rattle, and cough. In: Ferrell BR, Coyle N, eds. *Oxford Textbook of Palliative Nursing.* 3rd ed. Oxford, UK: Oxford University Press; 2010:303–320.
26. Downing GM, Wainwright W, eds. *Medical Care of the Dying.* 4th ed. Victoria, BC: Victoria Hospice Society; 2006.

27. Wang J, Nie B, Xiong W, Xu Y. Effect of long-acting beta-agonists on the frequency of COPD exacerbations: a meta-analysis. *J Clin Pharm Ther.* 2012;37(2):204–211.
28. Wee B, Hillier R. Interventions for noisy breathing in patients near to death. *Cochrane Database Syst Rev.* 2008;1:CD005177.
29. Levy MH, Cohen SD. Sedation for the relief of refractory symptoms in the imminently dying: a fine intentional line. *Semin Oncol.* 2005;32(2):237–246.
30. de Graeff A, Dean M. Palliative sedation therapy in the last weeks of life: a literature review and recommendations for standards. *J Palliat Med.* 2007;10(1):67–85.
31. Kirk TW, Mahon MM. National Hospice and Palliative Care Organization (NHPCO) position statement and commentary on the use of palliative sedation in imminently dying terminally ill patients. *J Pain Symptom Manage.* 2010;39(5):914–923.
32. Storey P, Knight, CF. *Unipac 6: Ethical and Legal Decision Making When Caring for the Terminally Ill.* 2nd ed. Glenview, IL: American Academy of Hospice and Palliative Medicine; 2003.
33. Leleszi JP, Lewandowski JG. Pain management in end-of-life care. *J Am Osteopath Assoc.* 2005;105(3 suppl 1):S6–S11.
34. Cherny NI, Radbruch L. European Association for Palliative Care (EAPC) recommended framework for the use of sedation in palliative care. *Palliat Med.* 2009;23(7):581–593.
35. Quill TE, Lo B, Brock DW, Meisel A. Last-resort options for palliative sedation. *Ann Intern Med.* 2009;151(6):421–424.
36. Morita T, Tsunoda J, Inoue S, Chihara S. Effects of high dose opioids and sedatives on survival in terminally ill cancer patients. *J Pain Symptom Manage.* 2001;21(4):282–289.
37. Swart SJ, van der Heide A, van Zuylen L, et al. Considerations of physicians about the depth of palliative sedation at the end of life. *CMAJ.* 2012;184(7):E360–E366.
38. Jackson WC. Palliative sedation vs. terminal sedation: what's in a name? *Am J Hosp Palliat Care.* 2002;19(2):81–82.
39. Mahon MM, McAuley WJ. Oncology nurses' personal understandings about palliative care. *Oncol Nurs Forum.* 2010;37(3):E141–E150.
40. Billings JA. Double effect: a useful rule that alone cannot justify hastening death. *J Med Ethics.* 2011;37(7):437–440.
41. Bakitas M. Self-determination: analysis of the concept and implications for research in palliative care. *Can J Nurs Res.* 2005;37(2):22–49.
42. *Palliative Sedation Policy.* Lebanon, NH: Dartmouth-Hitchcock Medical Center; 2010.
43. Shinjo T, Morita T, Hirai K, et al. Care for imminently dying cancer patients: family members' experiences and recommendations. *J Clin Oncol.* 2010;28(1):142–148.
44. Morita T, Akechi T, Ikenaga M, et al. Late referrals to specialized palliative care service in Japan. *J Clin Oncol.* 2005;23(12):2637–2644.
45. Morita T, Bito S, Kurihara Y, Uchitomi Y. Development of a clinical guideline for palliative sedation therapy using the delphi method. *J Palliat Med.* 2005;8(4):716–729.
46. Morrison LJ, Calvin AO, Nora H, Porter Storey C Jr. Managing cardiac devices near the end of life: a survey of hospice and palliative care providers. *Am J Hosp Palliat Care.* 2010;27(8):545–551.
47. Ghafoor VL, Silus LS. Developing policy, standard orders, and quality-assurance monitoring for palliative sedation therapy. *Am J Health Syst Pharm.* 2011;68(6):523–527.
48. Lo B, Rubenfeld G. Palliative sedation in dying patients: "we turn to it when everything else hasn't worked." *JAMA.* 2005;294(14):1810–1816.
49. Cohen LB, Delegge MH, Aisenberg J, et al. Aga Institute review of endoscopic sedation. *Gastroenterology.* 2007;133(2):675–701.
50. Rokach A, Matalon R, Safarov A, Bercovitch M. The dying, those who care for them, and how they cope with loneliness. *Am J Hosp Palliat Care.* 2007;24(5):399–407.
51. Byock I. *The Four Things That Matter Most: A Book About Living.* New York: Free Press; 2004.
52. Anderson JG, Taylor JG. Effects of healing touch ijn clinical practice: a systematic review of randomized clinical trials. *J Holist Nurs.* 2011;29(3):221–228.
53. Krout RE. Music therapy with imminently dying hospice patients and their families: facilitating release near the time of death. *Am J Hosp Palliat Care.* 2003;20(2):129–134.
54. Parik P, Brokaw F, Saggar S, et al. Has there been any progress in improving the quality of hospitalized death? Replication of a us chart audit study. *BMJ Support Palliat Care.* 2012;2:17–23.
55. Emanuel LL, Ferris FD, von Gunten CF. EPEC. Education for physicians on end-of-life care. *Am J Hosp Palliat Care.* 2002;19:17.
56. Running A, Tolle LW, Girard D. Ritual: the final expression of care. *Int J Nurs Pract.* 2008;14(4):303–307.
57. Sinclair HA, Hamill C. Does vicarious traumatisation affect oncology nurses? A literature review. *Eur J Oncol Nurs.* 2007;11(4):348–356.
58. Beck C. Secondary traumatic stress in nurses: a systematic review. *Arch Psychiatr Nurs.* 2011;25(1):1–10.
59. Quinal L, Harford S, Rutledge DN. Secondary traumatic stress in oncology staff. *Cancer Nurs.* 2009;32(4):E1–E7.
60. Abendroth M, Flannery J. Predicting the risk of compassion fatigue: a study of hospice nurses. *J Hosp Palliat Nurs.* 2006;8(6):346–356.

Understanding, Managing, and Coping with Delirium as Death Approaches

What Is Delirium?

Delirium can affect how a person thinks, remembers, and reasons. It usually comes on suddenly and can make the person either drowsy or agitated. A person with delirium may have difficulty thinking clearly, become forgetful, have hallucinations, or experience events that aren't really happening (e.g., behave as though he or she is at work or doing tasks such as sorting mail or making phone calls).

Why Is This Happening?

Illness can cause patients to not be able to think clearly. This symptom is very common in cancer patients with serious illness. Medications (including prescribed medications), the disease, and treatments can all cause confusion and interfere with a person's ability to think clearly.

Many times, if the problem is brought on by advanced cancer, it may not be able to be reversed. Your healthcare team can help you to know the best ways to deal with this symptom and can help determine if the cause can be reversed. Some cases of delirium at the end of life may result from a sense of "near death awareness." Your hospice or healthcare team can provide you with more information on this topic.

What Can I Do?

Reduce Environmental Distractions and Stimuli

If your loved one is overstimulated by noise, commotion, frequent visitors, and interruptions, you can help by reducing the stimulation in the environment:

- Turn off or turn down television sets.
- Close the door.
- Minimize the use of loud appliances (e.g., vacuums, dishwashers, clothes washers).
- Limit the number of visitors and enforce strict visitation hours.
- Keep conversations quiet and never discuss distressing things where he/she can hear you.
- If he/she has an oxygen concentrator, use extended-length tubing and move the concentrator to another room or put in a closet with the door closed.

Provide Reorientation

Disorientation to time and place (not knowing where you are or when it is) is very distressing and can contribute to delirium and terminal restlessness. If your loved one is confused and disoriented to time and place, try gently reminding where she or he is. Tell the date, including the year, and the time. If your attempts to reorient or correct cause your loved one more distress, just leave well enough alone. This is especially important for patients who are aware they are dying, and who become more restless when their loved ones don't understand what is happening to them.

(continued)

When All Else Fails

In the worst-case situations, delirium progresses to terminal restlessness. In this situation, despite the best care, your loved one's anguish, agitation, and distress cannot be controlled. If this happens to your dying loved one, palliative sedation may be a last resort. Palliative sedation consists of the use of sedatives to achieve a desired level of consciousness. Although rare, there are times when palliative sedation is the only way to bring comfort and rest.

Source: Adapted from www.cancer.net[14] and American Cancer Society, *Caring for the Patient with Cancer at Home: A Guide for Patients and Families.*[15]

Source: Bakitas M, Bishop MF, Hahn M. Symptoms When Death Is Imminent. In: Yarbro CH, Wujcik D, Gobel BH, eds. *Cancer Symptom Management.* 4th ed. Burlington, MA: Jones & Bartlett Learning; 2014.

Family Care Guide for Noisy Airway Secretions

Patient Name: ______________________________

This family care guide will help you with your loved one's experience of noisy airway secretions.

Symptom and Description

Noisy airway secretions can be heard when normal or extra secretions are no longer being completely swallowed or cleared by cough. What you are hearing is air moving over these secretions. It is important for you to know that your loved one is not drowning nor choking. Usually these sounds occur when someone is unconscious, the person's throat and mouth become very relaxed, and the individual has lost awareness of how he or she is breathing.

Management

- Remember that noisy secretions are not usually a sign of distress, discomfort, or suffering.
- Are there any other signs of discomfort:
  - o Vocal moaning?
  - o A furrowed brow?
  - o Tense or clenched lips, teeth, or jaw?
  - o Clenched hands?
  - o Restlessness or agitation?

If none of these are present, your loved one is likely not experiencing any discomfort from the noisy secretions.

- Consider repositioning your loved one onto one side, with the head slightly elevated. If you are worried the movement may be uncomfortable, and there are no other signs of discomfort, this is not necessary.
- Consider asking your medical team to stop any IV fluids. This sometimes contributes to secretions.
- Ask your medical team if there is any medication that might help dry up the secretions—but remember the sound usually bothers us more than our loved one.

Source: Bakitas M, Bishop MF, Hahn M. Symptoms When Death Is Imminent. In: Yarbro CH, Wujcik D, Gobel BH, eds. *Cancer Symptom Management.* 4th ed. Burlington, MA: Jones & Bartlett Learning; 2014.

Informed Consent for Palliative Sedation

Date: ____ Time: ________________

Palliative sedation is the use of sedating medications to bring about an uninterrupted sleep-like state in a terminally ill individual when symptoms and suffering have not responded to a variety of interventions and additional interventions are unlikely to provide relief. Once palliative sedation is begun, it is generally continued through the end of life.

The nature and purpose of palliative sedation, the previous attempts to control my symptoms, and the possible alternative methods of treatment have been explained to me. I have had an opportunity to ask questions and have had them answered to my satisfaction.

I understand that I may never regain consciousness once palliative sedation is initiated

I hereby authorize Dr. _________________________ and/or such designees as may be selected by him/her to initiate palliative sedation for control of my symptom ____________________.

I understand that I or my surrogate ____________________ can elect to discontinue palliative sedation at any time.

____ Date:________________

Signature of patient or person authorized to make decisions on patient's behalf

____ Date:________________

Witness signature

____ Date: ________________

Signature of person obtaining informed consent

Source: Dartmouth Hitchcock Medical Center[42].

Source: Bakitas M, Bishop MF, Hahn M. Symptoms When Death Is Imminent. In: Yarbro CH, Wujcik D, Gobel BH, eds. *Cancer Symptom Management.* 4th ed. Burlington, MA: Jones & Bartlett Learning; 2014.

Index

Figures and tables are indicated by *f* and *t* following page numbers.

A

B

C

D

E

J

O

Q

R

S

W

X

Y

Z